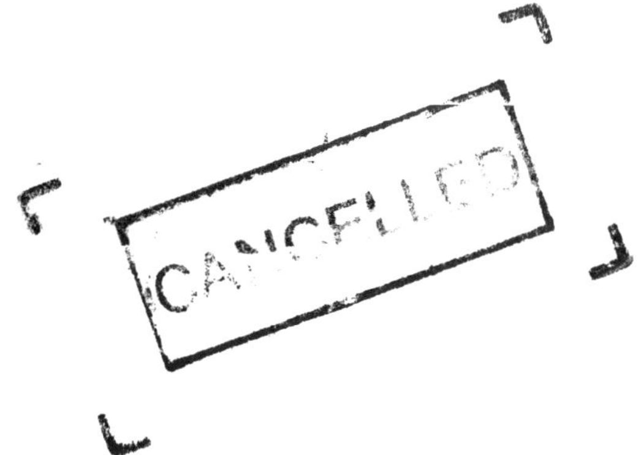

VETERINARY VIROLOGY

Third Edition

VETERINARY VIROLOGY

Third Edition

Frederick A. Murphy
School of Veterinary Medicine
University of California, Davis
Davis, California

E. Paul J. Gibbs
College of Veterinary Medicine
University of Florida
Gainesville, Florida

Marian C. Horzinek
Faculty of Veterinary Medicine
Utrecht University
Utrecht, The Netherlands

Michael J. Studdert
School of Veterinary Science
University of Melbourne
Melbourne, Victoria, Australia

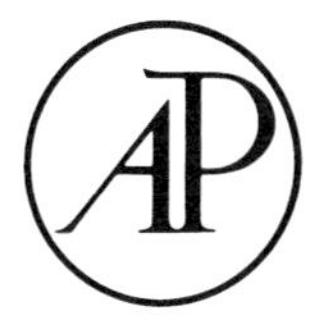

An Imprint of Elsevier
San Diego London Boston New York Sydney Tokyo Toronto

Cover illustration: Rabies encephalitis. Two hallmarks of street rabies virus infection are minimal cytopathology of infected neurons and minimal inflammatory infiltration into the neuropil. Here, in a thin section of part of the cytoplasm of a neuron in the hippocampus of a hamster inoculated intracerebrally 6 days earlier with a street rabies virus, the architecture of cellular organelles appears normal, but some of the cytosol has been displaced by aggregated viral nucleocapsids (smoothly granular areas; seen by light microscopy as Negri bodies). Large numbers of bullet-shaped virions are evident budding from adjacent endoplasmic reticulum membranes. Thin-section electron microscopy; uranyl acetate and lead citrate stain; magnification X 25,000.

This book is printed on acid-free paper. 

Academic Press
An Imprint of Elsevier
525 B Street, Suite 1900, San Diego, California 92101-4495, USA
http://www.academicpress.com

Academic Press
Harcourt Place, 32 Jamestown Road, London NW1 7BY, UK
http://www.academicpress.com

Library of Congress Catalog Card Number: 99-60582
ISBN-13: 978-0-12-511340-3
ISBN-10: 0-12-511340-4

PRINTED IN THE UNITED STATES OF AMERICA
08 09 10 EB 10 9 8

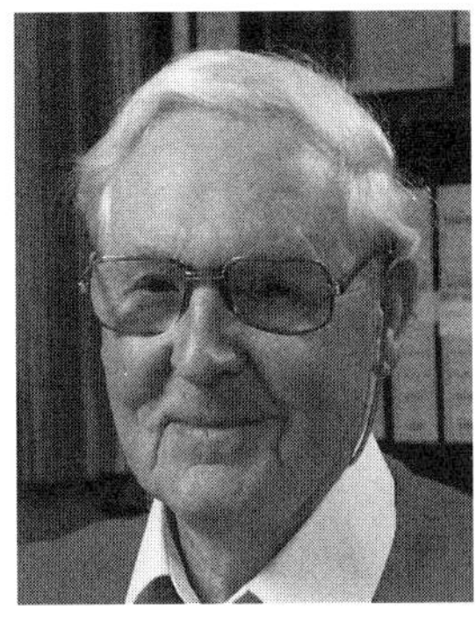

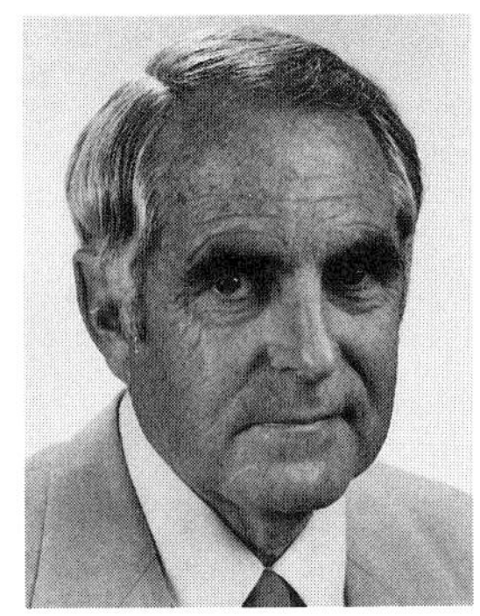

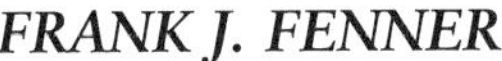

FRANK J. FENNER *DAVID O. WHITE*

This book is dedicated to our dear friends, Frank J. Fenner and David O. White, the founders of the series of books that now includes three editions of this book and four editions of "Medical Virology." They set a standard of scholarship that is impossible to match and a *joie de vivre* that made the writing and editing almost fun.

They taught us that the subject of virology must be seen within the context of society as a whole as well as within the context of science. They envisioned virology as being so broad as to extend from its roots as a microbiological science, a molecular and cell biological science, an infectious disease science, to become a major contributor to the overall advance of human and animal well-being. All this as a single seamless cloth. We hope our students will come to understand the "big picture" of veterinary and medical virology as well as Frank and David have throughout their amazing careers.

We would also like to dedicate this book to our families, our teachers and mentors, and our students, all of whom have shaped our thinking and provided our inspiration over the years in so many ways.

Frederick A. Murphy

E. Paul J. Gibbs

Marian C. Horzinek

Michael J. Studdert

Contents

PREFACE

The aim of "Veterinary Virology" is to present the fundamental principles of virology to students of veterinary medicine and related medical, biomedical, ecological, environmental, and comparative medical sciences. It will also serve as a useful resource for clinicians, teachers, and those involved in research in many related fields of comparative medicine. The pace of change since the previous edition has been so great that the book has been completely rewritten and greatly expanded. Coverage of zoonotic viruses and the diseases they cause has been expanded as has coverage of the viruses and viral diseases of laboratory animals, poultry, fish, and wildlife. We have tried to weave the concept of new, emerging, and reemerging viral diseases into the fabric of the book, reflecting the new perspective this concept has brought to veterinary and zoonotic virology and related fields.

The arrangement of the previous editions has been retained, but our account of the molecular biology of viral infections is much more detailed and more thoroughly integrated into the overall subject. Similarly, our account of viral genetics, phylogeny, and evolution has been expanded and has become a more integral part of the book. This, of course, is built on accurate and up-to-date viral taxonomic usage. The classification and nomenclature decisions of the International Committee on Taxonomy of Viruses, to May 1998, have been incorporated in this new edition.

Part I presents an overview of the principles of animal virology, starting with the viruses themselves and progressing to the infections they cause at the level of the cell, the individual animal host, and the host population. The emphasis is on pathogenesis, that is the events in the war between virus and host that we see as acute, chronic-persistent, and more subtle forms of disease. Our focus on pathogenesis naturally leads to emphasis on subjects pertaining to the host response to infection and to the means of intervening in the course of infection: immunology, diagnostics, vaccinology, epidemiology, prevention, and control.

Part II is arranged by virus family, with major subsections in each chapter providing more specific information about the viruses, their classification, their molecular properties and their replication, and on the important veterinary and zoonotic diseases caused by specific viruses. The diseases are covered from the perspective of their clinical features, their pathogenesis, pathology and immunity, their laboratory diagnosis, and their epidemiology, prevention, and control.

In order to focus on major virologic concepts and mechanisms that form the bases for our understanding of specific clinical diseases, minutiae have been omitted and much of the factual information is consolidated into tables and figures. Likewise, statements are not individually supported by citation of research papers; however, selective lists of authoritative books, reviews, and some key recent papers are provided at the end of each chapter to simplify the reader's entry into the virologic and infectious disease literature.

The pattern of producing "Veterinary Virology" and its companion volume "Medical Virology" involves alternating research, writing and editing between the two, with the authors' sense of the advances in the science pertaining to veterinary medicine being incorporated into one volume and at the same time into the files from which the next volume pertaining to human medicine is initiated; and, then, vice versa. Of course, this system pertains mostly to Part I and to the first part of each chapter in Part II of each book. We believe that this cross-fertilization between the veterinary and human medical sciences is a valuable and unique aspect of these volumes and a useful foundation for the concept of comparative medicine. Comparative medicine, in our view, is a powerful impetus in advancing both human and animal health. Thus, this book has as its base the fourth edition of "Medical Virology" published in 1994. In turn, this volume will serve as a foundation for the fifth edition of "Medical Virology."

We would like to acknowledge the help of the many colleagues who in so many ways have helped us in preparing this book: this has ranged from discussions on the qualities and shortcomings of the earlier editions and expectations for this edition, to the provision of new information from ongoing research work, to insights into the future of the science and its integration into clinical practice. We also acknowledge the help of many colleagues with the illustrations used throughout this book. Without all this help we would not have had the incentive to revise the book to the extent that we hope is evident. In this regard, we would also like to acknowledge the help of our teachers and our students who in their own ways have provided life-long incentives. Veterinary students, graduate students, and postdoctoral fellows were all in mind as we pondered questions of "too little" or "too much?"

Finally, we would like to acknowledge the devotion of Ms. Shirley Light of Academic Press in the preparation and production of this edition. Ms. Light has served in this role from the first edition and has played a central role in the continuing improvements in the style and layout that are evident as one looks at all the editions in the series.

Frederick A. Murphy
E. Paul J. Gibbs
Marian C. Horzinek
Michael J. Studdert

PART I

Principles of Virology

CHAPTER 1

The Nature of Viruses as Etiologic Agents of Veterinary and Zoonotic Diseases

Veterinary and Zoonotic Virology as Infectious Disease Sciences

> Infectious disease is one of the few genuine adventures left in the world. The dragons are all dead and the lance grows rusty in the chimney corner. . . . About the only sporting proposition that remains unimpaired by the relentless domestication of a once free-living human species is the war against those ferocious little fellow creatures, which lurk in the dark corners and stalk us in the bodies of rats, mice, and all kinds of domestic animals; which fly and crawl with the insects, and waylay us in our food and drink and even in our love.

This quote is taken from the book "Rats, Lice and History," written in 1935 by the great microbiologist Hans Zinsser as he reflected on his life in infectious disease science. Zinsser's thought has challenged generations of students and professionals ever since, and now it challenges those who use this book, those who, by their own clinical and scholarly experiences, understand that the infectious diseases of today are as demanding as those that faced Zinsser.

This book presents the subject of veterinary and zoonotic virology from the perspective of its traditional base as an infectious disease science. It is the perspective established by Frank Fenner and David White, who in 1970 conceived the venue for a book, "Medical Virology," now in its fourth edition, and in 1987 its complement, "Veterinary Virology," this being its third edition. It is the perspective that many others have used to teach medical and veterinary and zoonotic virology in many countries.

It seems fitting to start with a sense of the roots of the subject, with a sense of how the roots of veterinary and zoonotic virology are intertwined with those of all the other infectious disease sciences. The history of veterinary and zoonotic virology is brief, spanning only about a century, but it is crowded with wonderful discoveries and practical applications. It centers on the replacement of centuries-old beliefs, conceptions, and theories with scientific proofs. Scientific proofs established the concept of *specificity of disease causation;* i.e., particular viral diseases are caused not by some common miasma (a mysteriously poisonous substance), but rather by specific viruses. This concept led to the introduction of specific prevention and control strategies, specific diagnostic tests, and specific therapeutic approaches.

This concept and the reformation of thought that it caused involved bitter struggle against entrenched opposition, but in the end the scientific method, the evidence-based method, won out. In a larger sense, the infectious disease sciences have played a paramount role in the reformation of all veterinary and medical thought: the concept of specificity of disease causation and the requirement for verifiable scientific proofs have been extended universally throughout all medical and veterinary sciences. At the same time, the practical application of the infectious disease sciences has led to improvements in animal and human health and well-being that have exceeded the contribution of any other branch of science.

Proof of this practical value of the infectious disease sciences is seen in the momentous effects of scientific discoveries on animal productivity, life expectancy, and well-being, worldwide. For example, the great epidemics of foot-and-mouth disease, rinderpest, hog cholera, and fowl plague, to name a few, that were so common in the 19th century have been virtually eliminated from developed countries by the application of various prevention and control strategies. At the same time, many of the zoonotic and food-borne diseases that were the causes of many human deaths have largely been controlled in developed countries.

However, even as the great epidemic infectious diseases have been conquered, new diseases have emerged, in every case requiring increasing expertise and more complex technological solutions than ever imagined when diseases like foot-and-mouth disease and hog cholera were the primary targets of control efforts. Just a few years ago it was canine parvovirus disease that took center stage and today it is bovine spongiform encephalopathy that represents the need for advanced veterinary virologic expertise, technologies, and control strategies. Tomorrow it will be other diseases, their cause, nature, and means of control totally unpredictable. In any case, our virologic knowledge base, the stuff of this book, is the starting point for managing the viral diseases that affect domestic and wild animals and often humans in direct and indirect contact with animals. This is what the authors mean in presenting the subject of veterinary and zoonotic virology as an infectious disease science.

Discoverers and Discoveries

The foundation of the virologic/infectious disease sciences predates the concept of the specificity of disease causation and is heavily dependent on initial discoveries about bacteria. There are great names and discoveries to be remembered: Hippocrates, the Greek physician and father of medicine, who in the 4th century, made important epidemiologic observations on many infectious diseases, including rabies; Fracastoro, who theorized in 1546 that epidemic diseases were disseminated by minute particles carried over long distances; van Leewenhoek, who in 1676 first saw bacteria with his microscope; Spallanzani, who in 1775 first grew bacteria in culture; Jenner, who in 1796 introduced vaccination against the viral disease smallpox; Semmelweis and Holmes, who in the 1840s developed practical methods of cleanliness and antimicrobial disinfection; Davaine, who in 1850 first associated an infectious organism, the anthrax bacillus, with disease; and Darwin, Wallace, and Mendel, who from 1859 onward revolutionized thinking in genetics and evolution.

Pasteur's Influence

On this foundation, Pasteur (Figure 1.1) established the microbiologic/virologic/infectious disease sciences, first in 1857 by discovering the specificity of microbial fermentations (wine, beer, cheese), then in 1865 by extending the concept to infectious diseases of silkworms, and finally between 1877 and 1895 by extending the concept to animal and human infectious diseases. His early infectious disease work centered on septic war wounds; he then turned to anthrax and other bacterial diseases and finally to rabies. In each instance, he moved quickly from studies aimed at discovering the causative agent to the development of specific intervention. In 1885, Pasteur gave the first rabies vaccine to a boy, Joseph Meister, bitten severely by a rabid dog—that day marks the opening of the modern era of infectious disease science aimed at disease prevention and control. Clearly, Pasteur deserves his title of father of the microbiologic/virologic/infectious disease sciences.

Pasteur was joined by Koch, who discovered the causative agents of tuberculosis and cholera and contributed much to the development of laboratory methods in bacteriology. As a result, the identification of the causative agents of many important human bacterial diseases proceeded at breakneck pace around the turn of the 20th century. At the same time, the seminal work of Salmon, Smith, Kilborne, Curtice, and others identified the specific cause of many important animal pathogens, including the causative agent of Texas fever (*Babesia bigemina*, transmitted by the tick *Boophilus annulatus*—the first proof that arthropods can transmit infectious agents). These successes in turn nurtured the founding of the science of virology.

Founders of the Science of Virology

In the field of virology, there are great names and discoveries to be remembered: Beijerinck and Ivanovski, who in the 1890s discovered the first virus, tobacco mosaic virus, and Loeffler and Frosch, who in 1898, working

FIGURE 1.1.

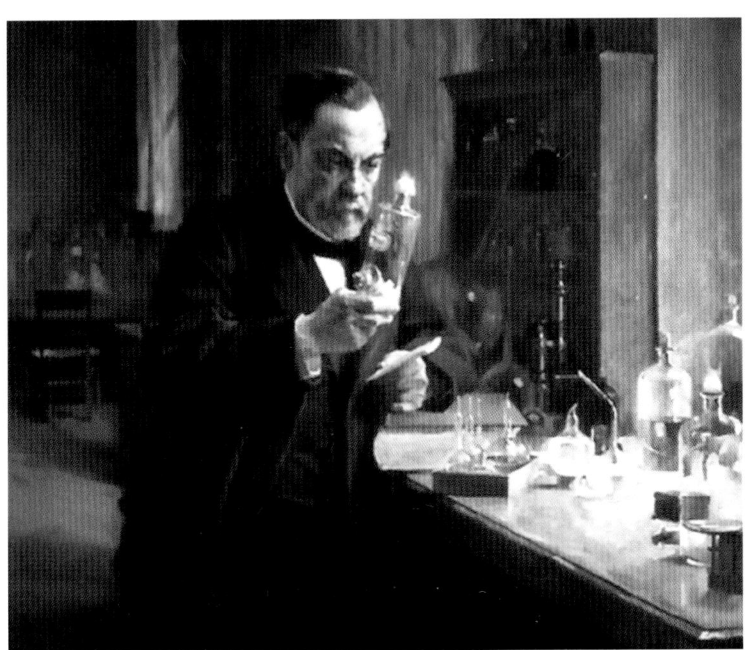

Louis Pasteur, 1822–1895, father of the microbiologic/virologic/infectious disease sciences.

FIGURE 1.2.

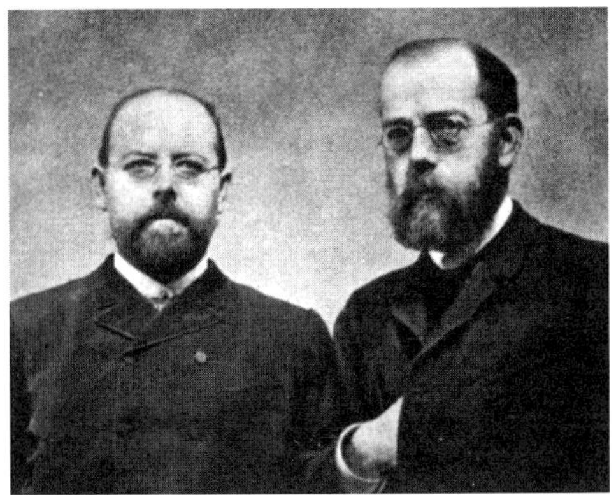

F. A. J. Loeffler (left) and P. Frosch, in 1898, working with Robert Koch (right), discovered the first virus of vertebrates, foot-and mouth disease virus.

with Koch (Figure 1.2), discovered the first virus of vertebrates, foot-and-mouth disease virus. They described the filterability of the virus, noting that "the filtered material contained a dissolved poison of extraordinary power or an as yet undiscovered agent that is so small that it is able to pass through the pores of a filter definitely capable of retaining the smallest known bacteria." On the basis of its virulence after successive dilutions in experimental animals, they concluded that the causal agent of foot-and-mouth disease was not soluble but "corpuscular." Loeffler and Frosch gave filtration a new emphasis by focusing attention on what passed through the filter rather than what was retained and establishing an experimental methodology that was adopted widely in the early 20th century in research on viral diseases.

There are other great names to be remembered: Sanarelli, who in 1898 discovered myxoma virus; Reed and Carroll, who discovered the first virus of humans, yellow fever virus, and who, influenced by the work of Salmon, Curtice, and their colleagues, also discovered its mosquito transmission cycle; M'Fadyean, who in 1900 discovered African horse sickness virus; Centanni, Lode, and Gruber, who in 1901 discovered fowl plague virus; Remlinger and Riffat-Bay, who in 1903 discovered rabies virus; DeSchweinitz and Dorset, who in 1903 discovered hog cholera virus; Arnold Theiler, who in the early 1900s made breakthrough discoveries concerning rinderpest, African horse sickness, and other animal diseases; Ellermann and Bang, who in 1908 discovered avian leukemia virus, the first cancer-causing virus; Landsteiner and Popper, who in 1909 discovered poliovirus; Rous, who in 1911 discovered the first solid tumor virus now known as Rous sarcoma virus; Laidlaw and Dunkin, who in 1926 discovered canine distemper virus; Shope, who in 1931 discovered swine influenza virus; Andrewes, Laidlaw, Smith, and Burnet, who in 1933 first isolated influenza virus, just 15 years after the great influenza pandemic of 1918–1919 in which 25 to 40 million people died; Max Theiler (Arnold Theiler's son), who in 1935 developed the yellow fever vaccine that is still in use today; Olafson, Pritchard, Gillespie, Baker, and colleagues, who in the 1940s–1950s determined the cause of bovine viral diarrhea; Sigurdsson, who in the 1950s in studies of scrapie and maedi/visna in sheep proposed the concept of slow infectious diseases; Salk and Sabin, who in 1954 and 1957 developed inactivated virus and attenuated virus polio vaccines; Montagnier and colleagues, who in 1984 discovered human immunodeficiency virus (HIV); Carmichael, Parrish, and colleagues, who in 1978 discovered canine parvovirus; Pedersen and colleagues, who in 1987 discovered feline immunodeficiency virus; the many British veterinary virologists, who in 1986 discovered the agent of bovine spongiform encephalopathy, and Prusiner, who discovered the nature of prions, the etiologic agents of bovine spongiform encephalopathy, scrapie, and similar diseases and who in 1997 was awarded the Nobel Prize in Medicine for his work.

The field of viral disease pathogenesis also celebrates great names and discoveries: the field was pioneered by Fenner, who in the 1940s in classical studies of ectromelia (mousepox) introduced viral quantitation methods for determining the sequential events in the course of infection, from portal of entry, viremic spread, seeding of target organs, to transmission. Fenner was followed by Mims, who starting in the 1960s used immunofluorescence to visualize the development of viral antigens in serially collected experimental animal tissues. In turn, Appel in the 1960s applied these methods to the study of canine distemper virus infection in dogs.

The sciences of immunology and cell and molecular biology have been intertwined with virology and the infectious disease sciences from their beginnings: these sciences also call to mind great names and discoveries that have influenced modern veterinary and zoonotic virology greatly. In immunology, we acknowledge Metchnikoff, Bordet, and Ehrlich, who by discoveries made between 1883 and 1909 outlined the nature of the immune system; Loeffler, Rous, Yersin, and Behring, who in 1888 discovered bacterial toxins and antitoxins; Avery and Lancefield, who between 1928 and 1933 developed the basic concepts of infectious disease diagnostics; Porter, Edelman, and Nisonoff, who in 1959 described the structure and molecular function of antibodies; Jerne and Burnet, who in 1974 conceived clonal selection as the basis of the immune response; Doherty and Zinkernagel, who in 1974 discovered how the cellular immune system recognizes virus-infected cells; and Kohler and Milstein, who in 1975 developed the first monoclonal antibodies. In cell biology we recognize Carrel, Steinhardt, Eagle, Puck, Dulbecco, Enders, and others, who from the 1910s to the 1960s invented cell culture methods, and Palade, Claude, Porter, and de Duve, who in the 1960s and 1970s described the fine structure of cells and organelles and their biochemical functions. In molecular biology we acclaim the work of Avery, Hershey, and Chase, who between 1944 and 1952 showed that DNA carries all hereditary specificity; Watson and Crick, who in 1953 discovered the structure of DNA and thereby the molecular basis for heredity; Nierenberg, Ochoa, Matthaei, and Khorana, who between 1961 and 1966 deciphered the genetic code; and Cohen and Boyer, who in 1973 developed recombinant-DNA technology.

From this brief, far from complete, history, it is clear that from its beginning veterinary and zoonotic virology has been intertwined with medical virology and the other infectious disease sciences. In fact, in the early 1900s, there did not seem to be any separation whatsoever, and today, in some areas of veterinary virology, notably those dealing with the zoonotic and arthropod-borne viruses, the seamless cloth is still intact. Even though this book now proceeds to deal with veterinary and zoonotic virology per se—the viruses infecting animals and the diseases they cause—understanding the full scope of the infectious diseases requires continuing integration of this subject with all the other infectious disease sciences—this is the perspective of "comparative medicine," "comparative virology," and the perspective of "lifelong learning." It is the perspective that all students and professionals who use this book will want to practice.

Viruses, "At the Edge of Life"

The unicellular *microorganisms* can be arranged in order of decreasing size and complexity: protozoa, fungi, and bacteria (the latter including mycoplasmas, rickettsiae, and chlamydiae). These microorganisms, however small and simple, are *cells*. They contain DNA as the repository of their genetic information; they also contain RNAs and they have most or all of their own machinery for producing energy and macromolecules. These microorganisms grow by synthesizing their own macromolecular constituents (nucleic acids, proteins, carbohydrates, and lipids), and most multiply by binary fission.

Viruses, however, are not cells, are not microorganisms. They possess no functional organelles and are completely dependent on their host for the machinery of energy production and synthesis of macromolecules. They contain only one type of functional nucleic acid, either DNA or RNA, never both, and they differ from microorganisms in having two clearly defined phases in their life cycle. Outside their host cell, the viruses are metabolically inert; this is the phase of their life cycle involved in transmission. Inside their host cell, the viruses are metabolically active; this is their replicative phase in which the viral genome exploits the machinery of the host cell to produce progeny genome copies, viral messenger RNA, and viral proteins (often along with carbohydrates and lipids) that assemble to form new virions (*virion,* the complete virus particle). Unlike any microorganism, many viruses can reproduce even if only their genomic DNA or RNA is introduced into the host cell. These qualities have been used to argue the question, "Are viruses alive?" One answer is to envision "*viruses, at the edge of life,*" in some ways fulfilling the criteria we use to define life, in some ways not. The key differences between viruses and microorganisms are listed in Table 1.1.

Given their unique characteristics, where might viruses have originated? There are two theories that have been argued for many years: viruses are either degenerate bacteria that have lost most of their cellular functions or they are escaped eukaryotic genes, i.e., nucleic acids that have learned to survive outside the environment of the cell. Viral genomic sequence analyses may at last resolve this question: for example, the genome of a plant viroid (a subviral agent composed of naked RNA), potato spindle tuber viroid, seems to be a self-replicating RNA copy of a bit of host DNA. Many of the genes of poxviruses are similar to those of eukaryotes. In any case, it seems certain from viral genomic sequence analyses that all the viruses did not evolve from a single progenitor; rather the different kinds of viruses likely arose independently and then continued to diversify and adapt their survival and transmission qualities to better fit particular niches by the usual Darwinian mutation/selection mechanisms. Some viruses have continued to evolve in long association with their evolving hosts (e.g., the herpesviruses); others have evolved by "host species jumping" (e.g., influenza viruses) and yet others by developing zoonotic transmission schemes (e.g., rabies virus).

Several important practical consequences follow from understanding that viruses are different from microorganisms and all other life forms: for example, (1) some viruses can persist for the lifetime of their host by the integration of their genomic DNA (or a DNA copy of their genomic RNA) into the genome of their host cell or by the carriage of their genomic DNA episomally in their host cell, and (2) most viruses have defied all antiviral drug development. Because viruses use the replicative machinery of their host cell, drugs that interfere

TABLE 1.1
Properties of Unicellular Microorganisms and Viruses

PROPERTY	BACTERIA	RICKETTSIAE	MYCOPLASMAS	CHLAMYDIAE	VIRUSES
>300 nm diameter[a]	+	+	+	+	−
Growth on nonliving media[b]	+	−	+	−	−
Binary fission	+	+	+	+	−
DNA and RNA	+	+	+	+	−
Infectious nucleic acid	−	−	−	−	−[c]
Functional ribosomes	+	+	+	+	−
Metabolism	+	+	+	+	−
Sensitivity to antibiotics	+	+	+	+	−[d]

[a]Some mycoplasmas and chlamydiae are less than 300 nm in diameter.
[b]Chlamydiae and most rickettsiae are obligate intracellular parasites.
[c]Some, among both DNA and RNA viruses.
[d]With very few exceptions.

with viral replication nearly always interfere with essential cell functions (bacteria have unique metabolic pathways, different from those of their host, and antibiotics are directed at these pathways).

The simplest viruses consist of a DNA or RNA genome contained within a protein coat, but there are classes of even simpler infectious agents: viroids, which as noted earlier consist of a naked RNA molecule that is infectious, and prions, the agents of the spongiform encephalopathies, which consist of an infectious protein, with no associated nucleic acid.

Viral Morphology

We know that viruses are smaller than microorganisms, but we forget how unbelievable this realization was at first and we forget just how small the viruses are—in fact, it is very difficult to understand from the perspective of direct human experience sizes of entities much smaller than we can see with the naked eye (Table 1.2). The first unequivocal discovery of an animal virus occurred in 1898, when Loeffler and Frosch demonstrated that the etiologic agent of foot-and-mouth disease, then an important disease of cattle throughout Europe and many other regions of the world, could be transferred by material that had been passed through a filter with pores too small to allow the passage of bacteria. The new infectious agents became known as *filterable viruses*, quickly shortened to *viruses*. Once the concept of filterability of viruses took hold, this experimental procedure was applied to many candidate infectious agents. The early discoveries of many important pathogenic viruses of animals and humans, as cited at the beginning of this chapter, were all made using ultrafiltration (together with animal inoculation of the filtrates).

Electron Microscopy of Viruses

For a time the viruses were also called "ultramicroscopic," as they are smaller than the limit of resolution of the light microscope (which is about 0.3 μm, i.e., 300 nm; poxviruses, the largest viruses, are just about this size but are visible in the light microscope using only dark-field optics or certain staining techniques). Only with the advent of the electron microscope was it possible to visualize the viruses. It then became apparent that the viruses range in size from about the size of the smallest microorganisms down to the size of large protein molecules.

Early electron microscopic studies of viruses by Ruska in 1939–1941, which employed metal shadowing of purified virus preparations, were expanded during the 1950s to include ultrathin sectioning of virus-infected cells. In 1959, visualization of viral ultrastructure was transformed when negative staining was developed. For negative staining, a solution of potassium phosphotungstate, which is electron dense, is added to a virus suspension on a coated specimen grid; it surrounds and fills the interstices in the surface of virions, giving a negative image of the virion, showing details not previously seen (Figure 1.3). The remarkable diversity of the viruses is evident when one compares the morphology of various viruses as they appear when negatively stained. This diversity is revealed in a different way when one com-

Table 1.2
Perspective on the Size of Viruses

10^{0}	1 m	1 m	Humans, adult males, are about 2 meters tall
10^{-1}	0.1 m		Human, adult, hand is about 10 cm wide
10^{-2}	0.01 m	1 cm	*Aedes aegypti,* adult, mosquito is about 1 cm long
10^{-3}	0.001 m	1 mm	*Ixodes scapularis* tick, nymphal stage, is about 1 mm long
10^{-4}	0.0001 m	100 μm	Smallest things visible to the naked eye
10^{-5}	0.00001 m	10 μm	Lymphocytes are about 20 μm in diameter
			Bacillus anthracis, among the largest of pathogenic bacteria, is 1 μm wide and 5–10 μm long
10^{-6}	0.000001 m	1 μm	Smallest things visible in light microscope are about 0.3 μm in size
			Poxviruses, the largest of the viruses of vertebrates, are 300 nm (or 0.3 μm) in their longest dimension
10^{-7}	0.0000001 m	100 nm	Influenza viruses and retroviruses, typical medium-sized viruses, are about 100 nm in diameter
			Pestiviruses, such as bovine viral diarrhea virus, typical smaller-sized viruses, are about 50 nm in diameter
10^{-8}	0.00000001 m	10 nm	Picornaviruses, such as foot-and-mouth disease viruses, typical small viruses, are about 30 nm in diameter
			Circoviruses, the smallest of the viruses of vertebrates, are 17–22 nm in diameter
10^{-9}	0.000000001 m	1 nm	Smallest things visible in transmission electron microscope; DNA double helix diameter is 2 nm
10^{-10}	0.0000000001 m	1 Å	Diameter of atoms is about 2–3 Å

pares the morphology of various viruses as they appear in ultrathin sections of infected cells (Figure 1.4).

Electron micrographs of virions and infected cells representing the families of viruses that cause animal and zoonotic diseases are shown in the chapters of Part II of this book. In the past few years, ultrathin sectioning of virus-infected cells and tissues and negative staining of purified virions have been complemented by several new microscopy technologies, particularly scanning electron microscopy and computer-based image constructions of frozen, unstained virions. It seems that each new technology reveals the viruses as more and more beautiful—but this is a terrible beauty (Figures 1.5A and 1.5B).

X-Ray Crystallography of Viruses

Electron microscopic approaches have added much to our understanding of the nature and structure of viruses, but in the past few years there has not been much improvement in their resolving power—for this, X-ray crystallography and computer analysis of resulting diffraction patterns have been employed to advance our knowledge of virion structural details at near atomic resolution (Figure 1.6A). X-ray crystallographic analyses of many important viruses have provided remarkable insight into virion organization and assembly, the location of antigenic sites on the surface of virions, and aspects of virion attachment and penetration into cells. For example, in several picornaviruses, the amino acids of each of the three larger structural proteins have been found to be packaged so as to form wedge-shaped, eight-stranded antiparallel β-barrel domains (Figures 1.6B and 1.6C). The overall contour of picornavirus virions reflects the packing of these domains. In the same way, other amino acid chains have been found to form loops that project from the main wedge-shaped domains. Some loops form flexible arms that interlock with the arms of adjacent wedge-shaped units, thereby providing physical stability to the virion. Other loops, those involved in virion attachment to the host cell, harbor the *antigenic sites (epitopes)* that are the targets of the host's neutralizing antibody response against the virus.

Larger viruses are much more complex in structure (Figures 1.3 and 1.4). To study the fine structure of the

FIGURE 1.3.

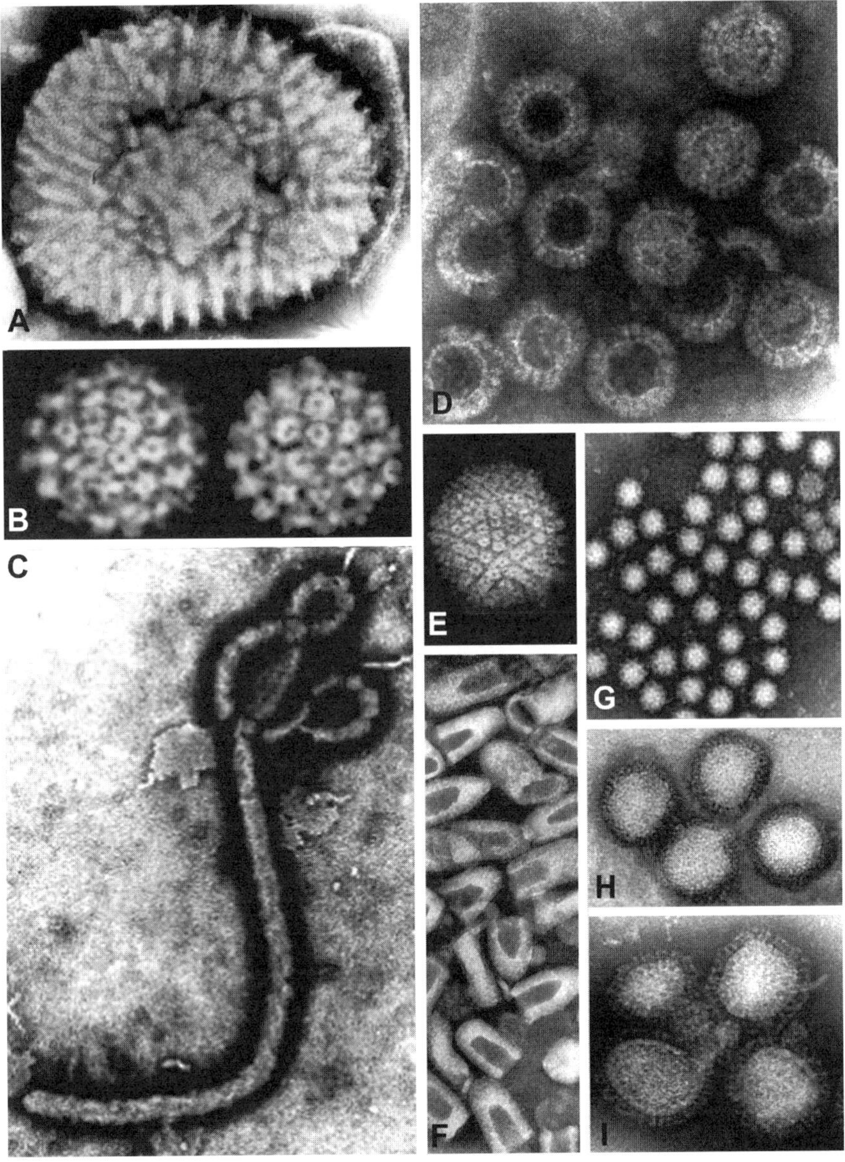

Negative contrast electron microscopy of selected viruses. The remarkable diversity of the viruses is revealed by all kinds of electron microscopic methods, but none better than by negative staining. (A) Family *Poxviridae*, genus *Orthopoxvirus*, vaccinia virus. (B) Family *Papovaviridae*, genus *Papillomavirus*, bovine papillomavirus 1. (C) Family *Filoviridae*, unnamed genus, Ebola virus. (D) Family *Reoviridae*, genus *Orthoreovirus*, a new reovirus isolated from colonized baboons with central nervous system disease. (E) Family *Herpesviridae*, genus *Simplexvirus*, human herpesvirus 1 (capsid only, envelope not shown). (F) Family *Rhabdoviridae*, genus *Lyssavirus*, rabies virus. (G) Family *Caliciviridae*, genus *Vesivirus*, feline calicivirus. (H) Family *Bunyaviridae*, genus *Phlebovirus*, Rift Valley fever virus. (I) Family *Orthomyxoviridae*, genus *Influenzavirus A*, influenza virus A/Hong Kong/1/68 (H3N2). These images represent various magnifications; sizes of the various viruses are given in Chapter 2 and in the chapters in Part II of this book.

more complex viruses, it is necessary to separate well-defined substructures, crystallize them, and subject the crystals to X-ray diffraction analysis. For example, bluetongue viruses are composed of a subcore and two capsid layers. The subcore structure, as determined by X-ray crystallography, is composed of 120 copies of VP3 that self-assemble and then seem to direct the assembly of the surrounding capsid layers (Figure 1.7). The structure of the entire bluetongue virus virion was determined by X-ray crystallography in 1997—intact virions are

FIGURE 1.4.

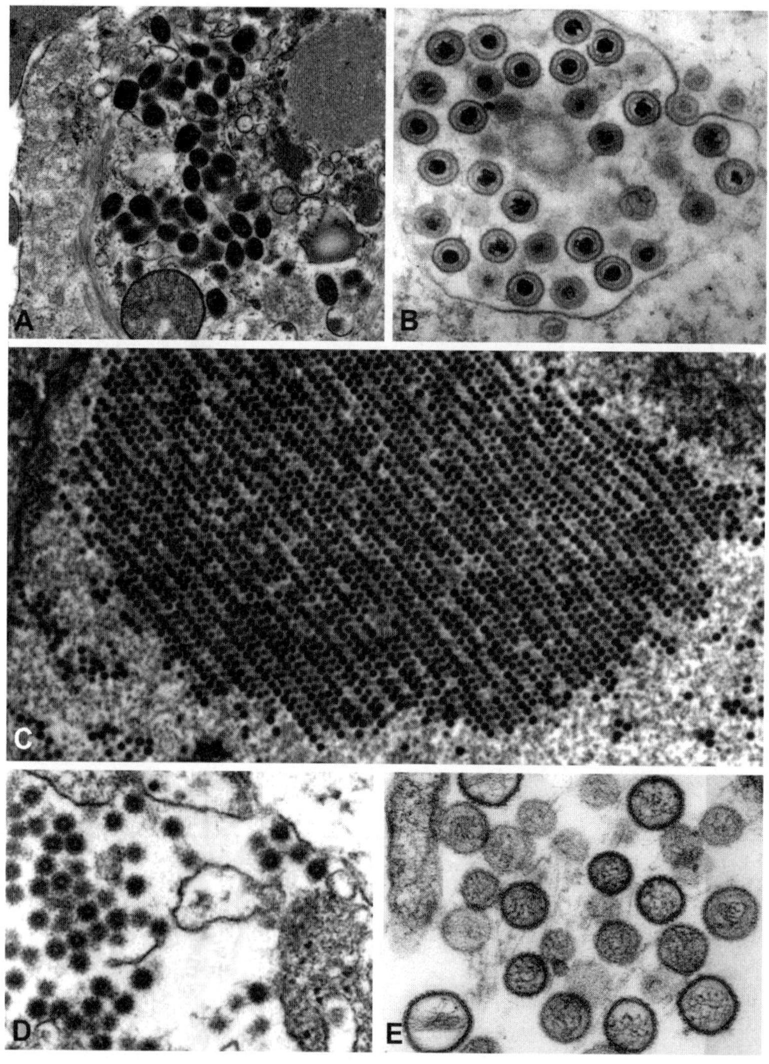

Thin-section electron microscopy of selected viruses. The remarkable diversity of the viruses is also revealed by thin-section electron microscopy of infected cells. (A) Family *Poxviridae*, genus *Orthopoxvirus*, variola virus. (B) Family *Herpesviridae*, genus *Simplexvirus*, human herpesvirus 1. (C) Family *Adenoviridae*, genus *Mastadenovirus*, adenovirus 5. (D) Family *Togaviridae*, genus *Alphavirus*, eastern equine encephalitis virus. (E) Family *Bunyaviridae*, genus *Hantavirus*, Sin Nombre virus. These images represent various magnifications; details of the morphogenesis of the various viruses are given in the chapters in Part II of this book.

composed of more than 1000 separate protein molecules (see Chapter 24).

One of the pioneering studies of viral structure was the determination by X-ray crystallography of the structure of the hemagglutinin molecule of influenza viruses and the placement and variation of neutralizing epitopes on this molecule. This has been described in exquisite detail (Figure 1.8). Today, the determination of new variations in the amino acid sequence and the structure of the influenza hemagglutinin are used in the development of updated vaccines and antiviral drugs. Of course the largest viruses, such as the poxviruses, asfarviruses, and herpesviruses, are even more complex and their study requires even more dissection of viral proteins and substructures (see Chapters 16, 17, and 18).

Capsid Structure

The *virion*, i.e., the complete virus particle, of the simplest viruses consists of a single molecule of nucleic acid (DNA or RNA) surrounded by a morphologically de-

FIGURE 1.5.

A

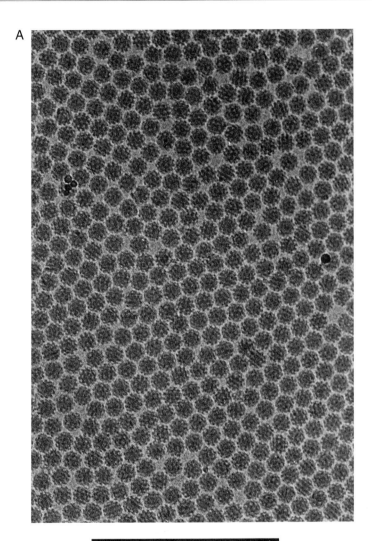

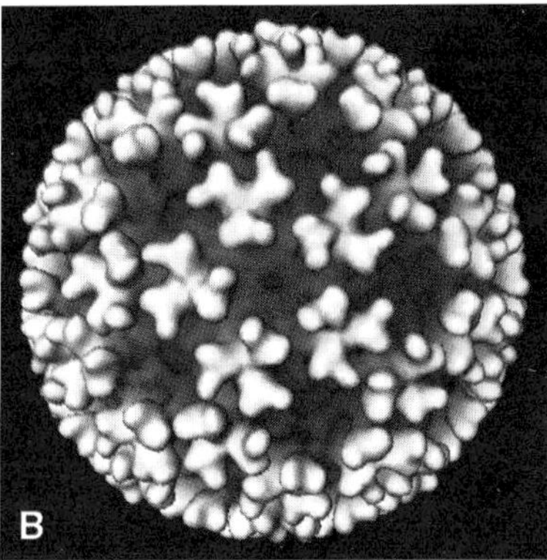

(A) Semliki Forest virus, a member of the family *Togaviridae*, genus *Alphavirus*. Purified virus was placed in a monolayer on a coated grid and frozen instantaneously in liquid helium; the unstained virus preparation, embedded in a microfilm of ice, was examined in an electron microscope equipped for cryoelectron microscopy. Details of virion structure are revealed that were never seen by other methods; such virion images are now digitized routinely and large numbers of such images are subjected to computer analysis. (B) The result of computer analysis of many cryoelectron microscopic images of the virus showing the arrangement of the structural units that make up the icosahedral capsid. [A, courtesy of C.-H. von Bonsdorff; B, from R. G. Webster and A. Granoff, eds., "Encyclopedia of Virology," 2nd ed. (CD-ROM). Academic Press, London, 1998.]

FIGURE 1.8.

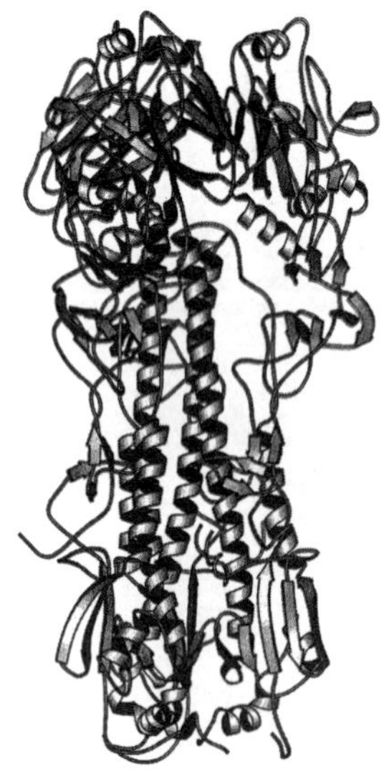

Classical schematic diagram of the three-dimensional structure of the influenza virus hemaglutinin trimer as determined from X-ray crystallography. Regions of β strands (flat, twisted arrows) and regions of α-helix (helices) are represented. (Courtesy of F. Hughson and D. Wiley.)

fined protein coat, the *capsid;* the capsid and enclosed nucleic acid constitute the *nucleocapsid.* The nucleocapsid of some viruses is surrounded by a lipoprotein *envelope* (Figure 1.3). There are many variations on these constructions and diverse additional components are found in the more complex viruses (Figure 1.9).

New information on the structure and organization of the components of the viral capsid obtained from X-ray crystallographic analyses requires a new synthesis of the terminology used to describe virions. Some features pertain to morphologically defined structures, others to molecular components themselves. *Capsomers* or *morphologic units* are discernible features (protrusions, depressions, etc.) seen on the surface of virions by electron microscopy (Figure 1.3). They may or may not correspond to individual molecular components. Folded polypeptide chains, specified by the viral genome, comprise *protein subunits;* assemblages of these protein subunits comprise *structural units* and in turn sets of these structural units comprise *assembly units,* which are the major intermediates in the formation of viral capsids. Only the simplest virions are assembled from the primary products of biosynthesis, i.e., protein subunits; in most cases, virions are constructed from distinct *subassemblies* by processes involving sequential synthesis and modification or cleavage of precursors. One crucial need in virion assembly is the incorporation of the viral nucleic acid into the nascent virion—several different mechanisms driving this process have been recognized, including the presence of *packaging signals* in the genomic nucleic acid sequence.

Virion Symmetry

For reasons of evolutionary progression and genetic economy, virions are assembled from multiple copies of one or a few kinds of protein subunits—the repeated occurrence of similar protein–protein interfaces leads to assembly of the subunits into symmetrical capsids. This efficiency of design also depends on principles of *self-assembly,* wherein structural units are brought into position through random thermal movement and are bonded in place through weak chemical bonds. Viruses come in a variety of shapes and sizes, depending on the shape, size, and number of their protein subunits and the nature of the interfaces between these subunits; however, only two kinds of symmetry have been recognized, *icosahedral* and *helical* (Figure 1.9).

Icosahedral Symmetry

The symmetry found in isometric viruses is invariably that of an icosahedron, one of the five classical *platonic solids* of geometry; virions with *icosahedral symmetry* have 12 vertices (corners), 30 edges, and 20 faces, each face an equilateral triangle. Icosahedra have axes of two-, three-, and fivefold rotational symmetry, which pass through their edges, faces, and vertices, respectively (Figure 1.10). The icosahedron is the optimum solution to the problem of constructing, from repeating subunits, a strong structure enclosing a maximum volume. The same principles were exploited by the architect Buckminster Fuller in his design of icosahedral buildings (geodesic domes). Only certain arrangements of structural units can form the faces, edges, and vertices of viral icosahedra. The structural units or capsomers on the faces and edges of adenovirus virions, for example, bond to six neighboring capsomers and are called *hexons;* those at the vertices bond to five neighbors and are called *pentons* (Figure 1.8). In the virions of some viruses, both *hexons* and *pentons* are composed of the same polypeptide(s), whereas in those of other viruses they are formed from different polypeptides. The arrangements of structural units on the surface of virions of three small icosahedral model viruses are shown in Figure 1.10. Because of variations in the arrangement of the structural units on different viruses, some appear rather hexagonal in outline and some appear nearly spherical. Even within rather smooth overall surface configurations, functional protrusions, bulges, and projections (often housing cellular attachment ligands and neutralizing epitopes) and depressions, clefts, and canyons

Figure 1.6.

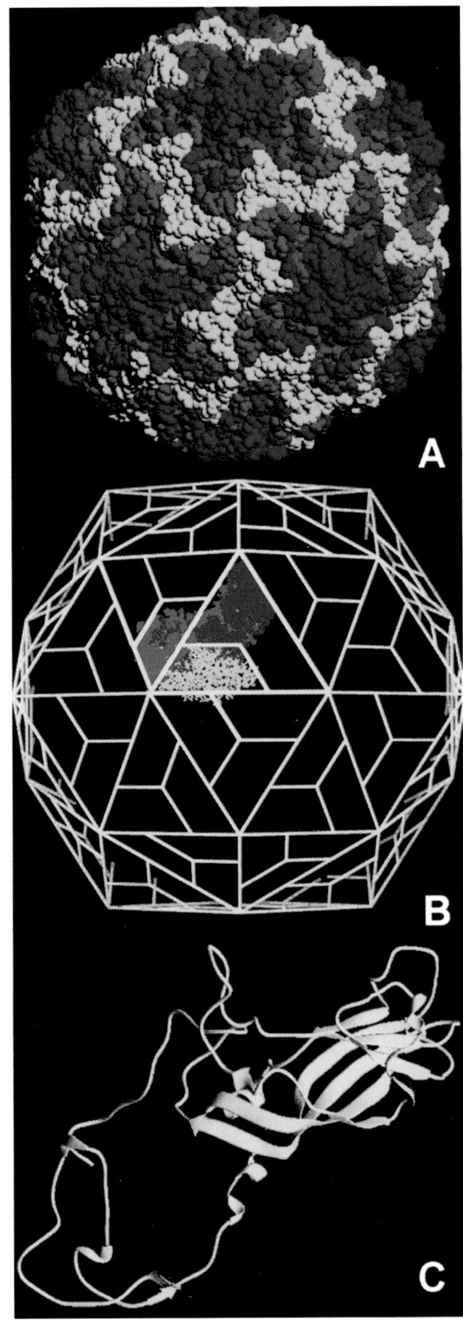

(A) Rhinovirus 14, a member of the family *Picornaviridae,* genus *Rhinovirus.* Depiction of a virion, as determined by X-ray crystallography; illustrated with VP1 in blue, VP2 in green, and VP3 in red (VP4 is inside and not visible). Each amino acid is represented by a 4-A sphere. (B) Model of a rhinovirus 14 virion, with VP1, VP2, and VP3 proteins (same colors as in A) placed diagrammatically on the icosahedral capsid. (C) VP1 of rhinovirus 14, with its atomic coordinates displayed using a ribbon program, which shows graphically the location of α helices and β barrels. Each of the viral structural proteins of this virus has an eight-stranded antiparallel β-barrel structure. (A, courtesy of S. Spencer and J.-Y. Sgro; see: http://www.bocklabs.wisc.edu. B and C, courtesy of M. G. Rossmann and R. R. Rueckert; see: http://www.bilbo.bio.purdue.edu/-viruswww.)

Figure 1.7.

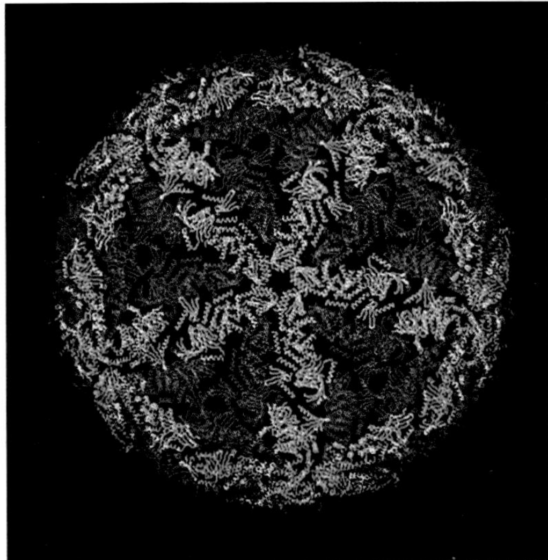

Bluetongue virus subcore structure, as determined by X-ray crystallography, illustrating the additional complexity of a larger virus. This subcore is composed of 120 copies of VP3 that self-assemble and then seem to direct the assembly of surrounding outer capsid layers. The structure of the entire bluetongue virus virion was determined by X-ray crystallography in 1997—intact virions are composed of more than 1000 separate protein molecules. (Courtesy of P. P. C. Mertens; see: http://www.iah.bbsrc.ac.uk.)

FIGURE 1.9.

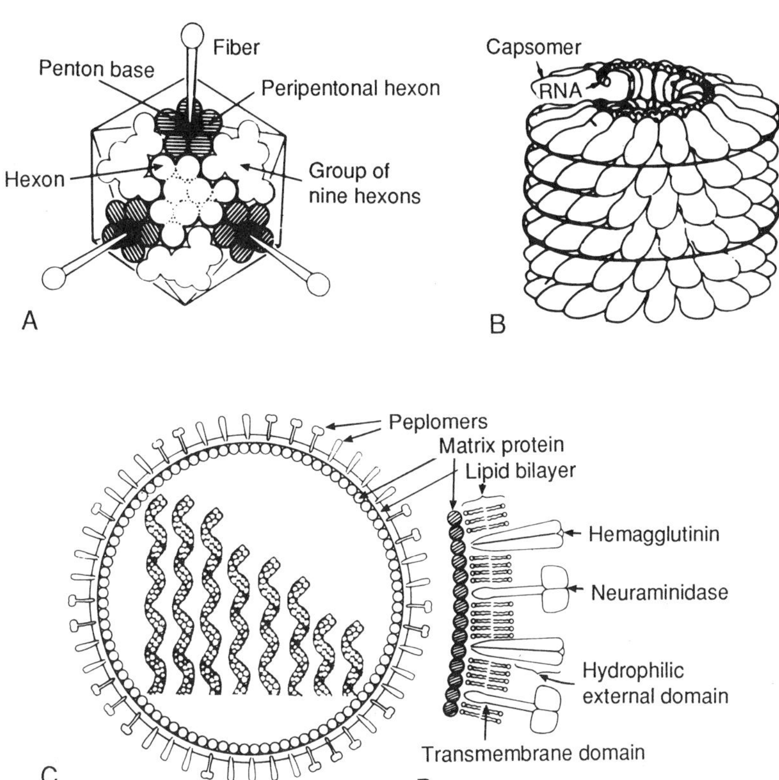

Features of virion structure, exemplified by adenovirus (A), tobacco mosaic virus (B), and influenza A virus (C, D). (A) Icosahedral structure of an adenovirus virion. All hexon capsomers are trimers of the same polypeptide, distinguished as peripentonal or group of nine by their location in the capsid. The penton base is a pentamer of another polypeptide; the fiber a trimer of a third polypeptide. (B) The structure of helical nucleocapsids was first elucidated by studies of a nonenveloped plant virus, tobacco mosaic virus, but the principles apply to animal viruses with helical nucleocapsids, all of which are enveloped. In tobacco mosaic virus, a single polypeptide forms a capsomer and 2130 capsomers assemble in a helix. The 6-kb RNA genome fits in a groove on the inner part of each capsomer and is wound to form a helix that extends the length of the virion. (C) Structure of virion of influenza A virus. All animal viruses with a helical nucleocapsid and some of those with an icosahedral capsid are enveloped. The nucleocapsids with helical symmetry are long and thin and in influenza A virus occur as eight segments, which may be connected loosely (not shown). The viral RNA is wound helically within the helically arranged capsomers of each segment, as shown for tobacco mosaic virus. (D) The envelope of influenza virus consists of a lipid bilayer in which several hundred glycoprotein peplomers or spikes are inserted; beneath the lipid bilayer there is a virus-specified matrix protein. The glycoprotein peplomers of influenza virus comprise two different proteins, hemagglutinin (a rod-shaped trimer) and neuraminidase (a mushroom-shaped tetramer), each of which consists of a hydrophobic internal domain, a transmembrane domain, and a hydrophilic external domain. Some 50 molecules of a small membrane-associated protein, M2 (not shown), form a small number of pores in the lipid bilayer. [A, from J. Mack and R. M. Burnett, *in* "Biological Macromolecules and Assemblies: Virus Structures" (F. Jurnak and A. McPherson, eds.), Vol. 1, p. 337. Wiley, New York; 1984; B, from C. F. T. Mattern, "Molecular Biology of Animal Viruses" (D. P. Nayak, ed.), p. 5. Dekker, New York, 1977.]

(also housing attachment ligands but usually not neutralizing epitopes) may be seen at higher resolution (Figures 1.11A and 1.11B).

Helical Symmetry

The nucleocapsid of several RNA viruses self-assembles as a cylindrical structure in which the protein structural units are arranged as a helix, hence the term *helical symmetry*. It is the shape and repeated occurrence of identical protein–protein interfaces on the structural units that lead to the symmetrical assembly of the helix. In helically symmetrical nucleocapsids the genomic RNA forms a spiral within the nucleocapsid (Figure 1.9). Many of the plant viruses with helical nucleocapsids are rod shaped, flexible or rigid, and nonenveloped. However, in all such animal viruses the helical nucleocapsid is wound into a secondary coil and enclosed within a lipoprotein envelope.

Viral Envelopes

The virions of the member viruses of many different virus families are enveloped, and in most cases the integrity of

FIGURE 1.10.

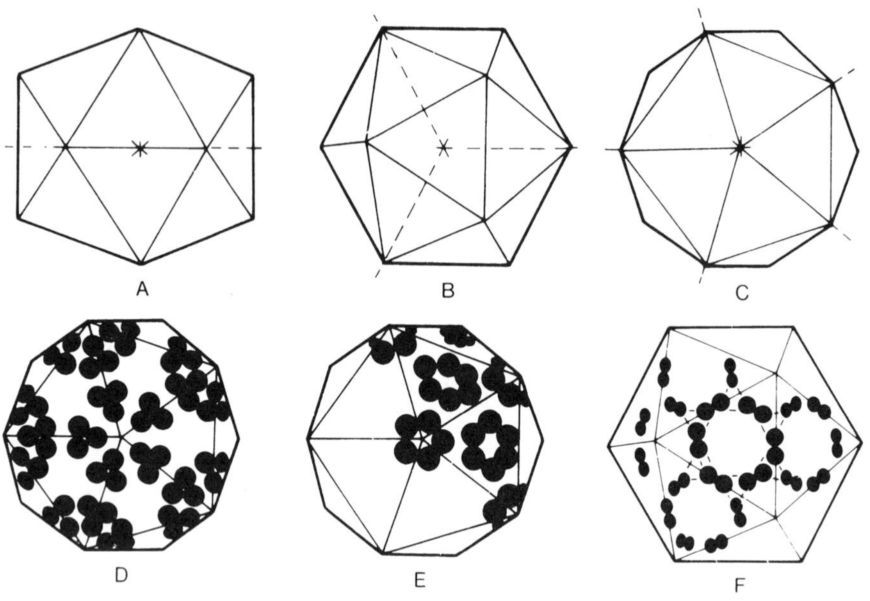

(Upper row) An icosahedron viewed along (A) twofold, (B) threefold, and (C) fivefold axes of symmetry. (Lower row) Differences in the clustering of capsid polypeptides are responsible for the characteristic appearances of particular viruses as seen by negative contrast electron microscopy. (D) When capsid polypeptides are arranged as 60 trimers, structural units themselves are difficult to see; this is the case with foot-and-mouth disease virus. (E) When capsid polypeptides are grouped as 12 pentamers and 20 hexamers they form bulky capsomers, as is the case with parvoviruses. (F) When capsid polypeptides form dimers on the faces, they produce ring-like features on the virion surface, as is the case with caliciviruses.

the envelope is necessary for viral infectivity. Enveloped virions acquire their outer layer when their nucleocapsid is extruded through one of the cellular membranes—this process is known as *budding*. The lipids of the viral envelope are derived directly from the cellular membrane, but the proteins associated with the envelope are virus coded. There are several kinds of envelope-associated proteins associated with at least four crucial activities: receptor binding, membrane fusion, uncoating, and receptor destruction. *Glycoproteins,* usually in the form of dimers or trimers, assemble into the virion peplomers (peplos = envelope) or spikes (Figure 1.9) seen in electron micrographs on the surface of orthomyxoviruses, paramyxoviruses, rhabdoviruses, filoviruses, coronaviruses, bunyaviruses, arenaviruses, and retroviruses. *Fusion proteins* are glycosylated and are also associated with peplomers; they are involved in key steps in viral entry and viral release. *Matrix proteins* are nonglycosylated and are found as a layer on the inside of the envelope of orthomyxoviruses, paramyxoviruses, rhabdoviruses, filoviruses, and retroviruses, but not coronaviruses, bunyaviruses, and arenaviruses. Matrix protein provides added rigidity to the virion; for example, the helical nucleocapsid of rhabdoviruses is closely apposed to a rather rigid layer of matrix protein, which in turn is tightly bound to the viral envelope and the internal domain of the surface glycoprotein peplomers.

Virion Structure/Function Relationships

Viral capsids and envelopes are not just packages—they must be stable enough in their expected environment to protect their contained nucleic acid, yet at the same time they must be in a primed status to facilitate uptake and infection of target cells. This primed status usually involves conformational rearrangements in virion surface structures in response to various triggers. For example, upon entry of the host, the hemagglutinin of influenza viruses is cleaved by extracellular enzymes, generating a primed modified structure. Upon entry of the host cell via endocytosis, the primed hemagglutinin is activated when exposed to the low pH within the endosome. This activated hemagglutinin mediates endosome membrane damage, thereby allowing viral RNA entry into the cytoplasm.

From this example, it is clear that knowledge of the fine structure of virions can shed light on practical matters: (1) the steps in virion attachment, penetration,

FIGURE 1.11.

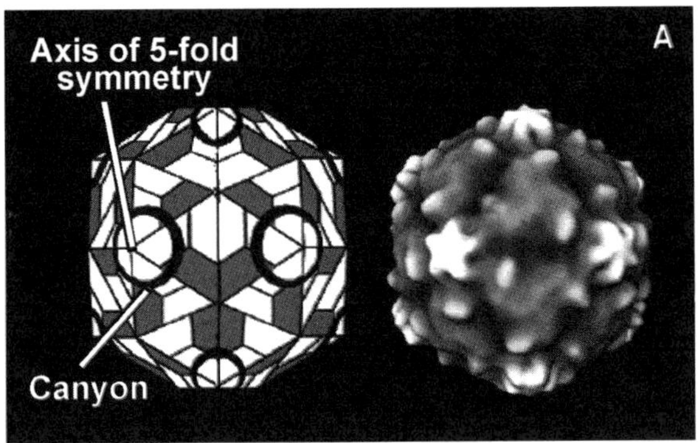

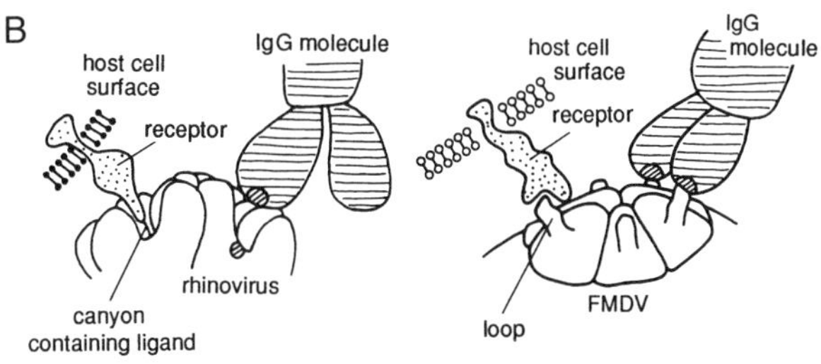

(A) The location of the canyon containing the cellular receptors surrounding the axes of fivefold symmetry on the rhinovirus virion. (B) Model of the interactions between receptors on host cells and ligands on virions, using rhinovirus and foot-and-mouth disease virus (FMDV) as examples. In the interaction of rhinovirus with its host cell, the ligands are situated within surface depressions ("canyons") near axes of fivefold symmetry. This location of the ligands serves to prevent antibody binding at those crucial sites. Antibodies specific for other antigenic sites on the surface of rhinoviruses do not necessarily block virion–cell receptor interaction. In the interaction of foot-and-mouth disease virus with its host cell, the ligands are situated on flexible, sequence-variable loops extending from the surface of the virion. These loops are not protected from antibody binding, which does block virion–cell interaction. (Courtesy of M. G. Rossmann and R. R. Rueckert.)

and uncoating as targets for antiviral drug design; (2) the steps in virion assembly, again as targets for antiviral drug design and use; (3) the bases for virion integrity as targets for disinfectant design; and (4) the mechanisms of viral shedding and the patterns of viral transmission as targets for vaccine development. In these ways, knowledge of virion structure contributes to the development of disease prevention and control strategies.

Perhaps most important of virion structure/function relationships and virus/host relationships are those that pertain to virion attachment and entry into the host cell. In this context the terms *receptor* and *ligand* have often been used in imprecise ways. In this book, the term receptor is used to designate specific molecule(s) or structure(s) on the surface of host cells that are involved in virus attachment. The term ligand is used for the receptor-binding molecule(s) on the surface of the virus. For example, the hemagglutinin of the influenza virus is the ligand that binds to the receptor on the host cell surface, in this case a glycoconjugate terminating in *N*-acetylneuraminic acid.

Chemical Composition of Virions

Viruses are distinguished from all other forms of life by their simple chemical composition, which includes a genome comprising one or a few molecules of either DNA or RNA, proteins that form the virion (i.e., structural proteins, including capsid proteins, in some cases tegument proteins, envelope proteins such as glycoproteins, fusion proteins, and matrix proteins), proteins that are needed for virion assembly (nonstructural proteins), proteins that facilitate the viral takeover of host cell machinery (enzymes involved in viral replication, including replicases, polymerases, transcriptases, etc.), some of which are incorporated in the virion, and in some viruses carbohydrates (mostly as side chains on glycoproteins) and lipids. The simplest virus (tobacco necrosis virus satellite, a defective virus that needs a helper virus to provide some of its functions) directs the synthesis of only one protein; many important viruses direct the synthesis of 5–10 proteins; and the largest viruses, such as poxviruses and herpesviruses, direct the synthesis of up to 200 proteins—still this is very few relative to the number of proteins involved in the life processes of bacteria (more than 5000 proteins) and eukaryotic cells (more than 100,000 proteins).

Viruses exhibit a remarkable variety of strategies for the expression of their genes and for the replication of their genomes. Knowledge of these schemes has much practical significance, especially in understanding infection and disease pathogenesis and the application of rational means of disease prevention and control. Many of the viruses discovered most recently have very limited host ranges and tissue tropisms (e.g., feline immunodeficiency virus). As more and more such viruses are discovered, we can expect to find additional novel genome replication and expression strategies, each of which will require new research approaches.

Viral Nucleic Acids

Viral genes are encoded in either DNA or RNA genomes; genomic DNA and RNA can be *double stranded* or *single stranded* and can be *monopartite* (all viral genes contained in a single molecule of nucleic acid) or *multipartite* (segmented: viral genes distributed in multiple molecules or segments of nucleic acid). For example, among the RNA viruses, only the member viruses of the families *Reoviridae* and *Birnaviridae* have a double-stranded RNA genome, and these genomes are segmented (*Reoviridae:* 10, 11, or 12 segments, depending on the genus; *Birnaviridae:* 2 segments). All viral genomes are haploid, i.e., they contain only one copy of each gene, except for retrovirus genomes, which are diploid. These characters, and others, have been used to order the presentation of the families of viruses containing pathogens of animals (and humans) in this book (Table 1.3).

When extracted carefully from the virion, the nucleic acid of viruses of certain families of both DNA and RNA viruses is itself infectious, i.e., when experimentally introduced into a cell it can initiate a complete cycle of viral replication, with the production of a normal yield of progeny virus. The essential features of the genomes of viruses of vertebrates are summarized in Table 1.4. Their remarkable variety is reflected in the diverse ways in which the information encoded in the viral genome is transcribed to RNA, then translated into proteins, and the ways in which the viral nucleic acid is replicated (see Chapter 3).

Viral Genomic DNA

The genome of all DNA viruses of vertebrates is monopartite, consisting of a single molecule which is double stranded, except in the case of the parvoviruses and the

TABLE 1.3
Families of Viruses Containing Pathogens of Animals and Humans

- DNA viruses
  - Double-stranded DNA
    - *Poxviridae*
    - *Asfarviridae*
    - *Iridoviridae*
    - *Herpesviridae*
    - *Adenoviridae*
    - *Papovaviridae*
  - Single-stranded DNA
    - *Parvoviridae*
    - *Circoviridae*
- DNA and RNA reverse-transcribing viruses
  - Double-stranded/single-stranded DNA
    - *Hepadnaviridae*
  - Single-stranded RNA
    - *Retroviridae*
- RNA viruses
  - Double-stranded RNA
    - *Reoviridae*
    - *Birnaviridae*
  - Single-stranded RNA
    - Negative sense,
      - Nonsegmented Order: *Mononegavirales*
        - *Paramyxoviridae*
        - *Rhabdoviridae*
        - *Filoviridae*
        - *Bornaviridae*
    - Negative sense, Segmented
      - *Orthomyxoviridae*
      - *Bunyaviridae*[a]
      - *Arenaviridae*[a]
    - Positive sense, Nonsegmented nested set transcription
      - Order: *Nidovirales*
      - *Coronaviridae*
      - *Arteriviridae*
    - Direct transcription
      - *Picornaviridae*
      - *Caliciviridae*
      - *Astroviridae*
      - *Togaviridae*
      - *Flaviviridae*
- Subviral agents: Satellites and prions
  - Single-stranded RNA (Negative sense, defective)
    - Floating genus: *Deltavirus*
  - No known nucleic acid, self-replicating protein
    - Prions

[a]Some member viruses of the family *Bunyaviridae* and all member viruses of the family *Arenaviridae* have ambisense genomes.

Table 1.4
Structure of Viral Genomes

Family	Structure of genome
Poxviridae *Asfarviridae* *Iridoviridae*	A single molecule of linear double-stranded DNA, both ends covalently closed, with inverted terminal repeats
Herpesviridae	A single molecule of linear double-stranded DNA, containing terminal and internal reiterated sequences, usually forming two covalently linked components (L and S) that result in the formation of two or four isomeric forms oriented differently in the various herpesviruses
Adenoviridae	A single molecule of linear double-stranded DNA with inverted terminal repeats and a covalently bound terminal protein
Papovaviridae	A single molecule of circular supercoiled double-stranded DNA
Parvoviridae	A single molecule of linear single-stranded DNA, negative or positive sense,[a] with palindromic sequences at ends that allow circularization of the DNA during replication
Circoviridae	A single molecule of circular single-stranded DNA, ambisense or positive sense
Hepadnaviridae	A single molecule of circular double-stranded DNA with a region of single-stranded DNA
Retroviridae	Diploid linear single-stranded RNA, positive sense, each molecule hydrogen bonded at 5′ end with 3′-termini polyadenylated and 5′ ends capped
Reoviridae	Ten, 11, or 12 molecules of linear double-stranded RNA (segmented genome)
Birnaviridae	Two molecules of linear double-stranded RNA (segmented genome)
Order: *Mononegavirales* *Paramyxoviridae* *Rhabdoviridae* *Filoviridae* *Bornaviridae*	A single molecule of linear single-stranded RNA, negative sense
Orthomyxoviridae	Eight, 7, or 6 molecules of linear single-stranded RNA, negative sense (segmented genome)
Bunyaviridae	Three molecules of linear single-stranded RNA, negative sense or ambisense, with "sticky ends" that allow circularization (segmented genome)
Arenaviridae	Two molecules of linear single-stranded RNA, negative sense or ambisense, with "sticky ends" that allow circularization (segmented genome)
Order: *Nidovirales* *Coronaviridae* *Arteriviridae*	A single molecule of linear single-stranded RNA, positive sense, with nested set transcription
Picornaviridae *Caliciviridae* *Astroviridae* *Togaviridae* *Flaviviridae*	A single molecule of linear single-stranded RNA, positive sense, 3′ end polyadenylated (except most member viruses of the family *Flaviviridae*), 5′ end capped, or protein covalently bound (*Picornaviridae, Caliciviridae, Astroviridae*)
Deltavirus	A single molecule of circular single-stranded RNA, negative sense
Prions	No nucleic acid, self-replicating infectious prion protein (PrP)

[a]Varying among the various parvoviruses.

circoviruses (Figure 1.12). DNA genomes may be linear or circular, depending on the virus family. The DNA of papovaviruses, hepadnaviruses, and circoviruses is circular. The circular DNA of hepadnaviruses is partially double stranded, partially single stranded. The circular DNA of the papovaviruses is also supercoiled.

Most of the linear viral DNAs have characteristics that enable them to adopt a circular configuration, which is a requirement for replication by what is called a rolling circle mechanism. The two strands of poxvirus DNA are covalently cross-linked at their termini (forming *hairpin ends*), so that on denaturation, the molecule becomes a large single-stranded circle. The linear double-stranded DNA of several DNA viruses (and the linear single-stranded RNA of retroviruses) contains repeat sequences at the ends of the molecule that permit circularization. In adenovirus DNA there are inverted terminal repeats; these are also a feature of the single-stranded DNA of

Figure 1.12.

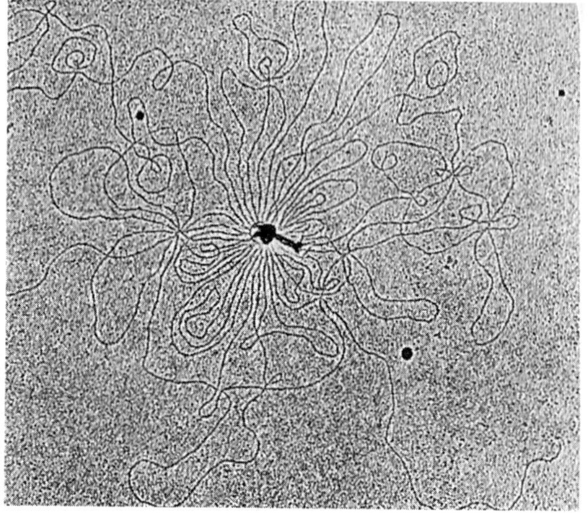

For this classical image, the DNA was released osmotically from a single T4 bacteriophage virion and floated on a liquid surface. From there, the spread-out DNA and the now empty virion head were transferred to a coated electron microscope grid and shadowed with atoms of a heavy metal. An amazing amount of DNA, up to 200 kbp, is coiled into the heads of the large DNA bacteriophages.

parvoviruses. Another type of terminal structure occurs in adenoviruses, hepadnaviruses, parvoviruses, and some single-stranded RNA viruses such as the picornaviruses and caliciviruses. In these viruses, a protein, which has an essential function in replication of the genome, is linked covalently to the 5′ terminus.

The size of viral DNA genomes ranges from 1.7 kb for some circoviruses, to over 200 kbp for the largest of the double-stranded DNA herpesviruses and poxviruses. As 1 kb or 1 kbp for double-stranded DNA contains enough genetic information to code for about one average-sized protein, it might be surmised that viral DNAs contain roughly between 2 and 200 genes, coding for some 2 to 200 proteins. However, the relationship between any particular nucleotide sequence and its protein products is not as straightforward as this. On the one hand, the DNA of most of the larger viruses, like that of mammalian cells, contains what appears to be redundant information in the form of repeat sequences, so the coding capacity of large viral genomes might be overestimated. On the other hand, the coding capacity might be underestimated: first, a given DNA or mRNA sequence may be read in up to three different reading frames, giving rise to two or three proteins with different amino acid sequences; second, either or both strands of double-stranded viral DNA may be transcribed, and in either direction, each yielding different proteins; third, genes may overlap, yielding various transcripts and protein products; and finally, a single primary RNA transcript may be spliced or cleaved in several different ways to yield several distinct mRNAs, each of which may be translated into a different protein.

Viral DNAs contain several kinds of noncoding sequences, some of which have been conserved throughout evolutionary time because they encode vital functions; these include DNA replication initiation sites, RNA polymerase recognition sites, translation initiation and termination sites, RNA splice sites, promoters, enhancers, and so on.

Viral Genomic RNA

With the exception of reoviruses and birnaviruses, the genomes of all vertebrate RNA viruses are single stranded. They can be monopartite or multipartite: for example, retroviruses, paramyxoviruses, rhabdoviruses, filoviruses, coronaviruses, arteriviruses, picornaviruses, togaviruses, and flaviviruses have monopartite genomes, whereas orthomyxoviruses, bunyaviruses, and arenaviruses have multipartite genomes. The genomes of arenaviruses consist of 2 segments, bunyaviruses 3, orthomyxoviruses 6, 7, or 8 (depending on the genus), birnaviruses 2, and reoviruses 10, 11, or 12 (depending on the genus). Each RNA molecule in these viruses is unique (often encoding a single protein). Except for the very small circular single-stranded RNA of delta hepatitis virus (the structure of which resembles that of viroids of plants), no animal virus RNA genome is a covalently linked circle. However, the single-stranded RNA of bunyaviruses and arenaviruses appears to be "circular" because of "sticky" hydrogen-bonded ends. The genomes of single-stranded RNA viruses have a considerable secondary structure, regions of base pairing causing the formation of loops, hairpins, and so on, which probably serve as signals controlling nucleic acid replication, transcription, translation, and/or packaging into the capsid.

Single-stranded genomic RNA can be defined according to its sense (also known as polarity). If it is of the same sense as mRNA, i.e., it can direct the synthesis of protein, it is said to be of *positive sense*. This is the case with the picornaviruses, caliciviruses, togaviruses, flaviviruses, coronaviruses, and retroviruses. If, however, the genomic nucleotide sequence is complementary to that of mRNA, it is said to be *negative sense*. Such is the case with paramyxoviruses, rhabdoviruses, filoviruses, orthomyxoviruses, arenaviruses, and bunyaviruses, all of which have an RNA-dependent RNA polymerase (transcriptase) in the virion, which in the infected cell transcribes positive-sense RNA using the viral genome as the template. With arenaviruses and at least one genus of bunyaviruses, one of the RNA segments is ambisense, i.e., part positive sense, part negative sense. Where the viral RNA is positive sense, it is usually polyadenylated at its 3′ end (in picornaviruses, caliciviruses, togaviruses, and coronaviruses, but not in flaviviruses) and capped at its 5′ end (togaviruses, flaviviruses, coronaviruses).

The size of single-stranded RNA viral genomes varies from 1.7 to 21 kb (M_r approximately 1–10 million) and that of double-stranded RNA viruses from 18 to 27 kbp, a much smaller range than found among double-stranded DNA viruses. Accordingly, these viruses encode fewer proteins than many DNA viruses, generally less than a dozen. Most of the segments of the genomes of orthomyxoviruses and reoviruses are individual genes, each coding for one unique protein.

Anomalous Features of Viral Genomes

Viral preparations often contain some particles with an atypical content of nucleic acid. Several copies of the complete viral genome may be enclosed within a single virion, or virions may be formed that contain no nucleic acid (empty particles) or that have an incomplete genome (defective interfering particles). Moreover, host cell DNA may sometimes be incorporated into virions (e.g., papovavirus), whereas fragments of ribosomal RNA have been found in orthomyxovirus and arenavirus virions.

Viral Proteins

The virions of all viruses of vertebrates contain several different proteins, the number ranging from 1 in the simplest virus to >100 in the most complex. Some virus-coded proteins are *structural,* i.e., they are used to construct the capsid and other components of the virion. Other proteins are *nonstructural;* some of these that are not part of the mature virion are involved in virion assembly whereas others are involved in the various aspects of viral replication processes. The latter are enzymes, most of which are involved in nucleic acid replication, transcription, and translation and in the shutdown of host cell functions and the subversion of its machinery to viral synthetic activities. These include various types of (1) replicases (e.g., DNA-dependent DNA replicases) and other enzymes involved in viral DNA replication, (2) transcriptases that transcribe mRNA from viral genomic double-stranded DNA or double-stranded RNA or negative-sense single-stranded RNA, and (3) various proteases, helicases, and ligases. Reverse transcriptase, which transcribes DNA from RNA, is found uniquely in retroviruses and hepadnaviruses. Other unique enzymes found in retroviruses are involved in the integration of the DNA product of reverse transcription into the cellular chromosomal DNA. Poxviruses, which replicate in the cytoplasm and therefore have less access to cellular machinery, carry a number of unique enzymes for processing RNA transcripts and replicating their DNA.

Viral Glycoproteins

Most viral glycoproteins occur as membrane-anchored peplomers (spikes) extending outward from the envelope of enveloped viruses, but the virions of some of the more complex viruses also contain glycosylated internal or outer capsid proteins. Oligosaccharide side chains (glycans) are attached by N-glycosidic or, more rarely, O-glycosidic linkages. Because they are synthesized by cellular glycosyl transferases, the sugar composition of these glycans corresponds to that of host cell membrane glycoproteins.

Viral Envelope Lipids

Most lipids found in enveloped viruses are present as a typical lipid bilayer in which the virus-coded glycoprotein peplomers (spikes) and, in some cases, other viral proteins are embedded. As a consequence, the composition of the lipids of particular viruses differs according to the composition of the membrane lipids of the host cells from which they came. The composition of the membrane lipids of viruses also varies with the particular membrane system employed for virion budding. For example, the lipids of paramyxoviruses that bud from the plasma membrane of host cells differ from those of bunyaviruses and coronaviruses, which bud from the membranes of intracytoplasmic organelles. Lipids constitute about 20–35% of the dry weight of most enveloped viruses; some 50–60% of viral envelope lipid is phospholipid and most of the remainder is cholesterol.

Stability of Viral Infectivity

In general, viruses are more sensitive than bacteria or fungi to inactivation by physical and chemical agents, but there are important exceptions. A knowledge of specific viral sensitivity to environmental conditions is therefore important for ensuring the preservation of the infectivity of viruses as reference reagents and in clinical specimens collected for diagnosis, as well as for their deliberate inactivation for such practical ends as sterilization, disinfection, and the production of inactivated vaccines.

Temperature

The principal environmental condition that may adversely affect the infectivity of viruses is temperature. Surface proteins are denatured within a few minutes at temperatures of 55–60°C, with the result that the virion is no longer capable of normal cellular attachment, penetration, and/or uncoating. At ambient temperature the rate of decay of infectivity is slower but significant, especially in the summer or in the tropics. To preserve infectivity, viral preparations must therefore be stored at low temperature; 4°C (wet ice or a refrigerator) is usually satisfactory for a day or so, but longer-term preservation requires much lower temperatures. Two convenient temperatures are −70°C, the temperature of solid CO_2 (dry ice) and of some mechanical freezers, or −196°C, the temperature of liquid nitrogen. As a rule of thumb, the half-life of most viruses can be measured in seconds at 60°C, minutes at 37°C, hours at 20°C, days at 4°C, and years at −70°C or lower. Enveloped viruses are more heat labile than nonenveloped viruses. Enveloped virions, e.g., those of the genus *Pneumovirus* in the family *Paramyxoviridae,* are also susceptible to repeated freezing and thawing, probably as a result of disruption of the virion by ice crystals. This poses problems in the collection and transportation of clinical specimens. The most practical way of avoiding such problems is to deliver specimens to the laboratory as rapidly as practicable, packed without freezing, on cold gel packs.

In the laboratory, it is often necessary to preserve virus stocks for years. This is achieved in one of two ways; (1) rapid freezing of small aliquots of virus suspended in medium containing protective protein and/or dimethyl sulfoxide, followed by storage at −70° or −196°C, or (2) freeze drying (lyophilization), i.e., dehydration of a frozen viral suspension under vacuum, followed by storage of the resultant powder at 4°C or −20°C. Freeze drying prolongs viability significantly even at ambient temperatures and is used universally in the manufacture of attenuated virus vaccines. The most prominent exception to this is the prions, which are amazingly stable under virtually all environmental conditions, surviving boiling, freezing, many physical and chemical insults, and even large doses of γ-irradiation (see Chapter 40).

Ionic Environment and pH

On the whole, viruses are best preserved in an isotonic environment at physiologic pH, but some tolerate a wide ionic and pH range. For example, whereas most enveloped viruses are inactivated at pH 5–6, rotaviruses and many picornaviruses survive the acidic pH of the stomach.

Lipid Solvents and Detergents

Because the infectivity of enveloped viruses is destroyed readily by lipid solvents such as ether or chloroform or detergents such as sodium deoxycholate, these agents must be avoided in laboratory procedures concerned with maintaining the viability of viruses. However, detergents are used commonly by virologists to solubilize viral envelopes and to liberate proteins for use as vaccines or for chemical analysis.

Further Reading

Alberts, B., Bray, D., Lewis, J., Raff, M., Roberts, K., and Watson, J. D. (1994). "Molecular Biology of the Cell," 3rd ed. Garland Publishing, New York.

Bhatt, P. N., Jacoby, R. O., Morse, H. C., and New, A. E. (1986). "Viral and Rickettsial Infections of Laboratory Rodents." Academic Press, Orlando, FL.

Branden, C., and Tooze, J. (1991). "Introduction to Protein Structure." Garland Publishing, New York.

Calnek, B. N., Barnes, H. J., Beard, C. N., McDougald, L. R., and Saif, Y. M., eds. (1997). "Diseases of Poultry," 10th ed. Iowa State University Press, Ames.

Carter, G. R., Chengappa, M. M., and Roberts, A. W. (1995). "Essentials of Veterinary Microbiology," 5th ed. Williams & Wilkins, Baltimore, MD.

Coetzer, J. A. W., Thompson, G. R., and Tustin, R. C., eds. (1994). "Infectious Diseases of Livestock with Special Reference to Southern Africa," 2 vols. Oxford University Press, Cape Town.

Darai, G., ed. (1987). "Virus Diseases in Laboratory and Captive Animals." Kluwer, Boston, MA.

Fenner, F. (1998). History of virology. *In* "Encyclopedia of Virology," (R. G. Webster and A. Granoff, eds.), 2nd ed. (CD-ROM). Academic Press, London.

Fowler, M. E., ed. (1986). "Zoo and Wild Animal Medicine," 2nd ed. Saunders, Philadelphia, PA.

Fraser, C. M. (1998). "The Merck Veterinary Manual: A Handbook of Diagnosis, Therapy, and Disease Prevention and Control for the Veterinarian," 8th ed. Merck, Rahway, NJ.

Gaskell, R. M., and Bennett, M. (1996). "Feline and Canine Infectious Diseases." Blackwell, London.

Greene, C. E., ed. (1998). "Infectious Diseases of the Dog and Cat," 2nd ed. Saunders, Philadelphia, PA.

Harrison, G. J., and Harrison, L. R. (1986). "Clinical Avian Medicine and Surgery." Saunders, Philadelphia, PA.

Harrison, S. C., Skehel, J. J., and Wiley, D. (1996). Virus structure. *In* "Fields Virology," (B. N. Fields, D. M. Knipe, P. M. Howley, R. M., Chanock, J. L. Melnick, T. P., Monath, B. Roizman, and S. E. Straus, eds.), 3rd ed., pp. 59–99. Lippincott-Raven, Philadelphia, PA.

Horzinek, M. C., ed. (1987–1996). "Virus Infections of Vertebrates," Book Series, vols. 1–6 Elsevier, Amsterdam.

Hugh-Jones, M. E., Hubbert, W. T., and Hagstad, H. V. (1995). "Zoonoses: Recognition, Control, and Prevention." Iowa State University Press, Ames.

Koprowski, H., and Oldstone, M. B. A. (1996). "Microbe Hunters, Then and Now." Medi-Ed Press, Bloomington, IN.

Leman, A. D., Straw, B. E., Mengeling, W. L., D'Allaire, S., and Taylor, D. J., eds., (1992). "Diseases of Swine." Iowa State University Press, Ames.

Levine, A. J. (1992). "Viruses." Scientific American Library Freeman, New York.

Levine, A. J. (1996). The origins of virology. *In* "Fields Virology," (B. N. Fields, D. M. Knipe, P. M. Howley, R. M., Chanock, J. L. Melnick, T. P. Monath, B. Roizman, and S. E. Straus, eds.), 3rd ed., pp. 1–14. Lippincott-Raven, Philadelphia, PA.

Lodish, H., Baltimore, D., and Berk, A. (1995). "Molecular Cell Biology," 3rd ed. CD ROM. Scientific American Books Freeman, New York.

Mahy, B. W. J. (1997). "A Dictionary of Virology." Academic Press, San Diego, CA.

Mahy, B. W. J., and Collier, L. H., eds., (1997). "Topley and Wilson's Microbiology and Microbial Infections," Vol. 1. Edward Arnold, London.

Martin, W. B., and Aitkin, I. D., eds. (1991). "Diseases of Sheep," 2nd ed. Blackwell, London.

Mims, C. A., Playfair, J. H., Roitt, I. M., Wakelin, D., and Williams, R. (1993). "Medical Microbiology." Mosby, St. Louis., MO.

National Research Council, National Academy of Sciences of the United States of America (1991). "Infectious Diseases of Mice and Rats." National Academy Press, Washington, DC.

Olsen, R. G., Krakowka, S., and Blakeslee, J. R., eds. (1985). "Comparative Pathobiology of Viral Diseases." CRC Press, Boca Raton, FL.

Pedersen, N. C. (1988). "Feline Infectious Diseases." American Veterinary Publications, Goleta, CA.

Radostits, O. M. Blood, D. C., and Gay, C. C. (1994). "Veterinary Medicine, a Textbook of the Diseases of Cattle, Sheep, Pigs, Goats and Horses," 8th ed. Baillière Tindall, London.

Rintoul, D., Welti, R., Storrie, B., and Lederman, M. (1995). "A Student's Companion in Molecular Cell Biology," 3rd ed. Scientific American Books Freeman, New York.

Spencer, S., and Sgro, J.-Y. (1998). "Multimedia Library, Computer Visualizations of Viruses and Viral Substructures, Access Point to Digitized Electron Micrographs of Viruses at Several Internet Websites." Institute for Molecular Virology, University of Wisconsin, Madison. Available at http://www.bocklabs.wisc.edu

Timoney, J. F., Gillespie, J. H., Scott, F. N., and Barlough, J. E. (1988). "Hagan and Bruner's Infectious Diseases of Domestic Animals," 8th ed. Cornell University Press, Ithaca, NY.

Waterson, A. P., and Wilkinson, L. (1978). "An Introduction to the History of Virology." Cambridge University Press, Cambridge, UK.

Webster, R. G., and Granoff, A., eds. (1998). "Encyclopedia of Virology," 2nd ed. (CD-ROM). Academic Press, London.

White, D. O., and Fenner, F. (1994). "Medical Virology," 4th ed. Academic Press, San Diego, CA.

Wolf, K. (1988). "Fish Viruses and Fish Viral Diseases." Cornell University Press, Ithaca, NY.

Zinsser, H. (1934). "Rats, Lice and History." The Atlantic Monthly Press/Little, Brown, Boston, MA.

CHAPTER 2

Viral Taxonomy and Nomenclature

There is evidence to indicate that all organisms may be infected by one virus or another: indeed, every organism that has been studied has yielded viruses. The number of different viruses existing as pathogens or silent passengers in animals, plants, invertebrates, protozoa, fungi, and bacteria is accordingly very large—more than 4000 different viruses and 30,000 different strains and subtypes have been recognized (particular strains and subtypes often have distinct health or economic significance). Several hundred different viruses are known to infect humans and somewhat fewer have been recovered from individual animals (livestock, companion animals and horses, laboratory animals, wild animals, birds, reptiles, amphibians, and fish). There is a sense that a significant proportion of all existing viruses of humans and domestic animals have now been isolated—this is certainly not true of the viruses infecting the myriad of other species populating the Earth.

Because all viruses, whatever their hosts, share the properties described in the preceding chapter, virologists have developed a single system of classification and nomenclature that covers all viruses—this is the system of the *International Committee on Taxonomy of Viruses* (ICTV). In this book we will be concerned primarily with the viruses that cause disease in animals; however, in some cases taxonomic categories blur among animal viruses, human viruses, viruses transmitted by arthropod vectors, and others.

Viral Taxonomy

The earliest efforts to classify viruses were based on common clinical and pathogenic properties, common organ tropisms, and common ecological and transmission characteristics. For example, viruses that cause hepatitis (e.g., canine hepatitis virus, an adenovirus, Rift Valley fever virus, a bunyavirus, and hepatitis B virus, a hepadnavirus) might have been brought together as "hepatitis viruses."

Subsequent taxonomic systems have focused on the viruses themselves and have been based on determinations of virion size, determined by ultrafiltration and electron microscopy; virion morphology, determined by electron microscopy; virion stability, determined by varying pH and temperature, exposure to lipid solvents and detergents, etc.; and virion antigenicity, determined by various serologic methods. This approach has worked because after large numbers of viruses had been studied and their characteristics used to build the overall taxonomic system, it was necessary in most cases only to measure a few characteristics in order to place an "unknown" in its proper taxon, and from there to identify it specifically. For example, an isolate from the respiratory tract of a dog, identified by negative contrast electron microscopy as an adenovirus, might be submitted immediately for serologic identification—it would certainly turn out to be a member of the family *Adenoviridae,* genus *Mastadenovirus* (the adenoviruses of mammals), and would be identifiable serologically as either canine adenovirus 1 or 2 or perhaps it would turn out to be a new adenovirus of dogs!

Today, the primary criteria for delineating the main viral taxa are: (1) the type and character of the viral genome, (2) the strategy of viral replication, and (3) the structure of the virion. Sequencing, or partial sequencing, of the viral genome provides powerful taxonomic information and now is often done very early in identification protocols. Reference genome sequences for all viral taxa are available in public databases (e.g., GenBank, National Center for Biotechnology Information, National Library of Medicine, National Institutes of Health, Bethesda, Maryland, United States: http://www.ncbi.nlm.nih.gov). Such an approach in most cases allows one to cut to specific taxonomic placement immediately, although traditional methods are often still used for reasons of economy.

The universal system of viral taxonomy is set at the levels of *order, family, subfamily, genus,* and *species.* The names of orders end with the suffix *-virales,* families with the suffix *-viridae,* subfamilies with the suffix *-virinae,* and genera with the suffix *-virus.* Lower levels, such as *subspecies, strains,* and *variants,* are established for practical purposes such as diagnostics and vaccine development, but this is not a matter of formal classification and there are no universal definitions or nomenclature at these lower levels.

Presently, the universal taxonomy system for viruses encompasses two orders, both of which contain animal and human pathogens, 54 families, 26 of which contain animal and human pathogens, and 184 genera (Table 2.1). Orders are only used to tie together families that exhibit distant phylogenetic relationships (e.g., ancient conserved genes, sequences, or domains) and because all viruses did not derive from a common ancestor, there is no intention to place all families into orders and fill in a single viral evolutionary tree. The universal taxonomy system is complete at the level of families and genera; i.e., virtually all of the viruses mentioned in this book have been placed in a family and genus. Subfamilies are used only where needed to deal with very complex interrelationships among the viruses in a family. Species is the most important taxon in all systems to classify life forms, but it is also the most difficult to define and apply—this is certainly the case in regard to the viruses. Virologists are still working on this; most of the viruses described in this book will stand as species, but a few may end up as subspecies or strains.

In the next section of this chapter, the 26 virus families that contain animal and human pathogens are outlined in the same order as the chapters in Part II of this book (see Table 1.3, Tables 2.1 and 2.2, and Figure 2.1[1]). The terms used reflect the system of the International Committee on Taxonomy of Viruses as of April 1998. The order of presentation is set by (1) nucleic acid type and strandedness (RNA or DNA, single or double stranded); (2) genome characteristics (e.g., segmentation, genome sense—positive, negative, or ambisense); and (3) replication and transcription strategy.

Families of DNA Viruses

Family: *Poxviridae*

Subfamily: *Chordopoxvirinae*
- Genus: *Orthopoxvirus* (vaccinia virus[2])
- Genus: *Capripoxvirus* (sheeppox virus)
- Genus: *Leporipoxvirus* (myxoma virus)
- Genus: *Suipoxvirus* (swinepox virus)
- Genus: *Molluscipoxvirus* (molluscum contagiosum virus)
- Genus: *Yatapoxvirus* (yabapox and tanapox viruses)
- Genus: *Avipoxvirus* (fowlpox virus)
- Genus: *Parapoxvirus* (orf virus)

Subfamily: *Entomopoxvirinae*
- Three genera: *Entomopoxvirus A, B,* and C (entomopoxviruses A, B, and C)

Characteristics: Poxviruses (*poc, pocc,* pustule) virions are brick shaped and complex in structure, measuring about 250 × 200 × 200 nm in size (except for the genus *Parapoxvirus* where virions are ovoid and 260 × 160 nm in size). The genome consists of a single linear molecule of double-stranded DNA, with covalently closed ends, 170–250 kbp in size. Virion formation involves coalescence of DNA within crescent-shaped immature particles, which then mature by the addition of outer coat layers. Replication and assembly occur in discrete sites within the cytoplasm (called *viroplasm* or *viral factories*), and virions are released by budding (enveloped virions) or by cell lysis (nonenveloped virions). Transmission is by direct contact (including wounds, abrasions), by fomites, by aerosol, or

1 For taxa that do not contain animal or human pathogens, see Murphy *et al.* (1995).

2 Throughout this chapter, names in parentheses are the type species of the taxon.

TABLE 2.1
Universal Taxonomy System for Taxa Containing Veterinary and Zoonotic Pathogens[a]

FAMILY (ORDER)	SUBFAMILY	GENUS	TYPE SPECIES (HOST IF NOT VERTEBRATE)
DNA viruses			
Double-stranded DNA viruses			
Poxviridae	*Chordopoxvirinae*	*Orthopoxvirus*	Vaccinia virus
		Capripoxvirus	Sheeppox virus
		Leporipoxvirus	Myxoma virus
		Suipoxvirus	Swinepox virus
		Molluscipoxvirus	Molluscum contagiosum virus
		Avipoxvirus	Fowlpox virus
		Yatapoxvirus	Yaba monkey tumor virus
		Parapoxvirus	Orf virus
	Entomopoxvirinae	*Entomopoxvirus genera A, B, C*	(Insect viruses, but likely also pathogens of fish)
Asfarviridae		*Asfivirus*	African swine fever virus
Iridoviridae		*Ranavirus*	Frog virus 3
		Lymphocystivirus	Flounder virus
Herpesviridae	*Alphaherpesvirinae*	*Simplexvirus*	Human herpesvirus 1
		Varicellovirus	Human herpesvirus 3
		Unnamed, Marek's disease-like viruses	Marek's disease virus
		Unnamed, infectious laryngotracheitis-like viruses	Gallid herpesvirus 1
	Betaherpesvirinae	*Cytomegalovirus*	Human herpesvirus 5
		Muromegalovirus	Mouse cytomegalovirus 1
		Roseolovirus	Human herpesvirus 6
	Gammaherpesvirinae	*Lymphocryptovirus*	Human herpesvirus 4
		Rhadinovirus	Ateline herpesvirus 2
	Unnamed, channel catfish herpesvirus-like viruses	Unnamed, channel catfish herpesvirus-like viruses	Ictalurid herpesvirus 1
Adenoviridae		*Mastadenovirus*	Human adenovirus 2
		Aviadenovirus	Fowl adenovirus 1
		Proposed, *Atadenovirus*[b]	Ovine adenovirus 287
Papovaviridae		*Polyomavirus*	Murine polyomavirus
		Papillomavirus	Cottontail rabbit papillomavirus
Single-stranded DNA viruses			
Parvoviridae	*Parvovirinae*	*Parvovirus*	Minute virus of mice
		Erythrovirus	B19 virus
		Dependovirus	Adeno-associated virus 2
Circoviridae		*Circovirus*	Chicken anemia virus

Table 2.1-Continued

Family (order)	Subfamily	Genus	Type species (host if not vertebrate)
DNA and RNA reverse-transcribing viruses			
Hepadnaviridae		*Orthohepadnavirus*	Hepatitis B virus
		Avihepadnavirus	Duck hepatitis B virus
Retroviridae		*Alpharetrovirus* (avian type C retroviruses)	Avian leukosis virus
		Betaretrovirus (mammalian type B and type D retroviruses)	Mouse mammary tumor virus
		Gammaretrovirus (mammalian and reptilian type C retroviruses)	Murine leukemia virus
		Deltaretrovirus (bovine leukemia and human T lymphotropic viruses)	Bovine leukemia virus
		Epsilonretrovirus (fish retroviruses)	Walleye dermal sarcoma virus
		Lentivirus	Human immunodeficiency virus 1
		Spumavirus	Human foamy virus 1
RNA viruses			
Double-stranded RNA viruses			
Reoviridae		*Orthoreovirus*	Reovirus 3
		Orbivirus	Bluetongue virus 1
		Rotavirus	Simian rotavirus SA11
		Coltivirus	Colorado tick fever virus
		Aquareovirus	Golden shiner virus
Birnaviridae		*Avibirnavirus*	Infectious bursal disease virus of fowl
		Aquabirnavirus	Infectious pancreatic necrosis virus of fish
Single-stranded negative-sense RNA viruses			
Order: *Mononegavirales*			
Paramyxoviridae	*Paramyxovirinae*	*Respirovirus*	Human parainfluenza virus 1
		Morbillivirus	Measles virus
		Rubulavirus	Mumps virus
		Possible new genus, Australian equine morbillivirus	Australian equine morbillivirus
	Pneumovirinae	*Pneumovirus*	Human respiratory syncytial virus
		Metapneumovirus	Turkey rhinotracheitis virus

TABLE 2.1-Continued

FAMILY (ORDER)	SUBFAMILY	GENUS	TYPE SPECIES (HOST IF NOT VERTEBRATE)
Order: *Mononegavirales*			
Rhabdoviridae		*Vesiculovirus*	Vesicular stomatitis Indiana virus
		Lyssavirus	Rabies virus
		Ephemerovirus	Bovine ephemeral fever virus
		Novirhabdovirus	Infectious hematopoietic necrosis virus of fish
Order: *Mononegavirales*			
Filoviridae		Unnamed, Marburg-like viruses	Marburg virus
		Unnamed, Ebola-like viruses	Ebola virus
Order: *Mononegavirales*			
Bornaviridae		*Bornavirus*	Borna disease virus
Orthomyxoviridae		*Influenzavirus A*	Influenza A virus
		Influenzavirus B	Influenza B virus
		Influenzavirus C	Influenza C virus
		Thogotovirus	Thogoto virus
Bunyaviridae		*Bunyavirus*	Bunyamwera virus
		Hantavirus	Hantaan virus
		Nairovirus	Nairobi sheep disease virus
		Phlebovirus	Sandfly fever Sicilian virus
Arenaviridae		*Arenavirus*	Lymphocytic choriomeningitis virus
Single-stranded positive-sense RNA viruses			
Order: *Nidovirales*			
Coronaviridae		*Coronavirus*	Avian infectious bronchitis virus
		Torovirus	Berne virus
Order: *Nidovirales*			
Arteriviridae		*Arterivirus*	Equine arteritis virus
Picornaviridae		*Enterovirus*	Poliovirus 1
		Rhinovirus	Human rhinovirus 1A
		Hepatovirus	Hepatitis A virus
		Cardiovirus	Encephalomyocarditis virus
		Aphthovirus	Foot-and-mouth disease virus O
		Parechovirus	Echovirus 22

Table 2.1-Continued

Family (order)	Subfamily	Genus	Type species (host if not vertebrate)
Caliciviridae		*Vesivirus*	Vesicular exanthema of swine virus
		Lagovirus	Rabbit hemorrhagic disease virus
		Unnamed, SRSV group 1 and 2 viruses	Norwalk virus
		Unnamed, classical human enteric caliciviruses	Sapporo virus
		Floating genus: Unnamed, hepatitis E-like viruses	Hepatitis E virus
Astroviridae		*Astrovirus*	Human astrovirus 1
Togaviridae		*Alphavirus*	Sindbis virus
		Rubivirus	Rubella virus
Flaviviridae		*Flavivirus*	Yellow fever virus
		Pestivirus	Bovine viral diarrhea virus
		Hepacivirus	Hepatitis C virus
Subviral agents: Viroids, satellites and prions (agents of spongiform encephalopathies)			
Satellites		*Deltavirus*	Hepatitis delta virus
Prions			Scrapie prion

[a]The terms used reflect the system of the International Committee on Taxonomy of Viruses as of April 1998.
[b]This proposed genus had not been approved by the International Committee on Taxonomy of Viruses as of the date of publication of this book.

mechanically by arthropods. The viruses generally have narrow host ranges, although there are some notable exceptions, including vaccinia virus and some of the avian poxviruses.

Pathogens: Genus *Orthopoxvirus:* variola (smallpox) virus, vaccinia virus (seen as rabbitpox in colonized rabbits and as buffalopox in buffaloes and cattle), cowpox virus, ectromelia (mousepox) virus, rabbitpox virus, monkeypox virus, camelpox virus, and raccoonpox virus. Genus *Capripoxvirus:* sheeppox virus, goatpox virus, and lumpy skin disease virus (cattle). Genus *Leporipoxvirus:* myxoma virus (rabbits), rabbit fibroma virus (Shope fibroma virus), hare fibroma virus, and squirrel fibroma virus. Genus *Suipoxvirus:* swinepox virus. Genus *Molluscipoxvirus:* molluscum contagiosum virus (humans). Genus *Yatapoxvirus:* tanapox virus and yabapox virus (monkeys). Genus *Avipoxvirus:* many specific bird poxviruses, including fowlpox virus, canarypox virus, and pigeonpox virus. Genus *Parapoxvirus:* orf virus (contagious pustular dermatitis virus), pseudocowpox virus, bovine papular stomatitis virus, and parapoxvirus of red deer. Subfamily: *Entomopoxvirinae:* entomopox-like virions, previously only associated with insects, have been found in lesions in commercially raised fish.

Family: *Asfarviridae*

Genus: *Asfivirus* (African swine fever virus)

Characteristics: (the family name *Asfarviridae* is derived from African Swine Fever And Related viruses; the genus name *Asfivirus* is derived from African Swine Fever) virions are enveloped, 175–215 nm in size and contain a complex icosahedral capsid composed of

TABLE 2.2
Viral Properties That Distinguish and Define Virus Families

	Virion		Nucleocapsid		Genome	
Family	**Diameter (nm)**	**Envelope**	**Symmetry**	**Structural Units**	**Nature**	**Size (kb, kbp)**
Poxviridae	250 × 200 ×200	±	Complex	NA	ds, linear	170–250
Asfarviridae	175–215	+	Icosahedral	≥1892	ds, linear	170–190
Iridoviridae	130–300	+	Icosahedral	1892	ds, linear	150–350
Herpesviridae	150	+	Icosahedral	162	ds, linear	125–235
Adenoviridae	80–100	−	Icosahedral	252	ds, linear	36–44
Papovaviridae	45–55	−	Icosahedral	72	ds, circular	5–8
Parvoviridae	25	−	Icosahedral	32	ss, (−), linear	5
Circoviridae	17–22	−	Icosahedral	32?	ss, (+), circular	1.7–2.3
Hepadnaviridae	42	−	Icosahedral	?	ds, circular	3.2
Retroviridae	80–100	+	Icosahedral	?	ss, (+), linear	7–11
Reoviridae	60–80	−	Icosahedral	92	ds, linear, 10, 11, or 12segments	16–27
Birnaviridae	60	−	Icosahedral	92	ds, linear, 2 segments	7
Paramyxoviridae	150–300	+	Helical	NA	ss, (−), linear	15–16
Rhabdoviridae	180 × 75	+	Helical	NA	ss, (−), linear	13–16
Filoviridae	790–970 × 80	+	Helical	NA	ss, (−), linear	19.1
Bornaviridae	50–60	+	Icosahedral	?	ss, (−), linear	8.9
Orthomyxoviridae	80–120	+	Helical	NA	ss, (−), linear, 6, 7, or 8 segments	10–13.6
Bunyaviridae	80–120	+	Helical	NA	ss, (−), linear, 3 segments	11–21
Arenaviridae	100–300	+	Helical	NA	ss, (−), linear, 2 segments	10–14
Coronaviridae	80–220	+	Helical	NA	ss, (+), linear	20–32
Arteriviridae	50–70	+	Icosahedral	?	ss, (+), linear	15
Picornaviridae	28–30	−	Icosahedral	60	ss, (+), linear	7.2–8.4
Caliciviridae	30–38	−	Icosahedral	32	ss, (+), linear	7.4–7.7
Astroviridae	28–30	−	Icosahedral	32	ss, (+), linear	7.2–7.9
Togaviridae	70	+	Icosahedral	60	ss, (+), linear	9.7–11.8
Flaviviridae	45–60	+	Icosahedral	?	ss, (+), linear	9.5–12.5
Deltavirus	36–43	+	?	?	ss, (−), circular	1.7
Prions (agents of spongiform encephalopathies)	Protein (PrP^{Sc})	NA	NA	NA	NA	M_r 33–35,000

FIGURE 2.1.

DNA VIRUSES

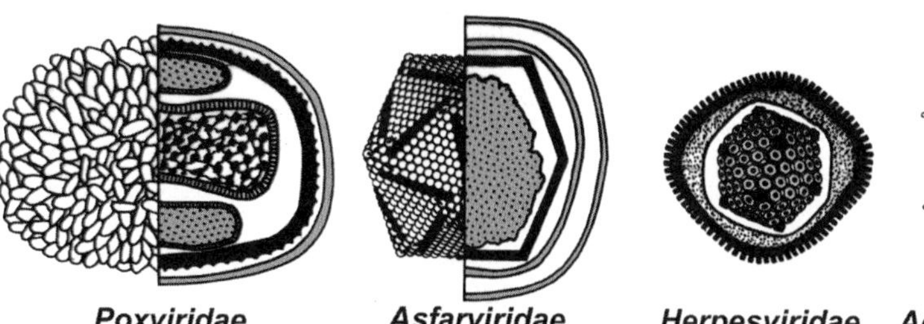

REVERSE-TRANSCRIBING VIRUSES

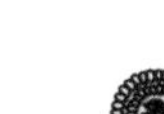

RNA VIRUSES

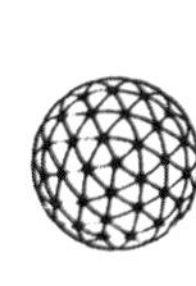

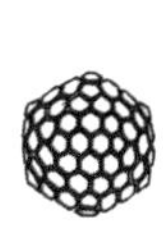

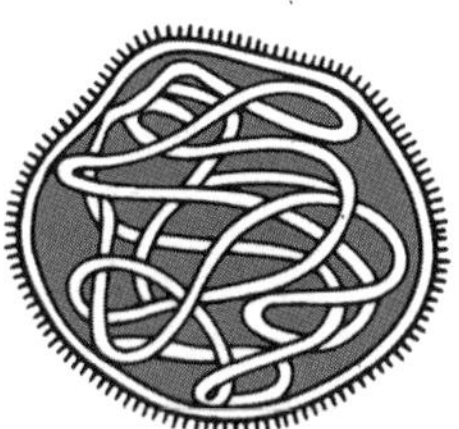

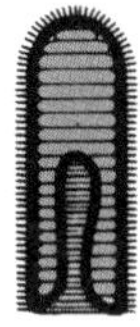

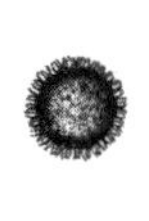

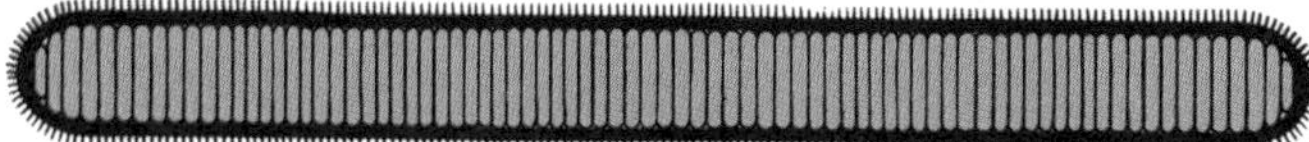

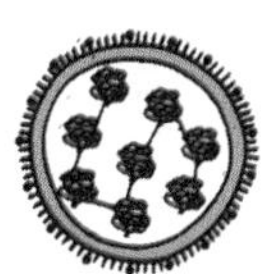

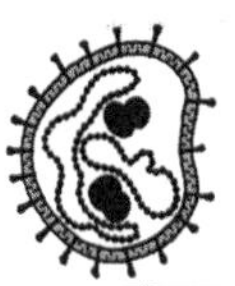

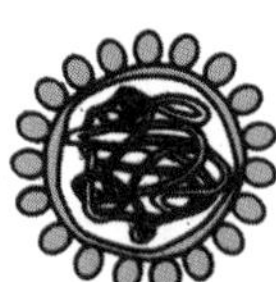

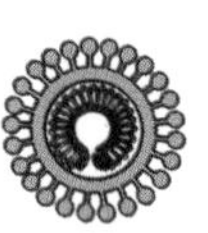

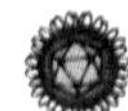

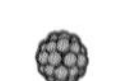

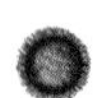

Diagram illustrating the shapes and sizes of viruses of families that include animal, zoonotic, and human pathogens. The virions are drawn to scale, but artistic license has been used in representing their structure. In some, the cross-sectional structure of capsid and envelope is shown, with a representation of the genome; with the very small virions, only their size and symmetry are depicted.

≥1892 capsomers and 180 nm in diameter. The genome consists of a single molecule of linear double-stranded DNA, 170–190 kbp in size. The DNA has covalently closed ends and encodes up to 200 proteins. Replication occurs primarily in the cytoplasm, although the nucleus is needed for viral DNA synthesis, and virions are released by budding or cell lysis. Virus strains differ in virulence; some strains cause severe disease and near 100% mortality, whereas others cause transient disease or even silent infection. The virus is transmitted by contact and also by soft ticks (genus *Ornithodoros*).

Pathogens: African swine fever virus is the only member of this taxon; it is an important pathogen of domestic swine, warthogs, bushpigs, and giant forest hogs.

Family: *Iridoviridae*

Genus: *Ranavirus* (frog virus 3)
Genus: *Lymphocystivirus* (flounder virus)
Genus: Unnamed (goldfish virus 1)

Characteristics: Iridovirus (*irido* iridescent) virions are enveloped, up to 300 nm in diameter, and contain a complex icosahedral capsid, 130–170 nm in diameter. The genome consists of a single linear molecule of double-stranded DNA, 150–350 kbp in size (mosquito iridescent virus has been reported to have a genome 440 kbp in size, the largest genome of any virus). The host cell nucleus appears to be required for transcription and replication of DNA, but some DNA synthesis and assembly of virions take place in the cytoplasm.

Pathogens: Genus *Ranavirus:* frog viruses 1-3, 5-24, L2, L4, L5, and several other viruses that affect amphibians. Genus *Lymphocystivirus:* flounder virus and many related viruses. Genus, unnamed: goldfish viruses 1–2.

Family: *Herpesviridae*

Subfamily: *Alphaherpesvirinae*
- Genus: *Simplexvirus* (human herpesvirus 1—herpes simplex virus 1)
- Genus: *Varicellovirus* (human herpesvirus 3—varicella-zoster virus)
- Genus: Unnamed (Marek's disease-like viruses) (Marek's disease virus)
- Genus: Unnamed (infectious laryngotracheitis-like viruses) (infectious laryngotracheitis virus)

Subfamily: *Betaherpesvirinae*
- Genus: *Cytomegalovirus* (human herpesvirus 5—human cytomegalovirus)
- Genus: *Muromegalovirus* (mouse cytomegalovirus 1)
- Genus: *Roseolovirus* (human herpesvirus 6)

Subfamily: *Gammaherpesvirinae*
- Genus: *Lymphocryptovirus* (human herpesvirus 4—Epstein–Barr virus)
- Genus: *Rhadinovirus* (ateline herpesvirus 2)

Subfamily: Unnamed (channel catfish herpesvirus-like viruses) (ictalurid herpesvirus 1)
- Genus: Unnamed (channel catfish-like herpesviruses) (ictalurid herpesvirus 1)

Characteristics: Herpesvirus (*herpes*, creeping) virions are enveloped, about 150 nm in diameter, and contain an icosahedral nucleocapsid about 100 nm in diameter. The genome consists of a single linear molecule of double-stranded DNA, 125–235 kbp in size. Viruses replicate in the nucleus and mature by budding through the nuclear membrane, thus acquiring an envelope. A feature of all herpesvirus infections is lifelong persistent infection, usually in latent form. Excretion, especially in saliva or genital secretions, may occur continuously or intermittently and with or without episodes of recurrent clinical signs. Some member viruses of the subfamily *Gammaherpesvirinae* cause tumors (e.g., herpesvirus ateles and herpesvirus saimiri in monkeys, and Epstein–Barr virus in humans, which is associated with nasopharyngeal cancer and Burkitt's lymphoma).

Pathogens: Subfamily *Alphaherpesvirinae,* genus *Simplexvirus:* human herpesviruses 1 and 2 (herpes simplex viruses 1 and 2), bovine herpesvirus 2 (bovine mammillitis virus), B-virus (macaques). Genus *Varicellovirus:* human herpesvirus 3 (varicella-zoster virus), bovine herpesvirus 1 (infectious bovine rhinotracheitis virus), equine herpesvirus 1 (equine abortion virus), equine herpesvirus 4 (equine rhinopneumonitis virus), and pseudorabies virus. Genus, unnamed (Marek's disease-like viruses): Marek's disease virus. Genus, unnamed (infectious laryngotracheitis-like viruses): gallid herpesvirus 1 (infectious laryngotracheitis virus) of fowl. Several animal pathogens have been placed in this subfamily, but not in genera: equine herpesvirus 3 (coital exanthema virus), feline herpesvirus 1 (feline rhinotracheitis virus), and canine herpesvirus. Subfamily *Betaherpesvirinae,* genus *Cytomegalovirus:* human herpesvirus 5 (human cytomegalovirus). Genus *Muromegalovirus:* mouse cytomegalovirus 1. Genus *Roseolovirus:* human herpesvirus 6. Several cytomegaloviruses of animals, including porcine cytomegalovirus, have been placed in this subfamily but not in genera. Subfamily *Gammaherpesvirinae,* genus *Lymphocryptovirus:* human herpesvirus 4 (Epstein–Barr virus). Genus: *Rhadinovirus:* ateline herpesvirus 2, equine herpesvirus 2, and equine herpesvirus 5. Several animal pathogens have been placed in this subfamily but not in genera. Subfamily, unnamed (channel catfish herpesvirus-like viruses): ictalurid herpesvirus 1 (channel catfish herpesvirus). Some important animal herpesvirus have not been classified beyond the family level.

Family: *Adenoviridae*

Genus: *Mastadenovirus* (human adenovirus 2)
Genus: *Aviadenovirus* (fowl adenovirus 1)
Genus (proposed): *Atadenovirus* (ovine adenovirus 287)[3]

Characteristics: Adenovirus (*adenos,* gland) virions are nonenveloped, hexagonal in outline, with icosahedral symmetry, 80–100 nm in diameter. The genome consists of a single linear molecule of double-stranded DNA, 36 to 44 kbp in size. Viruses replicate in the nucleus and their replication is facilitated by extensive modulation of the host immune response. The viruses have narrow host ranges. Many adenoviruses cause persistent infection and may be reactivated by immunosuppression—some viruses, such as equine adenovirus, cause severe disease in immunocompromised hosts. Some of the adenoviruses of humans, cattle, and chickens cause tumors when inoculated into newborn hamsters and have been used in experimental studies on oncogenesis, but none causes tumors in its natural host.

Pathogens: Genus *Mastadenovirus:* human adenoviruses 1-49, equine adenoviruses 1 and 2, canine adenovirus 1 (infectious canine hepatitis virus), canine adenovirus 2 (canine adenoviruses have also caused epidemics in foxes, bears, wolves, coyotes, and skunks), bovine adenoviruses 1, 2, 3, and 10, and ovine adenovirus 3. Genus *Aviadenovirus:* hemorrhagic enteritis virus (fowl, turkeys), marble spleen disease virus (fowl), unnamed viruses that cause pneumonitis and edema. Genus (proposed) *Atadenovirus:* ovine adenovirus 287, bovine adenoviruses 4, 5, 6, 7, and 8, and egg drop syndrome virus.

Family: *Papovaviridae*

Genus: *Polyomavirus* (murine polyomavirus)
Genus: *Papillomavirus* (cottontail rabbit papillomavirus)

Characteristics: Papovavirus [sigla, from *papilloma, polyoma, vacuolating* agent (early name for SV40)] virions are nonenveloped, spherical in outline, with icosahedral symmetry. Virions are 45 (genus *Polyomavirus*) and 55 (genus *Papillomavirus*) nm in diameter. The genome consists of a single molecule of circular double-stranded DNA, 5 (genus *Polyomavirus*) and 8 kbp (genus *Papillomavirus*) in size. Genomic DNA is infectious. Infection often is persistent, with the viral genome carried in an episomal form or integrated into the host cell DNA. Individual polyomaviruses and papillomaviruses have narrow host ranges.

Pathogens: Genus *Polyomavirus:* mouse polyoma virus, SV40 virus (both of which have been useful models for the study of viral oncogenesis), and budgerigar fledgling disease virus (the only papovavirus that causes an acute disease). Genus: *Papillomavirus:* human papillomaviruses (more than 70 types; cause of warts; particular types are associated with cancer of the cervix, anus, and pharynx), bovine papillomaviruses (cause of cutaneous papillomas in cattle), canine oral papillomatosis virus, and rabbit papillomavirus. Papillomaviruses cause lesions in many other species of mammals and birds.

Family: *Parvoviridae*

Subfamily: *Parvovirinae*
Genus: *Parvovirus* (minute virus of mice)
Genus: *Erythrovirus* (human parvovirus B19)
Genus: *Dependovirus* (adeno-associated virus 2)

Characteristics: Parvovirus (*parvus,* small) virions are nonenveloped, spherical in outline, with icosahedral symmetry, 25 nm in diameter. The genome consists of a single molecule of linear single-stranded DNA, 5 kb in size. Some parvoviruses encapsidate only negative-sense DNA strand (e.g., minute virus of mice), whereas others encapsidate different proportions of either strand (e.g., bovine parvovirus). DNA replication is complex, involving the formation of hairpin structures, extension to form a complete double-stranded DNA intermediate, and endonuclease cleavage of this intermediate. Replication and assembly take place in the nucleus; replication requires host cell functions of the S phase of the cell division cycle, indicating a viral requirement for host DNA replication machinery. Alternatively, some parvoviruses require coinfection with other viruses, such as adenoviruses or herpesviruses, for their replication. The viruses have narrow host ranges. Virions are very stable in the environment.

Pathogens: Genus *Parvovirus:* feline panleukopenia virus, canine parvovirus 1, 2a, and 2b, mink enteritis virus, Aleutian mink disease virus, bovine parvovirus, goose parvovirus, porcine parvovirus, murine parvovi-

[3] This proposed genus had not been approved by the International Committee on Taxonomy of Viruses as of the date of publication of this book.

rus, rat parvoviruses, and rabbit parvovirus. Genus *Erythrovirus:* human parvovirus B19 (the cause of an exanthem in children and hemolytic crisis in people with sickle cell disease). Genus *Dependovirus:* member viruses are defective, requiring an adenovirus for replication; they occur in birds, cattle, horses, dogs, and humans and may confound diagnostic test interpretation, but are not known to cause disease.

Family: *Circoviridae*

Genus: *Circovirus* (chicken anemia virus)

Characteristics: Circovirus (*circo,* circular) virions are nonenveloped, spherical in outline, with icosahedral symmetry, 17–22 nm in diameter. The genome consists of a single molecule circular (covalently closed ends) single-stranded DNA, 1.7–2.3 kb in size. Some viruses employ an ambisense transcription strategy, encoding some genes in the viral sense DNA strand and other genes in the complementary sense strand; other viruses encode all genes in the viral sense DNA. Replication occurs in the nucleus of cells in the S phase of the cell cycle. The viruses have narrow host ranges.

Pathogens: Genus *Circovirus:* chicken anemia virus (the cause of transient anemia and immunosuppression in baby chicks), psittacine beak and feather disease virus (the cause of chronic and ultimately fatal disease in psittacine birds), porcine circovirus (first isolated from cultures of pig kidney cells and later from a high proportion of swine in Germany; now being considered as the cause of postweaning multisystemic wasting syndrome in swine).

Families of Reverse-Transcribing Viruses

Family: *Hepadnaviridae*

Genus: *Orthohepadnavirus* (hepatitis B virus)
Genus: *Avihepadnavirus* (duck hepatitis B virus)

Characteristics: Hepadnavirus (*hepar,* liver; *dna,* sigla for DNA) virions are spherical, 42 nm in diameter, and consist of a 27-nm icosahedral core within a closely adherent outer capsid that contains cellular lipids, glycoproteins, and a virus-specific surface antigen (HBsAg). The genome consists of a single molecule of circular partially double-stranded, partially single-stranded DNA, consisting of a long (3.2 kb) and a short (1.7-2.8 kb) strand. Replication involves an RNA intermediate and requires a virus-coded reverse transcriptase. Hepadnaviruses replicate in the nucleus of hepatocytes and cause hepatitis, which may progress to chronic disease, cirrhosis, and primary hepatocellular carcinoma.

Pathogens: Genus *Orthohepadnavirus:* hepatitis B virus (humans), woodchuck hepatitis B virus, and ground squirrel hepatitis B virus. Genus *Avihepadnavirus:* duck hepatitis B virus, and heron hepatitis B virus (important causes of avian disease in some regions of the world).

Family: *Retroviridae*

Genus: *Alpharetrovirus* (avian type C retroviruses) (avian leukosis virus)
Genus: *Betaretrovirus* (mammalian type B and type D retroviruses) (mouse mammary tumor virus)
Genus: *Gammaretrovirus* (mammalian and reptilian type C retroviruses) (murine leukemia virus)
Genus: *Deltaretrovirus* (bovine leukemia and human T-lymphotropic viruses) (bovine leukemia virus)
Genus: *Epsilonretrovirus* (fish retroviruses) (walleye epidermal sarcoma virus)
Genus: *Lentivirus* (human immunodeficiency virus 1)
Genus: *Spumavirus* (human foamy virus 1)

Characteristics: Retrovirus (*retro,* backwards) virions are enveloped, 80–100 nm in diameter, with an icosahedral capsid, about 60 nm in diameter. The genome is diploid, consisting of two molecules of linear positive-sense single-stranded RNA, arranged as an inverted dimer; each monomer is 7–11 kb in size. Retrovirus replication is unique: replication starts with reverse transcription of virion RNA into double-stranded DNA by the enzyme reverse transcriptase. These linear double-stranded DNA intermediates are circularized, integrated into the host chromosomal DNA, and then used for transcription, including transcription of full-length genomic RNA and various mRNAs. Virion assembly occurs via budding from plasma membranes. The retroviruses are distributed widely in vertebrates. Endogenous proviruses (products of ancient retrovirus infections of germ line cells, inherited as Mendelian genes) also occur widely in vertebrates.

Pathogens: Retroviruses are associated with many different diseases, including leukemias, lymphomas, sarcomas, carcinomas, immunodeficiencies, autoimmune diseases, lower motor neuron diseases, and several acute diseases involving tissue damage. Genus *Alpharetrovirus:* Rous sarcoma virus, avian carcinoma viruses, avian sarcoma viruses, avian leukosis viruses, avian myeloblastosis viruses, and duck spleen necrosis virus. Genus *Betaretrovirus:* mouse mammary tumor virus, Mason–Pfizer monkey virus, simian type D virus 1, Langur type D virus, squirrel monkey type D virus, and ovine pulmonary adenomatosis virus (Jaagsiekte virus). Genus *Gammaretrovirus:* many murine leukemia viruses (e.g., Abelson, Friend, Moloney murine leukemia viruses), many murine sarcoma viruses (e.g., Harvey, Kirsten, Moloney murine sarcoma viruses), feline leukemia virus, feline sarcoma viruses, gibbon ape leukemia virus, woolly monkey sarcoma virus, porcine type C virus, guinea pig type C virus, viper type C virus, and avian reticuloendotheliosis viruses. Genus *Deltaretrovirus:* bovine leukemia virus, human T-lymphotropic viruses 1 and 2, and simian T lymphotropic viruses. Genus *Epsilonretrovirus:* walleye dermal sarcoma virus, walleye epidermal hyperplasia viruses 1 and 2, and similar viruses of fish. Genus *Lentivirus:* human immunodeficiency virus 1 and 2, simian immunodeficiency viruses (African green monkey, sooty mangabey, stump-tailed macaque, pig-tailed macaque, Rhesus, chimpanzee, and mandrill viruses), equine infectious anemia virus, maedi/visna virus, caprine arthritis–encephalitis virus, feline immunodeficiency virus, and bovine immunodeficiency virus. Genus *Spumavirus:* bovine, feline, simian, and human foamy viruses (which are a problem when they contaminate cultured cells but are not known to cause disease).

Families of RNA Viruses

Family: *Reoviridae*

Genus: *Orthoreovirus* (reovirus 3)
Genus: *Orbivirus* (bluetongue virus 1)
Genus: *Rotavirus* (simian rotavirus SA11)
Genus: *Coltivirus* (Colorado tick fever virus)
Genus: *Aquareovirus* (golden shiner virus of fish)

Characteristics: Reovirus (sigla, *r*espiratory *e*nteric *o*rphan virus[4]) virions are nonenveloped, appear nearly spherical in outline, and have a diameter of 60–80 nm. Virions have two or three shells (each with icosahedral symmetry), differing in morphologic details in each genus. The genome is linear double-stranded RNA, divided into 10 (genera *Orthoreovirus* and *Orbivirus*), 11 (genus *Rotavirus*), or 12 (genus *Coltivirus*) segments. The overall genome size is 23 (genus *Orthoreovirus*), 18 (genus *Orbivirus*), 16–21 (genus *Rotavirus*), or 27 (genus *Coltivirus*) kbp. Replication and assembly take place in the cytoplasm, often in association with granular or fibrillar inclusion bodies. Rotaviruses and reoviruses are spread by direct contact and indirectly by fomites (fecal–oral transmission); orbiviruses and coltiviruses are transmitted via arthropods (e.g., culicoides, mosquitoes, or ticks).

Pathogens: Genus *Orthoreovirus:* reoviruses 1, 2, and 3 (humans, mice, and other species; these viruses are isolated often but a causal relationship with disease is rare), avian reoviruses. Genus *Orbivirus:* bluetongue viruses 1-25, African horse sickness viruses 1-9, epizootic hemorrhagic disease of deer viruses 1-7, Ibaraki virus, equine encephalosis viruses 1-2, and other viruses affecting various animal species. Genus *Coltivirus:* Colorado tick fever virus and Eyach virus. Genus *Rotavirus:* group A rotaviruses (important pathogens of humans and other animals), group B rotaviruses (important pathogens of humans), group C rotaviruses (porcine pathogens), group D rotaviruses (fowl pathogens), group E rotaviruses (porcine pathogens), and group F rotaviruses (avian pathogens). Genus *Aquareovirus:* golden shiner virus, several salmon reoviruses, grass carp reovirus, chub reovirus, and channel catfish reovirus.

Family: *Birnaviridae*

Genus: *Avibirnavirus* (infectious bursal disease virus)
Genus: *Aquabirnavirus* (infectious pancreatic necrosis virus)

Characteristics: Birnavirus (sigla: bi-rna, two segments of RNA) virions are nonenveloped, hexagonal in outline, with icosahedral symmetry, 60 nm in diameter. The genome consists of two molecules of linear double-stranded RNA, 7 kbp in overall size. Virions assemble and accumulate in the cytoplasm and are released by cell lysis. Avian viruses are transmitted both vertically and horizontally; geographic distribution is worldwide. Natural hosts include chickens, ducks, turkeys, and other domestic fowl, salmonid fish, other fresh-water and marine fishes, and bivalve mollusks.

Pathogens: Genus *Avibirnavirus:* infectious bursal disease virus of chickens, ducks, and turkeys. Genus *Aquabirnavirus:* infectious pancreatic necrosis virus of salmonid fish.

4 The first reoviruses were found in both the respiratory and the enteric tract of humans and animals, but were not associated with any disease—"viruses in search of a disease" were called orphans.

(Order: *Mononegavirales*) Family: *Paramyxoviridae*

Subfamily: *Paramyxovirinae*
Genus: *Respirovirus* (human parainfluenza virus 1)
Genus: *Morbillivirus* (measles virus)
Genus: *Rubulavirus* (mumps virus)
Possible new genus: Unnamed (Australian equine morbillivirus)
Subfamily: *Pneumovirinae*
Genus: *Pneumovirus* (human respiratory syncytial virus)
Genus: *Metapneumovirus* (turkey rhinotracheitis virus)

Characteristics: Paramyxovirus [*para,* similar to (ortho)myxoviruses; *myxa,* mucus] virions are pleomorphic in shape (spherical as well as filamentous forms occur), 150–300 nm in diameter. Virions are enveloped, covered with large peplomers, and contain a herringbone-shaped helically symmetrical nucleocapsid. The genome consists of a single linear molecule of negative-sense, single-stranded RNA, 15–16 kb in size. The envelope contains two glycoproteins, a hemagglutinin (in most species with neuraminidase activity also) and a fusion protein. Replication takes place in the cytoplasm, and assembly occurs via budding on plasma membranes. The viruses have narrow host ranges and have only been identified in vertebrates, primarily in mammals and birds. Transmission is mainly by aerosol and droplets. Only morbilliviruses cause persistent infections, some with long-term clinical consequences.

Pathogens: Subfamily, *Paramyxovirinae,* genus *Respirovirus:* human parainfluenza viruses 1 and 3, bovine parainfluenza virus 3, mouse parainfluenza virus 1 (Sendai virus), and simian parainfluenza virus 10. Genus *Rubulavirus:* mumps virus (humans), human parainfluenza viruses 2, 4a, and 4b, Newcastle disease virus (avian paramyxovirus 1), avian paramyxovirus 2 (Yucaipa virus), avian paramyxoviruses 3, 4, 5 (Kunitachi virus), 6, 7, 8, 9, porcine paramyxovirus (la-Piedad-Michoacan-Mexico virus), and simian parainfluenza viruses 5 and 41. Genus *Morbillivirus:* measles virus, canine distemper virus, rinderpest virus, peste-des-petits-ruminants virus (goats and sheep), marine mammal morbilliviruses [porpoise distemper virus, phocine (seal) distemper virus, dolphin distemper virus, etc.]. Possible new genus: Australian equine morbillivirus. Subfamily *Pneumovirinae,* genus *Pneumovirus:* human respiratory syncytial virus, bovine respiratory syncytial virus, and pneumonia virus of mice. Genus *Metapneumovirus:* turkey rhinotracheitis virus.

(Order: *Mononegavirales*) Family: *Rhabdoviridae*

Genus: *Vesiculovirus* (vesicular stomatitis Indiana virus)
Genus: *Lyssavirus* (rabies virus)
Genus: *Ephemerovirus* (bovine ephemeral fever virus)
Genus: *Novirhabdovirus* (infectious hematopoietic necrosis virus)

Characteristics: Rhabdovirus (*rhabdos,* rod) virions are bullet shaped, about 180 × 75 nm, and consist of an envelope, covered with large peplomers surrounding a helically coiled cylindrical nucleocapsid. The genome consists of a single molecule of linear negative-sense, single-stranded RNA, 13–16 kb in size. Replication takes place in the cytoplasm, and assembly occurs via budding on plasma (vesiculoviruses) or intracytoplasmic (lyssaviruses) membranes. Rabies virus produces prominent cytoplasmic inclusion bodies (Negri bodies) in infected cells. The viruses have broad host ranges; many replicate in and are transmitted by arthropods. Rabies virus is transmitted by bite.

Pathogens: Genus *Vesiculovirus:* vesicular stomatitis-New Jersey virus, vesicular stomatitis-Indiana virus (VSV-I type 1), Cocal virus (VSV-I type 2), Alagoas virus (VSV-I type 3), Maraba virus (VSV-I type 4), Chandipura virus, Piry virus, Isfahan virus, pike fry rhabdovirus (grass carp rhabdovirus), spring viremia of carp virus. Genus *Lyssavirus:* rabies virus, Mokola virus, Duvenhage virus, Lagos bat virus, European bat viruses 1 and 2, Australian bat lyssavirus. Genus *Ephemerovirus:* bovine ephemeral fever virus, Adelaide River virus, and Berrimah virus. Genus *Novirhabdovirus:* infectious hematopoietic necrosis virus of fish. Many animal rhabdoviruses have not been classified beyond the family level [e.g., viral hemorrhagic septicemia virus of salmon (Egtved virus)].

(Order: *Mononegavirales*) Family: *Filoviridae*

Genus: Unnamed (Marburg-like viruses) (Marburg virus)
Genus: Unnamed (Ebola-like viruses) (Ebola virus)

Characteristics: Filovirus (*filo,* thread-like) virions are enveloped, pleomorphic, and appear as long filamentous forms, sometimes with extensive branching, and sometimes as "U"-shaped, "6"-shaped or circular forms. Virions have a uniform diameter of 80 nm and vary greatly in length (Marburg virus unit length is about 800 nm, Ebola virus 1000 nm; multimeric long forms are up to 14,000 nm in length). Virions consist of an envelope with large peplomers surrounding a rather rigid helical nucleocapsid. The genome consists of a single molecule of linear negative-sense, single-stranded RNA, 19.1 kb in size. Replication takes place in the cytoplasm, and assembly involves envelopment via budding of preformed nucleocapsids. Nucleocapsids accumulate in the cytoplasm, forming prominent inclusion bodies. The natural history of the viruses remains unknown. The viruses are Biosafety Level 4 pathogens; they must be handled in the laboratory under maximum containment conditions.

Pathogens: Genus, unnamed (Marburg-like viruses): Marburg virus, Genus, unnamed (Ebola-like viruses): Ebola virus (subtypes Zaire, Sudan, Reston, Côte d'Ivoire).

(Order: *Mononegavirales*) Family: *Bornaviridae*

Genus: *Bornavirus* (Borna disease virus)

Characteristics: Borna disease virus virions are spherical, enveloped, about 90 nm in diameter, and contain a core that is about 50–60 nm in diameter. The genome consists of a single molecule of linear negative-sense, single-stranded RNA, 8.9 kb in size. Most unusually, the genome is transcribed in the host cell nucleus into subgenomic mRNAs and produces high levels of polycistronic mRNAs. The genome contains three transcriptional units that code for five proteins through polymerase readthrough and posttranscriptional RNA splicing.

Pathogens: Borna disease virus is the only member of this taxon; it is the cause of meningoencephalomyelitis in a wide variety of vertebrates, including horses, sheep, cats, and birds, and has been transmitted experimentally to rodents, rabbits, and primates (macaques). Serologic and molecular evidence (polymerase chain reaction, using Borna virus primers, on human brain specimens) suggests that the virus may infect humans and cause neuropsychiatric disorders.

Family: *Orthomyxoviridae*

Genus: *Influenzavirus A* (influenza virus A/Pr8/8/34 H1N1)
Genus: *Influenzavirus B* (influenza virus B/Lee/40)
Genus: *Influenzavirus C* (influenza virus C/California/78)
Genus: *Thogotovirus* (Thogoto virus)

Characteristics: Orthomyxovirus (*orthos,* straight; *myxa,* mucus) virions are pleomorphic (often spherical but filamentous forms also occur), 80–120 nm in diameter. Virions consist of an envelope with large peplomers (that have either hemagglutinin or neuraminidase activities) surrounding helically symmetrical nucleocapsid segments of different sizes. The genome consists of eight (influenza viruses A and B) or seven (influenza virus C) or six (Thogoto virus) molecules of linear negative-sense, single-stranded RNA, 10–13.6 kb in overall size. Replication takes place in the nucleus and cytoplasm, and assembly occurs via budding from plasma membranes. Particular influenza A viruses infect humans and other mammalian and avian species; interspecies transmission coupled with mutation and genetic recombination accounts for the emergence of new human pandemic strains. Transmission is by aerosol and droplets and is water-borne among ducks. Thogoto and Dhori viruses are transmitted by ticks and replicate in both ticks and mammals.

Pathogens: Genus *Influenzavirus A:* influenza A viruses are pathogens of birds, horses, swine, mink, seals, and whales, as well as humans. Genus *Influenzavirus B:* influenza B viruses are human pathogens only. Genus *Influenzavirus C:* influenza C viruses infect humans and swine, but rarely cause serious disease.

Family: *Bunyaviridae*

Genus: *Bunyavirus* (Bunyamwera virus)
Genus: *Hantavirus* (Hantaan virus)
Genus: *Nairovirus* (Nairobi sheep disease virus)
Genus: *Phlebovirus* (sandfly fever Sicilian virus)

Characteristics: Bunyavirus (*Bunyamwera,* a locality in Uganda) virions are spherical or pleomorphic, 80–120 nm in diameter, and consist of an envelope with fine peplomers within which there are three circular helical nucleocapsid segments. The genome consists of three molecules (L, M, S) of "circular" negative- or ambisense, single-stranded RNA, 11–21 kb in overall size. Circular nucleocapsids are formed by base-paired terminal nucleotides, not by covalent bonds. Genome segments are negative sense except for the S RNA segment of phleboviruses, which encodes proteins in both viral and complementary strands. Viruses replicate in the cytoplasm and bud from Golgi membranes. Because of their segmented genomes, closely related viruses can undergo genetic reassortment. All members of the family except the hantaviruses are arboviruses (various viruses are transmitted by mosquitoes, ticks, phlebotomine flies, and other arthropods) and have wild animal reservoir hosts; some are transmitted transovarially in mosquitoes. Hantaviruses are transmitted by persistently infected rodents via aerosolization of urine, saliva, and feces. Some viruses have narrow host ranges, whereas others have wide host ranges. A few of the viruses are Biosafety Level 4 pathogens; they must be handled in the laboratory under maximum containment conditions (e.g., Rift Valley fever virus, Crimean-Congo hemorrhagic fever virus).

Pathogens: Genus *Bunyavirus:* Bunyamwera virus, Bwamba virus, Oriboca virus, Oropouche virus, Guama virus, LaCrosse virus, Jamestown Canyon virus, California encephalitis virus, snowshoe hare virus, Tahyna virus (all human pathogens), Akabane virus, and Aino virus (both livestock pathogens). Genus *Phlebovirus:* Rift Valley fever virus (livestock and human pathogen); sandfly fever Naples virus and sandfly fever Sicilian virus (both human pathogens). Genus *Nairovirus:* Nairobi sheep disease virus and Crimean-Congo hemorrhagic fever virus (sheep, humans). Genus *Hantavirus:* Hantaan virus, Seoul virus, Dobrava virus (all causing hemorrhagic fever with renal syndrome), Sin Nombre virus and several newly identified related viruses (causing acute respiratory distress syndrome in humans), and Puumala virus (nephropathia epidemica).

Family: *Arenaviridae*

Genus: *Arenavirus* (lymphocytic choriomeningitis virus)

Characteristics: Arenavirus (*arena,* sand, host cell ribosomes resembling grains of sand occur within virions) virions are pleomorphic, 100–300 nm in diameter, and consist of an envelope with large club-shaped peplomers enclosing two loosely helical circular nucleocapsid segments. The genome consists of two molecules (L and S) of "circular" negative- and ambisense, single-stranded RNA, 10–14 kb in overall size. Circular nucleocapsids are formed by base-paired terminal nucleotides, not by covalent bonds. Both RNA segments encode proteins in both viral and complementary strands. Replication takes place in the cytoplasm, and assembly occurs via budding from the plasma membrane. Arenaviruses cause chronic, often lifelong inapparent infections in specific rodent reservoir hosts; humans are infected via aerosol exposure to dried rodent urine, feces, and saliva and may develop serious generalized disease. The human pathogens, Lassa, Machupo, Junin, and Guanarito viruses, are Biosafety Level 4 pathogens and can be worked with in the laboratory only under maximum containment conditions.

Pathogens: Genus *Arenavirus:* Lymphocytic choriomeningitis (LCM) virus (reservoir is *Mus musculus,* globally; a human pathogen and an important laboratory model for the study of persistent infection and immunopathology), Lassa virus (Lassa fever, humans), Machupo virus (Bolivian hemorrhagic fever, humans), Junin virus (Argentine hemorrhagic fever, humans), and Guanarito virus (Venezuelan hemorrhagic fever, humans).

(Order: *Nidovirales*)
Family: *Coronaviridae*

Genus: *Coronavirus* (avian infectious bronchitis virus)
Genus: *Torovirus* (Berne virus)

Characteristics: Coronavirus (*corona,* crown) virions are enveloped, 80–220 nm in size, and roughly spherical in shape (coronaviruses) or 120–140 nm in size and disk, kidney, or rod shaped (toroviruses). Virions have large club-shaped peplomers enclosing what appears to be an icosahedral internal core structure within which is a helical nucleocapsid (coronaviruses) or a tightly coiled, doughnut-shaped nucleocapsid (toroviruses). The genome consists of a single molecule of linear positive-sense, single-stranded RNA, about 20 kb (toroviruses) or 27–32 kb (coronaviruses) kb in size, the latter being the largest RNA virus genomes known. Transcription of the genomic RNA yields full-length complementary RNA that acts as a template for the synthesis of a nested set of five to seven subgenomic mRNAs. Virions mature in the cytoplasm by budding through the endoplasmic reticulum and Golgi membranes. The viruses have narrow host ranges. Aerosol, fecal–oral, and fomite transmissions are common.

Pathogens: Genus *Coronavirus:* avian infectious bronchitis virus (fowl), turkey bluecomb virus, transmissible gastroenteritis virus (swine), hemagglutinating encephalomyelitis virus (swine), porcine epidemic diarrhea virus, calf coronavirus, feline infectious peritonitis virus, feline enteric coronavirus, canine coronavirus, mouse hepatitis viruses, rat coronavirus (sialodacryoadenitis virus), rabbit coronavirus, human coronaviruses 229-E, OC43, and others (causing the common cold, upper respiratory tract infection, probably pneumonia, and possibly gastroenteritis in humans). Genus *Torovirus:* Berne virus (horse), Breda virus (calves), porcine torovirus, human torovirus (recent evidence indicates that toroviruses infect humans and cause enteric and respiratory disease).

(Order: *Nidovirales*)
Family: *Arteriviridae*

Genus: *Arterivirus* (equine arteritis virus)

Characteristics: Arterivirus (from *arteritis*) virions are 50–70 nm in diameter and consist of an isometric nucleocapsid surrounded by a closely adherent envelope with ring-like surface structures. The genome consists of a single molecule of linear positive-sense, single-stranded RNA, 15 kb in size. Transcription of the genomic RNA yields full-length complementary RNA, which acts as a template for the synthesis of a nested set of six subgenomic mRNAs. Primary host cells are macrophages. Persistent infections are established regularly. Transmission is by contact (including sexual contact), fomites, and aerosol.

Pathogens: Genus *Arterivirus:* equine arteritis virus; lactate dehydrogenase-elevating virus (mice); simian hemorrhagic fever virus; Lelystad virus (porcine reproductive and respiratory syndrome virus); and VR2332 virus (swine). No known human pathogen.

Family: *Picornaviridae*

Genus: *Enterovirus* (poliovirus 1)
Genus: *Rhinovirus* (human rhinovirus 1A)[5]
Genus: *Hepatovirus* (hepatitis A virus)
Genus: *Cardiovirus* (encephalomyocarditis virus)
Genus: *Aphthovirus* (foot-and-mouth disease virus O)
Genus: *Parechovirus* (human echovirus 22 and 23)

Characteristics: Picornavirus ("*pico*" = "micro-micro," *rna,* sigla for RNA) virions are nonenveloped, 27 nm in diameter, and have icosahedral symmetry. The atomic structure of representative viruses of all genera has been solved; virions are constructed from 60 copies each of four capsid proteins and a single copy of the genome-linked protein. The genome consists of a single molecule of linear positive-sense, single-stranded RNA, 7.2–8.4 kb in size. Replication and assembly take place in the cytoplasm and the virus is released via cell lysis. Infection is generally acute and cytolytic, but persistent infections occur with some viruses. The viruses have narrow host ranges. Transmission is horizontal, mainly by contact, fecal–oral, or airborne routes.

Pathogens: Genus *Enterovirus:* polioviruses 1, 2, and 3; coxsackieviruses A1-22 and A24; coxsackieviruses B1-6; human echoviruses 1–7, 9, 11–21, 24–27, and 29–33; human enteroviruses 68–71; swine vesicular disease virus; Theiler's murine encephalomyelitis virus; porcine enteroviruses 1–8; bovine enteroviruses 1–7; and simian enteroviruses 1–18. Genus *Rhinovirus:* human rhinoviruses 1–100, 1A, 1B; bovine rhinoviruses 1–3. Genus *Hepatovirus:* hepatitis A virus and simian hepatitis A virus. Genus *Cardiovirus:* encephalomyocarditis virus. Genus *Aphthovirus:* foot-and-mouth disease viruses O, A, C, SAT 1–3, and Asia 1, equine rhinovirus 1. Genus *Parechovirus:* human echovirus 22 and 23. Ungrouped: equine rhinoviruses 2 and 3.

Family: *Caliciviridae*

Genus: *Vesivirus* (marine/vesicular disease viruses) (vesicular exanthema of swine virus)
Genus: *Lagovirus* (rabbit hemorrhagic disease virus)
Genus: Unnamed (SRSV group 1 and 2 viruses) (Norwalk virus)
Genus: Unnamed (classical human enteric caliciviruses) (Sapporo virus)
Floating genus: Unnamed (hepatitis E-like viruses) (hepatitis E virus)[6]

Characteristics: Calicivirus (*calix,* cup) virions are nonenveloped, 30–38 nm in diameter, and have icosahedral symmetry. By negative contrast electron microscopy, virions often have 32 symmetrically arranged cup-shaped depressions on their surface. The genome consists of a single molecule of linear positive-sense, single-stranded RNA, 7.4– 7.7 kb in size. Characteristically, capsids are constructed from 60 copies of a single large protein. Replication and assembly take place in the cytoplasm, and the virus is released via cell lysis. Viruses have narrow host ranges.

Pathogens: Genus *Vesivirus* (marine/vesicular disease viruses): vesicular exanthema viruses 1–13 of swine, San Miguel sea lion viruses 1–17, feline calicivirus, cetacean calicivirus (Tur-1), primate calicivirus (Pan-1),

[5] Evidence indicates that equine rhinoviruses 1 and 2 are not rhinoviruses; equine rhinovirus 1 has been placed in the genus *Aphthovirus;* equine rhinovirus 2 may be placed in a new genus.

[6] Hepatitis E-like viruses were members of the family *Caliciviridae,* but have been removed because of substantial genomic differences.

skunk calicivirus, and reptile calicivirus (Cro-1), Genus *Lagovirus:* rabbit hemorrhagic disease virus, European brown hare syndrome virus. Genus, unnamed (SRSV group 1): Norwalk virus, Southampton virus, Snow Mountain virus, Hawaii virus, and Taunton virus; (SRSV group 2): Toronto virus, Lordsdale virus and swine caliciviruses. Genus, unnamed (classical human enteric caliciviruses): Sapporo virus and Manchester virus. Unclassified caliciviruses: bovine enteric caliciviruses, canine calicivirus, mink calicivirus, porcine enteric calicivirus, walrus calicivirus, lion calicivirus, chicken calicivirus, and other caliciviruses of birds. Floating genus (removed from family): hepatitis E virus of humans and a similar virus of swine.

Family: *Astroviridae*

Genus: *Astrovirus* (human astrovirus 1)

Characteristics: Astrovirus (*astron,* star) virions are nonenveloped, 28–30 nm in diameter, and have icosahedral symmetry. By negative contrast electron microscopy, virions often appear to have a distinctive five- or six-pointed star on their surface. The genome consists of a single molecule of linear positive-sense, single-stranded RNA, 7.2–7.9 kb in size. Replication and assembly take place in the cytoplasm, and the virus is released via cell lysis. The viruses have narrow host ranges; transmission is by the fecal–oral route.

Pathogens: Genus *Astrovirus:* human astroviruses 1-5, bovine astroviruses 1-2, ovine astrovirus, porcine astrovirus, canine astrovirus, and duck astrovirus.

Family: *Togaviridae*

Genus: *Alphavirus* (Sindbis virus)
Genus: *Rubivirus* (rubella virus)

Characteristics: Togavirus (*toga,* cloak) virions are enveloped, spherical in outline, 70 nm in diameter, with an icosahedral nucleocapsid (50 nm in diameter). Virions have rather indistinct peplomers. The genome consists of a single molecule of linear positive-sense, single-stranded RNA, 9.7–11.8 kb in size. Viral replication involves the synthesis of a subgenomic mRNA, from which the structural proteins are synthesized. Replication takes place in the cytoplasm, and assembly involves budding through host cell membranes. Alphaviruses are transmitted between vertebrates by mosquitoes and certain other hematophagous arthropods; the infection of vertebrate cells is acute and cytolytic but the infection of mosquito cells is persistent and noncytolytic. Alphaviruses have a wide host range; the rubella virus infects only humans.

Pathogens: Genus *Alphavirus:* eastern equine encephalitis virus, western equine encephalitis virus, Venezuelan equine encephalitis virus, Sindbis virus (and variants Ockelbo and Babanki viruses), chikungunya virus, o'nyong-nyong virus, Igbo Ora virus, Ross River virus, Mayaro virus, Barmah Forest virus, and Getah virus. Genus *Rubivirus:* rubella virus.

Family: *Flaviviridae*

Genus: *Flavivirus* (yellow fever virus)
Genus: *Pestivirus* (bovine viral diarrhea virus)
Genus: *Hepacivirus* (hepatitis C virus)

Characteristics: Flavivirus (*flavus,* yellow) virions are enveloped, spherical in outline, and 45–60 nm in diameter. Virions have fine peplomers that do not show symmetrical placement. The viral core is spherical and is thought to have icosahedral symmetry, but its structure is unknown. The genome consists of a single molecule of linear positive-sense, single-stranded RNA, 10.7 (flaviviruses), 12.5 (pestiviruses), or 9.5 (hepatitis C virus) kb in size. Replication takes place in the cytoplasm, and assembly involves envelopment by internal host cell membranes (true budding is not seen). The infection of vertebrate cells is cytolytic, arthropod cells noncytolytic and persistent. Flaviviruses are transmitted between vertebrates by mosquitoes and ticks; some viruses have a limited vertebrate host range, whereas others have a wide host range and worldwide distribution. Pestiviruses infect only certain animals and are transmitted by direct and indirect contact (e.g., fecally contaminated food, urine, or nasal secretions); all pestiviruses are also transmitted transplacentally and congenitally. The hepatitis C virus is transmitted by close contact, sexual contact, and blood transfusion. A few of the viruses are Biosafety Level 4 pathogens; they must be handled in the laboratory under maximum containment conditions (e.g., members of the tick-borne encephalitis complex including Russian Spring-Summer encephalitis virus, Omsk hemorrhagic fever virus, and Kyasanur Forest virus).

Pathogens: Genus *Flavivirus:* yellow fever virus; dengue viruses 1-4; West Nile virus; St. Louis encephalitis virus; Japanese encephalitis virus; Murray Valley encephalitis virus; Rocio virus; tick-borne encephalitis virus complex (including European and far eastern tick-borne encephalitis viruses, Russian Spring Summer encephalitis virus, Kyasanur forest disease virus, Omsk hemorrhagic fever virus, louping ill virus, Powassan virus), Israel turkey meningoencephalitis virus, and Wesselsbron virus (sheep). Genus *Pestivirus:* bovine viral diarrhea virus (mucosal disease virus), hog cholera virus, and border disease virus of sheep. Genus *Hepacivirus:* hepatitis C virus and hepatitis G virus.

Subviral Agents: Defective Viruses, Satellites, and Prions (Agents of Spongiform Encephalopathies)

Defective Viruses and Satellites

Floating genus: *Deltavirus* (hepatitis D virus)

Characteristics: Hepatitis D virus, the only member of this genus, is a defective, satellite virus, the replication of which is dependent on simultaneous infection by the hepadnavirus hepatitis B virus (hence in nature it only occurs in humans). Virions are spherical, about 36–43 nm in diameter, and consist of a core encapsidated by helper hepadnavirus protein. The genome consists of a single molecule of circular negative-sense, single-stranded RNA, 1.7 kb in size. In humans infected simultaneously with the hepatitis B virus, the hepatitis D virus causes more severe disease, often progressing to cirrhosis. The genome structure and autocatalytic activities of hepatitis D virus closely resemble those of some viroids and satellite viruses found in plants.

Pathogens: Hepatitis D virus.

Prions (Agents of Spongiform Encephalopathies)

Characteristics: Prions are modified host protein molecules, not associated with detectable nucleic acid, that are transmissible and induce fatal neurologic disease. The modified protein, designated PrP^{Sc} (M_r 33,000–35,000), is generated from the normal isoform of the protein, PrP^{C}. Infecting PrP^{Sc} molecules are presumed to combine with PrP^{C} molecules, giving rise via abnormal protein folding to new PrP^{Sc} molecules. PrP^{Sc} molecules aggregate into fibrils that resist normal enzymatic degradation; their accumulation causes neurologic disease by unknown means. The mechanism of natural transmission of scrapie among sheep and goats is still unproved; transmission of the bovine spongiform encephalopathy agent has involved consumption of feed supplements contaminated with tissues of infected animals. Kuru in the New Guinea Fore people was transmitted by contact with brain tissue of infected people during rites of ritualistic cannibalism. Some cases of Creutzfeldt–Jakob disease are acquired iatrogenically, some are familial (with specific mutations in the PrP gene), but most are sporadic and of unknown origin.

Pathogens: Scrapie of sheep and goats, bovine spongiform encephalopathy (which has occurred in cats and captive exotic felids and ungulates), transmissible mink encephalopathy (scrapie in mink), chronic wasting disease of mule deer and elk, kuru (human), Creutzfeldt–Jakob disease (human), new variant Creutzfeldt–Jakob disease (human), Gerstmann–Sträussler–Scheinker syndrome (human), and fatal familial insomnia (humans).

Viral Nomenclature

Proper use of the specialized vocabulary of biological sciences and medicine, along with the additional vocabulary of veterinary medicine and veterinary and zoonotic virology, is key to accurate communication in all professional activities, whether these be clinical, research, or public program activities. The proper use of specialized virologic nomenclature is as indicative of one's understanding of the infectious diseases as is the proper use of the nomenclature of pathology, epidemiology, or clinical medicine.

In formal usage of virus nomenclature, the first letters of the virus family, subfamily, and genus names are capitalized and the terms are printed in italics. Species designations are not capitalized (unless they are derived from a place name) nor are they italicized. In formal usage, the identification of the taxon precedes the name; for example: ". . . the family *Paramyxoviridae*" or ". . . the genus *Morbillivirus.*" The following are examples of formal taxonomic terminology:

Order *Mononegavirales,* family *Rhabdoviridae,* genus *Lyssavirus,* rabies virus.
Family *Poxviridae,* subfamily *Chordopoxvirinae,* genus *Suipoxvirus,* swinepox virus.
Family *Herpesviridae,* subfamily *Alphaherpesvirinae,* genus *Simplexvirus,* bovine herpesvirus 2 (bovine mamillitis virus or pseudo-lumpy skin disease virus).
Family *Picornaviridae,* genus *Aphthovirus,* foot-and-mouth disease virus Asia 1.
Family *Parvoviridae,* subfamily *Parvovirinae,* genus *Parvovirus,* canine parvovirus 2.

In informal vernacular usage, all terms are written in lowercase script (except those derived from place names); they are not italicized, do not include the formal suffix, and the name of the taxon follows the name. For example, "... the picornavirus family" and "... the enterovirus genus." One particular problem in vernacular nomenclature lies in the common use of the same root terms in family and genus names—it is sometimes difficult to determine which level is being cited. For example, the vernacular name "bunyavirus" might refer to the family *Bunyviridae,* to the genus *Bunyavirus,* or to one particular virus, such as Bunyamwera virus. The solution is to add taxon identification, even some formal taxonomic identification. For example, when referring to Bunyamwera virus, one can say, "Bunyamwera virus, a member of the genus *Bunyavirus* in the family *Bunyaviridae*. . ."

Groupings of Viruses on the Basis of Epidemiologic Criteria

Separate from the formal universal taxonomic system and the formal and vernacular nomenclature that stems from it, there are other categorization of viruses that are practical and useful. These are based on virus tropisms and modes of transmission. Most viruses of animals are transmitted by inhalation, ingestion, injection (including via arthropod bites), close contact (including sexual contact), or congenitally.

Enteric viruses are usually acquired by ingestion (fecal–oral transmission) and replicate primarily in the intestinal tract. The term is usually restricted to viruses that remain localized in the intestinal tract, rather than causing generalized infections. Enteric viruses are included in the families *Picornaviridae* (genus *Enterovirus*), *Caliciviridae, Astroviridae, Coronaviridae, Reoviridae* (genera *Rotavirus* and *Reovirus*), *Parvoviridae,* and *Adenoviridae.*

Respiratory viruses are usually acquired by inhalation (respiratory transmission) or by fomites (inanimate objects carrying virus contagion) and replicate primarily in the respiratory tract. The term is usually restricted to viruses that remain localized in the respiratory tract, rather than causing generalized infections. Respiratory viruses are included in the families *Picornaviridae* (genus *Rhinovirus*), *Caliciviridae, Coronaviridae* (genus *Coronavirus*), *Paramyxoviridae* (genera *Paramyxovirus, Rubulavirus,* and *Pneumovirus*), *Orthomyxoviridae,* and *Adenoviridae.*

Arboviruses (from "*ar*thropod-*bo*rne viruses") replicate in their hematophagous (blood-feeding) arthropod vectors and are then transmitted by bite to vertebrate hosts, wherein virus replication produces viremia of sufficient magnitude to infect other blood-feeding arthropods. Thus, the cycle is perpetuated. Arboviruses are included in the families *Togaviridae, Flaviviridae, Rhabdoviridae, Bunyaviridae, Reoviridae* (genera *Orbivirus* and *Coltivirus*), and *Asfarviridae.*

Oncogenic viruses are acquired by close contact (including sexual contact), injection, fomites, and by unknown means. The viruses usually infect only specific cells in particular target tissues, where they usually become persistent and may evoke transformation of host cells, which may in turn progress to malignancy. Viruses that have demonstrated the capacity to be oncogenic, in experimental animals or in nature, are included in the families *Retroviridae, Hepadnaviridae, Papovaviridae, Adenoviridae,* and *Herpesviridae.*

Taxonomy and the Causal Relationship between Virus and Disease

One of the landmarks in the history of infectious diseases was the development of the Henle–Koch postulates, which established the evidence required to prove a causal relationship between a particular infectious agent and a particular disease. These simple postulates were originally drawn up for bacteria, but were revised in 1937 by Rivers and again in 1982 by Evans in attempts to accommodate the special problem of proving disease causation by viruses (Table 2.3). In many cases, virologists have had to rely on indirect evidence, "guilt by association," with associations based on epidemiologic data and patterns of serologic positivity in populations. The framework of virus taxonomy, again, plays a role, especially in trying to distinguish an etiological rather than a coincidental or opportunistic relationship between a virus and a given disease.

For example, early in the investigation of human acquired immunodeficiency syndrome (AIDS), before its etiology was established, many kinds of viruses were being isolated from patients and many candidate etiologic agents were being advanced. Prediction that the etiologic agent would turn out to be a member of the family *Retroviridae* was based on years of veterinary research on animal retroviruses and animal retroviral diseases. This prediction was based on the recognition of common biologic and pathogenetic characteristics of AIDS and animal retroviral diseases. This prediction guided many of the early experiments to find the etiologic agent of AIDS; later, after human immunodeficiency virus (HIV) was discovered, its morphological similarity to equine infectious anemia virus, a prototypic member of the genus *Lentivirus,* family *Retroviridae,* was the key

Table 2.3
Criteria for Disease Causation: A Unified Concept Appropriate for Viruses as Causative Agents of Disease, Based on Henle–Koch Postulates, Developed by A. S. Evans[a]

1. Prevalence of the disease is significantly higher in subjects exposed to the putative virus than in those not so exposed
2. Incidence of the disease is significantly higher in subjects exposed to the putative virus than in those not so exposed (prospective studies)
3. Evidence of exposure to the putative virus is present more commonly in subjects with the disease than in those without the disease
4. Temporally, the onset of disease follows exposure to the putative virus, always following an incubation period
5. A regular pattern of clinical signs follows exposure to the putative virus, presenting a graded response, often from mild to severe
6. A measurable host immune response, such as an antibody response and/or a cell-mediated response, follows exposure to the putative virus. In those individuals lacking prior experience, the response appears regularly, and in those individuals with prior experience, the response is anamnestic
7. Experimental reproduction of the disease follows deliberate exposure of animals to the putative virus, but nonexposed control animals remain disease free. Deliberate exposure may be in the laboratory or in the field, as with sentinel animals
8. Elimination of the putative virus and/or its vector decreases the incidence of the disease
9. Prevention or modification of infection, via immunization or drugs, decreases the incidence of the disease
10. "The whole thing should make biologic and epidemiologic-sense"

[a]A. S. Evans and R. A. Kaslow, eds., "Viral Infections of Humans: Epidemiology and Control," 4th ed. Plenum, New York, 1997.

to unraveling confusion over the fact that the human virus killed host lymphocytes rather than transforming them as typical oncogenic retroviruses would do. Ever since, this essential quality of *comparative medicine* has been guiding HIV/AIDS experimental design in many areas, including drug design, diagnostics, and vaccine development.

Further Reading

Ackermann, H.-W., and Berthiaume, L. (1995). "Atlas of Virus Diagrams." CRC Press, Boca Raton, FL.

American Type Culture Collection. (1996). "Reference Guide for Animal Viruses and Antisera, Chlamydiae, and Rickettsiae," 7th ed. American Type Culture Collection, Rockville, MD.

Büchen-Osmond, C., and Gibbs, A. J. (1998). "Index Virum (a collection of index files that list all names of virus families, genera and species)." Research School of Biological Science, Australian National University, Canberra. Available at: http://www.life.anu.edu.au/viruses/Ictv/fr-index.htm

Evans, A. S., and Kaslow, R. A., eds. (1997). "Viral Infections of Humans: Epidemiology and Control." 4th ed. Plenum, New York.

International Committee on Taxonomy of Viruses. (1998). Available at: http://www.ncbi.nlm.nih.gov/ICTV (constantly updated resource for the most up-to-date viral taxonomy and nomenclature).

Koonin, E. V., and Dolja, V. V. (1993). Evolution and taxonomy of positive-strand RNA viruses: implications of comparative analysis of amino acid sequences. *Crit. Rev. Biochem. Mol. Biol.* **28**, 375–430.

Murphy, F. A. (1996). Virus taxonomy. *In* "Fields Virology" (B. N. Fields, D. M. Knipe, P. M. Howley, R. M., Chanock, J. L. Melnick, T. P. Monath, B. Roizman, and S. E. Straus, eds.), 3rd ed., pp. 15–58. Lippincott-Raven, Philadelphia, PA.

Murphy, F. A., Fauquet, C. M., Bishop, D. H. L., Ghabrial, S. A., Jarvis, A. W., Martelli, G. P., Mayo, M. A., and Summers, M. D. (1995). "Virus Taxonomy: The Classification and Nomenclature of Viruses. The Sixth Report of the International Committee on Taxonomy of Viruses." Springer-Verlag, Vienna.

CHAPTER 3

Viral Replication

Unraveling the complexities of viral replication is a central focus of much of experimental virology. Studies with bacteriophages in the 1940s and 1950s provided the first insights. With the development of mammalian cell culture methods, the techniques used for the study of bacteriophages were adapted to animal viruses. Progress has been such that the basic mechanisms of transcription, translation, and nucleic acid replication have been characterized for all the major families of animal viruses and the strategies of gene expression and regulation have been clarified as well.

Our knowledge of viral replication continues to grow in complexity. It was easier to generalize when we knew less, but now we know that every family of viruses employs unique replication strategies. One important unifying and simplifying concept, as originally proposed by David Baltimore in 1978, is to assign all viruses to one of six classes based on the composition of their genomes and the pathway they use to produce their mRNAs (Figure 3.1). This chapter presents an overview of the subject, indicating similarities and differences in the replication strategies adopted by viruses of each family that contains pathogens of animals. Further information is provided in the viral replication sections of the chapters in Part II.

Viral Replication Cycle

One-Step Growth Curve

Most studies of the replication of animal viruses have been conducted using cultured mammalian cells growing either in suspension or as a monolayer adhering to a flat surface. Classic studies of this kind defined the *one-step growth curve,* in which cells in a culture are infected simultaneously using a high *multiplicity of infection,* and the increase in infectious virus over time is followed by sequential sampling and titration (Figure 3.2).

Virus that is free in the medium can be titrated separately from virus that remains cell associated. Shortly after infection, the inoculated virus "disappears"—infectious particles cannot be demonstrated, even intracellularly. This *eclipse period* continues until the first progeny virions become detectable some hours later. Nonenveloped viruses mature within the cell and may be detectable for some time as infectious intracellular virions before they are released by cell lysis. Many enveloped viruses, however, mature by budding from the plasma membrane of the host cell and are thus released immediately into the medium. The eclipse period generally ranges from 2 to 12 hours for viruses of different families (Table 3.1).

Early studies, relying on quantitative electron microscopy and assay of infectious virions, provided information about the early and the late events in the replication cycle (attachment, penetration, maturation, and release), but not about what happened during the eclipse period. Investigation of the expression and replication of the viral genome became possible only with the introduction of biochemical methods for the analysis of viral nucleic acids and proteins—now all of the sophisticated techniques of molecular biology are being applied to this aspect of the infection process.

FIGURE 3.1.

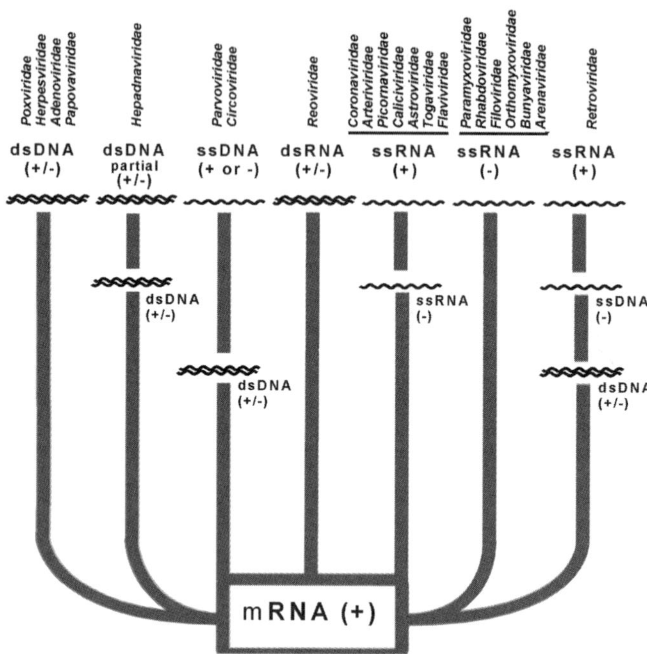

Animal virus replication strategies based on the composition of their genomes and the pathways of their mRNA synthesis. [Modified from D. Baltimore. Expression of animal virus genomes. *Bacteriol. Rev.* **35,** 235–241 (1971).]

FIGURE 3.2.

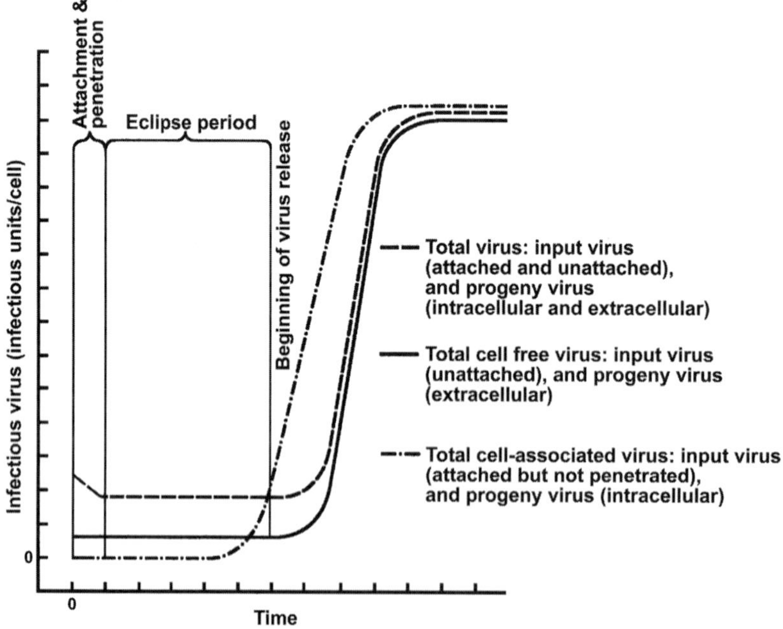

One-step growth curve of a nonenveloped virus. Attachment and penetration are followed by an eclipse period of 2 to 12 hours (see Table 3.1) during which cell-associated infectivity cannot be detected. This is followed by a period of several hours during which viral maturation occurs. Virions of nonenveloped viruses are often released late and incompletely, when the cell lyses. The release of enveloped virions occurs concurrently with maturation by budding from the plasma membrane.

Table 3.1
Characteristics of Replication of Viruses of Different Families

Family	Site of nucleic acid replication	Eclipse period (hours[a])	Budding site
Poxviridae	Cytoplasm	4	Golgi membrane
Asfarviridae	Cytoplasm	5	Plasma membrane
Herpesviridae	Nucleus	4	Nuclear membrane
Adenoviridae	Nucleus	10	None
Papovaviridae	Nucleus	12	None
Parvoviridae	Nucleus	6	None
Circoviridae	Nucleus	?	None
Hepadnaviridae	Nucleus	?	None
Retroviridae	Nucleus	10	Plasma membrane
Reoviridae	Cytoplasm	5	None[b]
Birnaviridae	Cytoplasm	4	None
Paramyxoviridae	Cytoplasm	4	Plasma membrane
Rhabdoviridae	Cytoplasm	3	Plasma membrane
Filoviridae	Cytoplasm	2	Plasma membrane
Bornaviridae	Nucleus	?	Enveloped but site unknown
Orthomyxoviridae	Nucleus	4	Plasma membrane
Bunyaviridae	Cytoplasm	4	Golgi membrane
Arenaviridae	Cytoplasm	5	Plasma membrane
Coronaviridae	Cytoplasm	5	Endoplasmic reticulum
Arteriviridae	Cytoplasm	5	Endoplasmic reticulum
Picornaviridae	Cytoplasm	2	None
Caliciviridae	Cytoplasm	3	None
Astroviridae	Cytoplasm	3	None
Togaviridae	Cytoplasm	2	Plasma membrane
Flaviviridae	Cytoplasm	3	Endoplasmic reticulum

[a]Differs with multiplicity of infection, strain of virus, cell type, and physiological condition.
[b]Pseudo-envelopes formed that are not essential for infectivity.

Events during Eclipse Period

Figure 3.3 illustrates in a greatly simplified fashion the major steps that occur during the eclipse period, using adenovirus as an example. Following attachment, the virion enters the cell and is partially uncoated to expose the viral genome. Certain *early viral genes* are transcribed into RNA, which may then be processed in a number of ways, including splicing. The early gene products translated from this *messenger RNA (mRNA)* are of three main types: proteins that shut down cellular nucleic acid and protein synthesis, proteins that regulate the expression of the viral genome, and enzymes required for the replication of the viral nucleic acid. Following viral nucleic acid replication, *late viral genes* are transcribed. The late proteins are principally viral structural proteins used for the assembly of new virions; some of these are subject to posttranslational modifications before use. Maturation occurs in the nucleus. Each infected cell yields thousands of virions that are free to infect other cells.

For most DNA viruses, transcription and DNA replication take place in the cell nucleus, using cellular RNA polymerase II and other cellular enzymes. Most RNA viruses replicate in the cytoplasm and, because cells lack enzymes to copy RNA from an RNA template, either the viral genome must itself function as mRNA or the virus must encode and carry its own RNA polymerase to transcribe RNA from the RNA genome.

Figure 3.3.

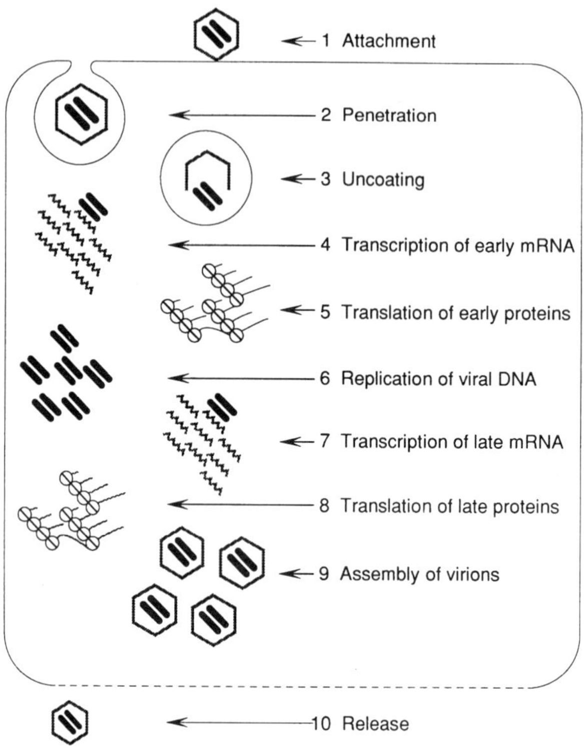

General features of the viral replication cycle, using adenovirus as a model. No topographic location for any step is implied. One step grades into the next such that, as the cycle progresses, several of these processes proceed simultaneously. Release occurs by cell lysis.

Attachment

In order to initiate infection, virions must be able to bind to cells. Binding occurs between ligands on the surface of the virion (*viral attachment proteins*) and receptors on the plasma membrane of the cell. Too often the illustrations used to describe this interaction make it seem too simple, but there are many variables and, *in vivo,* there are many different ligand–receptor pairings. In fact, the lack of correlation between attachment studies in cultured cells vs intact animals may be seen as an indication of this complexity. For example, with herpesviruses, several viral envelope glycoproteins may serve as attachment proteins and several cellular receptors may be involved, in sequential order, first achieving a loose attachment via one receptor, then irreversible binding via another. This multiple set attachment phenomenon provides redundancy and also facilitates the need that the herpesviruses have for invading epithelial and neural tissues so as to support their latent/recrudescent infection cycles. Other viruses do the same. Although there is a degree of specificity about the recognition of particular cellular receptors by particular viruses, quite different viruses (e.g., orthomyxoviruses and paramyxoviruses) may utilize the same receptor and, conversely, viruses in the same family or genus may use different receptors (see Chapter 7). All in all, viruses have evolved to make opportunistic use of a wide variety of host cell surface proteins as their receptors, in most cases using as receptors cellular proteins that are crucial for fundamental cellular functions—such cellular proteins are strongly conserved over evolutionary time so that viruses are rarely caught out by failure to find their favorite receptors.

The cellular receptor for most orthomyxoviruses is the terminal sialic acid on an oligosaccharide side chain of a glycoprotein (or glycolipid) exposed at the cell surface, whereas the viral ligand is in a cleft at the distal tip of each monomer of the trimeric viral hemagglutinin glycoprotein (see Chapter 1). The receptors for a number of other viruses are members of the immunoglobulin superfamily, such as ICAM-1 (intracellular adhesion molecule-1), which is the common receptor for many rhinoviruses. In the best-studied receptor–ligand interaction of all, that of human cells and human immunodeficiency virus (HIV), attachment initially involves

CD4 molecules on the surface of target cells, notably macrophages and T helper lymphocytes, via the viral gp120 envelope glycoprotein subunit termed SU. The CD4–SU complex then binds to a second cell receptor molecule, called fusin, which when sprung mousetrap fashion, displaces the SU subunit and brings the transmembrane (TM) subunit into direct contact with the cell membrane. A fusogenic domain of the transmembrane subunit then brings about the fusion of the viral envelope with the plasma membrane of the cell, permitting the viral nucleocapsid to enter the cytoplasm. Receptor–ligand interactions in other lentivirus infections are similar.

Uptake (Penetration)

Following attachment, virions can enter cells by one of two main mechanisms: receptor-mediated endocytosis or fusion.

Receptor-Mediated Endocytosis

The majority of mammalian cells are engaged continuously in receptor-mediated endocytosis for the uptake of macromolecules via specific receptors. Many enveloped and nonenveloped viruses use this essential cell function to initiate infection (Figure 3.4). Virion attachment to receptors, which cluster at *clathrin-coated pits,* is followed by endocytosis into clathrin-coated vesicles. Vesicles enter the cytoplasm and, after removal of the clathrin coat, fuse with endosomes (acidic prelysosomal vacuoles). Acidification within the vesicle triggers changes in virion proteins and surface structures. The configuration of capsid protein VP4 of picornaviruses, for example, leads to release of the viral RNA from the virion into the cytosol. Similarly, at the acidic pH of the endosome, the hemagglutinin molecule of influenza virus undergoes a conformational change, which enables fusion to occur between the viral envelope and the endosomal membrane, leading to release of the viral nucleocapsid into the cytoplasm. Many other nonenveloped and enveloped viruses undergo comparable changes.

Fusion with Plasma Membrane

The F (fusion) glycoprotein of paramyxoviruses causes the envelope of these viruses to fuse directly with the plasma membrane of the cell, even at pH 7. This allows the nucleocapsid to be released directly into the cytoplasm. A number of other enveloped viruses have the ability to fuse the host cell plasma membrane with their own envelope, thereby gaining entry of their nucleic acid.

Uncoating

For viral genes to become available for transcription, it is necessary that virions be at least partially uncoated. In the case of enveloped RNA viruses that enter by fusion of their envelope with either the plasma membrane or an endosomal membrane, the nucleocapsid is discharged directly into the cytoplasm and transcription commences from viral nucleic acid still associated with this structure. With the nonenveloped icosahedral reoviruses, only certain capsid proteins are removed and the viral genome expresses all its functions without ever being released from the virion core. For most other viruses, however,

FIGURE 3.4.

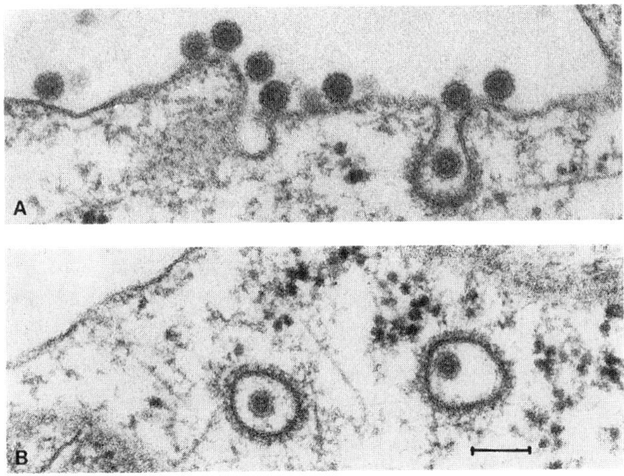

Receptor-mediated endocytosis: penetration by a togavirus. (A) Attachment and movement into a clathrin-coated pit; (B) endocytosis, producing a coated vesicle. (Courtesy of A. Helenius and K. Simons.)

uncoating proceeds to completion. For some viruses that replicate in the nucleus, the later stages of uncoating occur there rather than in the cytoplasm.

Strategies of Replication

Replication of most DNA viruses involves mechanisms that are familiar in cell biology; transcription of mRNA from double-stranded DNA and replication of DNA (Figure 3.3). The situation is quite different for RNA viruses, which are unique in having their genetic information encoded in RNA. RNA viruses with different types of genomes (single or double stranded, positive or negative sense, monopartite or segmented) have necessarily evolved different routes to the production of mRNA. In the case of positive-sense, single-stranded RNA viruses, the genomic RNA itself functions as messenger, whereas all other types of viral RNA must first be transcribed into mRNA. Because eukaryotic cells contain no RNA-dependent RNA polymerase, negative-sense, single-stranded RNA viruses and double-stranded RNA viruses must carry an RNA-dependent RNA polymerase in the virion.

Further, eukaryotic cells are not equipped to translate polycistronic mRNA into several individual species of protein, because in general they cannot reinitiate translation part way along the RNA molecule. DNA viruses overcome this limitation by using the cellular mechanism of cleavage (and sometimes splicing) of their polycistronic RNA transcripts to yield monocistronic mRNA molecules. RNA viruses, most of which replicate in the cytoplasm, do not have access to the RNA processing and splicing enzymes of the nucleus, have developed a remarkable diversity of solutions to the problem. Some have developed a segmented genome in which each molecule is, in general, a separate gene. Others have evolved a polycistronic genome but produce monocistronic RNA transcripts by termination and reinitiation of transcription. Yet others make use of a nested set of overlapping RNA transcripts each of which is translated into a single gene product. Finally, some have a polycistronic viral RNA that is translated into a polyprotein that is later cleaved proteolytically to yield the final products.

The diverse strategies followed by viruses of different families for transcription and translation are illustrated diagrammatically in Figure 3.5 (for DNA viruses) and Figure 3.6 (for RNA viruses) and are described as follows.

DNA Viruses

Poxviruses, Asfarviruses, and Iridoviruses

Poxviruses, asfarviruses, and iridoviruses, which replicate in the cytoplasm, carry their own transcriptase (DNA-dependent RNA polymerase) in the virion. Their

FIGURE 3.5.

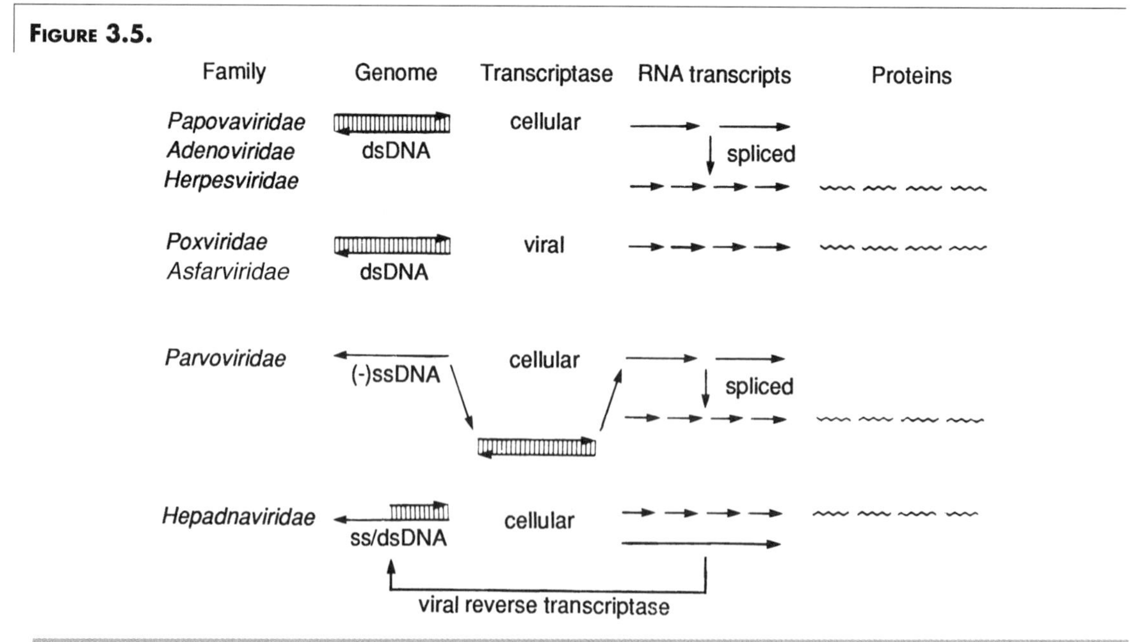

Simplified diagram showing the essential features of the replication of DNA viruses. The sense of each nucleic acid molecule is indicated by an arrow + to the right; − to the left). The number of mRNA and protein species for each virus has been shown arbitrarily as four. See text for details.

FIGURE 3.6.

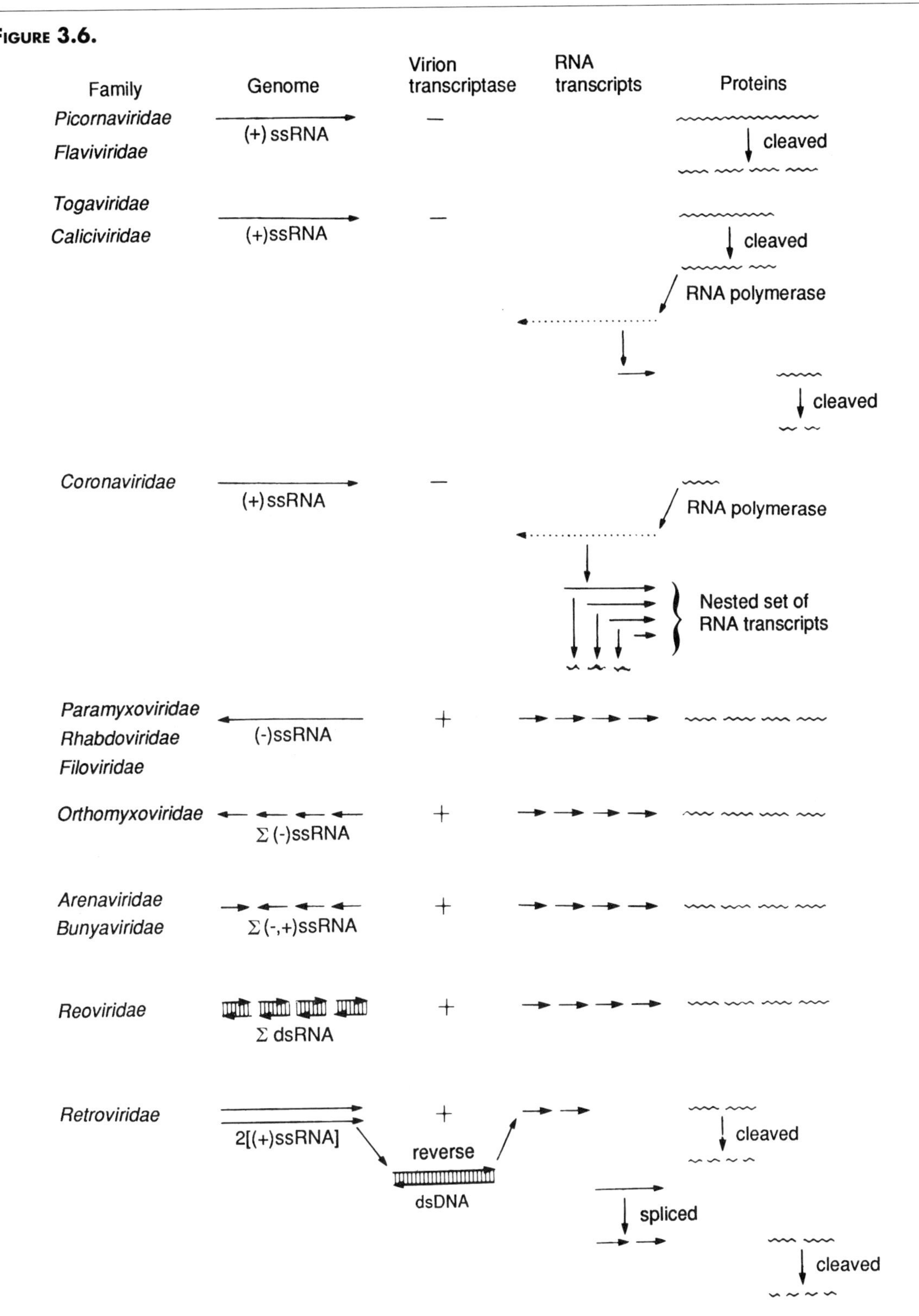

Simplified diagram showing the essential features of the replication of RNA viruses. The sense of each nucleic molecule is indicated by an arrow (+ to the right; − to the left; −, + for *Arenaviridae* and *Bunyaviridae*, indicating ambisense RNA). Σ, segmented genome; 2, diploid genome of *Retroviridae*. The number of mRNA molecules and protein molecules has been shown arbitrarily as four, as have the number of segments in viruses with segmented genomes (although less for *Arenaviridae* and *Bunyaviridae*). See text for details.

very large genomes encode numerous other enzymes that make them virtually independent of the cell nucleus. Monocistronic mRNAs are transcribed directly from the viral DNA.

Herpesviruses, Adenoviruses, and Papovaviruses

Herpesviruses, adenoviruses, and papovaviruses have, in one respect, the most straightforward strategy of replication: the viral DNA is transcribed within the nucleus by cellular DNA-dependent RNA polymerase II. There are two or more cycles of transcription, the various *transcription units* (groups of genes under the control of a single promoter) being transcribed in a given temporal sequence. Polycistronic, but subgenomic, RNA transcripts (corresponding to several genes but less than the whole genome) undergo cleavage and splicing to produce monocistronic mRNAs, with introns being removed in the process.

Parvoviruses and Circoviruses

Parvoviruses and circoviruses, with their single-stranded DNAs, use cellular DNA polymerases to synthesize double-stranded DNA, which is then transcribed in the nucleus by cellular DNA-dependent RNA polymerase II. Then, transcripts are processed by splicing to produce mRNAs.

Reverse-Transcribing Viruses

Hepadnaviruses

The single-stranded DNA portion of the partially double-stranded DNA genome of hepadnaviruses is first completed by a virion-associated DNA polymerase, and the DNA is converted into a supercoiled, double-stranded DNA. Transcription by cellular RNA polymerase II then occurs. Full-length, positive-sense RNA serves as a template for a viral reverse transcriptase and a negative-sense DNA strand, which in turn is the template for synthesis of the double-stranded DNA. The mRNA is transcribed from double-stranded DNA starting from various promoters.

Retroviruses

In retroviruses the viral RNA is positive sense, but instead of functioning as mRNA, it is transcribed by a viral RNA-dependent DNA polymerase (reverse transcriptase) to produce first an RNA–DNA hybrid molecule, which is in turn converted to double-stranded DNA (by another activity of the same enzyme) and inserted permanently into the cellular DNA genome. This integrated viral DNA (*provirus*) is subsequently transcribed by cellular RNA polymerase II, followed by splicing of the RNA transcript as well as cleavage of the resulting proteins. Some full-length, positive-sense RNA transcripts associate in pairs to form the diploid genomes of new virions.

RNA Viruses

Reoviruses and Birnaviruses

Reoviruses and birnaviruses have segmented double-stranded RNA genomes. The negative-sense strand of each segment is transcribed separately in the cytoplasm by a virion-associated transcriptase to produce mRNA. These positive-sense RNAs also serve as templates for replication. The resulting double-stranded RNA in turn serves as the template for further mRNA transcription.

Paramyxoviruses, Rhabdoviruses, Filoviruses, and Bornavirus

The nonsegmented negative-sense, single-stranded RNA of paramyxoviruses, rhabdoviruses, filoviruses, and Borna disease virus carries an RNA-dependent RNA polymerase (transcriptase), which transcribes five or more subgenomic positive-sense RNAs, each of which serves as a monocistronic mRNA. In contrast, transcription in the replication mode (by the same polymerase acting as a replicase) produces a full-length, positive-sense strand that is used as the template for the synthesis of new negative-sense viral RNA. The strategy of replication of Borna disease virus is somewhat more complex (see Chapter 29).

Orthomyxoviruses, Bunyaviruses, and Arenaviruses

Orthomyxoviruses, bunyaviruses, and arenaviruses have negative-sense RNA genomes that are segmented, with each segment being transcribed separately by a transcriptase carried in the virion. mRNAs transcribed from each segment are translated into one or more proteins. In the case of orthomyxoviruses, but not in the other two families, most of the segments encode single proteins. Furthermore, the S segment of arenaviruses and some bunyaviruses is ambisense, i.e., part positive sense and part negative sense. The replication strategy of ambisense RNA viruses, like the sense of their genomes, is mixed, with features of both positive-sense and negative-sense, single-stranded RNA viruses.

Coronaviruses and Arteriviruses

Coronaviruses and arteriviruses display an unusual transcriptional strategy: initially, part of the virion RNA acts as mRNA and is translated to produce an RNA polymerase, which then synthesizes a genome-length, negative-sense strand. From this RNA, a *nested set* of overlapping subgenomic mRNAs with a common 3′-termination site is transcribed. Only the 5′-terminal sequence of each successive member of this set of overlapping transcripts is translated.

Picornaviruses, Caliciviruses, Astroviruses, Togaviruses, and Flaviviruses

Picornaviruses, caliciviruses, astroviruses, togaviruses, and flaviviruses, i.e., positive-sense, single-stranded RNA viruses, replicate by the most straightforward means—their genomes function directly as mRNAs. Genomes of picornaviruses and flaviviruses acting as a single polycistronic mRNA, are translated directly into a single *polyprotein* that is subsequently cleaved to give the individual viral structural and nonstructural proteins. One of these proteins is an RNA-dependent RNA polymerase, which replicates the viral genome, transcribing viral RNA into a complementary (negative-sense) copy, which in turn serves as a template for the synthesis of positive-sense (viral) RNA. In togaviruses, only about two-thirds of the viral RNA (the 5′ end) is translated; the resulting polyprotein is cleaved into nonstructural proteins, all of which are required for RNA transcription and replication. Viral RNA polymerase makes a full-length, negative-sense strand, from which two species of positive-sense RNA are copied: full-length virion RNA destined for encapsidation and a one-third length RNA, which is collinear with the 3′ terminus of the viral RNA and is translated into a polyprotein from which the structural proteins are produced by cleavage. Caliciviruses produce both genome-length and subgenomic mRNA species.

Transcription

The viral RNA of most positive-sense, single-stranded RNA viruses binds directly to ribosomes and is translated in full or in part without the need for any prior transcriptional step. From all other classes of viral genomes, mRNA must be transcribed in order to begin the process of expression of the infecting viral genome. In the case of DNA viruses that replicate in the nucleus, cellular DNA-dependent RNA polymerase II performs this function. All other viruses require a unique and specific transcriptase that is virus coded and is an integral component of the virion. The double-stranded DNA viruses that replicate in the cytoplasm carry a DNA-dependent RNA polymerase, whereas double-stranded RNA viruses have a specific double-stranded RNA-dependent RNA polymerase and negative-sense single-stranded RNA viruses carry a specific single-stranded RNA-dependent RNA polymerase.

Regulation of Transcription from Viral DNA

In 1978 Fiers and colleagues presented the first complete description of the genome of an animal virus (Figure 3.7). Analysis of the circular double-stranded DNA molecule of the papovavirus SV40 and its transcription program revealed some remarkable insights, many of which can be generalized to other double-stranded DNA viruses. First, early genes and late genes are transcribed in opposite directions, from different strands of the DNA. Second, certain genes overlap, so that their protein products have some amino acid sequences in common. Third, some regions of the viral DNA may be read in different reading frames, so that quite distinct amino acid sequences are translated from the same nucleotide sequence. Fourth, certain long stretches of the viral DNA consist of introns, which are transcribed but not translated into protein because they are spliced out from the primary RNA transcript.

For many years a one-to-one relationship between a gene and its gene product (protein) was envisioned. Now, with overlapping reading frames, multiple splicing patterns of RNA transcripts, posttranslational cleavage of polyproteins, and so on, it is too simplistic to designate a particular nucleotide sequence as a gene encoding a particular protein. It is more appropriate to refer to the *transcription unit,* which is defined as a region of the genome beginning with the transcription initiation site and extending to the transcription termination site (including all introns and exons in between), the expression of which falls under the control of a particular promoter. *Simple transcription units* may be defined as those encoding only a single protein, whereas *complex transcription units* code for more than one.

Adenoviruses may be used to elucidate some of the mechanisms that regulate the expression of viral genomes—these operate principally, but not exclusively, at the level of transcription. There are several adenovirus transcription units; at different stages of the viral replication cycle, "pre-early," "early," "intermediate," and "late" transcription units are transcribed in a set temporal sequence. A product of the early region E1A induces transcription from the other early regions, including E1B, but following viral DNA replication there is a 50-fold increase in the rate of transcription from the major late promoter relative to early promoters such as E1B and a decrease in E1A mRNA levels. A second control operates at the point of termination of transcription. Transcripts that terminate at a particular point early in infection are read through later in infection to produce a range of longer transcripts with different polyadenylation sites and different functions. Again, we are reminded of the economy of

Figure 3.7.

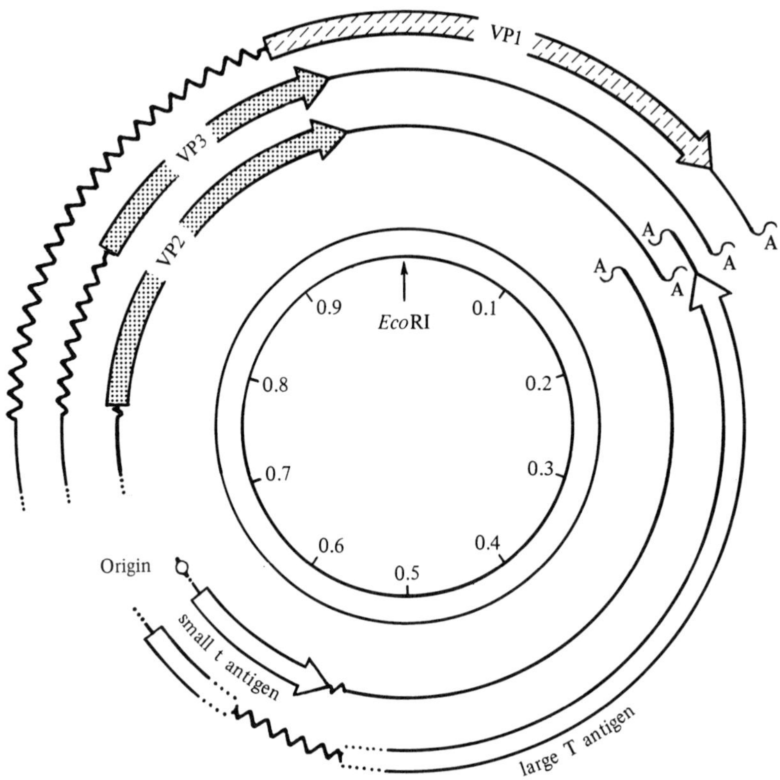

Transcription map of the DNA of the papovavirus SV40. The circular double-stranded DNA is oriented with the *Eco*RI restriction endonuclease cleavage site at zero and the origin of DNA replication (origin) at map position 0.66. The direction of transcription of the early genes is counterclockwise on one DNA strand (open arrows) and of the late genes is clockwise on the other strand (stippled and shaded arrows). The thin lines indicate regions of the primary RNA transcripts that are not translated into proteins, whereas the wavy lines indicate regions of the transcript that are spliced out (introns). The 3′-terminal poly(A) tail of each mRNA is labeled A. The coding regions of the primary transcript are shown as large arrows. The genes for the early proteins, small t and large T, overlap, as do those for the late proteins VP1, VP2, and VP3. Large T is coded by two noncontiguous regions of DNA. The amino acid sequence of VP3 corresponds with the C-terminal half of VP2. However, VP1 shares no part of its amino acid sequence with VP2 or VP3, even though the VP1 gene overlaps VP2 and VP3, because its mRNA is transcribed in a different reading frame. (Courtesy of W. Fiers.)

viral genomes in encoding complex functions in minimal nucleic acid sequences.

Regulation of Transcription from Viral RNA

In RNA viruses, the regulation of transcription is generally not as complex as in DNA viruses. In particular, the temporal separation into early genes transcribed before the replication of viral nucleic acid, and late genes thereafter, is not nearly so clear. In most families of viruses with positive-sense, single-stranded RNA genomes, which serve directly as messengers, transcription is required only to make the negative strand required for RNA replication.

However, other mechanisms of regulation are required for viruses with nonsegmented negative-sense RNA genomes. In cells infected by these viruses, once the nucleocapsid is released into the cytoplasm, the RNA polymerase initiates transcription from the 3′ end of the genome. Because there is only a single promoter, one might imagine that only full-length, positive-strand transcripts could be made. While some full-length, positive-sense strands are made as templates for RNA replication, mRNAs corresponding to each gene are also made, in the following fashion. The several genes along the viral RNA are each separated by a consensus sequence that includes termination and start signals as well as short intergenic sequences of U residues that enable the transcriptase to generate a long poly(A) tail for each mRNA by a process of reiterative copying (*stop–start transcrip-*

tion, also known as *stuttering*). Each completed mRNA is cleaved off, but the enzyme continues to transcribe the next gene, and so forth.

Paramyxovirus transcription also involves a process known as *editing*. The P gene encodes two proteins, P and V, which share a common N-terminal amino acid sequence but differ completely in their C-terminal sequences because of a shift in the reading frame brought about by the insertion of two uncoded G residues into the RNA transcript by transcriptase stuttering.

Regulatory Genes and Responsive Elements

In analyzing viral genomes and RNA transcripts derived from them, much attention has been given to identifying the open reading frames in order to derive the amino acid sequence of their gene products. There is also interest in the untranslated regions of the genome that contain numerous conserved (consensus) sequences, sometimes called motifs, which represent *responsive elements,* that play crucial roles in the regulation of transcription. For example, each transcription unit in viral genomes has near its 3′ end an mRNA transcription initiation site (*start site*), designated as nucleotide +1. Within the hundred or so nucleotides upstream of the start site lies the *promoter,* which up-regulates the transcription of that gene (or genes). Upstream or downstream from the start site there may be a long sequence with several, in some cases repeated, elements known as *enhancers,* which amplify transcription even further. These regulatory regions are activated by the binding of viral or cellular DNA-binding proteins. Several such proteins may bind to adjacent responsive elements in such a way that they also bind to one another or otherwise interact to facilitate attachment of the viral RNA polymerase. Viral regulatory genes that encode such regulatory proteins may act in *trans*, i.e., they may transactivate genes residing on a completely different molecule.

A description of the role of one of the six regulatory genes of human immunodeficiency virus 1 (HIV1) will illustrate the sophistication of such regulatory mechanisms. When a DNA copy of the viral genome is integrated into a chromosome of a resting T cell, it remains latent until a T-cell mitogen or a cytokine induces synthesis of the NF-κB family of DNA-binding proteins. NF-κB then binds to the enhancer present in the integrated provirus, thereby triggering transcription of the six HIV regulatory genes. One of these, *tat,* found in all lentiviruses, encodes a protein that binds to a responsive element, TAR, within the provirus, greatly augmenting (*trans*-activating) the transcription of all viral genes (including *tat* itself), thereby establishing a positive feedback loop that promotes the production of large numbers of progeny virions. Moreover, because TAR is present in all viral mRNAs, as well as in the proviral DNA, it is probable that *tat* enhances both transcription and translation. Although the control of lentivirus transcription may be unusually complex because of its complicated replication cycle and requirement for the establishment of latency, these viruses contain only nine genes, compared with 100 in the case of some DNA viruses.

Posttranscriptional Processing

Primary RNA transcripts from eukaryotic DNA are subject to a series of posttranscriptional alterations in the nucleus, known as *processing,* prior to export to the cytoplasm as mRNA. First a cap, consisting of 7-methylguanosine (m^7Gppp), is added to the 5′ terminus of the primary transcript; the cap facilitates the formation of a stable complex with the 40S ribosomal subunit, which is necessary for the initiation of translation. Second, a sequence of 50–200 adenylate residues is added to the 3′ terminus. This poly(A) tail may act as a recognition signal for processing and for transporting mRNA from the nucleus to the cytoplasm and it may stabilize mRNA against degradation in the cytoplasm. Third, a methyl group is added at the 6 position to about 1% of the adenylate residues throughout the RNA (methylation). Fourth, introns are removed from the primary transcript and the exons are linked together in a process known as *splicing*. Splicing is an important mechanism for regulating gene expression in nuclear DNA viruses. A given RNA transcript can have two or more splicing sites and be spliced in several alternative ways to produce a variety of mRNA species coding for distinct proteins; both the preferred poly(A) site and the splicing pattern may change in a regulated fashion as infection proceeds.

Special mention should be made of an extraordinary phenomenon known as *cap snatching*. The transcriptase of influenza virus, which also carries endonuclease activity, steals the 5′-methylated caps from newly synthesized cellular RNA transcripts in the nucleus and uses them as primers for initiating transcription from the viral genome.

The rate of degradation of mRNA provides another possible level of regulation. Not only do different mRNA species have different half-lives, but the half-life of a given mRNA species may change as replication progresses.

Translation

Capped, polyadenylated, and processed monocistronic viral mRNAs bind to ribosomes and are translated into protein in the same fashion as cellular mRNAs. The sequence of events has been studied closely in reovirus-infected cells. Each monocistronic mRNA molecule binds via its capped 5′ terminus to the 40S ribosomal subunit, which then moves along the mRNA molecule until stopped at the initiation codon. The 60S ribosomal subunit then binds, together with methionyl-transfer RNA and various initiation factors, after which translation proceeds.

In mammalian cells, mRNA molecules are *monocistronic* (encoding only one protein) and, with few exceptions, translation commences only at the 5′-initiation codon. However, with certain viruses, polycistronic mRNA can be translated directly into its several gene products as a result of initiation, or reinitiation, of translation at internal AUG start codons.

Where initiation of translation at an internal AUG is an option, a frameshift can occur. Another mechanism, known as ribosomal frameshifting, occurs fortuitously when a ribosome happens to slip one nucleotide forward or back along an RNA molecule. This phenomenon is exploited by retroviruses to access the reverse transcriptase reading frame hidden within the *gag* mRNA. Thus, taken together with the phenomenon of RNA splicing and RNA editing described earlier, it can be seen that there are several mechanisms of exploiting overlapping reading frames to maximize the usage of the limited coding potential of the small genomes of viruses.

Most viral proteins undergo various sorts of post-translational modification, such as phosphorylation (for nucleic acid binding), fatty acid acylation (for membrane insertion), glycosylation, myristylation, or proteolytic cleavage (see later). Newly synthesized viral proteins must also be transported to the various sites in the cell where they are needed, e.g., back into the nucleus in the case of viruses that replicate there. The sorting signals that direct this traffic are only now beginning to be understood, as are the polypeptide chain-binding proteins (*molecular chaperones*) that regulate folding, translocation, and assembly of oligomers of viral as well as cellular proteins.

Glycosylation of Envelope Proteins

Viruses exploit cellular pathways normally used for the synthesis of membrane-inserted and exported secretory glycoproteins (Figure 3.8). The programmed addition of sugars occurs sequentially as the protein moves in vesicles progressively from the rough endoplasmic reticulum to the Golgi complex and then to the plasma membrane. The side chains of viral envelope glycoproteins are generally a mixture of simple (high mannose)

FIGURE 3.8.

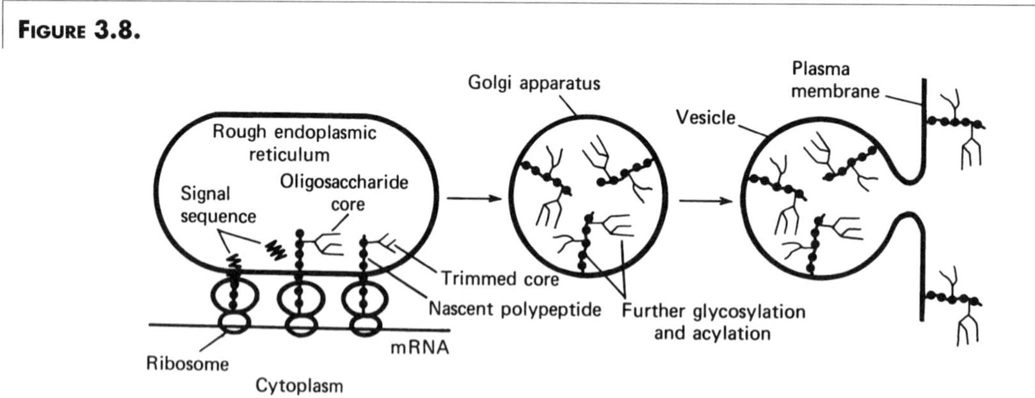

Glycosylation of viral protein. The amino terminus of viral envelope proteins contains an initial sequence of 15–30 hydrophobic amino acids, known as a signal sequence, which facilitates binding of the growing polypeptide chain (dotted) to a receptor site on the cytoplasmic side of the rough endoplasmic reticulum and its passage through the lipid bilayer to the lumenal side. Oligosaccharides are then added in N-linkage to certain asparagine residues of the nascent polypeptide by *en bloc* transfer of a mannose-rich core of preformed oligosaccharides, and glucose residues are removed by glycosidases (called *trimming*). The viral glycoprotein is then transported from the rough endoplasmic reticulum to the Golgi complex. Here the core carbohydrate is further modified by the removal of several mannose residues and by the addition of further *N*-acetylglucosamine, galactose, and the terminal sugars, sialic acid or fucose. The completed side chains are a mixture of simple oligosaccharides (also called high mannose oligosaccharides) and complex oligosaccharides. A coated vesicle then transports the completed glycoprotein to the cellular membrane from which the particular virus buds.

and complex oligosaccharides, which are usually N-linked (to asparagine) or, less commonly, O-linked (to serine or threonine). The composition of the oligosaccharides is determined not only by the amino acid sequence and tertiary structure of the proteins concerned, but more importantly by the particular cellular glycosyltransferases prevalent in the type of cell in which the virus happens to be growing at the time.

Posttranslational Cleavage of Viral Proteins

In the case of positive-sense picornaviruses and flaviviruses, the polycistronic viral RNA is translated directly into a single polyprotein, which carries protease activity that cleaves the polyprotein at defined recognition sites into smaller proteins. The first cleavage steps are carried out while the polyprotein is still associated with the ribosome. Some of the larger intermediates exist only fleetingly, whereas others are functional for a short period but are subsequently cleaved by additional virus-coded proteases to smaller proteins with alternative functions. Posttranslational cleavage occurs in several other RNA virus families, e.g., togaviruses and caliciviruses, in which polyproteins corresponding to large parts of the genome are cleaved. Some viruses encode several different proteases. Most are either trypsin-like (serine or cysteine proteases), pepsin-like (aspartyl proteases), or papain-like (thiol proteases).

Cellular proteases, present in organelles such as the Golgi complex or transport vesicles, are also vital to the maturation and assembly of many viruses. For example, cleavage of the hemagglutinin glycoprotein of orthomyxoviruses or the fusion glycoprotein of paramyxoviruses is essential for virion infectivity.

TABLE 3.2
Categories of Proteins Encoded by Viral Genomes

Structural proteins of the virion[a]

Virion-associated enzymes, especially polymerases (transcriptases)[b]

Nonstructural proteins, mainly enzymes, required for transcription, replication of viral nucleic acid, and cleavage of proteins[c]

Regulatory proteins that control the temporal sequence of expression of the viral genome[d]

Proteins down-regulating expression of cellular genes[e]

Oncogene products (oncoproteins) and inactivators of cellular tumor suppressor proteins[f]

Proteins influencing viral virulence, host range, tissue tropism, etc.[g]

Virokines, which act on noninfected cells to modulate the progress of infection in the body as a whole[h]

[a]Comprising capsid and (for some viruses) core and/or envelope.
[b]RNA viruses of positive sense and DNA viruses that replicate in the nucleus do not carry a transcriptase in the virion. Virions of some viruses, e.g., poxviruses, also contain several other enzymes.
[c]DNA and RNA polymerases, helicases, proteases, etc. DNA viruses with large complex genomes, notably poxviruses and herpesviruses, also encode numerous enzymes needed for nucleotide synthesis.
[d]Site-specific DNA-binding proteins (transcription factors) that bind to enhancer sequences in the viral genome or to another transcription factor. Some may act in trans (transactivators).
[e]Usually by inhibiting transcription, sometimes translation.
[f]Upgrade expression of certain cellular genes; may lead to cell transformation and eventually to cancer. Observed with herpesviruses, adenoviruses, papovaviruses, and retroviruses.
[g]Recorded so far mainly in the more complex DNA viruses (poxviruses, herpesviruses, adenoviruses) but may be more widespread.
[h]Mainly by subverting the immune response, e.g., by inhibiting cytokines, down-regulating MHC expression, and blocking the complement cascade.

Classes of Viral Proteins

Table 3.2 lists the various classes of proteins encoded by the genomes of viruses. In general, the proteins translated from the early transcripts of DNA viruses include enzymes and other proteins required for the replication of viral nucleic acid, as well as proteins that suppress host cell RNA and protein synthesis. The large DNA viruses (poxviruses and herpesviruses) also encode a number of enzymes involved in nucleotide metabolism.

The late viral proteins are translated from late mRNAs, most of which are transcribed from progeny viral nucleic acid molecules. Most of the late proteins are viral structural proteins and are often made in considerable excess.

Some viral proteins, including some with other important functions, serve as regulatory proteins, modulating the transcription or translation of cellular genes or of early viral genes. The large DNA viruses also encode numerous additional proteins, called *virokines,* which do not regulate the viral replication cycle itself but influence the host response to infection. Included in these are homologues of cellular cytokines.

For poxviruses and herpesviruses, it is possible to identify, using gene deletion studies, a significant number of genes (more than 40% of all genes) that are not essential for the replication of the virus in cultured cells. Of course, in the strict economy of viral genomes, it is likely that most or all of such genes are important in viral survival in nature.

Replication of Viral Nucleic Acids

Replication of Viral DNA

Different mechanisms of DNA replication are employed by each family of DNA viruses. Because cellular DNA polymerases cannot initiate synthesis of a new DNA strand but only extend synthesis from a short (RNA) primer, one end of newly synthesized viral DNA molecules might be expected to remain single stranded. Various DNA viruses have evolved different strategies for circumventing this problem. Viruses of some families have a circular DNA genome, others have a linear genome with complementary termini that serve as primers, while yet others have a protein primer attached covalently to each 5′ terminus.

Several virus-coded enzyme activities are generally required for the replication of viral DNA: a helicase (with ATPase activity) to unwind the double helix; a helix-destabilizing protein to keep the two separated strands apart until each has been copied; a DNA polymerase to copy each strand from the origin of replication in a 5′ → 3′ direction; an RNAse to degrade the RNA primer after it has served its purpose; and a DNA ligase to join the Okazaki fragments together (see later). Often a single large enzyme carries out two or more of these activities.

The papovavirus genome, with its associated cellular histones, morphologically and functionally resembles cellular DNA and utilizes host cell enzymes, including DNA polymerase A, for its replication. An early viral protein, large-T, binds to sites in the regulatory sequence of the viral genome, thereby initiating DNA replication. Replication of this circular double-stranded DNA commences from a unique palindromic sequence and proceeds simultaneously in both directions. As in the replication of mammalian DNA, both continuous and discontinuous DNA synthesis occurs (of leading and lagging strands, respectively) at the two growing forks. The discontinuous synthesis of the lagging strand involves repeated synthesis of short oligoribonucleotide primers, which in turn initiate short nascent strands of DNA (*Okazaki fragments*), which are then joined covalently by a DNA ligase to form one of the growing strands.

The replication of adenovirus DNA is quite different. Adenovirus DNA is linear, with the 5′ end of each strand being a mirror image of the other (terminally repeated inverted sequences) and each is linked covalently to a protein, the precursor of which serves as the primer for viral DNA synthesis. DNA replication proceeds from both ends, continuously but asynchronously, in a 5′ → 3′ direction, using a virus-coded DNA polymerase. It does not require the synthesis of Okazaki fragments.

Herpesviruses encode many or all of the proteins required for DNA replication, including a DNA polymerase, a helicase, a primase, a single-stranded DNA-binding protein, and a protein recognizing the origin of replication. Poxviruses and asfarviruses, which replicate entirely within the cytoplasm, are self-sufficient in DNA replication machinery. Hepadnaviruses, like retroviruses, utilize positive-sense, single-stranded RNA transcripts as intermediates for the production of DNA by reverse transcription. The single-stranded DNA parvoviruses use 3′-palindromic sequences that form a double-stranded hairpin structure as a primer for cellular DNA polymerase binding.

Replication of Viral RNA

The replication of RNA is a phenomenon unique to viruses. Transcription of RNA from an RNA template requires an RNA-dependent RNA polymerase, a virus-coded enzyme not found in uninfected cells. The replication of viral RNA requires first the synthesis of complementary RNA, which then serves as a template for making more viral RNA.

Where the viral RNA is of negative sense (orthomyxoviruses, paramyxoviruses, rhabdoviruses, filoviruses, bornavirus, arenaviruses, and bunyaviruses), the complementary RNA will be of positive sense and the RNA polymerase involved resembles the virion-associated transcriptase used for the primary transcription of mRNAs. However, whereas most transcripts from such negative-sense viral RNAs are subgenomic mRNA molecules, some full-length, positive-sense strands must also be made in order to serve as templates for viral RNA synthesis (replication). For some viruses there is good evidence that the RNA polymerases used for transcription and replication are distinct, whereas in others the same enzyme functions differently.

In the case of positive-sense RNA viruses (picornaviruses, caliciviruses, togaviruses, flaviviruses, coronaviruses, and arteriviruses), the complementary RNA is negative sense. Several viral RNA molecules can be transcribed simultaneously from a single complementary RNA template, with each RNA transcript being the product of a separately bound polymerase molecule. The resulting structure, known as the *replicative intermediate,* is therefore partially double stranded, with single-stranded tails. Initiation of replication of picornavirus and calicivirus RNA, like that of adenovirus DNA, requires a bound protein rather than an oligonucleotide as primer. This small protein is attached covalently to the 5′ terminus of nascent positive and negative RNA strands, as well as to virion RNA, but not to mRNA. Little is known about what determines whether a given picornavirus positive-sense RNA molecule will be directed (1) to a *replication complex* (a structure bound to smooth endoplasmic reticulum), where it serves as template for transcription by RNA-dependent RNA polymerase into negative-sense RNA, (2) to a *ribosome,* where it serves as mRNA for translation into protcin, or (3) to a *procapsid,* with which it associates to form a virion.

Retroviruses have a genome consisting of positive-sense, single-stranded RNA. Unlike other RNA viruses, they replicate via a DNA intermediate. The virion-associated reverse transcriptase, using a transfer RNA molecule as a primer, makes a single-stranded DNA copy. Then, functioning as a ribonuclease, the same enzyme removes the parental RNA molecule from the DNA:RNA hybrid and at the same time copies the negative-sense, single-stranded DNA strand to form a linear double-stranded DNA, which contains an additional sequence known as the *long terminal repeat* (*LTR*) at each end. This double-stranded DNA then circularizes and integrates into cellular chromosomal DNA. Transcription of viral RNA occurs from this integrated (proviral) DNA.

Assembly and Release

Maturation and Release of Nonenveloped Viruses

All nonenveloped animal viruses have an icosahedral structure. The structural proteins of simple icosahedral viruses associate spontaneously to form capsomers, which self-assemble to form capsids into which viral nucleic acid is packaged. Completion of the virion often involves proteolytic cleavage of one or more species of capsid protein. The best-studied example, that of the prototype picornavirus, poliovirus, is depicted in Figure 3.9.

The mechanism of packaging viral nucleic acid into a preassembled empty procapsid has been elucidated for adenovirus. A particular protein binds to a nucleotide sequence at one end of the viral DNA known as the *packaging sequence;* this enables the DNA to enter the procapsid bound to basic core proteins, after which some

FIGURE 3.9.

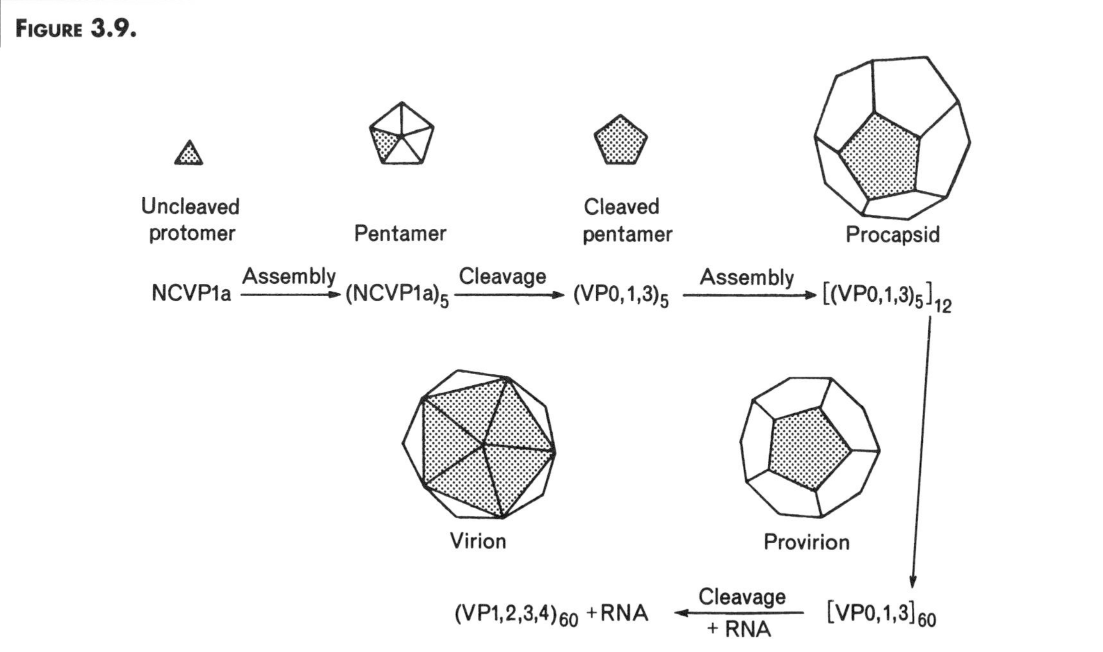

Overview of the assembly of a picornavirus. The capsomer precursor protein (NCVP1a) aggregates to form pentamers; each of the 5 NCVP1a molecules is then cleaved by viral protease into VP0, VP1, and VP3. Twelve such pentamers aggregate to form a procapsid. A final proteolytic event, which cleaves each VP0 molecule into VP2 and VP4, is required for RNA incorporation. The mature virion is a dodecahedron with 60 capsomers, each of which is made up of one molecule each of VP1, 2, 3, and 4. X-ray crystallography shows that the assembling units have extensions that reach across adjacent units to form second and third nearest neighbor relationships.

of the capsid proteins are cleaved to make the mature virion.

Most nonenveloped viruses accumulate within the cytoplasm or nucleus and are released only when the cell eventually lyses.

Maturation and Release of Enveloped Viruses

All mammalian viruses with helical nucleocapsids, as well as some with icosahedral nucleocapsids (e.g., herpesviruses, togaviruses, and retroviruses), mature by acquiring an envelope by budding through cellular membranes.

Budding from Cellular Membranes

Enveloped viruses bud from the plasma membrane, from internal cytoplasmic membranes, or from the nuclear membrane. Viruses that acquire their envelope within the cell are then transported in vesicles to the cell surface. Insertion of the viral glycoprotein(s) into the lipid bilayer of membranes occurs by lateral displacement of cellular proteins from that patch of membrane (Figure 3.10A). The monomeric cleaved viral glycoprotein molecules associate into oligomers to form the typical rod-shaped or club-shaped peplomer with a hydrophilic domain projecting from the external surface of the membrane, a hydrophobic transmembrane anchor domain, and a short hydrophilic cytoplasmic domain projecting slightly into the cytoplasm. In the case of icosahedral viruses (e.g., togaviruses), each protein molecule of the nucleocapsid binds directly to the cytoplasmic domain of the membrane glycoprotein oligomer, thus molding the envelope around the nucleocapsid. In the more usual case of viruses with helical nucleocapsids, it is the matrix protein that attaches to the cytoplasmic domain of the glycoprotein peplomer; in turn the nucleocapsid protein recognizes the matrix protein and this initiates budding. Release of each enveloped virion does not breach the integrity of the plasma membrane, hence thousands of virus particles can be shed over a period of several hours or days without significant cell damage (Figure 3.11). Many, but not all, viruses that bud from the plasma membrane are noncytopathogenic and may be associated with persistent infections.

Epithelial cells display *polarity,* i.e., they have an *apical* surface facing the outside world and a *basolateral* surface facing the interior of the body; the two are separated by lateral cell–cell tight junctions. These surfaces are chemically and physiologically distinct. Viruses that are shed to the exterior (e.g., influenza virus) tend to bud from the apical plasma membrane, whereas others (e.g., C-type retroviruses) bud through the basolateral membrane (see Chapter 5).

Exocytosis

Flaviviruses, coronaviruses, arteriviruses, and bunyaviruses mature by budding through membranes of the Golgi complex or rough endoplasmic reticulum; vesicles containing the virus then migrate to the plasma membrane with which they fuse, thereby releasing the virions by

FIGURE 3.10.

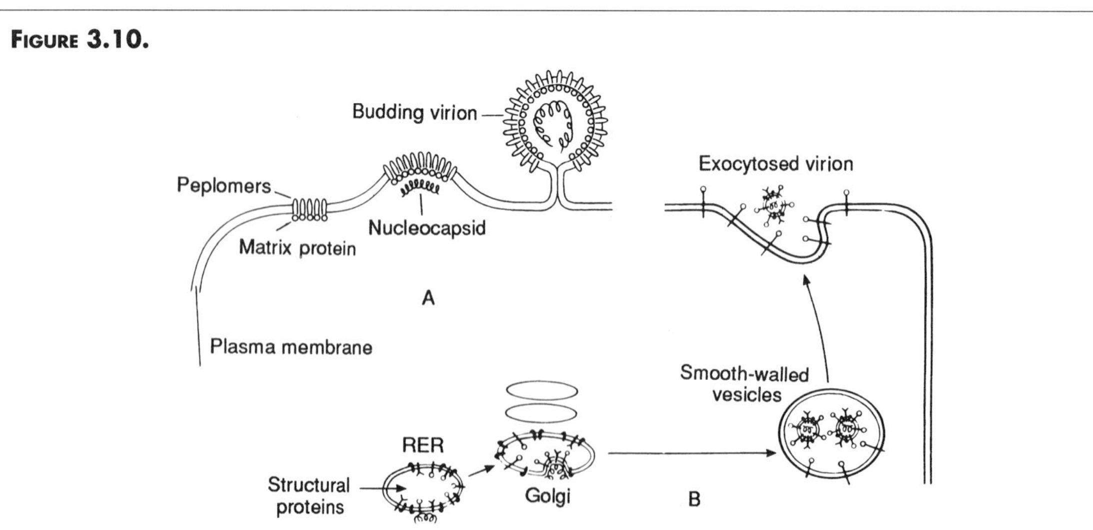

Maturation of enveloped viruses. (A) Viruses with a matrix protein (and some viruses without a matrix protein) bud through a patch of the plasma membrane in which glycoprotein peplomers have accumulated over matrix protein molecules. (B) Most enveloped viruses that do not have a matrix protein bud into cytoplasmic vesicles [rough endoplasmic reticulum (RER) or Golgi], then pass through the cytoplasm in smooth vesicles and are released by exocytosis.

FIGURE 3.11.

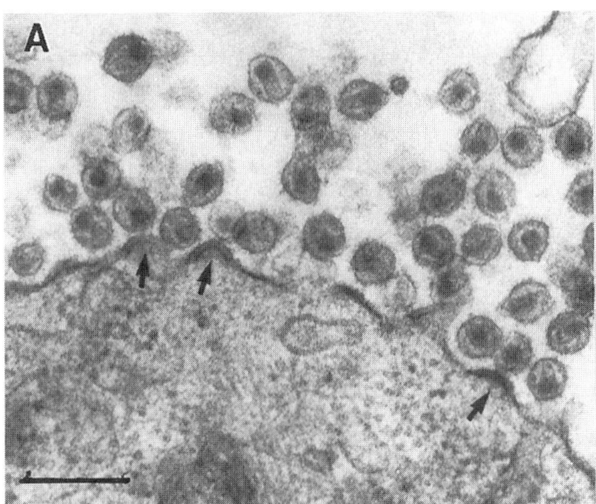

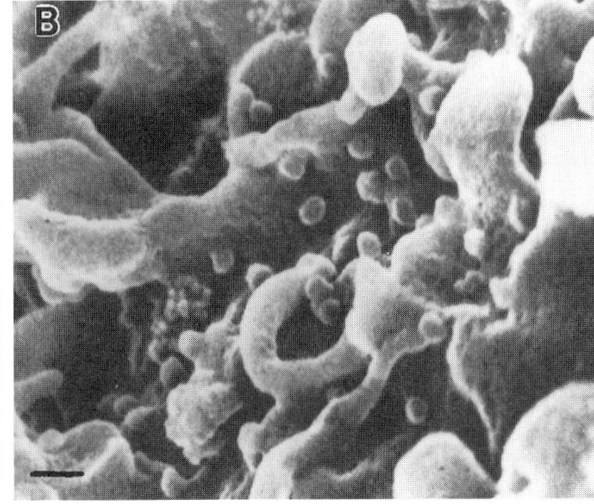

Lentivirus virions budding from the plasma membrane. (A) Feline immunodeficiency virus budding from the plasma membrane of a feline T lymphocyte. Retroviruses have no matrix protein; the arrows indicate accumulations of patches of viral glycoprotein peplomers in the plasma membrane. (B) Scanning electron micrograph of human immunodeficiency virus 1 budding from the plasma membrane of a human T lymphocyte. Bars: 100 nm. [(A) courtesy of J. A. Marshall; (B) courtesy of C. S. Goldsmith.]

exocytosis (Figure 3.10B). Uniquely, the envelope of the herpesviruses is acquired by budding through the inner lamella of the nuclear membrane; the enveloped virions then pass directly from the space between the two lamellae of the nuclear membrane to the exterior of the cell via the cisternae of the endoplasmic reticulum.

Further Reading

Fields, B. N., Knipe, D. M., Howley, R. M., Chanock, R. M., Melnick, J. L., Monath, T. P., Roizman, B., and Straus, S. E., eds. (1996). "Fields Virology," 3rd ed. Lippincott-Raven, Philadelphia, PA.

Joklik, W. K. (1992). The viral multiplication cycle. *In* "Zinsser's Microbiology" (W. K. Joklik, H. P. Willett, and D. B. Amos, eds.) 20th ed. pp. 789–835. Appleton & Lange, CT.

Lodish, H., Baltimore, D., and Berk, A. (1995). "Molecular Cell Biology," 3rd ed. with CD ROM. Scientific American Books Freeman, New York.

Marsh, M., and Helenius, A. (1989). Virus entry into cells. *Adv. Virus Res.* **36,** 107–152.

Pennington, T. H. (1998). The replication of viruses. *In* "Topley and Wilson's Microbiology and Microbial Infections" (B. W. J. Mahy and L. H. Collier, eds.), Vol. 1, pp. 23–32. Edward Arnold, London.

Peterlin, B. M. ed. (1993). Transcriptional regulation of viruses. *Semin. Virol.* **4,** 1–150.

Roizman, B., and Palese, P. (1996). Multiplication of viruses: An overview. *In* "Fields Virology" (B. N. Fields, D. M. Knipe, P. M. Howley, R. M., Chanock, J. L. Melnick, T. P. Monath, B. Roizman, and S. E. Straus, eds.), 3rd ed., pp. 101–112. Lippincott-Raven, Philadelphia, PA.

Stephens, E. B., and Compans, R. W. (1988). Assembly of viruses at cellular membranes. *Annu. Rev. Microbiol.* **42,** 489–525.

Strauss, J. H. (1990). Viral proteases. *Semin in Virol.* **1,** 307–336.

Watson, J. D., Hopkins, N. H., Roberts, J. W., Steitz, J. A., and Weiner, A. M. (1987). "Molecular Biology of the Gene," 4th ed., Vol. 2. Benjamin-Cummins, Menlo Park, CA.

Wimmer, E. (1994). "Cellular Receptors for Animal Viruses." American Society for Microbiology, Washington, DC.

CHAPTER 4

Viral Genetics and Evolution

In nature, viruses undergo an infinitely long series of replication cycles as they are transmitted from host to host. During this process, spontaneous mutants are continually generated, some of which will have different biological properties than the parent virus from which they arise. The *in vivo* environment brings pressures to bear which favor the selection of certain of these biological variants, primarily because of their preferential ability to be transmitted serially. Properties important in the survival and evolutionary progression of various viruses in nature include:

1. *The capacity to replicate rapidly.* In many instances, the most virulent strains of a virus replicate faster than more temperate strains. However, if replication is too rapid, it can be self-defeating—extremely rapid viral growth may not allow time enough for transmission before the host is removed by death or severe illness.

2. *The capacity to replicate to high titer.* A very high vertebrate host viremia titer is employed as a survival mechanism by arthropod-borne viruses to favor infection of the next arthropod. The same viruses produce very high titers in the salivary glands of their arthropod hosts so as to favor infection of the next vertebrate host. Such very high virus titers can be associated with silent infections in some natural vertebrate hosts (e.g., reservoir avian hosts), but in vertebrate hosts the evolution of this capacity is most often associated with severe, even fatal, illness.

3. *The capacity to replicate in certain key tissues.* This quality is often important for the completion of the viral transmission cycle. For example, the evolution of viral tropisms and the employment of specific host cell receptors define many disease patterns. Further, the evolution of the capacity to grow in immunologically sequestered sites (such as brain or kidney) or in cells of the immune system itself provides great survival advantage.

4. *The capacity to be shed for long periods of time.* The evolution of the capacity for chronic shedding offers exceptional opportunity for virus survival and entrenchment (e.g., in maedi/visna virus infection, persistence is so sustained that disease control has required slaughter of sheep over large areas). Recrudescence and intermittent shedding add additional survival advantages to the virus (e.g., herpesvirus infections in all animals).

5. *The capacity to elude host defenses.* Animals have evolved elaborate immune systems to defend themselves against the viruses, but the viruses in turn have evolved equally elaborate systems to evade host defenses. Viruses, particularly those with large genomes, have genes that encode proteins that interfere with specific host antiviral activities. The capacity to cause immunologically tolerant infection represents an evolutionary progression that gives the virus an extreme survival advantage (e.g., bovine viral diarrhea virus infection in calves, feline immunodeficiency virus infection in cats, lymphocytic choriomeningitis virus infection in mice).

6. *The capacity to survive after being shed into the external environment.* All things being equal, a virus that has evolved a capsid that is environmentally stable must have an evolutionary advantage. For example, because of its stability, canine parvovirus was transported around the world within 2 years of its emergence, mostly by carriage on human shoes and clothing, cages, etc.

7. *The capacity to be transmitted vertically.* Viruses that employ vertical transmission and survive without ever confronting the external environment represent another evolutionary progression.

Knowledge of the genetic bases for many of these viral survival strategies expanded greatly following the inception of recombinant DNA technology by Berg, Boyer, and Cohen in 1972. During the 1980s molecular cloning and nucleotide sequencing methods became generally available in many veterinary and zoonotic virology laboratories. Another quantum leap followed the introduction of the polymerase chain reaction in the mid-1980s. It was found that viruses, overall, employ remarkably diverse and seemingly clever molecular mechanisms to assure their survival. It was also found that they have evolved intricate ways to maximize their limited coding capacity. For example, even a small single-stranded RNA virus may encode genes (1) in different reading frames, (2) in reading frames that are encoded in opposite directions, (3) in overlapping reading frames, or (4) in reading frames that are read by frameshifting or with alternating splicing patterns of the transcribed mRNAs. The large double-stranded DNA viruses employ even more complex schemes to synthesize all the proteins they need to succeed in their Darwinian battle for survival. Clearly, an understanding of viral genetics is central to the study of veterinary and zoonotic virology and to understanding how to interfere with viral transmission cycles, whether this be for the prevention, control, or treatment of viral diseases or for more basic or comparative purposes.

Mutation

In productive virus infections of animals, a few virions gain entry and replicate through many cycles to generate millions or billions of progeny. During such replication cycles, errors in copying the viral nucleic acid inevitably occur; these are called *mutations*. Most mutations are lethal because the mutated virus has lost some vital information and can no longer replicate or compete with the wild-type virus. Whether a particular nonlethal mutation survives depends on whether the resultant phenotypic change in its gene product is disadvantageous, neutral, or affords the mutant virus some selective advantage. In the laboratory, genetic variants are obtained by subjecting a virus population to some selective condition and isolating a *clone*, i.e., a population of virions originating from a single virion, in this case a variant virion. A clone is usually obtained by picking a single viral plaque in a cell monolayer, followed by replaquing or other means to assure that only one genotype has been isolated.

Types of Mutations

Mutations can be classified according to the kind of change they produce in the viral genome or the kind of change they produce in the properties of the virus or the infection it causes. The former pertains to change in the viral genotype, the latter in the viral phenotype. Phenotypic change may be evidenced by a change in a physical characteristic of the virion, by a change in a replicative characteristic seen during infection in cell culture, or by a change in a pathogenetic property in an infected animal.

Genotypic Classification of Mutants

The most common mutations are single nucleotide substitutions—these are called *point mutations*. Mutations may also involve deletions or insertions of single nucleotides or small or large blocks of nucleotides. The phenotypic expression of a mutation may be reversed not only by a back-mutation in the affected nucleotide(s) but also by a *suppresser mutation* occurring elsewhere in the same gene, or even in a different gene, which leads to the reappearance of the wild-type phenotype. For example, some temperature-sensitive mutants of influenza virus developed as potential attenuated virus vaccines have reverted to virulence because of independent suppresser mutations in apparently unrelated genes. Mutations based on nucleotide substitutions revert most frequently, those based on small deletions or insertions less frequently, and those based on large deletions rarely if ever. Various other sorts of viral gene rearrangements also occur that mimic simple mutations; these occur especially in DNA viruses and retroviruses and include large duplications, inversions, and the incorporation of foreign viral or cellular nucleic acid sequences by recombination. Such genomic changes often have important biological consequences.

Phenotypic Classification of Mutants

The phenotypic expression of a mutation may be seen in various ways: relative to the wild type a mutant may produce a different type of plaque in a cell monolayer (*plaque mutants*), may become resistant to neutralization by antibody raised against the wild type (*antibody escape mutants*), or may exhibit any of many other variant properties. Mutations affecting antigenic determinants on virion surface proteins are strongly favored when viruses replicate in the presence of an antibody. Such mutants are of importance in persistently infected animals (e.g., in sheep infected with maedi/visna virus and horses infected with equine infectious anemia virus). They are also important epidemiologically (e.g., in swine infected with vesicular exanthema viruses where antibody escape mutants emerged very often and in sea lions infected with San Miguel sea lion viruses where the same phenomenon occurs). Perhaps the most prominent example of the importance of mutations affecting viral antigenicity is influenza viruses, where antigenic drift occurs constantly.

Conditional lethal mutants cannot grow under certain (restrictive) experimental conditions but can replicate under other (permissive) conditions. When a particular growth condition is chosen that allows only such mutants to replicate, usually several different genotypic variants are present, each adapting to the restrictive growth conditions via different mutations, even mutations in different genes. The conditional lethal mutants studied most commonly are those whose replication is blocked in certain host cells (*host range mutants*) or at certain defined temperatures (*temperature-sensitive mutants, cold-adapted mutants*). With the latter, the selective condition used is the temperature of incubation of infected cells. Mutation results in a structurally abnormal protein which—although functional at the *permissive temperature*—cannot maintain its structural integrity and functional conformation when the temperature is changed by a few degrees. Temperature-sensitive mutants and cold-adapted mutants have been used extensively in attempts to produce attenuated virus vaccines; there has been exceptional success in the development of cold-adapted influenza vaccines.

Special Case of Defective Interfering Mutants

Defective interfering (DI) mutants have been demonstrated in most families of viruses; these mutants cannot replicate by themselves but need the presence of the parental wild-type virus; at the same time they interfere with and usually decrease the yield of the parental virus. All DI particles of RNA viruses that have been characterized are deletion mutants. In influenza viruses and reoviruses, which have segmented genomes, defective virions lack one or more of the larger segments and contain instead smaller segments consisting of an incomplete portion of the encoded gene(s). In the case of viruses with a nonsegmented genome, defective interfering particles contain RNA that is shortened, as much as two-thirds of the genome may have been deleted in the defective interfering particles of vesicular stomatitis viruses. Morphologically, defective interfering particles usually resemble the parental virions; however, in vesicular stomatitis viruses, with their normally bullet-shaped virions, they are shorter than wild-type virions. In the jargon used to describe these particles, normal vesicular stomatitis virions are called *B particles* and the defective interfering particles are called truncated or *T particles*. Sequencing studies of the RNA of these defective interfering particles have revealed massive deletions and a great diversity of genomic rearrangements.

In cell culture, the concentration of DI particles increases greatly with serial passage at high multiplicity. This is due to several mechanisms: (1) their shortened genomes require less time to be replicated; (2) they are less often diverted to serve as templates for transcription of mRNA; and (3) they have enhanced affinity for the viral replicase, giving them a competitive advantage over their full-length counterparts. These features also explain why defective interfering particles interfere with the replication of infectious virions with full-length RNA genomes with progressively greater efficiency on serial passage.

The generation of other defective DNA virus genomes can occur by any of a great variety of modes of DNA rearrangement. For example, papovavirus defective interfering particles usually contain reiterated copies of the genomic origins of replication, sometimes interspersed with DNA of host cell origin.

Our knowledge of DI particles derives mostly from studies in cultured cells, but they may also play a role in the animal: by interfering with the replication of an otherwise lethal standard virus they may attenuate its virulence. This may explain "zone phenomena," where virus preparations cause disease only when diluted, while concentrated stock virus is attenuated. Defective interfering mutants may be involved in a variety of chronic animal diseases. However, because their defective and variable nature makes them difficult to detect in animals, their role in disease is still obscure.

Mutation Rates

Replication of cellular DNA in eukaryotic cells is subject to *proofreading,* an error-correction mechanism involving exonuclease activity. Because the replication of those DNA viruses that replicate in the nucleus is subject to the same proofreading, their mutation rates are probably similar to that of host cell DNA. Errors occur at a rate of 10^{-10} and 10^{-11} per incorporated nucleotide (i.e., per nucleotide per replication cycle). Point mutations in the third nucleotide of a codon are often silent, i.e., do not result in an altered amino acid, because of redundancy in the genetic code and some point mutations are lethal because they produce nonfunctioning gene products, a stop codon, or other aberrant regulatory sequences. Viable mutations that are neutral or deleterious in one host may provide a selective advantage in a different host.

Because of the absence of a cellular proofreading mechanism for RNA, error rates during the replication of viral RNAs are much higher than those of viral DNA. For example, the nucleotide substitution rate in the 11-

kb genome of the vesicular stomatitis virus is 10^{-3} to 10^{-4} per nucleotide per replication cycle, so that in an infected cell nearly every progeny genome will be different from the parental genome and from every other progeny genome in at least one nucleotide. This rate of nucleotide substitution is about one million times higher than the average rate in eukaryotic DNA. Of course, most of the nucleotide substitutions are deleterious and the genomes containing them are lost. However, nonlethal mutations in the genome of RNA viruses accumulate very rapidly. For example, genomic sequence comparison of two hepatitis C virus isolates obtained from a chronically infected person at an interval of 13 years showed that the mutation rate was about 2×10^{-3} nucleotide substitutions per genome nucleotide per year. The changes found were distributed unevenly throughout the genome, which means that genes coding for different proteins evolved at different rates. This uneven rate is most probably a consequence of selection of certain mutants over others. As another example, in 1978–1979 outbreaks of human poliomyelitis caused by poliovirus 1 were traced from the Netherlands to Canada and then to the United States. Viral RNA obtained from patients in each country showed that over a period of 13 months of epidemic transmission there were about 100 nucleotide changes in the genome of 7441 nucleotides.

Viral Quasispecies Concept

Every virus species, as defined by conventional phenotypic properties, exists as a genetically dynamic, diverse population of virions in which individual genotypes have only a fleeting existence. Most individual viral genomes differ in one or more nucleotides from the consensus or average sequence of the population and over relatively short times genotypic drift occurs as particular variants gain advantage. Genotypic drift over longer times leads to the evolution of substantially different viruses. Manfred Eigen, John Holland, and their colleagues introduced the term *quasispecies* to describe such diverse, rapidly evolving and competing viral populations.

The evolution of quasispecies would be expected to be most conspicuous in viruses with large RNA genomes, where nonlethal changes may accumulate rapidly. Indeed, the genomes of coronaviruses, the largest RNA genomes known, are fraught with "genetic defects." At the mutation rates noted earlier, 1 out of 3000 nucleotides in every coronavirus genome would be changed in every round of replication; because coronavirus genomes contain about 30,000 nucleotides, every genome must differ from the next by at least one nucleotide. Further, coronavirus genomes undergo other more substantial mutations, including massive deletions, which affect their pathogenicity. From this, one might wonder how coronaviruses or other RNA viruses can maintain their identities as pathogens over any evolutionarily significant period of time; why have these viruses not mutated out of existence? The answer lies in the quasispecies concept, which is not just an abstraction but a proven reality in vesicular stomatitis viruses, foot-and-mouth disease viruses, influenza viruses, and others.

If viral nucleic acid replication was without error, all progeny would be the same and there would be no evolution of phenotypes. If the error rate was too high, mutants of all sorts would appear and the viral population would lose its integrity. However, at an intermediate error rate such as is seen with RNA viruses, the viral population becomes a coherent, self-sustaining entity that resembles a metaphorical cloud of variants centered around a consensus sequence, but capable of continuous expansion and contraction in different directions as new mutants continue to emerge and others disappear within the population. Darwinian selection limits the survival of the most extreme mutants—extreme outliers do not survive—and favors variants near the center of the cloud as these best achieve environmental "fit." Just as the center of a cloud is unclear, so the consensus sequence at the heart of the quasispecies is inscrutable. Any published viral genomic nucleotide sequence reflects a random choice of starting material, one biological clone among many, more or less representative of the consensus sequence of the genome of the population as a whole, the cloud as a whole. In Eigen's metaphor, the cloud is the quasispecies—a graphic depiction has been used to try to make this concept more understandable (Figure 4.1).

To return to the example of the coronaviruses as highly mutable pathogens, studies on the pathogenesis of the coronavirus, feline infectious peritonitis virus, have shown that every cat harbors its own unique coronavirus quasispecies cloud that persists at low levels of replication in the gut, kept in check by an efficient immune system. The fatal disease is the result of mutants arising in large numbers when a burst of replication activity occurs (e.g., after immunosuppression); among these are mutants that grow to high titers in macrophages, inducing a cascade of immunosuppressive and immunopathologic events.

Mutagenesis

Spontaneous mutations occur because of errors during replication. Their frequency can be enhanced by the treatment of virions or isolated viral nucleic acid with physical agents such as UV- or X-irradiation or with

FIGURE 4.1.

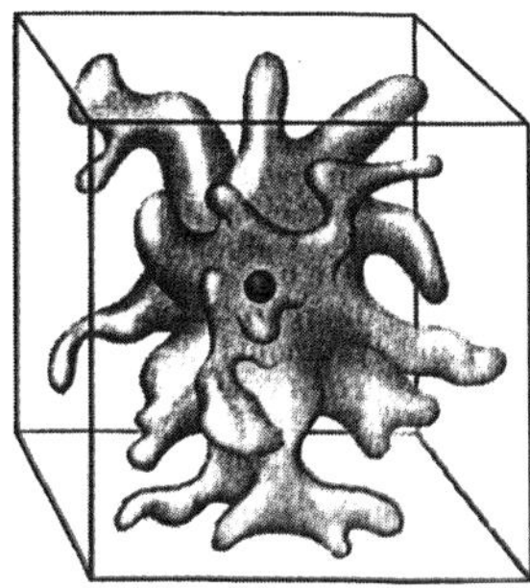

Depiction of the quasispecies concept of Manfred Eigen. The box represents "sequence space," i.e., the confines of all possible variants that might occur when a virus replicates through many infection cycles. The central spot represents the lack of variance that would follow if the replication process of the virus was perfectly accurate and environmental selective pressures were constant. The *cloud* (also called the *swarm*) represents the viral population diversity that actually follows on an intermediate error rate in replication. The population, overall, becomes a coherent, self-sustaining entity that metaphorically resembles a cloud in that its center, the original consensus sequence, is inscrutable, whereas its edges represent probes pushing into the environment seeking a better-and-better "fit." Viral evolution operates at the level of the quasispecies as a whole, not individual genotypes, and the result is the continuing emergence of new viral phenotypes, some of which cause new or more severe disease. (From M. Eigen, Viral quasispecies. *Sci. Am.* **269,** 42–49 (1993)).

chemicals such as nitrous acid or nitrosoguanidine. Nucleotide analogs such as 5-fluorouracil (for RNA viruses) or 5′-bromodeoxyuridine (for DNA viruses) are mutagenic only when virus replicates in their presence, because they are incorporated into the viral nucleic acid and produce mutations by miscoding during replication.

Site-Directed Mutagenesis

Instead of relying on chance mutations anywhere in the genome, recombinant DNA technology makes it possible to introduce mutations at any site of interest and to test their effects on the viral phenotype. That is, using site-directed mutagenesis the nucleotide at any prescribed position in a DNA genome or complementary DNA (cDNA) transcribed from an RNA genome can be changed to any other nucleotide or it can be deleted or affected by the nearby insertion of an additional nucleotide(s). There are many variations in the methods used to carry out these manipulations, especially in the host chosen to accept the manipulated gene. In general the technology involves (1) the synthesis of cloned copies of the DNA of interest, usually in a bacteriophage vector such as M13; (2) the denaturation of this DNA to yield single-stranded molecules; (3) the hybridization of this single-stranded DNA with chemically synthesized oligonucleotides (short sequences of DNA) containing the nucleotide substitution or deletion or addition of interest; (4) the extension of this partial hybrid containing the mutation of interest, using a DNA polymerase and ligase, to form a complete double-stranded DNA copy; (5) the transfer of this DNA to an appropriate host system such as *Escherichia coli* or any of several vertebrate viruses, where millions of copies of the mutant may be produced; and (6) screening for the mutant of interest using selective conditions favoring the replication of the mutant (called marker rescue). The polymerase chain reaction followed by sequence analysis may be used to verify success in introducing the mutation of interest (Figure 4.2).

The ability to isolate infectious viral DNA clones and infectious complementary DNA clones of RNA viruses and to manipulate these clones have been complemented by the development of several viral vectors, i.e., vertebrate viruses with desired tropisms and infection characteristics that make them valuable in carrying foreign genes. Poxviruses, adenoviruses, herpesviruses, parvoviruses, enteroviruses, togaviruses, and other viruses have been advanced as vectors, each for particular purposes. The power of this approach is that without knowing the role of a particular sequence beforehand, it is possible to determine the protein(s) it encodes and its function(s) by altering its sequence and reintroducing all variants back into host cells (or even host animals). This approach has been called *reverse genetics,* i.e., genetic investigation proceeding from genotype to phenotype. Site-directed mutagenesis has opened other new research avenues in veterinary and zoonotic virology; for example, mutations can be introduced into genes suspected of having roles in viral pathogenicity and mutations can be introduced to produce attenuated virus vaccines that may also carry an immunological marker.

Genetic Analysis of Noncultivable Viruses

Growth in cell culture is no longer a precondition for the study of viruses as virtually unlimited quantities of any required viral nucleic acid can be produced using polymerase chain reaction or cloning. Remarkable progress has been made in the genetic analysis of pathogens that cannot be grown in cell culture or experimental animals: for example, noncultivable bovine papillomaviruses have been analyzed using DNA extracted directly from papillomas collected at abattoirs. The complete nucleotide sequences of rabbit hemorrhagic disease virus, a calicivirus that cannot be cultivated in cell culture, has been determined, starting with virus obtained from the livers of infected rabbits. Similarly, the genomes of

Figure 4.2.

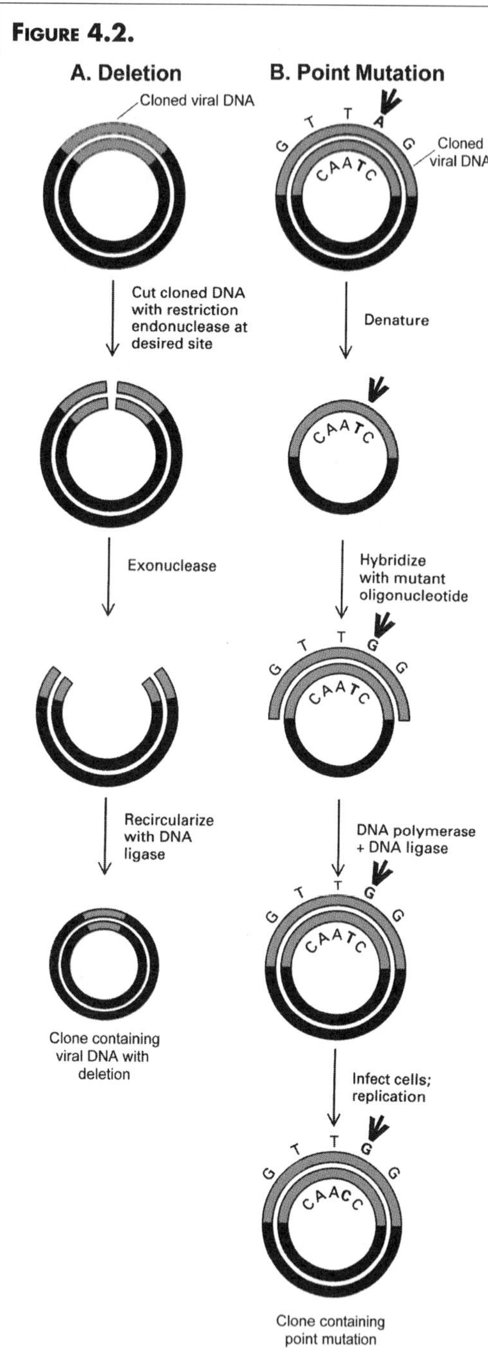

Site-directed mutagenesis. (A) Deletions may be made in cloned viral DNA (or complementary DNA obtained by reverse-transcribing viral RNA) by inserting the DNA in a plasmid and removing whole blocks of DNA between two restriction endonuclease cutting sites or by cutting at a single restriction site and using an exonuclease to remove nucleotides from both cut ends. Deletions of various sizes may be selected from a collection of such clones. (B) Point mutations may be inserted in cloned viral DNA by (1) denaturing the DNA to obtain single-stranded molecules, (2) hybridizing these molecules to a chemically synthesized oligonucleotide primer that is mismatched at a desired site (arrow), (3) extending the double-stranded DNA using a DNA polymerase, and (4) cloning the resulting DNA and selecting clones containing the mutant of interest.

human hepatitis C virus and hepatitis G virus, both uncultivable flaviviruses, have been sequenced and the sequences used to produce synthetic diagnostic antigens.

Genetics of Viral Adaptation to Cell Cultures or Laboratory Animals

Although experiments with viruses of veterinary importance can often be carried out in their natural hosts, growing the viruses in cultured cells or small laboratory animals offers great advantages. Many wild-type viruses initially grow poorly in cell cultures or laboratory animals, but can be adapted by serial passage. Such adaptation depends on the spontaneous generation of mutations and progressive selection of the best growing mutants. These host-range variants may contain mutations in any of several genes, but most often in genes encoding the virion surface proteins. Adapted variants often have modified attachment domains on their surface proteins that bind better to the different receptors on cultured cells or key cells in experimental animals. For example, influenza viruses may acquire the capacity to grow well in the lungs of mice or in cultured mammalian or avian cells via point mutations affecting their hemagglutinin. Often such mutations affect the proteolytic cleavage of the hemagglutinin, which is essential for viral infectivity.

Some viruses produce a cytopathic effect or disease the first time they are inoculated into cell cultures or experimental animals [e.g., Eastern equine encephalitis virus in BHK-21 (baby hamster kidney) cells or suckling mice]. In other cases, a minimal cytopathic effect or disease may be observed at first, but may be produced regularly after serial passage, even prolonged blind passage (e.g., bluetongue viruses in mice and various cell cultures; street rabies virus in mice, hamsters and neuroblastoma cells). Likewise, newly isolated viruses at first often fail to grow well in certain kinds of cultured cells, but can be adapted by serial passage. Most modern virologic research is performed with virus strains highly adapted to a given host system, usually a particular cell culture system that provides a maximum virus yield. A frequent by-product of such adaptation is a loss of virulence for the natural host species; thus adaptation of infectious canine hepatitis virus (an adenovirus) to pig kidney cell cultures results in its attenuation for the dog—this was the basis for the development more than 40 years ago of the most widely used attenuated virus vaccine for dogs.

Although such adaptations of viruses to cultured cells and laboratory animals have been practiced for many years, leading to many practical vaccine products, until recently little was known of the nature of the mutations involved. Now, using site-directed mutagenesis and other molecular genetic methods, the key viral genes, their gene products, and their infection strategies are being revealed. Seemingly, the more we study attenuating mutations the more complex they become; however, at the same time, more and more practical products are coming from our increased genetic understanding.

Genetic Recombination between Viruses

When two different viruses simultaneously infect the same cell, genetic recombination may occur between the nucleic acid molecules during or after their synthesis; this may take the form of *intramolecular recombination, reassortment,* or *reactivation* (the latter if one of the viruses had been inactivated) (Figure 4.3).

Intramolecular Recombination

Intramolecular recombination involves the exchange of nucleotide sequences between different—but usually closely related—viruses during replication (Figure 4.3A). It occurs with all double-stranded DNA viruses, presumably because of template switching by the polymerase. Intramolecular recombination also occurs among RNA viruses (e.g., picornaviruses, coronaviruses and togaviruses); western equine encephalitis virus arose as a result of intramolecular recombination between an ancient Sindbis-like virus and eastern equine encephalitis virus. Such phenomena are likely more widespread among RNA viruses than has been appreciated because the detection of recombinants has been difficult. Now, use of the reverse-transcriptase polymerase chain reaction has overcome earlier technical problems.

Under experimental conditions, intramolecular recombination may even occur between viruses belonging to different families; the best example is the now classical discovery of recombination between SV40 (a papovavirus) and adenoviruses. Both SV40 and adenovirus DNAs occasionally become integrated into cellular DNA, so it is perhaps not surprising to find that when rhesus monkey cells that harbor a persistent SV40 infection are superinfected with an adenovirus, not only does *complementation* occur, the SV40 acting as a helper in an otherwise abortive adenovirus infection, but recombination occurs between SV40 DNA and adenovirus DNA to yield hybrid (recombinant) DNA, which is packaged into adenovirus capsids. Integration of viral DNA into cellular DNA by intramolecular recombination occurs in cells transformed by adenoviruses, hepadnaviruses, and polyomaviruses, but not always in cells transformed by papillomaviruses or certain herpesviruses, in which transformation may occur, although the viral DNA usually remains episomal.

Recombination between viral and cellular genetic information has been established and, for at least some viruses, is also important in virus evolution. After all, viruses have access to the almost unlimited gene pool of their host cells and certainly have the capacity to incorporate and exploit genes that favor their growth and survival. The presence of cellular genes or pseudogenes within the genomes of retroviruses is well established, and the same has now been found for other RNA viruses. For example, in influenza virus infections, proteolytic cleavage of the viral hemagglutinin by cellular proteases is essential for the production of infectious progeny. During the adaptation of nonvirulent influenza virus strains to chicken cells (which are nonpermissive for hemagglutinin cleavage), a pathogenic variant was isolated that contained an insertion of 54 nucleotides that was complementary to a region of host cell 28S ribosomal RNA. This suggests template switching by the viral polymerase during viral RNA replication. This insertion seems to have changed the conformation of the viral gene product, the hemagglutinin, rendering it accessible to cellular proteases and thereby producing infectious virions in previously nonpermissive cells.

The pathogenetic consequences of cellular information being inserted into viruses by intramolecular recombination can be dramatic. The discovery that Marek's disease virus, an oncogenic herpesvirus of chickens, had been misclassified because it carries extra genes was particularly surprising. This virus had been considered a gammaherpesvirus, partly because all other oncogenic herpesviruses are members of this subfamily. Subsequently, as the genome of the virus was partially sequenced it was realized that it is an alphaherpesvirus—oncogenic strains of the virus had acquired oncogenic genes either from avian retroviruses or from the cellular homologues of retrovirus genes.

Equally surprising was the discovery of the molecular basis for the progression of bovine viral diarrhea to mucosal disease. When a cellular ubiquitin gene is inserted into a nonstructural gene of noncytopathic bovine viral diarrhea virus strains they become cytopathic and gain the capacity to cause persistent infection. Severe disease, i.e., mucosal disease, occurs when such mutant viruses infect bovine fetuses previously infected with noncytopathic, nonpersistent virus strains during the first 80 to 100 days of gestation. This complex infection and mutation pattern explains the sporadic occurrence of universally fatal mucosal disease in calves and, in some cases, older animals.

Figure 4.3.

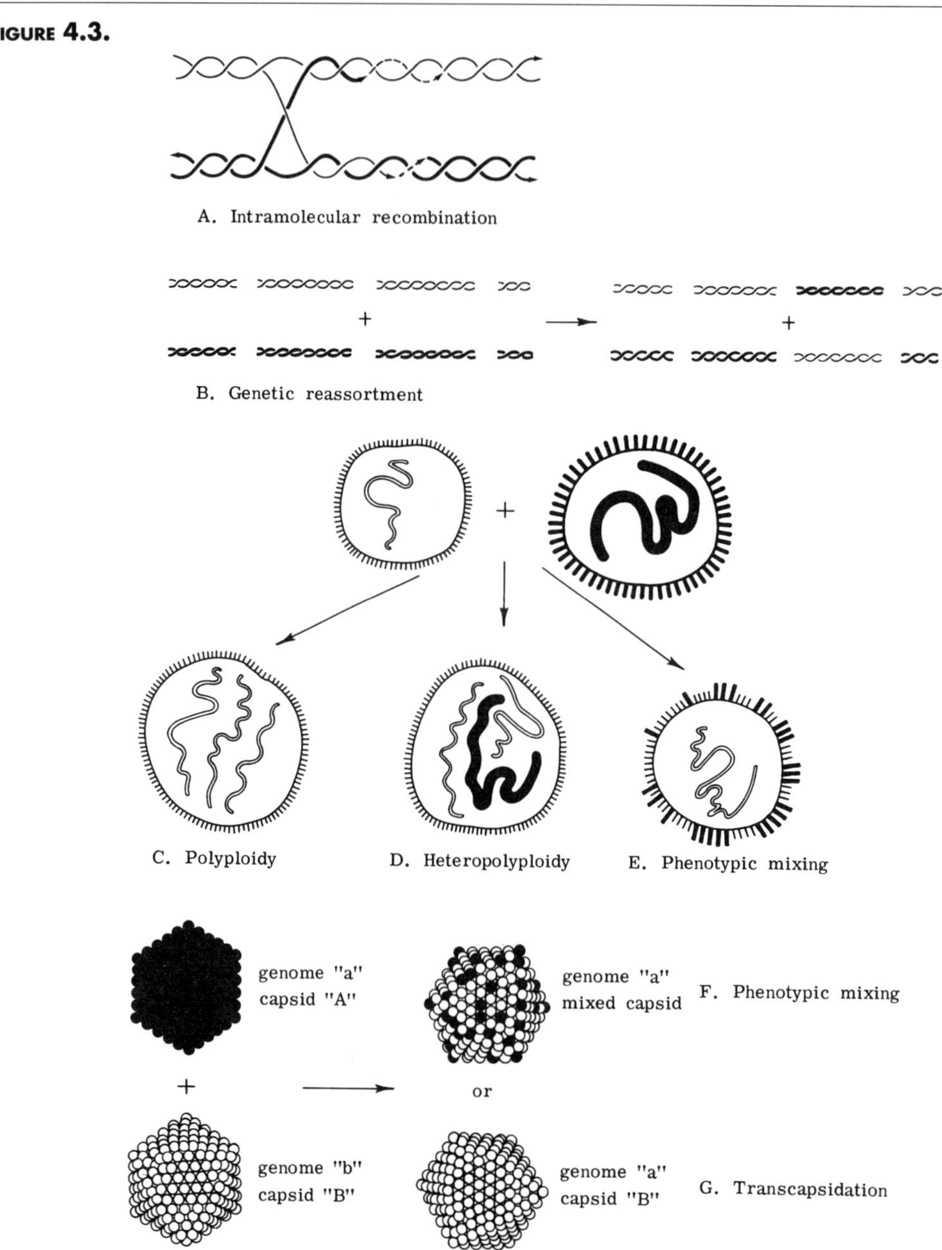

Genetic recombination, polyploidy, phenotypic mixing, and transcapsidation. (A) Intramolecular recombination, as occurs with double-stranded DNA viruses. (B) Reassortment of genome fragments, as occurs in mixed infections with reoviruses and orthomyxoviruses. (C) Polyploidy, as seen in unmixed infections with paramyxoviruses; (D) Heteropolyploidy, as may occur in mixed infections with paramyxoviruses and other enveloped RNA viruses. (E–G) Phenotypic mixing: (E) with enveloped viruses, (F) viruses with icosahedral capsids, (G) transcapsidation.

Unlike other RNA viruses, retroviruses have no replicating pool of viral RNA. Although the genome of retroviruses is positive-sense, single-stranded RNA, replication does not occur until the genomic RNA is transcribed into DNA by the virion-associated reverse transcriptase and the resultant double-stranded DNA is integrated into the DNA of the host cell. However, both negative-strand and positive-strand recombinations occur between the two DNA copies of the diploid retrovirus genome, as well as between the DNA provirus and cellular DNA. In the latter instance, the retrovirus may pick up a *cellular oncogene;* such oncogenes are incorporated into the viral genome to become *viral oncogenes,* which confer the property of rapid oncogenicity on the retrovirus concerned (see Chapters 11 and 23).

Reassortment

Reassortment is a form of genetic recombination observed in RNA viruses with segmented genomes, whether these be single or double stranded and whether these involve few or many segments. Reassortment has been documented in families with 2 (*Arenaviridae* and *Birnaviridae*), 3 (*Bunyaviridae*), 6, 7, or 8 (*Orthomyxoviridae*), or 10, 11, or 12 (family *Reoviridae*) genome segments (Figure 4.3B). In a cell infected with two related viruses within each of these families, an exchange of segments may occur, with the production of viable and stable reassortants. Such reassortment occurs in nature and is an important source of genetic variability; for example, bluetongue virus isolates have been found in cattle that are reassortants of two parental viruses.

Reactivation

The term *multiplicity reactivation* is applied to the production of infectious virus by a cell infected with two or more virus particles of the same strain, each of which had suffered a lethal mutation in a different gene. Multiplicity reactivation could theoretically lead to the emergence of infectious virus if animals were inoculated with vaccines produced by UV-irradiation or chemical mutagenesis; these methods are therefore not used for vaccine production. *Cross-reactivation, genome rescue,* and *DNA fragment rescue* are terms used to describe genetic recombination between infectious and inactivated viruses of related but distinguishable genotypes (or a DNA fragment from such a virus). Appreciation of such phenomena was important in the development of viral vectors as vaccines.

Interactions between Viral Gene Products

The interaction between viruses may involve not only their nucleic acids but also their proteins, and the products of such interactions may affect the viral phenotype. For the most part, such interactions are laboratory phenomena, but some may operate in nature and some have proven useful in practical ways.

Complementation

The term complementation is used to describe interactions between viral proteins in doubly infected cells that result in rescue or increased yields of one or both viruses. This can occur between two strains of the same virus, two related viruses, or two unrelated viruses [e.g., between an adenovirus and an adeno-associated virus (a parvovirus) or between an adenovirus and SV40 virus (a polyomavirus)]. One virus provides a gene product that the other cannot make, thereby allowing the latter to replicate in the mixedly infected cell. Of course, because neither genome is involved, nothing permanent comes of this. Genes can be localized by complementation analysis, as viruses with mutations in identical genes do not complement each other.

Phenotypic Mixing

Following infection of cells by two viruses, progeny virions may be found that have acquired phenotypic characteristics from both parents. For example, when cells are coinfected with an influenza virus and a paramyxovirus, the envelopes of some of the progeny particles display antigens derived from both parents. However, each virion contains the genome of only one parent and on passage produces only virions resembling that parent (Figures 4.3E and 4.3F). Phenotypic mixing plays an essential part in the replication cycle of envelope-defective retroviruses. The progeny virions are called pseudotypes and contain the genome of the defective parental virus enveloped by host cell membrane containing the glycoproteins of the helper retrovirus, in whose company it will always be found.

Experimentally, and in nature with some viruses, phenotypic mixing of nonenveloped viruses can take the form of transcapsidation (Figure 4.3G), in which there is partial or usually complete exchange of capsids. For example, poliovirus nucleic acid may be enclosed within a coxsackievirus capsid or the adenovirus 7 genome may be enclosed within an adenovirus 2 capsid. Because the viral ligands that govern cellular attachment reside in the capsid, transcapsidation can change the tropism of a virus.

Polyploidy

With the exception of the diploid retroviruses, vertebrate viruses are haploid, i.e., they contain only a single copy of each gene. Even with the retroviruses, diploidy is in no sense comparable to that seen in eukaryotic cells, as both copies of the genome are essentially identical and derived from the same parental virus. Among viruses that mature by budding from the plasma membrane, e.g., paramyxoviruses, several nucleocapsids (and thus genomes) may be found enclosed in a single envelope (*polyploidy* or *heteropolyploidy,* Figure 4.3C and 4.3D).

Mapping Viral Genomes

Viral genomes have been mapped in many ways. Since the early 1980s, partial or complete sequencing has largely replaced all older methods for analyzing viral genomes, especially smaller viral genomes. Methods have become simpler, cheaper, more automated, and more accessible to the average virology laboratory. The complete sequences for prototypic members of every family containing animal or zoonotic pathogens are now available and retrievable from international databanks, and partial sequences are being used in many genetic studies and reference identification schemes. Restriction endonuclease analysis is still useful for characterizing viruses with large genomes, but most other older methods, such as oligonucleotide fingerprinting using T1 ribonuclease digestion followed by two-dimensional electrophoresis, have fallen by the wayside.

Viral Genomic DNA and RNA Sequence Analysis

There are two basic sequencing techniques, known as the Maxam–Gilbert and Sanger methods. Maxam–Gilbert sequencing is based on the chemical degradation of the fragment to be sequenced and Sanger sequencing (also called the dideoxy method) is based on the enzymatic synthesis of the DNA strand to be sequenced. Both methods work because gel electrophoresis produces very high-resolution separations of DNA molecules; fragments of DNA that differ in size by only a single nucleotide can be resolved. Variations on the Sanger method are used most commonly today—they are often automated, allowing high throughput and computer-based management and interpretation of data.

The Maxam–Gilbert Method

Walter Gilbert's knowledge of organic chemistry allowed him to select a set of chemicals that specifically break DNA at A's, G's, or T's. By separating the fragments of DNA that result from such chemical treatment it was possible to infer the order in which each of the nucleotides was present in the fragment of DNA.

In this method, individual fragments are first isolated by treating the DNA with a restriction endonuclease; these fragments are then radioactively 5′ end labeled with ^{32}P or ^{35}S. The fragments are then cut with a second restriction enzyme and the resulting fragments are subjected to chemical treatments to modify and remove specific nucleotides. For example, in one reaction mixture, chemicals are chosen that break the DNA fragments at G residues. Reaction mixtures specific for the other nucleotides are run in parallel. The length of each DNA fragment, from the labeled 5′ end to the break point, indicates the location of a G residue in the original DNA. To visualize the sequence, the degraded fragments from each reaction mixture are separated by gel electrophoresis. The gel is then exposed to X-ray film where only the products containing the radioactively labeled 5′ end become visible (Figure 4.4). This method allows detection of up to 1000 bp of DNA from a single gel. Unfortunately, fragment preparation is tedious and the chemical base digestions are difficult to control. Because of these difficulties, this method is no longer widely used.

Sanger Method

In 1977 Fred Sanger described a DNA sequencing method based on the enzymatic synthesis of complemen-

FIGURE 4.4.

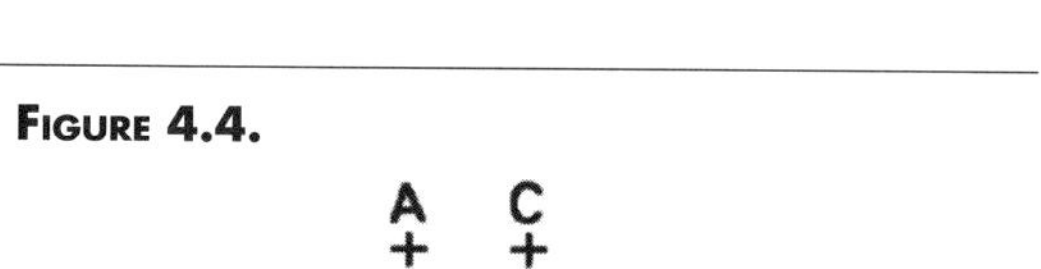

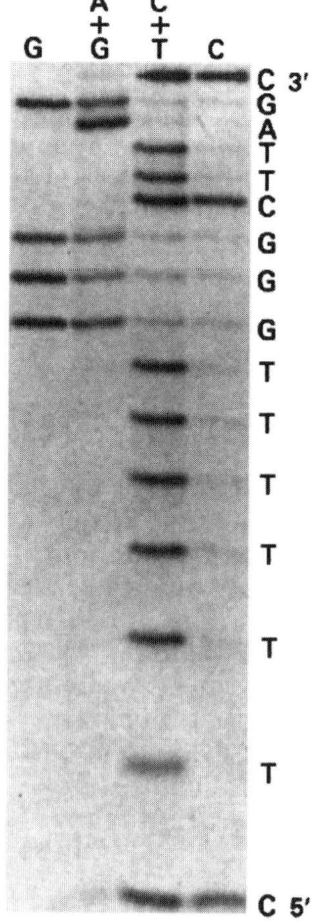

Maxam–Gilbert method of sequencing DNA (see text for details). Chemicals are used that specifically break fragments of DNA at either A's, G's, or T's. The radioactively labeled fragments are separated by gel electrophoresis and the gel is exposed to X-ray film. The heading of the lanes of the gel indicates the product of each reaction; the nucleotide sequence is shown at the side.

tary strands of DNA using the DNA of interest as the template. Synthesis of these complementary strands is terminated by the incorporation of nucleotide analogues, referred to as dideoxynucleotides (ddNTP). In the reaction mixtures the DNA polymerase incorporates normal dNTPs to form the growing chains until it uses a ddNTP, which forces chain termination.

By performing four reactions, each containing a single dideoxynucleotide (ddATP, ddCTP, ddGTP, or ddTTP), along with all four normal dNTPs, four sets of DNA fragments are generated. To visualize the products of the polymerase reaction, either the primer or the normal nucleotides are radiolabeled ([^{32}P]- or [^{35}S]dNTP). Newly synthesized fragments are denatured from their templates and resolved according to size by electrophoresis in a denaturing polyacrylamide gel. The resulting gel is then exposed to X-ray film (Figure 4.5). The DNA sequence is determined by reading the order of bands in the four lanes representing each nucleotide. These bands form a ladder corresponding to the size of the specifically terminated fragments. The fastest migrating bands (from all four reactions) represent the shortest fragments synthesized. The sequence can be interpreted by reading up the four lanes of the autoradiogram in order of the occurrence of the bands on the ladder. Using this method, 300–500 nucleotides can be sequenced per set of reactions. This is far fewer than the Maxam–Gilbert method, but far more runs can be managed per day; without automated equipment, one person can sequence about 25,000 bp per week.

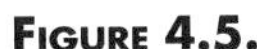

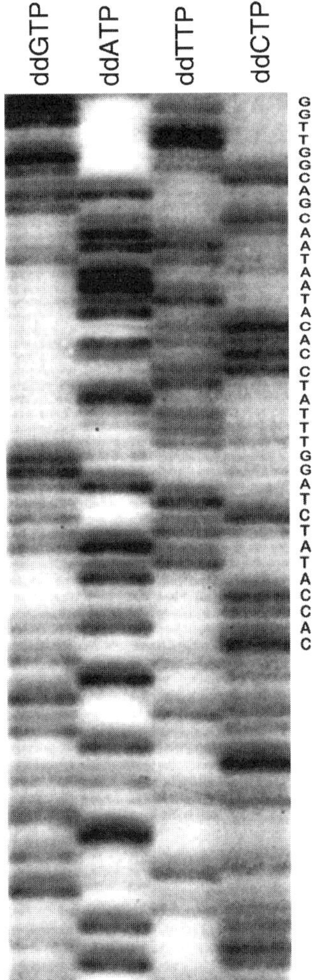

Sanger (dideoxy) method of sequencing DNA (see text for details). The products of four reactions, each containing radiolabeled normal dNTP and a single dideoxynucleotide (ddATP, ddCTP, ddGTP, or ddTTP) to specifically terminate DNA fragment synthesis, are placed in adjacent lanes and electrophoresed. The bands form a ladder in the autoradiograph corresponding to the size of the specifically terminated fragments. The sequence is read from the bottom up by identifying which of the four lanes contains each sequential signal because it is the newly synthesized DNA fragments that provide the signals, the nucleotide identified at each place in the ladder is the complement (A = T, G = C) of that in the viral DNA of interest. This small part of a sequencing gel is from a study of the genome of equine arteritis virus. (Courtesy of N. J. MacLachaln.)

Automated Fluorescence Sequencing

The Sanger method requires four lanes per sample, one for each of the bases (A, C, T, G). In automatic sequencing, each dideoxy terminator or primer is marked with a different fluorochrome (conventionally, red for T, green for A, blue for C, and black for G). The sample is loaded in a single lane on the gel and separated by electrophoresis, but the gel is housed in a complex detector that discriminates the four different fluorochrome signal emissions using a laser to scan across the bottom of the gel as the labeled fragments pass by. Software then superimposes the four readings, producing an integrated readout (Figure 4.6). The software provides an interpretation of the colorimetric data—it determines the maximum color intensity at each position and indicates over the peak the corresponding nucleotide. Another technical improvement involves the use of *Taq* polymerase instead of *E. coli* DNA polymerase—this allows multiple cycles of termination reactions to occur, as is done in the polymerase chain reaction, greatly amplifying sequence signal from limiting quantities of template DNA. Using automated fluorescence sequencing equipment, it is possible for a single person to process 32 DNA samples per day, sequencing about 600 nucleotides per sample, i.e., 96,000 nucleotides per week. A major focus of the Human Genome Project is the development of even better automated sequencing technology—one goal is to be able to accurately and economically sequence 100,000 or more nucleotides per day per person.

Uses of Sequencing in Veterinary and Medical Virology

Viral genome sequencing is yielding an ever increasing body of genetic information. The field of *molecular epidemiology* has blossomed, based on sequencing (usually partial sequencing) of large numbers of isolates obtained in the course of investigating outbreaks, epidemics, or endemic viral disease problems. For example, in medical/public health virology, nearly all poliovirus isolates are partially sequenced as the basis for identifying them as (1) poliovirus 1, 2, or 3; (2) wild or vaccine genotype; (3) endemic or imported genotype; (3) a traceable imported genotype, providing clues for guiding intensified vaccine usage; and (4) evidence in the global surveillance being done as part of the WHO Polio Eradication Program. Similar partial sequencing of large numbers of isolates is being done as part of regional dengue surveillance programs—in this case the finding of newly introduced genotypes is the basis for intensified mosquito control programs. In the major epidemic of Venezuelan equine encephalitis in Columbia and Venezuela in 1995, the partial sequencing of large numbers of isolates was crucial in establishing the source of the epidemic virus as a mutant of an endemic virus genotype.

Sequencing is also proving to be of great value in more basic virologic studies. Open reading frames (ORFs) in viral genomes are identified easily [translatable sequences start with the methionine codon (AUG) and are uninterrupted by stop codons (UAA, UAG, UGA)]. This is the first step in identifying the viral structural or nonstructural protein encoded by each open reading frame. The function of viral proteins can often be surmised by comparing the sequence of the genes that encode them to those of known proteins with established functions from other viruses or eukaryotic organisms. Such comparisons are carried out by searching international computer databases. It is also possible from an examination of viral genome sequences to find characteristic groups of amino acids, called *motifs,* that indicate particular functions of encoded proteins. For example, particular motifs indicate (1) *signal sequences,* i.e., sequences that target a given protein to the endoplasmic reticulum or the plasma membrane; (2) *transmembrane sequences* and *glycosylation sequences,* i.e., sequences that indicate that the protein is a peplomer or other virion surface protein that may contain epitopes that are targets of the immune response; (3) *protein–nucleic acid* or *protein–protein-binding sequences,* i.e., sequences that indicate that the protein is involved in viral synthetic or regulatory processes; and (4) *short sequence motifs,* i.e., sequences involved in viral gene expression (e.g., sites of mRNA polyadenylation, often indicated by AAUAAA, indicate the 3′ end of a viral protein). This kind of genetic information is becoming crucial in the logical design of vaccines, diagnostic reagents, and antiviral drugs.

The pace and scale of progress in viral genomics is leading, as it is in the Human Genome Project, to the emergence of a new field, that of *functional genomics,* i.e., is the linking of phenotypic characters to specific genes. This field promises much further progress that will advance the standard of practice in veterinary and zoonotic virology laboratories and clinics.

Restriction Endonuclease Mapping

Several hundred sequence-specific DNases, called *restriction endonucleases,* have been identified and purified from various bacteria. Each recognizes a unique *palindromic sequence* of nucleotides (a sequence that reads the same backward as forward), four to nine nucleotide pairs long. Depending on the location and frequency of its target sequence in the DNA molecule of interest a given restriction endonuclease cleaves DNA into a determinate number of fragments of precise sizes. Different endonucleases, recognizing different sequences, cleave the same DNA into different numbers and sizes of fragments, all of which may be separated by gel electrophoresis. The pattern of these fragments in gels is also referred to as restriction fragment length polymorphism (RFLP) or as a DNA fingerprint.

Different viruses, along with closely related strains of the same virus yield characteristically different restriction endonuclease fragment patterns or fingerprints. Restriction endonuclease mapping has been invaluable for distinguishing viruses or strains of large genomes, e.g., orthopoxviruses and herpesviruses. Further, with considerably more effort, depending on the size of the genome, the order of the restriction fragments can be determined, and when large numbers of such fragments are laid out they can provide a physical map of the entire viral genome. By convention the genome of a virus represents 100 map units so that the coordinates of individual restriction fragments can be given. Restriction enzymes can also be used to analyze the molecularly cloned complementary DNA copies of genomes or individual genes of RNA viruses and to identify specific map locations of various genetic markers in the viral genome sequence. Similarly, mRNAs of both DNA and RNA viruses can be analyzed by these procedures.

Recombination Mapping

Among viruses that undergo intramolecular recombination, the probability of recombination occurring be-

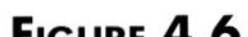

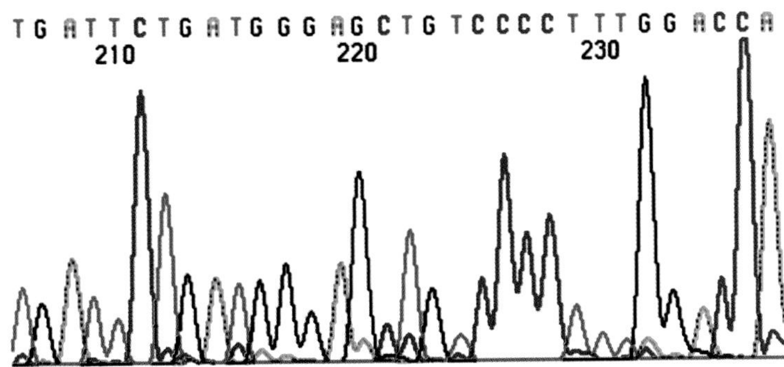

Automated fluorescence sequencing. Each dideoxy terminator is marked with a different fluorochrome (conventionally, red for T, green for A, violet for C, and black for G). The sample is loaded in a single lane of a gel and electrophoresed. A laser detector discriminates the four different fluorochrome signal emissions as it scans continuously across the bottom of the gel as the reaction products move past. Software then superimposes the four readings and interprets colorimetric data—the nucleotide at each position is indicated over the colorimetric peak.

tween two markers reflects the distance between them, and recombination frequencies in adjacent intervals are approximately additive. Two-factor crosses are used to determine recombination frequencies between pairs of mutants; for very close or distant markers, three-factor crosses are used to resolve ambiguities. Recombination maps have been made for several large DNA viruses, notably herpesviruses, and for poliovirus. With the determination of nucleotide sequences, the genetic markers of a number of viruses have been located on the relevant physical maps. For viruses that have segmented genomes, reassortant maps can be constructed by crossing mutants of different serotypes that have electrophoretic polymorphisms for each of the genome segments. They have confirmed that mutants able to recombine reside on different genome segments.

Recombinant DNA Technology

The discovery of restriction endonucleases and the recognition of other enzymes involved in DNA synthesis (polymerases, ligases, transferases) opened up the possibility of deliberately introducing foreign genetic information into the DNA of viruses, bacteria, yeast, and vertebrate cells. The discovery that such foreign DNA can be amplified greatly by coreplicating along with the DNA of its host opened up many other possibilities, including novel vaccines (e.g., DNA vaccines) and diagnostic reagents (e.g., hybridization probes). Overall, the technology is called *molecular cloning* or, in lay terms, *genetic engineering*.

When a foreign DNA segment is inserted into an appropriate vector in frame and with appropriate upstream and downstream regulatory sequences and the recombinant plasmid is introduced into a host cell, the foreign DNA may be expressed, i.e., the protein it specifies may be produced in large amounts. This technology is called *expression*. The vector used may be a bacteriophage (a virus of bacteria) or a bacterial plasmid so that the protein is expressed in bacteria (Figure 4.7). Similarly, the foreign DNA may be incorporated into a yeast plasmid or virus so that it may be expressed in yeast, insect cells, or mammalian cells. The bacteriophage or plasmid or virus serve as *cloning vectors* (to amplify the foreign DNA) and/or *expression vectors* (to produce gene products). Some vectors have been engineered to replicate in different host cells and are called *shuttle vectors*. Some eukaryotic vectors allow the introduction and expression of foreign genes in intact animals—these are called *transgenic vectors*.

Role of Vectors in Recombinant DNA Technology

The use of animal viruses and vertebrate and insect cells for the expression of foreign genes was developed early in the evolution of molecular cloning techniques. Papovaviruses were first utilized to introduce foreign genes into mammalian cells: early understanding of the nature of the genomes of these viruses and their capacity to incorporate rather large amounts of foreign DNA underpinned this breakthrough research. Success in developing full-length infectious clones of DNA viruses used as vectors and full-length complementary DNA clones from RNA viruses, used as vectors, has opened the door for many new ways to produce valuable proteins (for vaccines and diagnostic reagents) and nucleic acids (for diagnostic probes and DNA vaccines).

Poxviruses as Vectors

Among the DNA viruses, poxviruses have been prototypes as cloning and expression vectors, delivering foreign genes of interest into many kinds of cultured cells and into mammals and birds. The large genomes of the poxviruses have allowed the insertion of large amounts of foreign DNA into nonessential genome regions. Vaccinia virus has become a workhorse of recombinant DNA technology; hundreds of foreign proteins of biological and medical importance have been vectored by the vaccinia virus system. When engineered properly, the proteins vectored by vaccinia virus and expressed in mammalian cells or animals have had the predicted molecular mass, have undergone proper posttranslational modifications required for biological activity (proteolytic cleavage, glycosylation, phosphorylation, myristylation), and have been transported to the proper intracellular or extracellular compartment. Because of the broad host range of vaccinia virus, many cell-type specific products have been vectored successfully.

Vaccinia virus recombinant vectors are generated by incorporating the foreign DNA into the intact viral genome via homologous recombination. This is facilitated by adding vaccinia DNA flanking sequences to the foreign DNA. In infected cells, recombinant, chimeric vaccinia genomes are packaged faithfully into infectious progeny. In contrast to procedures used with other DNA viruses, the transfected foreign DNA can only be rescued by infectious vaccinia virus. This is due to the noninfectious nature of isolated poxvirus DNA, which replicates in the cytoplasm and requires many virion-associated enzymatic functions. One particular advantage of vaccinia virus recombinants is their very large carrying capacity—it has been estimated that the vaccinia virus can carry over 25 kbp of foreign DNA without its infectivity being affected. This allows the simultaneous expression

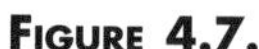

FIGURE 4.7.

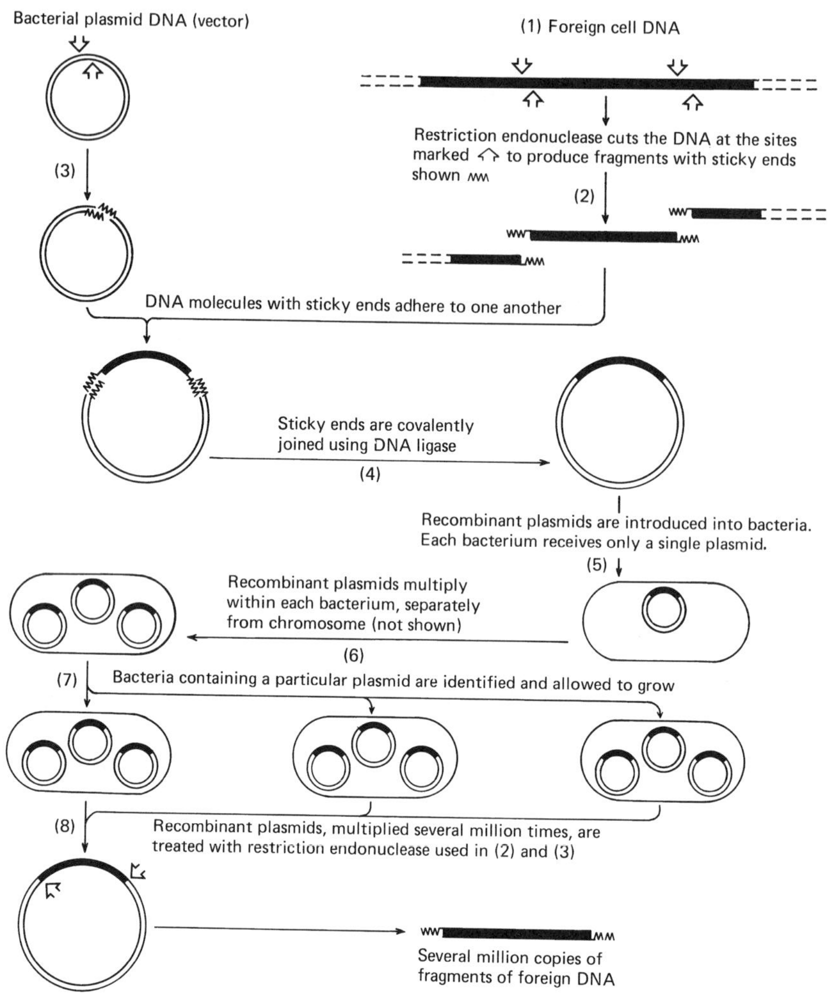

Steps in obtaining large amounts of recombinant DNA. In parallel, DNA (genome DNA or complementary DNA from virion RNA or mRNA) from a virus (1) is cut into fragments by a selected restriction endonuclease (2), and the circular DNA molecule of the plasmid vector is cut with the same endonuclease (3). The viral DNA is inserted and ligated into the plasmid DNA, which is thus circularized again (4). The plasmid is then introduced into the host bacterium by transfection (5). Replication of the plasmid as an episome may produce many copies per bacterial cell (for small plasmids) or there may be only one copy (for large plasmids) (6). Bacteria containing the desired plasmid are identified, cloned, and allowed to grow (7). The plasmids are isolated from the bacteria and the viral DNA insert is excised (8) using the same restriction endonuclease as was employed in steps (2) and (3). In this way a specified gene may be replicated several millionfold. With the appropriate addition of regulatory and termination sequences, the protein product of the inserted gene may be expressed in prokaryotic or eukaryotic cells in very large amounts.

of multiple foreign proteins and offers promise for the development of multivalent vaccines.

Vaccinia virus-vector technology has been extended to other poxviruses, providing vectors and candidate vectored vaccines with desired limited host ranges (avipoxviruses, capripoxvirus, raccoonpoxvirus, suipoxvirus, etc.). The practical application of poxvirus-vectored vaccine candidates has been demonstrated for the control of several veterinary and zoonotic diseases: extensive field testing has been carried out with a vaccinia-based rabies glycoprotein G recombinant, and its safety and efficacy have been ascertained. A similar construct in raccoonpox virus for the control of the large raccoon rabies epidemic in eastern regions of the United States has also been proven in field trials. Vaccinia recombinants expressing the H and/or F protein of rinderpest virus have been shown to protect cattle and are being tested in large open field trials in Africa. In addition to being efficacious, safe, and inexpensive, these vaccines have the added advantage of being very stable at elevated ambient temperatures, a great advantage in the tropics and in bait-delivered vaccines.

Other Viruses as Vectors

Viruses that have been used in research toward the goal of developing vectored vaccines to carry genes for antigens of viruses for which no vaccines exist include baculoviruses, herpesviruses, adenoviruses, papillomaviruses, SV40 (a polyomavirus), enteroviruses, togaviruses, flaviviruses, and influenza viruses. Because many attenuated virus vaccines have been so successful there is also a potential for using them as vectors for veterinary vaccines—it seems likely that every licensed attenuated virus vaccine used in veterinary practice is being considered for such use in one laboratory or another.

Transgenic Mice and Recombinant DNA Technology

Transgenic mice provide a valuable tool for investigating many problems in virology, immunology, and developmental biology. They are produced by injecting selected cloned fragments of DNA into the nuclei of fertilized eggs washed out of the mouse oviduct. After replacement, some ova develop normally to form the base of a colony of transgenic mice. The technique provides insights into the potential role in viral pathogenesis of individual viral genes and gene products in the context of the intact animal. For example, transgenic mice have been produced in which every cell contained genome length hepatitis B DNA sequences. All of these mice had viral antigen in their plasma, but the viral genes were selectively expressed only in cells of the liver, kidney, and pancreas. Likewise, transgenic mice containing the DNA for the early region of bovine papillomavirus developed skin tumors at 8–9 months of age. In these mice, episomal viral DNA was detected in tumor cells and integrated viral DNA in normal tissues.

Practical Achievements of Recombinant DNA Technology

Practical applications of genetic engineering of viruses include the development of nucleic acid probes for diagnosis and novel methods for the production of vaccines, such as the use of vaccinia virus as a vector. Combined with the availability of simple and fast methods of sequencing nucleic acids, genetic engineering has also led to studies of animal virus genomes that could not be contemplated before it became possible to produce large quantities of selected fragments of viral nucleic acid by the use of the polymerase chain reaction. Among the achievements so far are:

1. Complete sequencing of the genomes of representative viruses of all the families of DNA viruses containing animal pathogens, including the 230-kbp genome of a cytomegalovirus and the 192-kbp genome of vaccinia virus.
2. Complete sequencing of the complementary DNA corresponding to the genomes of representative viruses of most of the families of RNA viruses containing animal pathogens.
3. Characterization of the viral or proviral DNAs that are integrated into the DNA of transformed cells and animals infected with retroviruses and papillomaviruses.
4. Development of probes for use in rapid diagnostic assays, including hybridization assays (dot-blot assays).
5. Application of the polymerase chain reaction to amplify specific viral genome sequences for diagnostic and research purposes.
6. Development of marker rescue by transfection with gene fragments as a method for genetic mapping.
7. Production of proteins coded by specific viral genes, using bacterial, yeast, baculovirus, and animal cell expression systems and by cell-free translation systems.
8. Production of peptides based on DNA sequence data for use in diagnostics and immunotherapeutics.

Genetic Variation and Viral Evolution

Because viruses leave no fossils (except perhaps within frozen bodies, within formalin-fixed pathology specimens, or within arthropods and other creatures and their blood meals embedded in amber), it was presumed that there never would be enough evidence to prove whether different viruses had common evolutionary roots. Some scientists regarded it as axiomatic that viruses evolved originally from DNA or RNA already present in a cellular organelle or chromosome or from some form of intracellular parasite such as a bacterium. Others pictured a primeval "RNA world" in which a form of self-replicating RNA akin to modern viroids predated DNA, proteins, and cells. In either case, most virologists agreed that it would be foolish to consider any idea of a single evolutionary "tree" for all the viruses. The generally very different morphological and physicochemical characteristics of the member viruses of many different families supported this view.

Now, as genome sequencing is revealing many conserved functional or nonfunctional "fossil" domains of ancient lineage, for the first time the archaeology of the viruses is being explored from the perspective of data, not just "armchair theory." We now know that many viruses have gained some functional genes from their hosts (and hosts have gained some genes from their viruses) and have gained other genes from other viruses, i.e., viral genomes seem to represent more-or-less ancient "grab bags" of genes, fine-tuned by the Darwinian forces of selection into replicative machines with extraordinary functional economy.

We now know that the genomes of viruses in different families, in most cases, are extremely different from each other, but we also know that in some cases seemingly unrelated viruses are similar—similar in gene order and arrangement, fine points of strategy of replication, and even in conserved sequence domains encoding similarly functioning proteins. Overall, the differences between most kinds of viruses are so great that it still seems foolish to think of building a monophyletic tree uniting all the viruses. However, unexpected similarities have prompted new considerations for a small set of independent trees. One example has been the construction of the order *Mononegavirales,* comprising the families *Paramyxoviridae, Rhabdoviridae, Filoviridae,* and *Bornaviridae.* This order was formed in recognition that the member viruses have similar gene arrangements, similar gene products, and some common sequences in their nucleocapsid genes, all perhaps indicating an ancient common ancestor. The order *Nidovirales,* comprising the families *Coronaviridae* and *Arteriviridae,* was formed for similar reasons, especially in recognition of the common nested-set transcription strategy used by all member viruses and some common sequences, again perhaps indicative of a common ancestor.

There is a further occasion for considering ancient common roots: many of the positive-sense, single-stranded RNA viruses have the same genome organization, gene order, and sequence similarities in domains encoding their RNA-dependent RNA polymerases, their proteases, and their helicases. These viral proteases and helicases display sufficient resemblance to their cellular homologues to indicate that they might originally have been acquired from cellular genes by recombination. Indeed, there is much evidence to suggest that genetic recombination among viruses has been a more important evolutionary mechanism than point mutation. Minor changes continue to occur at a very high frequency as a result of point mutations or less frequently nucleotide insertion or deletion. Such mutations do not appear at the same rate in all genes. Many of these single-stranded RNA viruses also have a similar 5′-terminal covalently linked polypeptide, a 3′-terminal poly(A) tract, a 5′-terminal cap, and employ a subgenomic RNA to assure the production of very large amounts of their capsid proteins. Even though there are many hundreds of these single-stranded RNA viruses, they seem to fall into only three clusters; *picorna-like viruses, toga-like viruses,* and *flavi-like viruses.* So, even though these viruses infect hosts as different as vertebrates, invertebrates, plants, and bacteria, again it would seem that all may have derived from a common ancestor and diverged along only three lines.

Within this subject of viral archeology, one of the most interesting debates centers on which characteristics of a virus are most ancient, which are most recent, which are most stable, and which are most changing. Many virologists had considered that virion structural elements were most ancient; after all, cumulative mutations in icosahedral capsids could only lead to lethal instability. Other virologists had considered that viral genome expression strategies were most ancient; again, even if a virus were able to reinvent its capsid, changes in integrated multigenic replication steps would certainly be lethal. At present, however, the finding of conserved sequence domains in polymerases, helicases, and proteases, but not in structural or other genes of single-stranded RNA viruses, suggests that the answer to this question is not yet at hand. It is unfortunate that viruses have such small genomes, so that there will not be an opportunity to find confirmatory evidences of relationships by analyzing additional genes.

The genetic mechanisms described in this chapter, operating under the pressure of Darwinian forces of variation (mutation) and the fixation of traits under the pressure of selection, have been incriminated clearly in several recent important examples of viral evolution (Table 4.1). Here we shall content ourselves with a description of two viruses that illustrate particularly well the dramatic impact of evolution, even over a relatively short time span. One, myxoma virus, highlights the coevolution of viral virulence and host resistance. The other, influenza A viruses, illustrates how effectively viruses can evolve in horses, birds, swine, and humans to avoid the host's immune response.

Coevolution of Virus and Host in Myxomatosis

Myxoma virus (family *Poxviridae,* genus *Leporipoxvirus*) occurs naturally as a mild infection of rabbits in South America and California (*Sylvilagus* spp.), in which

Table 4.1
Genetic Changes and Recent Evidences of Viral Evolution

Mechanism	Example
Point mutation	Avian influenza virus (H5N2), minimally pathogenic strain changed into lethal epidemic strain by just a few point mutations
Point mutation	Canine parvovirus, host range mutation of feline panleukopenia virus leading to the emergence of a new global pathogen
Intramolecular recombination	Western equine encephalitis virus, originated by recombination between Eastern equine encephalitis virus and a Sindbis-like alphavirus that no longer exists
Genetic reassortment (shift)	Pandemic human influenza A subtypes H1N1 (1918), H2N2 (1957), and H3N2 (1968), each originated by gaining genes from avian viruses, in each case after passage through swine
Intramolecular recombination and mutation	Polio vaccine viruses, reversion of attenuated viruses to virulence following vaccination
Probable mutation in individual host	Feline infectious peritonitis virus, evolution of lethal virus from temperate feline coronavirus
Possible mutation	Lelystad virus (porcine reproductive and respiratory syndrome virus) may have emerged via host range mutation of a rodent arterivirus
Possible mutation	Equine morbillivirus, the cause of acute respiratory distress syndrome in horses and humans in Australia, may have required a host range mutation to jump from its reservoir in bats

it produces a benign fibroma from which virus is transmitted mechanically by biting insects. However, in laboratory (European) rabbits (*Oryctolagus cuniculus*), the virus causes a lethal infection, a finding that led to its use for the biological control of wild European rabbits in Australia.

The wild European rabbit was introduced into Australia in 1859 for sporting purposes and rapidly spread over the southern part of the continent, where it became the major animal pest of agricultural and pastoral industries. Myxoma virus from South America was successfully introduced into the rabbit population in 1950; when originally liberated, the virus produced case-fatality rates of over 99%. This highly virulent virus was transmitted readily by mosquitoes. Farmers undertook "inoculation campaigns" to introduce virulent myxoma virus into wild rabbit populations.

It might have been predicted that the disease—and with it the virus—would disappear at the end of each summer, due to the greatly diminished numbers of susceptible rabbits and the greatly lowered opportunity for transmission by mosquitoes during the winter. This must often have occurred in localized areas, but it did not happen over the continent as a whole. The capacity of the virus to survive the winter conferred a great selective advantage on viral mutants of reduced lethality, since during this period, when mosquito numbers were low, rabbits infected by such mutants survived in an infectious condition for weeks instead of a few days. Within 3 years such attenuated mutants became the dominant strains throughout Australia. Some inoculation campaigns with the virulent virus produced localized highly lethal outbreaks, but in general the viruses that spread through the rabbit populations each year were the attenuated strains, which because of the prolonged illness in their hosts provided a greater opportunity for mosquito transmission. Thus the original highly lethal virus was progressively replaced by a heterogeneous collection of strains of lower virulence, but most of them still virulent enough to kill 70–90% of genetically unselected rabbits.

Rabbits that recover from myxomatosis are immune to reinfection. However, because most wild rabbits have a lifespan of less than 1 year, herd immunity is not so critically important in the epidemiology of myxomatosis as it is in infections of longer lived species. The early appearance of viral strains of lower virulence, which allowed 10% of genetically unselected rabbits to recover, allowed selection for genetically more resistant animals to occur. In areas where repeated outbreaks occurred, the genetic resistance of the rabbits increased steadily such that the case-fatality rate after infection under laboratory conditions with a particular strain of virus fell from 90% to 50% within 7 years. Subsequently, in areas where there were frequent outbreaks of myxomatosis, somewhat more virulent strains of myxoma virus became dominant, because they produced the kind of disease that was best transmitted in populations of genetically resistant rabbits. Thus, the ultimate balance struck between myxoma virus and Australian rabbits involved adaptations of both the virus and host populations, reaching a dynamic equilibrium that finds rabbits greatly reduced compared with their premyxomatosis numbers (600 million to 1 billion), but still too numerous for the wishes of farmers and conservationists. Now, rabbit hemorrhagic disease virus is being used across Australia to complement the effects of myxoma virus.

Genetic Shift and Drift and the Evolution of Influenza A Viruses

Influenza A viruses produce important diseases in birds, horses, swine, mink, marine mammals, and humans. Because of the importance of human influenza, detailed long-term studies of the evolution of the viruses have been carried out, often in the vain hope of predicting future epidemics. Since the first isolation of an influenza virus in 1933, many strains have been obtained from all parts of the world and their antigenic properties studied in detail. In recent years their genetic properties have been studied in parallel, thus revealing the molecular bases for their remarkable evolutionary progression.

Influenza A viruses are classified according to epitopes on their two envelope proteins, the hemagglutinin (H) and neuraminidase (N). All 15 subtypes of the hemagglutinin have been found in birds, 3 of them also in humans, 2 each in pigs, horses, seals, and whales, and 1 in mink. The 9 N subtypes show a similar distribution. An outstanding feature of influenza A viruses is the antigenic variability of these two proteins as a result of two types of changes, *genetic* or *antigenic drift* and *shift*. Antigenic drift occurs within a subtype and involves a gradual accumulation of point mutations; those affecting neutralizing epitopes produce strains each antigenically slightly different from its predecessor. In contrast, antigenic shift involves the sudden acquisition of the gene for a completely new hemagglutinin or neuraminidase, giving rise to a novel subtype that may spread rapidly around the world, unencumbered by any herd immunity.

Genetic/Antigenic Shift

During the past century there have been five pandemics of human influenza: in 1890, 1900, 1918, 1957, and 1968. The pandemic at the end of the first World War killed over 20 million people—more than the war itself. In 1957 the H1N1 subtype was suddenly replaced by a new subtype, A/H2N2, known as "Asian flu" because it originated in China. Within a year over a billion people had been infected, but fortunately the mortality was much lower than in 1918, probably because the strain was intrinsically less virulent, although the availability of antibiotics to treat secondary bacterial infection undoubtedly saved many lives. In 1968 this subtype was in turn replaced by another subtype, A/H3N2, known as the "Hong Kong flu." In 1977 the A/H1N1 subtype mysteriously reappeared, and since then the two subtypes, A/H3N2 and A/H1N1, have cocirculated.

Clear evidence that distinct mechanisms are involved in the processes of antigenic shift and drift have come from sequencing of hemagglutinin genes of representative isolates; sequencing has shown relatively close relationships between strains within each of the three human subtypes, H1, H2, and H3, but major differences between subtypes, indicating that a sharp discontinuity in the evolutionary pattern had occurred with the emergence of H2 viruses in 1957 and H3 viruses in 1968. As data from sequencing all eight gene segments of many strains of influenza viruses isolated from several species of animals and birds became available, it became clear that all of the influenza viruses of mammals, including humans, originated from the avian influenza gene pool, which itself presumably evolved from a common ancestral avian influenza virus. In 1957, five of the eight gene segments of the prevalent human H1N1 subtype were replaced by Eurasian avian influenza genes to produce the human H2N2 subtype; then, in 1968 the human H2N2 subtype acquired two gene segments, including the hemagglutinin gene from another avian influenza virus to produce the human H3N2 subtype. Moreover, retrospective serological studies have indicated that the 1890 human pandemic subtype was H2N8, the 1900 subtype H3N8, and the 1918 subtype H1N1, suggesting a pattern of recycling of the three human H subtypes (H1, H2, H3) and suggesting the origin of the virus that caused the 1918 pandemic in swine.

Influenza A viruses from birds grow very poorly in humans, and vice versa; indeed, reassortants containing avian genes have been tested as experimental vaccines because of their avirulence and their inability to spread from human to human. However, both avian and human influenza viruses can replicate in swine, and genetic reassortment between them can be demonstrated experimentally in that host. It has now been shown quite certainly that an antigenic shift in nature occurs when the prevailing human strain of influenza A virus and an avian influenza virus concurrently infect a pig, which serves as a "mixing vessel." Every 10–20 years a reassortant virus from the pig, containing genes encoding replicative functions from a human virus and a hemagglutinin gene derived from an avian virus, emerges. It might be argued that the chances of this happening again must be vanishingly small, but it must be appreciated that in rural southeast Asia, the most densely populated area of the world, hundreds of millions of people live and work in close contact with domesticated pigs and ducks. It is no coincidence that the last two antigenic shifts that have produced major pandemics in humans emanated from China.

However, not all new influenza viruses in mammals arise by reassortment between a preexisting mammalian strain and an avian virus. For example, the H1N1 swine influenza virus strain that appeared in Europe in 1979 was derived directly from birds, and the equine H3N8 influenza virus that appeared in northern China in 1989 was very different from the H3N8 equine influenza virus currently found elsewhere in the world, but very similar to an avian H3N8 influenza A virus. An important additional example of *host species jumping* without genetic reassortment occurred in 1997 in Hong Kong (see later).

Genetic/Antigenic Drift

After a new pandemic influenza virus strain has emerged as a consequence of genetic reassortment, antigenic drift begins when point mutations accumulate in all of its RNA segments (Figure 4.8). Mutations in the gene encoding the hemagglutinin sometimes alter its antigenic sites. When antiserum against the formerly prevalent strain no longer neutralizes the variant, a new strain has emerged. Changes in the hemagglutinin are clustered in five regions of the molecule, which correspond to important antigenic sites. Substitution of a single amino acid in a critical antigenic site may abolish the capacity of the antibody to bind to that site. However, some regions of the hemagglutinin protein are conserved in all human and avian strains, presumably because they are essential for the maintenance of the structure and function of the molecule. The important feature of antigenic drift in human influenza viruses is that in immune populations the new strains have a selective advantage over their predecessors and tend to displace them. Although minor variants may cocirculate, a novel strain usually supplants previous strains of that subtype in a particular region.

Figure 4.8.

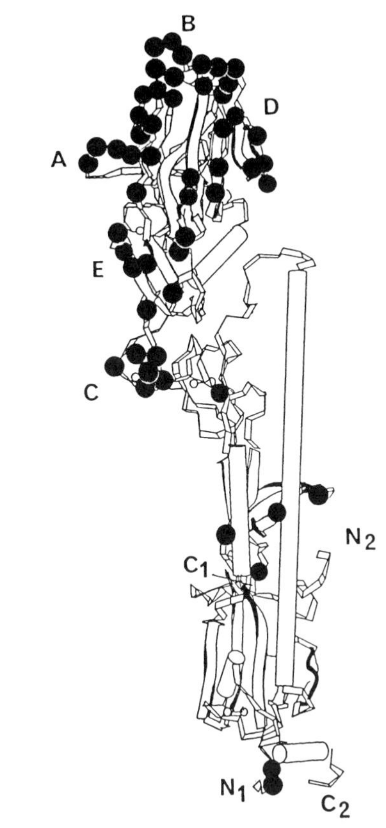

Diagram of the same influenza virus hemagglutinin monomer that is shown in more detail in Figure 1.8, but showing as black dots the location of all the amino acid positions that changed in the A/Hong Kong/1968 (H3N2) subtype during natural drift between 1968 and 1986. Most of the changes are concentrated near the receptor-binding pocket at the center of the tip of the molecule. These sites include the two immunodominant antigenic sites, A and B, with fewer changes at sites C, D, and E. When the antibody, evoked by prior infection or vaccine, binds to epitopes in sites A and B, it can sterically hinder attachment of the virus to its cellular receptor. When the virus drifts, antibody specific for earlier virus strains no longer binds to these epitopes and the virus is free to cause infection, transmission chains, and epidemics. (From J. J., Skehel, D. C., Wiley, E., Domingo, J. J., Holland, and P. Ahlquist, eds., "RNA Genetics." Vol. 3, p. 142. CRC Press, Boca Raton, FL 1988.)

Avian Influenza

In April 1983, a H5N2 influenza virus appeared in chickens in Pennsylvania, producing a mortality of less than 10%. Comparison of the genome segments of this isolate with other influenza A isolates by RNA hybridization indicated that all of its genes were closely related to the genes of H5N2 isolates from wild birds in the eastern United States at the time. Then, suddenly, in October 1983, mortality rose to over 80%. Comparison of individual RNA segments of the April and October isolates showed that reassortment (shift) had not occurred, suggesting that the change in virulence had been due to point mutations, i.e., to genetic drift. Previous studies had shown that virulence for birds is polygenic but that the hemagglutinin gene is of major importance. Sequencing of the hemagglutinin genes from the April and October isolates revealed seven nucleotide differences, resulting in four predicted amino acid changes in the hemagglutinin protein. One of these changes indeed removed a glycosylation site, thereby facilitating the cleavage and activation of the hemagglutinin. The importance of this critical single nucleotide change may be measured in practical terms: measures to control the epidemic and protect the poultry industry of the United States involved the slaughter of more than 17 million chickens at a cost of about $60 million.

In August 1997, an H5N1 avian influenza virus not previously known to infect humans and without the intermediary cycle through swine infected humans in Hong Kong, four of whom died. The end of British rule in Hong Kong had resulted in the shipment of many chickens from mainland China to Hong Kong. The H5N1 virus, which had been causing an epidemic in chickens in China, was transported into a setting where viral genetic analysis was being done as part of a global surveillance system to identify new human strains. A decision was made to destroy all chickens in Hong Kong—some 1.2 million birds—at a cost of $4 million (see Chapter 30). As this happened, further genetic analysis of the virus showed (1) that the human pathogen had retained all of its avian virus genes; (2) that the virus retained its extreme virulence for chickens while at the same time gaining the capacity to infect humans (this was the first time this had been proven); and (3) that there was some human-to-human transmission, raising concern that the virus might be introduced into other human and poultry populations by the travel of infected humans (see Chapter 30).

Further Reading

Bangham, C. R., and Kirkwood, T. B. (1993). Defective interfering particles and virus evolution. *Trends Microbiol.* **1**, 260–264.

Barrett, A. D., and Dimmock, N. J. (1986). Defective interfering viruses and infections of animals. *Curr. Top. Microbiol. Immunol.* **128**, 55–84.

Burden, D., and Whitney, D. B. (1995). "Proteins to PCR: A Course in Strategies and Lab Techniques." Birkhaeuser, Boston, MA.

Coen, D. M., and Ramig, R. F. (1996). Viral genetics. *In* "Fields Virology," (B. N. Fields, D. M. Knipe, P. M. Howley, R. M., Chanock, J. L. Melnick, T. P. Monath, B. Roizman, and S. E. Straus, eds.), 3rd ed., pp. 113–153. Lippincott-Raven, Philadelphia, PA.

Duarte, E. A., Novella, I. S., Weaver, S. C., Domingo, E., Wain-Hobson, S., Clarke, D. K., Moya, A., Elena, S. F., de la Torre, J. C., and Holland, J. J. (1994). RNA virus quasispecies: Significance for viral disease and epidemiology. *Infect. Agents Dis.* **3**, 201–214.

Eigen, M. (1993). Viral quasispecies. *Sci. Amer.* **269**, 42–49.

Fenner, F., and Ross, J. (1993). Myxomatosis. *In* "The European Rabbit. The History and Biology of a Successful Colonizer," (H. V. Thompson, and C. M. King, eds.) pp. 205–245. Oxford University Press, Oxford.

García-Sastre, A., and Palese, P. (1993). Genetic manipulation of negative-strand RNA virus genomes. *Annu. Rev. Microbiol.* **47**, 765–790.

Gibbs, A. J., Calisher, C. H., and García-Arenal, F., eds. (1995). "Molecular Basis of Virus Evolution." Cambridge University Press, Cambridge, UK.

Holland, J. J., de la Torre, J. C., and Steinhauer, D. A. (1992). RNA populations as quasispecies. *Curr. Top. Microbiol. Immunol.* **176**, 1–20.

Jarvis, T. C., and Kirkegaard, K. (1991). The polymerase in its labyrinth: Mechanisms and implications of RNA recombination. *Trends Genet.* **7**, 186–202.

Klenk, H.-D., and Rott, R. (1989). The molecular biology of influenza virus pathogenicity. *Adv. Virus Res.* **34**, 247–282.

Koonin, E. V. ed. (1992). Evolution of viral genomes. *Semin. Virol.* **3**, 311–450.

Lodish, H., Baltimore, D., and Berk, A. (1995). "Molecular Cell Biology," 3rd ed. with CD ROM. Scientific American Books. Freeman, New York.

Nathanson, N., and Murphy, F. A. (1997). Evolution of viral diseases. *In* "Viral Pathogenesis" (N. Nathanson, R. Ahmed, F. Gonzalez-Scarano, D. E. Griffin, K. V. Holmes, F. A. Murphy, and H. L. Robinson, eds.), pp. 353–370. Lippincott-Raven, Philadelphia, PA.

Rice, C. M., ed. (1992). Animal virus expression vectors. *Semin. Virol.* **3**, 235–370.

Roux, L., Simon, A. E., and Holland, J. J. (1991). Effects of defective interfering viruses on virus replication and pathogenesis *in vitro* and *in vivo*. *Adv. Virus Res.* **40**, 181–212.

Sambrook, J., Fritsch, E. F., and Maniatis, T., eds. (1989). "Molecular Cloning: A Laboratory Manual," 2nd ed. Cold Spring Harbor Laboratory Press, Cold Spring Harbor, NY.

Strauss, E. G., Strauss, J. H., and Levine, A. J. (1996). Virus evolution. *In* "Fields Virology" (B. N. Fields, D. M. Knipe, P. M. Howley, R. M., Chanock, J. L. Melnick, T. P. Monath, B. Roizman, and S. E. Straus, eds.), 3rd ed., pp. 153–172. Lippincott-Raven, Philadelphia, PA.

Tartaglia, J., Gettig, R., and Paoletti, E. (1996). Vectors, animal viruses. *In* "Encyclopedia of Virology" (R. G. Webster and A. Granoff, eds.), 2nd ed. (CD-ROM). Academic Press, London.

Webster, R. G., and Kawaoka, Y. (1994). Influenza—an emerging and re-emerging disease. *Semin. Virol.* **5**, 103–111.

White, B. A., and Totowa, N. J. eds. (1997). "PCR Cloning Protocols: From Molecular Cloning to Genetic Engineering, Methods Mol. Biol., Vol. 67. Humana Press, Clifton, NJ.

CHAPTER 5

Virus–Cell Interactions

Just as understanding of the nature of a viral infection in the individual host animal is key to understanding infection in the whole host population, so understanding of the nature of infection in the individual cell is key to understanding infection in complex tissues, organs, and the whole host animal. The range of changes induced in the more than 200 different kinds of cells in the typical animal host by different viruses is remarkably diverse. Viruses often encode genes that induce, mimic, or shut down host cell functions for their own benefit and, of course, the host has elaborate systems to shut down viral functions. The outcome of infection may vary from essentially benign and undetectable, to tolerated, to lethal. The viral and cellular factors that influence the outcome of infection are often in delicate balance, easily shifted one way or the other, e.g., by the physiologic, immune, or inflammatory responses of the host or by the expression of virulence factors by the virus. The disruption of cellular functions, the induction of cell death or transformation, or the activation of an inappropriate immune response are manifested as *disease*. Although virus-induced changes at the cellular, subcellular, and molecular levels are most commonly studied in cultured cells, in recent years the use of explant and organ cultures and transplantation of infected cells and tissues back into experimental animals have brought research findings in cellular pathology closer to the whole animal and clinical practice.

Types of Virus–Cell Interactions

Viral infections may be categorized as *cytocidal* (*cytolytic, cytopathic*) or *noncytocidal*. Further, not all viral infections are *productive*, i.e., not all infections lead to the production and release of new virions. Host cell changes of a profound nature, leading to cell death in some instances and cell transformation in others, may also occur in *nonproductive (abortive)* infections. Certain kinds of cells are *permissive*, i.e., they support complete replication of a particular virus, whereas others are *nonpermissive* i.e., viral replication may be blocked at any point from viral attachment through to the final stages of virion assembly and release. Cytopathic changes can occur in both permissive and nonpermissive cells. Often a virus that replicates perfectly well in a particular cell type finds a similar cell type nonpermissive or nonproductive; in such cases it may be impossible to trace the defect to the cell or the virus—it often is the combination that is unproductive. For example, if there is a defect in the viral genome, replication may be nonproductive even within an otherwise fully permissive cell. Two particular examples of such viral defects are the deletion mutants known as defective interfering (DI) mutants and the point mutants known as conditional lethal mutants (see Chapter 4).

Some of the most important of all nonproductive virus cell interactions are those associated with *persistent infections* or *latent infections.* The term persistent infection simply describes an infection that lasts a long time. The term latent infection describes an infection that "exists but is not exhibited," i.e., an infection in which infectious virions are not formed. In either case, the virus or its genome is maintained indefinitely in the cell, either by the integration of the viral nucleic acid into the host cell DNA or by carriage of the viral nucleic acid in the form of an *episome.* In these instances, the cell survives, indeed may divide repeatedly. In some instances such cells never release virions, in others the infection may become productive when induced by an appropriate stimulus (see Chapter 10). Persistent or latent infections may also be associated with cell *transformation;* the transformation of cells by oncogenic viruses is described in Chapter 11. The various types of interaction that can occur between virus and cell are summarized in Table 5.1.

Cytocidal Changes in Virus-Infected Cells

Cytopathic viruses kill the cells in which they replicate. When a monolayer of cultured cells is inoculated with a cytopathic virus, the first round of infection yields progeny virus that spreads through the medium to infect adjacent as well as distant cells—eventually all cells in the culture may become infected. The resulting cell damage is known as a *cytopathic effect* (CPE). Cytopathic effect, can usually be observed by low-power light microscopy of unstained cell cultures (Figures 5.1 and 5.2A–5.2C). The nature of the cytopathic effect is often characteristic of the particular virus involved and is therefore an important preliminary clue in the identification of clinical isolates (see Chapter 12). Fixation and staining of infected cell monolayers may reveal further diagnostic details.

Mechanisms of Cell Damage

So many pathophysiologic changes occur in cells infected with cytopathic viruses that the death of the cell usually cannot be attributed to any particular event; rather, cell death may be the final result of the cumulative action of many insults. Nevertheless, in recent years several specific mechanisms have been discovered, some of which are becoming targets of therapeutic drugs. Particular viruses can cause host cell damage by many different means.

Table 5.1
Types of Virus–Cell Interaction

Type of infection	Effects on cell	Production of infectious virions	Examples
Cytocidal	Morphologic changes in cells (cytopathic effects); inhibition of protein, RNA and DNA synthesis; cell death	Yes	Alphaherpesviruses, enteroviruses, reoviruses
Persistent, productive	No cytopathic effect; little metabolic disturbance; cells continue to divide; may be loss of the special functions of some differentiated cells	Yes	Pestiviruses, arenaviruses, rabies virus, most retroviruses
Persistent, nonproductive	Usually nil	No, but virus may be induced[a]	Canine distemper virus in brain
Transformation	Alteration in cell morphology; cells can be passaged indefinitely; may produce tumors when transplanted to experimental animals	No, oncogenic DNA viruses	Polyomavirus, adenoviruses
		Yes, oncogenic retroviruses	Murine, avian leukosis, and sarcoma viruses

[a]By cocultivation, irradiation, or chemical mutagens.

FIGURE 5.1.

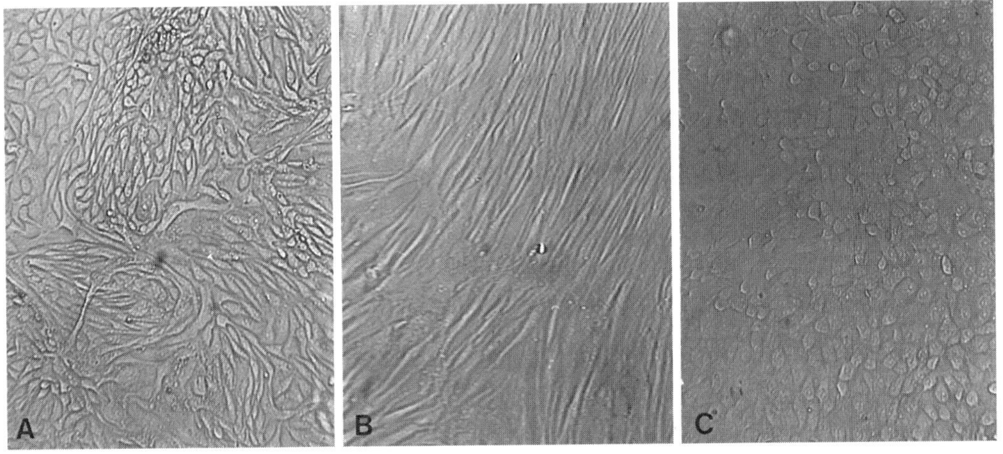

Unstained confluent monolayers of the three main types of cultured cells as they appear by low-power light microscopy through the wall of the glass or plastic flask in which they form a monolayer. (A) Primary monkey kidney epithelial cells obtained directly by the dissociation of cells from a kidney; this produces a mixed population of mainly epithelial cells. (B) Diploid cell line of fetal fibroblasts. (C) Continuous line of malignant epithelial cells. Magnification: ×60. (Courtesy of I. Jack.)

Inhibition of Host Cell Nucleic Acid Synthesis

Inhibition of host cell DNA synthesis is common in viral infections. It is an inevitable consequence of viral inhibition of host cell protein synthesis and its effect on the machinery of DNA replication, but some viruses employ more specific mechanisms. For example, poxviruses produce a DNase that degrades cellular DNA, and herpesviruses specifically displace the synthesis of host cell DNA with their own synthetic processes.

Inhibition of Host Cell RNA Transcription

Many different classes of viruses, including poxviruses, rhabdoviruses, reoviruses, paramyxoviruses, and picornaviruses, inhibit host cell RNA transcription. In some instances, this inhibition may be the indirect consequence of viral effects on host cell protein synthesis, which decreases the availability of transcription factors required for RNA polymerase activity. In other instances, viruses encode specific transcription factors for the purpose of regulating the expression of their own genes and, in some instances, these factors modulate the expression of cellular genes as well. For example, herpesviruses encode proteins that bind directly to specific viral DNA sequences, thereby regulating the transcription of viral genes.

Inhibition of Processing of Host Cell mRNAs

Many viruses, including vesicular stomatitis viruses, influenza viruses, and herpesviruses, interfere with the splicing of cellular primary mRNA transcripts that are needed to form mature mRNAs. In some instances, spliceosomes are formed, but subsequent catalytic steps are inhibited. For example, a protein synthesized in herpesvirus-infected cells suppresses RNA splicing and leads to reduced amounts of cellular mRNAs and the accumulation of primary mRNA transcripts.

Inhibition of Host Cell Protein Synthesis

The shutdown of host cell protein synthesis, while viral protein synthesis continues, is a characteristic of many virus infections. This shutdown is particularly rapid and profound in picornavirus infections, but it is also pronounced in togavirus, influenzavirus, rhabdovirus, poxvirus, and herpesvirus infections. With some other viruses, the shutdown occurs late in the course of infection and is more gradual, whereas with noncytocidal viruses, such as pestiviruses, arenaviruses, and retroviruses, there is no shutdown and no cell death. The mechanisms underlying the shutdown of host cell protein synthesis are varied: some are as mentioned earlier, whereas others include (1) the production of viral enzymes that degrade cellular mRNAs, (2) the production of factors that bind to ribosomes and inhibit cellular mRNA translation, and (3) the alteration of the intracellular ionic environment favoring the translation of viral mRNAs over cellular mRNAs. Most importantly, some viral mRNAs simply outcompete cellular mRNAs for cellular translation machinery by mass action; i.e., the large excess of viral mRNA outcompetes cellular mRNA for host ribosomes. Viral proteins may also inhibit the processing and transport of cellular proteins from the

FIGURE 5.2.

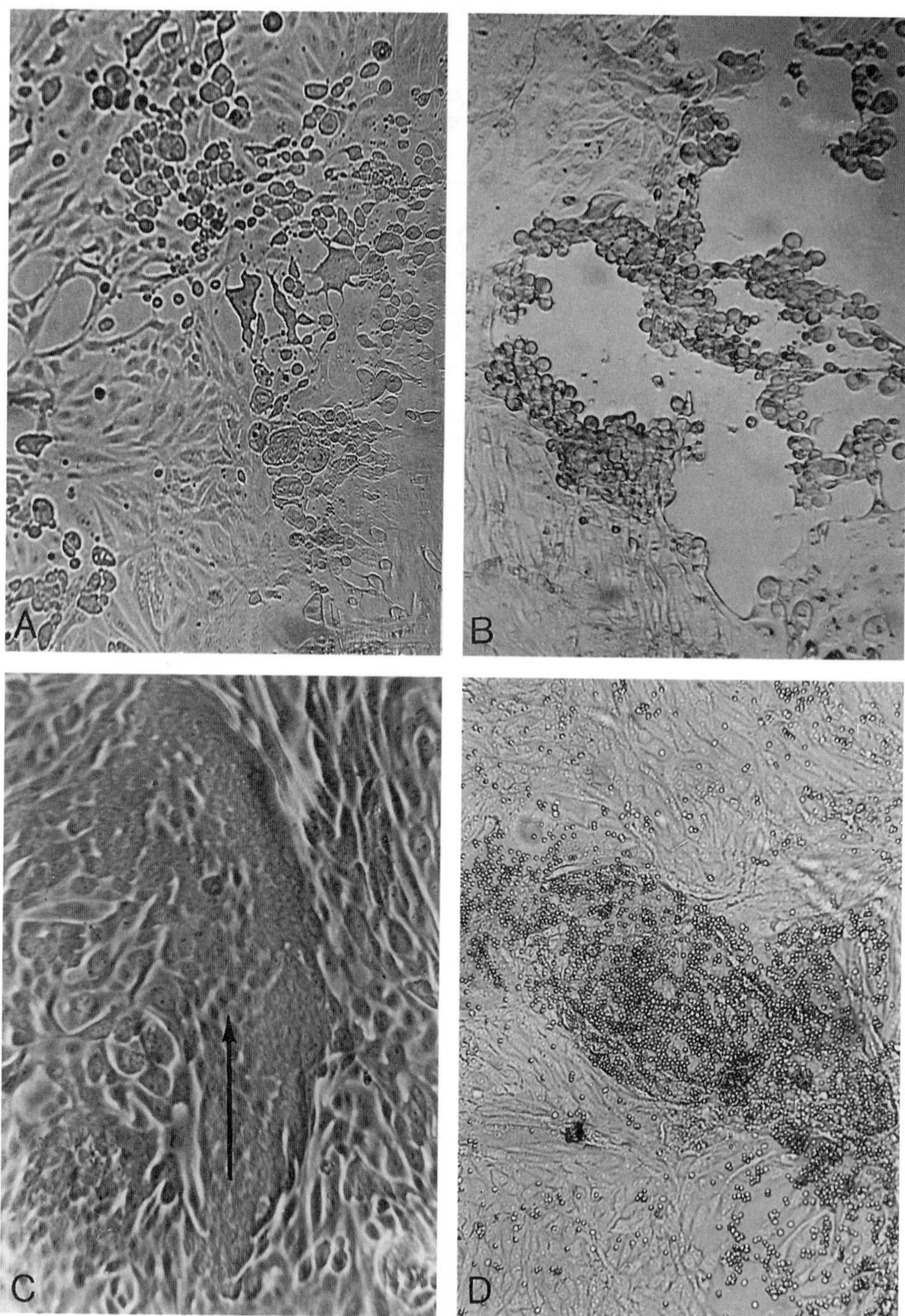

Cytopathic effects produced by different viruses. The cell monolayers are shown as they would normally be viewed in the laboratory, unfixed and unstained. (A) Typical cytopathology of an enterovirus: rapid rounding of cells, progressing to complete cell lysis. (B) Typical cytopathology of a herpesvirus: focal areas of swollen rounded cells. (C) Typical cytopathology of a paramyxovirus: focal clusters of cells are fused to form syncytia. (D) Hemadsorption: erythrocytes adsorb to infected cells that have incorporated hemagglutinin into the plasma membrane. Magnification: ×60. (Courtesy of I. Jack.)

endoplasmic reticulum, and this inhibition may lead to their degradation. This effect is seen in lentivirus and adenovirus infections.

Cytopathic Effects of Toxic Viral Proteins

Large amounts of various viral components may accumulate in the cell late in infection. In the past, it was thought that the cytopathic effect was simply a consequence of the intrinsic toxicity of these proteins, but in recent years most cell damage has been recognized as the supervening of viral replication events on cellular events. Hence, the list of "toxic proteins" has been shortened, but some remain. For example, the toxicity of adenovirus penton and fiber proteins seems direct and independent of adenovirus replication.

Cytopathic Changes Involving Cell Membranes

Cellular membranes participate in many phases of viral replication, from viral attachment and entry, to the formation of replication complexes, to virion assembly. Viruses may alter plasma membrane permeability, affect ion exchange and membrane potential, induce the synthesis of new intracellular membranes, and induce the rearrangement of previously existing membranes. A generalized increase in membrane permeability, detected by entry into cells of normally excluded macromolecules or escape of intracellular molecules, occurs early during picornavirus, alphavirus, reovirus, rhabdovirus, and adenovirus infections. Most importantly, enveloped viruses also direct the insertion of their surface glycoproteins, including fusion proteins, into host cell membranes as part of their budding process, often leading to membrane fusion and syncytium formation.

Cell Membrane Fusion and Syncytium Formation

A conspicuous feature of infection of cell monolayers by lentiviruses, paramyxoviruses, morbilliviruses, pneumoviruses, some herpesviruses, and some other viruses is the production of *syncytia* (Figures 5.2C and 5.3C), which result from the fusion of an infected cell with neighboring infected or uninfected cells. Such multinucleate syncytia may also be seen in the tissues of animals infected with these viruses; for example, in horses fatally infected with the Australian equine morbillivirus, a prominent feature of the interstitial pneumonia has been alveolar epithelial syncytia (also called multinucleate giant cells). Such syncytia may represent an important mechanism of viral spread in tissues: fusion bridges may allow subviral entities, such as viral nucleocapsids and nucleic acids, to spread while escaping the effects of host defenses. Cell membrane fusion is mediated by viral fusion proteins or fusion domains

FIGURE 5.3.

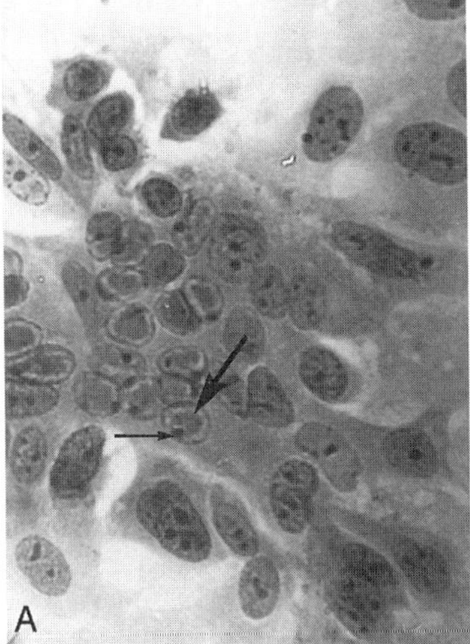

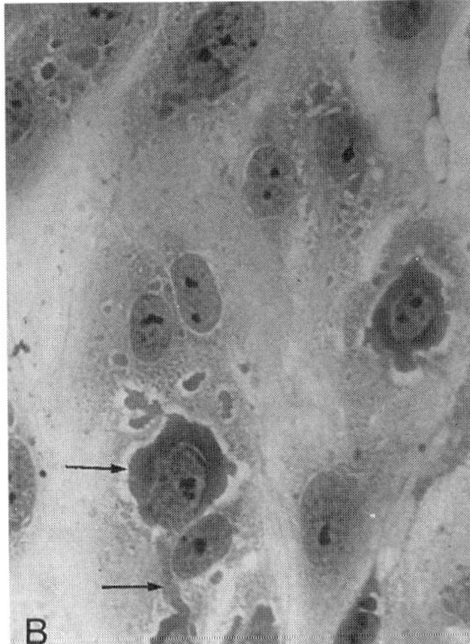

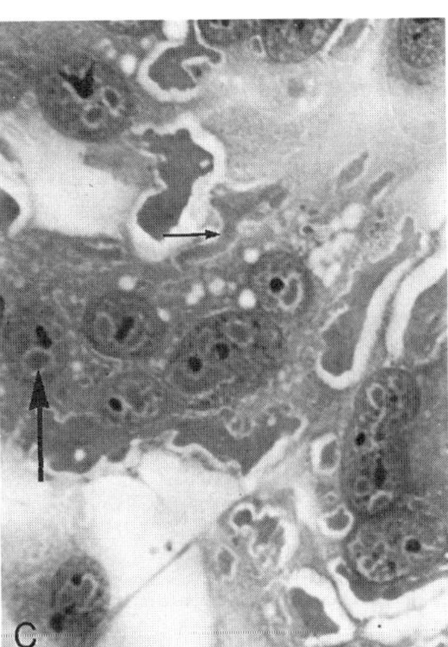

Types of viral inclusion bodies (hematoxylin and eosin stain). (A) Intranuclear inclusions and syncytium formation (herpesvirus). Small arrow, nucleolus; large arrow, inclusion body. The characteristic appearance of this kind of inclusion body is caused by chromatin condensation and a fixation artifact that results in the formation of a clear zone between centrally condensed chromatin and marginated chromatin. (B) Intracytoplasmic inclusions (reovirus). Arrows indicate inclusion bodies, mainly in perinuclear locations. (C) Intranuclear and intracytoplasmic inclusions and syncytium formation (typical of all morbilliviruses). Small arrow, intracytoplasmic inclusion body; large arrow, intranuclear inclusion body. Magnification: ×200. (Courtesy of I. Jack.)

on other viral surface proteins. For example, the fusion activity of influenza viruses is carried on hemagglutinin peplomers (spikes), whereas the fusion activity of many paramyxoviruses, such as parainfluenza virus 3, is carried on separate peplomers composed of fusion (F) protein.

At high multiplicity of infection, paramyxoviruses may cause a rapid fusion of cultured cells without any requirement for viral replication—this occurs simply as a result of the action of fusion protein activity of input virions as they interact with plasma membranes. This phenomenon has been used to produce functional *heterokaryons* by fusing different types of cells. In the pioneering experiments by Milstein and Köhler that produced the first monoclonal antibodies, parainfluenza virus inactivated by irradiation with ultraviolet light was used to produce *hybridoma* cells by the fusion of antibody-producing B lymphocytes with myeloma cells.

Hemadsorption and Hemagglutination

Cells in monolayer cultures infected with orthomyxoviruses, paramyxoviruses, and togaviruses, all of which bud from the plasma membrane, acquire the ability to adsorb erythrocytes. This phenomenon, known as *hemadsorption* (Figure 5.2D), is due to the incorporation of viral glycoprotein peplomers into the plasma membrane of infected cells where they serve as receptors for ligands on the surface of erythrocytes. The same glycoprotein peplomers are responsible for *hemagglutination, in vitro,* i.e., the agglutination of erythrocytes. In this instance, virions added to an erythrocyte suspension form cell–virus–cell bridges involving large numbers of erythrocytes. Although hemadsorption and hemagglutination are not known to play a role in the pathogenesis of viral diseases, both phenomena are used extensively in laboratory diagnostics (see Chapter 12).

Cytolysis by Immunologic Mechanisms

Viral proteins (antigens) inserted into the host cell plasma membrane may constitute targets for specific humoral and cellular immune responses that may cause the lysis of the cell. This may happen before significant progeny virus is produced, thus slowing or arresting the progress of infection and hastening recovery (see Chapter 8). Alternatively, in some instances the immune response may precipitate immunopathologic disease (see Chapter 9) and, in cells that are transformed by viruses, viral antigens incorporated in the cell membrane may behave as *tumor-specific transplantation antigens* (see Chapter 11).

Cytopathic Changes Involving the Cytoskeleton

Changes in cell shape are one of the common characteristics of virus infection in cultured cells. Such changes are caused by damage to the cytoskeleton, which is made up of several filament systems, such as microfilaments (e.g., actin), intermediate filaments (e.g., vimentin), and microtubules (e.g., tubulin). The cytoskeleton is responsible for the structural integrity of the cell, for the transport of organelles through the cell, and for certain cell motility activities. Particular viruses are known to damage specific filament systems: for example, canine distemper virus, vesicular stomatitis viruses, vaccinia virus, and herpesviruses cause a depolymerization of actin-containing microfilaments and enteroviruses induce extensive damage to microtubules. Such damage contributes to the drastic cytopathic changes that precede cell lysis in many infections. The elements of the cytoskeleton are also employed by many viruses in the course of their replication: in viral entry, in the formation of replication complexes and assembly sites, and in virion release.

Noncytocidal Changes in Virus-Infected Cells

Noncytocidal viruses usually do not kill the cells in which they replicate. On the contrary, they often cause persistent infection, in which infected cells produce and release virions but overall cellular metabolism is little affected. In many instances, infected cells even continue to grow and divide. This type of virus–cell interaction is found in cells infected with several kinds of RNA viruses: pestiviruses, arenaviruses, retroviruses, and some paramyxoviruses, in particular. Nevertheless, with few exceptions (e.g., some retroviruses), there are slowly progressive changes that ultimately lead to cell death. In the host animal, cell replacement occurs so rapidly in most organs and tissues that the slow fallout of cells due to persistent infection may have no effect on overall function; however, neurons, once destroyed, are not replaced and persistently infected differentiated cells may lose their capacity to carry out specialized functions.

Effects of Noncytocidal Viral Infection on Functions of Specialized Cells

Some viruses, such as pestiviruses, arenaviruses, and retroviruses, that do not shut down host cell protein, RNA, or DNA synthesis and do not kill their host cells produce important pathophysiologic changes in their hosts by affecting crucial functions that are neither associated with the integrity of cells nor their basic housekeeping functions. Damage to the specialized functions of differentiated cells may affect the regulatory and homeostatic functions of endocrine organs, the digestive and metabolic functions of exocrine organs, the locomotor and circulatory functions of muscles, the "fight-or-flight" behavioral functions of neuroendocrine systems, and the protective functions of the immune system. The effects of viral infections on these organs and tissues, affecting hormonal levels, enzyme activities, chemical and electrical neurotransmitter functions, and other higher functions, are just beginning to be appreciated, yet there is already a sense that this will be a major extension from research into clinical practice in the future.

To date, much of the basis for considering the importance of this subject stems from experimental models in laboratory rodents. For example, lymphocytic choriomeningitis virus replicating in somatotropic cells of the pituitary gland of the persistently infected mouse lowers the production of the mRNA for growth hormone in infected cells, thus impeding the growth and development of the animal. Similarly, lymphocytic choriomeningitis virus replicating in β cells of the islets of Langerhans in the pancreas of the mouse can induce hyperglycemia that is not dissimilar to insulin-dependent diabetes in dogs or humans. Neuropsychiatric effects may follow persistent viral infection of particular neuronal tracts: for example, Borna disease virus induces bizarre changes in the behavior of rats, cats, and horses and is now being studied as the possible cause of depression and other bipolar neuropsychiatric illnesses in humans.

When the pathophysiologic effects of persistent viral infection are manifested through influences on the immune system, we do not usually think about the infection of individual cells, but rather about infection in the whole organ system, the whole host animal. Viruses that infect lymphocytes may induce a generalized immunosuppression or more subtle dysfunctions in particular immune responses. The complexity of the infection caused by feline immunodeficiency virus is a case in point. Similarly, when persistent infection involves muscle cells, we usually focus on system dysfunctions, such as changes in cardiac capacity or rhythm or gastrointestinal motility. When infection involves respiratory epithelial cells, we focus not on these cells but on cilial stasis, airway congestion, and the likelihood of bacterial superinfection and secondary pneumonia (Figure 5.4). Nevertheless, in each case it is damage to specialized functions of differentiated cells that underlies the complex pathophysiologic effect and the disease.

Inclusion Bodies

A characteristic morphological change in cells infected by certain viruses is the formation of *inclusion bodies* (or *inclusions*), which may be recognized by light microscopy following fixation and staining (Figures 5.3A, 5.3B, 5.3C). Depending on the virus, inclusion bodies may be intranuclear or intracytoplasmic, single or multiple, large or small, round or irregular in shape, and acidophilic (pink, stained by eosin) or basophilic (blue, stained by hematoxylin).

The most striking viral inclusion bodies are the intracytoplasmic inclusions found in cells infected with poxviruses, reoviruses, paramyxoviruses, and rabies virus and the intranuclear inclusion bodies found in cells infected with herpesviruses, adenoviruses, and parvoviruses. Some viruses, e.g., canine distemper virus and porcine cytomegalovirus, may produce both nuclear and cytoplasmic inclusion bodies in the same cell.

Inclusion bodies are diverse in nature: some inclusions are accumulations of viral components. For example, the intracytoplasmic inclusions in cells infected with rabies virus, known as Negri bodies, are actually masses of viral nucleocapsids, and the intracytoplasmic inclusions found in cells infected with poxviruses are actually sites of viral synthesis (*viroplasm,* also called viral factories). Other inclusions are composed of crystalline aggregates of virions; for example, adenovirus inclusions in the nucleus and reovirus inclusions in the cytoplasm of infected cells represent large accumulations of virions. Still other inclusion bodies are the result of degenerative cellular changes. In fixed, stained cells, herpesvirus intranuclear inclusions are often striking in appearance—they often appear as "owl's eyes." This is because of viral-induced chromatin condensation and a fixation artifact that results in the formation of a clear zone between centrally condensed nucleoplasm and marginated chromatin (Figure 5.3A).

Polarity of Viral Budding

In the course of their replication, viruses belonging to several families of enveloped viruses insert their glycoproteins into the plasma membrane of their host cells; as discussed in Chapter 3, this insertion is not a random matter. Viruses that mature at the apical surface of epithelial cells may be shed into the environment, whereas those maturing at the basolateral surface are free to proceed to other sites in the body, sometimes entering the bloodstream and establishing systemic infection (Figure 5.5). For example, in reservoir host species, rabies virus

FIGURE 5.4.

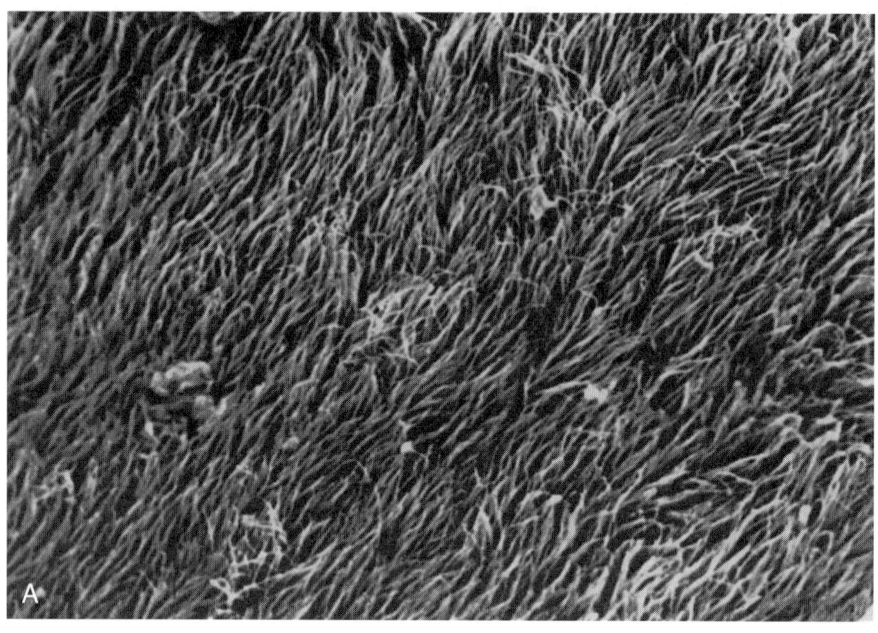

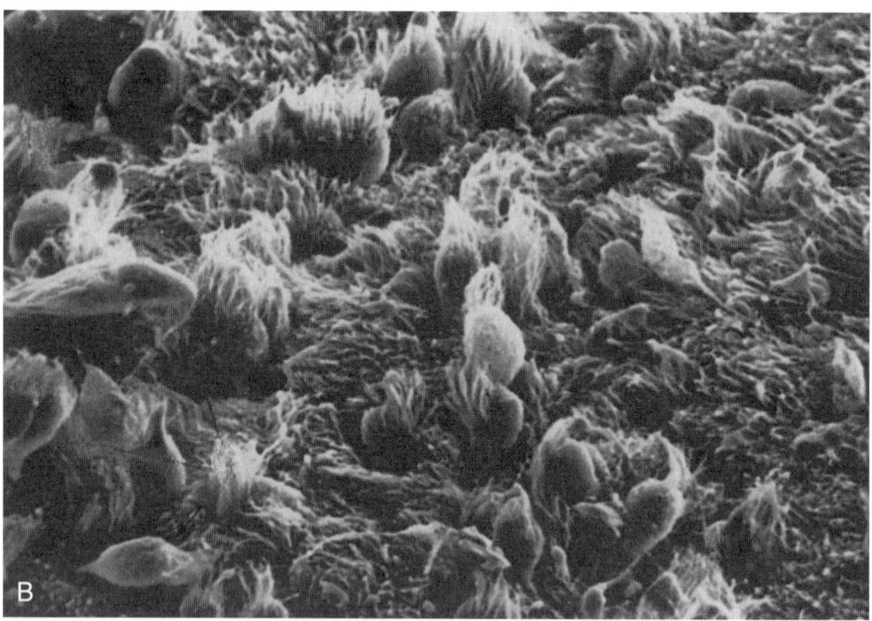

Effect of a rhinovirus on bovine tracheal epithelium grown *in vitro* as an explant culture (also called organ culture), as shown by scanning electron microscopy. (A) Normal appearance of ciliated cells. (B) Six days after infection; many cells are rounded up or detached. (Courtesy of S. E. Reed and A. Boyde.)

is shed from the apical surface of salivary gland epithelial cells where it enters the saliva and is transmitted by bite. However, lentiviruses bud from basolateral plasma membranes and pass directly from cell to cell or become disseminated through tissue spaces and the bloodstream. Wild-type parainfluenza virus 1 (Sendai virus), which causes respiratory disease in several animal species, buds apically into airways and is transmitted by aerosol, whereas a variant that causes generalized disease buds basolaterally.

FIGURE 5.5.

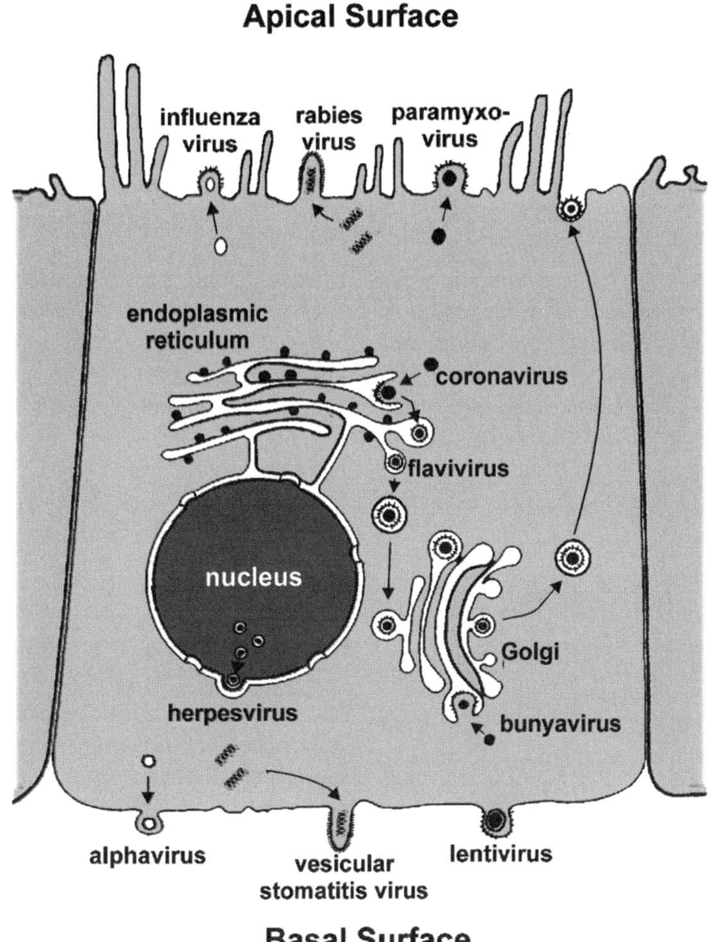

Sites of budding of various enveloped viruses. Viruses that bud from apical surfaces of epithelial cells at body surfaces are in position to be shed in respiratory or genital secretions or intestinal contents. Viruses that bud from basal surfaces are in position for systemic spread via viremia or lymphatics. Some viruses, such as flaviviruses, bunyaviruses, and coronaviruses, take a more circuitous route in exiting the cell (see specific chapters in Part II). Viruses that do not bud usually are released only via cell lysis.

Ultrastructural Changes in Virus-Infected Cells

As seen at the higher resolution provided by the electron microscope, specific and nonspecific changes in virus-infected cells are varied and may be dramatic. Early changes in cell structure often are dominated by proliferation of various cell membranes: for example, herpesviruses cause increased synthesis, even reduplication, of nuclear membranes; flaviviruses cause proliferation of the endoplasmic reticulum; picornaviruses and caliciviruses cause a distinctive proliferation of vesicles in the cytoplasm; and many retroviruses cause peculiar fusions of cytoplasmic membranes. Other ultrastructural changes that are prominent in many viral infections include disruption of cytoskeletal elements, mitochondrial damage, and changes in the density of the cytosol. Late in the course of infection, many cytolytic viruses cause nuclear, organelle, and cytoplasmic rarefaction and/or condensation, with terminal loss of host cell membrane integrity. In many instances the inevitability of cell death is obvious, but in others host cell functional loss is subtle and cannot be attributed to particular ultrastructural pathologic changes. In noncytolytic infections, most functional losses cannot be attributed to damage that is morphologically evident. Specific examples reflecting the range of host cell changes occurring in virus-infected cells are included in many of the chapters in Part II of this book.

In addition to changes directly attributable to viral replication, most virus-infected cells also show nonspecific changes, very much like those induced by physical or chemical insults. The most common early and potentially reversible change is what pathologists call *cloudy swelling.* This change is associated with increasing permeability of the plasma membrane. Electron microscopic study of such cells reveals diffuse swelling of the nucleus, distention of the endoplasmic reticulum and mitochondria, and rarefaction of the cytoplasm. Later in the course of many viral infections the nucleus becomes condensed and shrunken, and cytoplasmic density increases. Cell destruction can be the consequence of further loss of osmotic integrity and leakage of lysosomal enzymes into the cytoplasm. This progression, overall, is called by pathologists the *common terminal pathway* to cell death.

Virus-Induced Cell Death: Apoptosis Versus Necrosis

It had long been assumed that viruses kill cells by direct means, by usurping cellular machinery, disrupting membrane integrity, etc. That is, it was thought that the level of insult was such that the cell could not go on living—that in thc words of the virologist Kay Holmes, "the cell dies by *necrosis,* or 'murder.'" In recent years, however, it has been found that although some viruses do cause the necrosis of their host cell, many others kill their host cell by triggering cellular "suicide," or *programmed cell death.* Cells that have activated their programmed cell death pathway undergo characteristic morphologic changes referred to as *apoptosis.* The striking morphologic changes that occur during apoptosis are distinguishable from those of necrosis. Cells dying by apoptosis exhibit chromatin condensation and margination and eventually break up into membrane-bound bodies that contain dense cytoplasmic and nuclear debris. Also, characteristically, a cellular endonuclease is activated during apoptosis that cleaves cellular DNA into 180- to 200-bp fragments. These are seen in agarose gels as many rather evenly spaced bands, called "ladders." This endonuclease-induced change is not seen in cellular necrosis.

There are several potential mechanisms by which cells are induced to activate their apoptotic pathway; some viruses induce apoptosis by the direct action of a specific protein—adenoviruses, alphaviruses, and the circovirus, chicken anemia virus, have proteins that by themselves are sufficient to induce apoptotic cell death. In other cases, viruses induce apoptosis indirectly through their effects on cellular processes. Conversely, some viruses have acquired one or more antiapoptotic genes and gene products to prolong cell survival until their replication cycle is complete and progeny virions have been released.

All in all, programmed cell death, i.e., apoptosis, seems to be an important host defense mechanism. When a virus induces cell death by necrosis, it usually does so late, after progeny virus production is complete. In many cases, e.g., with picornaviruses, lysis of the host cell by necrosis is part of the viral strategy to effect virion release. However, when a cell induces its own death, by apoptosis, it usually does so early, before progeny virus production is complete. Paradoxically, this early elimination of virus-infected cells that occurs before the release of progeny virus may arrest or at least slow the spread of virus throughout the body enough such that other host defenses can be marshaled.

Interferons

Viral *interference* is said to occur when a virus-infected cell resists superinfection with the same or a different virus. The interfering virus does not necessarily have to replicate to induce interference, and the ability of the challenge virus to replicate may be completely or only partially inhibited. Two main mechanisms have been demonstrated: (1) interference mediated by defective interfering mutants, operating only against the homologueous virus (see Chapter 4), and (2) interference mediated by *interferons.*

Properties of Interferons

In 1957 Isaacs and Lindenmann reported that cells of the chorioallantoic membrane of embryonated hen's eggs infected with influenza virus release into the medium a nonviral protein, "interferon," that protects uninfected cells against infection with the same or unrelated viruses. This discovery raised hopes that this substance would become a safe, nontoxic, broad-spectrum antiviral chemotherapeutic agent. Despite an enormous amount of work since then, and the capacity to produce large amounts by recombinant DNA technology, its usefulness as a therapeutic agent for the treatment of viral diseases remains an unfulfilled dream.

Today we know that there are about 24 interferons in humans, and fewer in animals probably only because of less research. We know that interferons are typical

TABLE 5.2
Properties of Interferons

PROPERTY	INTERFERON α	INTERFERON β	INTERFERON γ
Principal source	Leukocytes, many other cells	Fibroblasts Epithelial cells	T lymphocytes, NK cells
Inducing agent	Virus infection	Virus infection	Antigen (or mitogen)
Number of subtypes	At least 22 in humans, fewer identified in animals	1	1
Glycosylation	No (most subtypes)	Yes	Yes
Functional form	Monomer	Dimer	Tetramer
Principal activity	Antiviral	Antriviral	Immunomodulation
Mechanism of action	Inhibits protein synthesis	Inhibits protein synthesis	Enhances MHC antigens; activates cytotoxic T cells, macrophages, and NK cells

members of the large family of normal cellular regulatory proteins called *cytokines*. They fall into three chemically distinct types, known as interferon α (which occurs as at least 22 subtypes in humans), interferon β, and interferon γ—some of their properties are listed in Table 5.2.

Interferons are not synthesized by cells constitutively, rather they are produced and secreted transiently in response to external stimuli, such as viral infections. Any virus, especially RNA viruses, multiplying in almost any type of cell, in any vertebrate species, induces interferons α and β. Interferon γ is made only by T lymphocytes (and natural killer cells) and only following antigen-specific or mitogenic stimulation; it is a *lymphokine*, with immunoregulatory functions. Some interferons, especially β and γ, display a degree of host species specificity; for instance, mouse interferons are ineffective in humans, and vice versa. However, there is little or no viral specificity, i.e., interferons α, β, or γ induced by, say, a paramyxovirus infection are fully effective against a togavirus infection. Secreted interferons are distributed locally or carried by the circulation throughout the body. Usually, virus-induced interferons are produced early in the course of infection, as early as the time viral progeny are first released by infected cells; thus, they can have a very important effect in protecting neighboring cells and inhibiting the early spread of virus locally and the early dissemination of virus throughout the body.

The important role played by interferons as a defense mechanism has been documented by three types of experimental and clinical observations: (1) in many viral infections, interferon production correlates with recovery; (2) inhibition of interferon production, such as in knockout mice, enhances the severity of infection; and (3) treatment with interferons protects against infection.

Antiviral Actions of Interferons

Following their induction by viral infection, interferons are released from the infected cell and bind to specific receptors on the plasma membrane of other cells. There appears to be one receptor for interferons α and β and another for interferon γ. Binding of interferons α and β to their receptor activates a complex transcriptional cascade by signal transduction, which in turn leads to the synthesis of many cellular proteins—over 20 cellular genes are up-regulated. Binding of interferon γ to its receptor triggers a different cascade, a different set of genes and proteins. Many of the induced proteins directly or indirectly inhibit the replication of virus, each in a different way. The mechanisms involved are beyond the scope of this book, but one example will be used to illustrate the complexity of mechanisms involved in interferon-mediated interference.

P1/eIF-2a kinase, which is made constitutively at low levels in untreated cells, is up-regulated by interferon α, β, or γ. Following binding of double-stranded RNA, which is an intermediate or by-product formed in the course of RNA virus replication, this protein kinase phosphorylates its own P1 subunit, thus activating the enzyme to phosphorylate the α subunit of the eukaryotic protein synthesis initiation factor eIF-2, thereby inactivating it. Because eIF-2 is required to initiate the synthesis of all polypeptides, interferon-induced P1/eIF-2a kinase inhibits the synthesis of all proteins of any virus that has stimulated its activation.

Interferons and Resistance/Susceptibility to Viral Infections

It is difficult to determine which cell types are responsible for interferon production in particular viral infections *in vivo*. Certainly, interferons can be found in the fluids bathing most infection sites, e.g., in the mucus bathing airway epithelial surfaces during respiratory infections and in the blood in systemic infections. These interferons are produced by epithelial and mesenchymal cells as well as by T cells, natural killer cells, killer cells, and macrophages in infection sites.

Compelling evidence that interferons can be instrumental in deciding the fate of the animal following viral infection was provided in the early 1970s by Gresser and colleagues, who showed that mice infected with any of several nonlethal viruses, or with sublethal doses of more virulent viruses, die if anti-interferon globulin is administered. In studies with transgenic mice carrying multiple copies of the gene for human interferon β, enhanced resistance to pseudorabies virus was found that was proportional to the resulting concentration of circulating interferon evoked by the transgene.

Although it is widely thought that interferons play an important role in recovery from viral infections, data are less certain. If interferons were key, one might expect that infection caused by any virus or indeed immunization by any attenuated virus vaccine might protect an animal against challenge with an unrelated virus, yet this cannot be demonstrated. The evidence is somewhat stronger that infection of the respiratory tract with one virus will provide temporary, local protection against others. Perhaps this distinction provides a clue that the antiviral effect of interferons is limited in both time and space. Their main antiviral effect in natural infections may be local, protecting cells in the immediate vicinity of the initial focus of infection, slowing down the movement of virus during crucial early stages of infection.

Actions of Viruses to Combat Effects of Interferons

Because of its early induction and broad effectiveness, many viruses have evolved defense mechanisms for circumventing the host's interferon system. For example, adenoviruses encode RNAs that bind to P1/eIF-2a kinase, preventing its activation by double-stranded RNA. Reoviruses, which might be expected to be exceptionally susceptible to interferons because they have double-stranded RNA genomes, are not because one of their capsid proteins binds more strongly to viral double-stranded RNA than P1/eIF-2a kinase.

Further Reading

Alberts, B., Bray, D., Johnson, A., and Lewis, J., eds. (1997). "Essential Cell Biology: An Introduction to the Molecular Biology of the Cell." Garland Publishers, New York.

Ball, L. A. (1998). Virus-host cell interactions. *In* "Topley and Wilson's Microbiology and Microbial Infections" (B. W. J. Mahy and L. H. Collier, eds.), Vol. 1, pp. 115–146. Edward Arnold, London.

Benz, J. (1993). "Viral Fusion Mechanisms." CRC Press, Boca Raton, FL.

Carrasco, L. (1987). "Mechanisms of Viral Toxicity in Animal Cells." CRC Press, Boca Raton, FL.

Carrasco, L. (1994). Entry of animal viruses and macromolecules into cells. *FEBS Lett.* **350,** 151–154.

Greber, U. F., Singh, I., and Helenius, A. (1994). Mechanisms of virus uncoating. *Trends Microbiol.* **2,** 52–56.

Helenius, A. (1992). Unpacking the incoming influenza virus. *Cell* **69,** 577–578.

Johnson, H. M., Bazer, F. W., Szente, B. E., and Jarpe, M. A. (1994). How interferons fight disease. *Sci. Am.* **270,** 68–75.

Knipe, D. M. (1996). Virus-host cell interactions. *In* "Fields Virology" (B. N. Fields, D. M. Knipe, P. M. Howley, R. M., Chanock, J. L. Melnick, T. P. Monath, B. Roizman, and S. E. Straus, eds.), 3rd ed., pp. 273–299. Lippincott-Raven, Philadelphia, PA.

Lodish, H., Baltimore, D., and Berk, A. (1995). "Molecular Cell Biology," 3rd ed. with CD ROM. Scientific American Books Freeman, New York.

Oldstone, M. B. A. (1989). Viral alteration of cell function. *Sci. Am.* **261,** 34–39.

Tucker, S. P., and Compans, R. W. (1993). Virus infection of polarized epithelial cells. *Adv. Virus Res.* **42,** 187–214.

Welsh, R. M., and Sen, G. C. (1997). Nonspecific host responses to viral infections. *In* "Viral Pathogenesis" (N. Nathanson, R. Ahmed, F. Gonzalez-Scarano, D. E. Griffin, K. V. Holmes, F. A. Murphy, and H. L. Robinson, eds.), pp. 109–142. Lippincott-Raven, Philadelphia, PA.

Williams, G. T. (1994). Programmed cell death: A fundamental protective response to pathogens. *Trends Microbiol.* **2,** 463–464.

CHAPTER 6

Mechanisms of Infection and Viral Spread through the Body

At the level of the cell, infection by viruses is quite different from that caused by bacteria and other microorganisms. However, at the level of the whole animal and animal populations there are more similarities than differences. Like microorganisms, viruses must gain entry into their host's body, replicate, and spread, either locally or systemically, and in generalized infections they must localize in appropriate target organs (Table 6.1). Further, to survive in nature, viruses must be transmitted, i.e., they must be shed with secretions or excretions into the environment, be taken up by a host or a vector, or be passed congenitally from mother to offspring.

Routes of Entry

To infect its host, a virus must first attach to and infect cells of one of the body surfaces, i.e., unless the body surfaces are bypassed by parenteral inoculation via a wound, needle, or the bite of an arthropod or vertebrate. The animal body may be represented by Cedric Mims' now classic diagram of a set of surfaces, each covered by a sheet of epithelial cells separating host tissues from the outside world (Figure 6.1).

The outer surface of the body proper, the skin, has a relatively impermeable, dry, outer layer of dead, keratinized cells. In the respiratory tract and in the intestinal tract, the surface lining consists of one or more layers of nonkeratinized epithelial cells. In the urogenital tract, where urine and sexual fluids are produced and excreted, there is another discontinuity in the body's protective covering, and in the eye the skin is replaced by a layer of living cells to form the conjunctiva and cornea. Each of these sites is the target for invasion by one or more viruses.

Entry via the Respiratory Tract

The mucosal surfaces of the respiratory tract have living cells at their surfaces; these cells can support the replication of many viruses so safeguards are necessary to minimize the risk of infection. The respiratory tract is ordinarily protected by two effective cleansing systems: (1) a blanket of mucus produced by goblet cells that is kept in continuous flow by (2) the coordinated beating of ciliated epithelial cells lining the upper and much of the lower respiratory tract. Most inhaled virions are trapped in mucus, carried by ciliary action from the nasal cavity and airways to the pharynx, and then swallowed or coughed out. Particles that are 10 μm or more in diameter are usually trapped on the nasal mucosa over the turbinate bones, which project into the nasal cavity and act as baffle plates. Particles 5–10 μm in diameter may be carried to the trachea and bronchioles, where they are usually trapped in the mucus blanket. Particles 5 μm or less in diameter are often inhaled directly into the lungs and some may reach the alveoli where they may be ingested by alveolar macrophages. At each of these levels, virus may infect epithelial cells.

Despite its protective systems, the respiratory tract is, overall, the most common portal of viral entry into

Table 6.1
Obligatory Steps in Viral Infection

Step in infection process	Requirement for viral survival and progression of infection
Entry into host and primary viral replication	Evade host's natural protective and cleansing mechanisms
Local or general spread in the host, cell and tissue tropism, and secondary viral replication	Evade immediate host defenses and natural barriers to spread; at the cellular level the virus takes over necessary host cell functions for its own replication processes
Evasion of host inflammatory and immune defenses	Evade host inflammatory, phagocytic, and immune defenses long enough to complete the viral transmission cycle
Shedding from host	Exit host body at site and at concentration needed to ensure infection of the next host
Cause damage to host	Not necessary, but this is the reason we are interested in the virus and its pathogenetic processes

the body (Table 6.2). All viruses that infect the host via the respiratory tract probably do so by attaching to specific receptors on epithelial cells. Following respiratory invasion, many viruses remain localized (e.g., rhinoviruses, adenoviruses, and influenza viruses of mammals) whereas others become systemic (e.g., foot-and-mouth disease viruses, canine distemper virus, rinderpest virus, hog cholera virus, and Newcastle disease virus).

Entry via the Oropharynx and Intestinal Tract

Many viruses are acquired by ingestion. They may either be swallowed and reach the stomach and intestine directly or they may first infect cells in the oropharynx, their progeny being eventually carried into the intestinal tract. The esophagus is rarely infected, probably because of its tough stratified squamous epithelium and the rapid passage of swallowed material over its surface. The intestinal tract is protected by mucus, which may contain specific secretory antibodies (IgA), but the directional peristaltic movement of gut contents provides many opportunities for virions to contact susceptible epithelial cells. Virions may also be taken up by M cells that overlie Peyer's patches in the ileum, from where they may be passed to adjacent mononuclear cells where they may replicate.

Figure 6.1.

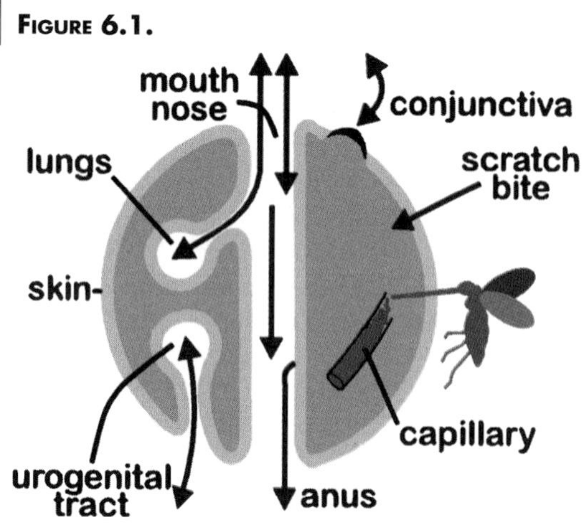

The surfaces of the body in relation to the entry and shedding of viruses. (Courtesy of C. A. Mims.)

Other protective mechanisms may inactivate viruses in the intestinal tract: acid in the stomach and bile and proteolytic enzymes in the small intestine. In general, viruses that cause intestinal infection, such as rotaviruses, caliciviruses, and enteroviruses (Table 6.3), are acid and bile resistant. However, there are acid- and bile-labile viruses that cause important intestinal infections; for example, bovine, porcine, and murine coronaviruses are protected during passage through the stomach of young animals by the buffering action of milk. Some enteric viruses not only resist inactivation by proteolytic enzymes in the stomach and intestine, their infectivity may actually be increased by such exposure. Thus, cleavage of an outer capsid protein by intestinal proteases enhances the infectivity of rotaviruses and some coronaviruses.

Rotaviruses, caliciviruses, toroviruses, and astroviruses are now recognized as major causes of viral diarrhea in animals, whereas the great majority of intestinal infections caused by enteroviruses (e.g., porcine, avian, and murine encephalomyelitis viruses) and adenoviruses are asymptomatic. Parvoviruses cause di-

Table 6.2
Viruses of Animals That Initiate Infection by Entry through the Respiratory Tract

Family/Genus	Virus
Producing respiratory disase	
Herpesviridae/several genera	Herpesviruses of many animals
Adenoviridae/*Mastadenovirus* and *Aviadenovirus*	Adenoviruses of many animals
Paramyxoviridae/several genera	Parainfluenza and respiratory syncytial viruses
Orthomyxoviridae/*Influenzavirus A*	Influenza viruses of swine and horses
Coronaviridae/*Coronavirus*	Infectious bronchitis virus of chickens
Picornaviridae/*Rhinovirus* and *Aphthovirus*	Rhinoviruses of many animals, foot-and-mouth disease viruses
Caliciviridae/*Vesivirus*	Feline calicivirus
Producing systemic disease, usually without initial respiratory signs	
Herpesviridae/several genera	Pseudorabies, bovine malignant catarrhal fever, Marek's disease viruses
Paramyxoviridae/*Morbillivirus*	Canine distemper, rinderpest viruses
Orthomyxoviridae/*Influenzavirus A*	Avian influenza viruses (fowl plague viruses)
Arenaviridae/*Arenavirus*	Lymphocytic choriomeningitis virus
Flaviviridae/*Pestivirus*	Hog cholera virus

arrhea after reaching cells of the intestinal tract via viremic spread.

Entry via the Skin

The skin is the largest organ of the body, and because its outer layer consists of keratinized cells, it provides a tough and usually impermeable barrier to the entry of viruses. Breaches in skin integrity such as cuts, punctures, abrasions, or wounds expose deep epidermal layers that contain few blood vessels and lymphatics and therefore are rather remote from host inflammatory defenses. Viruses that enter these layers, such as the papillomaviruses, typically induce local pathology (Table 6.4). Deeper trauma may introduce viruses into the dermis,

Table 6.3
Viruses of Animals That Initiate Infection by Entry through the Intestinal Tract

Family/Genus	Virus
Producing diarrhea	
Parvoviridae/*Parvovirus*	Feline panleukopenia virus, canine parvovirus
Reoviridae/*Rotavirus*	Rotaviruses of many animals
Coronaviridae/*Coronavirus*	Enteric coronaviruses of many animals, mouse hepatitis virus
Coronaviridae/*Torovirus*	Breda virus
Astroviridae/*Astrovirus*	Astroviruses of many animals
Flaviviridae/*Pestivirus*	Bovine viral diarrhea virus
Producing systemic disease, usually without diarrhea	
Adenoviridae/*Mastadenovirus* and *Aviadenovirus*	Adenoviruses of many animals
Picornaviridae/*Enterovirus*	Enteroviruses of many animals
Caliciviridae/*Vesivirus*	Vesicular exanthema of swine virus

TABLE 6.4
Viruses That Initiate Infection by Entry through the Skin, Oral Mucosa, Genital Tract, or Eye

ROUTE	FAMILY/GENUS	VIRUS
Minor abrasions (skin or mucosa)	*Papovaviridae/Papillomavirus*	Papillomaviruses of many animals
	Herpesviridae/several genera	Herpesviruses of many animals
	Poxviridae/several genera	Cowpox, swinepox, orf, bovine papular stomatitis, pseudocowpox, fowlpox viruses
	Picornaviridae/Enterovirus	Swine vesicular disease virus
	Rhabdoviridae/Vesiculovirus	Vesicular stomatitis viruses
Arthropod bite (mechanical transmission)	*Poxviridae*/several genera	Fowlpox, swinepox, myxoma viruses
	Retroviridae/Lentivirus	Equine infectious anemia virus
	Rhabdoviridae/Vesiculovirus	Vesicular stomatitis viruses
Arthropod bite (biological transmission, i.e., with viral replication in the arthropod)	*Asfarviridae/Asfivirus*	African swine fever virus
	Reoviridae/Orbivirus	Bluetongue viruses, African horse sickness viruses
	Rhabdoviridae/Ephemerovirus	Bovine ephemeral fever
	Rhabdoviridae/Vesiculovirus	Vesicular stomatitis viruses
	Bunyaviridae/Phlebovirus	Rift Valley fever virus
	Bunyaviridae/Nairovirus	Nairobi sheep disease virus
	Togaviridae/Alphavirus	All member viruses
	Flaviviridae/Flavivirus	Nearly all member viruses
Bite of vertebrate	*Retroviridae/Lentivirus*	Feline immunodeficiency virus
	Rhabdoviridae/Lyssavirus	Rabies virus
Contaminated needles or equipment	All viruses causing systemic infection, e.g., *Papovaviridae/Papillomavirus*	Papillomaviruses of many animals
	Retroviridae/Lentivirus and *Deltaretrovirus*	Equine infectious anemia, bovine leukemia virus
	Flaviviridae/Pestivirus	Hog cholera, bovine viral diarrhea viruses
Genital contact	*Herpesviridae*/several genera	Herpesviruses of many animals
	Papovaviridae/Papillomavirus	Bovine papillomaviruses
	Arteriviridae/Arterivirus	Equine arteritis virus
Conjunctival contact	*Herpesviridae*/several genera	Infectious bovine rhinotracheitis virus, equine herpesvirus 1
	Adenoviridae/Mastadenovirus	Canine adenoviruses 1 and 2

with its rich supply of vessels, lymphatics, and nerves, or even into the underlying subcutaneous tissue and muscle. These tissues often provide fertile ground for viral replication and subsequent dissemination. Generalized infections of the skin with exanthema, such as in lumpy skin disease, sheeppox, and swine vesicular disease, are due to viral spread via viremia.

One of the most efficient ways by which viruses are introduced through the skin is via the bite of arthropods, such as mosquitoes, ticks, *Culicoides* spp., or sandflies. Insects, especially flies, may act as simple mechanical vectors ("flying needles"); for example, equine infectious anemia virus is spread among horses, rabbit hemorrhagic disease virus and myxoma virus are spread among rabbits, and fowlpox virus among chickens in this way. However, most viruses that are spread by arthropods replicate in their vector. Viruses that are transmitted by and replicate in arthropod vectors are called *arboviruses* (from *ar*thropod-*bo*rne).

Infection can also be acquired through the bite of an animal, as in rabies. Finally, introduction of a virus by skin penetration may be *iatrogenic,* i.e., the result of veterinary care or related husbandry practices. For example, equine infectious anemic virus has been transmitted via contaminated needles, twitches, ropes, and harnesses and orf virus and papillomaviruses have been transmitted via ear tagging or tattooing.

Entry via Other Routes

The urogenital tract is the route of entry of several important pathogens (e.g., bovine herpesvirus 1, equine herpesvirus 3, and porcine papillomavirus). Small tears or abrasions in the penile mucosa and the epithelial lining of the vagina may occur during sexual activity and permit the entry of virus. The conjunctiva, although much less resistant to viral invasion than the skin, is constantly cleansed by the flow of secretion (tears) and is wiped by the eyelids; some adenoviruses and enteroviruses gain entry in this way.

Host Specificity and Tissue Tropism

The capacity of a virus to selectively infect cells in particular organs is referred to as *tropism* (see Chapter 7). Viral tropism depends on viral and host factors. At the cellular level, there must be an interaction between viral attachment proteins and matching cellular receptors. Although such interactions are usually studied in cultured cells, the situation *in vivo,* where heterogeneous cell populations are involved, is much more complex. If, for example, experimental animals are treated with neuraminidase intranasally, there is substantial protection against intranasal infection with influenza virus that lasts until the neuraminidase-sensitive receptors have regenerated. Receptors for a particular virus are usually restricted to certain cell types in certain organs; only these cells can be infected. In large part, this accounts for both the tissue and organ tropism of a given virus and the pathogenesis of the disease caused by the virus. Of course, the presence of receptor is not the only factor that determines whether the cell may become infected—other, intracellular factors, such as enhancers, are required for productive infection.

Viral enhancers are short, often tandem-repeated sequences of nucleotides that can regulate tissue-specific transcription. Papillomavirus DNA contains such enhancers, which are active only in keratinocytes and indeed only in the subset of these cells where papillomavirus replication occurs. Enhancer sequences have also been defined in the genomes of retroviruses and several herpesviruses, where they appear to influence tropism by regulating the expression of viral genes in specific cell types. For example, certain strains of avian leukosis virus induce lymphomas, whereas others cause osteoporosis.

Mechanisms of Spread in the Body

Viruses may replicate only at or near the body surface through which they entered, whether this be the respiratory tract, intestine, skin, genital tract, or conjunctiva; alternatively, they may cause generalized infections or infections in specific organs following lymphatic and hematogenous spread from entry sites.

In pioneering experiments that first revealed the pathogenetic events leading to systemic infection and disease, Frank Fenner used ectromelia (mousepox) virus as a model system. Groups of mice were inoculated in the footpad of a hind limb and at daily intervals their organs were titrated to determine the amount of virus present. Fenner showed that during the incubation period, infection spread through the mouse body in a stepwise fashion (Figure 6.2). The virus first replicated locally in tissues of the footpad and then in local lymph nodes. Virus produced in these sites gained entry into the bloodstream, causing a primary viremia, which brought the virus to its ultimate target organs, especially lymphoreticular organs and the liver. This stage of infection was accompanied by the development of focal necrosis, first in the skin and draining lymph nodes in the inoculated hind limb and then in the spleen and liver. Within days there was massive necrosis in the spleen and liver leading to death. However, this was not the whole pathogenetic sequence—to complete the viral life cycle, shedding and infection of the next host had to be explained. Fenner found that the virus produced in the major target organs, i.e., the spleen and liver, caused a secondary viremia, bringing the virus back to the skin. Infection in the skin caused a macular and papular rash from which large amounts of virus were shed, leading to contact exposure of other mice. These experiments led to many more studies, of many other viruses in many different animal species, cumulatively bringing us to our present state of knowledge of the pathogenesis of viral diseases in ani-

FIGURE 6.2.

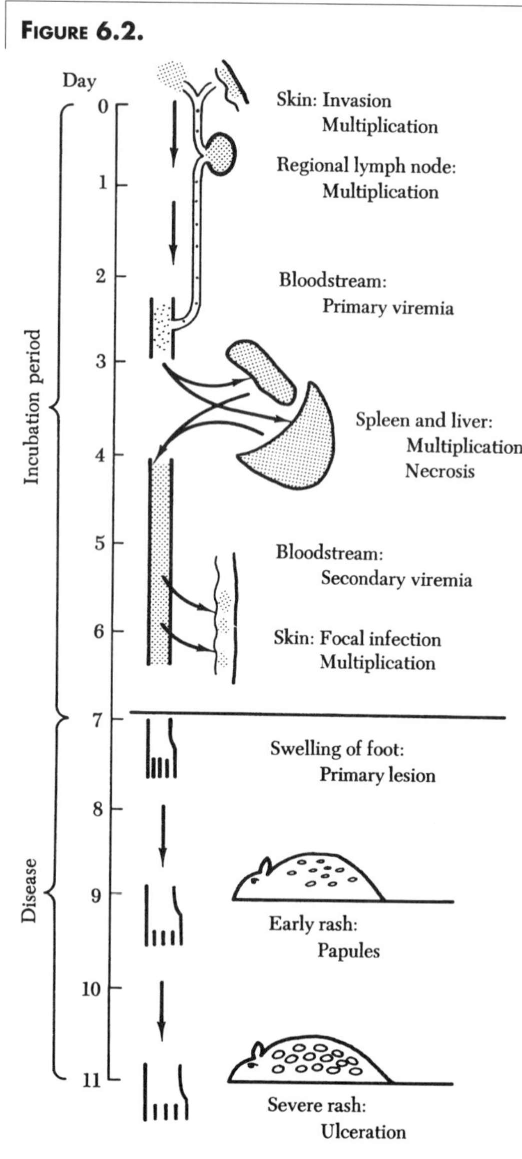

Frank Fenner's classic study of the pathogenesis of ectromelia (mousepox) virus infection. This was the first study ever done using serial (daily) titration of the virus content of organs and tissues and the model for many studies that have since advanced knowledge of the pathogenesis of systemic viral infections. [From F. Fenner, Mousepox (infectious ectromelia of mice): A review. *J. Immunol.* **63,** 341–373 (1949).]

mals infected in nature and underlining the importance and general applicability of the ectromelia model.

Local Spread on Epithelial Surfaces

Many viruses replicate in epithelial cells at the site of entry and produce a localized or spreading infection in the epithelium—some are then shed directly into the environment from these sites. The spread of infection along epithelial surfaces usually occurs by the sequential infection of neighboring cells. Many poxviruses produce infection via the skin, but in addition to spreading from cell to cell, there is usually also local subepithelial and lymphatic spread. For example, in myxoma virus infection in rabbits, a few epidermal cells are usually infected by scarification (or by a biting arthropod) and the virus spreads locally from cell to cell, primarily in the epidermis, before spreading to the local lymph nodes. The poxviruses that cause molluscum contagiosum, orf, and tanapox remain localized in the skin and produce an overgrowth of cells and inflammatory infiltration. In the skin, papillomaviruses initiate infection in the basal layer of the epidermis, but the maturation of virions occurs only in cells as they move toward the skin surface and become keratinized. Because this is a slow process, taking several weeks, papillomas develop slowly.

Viruses that enter the body via the respiratory or intestinal tracts can spread rapidly in the layer of fluid that covers epithelial surfaces; consequently, such infections often progress rapidly. Usually these viruses have a short incubation period as well. After infections of the respiratory tract by paramyxoviruses and influenza viruses or the intestinal tract by rotaviruses or coronaviruses, there is little or no invasion of subepithelial tissues. Although these viruses usually enter lymphatics and thus have the potential to spread, they usually do not replicate well in deeper tissues, possibly because appropriate virus receptors or other permissive cellular factors, such as cleavage-activating proteases, are restricted to epithelial cells or because the temperature of deeper tissues is higher than the optimal temperature for viral replication.

Restriction of infection to an epithelial surface cannot be equated with a lack of severity of disease. Large areas of intestinal epithelium may be damaged by rotaviruses and coronaviruses, causing severe diarrhea. The severity of localized infections of the respiratory tract depends on their location: infections of the upper respiratory tract may produce severe rhinitis but few other signs, whereas infection of the bronchioles or alveoli may produce more severe respiratory distress. The whole tracheal epithelial and bronchial lining may be destroyed in influenza or parainfluenza virus infections, causing extravasation of fluids and hypoxia, especially in young animals. Fluid buildup in airways may predispose to secondary bacterial invasion—shipping fever in cattle is often a consequence of parainfluenza virus 3 infection followed by *Pasteurella hemolytica* superinfection. The generalized signs of fever, chills, malaise, fatigue, and anorexia accompanying localized respiratory infections are generally the result of induced circulating cytokines.

Subepithelial Invasion and Lymphatic Spread

The factors that direct some viruses to invade subepithelial tissues are poorly understood. In addition to the distribution of viral receptors and the differences between body core and surface temperatures, as discussed earlier, directional shedding of viruses from infected epithelial layers may be crucial. Release of virus into the lumen of the respiratory or intestinal tracts facilitates local spread to contiguous epithelial surfaces and immediate shedding into the environment, but does not favor invasion of subepithelial tissues. Conversely, shedding from the basolateral cell surface of epithelial cells facilitates the invasion of subepithelial tissues and the subsequent dissemination of virus through lymphatics, blood vessels, or nerves.

Paramyxoviruses and orthomyxoviruses are released preferentially from lumenal (or apical) surfaces of epithelial cells, whereas rhabdoviruses (except rabies virus in salivary glands) are shed from basolateral surfaces into subepithelial spaces. Within the family *Coronaviridae,* transmissible gastroeneteritis virus is shed from lumenal surfaces of infected cells from where it enters body excretions, whereas strains of mouse hepatitis virus that cause generalized disease are shed from basolateral membranes from where they can enter the circulation and be carried to other target organs. These shedding patterns are determined by the localization of the insertion of viral surface glycoproteins in the plasma membrane of the host cell; in turn, viral glycoprotein localization is determined by specific signaling sequences within the glycoproteins themselves.

After traversing the epithelium and its basement membrane to reach subepithelial tissues, virions can enter lymphatics that form a network beneath all cutaneous and mucosal epithelia (Figure 6.3). Virions that enter lymphatics are carried to local lymph nodes. As they enter, virions are exposed to macrophages lining marginal sinuses and may be engulfed. Virions may be inactivated and processed by macrophages and dendritic cells so that their component antigens are presented to adjacent lymphocytes in such a way that an immune response is initiated (see Chapter 8). Some viruses, however, also replicate in macrophages (e.g., many retroviruses, canine distemper virus, feline infectious peritonitis virus, Borna disease virus, arteriviruses, some adenoviruses, and some herpesviruses), whereas other viruses are able to replicate in lymphocytes or dendritic cells. Some virions may pass directly through lymph nodes to enter the bloodstream. Monocytes and lymphocytes circulate through the blood, lymphatics, and lymph nodes; this circulation is an effective means of disseminating viruses throughout the body.

Normally, there is a local inflammatory response at the site of viral invasion, the extent of which depends on the extent of tissue damage. Local blood vessels become dilated and rendered more permeable so that monocytes and lymphocytes, cytokines, immunoglobulins, and complement components may be delivered directly to the site of infection. These events are especially vigorous once the immune response has been initiated. In some cases, viruses take advantage of these events to infect involved cells and spread locally or systemically.

Spread via the Bloodstream: Viremia

In veterinary medicine, unintentional inoculation of a virus into the bloodstream is rare, but it may occur during the transfusion of infected blood (e.g., transmission of feline immunodeficiency virus) or by use of nonsterile instruments (e.g., transmission of many viruses by reuse of disposable syringes and needles or improperly

FIGURE 6.3.

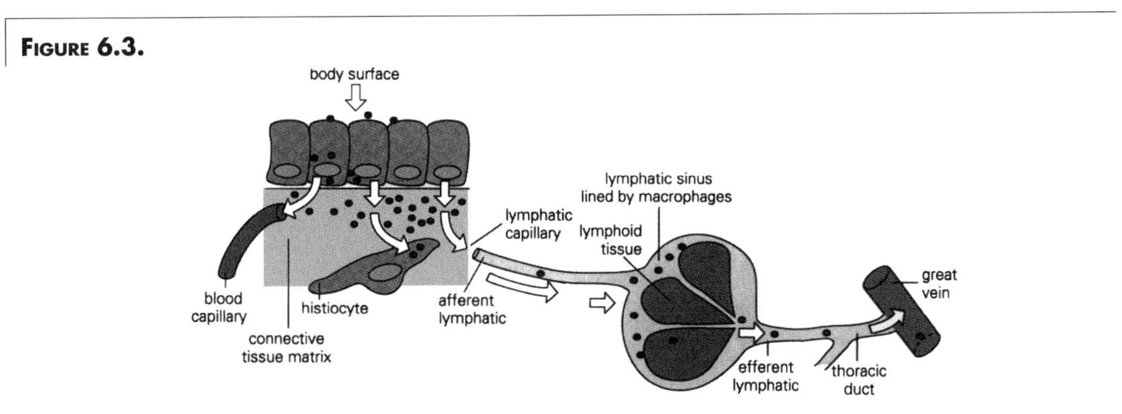

Subepithelial invasion and lymphatic spread of infection. (Courtesy of C. A. Mims.)

sterilized multiuse syringes and needles). The bite of arthropod vectors also allows direct entry of virus into the bloodstream.

The blood is the most effective and rapid vehicle for the spread of virus through the body. Once a virus has reached the bloodstream, usually via the lymphatic system (Figure 6.3), it can localize in any part of the body within minutes. The first entry of virus into the blood is called *primary viremia*. This early viremia may be clinically silent, known to have taken place only because of the invasion of distant organs. Virus replication in major target organs leads to the sustained production of much higher concentrations of virus, producing a *secondary viremia* (Figure 6.4), which can in turn lead to the establishment of infection in yet other parts of the body.

In the blood, virions may be free in the plasma or may be contained in, or adsorbed to, leukocytes, platelets, or erythrocytes. Parvoviruses, enteroviruses, togaviruses, and flaviviruses circulate free in the plasma. Viruses carried in leukocytes, generally lymphocytes or monocytes, are not cleared as readily or in the same way as viruses circulating free in the plasma. Being protected from antibodies and other plasma components, they can be carried to distant tissues. Monocyte-associated viremia is a feature of canine distemper, bluetongue, feline leukemia, and of beta- and gammaherpesvirus infections; lymphocyte-associated viremia is a feature of Marek's disease, lymphocytic choriomeningitis, and feline immunodeficiency virus infections. In infections caused by African swine fever virus, Rift Valley fever virus, Colorado tick fever virus, and bluetongue viruses, virions are asso-

Figure 6.4.

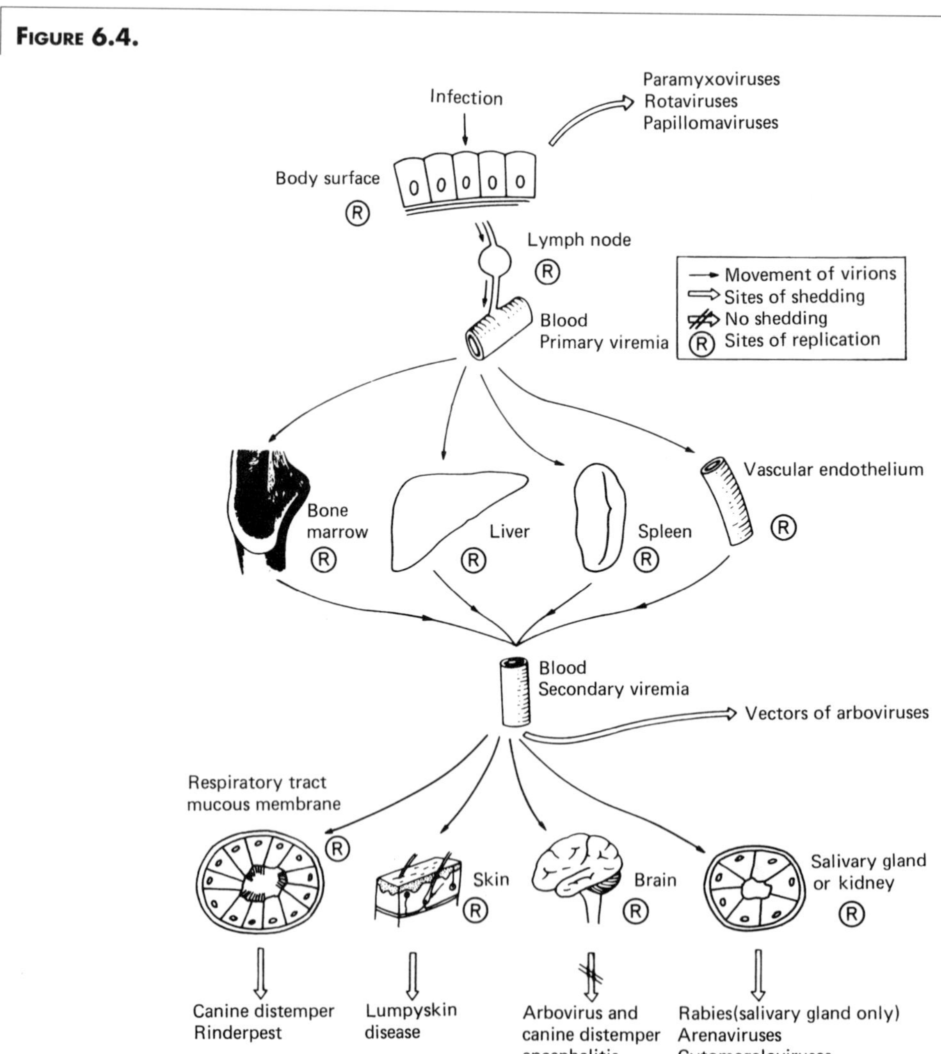

The role of viremia in the spread of viruses through the body, indicating sites of replication and important routes of shedding of various viruses. (Adapted from the work of C. A. Mims and D. O. White.)

ciated with erythrocytes—in bluetongue and Colorado tick fever virus infections, the virus replicates in erythrocyte precursors in the bone marrow, producing a viremia that lasts for the life span of erythrocytes. Certain mouse leukemia viruses and arenaviruses infect megakaryocytes and thereby are present in circulating platelets, but this does not appear to be important in the pathogenesis of diseases caused by these viruses. Neutrophils have a very short life span and powerful antimicrobial mechanisms; they are rarely infected, although they may contain phagocytosed virions.

Viruses circulating in the plasma encounter many kinds of cells, but two play special roles in determining the subsequent fate of infection: macrophages and vascular endothelial cells.

Virus Interactions with Macrophages

Macrophages are very efficient phagocytes and are present in all compartments of the body: free in plasma, in alveoli, subepithelial tissues, sinusoids of the lymph nodes, and above all the sinusoids of the liver, spleen, and bone marrow. Together with dendritic cells and B lymphocytes, macrophages are antigen-processing and antigen-presenting cells and therefore play a pivotal role in initiation of the primary immune response (see Chapter 8). The antiviral action of macrophages depends on the age and genetics of the host and their site of origin in the body; indeed, even in a given site there are subpopulations of macrophages that differ in phagocytic competence and in susceptibility to infection. Their state of activation is also important. The various kinds of interactions that can occur between macrophages and virions may be described in relation to Kupffer cells, the macrophages that line the sinusoids of the liver, as shown in Figure 6.5. Not shown in this model is tissue invasion via carriage of virus inside mobile monocytes/macrophages as they emigrate across capillary or sinusoidal walls (diapedesis). Such transport of viruses inside infected cells has been referred to as the "Trojan Horse" mechanism of invasion; it is especially important in the pathogenesis of lentivirus infections.

Differences in virus–macrophage interactions may account for differences in the virulence of virus strains and differences in host resistance. Even though they are innately efficient phagocytes, this capacity is enhanced greatly during an immune response in response to the

FIGURE 6.5.

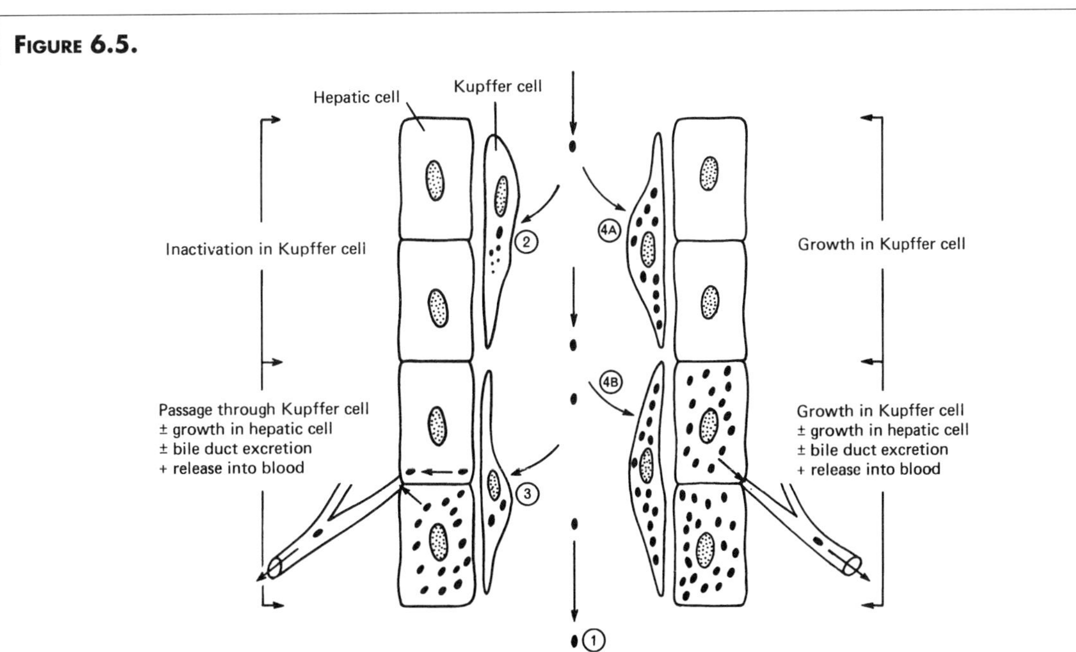

Types of interaction between viruses and macrophages, exemplified by Kupffer cells, the macrophages that line the sinusoids in the liver. (1) Macrophages may fail to phagocytose virions; e.g., in Venezuelan equine encephalitis virus infection this is an important factor favoring prolonged high viremia. (2) Virions may be phagocytosed and destroyed: because the macrophage system is so efficient, viremia can be maintained only if virions enter the blood as fast as they are removed. (3) Virions may be phagocytosed and then transferred passively to adjacent cells (hepatocytes in the liver); e.g., in Rift Valley fever virus infection, the virus replicates in hepatocytes and causes severe hepatitis—the virus produced in the liver sustains the high viremia. (4) Virions may be phagocytosed by macrophages and then may replicate in them: (4A) with some viruses, such as lactate dehydrogenase elevating virus in mice, only macrophages are infected and progeny from that infection are the source of the extremely high viremia. (4B) More commonly, as in infectious canine hepatitis, the virus replicates in both macrophages and hepatocytes, producing severe hepatitis. (Adapted from the work of C. A. Mims and D. O. White.)

release of cytokines, notably from T helper lymphocytes. Macrophages also have Fc receptors and C3 receptors in their plasma membranes, which further enhance their ability to ingest virions, especially when they are coated with antibody or complement. Certain togaviruses, flaviviruses, coronaviruses, arenaviruses, reoviruses, and especially retroviruses are capable of replicating in macrophages—when virus uptake is facilitated by bound antibody, antibody-mediated enhancement of infection may occur. This is a major pathogenetic factor in human dengue, feline infectious peritonitis, and many retrovirus infections.

Virus Interactions with Vascular Endothelial Cells

The vascular endothelium with its basement membrane and tight cell junctions constitutes the blood–tissue interface and for particles such as virions, often a barrier. Parenchymal invasion by circulating virions depends on crossing this barrier, usually in capillaries and venules where blood flow is slowest and the barrier is thinnest. Virions may move passively between or through endothelial cells and basement membranes or they may infect endothelial cells and "grow" their way through this barrier. This subject has been studied most intensively in relation to viral invasion of the central nervous system (see later), but it also applies to secondary invasion of the skin, respiratory tract, salivary glands, intestine, kidney, and placenta.

Maintenance of Viremia

Because virions circulating in the blood are removed continuously by macrophages, viremia can be maintained only if there is a continuing introduction of virus into the blood from infected tissues or if clearance by macrophages is impaired. Although circulating leukocytes can themselves constitute a site for viral replication, viremia is usually maintained by infection of the parenchymal cells of target organs such as the liver, spleen, lymph nodes, and bone marrow. In some infections, such as in hog cholera, the viremia is partly maintained by the infection of endothelial cells. Striated and smooth muscle cells may be an important site of replication of some enteroviruses, togaviruses, and rhabdoviruses, with virions reaching the blood via the lymph circulation.

There is a general correlation between the magnitude of viremia generated by blood-borne viruses and their capacity to invade target tissues. However, the failure of some attenuated vaccine viruses to generate a significant viremia may account for their lack of invasiveness. Certain neurotropic viruses are virulent after intracerebral inoculation, but avirulent when given peripherally because they do not attain viremia titers high enough to allow invasion of the nervous system. The capacity to produce viremia and the capacity to invade tissues from the bloodstream are thus two different properties of a virus. For example, some strains of Semliki Forest virus, an alphavirus, have lost the capacity to invade the central nervous system while retaining the capacity to generate a viremia equivalent in duration and magnitude to that produced by neuroinvasive strains.

Spread via Nerves

An important route of infection of the central nervous system is via the peripheral nerves, as seen, for example, in rabies, Borna disease, B virus encephalitis, pseudorabies, and bovine herpesvirus 5 encephalitis. Herpesvirus capsids travel to the central nervous system in axon cytoplasm and while doing so also sequentially infect the Schwann cells of the nerve sheath. Rabies virus and Borna disease virus also travel to the central nervous system in axon cytoplasm, but usually do not infect the nerve sheath. Sensory, motor, and autonomic nerves may be involved in the neural spread of these viruses. As these viruses move centripetally, they must cross cell–cell junctions. Rabies virus and pseudorabies virus are known to cross at synaptic junctions (Figure 6.6).

In addition to passing centripetally from the body surface to the sensory ganglia and from there to the brain, herpesviruses, such as pseudorabies virus and bovine herpesvirus 1, can move through axons centrifugally from ganglia to the skin or mucous membranes. This is what happens in the reactivation of latent infections and in the production of recrudescent epithelial lesions.

Rabies virus, Borna disease virus, and some togaviruses are able to use olfactory nerve endings in the nares as sites of entry. They gain entry in the special sensory endings of the olfactory neuroepithelial cells, cause local infection and progeny virus (or subviral entities containing the viral genome) then travels in axoplasm of olfactory nerves directly to the olfactory bulb of the brain.

Mechanisms of Infection of Major Target Organs and Tissues

Infection of the Respiratory Tract

The frequency and diversity of clinical respiratory infection episodes are only the "tip of the iceberg" in relation to the number of viral assaults occurring in the close-

FIGURE 6.6.

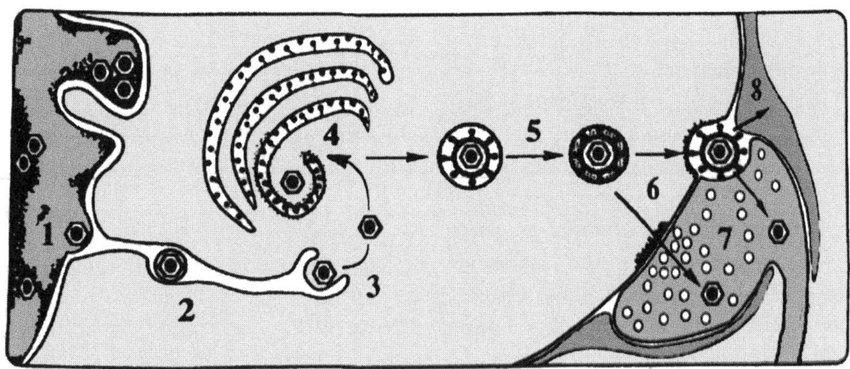

Events leading to the passage of pseudorabies virus across the junction between nerve cells on its centripetal intraaxonal transit to the brain: (1) Virions replicate in the nucleus of a peripheral nerve cell, acquiring an envelope as they bud from the inner lamella of the nuclear envelope. (2) Virions traverse the endoplasmic reticulum. (3) Virions are subsequently released into the cytoplasm after a fusion event between the virion envelope and endoplasmic reticulum membrane. (4) Virions acquire another envelope at the Golgi apparatus. (5) Virions are transported across the cytoplasm in vacuoles. (6) Virions enter the next neuron by fusion of the viral envelope and plasma membrane at a synaptic terminus. (7) Virions, now without their envelope, are carried centrally by retrograde axoplasmic flow, reaching the cell body and nucleus of the neuron where further replication occurs. The process continues, eventually bringing the virus to the brain where necrotizing encephalitis follows. (8) Some virions invade and replicate in the Schwann cells of the myelin sheaths surrounding neurons, thereby amplifying the amount of virus available to invade neurons. [From J. P. Card, L. Rinaman, R. B. Lynn, B. H. Lee, R. P. Meade, R. R. Miselis, and L. W. Enquist. Pseudorabies virus infection of the rat central nervous system: Ultrastructural characterization of viral replication, transport and pathogenesis. *J. Neurosci.* **13,** 2515–2539 (1993). With permission.]

contact environment of many animals. It is estimated that viruses are the cause of more than 90% of upper respiratory infections and the predisposing trigger for many "mixed etiology" lower respiratory infections. Different viruses are considered to favor different levels in the respiratory tract, from the nasal turbinates to the alveoli, but there is more overlap than is usually appreciated. For example, influenza viruses primarily cause tracheitis, bronchitis, and only to a lesser extent alveolar infection and pneumonia in mammals, whereas bovine respiratory syncytial virus primarily causes bronchiolitis. At whatever level of the respiratory tree that is involved, infection leads to (1) local cessation of cilial beating, (2) local loss of integrity of the overlying mucus layer, and (3) multifocal destruction of small numbers of epithelial cells. There is progressive infection of epithelial cells at the edges of such lesions; more and more cells are invaded until there are large denuded patches. The coincident influx of inflammatory cells and transudated fluid continues to damage the mucous protective layer and lay bare more and more epithelial cells and eventually in the most severe infections there is acidosis, edema, and massive epithelial sloughing.

Accumulation in the airways, especially in the narrow-diameter airways of small animal species and newborns, of transudates, exudates, inflammatory infiltrates, and necrotic epithelial cell debris leads to a local state of anoxia and respiratory distress. Total plugging of small airways can cause anoxic death, again, especially in animals with the narrowest airways and least lung capacity to dislodge debris. In animals that survive, at this stage of infection airways are lined by a layer of flat, undifferentiated basal epithelial cells that are resistant to further progression of the infection. These cells lack viral receptors and likely are temporarily protected by interferons. By the time these cells differentiate into ciliated and mucus-secreting columnar epithelial cells, the evolving host immune response protects them from continuing rounds of infection.

Infection of the Intestinal Tract

The intestinal epithelium is usually infected directly by ingested virions, but sometimes viremic infections reach the intestinal epithelium, also causing enteritis and diarrhea. The pathophysiologic effects of viral diarrhea are a consequence of rapid destruction of epithelial cells and their replacement by immature, transitional cells that cannot carry out normal absorptive, resorptive, and enzyme secretory functions. Glucose-coupled sodium transport is impaired, disaccharidase (lactase, sucrase) activities are diminished, and, in some cases, adenylate cyclase and cyclic AMP levels are increased (the latter causing a hypersecretion of water and chlorides). The disturbance to the osmotic equilibrium is most severe in newborns because of the normal presence of high concentrations of milk lactose in the intestinal lumen.

Osmotic equilibrium returns when the regenerating intestinal epithelium matures sufficiently to produce lactase and to absorb the hexoses resulting from the enzymatic breakdown of milk lactose.

Although the pathophysiologic mechanism of diarrhea is similar whatever the etiologic agent, there are differences in clinical and epidemiologic manifestations of disease caused by each of the important groups of diarrhea viruses, namely rotaviruses, caliciviruses, coronaviruses, toroviruses, and parvoviruses (see Chapters 9 and 10). In infections caused by most of these viruses, it is the differentiated cells at the tips and upper parts of villi that are involved primarily. In feline and canine parvovirus enteritis, it is the cells in the crypts that are in S phase of the cell division cycle that are destroyed. The destruction of crypt cells and the consequent failure of the process of replacement of cells lost by normal sloughing at the tips of villi leads to the same sort of imbalance in the absorptive and secretory functions of villus epithelium as occurs when cells at the tips of villi are infected—in some cases repair takes longer when crypt cells are destroyed (the cell division cycle of crypt cells is about 8 hours). In all cases, villi become blunted and club shaped and there is progressive further epithelial necrosis and desquamation.

Nearly all intestinal viral infections are localized to the intestinal epithelium (and to a lesser extent to cells of the lamina propria). The failure to penetrate further may represent an evolutionary progression on the part of the viruses that maximizes the shedding capacity and transmissibility without destroying the host population.

Infection of the Skin

As well as being a site of initial infection, the skin may be invaded secondarily via the bloodstream, producing erythema (inflammation), which may be generalized but more often is localized and seen readily on exposed, hairless, nonpigmented areas such as the snout, ears, paws, scrotum, and udder. Infection of the skin may also result in a rash. Individual lesions in generalized rashes are described as *macules, papules, vesicles,* and *pustules.* Lasting localized dilation of dermal blood vessels produces macules. Macules become papules if there is also localized edema and infiltration of cells into the area. Primary localized involvement of the epidermis or separation of the epidermis from the dermis by fluid pressure results in the formation of vesicles. Localized erosion or sloughing of epithelium results in ulceration and scabbing, but prior to this vesicles may be converted to pustules by neutrophil infiltration. More severe involvement of the dermal vessels may lead to petechial or hemorrhagic lesions, although coagulation defects and thrombocytopenia may also be important in the genesis of such lesions. Viral exanthems, such as those caused by poxviruses in various animals, usually present a progression through these lesions, in most cases terminating with full resolution or fatal progressive systemic disease.

Infection of the Central Nervous System

Because of the controlling physiologic importance of the central nervous system and its vulnerability to damage by any process that damages neurons directly or indirectly via increased intracranial pressure, viral invasion of the central nervous system is always a serious matter. Viruses can spread from distal sites to the brain via nerves, as already described. Viruses can also spread from the blood to the brain, but first they must overcome the obstacle of the blood–brain barrier. This anatomic and functional barrier is made up of capillary endothelial cells with tight junctions, vascular basement lamina, and choroid plexus and ependymal epithelia with tight junctions. However, despite knowledge of this microanatomy, little is known about how most viruses transit this barrier and gain entrance into the parenchyma of the central nervous system. Studies using inert particles the same size as viruses have shown that there is no absolute hindrance to direct movement across capillary walls, yet some small viruses seem to penetrate this barrier whereas others do not. Some viruses are able to infect the endothelium of deep capillaries and "grow across" the barrier; others localize in blood vessels in the meninges and invade by progressive extension from that site, and yet others infect the choroid plexus and ependyma, with invasion of the brain parenchyma then occurring via the cerebrospinal fluid. Rarely, virus may be carried across capillary walls into the brain parenchyma via carriage in infected leukocytes (Figure 6.7).

Subsequent spread in the central nervous system can take place via intercellular spaces or by the sequential infection of neural cells. Lytic infections of neurons, whether due to togaviruses, herpesviruses, or other viruses, lead to the three histologic hallmarks of encephalitis; neuronal necrosis, phagocytosis of neurons (neuronophagia), and perivascular infiltrations of mononuclear cells (perivascular cuffing), the latter two reflecting the immune response to infection. In some infections these hallmarks are not seen and the cause of clinical neurologic signs is more obscure. For example, although street rabies virus infection of neurons is noncytocidal and evokes little inflammatory reaction, it is uniformly lethal for most mammalian species.

FIGURE 6.7.

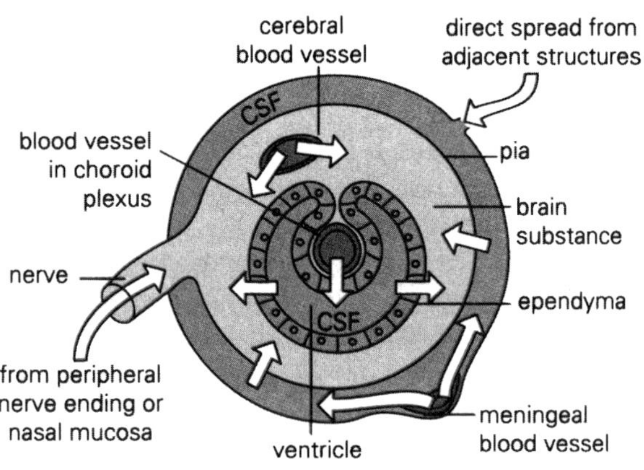

Routes of viral invasion of the central nervous system. [From C. A. Mims, J. H. Playfair, I. M. Roitt, D. Wakelin, and R. Williams, "Medical Microbiology." Mosby, St. Louis, MO, 1993.]

Other characteristic pathologic changes are produced by various viruses and prions that cause slowly progressive diseases of the central nervous system. In bovine spongiform encephalopathy in cattle and scrapie in sheep, for example, there is slow progressive neuronal degeneration and vacuolization, and in maedi/visna virus infection of sheep there are changes in glial cells that lead to demyelination.

In most cases, central nervous system infection seems to be a dead end in the natural history of viruses, i.e., shedding and transmission of most neurotropic viruses do not depend on pathogenetic events in the nervous system. For example, in the encephalitis caused by canine distemper virus (and its late manifestation, old dog encephalitis), virus may be recovered from brain tissue long after the acute phase of infection, but only by methods such as cocultivation and explant culture and never under circumstances where transmission might occur.

Togavirus, flavivirus, and bunyavirus encephalitides represent dead ends also; in these cases, it is the extraneural sites of virus replication that generate the viremia and thereby sustain transmission by allowing the infection of the next arthropod host. The exceptions to this generalization are important, however. Alphaherpesviruses depend on the delivery of virus from cranial and spinal sensory ganglia to epithelial sites. Epithelial shedding, which follows on recrudescent virus emergence from ganglia, is important because it offers the opportunity for transmission long after primary lesions have resolved. There are other examples where virus seemingly trapped in the nervous system may become the source for transmission. For example, in the epidemic of bovine spongiform encephalopathy in the United Kingdom, transmission occurred through inclusion of sheep and subsequently cattle central nervous system tissue in meat and bone meal fed to cattle. Transmission of rabies and other neurotropic viruses to humans has occurred via laboratory aerosolization of animal brain material. All in all, it seems anomalous that neurotropism should be the outstanding characteristic of so many of the most notorious pathogens of animals and zoonotic pathogens of humans and yet be the pathogenetic characteristic least related to virus perpetuation in nature. The irreparable damage that is of such grave consequence to the host is of such little consequence to the virus.

Infection of the Lymphoreticular and Hematopoietic Systems

Most cell types in the lymphoreticular and hematopoietic lineages are the targets of one or more viral pathogens. In every case the interaction between cell and virus is complex and intertwined with the immune response. Infection and damage of reticuloendothelial and lymphoid tissues assures an invading virus protection from phagocytic removal and from inflammatory or immunological inactivation. Some of the most destructive and lethal viruses known exhibit this tropism: filoviruses, arenaviruses, hantaviruses, certain bunyaviruses such as Rift Valley fever virus, Venezuelan equine encephalitis virus, and yellow fever virus. Commonly, invasion starts with phagocytic viral uptake by dendritic macrophages, such as occurs in the marginal zones of lymph nodes, thymus, bone marrow, Peyer's patches, and the white pulp of the spleen. Later, virus shed from these cells infects nearby lymphoid cells, leading to overwhelming lymphoid dysfunction and destruction. In the course of these destructive events, nearby hematopoietic cells are often caught up and destroyed as well. These events are becoming more appreciated; for example, they are now recognized in the progression that is operative in the early stages of several retrovirus infections (feline leukemia virus infection, maedi/visna virus infection).

Infection of the Fetus

Most viral infections of the dam have no harmful effect on the fetus, but some blood-borne viruses cross the placenta to reach the fetal circulation, sometimes after establishing foci of infection in the placenta (Table 6.5).

Severe cytolytic infections of the fetus cause fetal death and resorption or abortion; these outcomes

Table 6.5
Viral Infections of the Fetus or Embryo

Animal	Family/Genus	Virus	Syndrome
Cattle	*Herpesviridae/Varicellovirus*	Infectious bovine rhinotracheitis virus	Fetal death, abortion
	Retroviridae/Deltaretrovirus	Bovine leukemia virus	Inapparent infection, leukemia
	Reoviridae/Orbivirus	Bluetongue virus	Fetal death, abortion, congenital defects
	Bunyaviridae/Bunyavirus	Akabane virus	Fetal death, abortion, stillbirth, congenital defects
	Flaviviridae/Pestivirus	Bovine viral diarrhea virus	Fetal death, abortion, congenital defects, inapparent infection with lifelong carrier state and shedding
Horses	*Herpesviridae/Varicellovirus*	Equine herpesvirus 1	Fetal death, abortion, neonatal disease
	Arteriviridae/Arterivirus	Equine arteritis virus	Fetal death, abortion
Swine	*Herpesviridae/Varicellovirus*	Pseudorabies virus	Fetal death, abortion
	Parvoviridae/Parvovirus	Swine parvovirus	Fetal death, abortion, mummification, stillbirth, infertility
	Flaviviridae/Flavivirus	Japanese encephalitis virus	Fetal death, abortion
	Flaviviridae/Pestivirus	Hog cholera virus	Fetal death, abortion, congenital defects, inapparent infection with lifelong carrier state and shedding
Sheep	*Reoviridae/Orbivirus*	Bluetongue viruses	Fetal death, abortion, congenital defects
	Bunyaviridae/Phlebovirus	Rift Valley fever virus	Fetal death, abortion
	Bunyaviridae/Nairovirus	Nairobi sheep disease virus	Fetal death, abortion
	Flaviviridae/Pestivirus	Border disease virus	Congenital defects
Dogs	*Herpesviridae*/ungrouped	Canine herpesvirus	Perinatal death
Cats	*Parvoviridae/Parvovirus*	Feline panleukopenia virus	Cerebellar hypoplasia
	Retroviridae/Gammaretrovirus	Feline leukemia virus	Inapparrent, leukemia, fetal death
Mice	*Parvoviridae/Parvovirus*	Rat virus	Fetal death
	Arenaviridae/Arenavirus	Lymphocytic choriomeningitis virus	Inapparent, with lifelong carrier state and shedding
Chicken	*Picornaviridae/Enterovirus*	Avian encephalomyelitis virus	Congenital defects, fetal death
	Retroviridae/Alpharetrovirus	Avian leukosis/sarcoma viruses	Inapparent, leukemia, other diseases

are common in, for example, pseudorabies and parvovirus infections in swine. Also important are the teratogenic effects of less lethal viruses such as bovine viral diarrhea virus and Akabane virus infections in cattle and sheep.

The outcome of infections of pregnant animals with teratogenic viruses is influenced to a great extent by gestational age. Generally, infection in the early period of gestation is most damaging, usually leading to fetal death and abortion. Maternal infection with viremia, often subclinical in nature, leads to the subsequent transplacental passage of virus. Later in pregnancy the outcome of infection is influenced by the developing fetal immune response. For example, infection of piglets with porcine parvovirus after days 65 to 70 of gestation does not result in death but in fetal antibody production and normal birth. When bovine viral diarrhea virus infects the fetus in the first half of gestation, immune tolerance is established, leading to lifelong virus persistence and chronic disease. When the infection occurs late in gestation, an effective immune response usually eliminates the virus and there is no disease. When viral replication in the fetus is rapid, as in alphaherpesvirus infections in horses, cattle, swine, and dogs, fetal death and abortion can occur, even during the last trimester of pregnancy.

Infection of Other Organs

Almost any organ may be infected via the bloodstream with one or another kind of virus, but most viruses have well-defined organ and tissue tropisms. The clinical importance of infection of various organs and tissues depends, in part, on their role in the physiologic well-being of the animal. The critical importance of the brain, heart, and lungs is self-evident, and invasion of the liver, causing severe hepatitis, as in Rift Valley fever and infectious canine hepatitis, is also usually a life-threatening situation. Infection of muscle cells occurs with several togaviruses and coxsackieviruses, whereas infection of the synovial cells of goats by caprine arthritis–encephalitis virus produces arthritis. Infection of the salivary glands or mammary glands may lead to lesions in those organs and excretion of virus in saliva or milk. One virus or another employs virtually every organ and tissue in the animal body as its primary target—given the harsh Darwinian selective pressures that drive viral evolution, there is likely to be survival value and purpose in every viral tropism and pathogenetic mechanism that we uncover. Here is an area of veterinary medical research that still has far to go before we have adequate understanding.

Mechanisms of Virus Shedding

Shedding of infectious virions is crucial to the maintenance of infection in populations (see Chapter 14). Exit usually occurs from one of the body openings or surfaces that are involved in viral entry. With viruses that cause infection only in cells at one or another body surface (particularly respiratory and intestinal epithelium), the same body opening is involved in entry and exit (Figure 6.1); in generalized infections, a greater variety of sites of shedding is recognized (Figure 6.4), and some viruses are shed from multiple sites. The amount of virus shed in an excretion or secretion is important in relation to transmission. Very low concentrations may be irrelevant unless very large volumes of infected material are involved; however, some viruses occur in such high concentrations that a minute quantity of virus-laden secretion or excretion can lead to transmission to the next animal host.

Viral Shedding from the Respiratory Tract

Many different viruses that cause localized disease of the respiratory tract are shed in mucus or saliva and are expelled from the respiratory tract during coughing, sneezing, eating, and drinking. Respiratory viruses, such as bovine herpesvirus 1, paramyxoviruses, some coronaviruses, and bovine respiratory syncytial virus, are excreted in both nasal and oral secretions. Viruses are also shed from the respiratory tract in several systemic infections.

Viral Shedding from the Oropharynx and Intestinal Tract

Enteric viruses are shed in the feces, and the more voluminous the fluid output the greater is the environmental contamination they cause. Enteric viruses are in general more resistant to inactivation by environmental conditions than respiratory viruses; especially when suspended in water, such viruses can persist for some time.

A few viruses are shed into the oral cavity from infected salivary glands (e.g., rabies virus and cytomegaloviruses) or from the lungs or nasal mucosa. Salivary spread depends on activities such as licking, nuzzling, grooming, or biting. Viral shedding in saliva may continue during convalescence or recurrently thereafter, especially with herpesviruses.

Viral Shedding from the Skin

The skin is an important source of virus in diseases in which transmission is by direct contact or via small abrasions: cowpox, vaccinia, orf, pseudocowpox, and molluscum contagiosum viruses, as well as papillomaviruses and herpesviruses employ this mode of transmission. Although skin lesions are produced in several generalized diseases, in only a few are viruses shed from skin lesions. However, foot-and-mouth disease viruses and vesicular stomatitis viruses and swine vesicular disease virus are produced in great quantities in vesicular mucosal lesions and are then shed as vesicles break. Localization of virus in the feather follicles is important in the shedding of Marek's disease virus by infected chickens.

Viral Shedding from the Urinary Tract

Urine, like feces, tends to contaminate food supplies and the environment. A number of viruses (e.g., rinderpest virus, infectious canine hepatitis virus, foot-and-mouth disease viruses, and arenaviruses) replicate in tubular epithelial cells in the kidney and are shed in urine. Viruria is prolonged and common in equine rhinovirus 1 infection and lifelong in arenavirus infections of reservoir host rodents and constitutes the principal mode of contamination of the environment by these viruses.

Viral Shedding from the Genital Tract

Several viruses that cause important diseases of cattle, horses, and sheep are excreted in the semen and are transmitted during coitus. For example, equine arteritis virus persists for long periods in the accessory sexual glands of fertile stallions. Viruses shed from the genital tract depend on mucosal contact for successful transmission.

Viral Shedding in Milk

Several viruses replicate in the mammary gland and are excreted in milk, which may serve as a route of transmission, e.g., caprine arthritis–encephalitis virus, mouse mammary tumor virus, and some of the tick-borne flaviviruses.

Viral Shedding via Blood and Tissues

Although not "shedding" in the usual sense of the word, blood and tissues from slaughtered animals must be considered important sources of viral contagion. Blood is the usual source from which arthropods acquire viruses, and blood may also be the source of viruses transferred to the avian egg or mammalian fetus. As noted earlier, mechanical transmission by arthropods ("flying needles") is important in veterinary medicine: equine infectious anemia virus and bovine leukemia virus may be transmitted by biting flies that feed intermittently on animals. Virus-laden blood is also the basis for transmission when it contaminates needles and other equipment used by veterinarians and others treating or handling sick animals.

Infection without Shedding

Many sites of viral replication might be considered "dead ends" from the point of view of natural transmission to the next host. One might question the role of any target organ not connected with a body surface, but on further reflection it becomes clear that viral replication in many organs can contribute indirectly to viral transmission. For example, carnivores and omnivores may be infected by consuming virus-laden meat or tissues. In the past, hog cholera, African swine fever, and vesicular exanthema of swine viruses were often transmitted through feeding garbage containing contaminated pork scraps. The epidemic of bovine spongiform encephalopathy in the United Kingdom was most likely triggered by the feeding of meat and bone meal containing scrapie-infected sheep offal to cattle; it clearly then was transmitted widely among cattle by the feeding of meat and bone meal containing bovine offal.

Many retroviruses are not shed at all, but instead are transmitted directly in the germplasm or by infection of the avian egg or developing mammalian embryo—these viruses accomplish the same ends as those shed into the environment, i.e., transmission to new hosts and perpetuation in nature.

Further Reading

Collier, L. H. ed. (1997). "Topley and Wilson's Microbiology and Microbial Infections," 6 vol. Edward Arnold, London.

Connor, D. H., Chandler, F. W., Schwartz, D. A., Manz, H. J., and Lack, E. E. (1997). "Pathology of Infectious Diseases." Appleton & Lange, Stamford, CT.

Fenner, F. (1949). Mousepox (infectious ectromelia of mice): A review. *J. Immunol.* **63**, 341–373.

Johnson, R. T. (1982). "Viral Infections of the Nervous System." Raven, New York.

Jubb, K. V. F., Kennedy, P. C., and Palmer, N., eds. (1993). "Pathology of Domestic Animals," 4th ed. Academic Press, San Diego, CA.

Knipe, D. M. (1996). Virus-host cell interactions. *In* "Fields Virology" (B. N. Fields, D. M. Knipe, P. M. Howley, R. M., Chanock, J. L. Melnick, T. P. Monath, B. Roizman, and S. E. Straus, eds.), 3rd ed., pp. 273–299. Lippincott-Raven, Philadelphia, PA.

Mims, C. A. (1989). The pathogenetic basis of viral tropism. *Am. J. Pathol.* **135**, 447–488.

Mims, C. A., and White, D. O. (1984). "Viral Pathogenesis and Immunology." Blackwell Scientific Publications, Oxford.

Mims, C. A., Dimmock, N., Nash, A., and Stephen, J. (1995). "Mims' Pathogenesis of Infectious Disease," 4th ed. Academic Press, London.

Nathanson, N., Ahmed, R., Gonzalez-Scarano, F., Griffin, D. E., Holmes, K. V., Murphy, F. A., and Robinson, H. L., eds. (1997). "Viral Pathogenesis." Lippincott-Raven, Philadelphia, PA.

Tyler, K. L. (1998). Pathogenesis. *In* "Encyclopedia of Virology" (R. G. Webster and A. Granoff, eds.), 2nd ed. (CD-ROM). Academic Press, London.

Tyler, K. L., and Fields, B. N. (1996). Pathogenesis of viral infections. *In* "Fields Virology" (B. N. Fields, D. M. Knipe, P. M. Howley, R. M. Chanock, J. L. Melnick, T. P. Monath, B. Roizman, and S. E. Straus, eds.), 3rd ed., pp. 173–218. Lippincott-Raven, Philadelphia, PA.

CHAPTER 7

Determinants of Viral Virulence and Host Resistance/Susceptibility

Infection is not synonymous with disease. Many infections are *subclinical (asymptomatic, inapparent),* whereas others result in *disease,* with varying degrees of severity and characteristic, identifiable clinical signs (Figure 7.1). The outcome of the virus–host encounter is the product of the *virulence* of the infecting virus on the one hand and the susceptibility of the host on the other. The term virulence is used as a quantitative or relative measure of the *pathogenicity* of the infecting virus, i.e., a virus is said to be *pathogenic* or *nonpathogenic,* but its virulence is stated in relative terms ("virus A is more virulent than virus B" or "virus strain A is more virulent in animal species Y than species Z"). The terms pathogenicity and virulence refer to the capacity of a virus to cause disease in the host animal, not to the properties of *infectiousness* or *transmissibility,* properties that are discussed in Chapter 14.

Interplay of Viral Virulence and Host Resistance/Susceptibility Factors

Viruses may differ greatly in their virulence; conversely, within an animal population infected by a particular virus there are often striking differences in the outcome of infection depending on resistance/susceptibility factors operating at the level of the individual animal. The determinants of viral virulence are usually *multigenic,* and the determinants of host resistance/susceptibility are usually *multifactorial.* In recent years, the application of molecular genetic technologies has made it possible to map virulence determinants in the viral genome (e.g., by site-directed mutagenesis, recombination, reassortment) and resistance determinants in the host experimental animal genome (e.g., by use of knockout mice, chimeric mice), thereby adding a new level of analysis of these determinants. Virus strain differences may be *quantitative,* involving the rate and yield of virus replication, the number of cells infected in a given organ, or they may be *qualitative,* involving organ or tissue *tropism,* level of host cell damage, mode and efficacy of spread in the body, and character of the disease (disease pathogenesis, see Chapters 6 and 9). Virus strain differences, usually multigenic in nature, are of course also the basis of attenuated virus vaccines.

Within a susceptible outbred population in nature, the resistance or susceptibility of individual animals varies not only with their genetic constitution (which may affect, among other things, their capacity to mount a rapid immune response), but also with their age, nutritional status, level of stress, other hormonal factors, and many other factors. Together, these genetic and physiologic factors determine what is called the *nonspecific (natural, innate)* resistance of the host, in contrast to the

FIGURE 7.1.

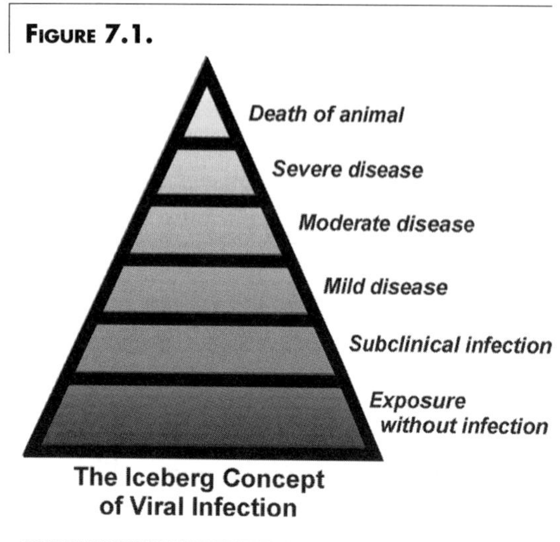

The iceberg concept of viral infection and disease.

specific (acquired) resistance to infection and reinfection that results from the intervention of the specific immune response, as described in Chapter 8.

Assessment of Viral Virulence

In nature, viral virulence may vary over a wide range, from strains of virus that almost always cause inapparent infections, to those that usually cause disease, to those that usually cause death. Meaningful comparison of the virulence of viruses requires that factors such as the infecting viral dose, the age, sex, and condition of the host animals and their specific immune status be equal; however, these conditions are never met in nature or in clinical practice where heterogeneous outbred animal populations are the rule and viral exposure and infection dynamics are incredibly varied. Hence, qualities describing the virulence of particular viruses in domestic and wild animals are usually stated in vague terms—precise measures of virulence are usually derived from assays in inbred animals, such as inbred strains of mice. Of course, such assays are only feasible for those viruses of clinical interest that grow in mice, and when this approach is employed, care must be taken in extrapolating from mice to the host species of interest.

The virulence of a particular strain of virus administered in a particular dose, by a particular route, to a particular age and strain of a laboratory animal may be assessed in various quantitative ways. Measures of the capacity of the virus to produce disease, death, specific clinical signs, or particular histopathologic lesions have been used for many years. The dose of the virus required to cause death in 50% of animals (lethal dose 50, LD_{50}) is a valuable measure of the character of the virus. For example, in the susceptible BALB/c strain of mouse, the LD_{50} of a virulent strain of ectromelia virus is 5 virions, compared with 5000 for a moderately attenuated strain and about 1 million for a highly attenuated strain.

Viral virulence can also be measured in experimental animals by determining the ratio of the dose of a particular strain of virus that causes infection in 50% of individuals (infectious dose 50, ID_{50}) to the dose that kills 50% of individuals (the ID_{50}/LD_{50} ratio). Thus with a virulent strain of ectromelia virus, tested in highly susceptible BALB/c mice, the ID_{50} is 1–2 virions and the LD_{50} about 5 virions, whereas for resistant C57BL strain mice the ID_{50} is the same but the LD_{50} is 1 million virions. The severity of an infection, therefore, depends on the interplay between the virulence of the virus and the resistance of the host.

Assessment of histopathologic lesions can also be a valuable measure of viral virulence—the severity and location of lesions, even ultrastructural pathologic changes, have provided valuable insight in many instances where the virulence of a virus has been in question. For example, the virulence of various rabies virus strains that had been used in attenuated virus vaccines for dogs and cats were compared and although their occasional lethality was difficult to assess, some were found to cause necrotic, inflammatory lesions in the brains of intracerebrally inoculated mice. These strains were reviewed more carefully and found to be the most troublesome in clinical use—vaccines containing these viruses were removed from the marketplace.

Variability in the response of individual animals to infection is observed regularly during epidemics. For example, during an outbreak of Venezuelan equine encephalitis, some horses die, whereas others suffer a brief illness but quickly recover. The great majority of arbovirus and many other viral infections are subclinical; for every individual animal that develops encephalitis during an epidemic, many more will have no clinical signs and the only evidence of infection will be a sharp rise in antibody titer. The dose of infecting virus may play a part in determining such differences, but genetic and physiologic factors in the host seem to be more important. Certainly in instances like this, caution is called for in attributing epidemic characteristics to viral virulence.

One can regard an acute infection as a race between the capacity of the virus to replicate, spread in the body, and cause disease versus the capacity of the host to curtail and control these events (see Chapter 6). Because of the variables in this race, one individual animal may not be seriously affected even by a virulent strain of virus, whereas another animal, usually one with a low level of innate or acquired resistance, may be endangered by a relatively avirulent strain of virus.

Determinants of Viral Virulence

Unraveling the genetic basis of viral virulence has long been one of the major goals of animal virology, and also one of the most difficult to achieve, as many viral genes are involved in the course and outcome of infection. With advances in molecular genetics it has been possible to dissect the problem in a more precise way. Of necessity, most experimental work has been carried out in inbred laboratory animals.

With viruses causing acute infections, those with segmented genomes (orthomyxoviruses, bunyaviruses, arenaviruses, reoviruses, birnaviruses) have provided the most easily manipulated experimental models. Each segment of the genome of these viruses is equivalent to one gene (in most cases) and reassortants between strains can be obtained readily. Study of large numbers of reassortant viruses carrying different combinations of genome segments from parental viruses with known phenotypic characters allows the functions that relate to virulence to be assigned to particular genes. For example, the function of each gene of reovirus 1 and 3 has been determined, virulence characters assigned, and differences in the pathogenesis of infections caused by the two viruses explained.

Using a different approach, the basis of canine parvovirus virulence has been explained in great detail: in this case, nucleotide sequence comparisons of the genomes of different wild-type viruses with those of avirulent vaccine strains have allowed identification of nucleotide changes (and by extension amino acid changes) responsible for virulence and attenuation. Investigations with poxviruses have revealed the complexity of the armamentarium of viral gene products directed against various components of innate and acquired host resistance. Investigations of herpesvirus infections of several animal species have gone a long way to explain the complex genetic basis of persistent infection, latency, and recrudescence that has made these infections so difficult to deal with in veterinary practice (see Chapter 10). Studies have been conducted with retroviruses to explain the genetic basis of cellular transformation and oncogenicity (see Chapter 11). Further examples are provided at the end of this chapter to illustrate how molecular biology has opened up the new field of *molecular pathogenesis.*

Most viral genes encode proteins that are essential for viral replication, notably those required for viral entry into the principal host cells, replication of the viral genome, production of viral proteins, and assembly/release of new virions. A second class of viral genes has evolved to maximize the yield of virions by down-regulating the expression of cellular genes and up-regulating the expression of particular viral genes at appropriate times in the replication cycle. A third class of viral genes (*virokines,* see later) has been recognized, which is not involved in viral replication per se, but which enhances the spread and ultimate titer of virus in the body as a whole, principally by suppressing the host's immune response.

Viral Tropism and Dissemination and Resistance/Susceptibility to Viral Infections

All viruses exhibit host and tissue specificity (tropism), usually more than is appreciated clinically. Mechanistically, the organ or tissue tropism of the virus is an expression of all the steps in cellular infection: the correspondence between viral attachment molecules *(ligands)* and cellular receptors (see later); the viral functions that assure penetration of the cell and viral uncoating; the efficacy of the viral replicative machinery; and other factors that govern successful viral infection of the host cell (see Chapter 3). Organ and tissue tropisms also involve all stages in the course of infection in the whole host animal, from the site of entry, to the major target organs responsible for the clinical signs, to the site involved in shedding. Tropisms of the viruses that are important in veterinary medical practice are described throughout Part II of this book; an illustration of the diversity and precision of tropism of specific viruses for particular cells in one tissue/organ system, the immune system, is provided in Table 7.1.

Mouse hepatitis virus, the cause of the most important disease in mouse colonies worldwide, provides an example of the effect of organ and tissue tropism as a determinant of viral virulence. Particular strains of wild-type mouse hepatitis virus replicate in intestinal epithelial cells and cause lethal diarrhea—this is the tropism that is most devastating in mouse colonies because so much virus is shed that spread is very efficient. Other strains replicate mainly in hepatocytes, the tropism that originally gave the virus its name. Yet other strains replicate in both neurons and oligodendroglia and cause acutely fatal encephalomyelitis as a result of neuronal destruction. Variant substrains, however, show marked reduction in their neuronotropism and do not kill their hosts acutely, but rather produce persistent infection of oligodendroglia leading to demyelination and hind limb paralysis. This range of clinical presentations, the cause of many diagnostic puzzles over the years, is simply a matter of viral variants exhibiting different tropisms.

Table 7.1
Viruses That Infect Cells of the Immune System

Cell	Virus
T lymphocytes	Feline leukemia virus
	Feline immunodeficiency virus
	Simian immunodeficiency virus
	Human immunodeficiency viruses 1 and 2
B lymphocytes	Equine herpesvirus 2
	Simian type D retrovirus
	Murine leukemia virus
	Infectious bursal disease virus (fowl)
	Infectious pancreatic necrosis virus (fish)
	Epstein–Barr virus (human)
Monocytes	Canine distemper virus
	Influenza viruses (horse, fowl, human)
	Venezuelan equine encephalitis virus (horse, human)
	Parainfluenza viruses (cattle, human, several host species)
	Maedi/visna virus (sheep)
	Caprine arthritis–encephalitis virus
	Lymphocytic choriomeningitis virus (mouse, hamster)
	Lactate dehydrogenase elevating virus (mouse)
	Cytomegaloviruses (many host species)
Dendritic cells	Venezuelan equine encephalitis virus (horse, human)
	Lymphocytic choriomeningitis virus (mouse, hamster)
	Human immunodeficiency viruses 1 and 2
Stromal cells of lymphoreticular tissues	Borna disease virus (horse, rabbit, cat)
	Cytomegalovirus (many host species)

Viral *dissemination* from primary sites of replication represents an extension of the concept of tropism. Viremia, either as free extracellular virions or as virus-infected circulating cells, is a crucial step in the dissemination of many viruses that cause systemic disease. It can be a key virulence determinant. Reduction in the titer or duration of viremia can have a major influence on the outcome of infection, which is especially important in central nervous system infections. Here, the outcome of the viral assault on the blood–brain barrier is often determined by the concentration of virus present in brain capillaries. The same is true for viruses such as rabies and herpesviruses (e.g., pseudorabies virus and B virus) that are disseminated by the neural route—the more virus present at peripheral nerve endings the more nerve fibers that become involved in transporting virus to the brain.

Viral Enhancers, Promoters, and Transcription Factors and Resistance/Susceptibility to Viral Infections

Enhancers are a class of gene activators that increase the efficiency of transcription of viral or cellular genes. These nucleotide sequences often contain a number of motifs representing DNA-binding sites for various cellular or viral site-specific DNA-binding proteins (transcription factors). They bring about augmented binding of DNA-dependent RNA polymerase II to promoters, thereby accelerating transcription. Because many of the transcription factors affecting particular enhancer sequences in viral genomes as well as cellular genomes are restricted to particular cells, tissues, or host species, they can determine the tropism of viruses and can act as specific virulence factors. Enhancer sequences have been defined in the genomes of retroviruses, herpesviruses, and hepadnaviruses, and in all cases these appear to influence the tropism of the viruses by regulating the expression of viral genes in specific types of cells.

Virokines and Resistance/Susceptibility to Viral Infections

Virokines comprise a class of virus-coded proteins that are not required for viral replication *in vitro,* but influence the pathogenesis of infection *in vivo* by sabotaging the body's innate resistance or immune response. Virokines can be grouped as (1) inhibitors of T cell cytotoxicity that bind nascent class I MHC protein; (2) inhibitors of cytokines, such as interleukin 1, interferon γ and tumor necrosis-factor α; (3) inhibitors of the complement cascade; (4) inhibitors of antibody-mediated cytolysis; and (5) cytokine mimics, e.g., interleukin 10. Many virokines mimic normal cellular molecules involved in the immune response, such as cytokines and cytokine receptors. For example, three virokines encoded by poxviruses closely resemble the receptors for tumor necrosis factor α, interferon γ, and interluekin 1. So far, virokines seem to be confined to large DNA viruses—poxviruses, herpesviruses, and adenovirus—and to retroviruses. The number of genes involved is considerable; more than a quarter of all the genes of vaccinia virus can be deleted without impeding its replication in cell culture, although such deletion mutants are attenuated *in vivo*. Currently only a few vaccinia virus genes have been identified as virokines, but their diversity already indicates that we may have only begun to unravel this important new area of molecular pathogenesis.

Determinants of Host Resistance/Susceptibility

Genetic differences in resistance/susceptibility to viral infections are most obvious when different animal species are compared. Common viral infections often tend to be less pathogenic in their natural host species than in exotic or introduced species. For instance, myxoma virus produces a small benign fibroma in its natural host, the wild rabbit of South America, *Sylvilagus brasiliensis,* but an almost invariably fatal generalized infection in the European domestic rabbit, *Oryctolagus cuniculus.* Likewise, most *zoonoses* (diseases caused by viruses transmitted from animals to humans), such as arenavirus, filovirus, and various arbovirus diseases, are more severe in humans than in their reservoir hosts.

Accurate data on the bases of variations in resistance to infection are difficult to obtain from outbred animal populations in nature, largely because genetic, physiologic, and environmental differences are generally confounding. With inbred strains of mice, however, it has been possible to study the genetics of resistance to viral infection in some detail. Having identified a susceptible (S) and a resistant (R) mouse strain, the LD_{50} assay is repeated in (S × R) F1 and F2 backcrossed mice to determine whether a single gene is responsible and whether susceptibility or resistance is dominant. Then, recombinant or congenic strains can be constructed, with a common genetic background differing only in the gene in question. In this way, resistance/susceptibility to a few viruses has been mapped to particular genes. Often such experiments become quite complicated as additional genes that influence resistance/susceptibility in quite different ways have been found. For example, the response of mice to murine leukemia viruses is influenced by over a dozen genes, whereas the response to murine cytomegalovirus is influenced secondarily by one gene that maps to the major histocompatibility complex (MHC) region and a second gene that determines by unknown means the titer of virus in the spleen.

Immune Response Genes and Resistance/Susceptibility to Viral Infections

Immune responsiveness to particular viral infections differs greatly from one individual animal to another, being under the control of specific *immune response (Ir)* genes. There are many of these antigen-specific immunoregulatory genes, most of them situated in the MHC. Susceptibility of mice to infection with some viruses, e.g., cytomegaloviruses, retroviruses and lymphocytic choriomeningitus virus, has been linked to particular MHC genotypes. Particular Ir genes encode class II MHC proteins on the surface of macrophages and B lymphocytes and are needed to present immunogenic peptides to the receptors carried by helper T cells. Presentation of these peptides to receptors on B cells initiates antibody synthesis (see Chapter 8). Nonresponsiveness of an animal host to a particular virus may be caused by a lack of class II MHC molecules capable of binding an important epitope on the virus. Even when a viral epitope is presented satisfactorily by antigen-presenting cells, there will be no response if the animal does not possess a clone of T cells with a receptor capable of recognizing that particular epitope. Such "holes" in the MHC and T cell receptor repertoires occur with both MHC class II-restricted $CD4^+$ (helper) T cells and MHC class I-restricted $CD8^+$ (cytotoxic) T cells. While the number of immunogenically important peptides derived from even the simplest viruses is not known, nor for the most part is the importance of particular peptides, it will seldom be the case that the hole in the MHC peptide-binding repertoire will not be compensated for by other peptides that are bound. The reactivity of antigen-specific receptors on the surface of B and T lymphocytes may be defeated only rarely in an otherwise immunocompetent animal, but when this does happen, infection may resemble that in a profoundly immunosuppressed animal.

A variety of inherited defects leading to immunologic nonresponsiveness have been identified in humans and mice and a few have been identified in domestic animals. These include agammaglobulinemia, where functional B cells are reduced greatly in number or are entirely absent and thymic aplasia where T cells responsible for cell-mediated immunity are absent. There are also conditions where there are defects in the cells responsible for both humoral and cellular immune responses. These "experiments of nature" are instructive in indicating which arms of the immune response are crucial in infections with particular viruses—some infections are fought primarily by the humoral immune arm, some by the cellular immune arm. For example, certain Arabian foals that suffer from primary severe combined immunodeficiency disease, in which there is an almost total absence of both T and B cells, are particularly susceptible to adenovirus infections—as maternal antibody levels wane, these foals die of fulminant systemic disease.

In a similar fashion, acquired defects in immune responsiveness, including various forms of immunologic tolerance, can also be considered determinants of host resistance/susceptibility. For example, the congenital infection of bovine fetuses by bovine viral diarrhea virus leads to persistent viral carriage and shedding and is the key to the success of this virus as a pathogen in cattle worldwide. As in this example, it is clear that immune response defects (whether inherited or acquired) are not only important in regard to the outcome of infection in the individual affected animal, they can also be important epidemiologically, as affected animals may shed high titers of virus over very long periods.

Other Genes Influencing Resistance/ Susceptibility to Viral Infections

Many genes affecting resistance/susceptibility to particular viruses do not map to the MHC region of the genome and presumably operate via any of a wide range of nonimmunologic mechanisms. For example: (1) cellular genes turned on by interferons that encode proteins that inhibit the replication of viruses; (2) cellular genes turned on by interferons that encode proteins that are required for the replication of particular viruses; (3) cellular genes turned on by interferons that encode the various receptors that are needed for entry of viruses; and (4) certain cellular genes turned on by interferons that determine whether particular viruses can infect macrophages or can resist destruction by macrophages. Clearly, such qualities may be major determinants in the overall success or failure of a virus as a pathogen.

Macrophages and Resistance/ Susceptibility to Viral Infections

Macrophages play a central role as determinants of host resistance/susceptibility, in part because of their role in inflammatory and immune responses and in part because of their intrinsic susceptibility to infection. Macrophages are concentrated at natural portals of viral entry, such as in alveoli in the lungs, and respond quickly following viral entry. Nevertheless, some viruses replicate preferentially in macrophages, in fact in some diseases they appear to be the only cells infected. In some diseases, viral replication in macrophages is the basis for clinical signs.

Ectromelia virus, injected intravenously into nonimmune mice, is cleared rapidly from the blood by the resident macrophages of the liver, the Kupffer cells. The outcome of the infection depends entirely on the battle fought between virus and macrophages (macrophages activated by T cells, mediating antiviral activity partly by secretion of interferons α and β). Macrophages/monocytes play a major role in the pathogenesis of retroviruses, especially lentivirus infections in animals. In some lentivirus infections, macrophages are the first cells infected, whereas in others they are the only cells infected. In all cases they are the major reservoirs of virus, providing virus for viremia and spread of infection to different tissues within the body. In many other acute viral infections of animals, including those caused by herpesviruses, vesiculoviruses, coronaviruses (mouse hepatitis virus in particular), arenaviruses, bunyaviruses (Rift Valley fever virus in particular), flaviviruses, and pestiviruses, macrophages are central to host resistance.

Cellular Receptors and Resistance/ Susceptibility to Viral Infections

A cell cannot be infected by a particular virus unless it expresses on its plasma membrane the molecule that serves as the *receptor* for that virus. Viral receptors are usually proteins, but carbohydrates and occasionally glycolipids are employed as well. Receptors are molecules essential to the normal functioning of the cell, usually molecules that are highly conserved over time. Viruses have evolved so that their surfaces are studded with *viral attachment proteins,* i.e., ligands that have high affinity for binding with specific cellular receptors so as to initiate viral attachment. Viruses have evolved to take advantage of the unfailing presence of their specific receptors at entry sites and in target tissues of their usual hosts; many viruses have no fallback means to bypass this crucial step in their life cycle. Theoretically, any cellular membrane component might serve as a receptor for one virus or another; in fact, the variety of molecules used as receptors by different viruses is remarkable (Table 7.2; Figure 7.2).

Good evidence exists that receptor expression on candidate target cells is a fundamental determinant of host resistance/susceptibility to the particular virus. The first indication came from studies of influenza virus infection. It was shown in the late 1940s that intranasal pretreatment of mice with neuraminidase conferred temporary protection against intranasal virus challenge. Subsequently, it was shown that influenza viruses attach to various sialic acid (*N*-acetyneuraminic acid) residues on the apical surface of respiratory epithelial cells, the

Table 7.2
Cellular Receptors for Animal Viruses

Virus family	Virus	Receptor on target cells
Poxviridae	Vaccinia virus	Epidermal growth factor receptor 1
Herpesviridae	Bovine herpesviruses 1 and 4	Heparan sulfate
	Pseudorabies virus	Heparan sulfate
	Murine cytomegalovirus	Major histocompatibility complex I
	Herpes simplex virus 1	Heparan sulfate
Adenoviridae	Human adenovirus 2	Specific integrins
Papovaviridae	Polyomavirus	Sialic acid-containing oligosaccharides
Parvoviridae	Canine parvovirus 2	Sialic acid-containing oligosaccharides
Retroviridae	Feline immunodeficiency virus	CD4 and an unknown number of coreceptors
	Human immunodeficiency virus 1	CD4 and more than 10 coreceptors
Reoviridae	Reovirus 3	β-Adrenergic receptor and sialic acid-containing oligosaccharides
	Rotavirus SA11 (vaccine strain)	Sialic acid-containing oligosaccharides
Paramyxoviridae	Parainfluenza viruses	Sialic acid-containing oligosaccharides, gangliosides GD1a, GQ16
Rhabdoviridae	Rabies virus	Acetylcholine receptor, gangliosides, phospholipids
Orthomyxoviridae	Influenza A viruses	Sialic acid-containing oligosaccharides
Arenaviridae	Lymphocytic choriomeningitis virus	100 kDa glycoprotein
Coronaviridae	Transmissible gastroenteritis virus	Porcine aminopeptidase N
	Bovine coronavirus	Sialic acid-containing oligosaccharides
	Mouse hepatitis virus	Carcinoembryonic antigen family (immunoglobulin superfamily)
Picornaviridae	Foot-and-mouth disease viruses	Integrins
	Polioviruses	Poliovirus receptor (immunoglobulin superfamily)
	Coxsackie B viruses	Decay-accelerating factor
	Echoviruses	Decay-accelerating factor and integrins
	Rhinoviruses (major group)	ICAM-1
Togaviridae	Sindbis virus	Laminin receptor
	Semliki Forest virus	HLA H2-K, H2-D protein

same residues removed by neuraminidase treatment. Neuraminidase became known as the *receptor destroying enzyme*. Then, in 1981, the structure of the influenza hemagglutinin was determined by X-ray crystallography and a few years later the structure of its cellular receptor complex was determined by the same means—this was the first virus attachment protein/receptor complex combination to be resolved at very high resolution. These studies showed that there is a conserved pocket near the tip of the viral hemagglutinin molecule that engages the terminal sialic acid on an oligosaccharide side chain protruding from the receptor complex—the two fit together as lock and key. On the surface of respiratory epithelial cells sialic acid occurs in numerous combinations with other sugars, and different combinations have different affinities for different influenza virus strains. Avian, equine, and human influenza viruses bind preferentially to cells with different sialic acid/sugar combinations—this may play an important role in determining the host range of each virus. Influenza viruses also bind to the same receptors on erythrocyte membranes, causing hemagglutination.

FIGURE 7.2.

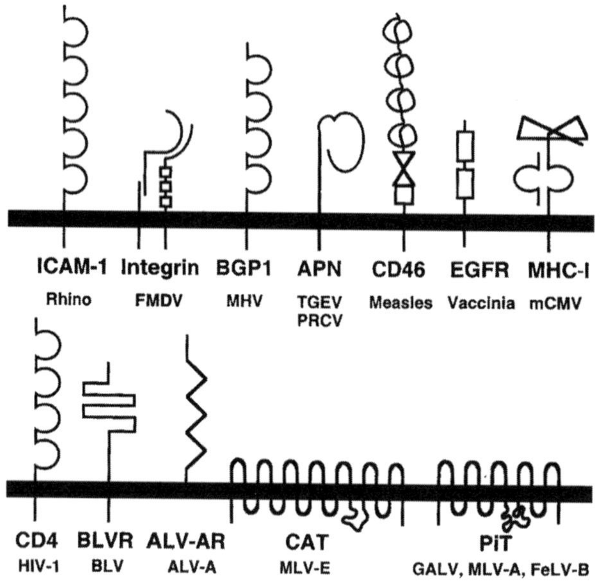

Many different types of cell surface proteins serve as specific receptors for viruses; some of these are illustrated schematically. In some cases, several isoforms of a glycoprotein can have virus receptor activity or the receptor may be expressed on the membrane as an oligomer (not shown). Many of these cell surface proteins have known functions, such as the intercellular adhesion molecule (ICAM-1), integrins, biliary glycoprotein (BGP1), aminopeptidase N (APN), MHC class 1 protein, and CD4. Virus receptors can be ligands for growth factors, such as epidermal growth factor receptor (EGFR), or for complement proteins, such as CD46. The receptors are identified in large type and examples of viruses that use the receptor are abbreviated in smaller type: BLVR, receptor for bovine leukemia virus; ALV-AR, receptor for avian leukosis virus A; CAT, cationic amino acid transporter; PIT, inorganic phosphate transporter; rhino, rhinovirus; FMDV, foot-and-mouth disease virus; MHV, mouse hepatitis virus; TGEV, transmissible gastroenteritis virus; PRCV, porcine respiratory coronavirus; measles, measles virus, as an example of a morbillivirus; vaccinia, vaccinia virus, as an example of a poxvirus; mCMV, murine cytomegalovirus; HIV-1, human immunodeficiency virus 1; BLV, bovine leukemia virus; ALV-A, avian leukosis virus A; MLV-E, murine leukemia virus E; GALV, Gibbon ape leukemia virus; MLV-A, murine leukemia virus A; FeLV-B, feline leukemia virus B. Semicircles, immunoglobulin-like domains; boxes, serine–threonine-rich domains; rectangles, cysteine-rich domains; thick black line, plasma membrane. [Adapted from D. M. Knipe, Virus-host cell interactions. *In* "Fields Virology" (B. N. Fields, D. M. Knipe, P. M. Howley, R. M. Chanock, J. L. Melnick, T. P. Monath, B. Roizman, and S. E. Straus, eds.), 3rd ed., pp. 273–299. Lippincott-Raven, Philadelphia PA, 1996.]

The more conserved or ubiquitous the receptor, the wider the host range of the virus that exploits it; for example, rabies virus, which uses sialylated gangliosides as well as the acetylcholine receptor, has a very wide host range. However, rabies virus infection is restricted narrowly to few host cell types, such as striated muscle cells, neurons, salivary gland, and a few other glandular epithelial cells.

Some viruses utilize alternative receptors to enter different cells in different tissues and in different hosts. For example, the life cycle of Sindbis virus requires that it alternates between mosquito and vertebrate hosts. The virus has a wide vertebrate host range, including birds and mammals, but a narrow arthropod host range, primarily *Aedes* spp. mosquitoes. The vertebrate receptor is the laminin receptor, a membrane protein that is very highly conserved and present in many different vertebrates; the arthropod receptor remains unknown.

Some of the larger, more complex viruses use two or more distinct attachment proteins in concert or sequentially, seemingly for tighter binding or for more complex mechanisms for viral attachment. Herpesviruses bind initially to low-affinity receptors, then move to secondary higher-affinity receptors that better facilitate viral entry by fusion. Human immunodeficiency virus 1 uses CD4 as its primary receptor, but it has several secondary coreceptors (fusin and other molecules), each of which is now the target of antiviral drug research.

When variant viruses are found that cause new disease patterns, changes in viral attachment proteins and the specificity of cellular receptors must be suspected. For example, transmissible gastroenteritis virus has long been the cause of enteric disease in piglets; it replicates in epithelial cells of the small intestine and in the lung. In the 1980s, a variant virus was discovered in Europe that caused only respiratory infection. This virus, which spread rapidly and caused severe economic losses, was found to be very closely related to transmissible gastroenteritis virus but had specific mutations in genes encoding the viral attachment protein and one other protein. These mutations affected the tropism of the virus as well as its transmissibility. Variant viruses can even appear expressing changes in host range. For example, the explosive emergence of canine parvovirus in 1978 was the consequence of specific attachment protein mutations of an ancestral felid virus (see Chapter 21).

Tumor Necrosis Factors, Interferons, and Other Cytokines and Resistance/Susceptibility to Viral Infections

The role of interferons as cytokines that are important in the host response to viral infections is covered in Chapter 5. Tumor necrosis factors α and β are cytokines that also have direct antiviral and immunomodulatory activities. Tumor necrosis factor α is produced by macrophages, natural killer (NK) cells, and other cell types; tumor necrosis factor β is produced mainly by T cells. Tumor necrosis factors have many functions: they can act as cellular growth factors and differentiation factors, but they can also act synergistically with the antiviral actions of interferons, inhibit viral synthetic activities, and induce cell death by apoptosis.

The discovery of so many other cytokines makes it clear that there are many more such antiviral effectors active within host cells. It is clear that the degree of sensitivity of any particular virus to any particular interferon or other cytokine represents only one small facet in the overall virus–cell interaction. As we learn how particular viruses have developed different mechanisms for circumventing the antiviral actions of interferons and other cytokines, we can see the intricacy of the web of biochemical pathways involved and we can appreciate better how much more there is to learn about virus cell interactions and the means to interfere with virus replication. We can also see the role of continuing evolution in the never-ending battle for survival between host and virus.

Physiologic Factors Affecting Host Resistance/Susceptibility

A great variety of physiologic factors affect host resistance/susceptibility, the most important being the immune response, which is described in detail in Chapter 8. Little is known of many of the nonspecific factors in resistance, but age, nutritional status, levels of certain hormones, especially as affected by pregnancy, and cell differentiation play roles in a variety of viral diseases.

Age and Resistance/Susceptibility to Viral Infections

Viral infections tend to be most serious at the extremes of life. The extreme susceptibility of neonates to many viral infections is a major concern in clinical practice. In the newborn, even a few days matter, as very rapid physiologic changes occur during the postpartum period and resistance to the most severe manifestations of many intestinal and respiratory infections builds quickly. The basis for this change lies mainly in the maturation of the immune system, but anatomic and physiologic changes are involved as well. The best-studied model of this is lymphocytic choriomeningitis virus infection in inbred mice. In the days after birth, mice pass from a stage of nearly complete immunologic nonreactivity to immunologic maturity. Lymphocytic choriomeningitis virus induces a persistent tolerated infection, free of clinical signs, when inoculated into newborn mice, but a fulminant fatal meningoencephalitis in mice infected when over 1 week old. The virus is the cause of the classic immunopathologic disease—the infection itself causes no acute damage, as evidenced in the survival of newborns, but the infection evokes an exuberant host immune response that destroys crucial cells and upsets homeostasis in the brain. Mice often die in convulsion.

Most domestic animals are reasonably mature immunologically at the time of birth; nevertheless, newborns are particularly vulnerable to infections with viruses such as canine distemper virus, canine parvovirus, transmissible gastroenteritis virus (swine), hog cholera virus, bovine viral diarrhea virus, enteropathogenic coronaviruses (many animals), rotaviruses (many animals), and various herpesviruses (many animals). In mammalian and avian species, an umbrella of maternal antibody protects newborns against many viruses for the first few months of life. The importance of this protection is seen in individual animals that are born without maternal antibodies or fail to receive such antibodies in colostrum or yolk (see Chapter 8).

Nutritional Status and Resistance/Susceptibility to Viral Infections

Malnutrition can interfere with any of the mechanisms that act as barriers to the replication or progress of viruses through the body. It has been demonstrated repeatedly that severe nutritional deficiencies interfere with the generation of antibody and cell-mediated immune responses, with the activity of macrophages, and with the integrity of skin and mucous membranes. However, often it is impossible to disentangle adverse nutritional effects from other factors found in animals living in extremely harsh environments. Moreover, just as malnutrition can exacerbate viral infections, so can viral infections exacerbate malnutrition, especially when severe diarrhea is present. Thus, starvation and malnutrition and viral diseases can create a vicious circle.

Animals with a general protein deficiency or deficiencies in certain key amino acids may be highly susceptible to particular viruses. Viruses that cause epithelial infections, especially respiratory and intestinal infections, become particular problems. Secondary bacterial infections are common as the cause of life-threatening pneumonia and enteritis.

Hormones and Pregnancy and Resistance/Susceptibility to Viral Infections

During pregnancy certain infections of the dam can be more severe or can be reactivated (e.g., Rift Valley fever virus infection in sheep). In addition a novel set of potentially susceptible tissues appear, including the fetus, the placenta, and the lactating mammary gland. Herpesvirus infections may be reactivated during pregnancy, leading to abortion or perinatal infection.

The immunosuppressive effects of therapeutic doses of corticosteroids exacerbates many viral infections (e.g., infectious bovine rhinotracheitis and pseudorabies). The precise mechanisms have not been determined, but corticosteroids reduce inflammatory and immune responses, dampen macrophage action, and depress interferon synthesis. It is also clear that adequate levels of these hormones are vital for the maintenance of normal resistance to infection. Stress causes adrenocortical immunosuppression, which is seen in many settings where animals are transported or brought into crowded environments. For example, stress contributes to the prevalence and severity of shipping fever in cattle.

Fever and Resistance/Susceptibility to Viral Infections

Almost all viral infections are accompanied by fever. The principal mediator of the febrile response is the cytokine interleukin 1, which is produced in macrophages and is induced during immune responses. Interleukin 1 is found in inflammatory exudates and acts on the temperature-regulating center in the anterior hypothalamus. The increased metabolic rate augments the metabolic activity of phagocytic cells and the rate at which inflammatory responses are induced. Of course these effects might be expected to have antiviral effects.

In classic studies of myxoma virus infection in rabbits it was demonstrated that increasing body temperature increased protection against infection whereas decreasing temperature increased the severity of infection. Blocking the development of fever with drugs (e.g., salicylates) increased mortality. Similar results have been obtained with ectromelia and coxsackievirus infections in mice.

Cell Differentiation and Resistance/Susceptibility to Viral Infections

The replication of some viruses is determined by the state of differentiation of the cell. The warts produced by papillomaviruses in many species of animals provide a classic example. Productive infection is not seen in the deeper layers of the epidermal tumor, but occurs only when the cells become keratinized as they move to the surface layers. Basal cells contain 50–200 copies of viral DNA, but viral antigens and finally viral particles are produced only as the cells differentiate when they approach the surface of the skin. Other examples involve cells of the immune system. For example, vesicular stomatitis and distemper viruses, which do not replicate in normal (resting) peripheral blood lymphocyte cultures, do so when cells differentiate after activation by mitogen. Likewise, maedi/visna virus infects monocytes abortively with low levels of transcription of viral RNA, but the infection becomes productive as the cells differentiate into macrophages.

The stage of the cell cycle may affect susceptibility. Parvoviruses replicate only in cells that are in the late S phase of the cell cycle. Most vulnerable are the rapidly dividing cells of bone marrow, intestinal epithelium, and the developing fetus. In the feline fetus, the parvovirus, feline panleukopenia virus, infects the rapidly dividing cells of the germinal layer of the cerebellum, destroying some of them and arresting the normal migration of others to their final locations in the mature brain—this results in cerebellar hypoplasia, clinical ataxia, and severe neurological disease. In newborn cats the same virus infects rapidly dividing cells in the bone marrow and intestinal epithelium, producing severe leukopenia and diarrhea. The same virus is much less virulent when it infects adult cats where fewer cells in these tissues are in the late S phase and dividing.

Natural Inhibitors of Attachment of Virions to Cells

Blood, mucus, milk, and other body fluids contain a wide range of substances that can coat particular viruses and impede their attachment to cells. For example, influenza virions can be neutralized by mannose-binding lectins (conglutinin and "mannose-binding protein," MBP) found in the plasma of a number of animal species and in the lungs as pulmonary surfactant proteins, as well as by sialylated glycoproteins found in plasma and respiratory mucus. Cytomegaloviruses are often coated with β_2-microglobulin, a component of plasma. Antiviral fatty acids derived from lipids in colostrum and milk have also been described. The relative importance of such inhibitors remains unknown, but given the range of normal plasma and tissue proteins, carbohydrates, lipids, and more complex substances, the ones we know about may represent the tip of an iceberg of innate natural defense mechanisms, which through recombinant DNA technology might be exploited for chemotherapeutic purposes.

Multiple Infections

Under intensive management systems, such as cattle feedlots, swine farrowing units, and broiler houses, multiple infections are common and can be difficult to analyze as to primary and secondary etiologic agents. Such multiple infections with two or more viruses or a virus and one or more bacteria are important as the cause of severe respiratory and intestinal diseases.

Viral infections of the respiratory tract often predispose animals to bacterial superinfection; for example, shipping fever may be initiated by a variety of respiratory viruses and other stressors, but its serious consequences are due to secondary infection with *Pasteurella multocida* or *hemolytica* (see Chapter 10). Alternately, primary bacterial respiratory infection may increase the severity of secondary avian and equine influenza virus infections. In the course of such dual infections, the bacteria (any one of several different bacteria) produce proteases that cleave the influenza virus hemagglutinin, thereby activating its viral attachment domain and facilitating viral entry into airway epithelial cells.

Secondary opportunistic infections, viral, bacterial, or fungal, are particular problems when the primary infection is caused by a virus that is immunosuppressive. Today, the classic example is HIV infection, which so profoundly depletes the infected person's $CD4^+$ cell population that any of a number of secondary infections may be lethal: clinical management problems are caused by herpesviruses (especially cytomegaloviruses), papillomaviruses, polyomaviruses, adenoviruses, and hepatitis viruses B and C, as well as *Salmonella, Shigella,* and *Campylobacter* spp., *Pneumocystis carinii, Toxoplasma gondii, Mycobacterium avium-intracellulare, Candida albicans,* and *Cryptococcus neoformans.* Although the list of secondary opportunistic infections may be shorter, the same sort of clinical management problems occur in veterinary medical practice, e.g., when cats are infected initially with feline immunodeficiency virus, feline leukemia virus, or feline panleukopenia virus, or when puppies are infected with canine parvovirus or canine distemper virus.

Model Studies of Bases for Viral Virulence and Host Resistance/Susceptibility

Canine Parvovirus as a Model of Viral Determinants Affecting Host Range and Susceptibility

A dramatic example of the emergence of a new virulent virus by mutation is afforded by canine parvovirus. Serological evidence suggests that this virus made its first appearance as a new pathogen of dogs in 1976. The virus was isolated in 1978 as the cause of severe enteritis, sometimes fatal, that occurred in dogs in the United States, Europe, and Australia (see Chapter 21). Outbreaks of sudden death in puppies due to myocarditis were also linked to the new virus. Soon after its isolation, it became clear from antigenic analysis and restriction endonuclease mapping that the canine virus was related closely to feline panleukopenia virus, a pathogen that had been recognized at least since the 1920s. Sequence analysis of the canine virus by C. R. Parrish, L. E. Carmichael, and colleagues at the James A. Baker Institute for Animal Health at Cornell University and others showed that the canine virus differed from the feline panleukopenia virus in only a few nucleotides and probably originated as a result of only two amino acid substitutions in the viral capsid. These changes allowed the virus to attach to and replicate in dog cells (Figure 7.3). The rapidity with which canine parvovirus disease spread around the world has not been explained, but the extreme physical stability of parvoviruses makes fomite carriage very likely.

Avian Influenza Viruses as a Model of the Multigenic Nature of Viral Virulence Determinants

The great pioneer in experimental virology, F. M. Burnet, first suggested that influenza virus virulence is

FIGURE 7.3.

Virus (wild type or mutant)	VP2 nucleotide # 93	103	323	Virus titer (PFU in cat cells / PFU in dog cells; 10^1 10^2 10^3 10^4 10^5 10^6 10^7)	CPV-specific epitope
Canine parvovirus (wild type, CPV-d)	N	A	N		+
Feline panleukopenia virus (wild type, FPV-b)	K	V	D	<	-
Canine parvovirus (mutant, vB1280)	K	A	N	<	-
Canine parvovirus (mutant, vB1279)	N	A	D	<	+
Feline panleukopenia virus (mutant, vB1319)	N	A	N		+
Feline panleukopenia virus (mutant, vB1340)	N	V	N		+
Feline panleukopenia virus (mutant, vB1339)	N	A	D	< < not viable	ND

Analysis of the sequence differences between canine parvovirus (CPV) (solid bars) and feline panleukopenia virus (FPV) (hatched bars), which determine the ability of the canine virus to infect dogs and dog cells. A series of mutants of the two viruses was prepared and tested for their ability to infect canine cells or feline cells. Changing either nucleotide 93 or nucleotide 323 in the canine parvovirus genome to the feline panleukopenia sequence [93 lysine (K) to asparagine (N); 323 aspartic acid (D) to asparagine (N)] resulted in a virus that was not able to infect dog cells. When both nucleotides 93 and 323 of feline panleukopenia virus were changed to the nucleotides found in canine parvovirus the resulting virus gained the ability to efficiently infect dog cells. In addition, changing nucleotide 93 in feline panleukopenia virus to asparagine (N) gave the resulting virus a canine parvovirus-specific epitope. Thus, in this case, important biologic, antigenic, and pathogenic qualities were found to be the product of very small genetic differences between viruses as they exist in nature. This is not always the case—host range differences between various strains of some other viruses are founded in complex genetic differences involving multiple genes. (Courtesy of C. R. Parrish.)

multigenic, i.e., no one gene determines its virulence. Subsequent studies by R. Rott, C. Scholtissek, and colleagues at the veterinary faculty in Giessen, Germany, proved this point: they made reassortants between highly virulent and avirulent strains of avian influenza virus, exchanging separately each of the eight genome segments of each strain. The virulence of the progeny viruses they obtained varied in complex patterns. They showed that some genes worked better together than others, that there was an optimal combination of genes, an optimal *gene constellation,* that favored viral survival in nature and determined virulence.

Despite this proof that all influenza genes are important in determining virulence in the chicken (and in horses and humans), the gene encoding the viral hemagglutinin is preeminent—more specifically, the essential virulence determinant is the cleavability of the hemagglutinin. In relatively nonpathogenic strains of avian influenza virus, the HA1 and HA2 polypeptide chains of the hemagglutinin are linked by a single arginine residue, whereas in virulent strains the linker is a sequence of several basic amino acids that is cleaved more readily by available cellular or bacterial protease(s). Cleavage activates the hemagglutinin, making it ready to attach to receptors on target cells. The most striking lesson of how easily hemagglutinin cleavability can be altered and virulence changed comes from analysis of an outbreak of avian influenza in Pennsylvania in 1983. Early in the year, a virus (H5/N2) was introduced from wild birds into chicken flocks, producing a mortality of less than 10%. However, in October 1983, the accumulation of about seven point mutations in the hemagglutinin gene of this virus resulted in an increase in mortality to over 80% and a coincident increase in viral transmissibility—all contributing to an epidemic that cost the regional poultry industry more than $60 million. One of the mutations abolished a glycosylation site on the viral hemagglutinin molecule, thus exposing the HA1/HA2 cleavage site that had previously been concealed by a carbohydrate side chain.

Reoviruses as Model for Associating Viral Virulence Determinants with Clinical and Pathological Characteristics of Disease

Now classic studies of the genetic bases for the virulence of reoviruses for mice were carried out over many years by B. N. Fields and colleagues at Harvard University. Many of the pathogenetic principles that are now being extended to other viruses, to other host animals, and to clinical practice stem from these studies. This is the case

Table 7.3
Reovirus Genes and Proteins and Their Functions

Genome segment	Specified protein	Copies/ virion	Location in virion	Function (effect of mutation on pathogenesis in mice)
L1	λ3	12	Inner capsid	RNA-dependent RNA polymerase (neonatal myocarditis)
L2	λ2	60	Outer capsid, core spike	Guanyl transferase (efficiency of horizontal spread)
L3	λ1	120	Inner capsid	Binds double-stranded RNA, zinc metalloprotein (unknown)
M1	μ2	12	Inner capsid	RNA synthesis (unknown)
M2	μ1	600	Outer capsid	Cleaved in intestine yielding ISVP (determines invasion by the intestinal route and neurovirulence)
M3	μNS	0	Nonstructural	Binds single-stranded RNA, associates with cytoskeleton, role in gene assortment (unknown)
S1	σ1	36–48[a]	Outer capsid	Cell attachment protein, primary serotype determinant, hemagglutinin (neurotropism, oily-fur syndrome)
	σ1s	0	Nonstructural	Unknown
S2	σ2	120–180[a]	Inner capsid	Binds double-stranded RNA (unknown)
S3	σNS	0	Nonstructural	Binds single-stranded RNA, role in assortment (unknown)
S4	σ3	600	Outer capsid	Major outer capsid protein; inhibitor of host cell protein and RNA synthesis; cleaved yielding ISVP (virion stability in the environment)

[a]Number uncertain.

despite the fact that reoviruses are not important pathogens in nature. At the heart of these studies has been the manipulation by reassortment of the 10 genome segments of reoviruses 1 and 3 and the functional characterization of the protein product of each gene of each of these viruses. In turn, the role of each protein in the pathogenesis of reovirus disease has been unraveled. The overall account is complex, indeed, especially since most reovirus proteins have more than one function. The following is just a sampling of the associations between viral genes, their gene products, and their pathogenetic functions.

Four genes (S1, S4, M2, and L2) encode four proteins that make up the outer capsid of reoviruses (Table 7.3 and Figure 7.4). Each of these proteins has specific functions in the interaction of the virus with target cells and animal hosts:

1. Gene S1 encodes protein σ1, which is located at the end of the stalks that are extended at each of the 12 vertices of infectious subviral particles (ISVPs)—there are 36 or 48 copies of this protein in each virion. This protein mediates the attachment of the virion to the host cell receptor and therefore directs cellular and tissue tropism. Reovirus 1 and 3 differ in their tropism in the mouse central nervous system, the former infecting ependymal cells, the latter neurons. Studies with reassortants of these two viruses indicate that the S1 gene determines this pattern—differences in virulence between the two viruses conform to the same pattern, with neuronal infection and encephalitis being associated with enhanced mortality compared with ependymal infection.

2. Gene S4 encodes protein σ3, which is the major outer capsid protein—there are 600 copies of this protein in each virion. Proteolytic enzymes, either in the intesti-

FIGURE 7.4.

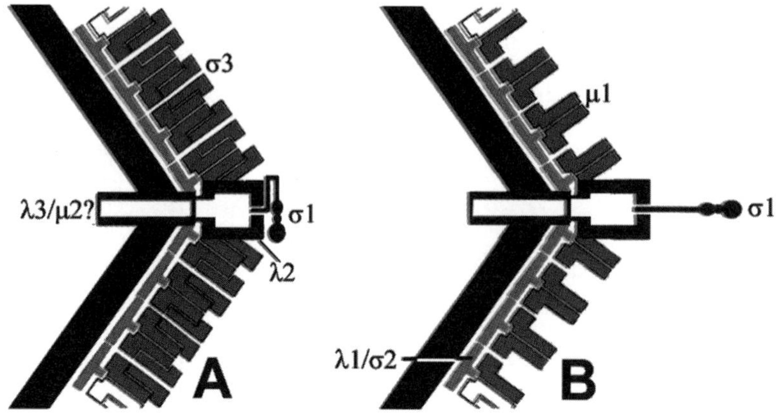

Schematic representation of part of the reovirus capsid, showing the location of some proteins that play major roles in infection and virulence. (A) Intact virion, showing protein $\sigma 1$, which forms the spike that mediates attachment, located at each vertex of the viral icosahedron. In the intact virion the spike is not exposed at the virion surface. This representation also shows protein $\sigma 3$, which is the major outer capsid protein and is responsible for the extreme environmental stability of the virion. (B) Infectious subvirion particle (ISVP), formed in the intestinal lumen by the action of chymotrypsin (or within endosomes by the action of cellular proteases). Enzymatic action causes the removal of protein $\sigma 3$ and the cleavage of protein $\mu 1$, leaving the structure that enters the host cell and initiates replication. The removal of $\sigma 3$ also causes the extension and activation of the viral attachment protein $\sigma 1$, which then directs the cellular and tissue tropism of the virus. [Adapted from M. L. Nibert, L. A. Schiff, and B. N. Fields, *In* "Fields Virology" (B. N. Fields, D. M. Knipe, P. M. Howley, R. M. Chanock, J. L. Melnick, T. P. Monath, B. Roizman, and S. E. Straus, eds.), 3rd ed., pp. 1557–1596. Lippincott-Raven, Philadelphia PA, 1996.]

nal lumen or within endosomes, remove this protein (and also cleave $\mu 1$), leaving infectious subviral particles, which are the structures that enter host cells and initiate replication. The removal of $\sigma 3$ also causes the extension of the viral attachment protein $\sigma 1$, thereby activating it. This protein is a major determinant of virion stability in the environment and because it also inhibits cellular protein and RNA synthesis, it plays a role in establishing persistent infection.

3. Gene M2 encodes protein $\mu 1$ (and $\mu 1C$), which is another major outer capsid protein that, along with protein $\sigma 3$, determines the capacity of the virus to invade by the intestinal route—there are 600 copies of this protein in each virion. The $\mu 1$ protein (and $\sigma 3$ protein) is cleaved by chymotrypsin in the intestine; the resulting ISVPs, but not intact virions, adhere to and enter M cells overlying lymphoid tissues of the intestine. From here, infection spreads to intestinal epithelial cells.

4. Gene L2 encodes protein $\lambda 2$, which are arranged at each of the 12 vertices of the outer capsid and are involved in the extension of the receptor-bearing stalk when ISVPs are activated—there are 60 copies of this protein in each virion.

Reovirus molecular pathogenesis provides a sense of balance in our understanding of the importance of various viral genes and gene products. Although a great deal of attention is given to genes encoding viral attachment proteins as determinants of tropism and disease patterns, the reovirus model makes it clear that many other factors determine the course and outcome of infection in the whole animal.

Rabies as Model of Interaction of Viral Virulence Determinants with Host and Ecologic Determinants

Rabies can serve to illustrate host and ecologic determinants as keys to viral adaptations and changing transmission patterns. The ongoing epidemic of raccoon rabies in the northeastern United States has brought these determinants into focus. The epidemic has been traced to the importation of raccoons from an old rabies endemic area in Florida to West Virginia in 1977. Its continuing spread, as far as eastern Canada and across the Appalachian mountains into Ohio, is the cause of massive prevention and control efforts. One key to our understanding of this epidemic was the discovery some years ago that rabies virus is not a single invariant virus, rather it is a set of different variants or genotypes, each transmitted within a separate reservoir host niche. In North America, there are six genotypes in terrestrial animals (and many more in various species of bats): one genotype involves the skunk in the north-central United States and south-central Canada, one the skunk in the south-central United States, one the Arctic fox and red fox in Alaska and Canada, one the gray fox in Arizona and western Texas, one the coyote in southern Texas and northern Mexico, and one the raccoon as cited earlier. "Raccoons-bite-raccoons-bite-raccoons," and after an unknown time their virus becomes a distinct genotype, highly adapted to the host and inefficiently transmitted if introduced into another host. When this discovery was made (using monoclonal antibodies and partial genomic sequencing of isolates), many mysteries of rabies ecology were clarified. Now, even finer variations in genotypes are being analyzed to determine virus transmission patterns within the major host animal niches and likely sites of future epidemic spread. Here, modern virologic, epidemiologic, and ecologic sciences are coming together around the common need to understand virus and host variables.

Further Reading

Baron, S., Coppenhaver, D. H., Dianzani, F., Fleischman, W. R., Hughes, T. K., Klimpel, G. R., Niesel, D. W., Stanton, G. J., and Tyring, S. K. (1992). "Interferon: Principles and Medical Applications." University of Texas Medical Branch Press, Galveston.

Knipe, D. M. (1996). Virus-host cell interactions. *In* "Fields Virology" (B. N. Fields, D. M. Knipe, P. M. Howley, R. M. Chanock, J. L. Melnick, T. P. Monath, B. Roizman, and S. E. Straus, eds.), 3rd ed., pp. 273–299. Lippincott-Raven, Philadelphia, PA.

Mims, C. A., Playfair, J. H. L., Roitt, I. M., Wakelin, D., and Williams, R. (1993). "Medical Microbiology." Mosby-Year Book, St. Louis, MO.

Mims, C. A., Dimmock, N., Nash, A., and Stephen, J. (1995). "Mims' Pathogenesis of Infectious Disease," 4th ed. Academic Press, London.

Nathanson, N., Ahmed, R., Gonzalez-Scarano, F., Griffin, D. E., Holmes, K. V., Murphy, F. A., and Robinson, H. L., eds. (1997). "Viral Pathogenesis." Lippincott-Raven, Philadelphia, PA.

Nomoto, A., ed. (1992). Cellular receptors for virus infection. *Semin. Virol.* **3**, 77–186.

Roitt, I. M., Male, D., and Bonstoff, J. (1996). "Immunology," 4th ed. Mosby-Year Book, St. Louis, MO.

Tyler, K. L., and Fields, B. N. (1996). Pathogenesis of viral infections. *In* "Fields Virology" (B. N. Fields, D. M. Knipe, P. M. Howley, R. M. Chanock, J. L. Melnick, T. P. Monath, B. Roizman, and S. E. Straus, eds.), 3rd ed., pp. 173–218. Lippincott-Raven, Philadelphia, PA.

Welsh, R. M., and Sen, G. C. (1997). Nonspecific host responses to viral infections. *In* "Viral Pathogenesis" (N. Nathanson, R. Ahmed, F. Gonzalez-Scarano, D. E. Griffin, K. V. Holmes, F. A. Murphy, and H. L. Robinson, eds.), pp. 109–142. Lippincott-Raven, Philadelphia, PA.

CHAPTER 8

Immune Response to Viral Infections

In response to the constant threat of invasion by infectious agents, including viruses, vertebrates have evolved an elaborate set of defensive measures, called, collectively, the immune system. During the initial encounter with a virus, the immune system of the host recognizes certain viral macromolecules (proteins, carbohydrates) called *antigens* as foreign which elicit several kinds of responses to eliminate the virus and to prevent reinfection. B lymphocytes respond (the humoral immune response) to an antigenic stimulus by producing and secreting *immunoglobulins* or *antibodies.* T lymphocytes respond (the cell-mediated immune response) by secreting cytokines that regulate the immune response by coordinating the activities of the various types of cells involved, including antibody production by B lymphocytes; T lymphocytes also have direct effector functions, such as cytotoxic functions. Both B and T lymphocytes bear highly specific receptor molecules that recognize discrete regions on viral proteins, known as *antigenic determinants* or *epitopes.*

Antigen-specific immune responses in concert with innate defense mechanisms terminate many viral infections before much damage has been done; this results in mild disease or even subclinical infection. This chapter deals with the role of the immune response in recovery from viral infection and resistance to reinfection. Later chapters address situations where the immune system does not function so effectively, where the immune response is actually harmful and a significant component in the pathogenesis of disease, and where the virus evades the immune system and establishes a persistent infection.

Cellular Components of the Immune System

The cells of the immune system include B and T lymphocytes, cells of the monocyte/macrophage lineage, dendritic cells, and natural killer (NK) cells (Figure 8.1). Lymphocytes have antigen-specific receptors on their surfaces, which are the basis for immunologic specificity. Any given T or B lymphocyte possesses receptors with specificity for a single epitope. When T or B lymphocytes bind antigen they signal the cell to divide to form an expanded clone of cells (*clonal expansion*). B lymphocytes differentiate into plasma cells, which are end cells that produce and secrete antibody. T lymphocytes secrete soluble factors known as *lymphokines* or *interleukins,* which are representatives of a large family of hormone-like molecules, known generically as *cytokines*; these molecules modulate the activities of the cells involved in the immune response. Some T and B cells revert to long-lived small lymphocytes responsible for *immunologic memory.* Whereas antibodies and the receptors on B cells recognize epitopes on foreign antigens in their native conformation, T cell receptors recognize small

FIGURE 8.1.

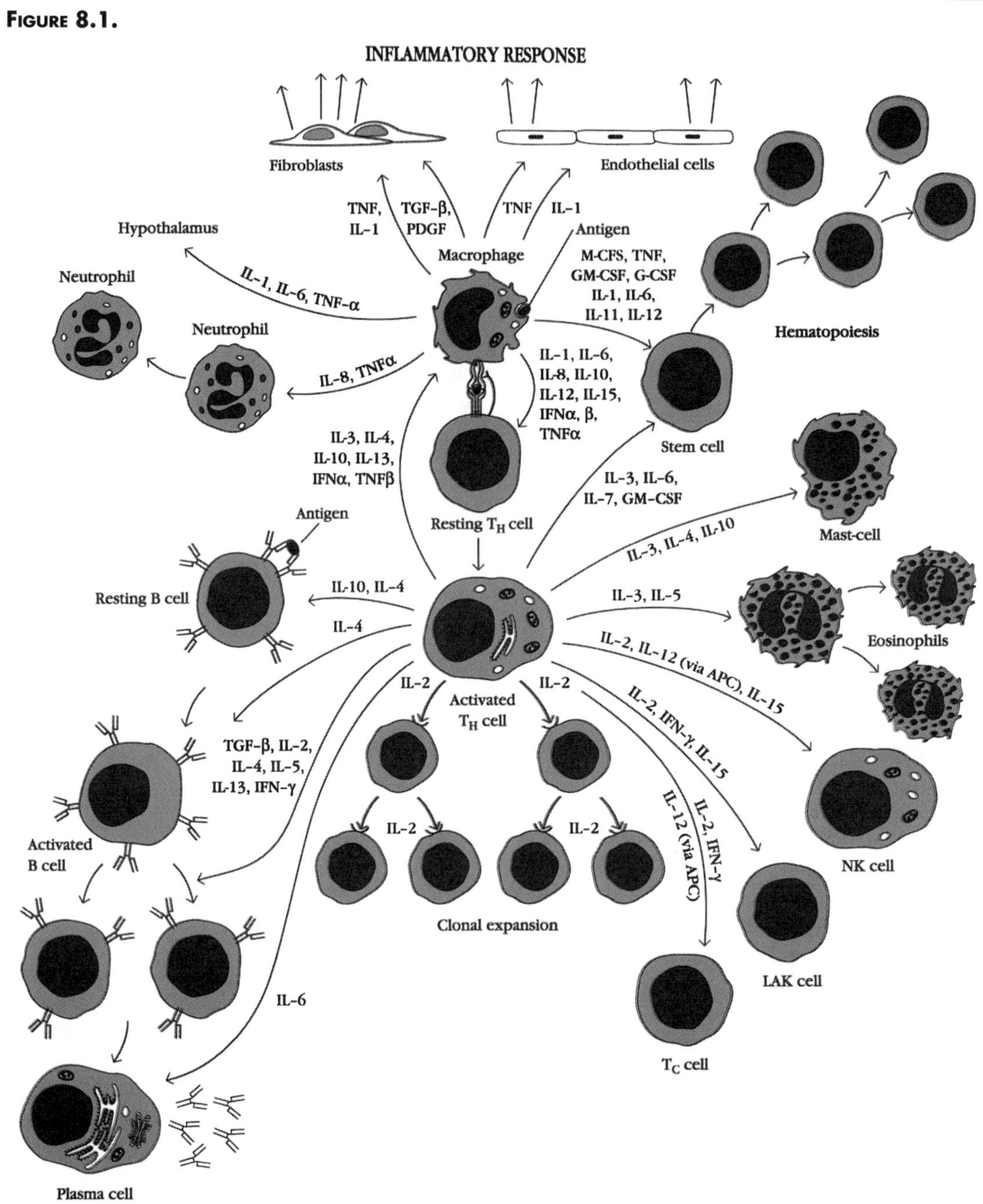

An overview of the complex network of interactions of the immune system following a virus infection. The process begins with the interaction of extracellular viral antigen with macrophages, which process and present peptide cleavage products of the antigen in association with the MHC class II complex to resting Th cells that bear T cell receptors that specifically recognize the peptide and the MHC complex. The interaction induces signal transduction pathways that lead to the synthesis and release of a particular suite of cytokines, each of which then binds to its specific receptor on the surface of other cells and signals those cells to respond either by also releasing other cytokines or by more direct effector actions such as cell lysis of virus-infected target cells by Tc cells. (From J. Kuby, "Immunology," 3rd ed. Freeman, New York, 1997).

peptides that are formed by the cleavage of viral proteins; they do this only when the foreign peptides are presented to them in association with membrane glycoproteins known as *major histocompatibility complex (MHC) proteins*.

Antigen-Specific Receptors

The antigen-specific receptors on the surface of B lymphocytes are modified immunoglobulin molecules composed of four polypeptides: two light (L) and two heavy (H) chains termed surface immunoglobulin (sIg). They are modified at the C terminus of the H chains to have a transmembrane domain that anchors them in the cell membrane where they serve their receptor function. Prior to primary antigen stimulation the sIg molecules are sIgM; after class switching (see later) the Ig of the class switch becomes the sIg antigen-specific receptor.

The T cell antigen-specific receptor (TCR) is quite distinct; it is a two polypeptide heterodimer and although immunoglobulin like, it is encoded by an entirely different set of genes. The two polypeptides of the most common T cell receptors are designated α/β. A second T lymphocyte population bears a different T cell receptor designated γ/δ.

Specific recognition and binding of either sIg or a T cell receptor to its epitope triggers, by signal transduction across the plasma membrane of the lymphocyte, a wide range of effector processes that attack and remove the invading virus and/or virus-infected cells (Figure 8.1). The resulting cascade of cell–cell interactions and cytokine secretion amplifies the immune response to match the scale of the virus infection and, in addition, establishes a long-lived memory that enables the immune system to respond more quickly (secondary or anamnestic response) to reinfection with the same virus.

B Lymphocytes

Some of the pluripotent hematopoietic stem cells originating from fetal liver and later from bone marrow differentiate into B lymphocytes in the bursa of Fabricius in birds or its equivalent, the bone marrow, in mammals. They are characterized by the presence of specific antigen-binding receptors on their surface, plus receptors for complement (C3) and receptors for the Fc portion of immunoglobulin. During ontogeny, several hundred inherited V (variable) L and H chain immunoglobulin gene segments undergo somatic recombination. There are also multiple copies of J (joining) gene segments in the case of light chains and J and D (diversity) gene segments in the case of heavy chains that also somatically recombine with V genes. Somatic mutation (see later) also adds to the generation of antibody diversity to yield potentially more than 10^7 unique specificities.

Each individual B lymphocyte and its progeny express a set of immunoglobulin genes that are specific for a single epitope. During development such cells have three possible fates: (1) they may react with a self-antigen and be eliminated, (2) they may be nonviable and be eliminated, or (3) they may react with a foreign antigen and proliferate.

In contrast to T cells, the sIg receptors of B cells recognize antigens in their native and soluble state rather than as peptide–MHC complexes on the surface of cells, hence B cells interact directly with viral proteins or virions. When the particular clones of B cells bearing receptors complementary to any one of the several epitopes on an antigen bind that antigen, they respond, after receiving the appropriate signals from helper T cells, by division and differentiation into antibody-secreting plasma cells.

Each plasma cell secretes antibody of a single specificity, corresponding to the particular V (variable) region of the sIg receptor it expresses. Initially, this antibody is of the IgM class, but somatic genetic recombination (translocation) then brings about a class switch by associating V gene segments with different H chain constant domains. Various cytokines play an important role in isotype switching. Thus, after a few days, IgG, IgA, and sometimes IgE antibodies of the same specificity begin to dominate the immune response. Early in the immune response, when large amounts of antigen are present, antigen-reactive B cells may be triggered even if their receptors fit the epitope with relatively poor affinity; the result is the production of antibody that binds the antigen with low affinity. Later on, when only small amounts of antigen remain, B cells that have evolved by hypermutation in their V region genes to produce receptors that bind the antigen with high affinity are selected (*affinity maturation*) and the affinity of the antibody secreted increases correspondingly.

T Lymphocytes

T lymphocytes are so named because of their dependence on the thymus for their maturation from pluripotent hematopoietic stem cells. Within the thymus there is positive selection for those cells able to recognize appropriate peptides on the surface of cells and negative selection to eliminate those T cells that recognize self antigens with possible autoimmune disease as a consequence. Only 1 or 2% of the lymphocytes that are produced in the thymus leave and populate the secondary lymphoid tissues. Functionally, T lymphocytes are classified into two subsets: *T helper (Th) lymphocytes,* which are further divided into Th1 and Th2 cells, and *cytotoxic T (Tc) lymphocytes (CTLs).* Th cells are generally considered to have a regulatory function and Tc cells a direct effector function, i.e., target cell lysis. Close examination of T cell clones indicates that a single cell type can discharge both regulatory and effector functions and secrete a range of different lymphokines.

T Helper Lymphocytes

T helper cells carry a surface marker known as CD4. They recognize viral peptides in association with class II MHC protein, usually on the surface of an *antigen-presenting cell* (APC). They then secrete cytokines that further activate themselves and subsequently activate other cells, including other Th, Tc, and B lymphocytes, in the process helping Tc lymphocytes to become cytotoxic and B cells to produce antibody.

Th1 cells (*inflammatory* T cells) are defined as typically (1) secreting the cytokines IL-2, IFN-γ, and TNF-β [plus granulocyte–macrophage colony-stimulating factor (GM-CSF) and IL-3]; (2) mediating delayed-type hypersensitivity; and (3) promoting IgG2a production. Th2 cells are defined as typically (1) secreting IL-4, IL-5, and IL-6 (plus GM-CSF and IL-3); (2) providing help, but not directly mediating delayed-type hypersensitivity responses; and (3) promoting the switch by B cells from IgG2 to IgG1 production in some species. Individual $CD4^+$ T cell clones vary widely in the particular combinations of cytokines they produce; the two dominant patterns described earlier tend to emerge in chronic persisting infections.

Th1 cells, i.e., cells expressing CD4 (and some expressing CD8), secrete lymphokines that set up the inflammatory response and greatly augment the immune response by attracting both monocytes/macrophages and other T cells to the site of the viral infection. These same lymphokines are self-activating, causing the cells that secrete them to be activated, to proliferate, to differentiate, and to secrete other cytokines. This response is the basis for delayed-type hypersensitivity responses that are a recognized part of the pathogenesis of many viral infections. The same response occurs when an antigen is injected intradermally—this is the basis for skin tests wherein a localized reaction is elicited in previously infected animals.

Some T cells can be demonstrated to down-regulate other T cell and/or B cell responses, which at one time suggested that there may be a further class of cell, once referred to as T suppressor cells. However, it has proved difficult to clone T cells that display this property and the view now is that suppressor functions are subsumed by Th and Tc cells. T cells may suppress various arms of the immune response in a variety of ways; e.g., by direct interaction with lymphocytes or via the production of immunosuppressive cytokines.

Cytotoxic T Lymphocytes

Cytotoxic T lymphocytes carry the CD8 surface marker and possess T cell receptors that recognize viral peptides presented on the surface of virus-infected target cells in association with class I MHC molecules. Activation and subsequent cytolysis of target cells by Tc cells require direct Tc–target cell contact in a manner reminiscent of a synapse (this contact has been called "the kiss of death"). Granules within the cytoplasm of the Tc cell polarize toward the target cell plasma membrane and their contents are released. A monomeric protein called perforin is secreted and polymerizes to form ~17-mer mushroom-shaped structures that insert themselves into the target cell plasma membrane, creating a pore that brings about the lysis of the cell. Perforin is structurally and functionally very similar to C9, which is responsible for complement-mediated lysis (see later). There is also evidence that both Tc and NK cells release lymphocyte-specific granules that have serine esterase activity (granzymes); these granules induce apoptosis in target cells.

The effector response of T cells is generally transient: in certain acute infections, Th and Tc activities peak about 1 week after the onset of viral infection and disappear by 2 to 3 weeks. It is not yet clear whether this is attributable to the destruction of infected cells with consequential removal of the antigenic stimulus or whether it is due to suppressor functions of T cells.

γ/δ T Lymphocytes

An entirely different class of T cells with a different type of T cell receptor composed of polypeptide heterodimers designated γ and δ (rather than the conventional α and β chains) is found principally in epithelia such as the skin, intestine, and lungs. In mice and humans this class constitutes a small minority (about 5%) of the T cell population. These cells appear to display a relatively limited immunologic repertoire, reflecting highly restricted V (variable) gene usage. There is emerging evidence, however, that these T cells are involved in the immune responses to viral infections that enter through those portals at which they are localized and there is evidence that they may recognize antigen in a non-MHC-restricted manner. These characteristics suggest that these cells may be more important than previously recognized, but their precise role and importance in specific infections have not been established. In swine, ruminants, and chickens, γ/δ cells represent about 30% of T lymphocytes and are distributed more widely in the body.

Monocytes, Macrophages, and Dendritic Cells

Monocytes, because of their mobility and homing capacity, and macrophages and dendritic cells, because of their key locations in various tissues (e.g., alveolar macrophages in the lung, Kupffer cells in the liver, Langerhans dendritic cells in the skin), are important initiators of the immune response against viral invasion. They are involved early in the host's response: (1) monocytes infiltrate tissue and differentiate to become macrophages, (2) macrophages often become the predominant cell in an infection focus by 24 hours after viral invasion, and (3) dendritic cells carry out afferent immune functions at all body surfaces and in key organs such as lymph nodes, spleen, and liver, where most phagocytic removal of foreign particles occurs. All three cell types bear immunoglobulin Fc and C3b receptors on their surfaces, which promotes the phagocytosis of immune complexes, i.e., virions coated with antibody. By serving as "professional" antigen-presenting cells, these cells exercise a controlling influence over the rapidity, magnitude, and dynamics of the immune response.

Macrophages then also give expression to the efferent limb of the immune response: cytokines secreted by activated T cells bring more monocytes into the infection focus and activate them as they differentiate into macrophages. Activated macrophages have increased chemotactic activity, phagocytic activity, and digestive powers.

Natural Killer Cells

Natural killer (NK) cells are a heterogeneous group of $CD3^-$, $CD16^+$, $CD56^+$ large granular lymphocytes of uncertain lineage that have the capacity to kill virus-infected cells and tumor cells. The basis for their selectivity for virus-infected cells is related to the down-regulation of the synthesis and expression of MHC class I proteins ("missing self-hypothesis"), which is an early feature of many virus-infected cells. They display no immunologic specificity for particular viral antigens, no memory, no MHC restriction, and no dependence on antibody. They are an important early defense mechanism, as their activity is enhanced greatly within 1 or 2 days of viral infection. Virus-induced activation of NK cells is mediated by interferons, acting synergistically with IL-2, and NK cells themselves secrete several cytokines, including interferon γ and tumor necrosis factor α.

Subcellular Components of the Immune System

Major Histocompatibility Complex

To understand antigen processing and presentation, one must first know something about the structure and intracellular production of MHC proteins. During ontogeny, the positive selection of developing T cells in the thymus by "self" MHC molecules results in mature T cells that can recognize foreign peptides, but only if they are located in the peptide-binding cleft of "self" MHC protein molecules—not when they are free in the extracellular space and not when they are associated with non-self MHC molecules (Figure 8.2). This phenomenon is known as *MHC restriction.*

There are two classes of MHC molecules, class I and class II; their structure is shown in Figure 8.3A. The two classes of T lymphocytes namely, Th and Tc, are defined by their interactions with class I or class II MHC proteins, respectively. The pathways used by cells to process and present antigenic peptides to Th and Tc cells are fundamentally different: they are referred to as the *exogenous pathway* for those peptides presented in association with MHC class II molecules and as the *endogenous pathway* for those peptides presented in association with MHC class I molecules.

The MHC is a genetic locus encoding three MHC class I proteins and up to 12 MHC class II proteins, each of which occurs in from 50 to 100 alternative allelic forms. Class I glycoproteins can be expressed on the plasma membrane of most types of cells (neurons are an exception), although they are not expressed constitutively, class II glycoproteins are expressed principally by "professional" antigen-presenting cells. At the distal tip of each class of MHC protein there is a cleft in which the antigenic peptide is bound and presented (Figures 8.3A and 8.3B). Peptide binding is determined by only two or three hydrophobic amino acids, called anchor residues, in a particular peptide and accordingly a particular MHC protein can bind numerous different peptides and some peptides can bind to several different MHC molecules. Peptides presented by class I molecules are usually 9 amino acids long (range 8- to 11-mers), whereas peptides binding to class II proteins range from 13 to 18 amino acids. The peptide-binding cleft in the case of class II is open at the ends whereas that of class I is closed. Specific amino acids that form pockets on the floor of the cleft of any particular MHC protein determine the particular range of peptides that can bind (Figure 8.3B). The peptide–MHC complex is in turn recognized, with absolute specificity, by the T cell receptor of the appropriate clone of T cells. Amino acid resi-

FIGURE 8.2.

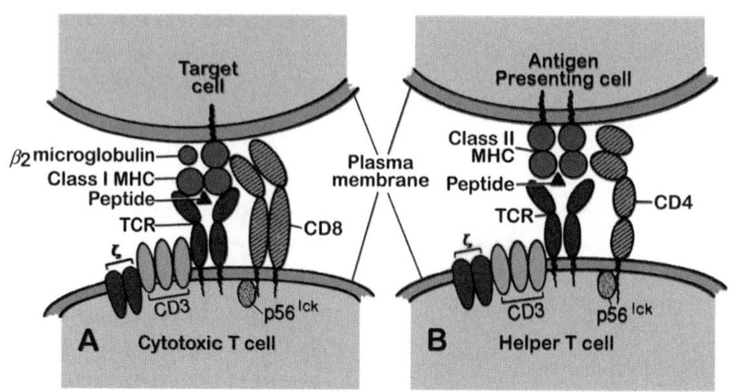

Model for the interaction among MHC proteins, T cell receptors, and CD4 or CD8 molecules. (A) CD8 on a cytotoxic T cell binds to a class I MHC protein on a target cell and interacts with a T cell receptor (TCR) molecule that is binding both to the same class I MHC protein and to the viral peptide it is presenting. (B) CD4 on a helper T cell binds to a class II MHC protein on an antigen-presenting cell and interacts with a TCR molecule that is binding both to the class II MHC protein and to the peptide it is presenting. The TCR is a heterodimer of two polypeptide chains, α and β, each with a constant domain spanning the plasma membrane of the cell and a variable region containing the peptide-binding groove. The TCR is associated with the accessory molecule CD3, a complex of three polypeptides (γ, δ, ε), plus a homodimer of ζ, which is thought to serve as a signal transducer for the TCR, being phosphorylated by the tyrosine kinase p56^{lck}, which is associated with the accessory molecules CD4 or CD8. The class I MHC protein is a polypeptide chain with three extracellular domains, associated with β_2-microglobulin; the class II MHC protein is composed of two polypeptide chains, each having two extracellular domains. Additional pairs of complementary adhesion molecules of different types (not shown) contribute to establishing and stabilizing close contact between T cells and antigen-presenting cells (including B cells). [Adapted from J. R. Parnes, Immunology. *In* "Encyclopedia of Human Biology" (R. Dulbecco, ed), Vol. 2, P. 225. Academic Press, San Diego, CA, 1991.]

dues that do not bind in the MHC cleft are hydrophobic and project outward, inviting recognition by T cell receptors.

Although there is extensive polymorphism of MHC genes between individual animals, any individual has only a limited number of different MHC proteins and any given antigenic peptide binds only to certain MHC molecules. If certain peptide–MHC complexes are important in eliciting a protective immune response to a serious viral infection, animals lacking suitable MHC proteins will be genetically more susceptible to that disease. A further cause of increased susceptibility lies in the possible absence from an individual animal's T cell repertoire of lymphocytes bearing receptors for that particular MHC–peptide complex.

Antigen Presentation by Cells Expressing MHC Class II: The Exogenous Pathway

Only a restricted range of cells, defined as antigen-presenting cells, process and present antigens in association with MHC class II to Th cells. Antigen-presenting cells include dendritic cells, monocyte/macrophages, and, later in the immune response, B lymphocytes. Dendritic cells, including Langerhans cells of the skin and the dendritic cells of lymph nodes and the splenic red pulp and marginal zones, are so named because they form long finger-like processes that interdigitate with lymphocytes, thereby favoring antigen presentation. Unlike dendritic cells, macrophages express relatively low levels of MHC class II protein while resting, but more following activation, particularly by interferon γ. After primary activation, B lymphocytes become important antigen-presenting cells; they are especially important during the latter stages of an infection and during reinfection. Memory B cells serve as very efficient antigen-presenting cells. Viral antigen, or the virion itself, binds to the specific immunoglobulin receptors on the B lymphocyte and is endocytosed, cleaved into peptides that are presented on the surface of the B cell in association with class II MHC proteins. These peptides generally represent different epitopes from those of the same antigen recognized by the B cell for the production of antibody. CD4$^+$ Th cells to which B cells present antigen respond by secreting cytokines that stimulate B cells to make antibody. Such *cognate* interaction, involving close physical association of T and B cells, ensures very efficient delivery of "helper factors" (cytokines) from the Th cell to the relevant primed B cell.

Virus or viral proteins taken up from an external source by antigen-presenting cells are said to enter the exogenous pathway; they pass progressively through early endosomes to late (acidic) endosomes and prelysosomes, where they are cleaved by proteolytic enzymes (Figure 8.4). Some of the resulting viral peptides are able to bind to class II MHC α and β polypeptides to form a trimeric complex that is then transported to the plasma membrane where they are recognized by CD4$^+$ T cells, leading to a Th cell response.

Antigen Presentation by Cells Expressing MHC Class I: The Endogenous Pathway

Almost all cells can be induced to synthesize MHC class I proteins following virus infection; neurons are an exception. After synthesis, MHC class I α- and β-microglobulin polypeptides are transported to the endoplasmic reticulum where they assemble to form a stable complex in association with a molecular chaperone protein called calnexin (Figure 8.4). In virus-infected cells, some viral protein molecules are degraded (cleaved) in the cytoplasm by the large (26S) LMP-containing proteosome complex—these viral proteins are said to enter the endogenous pathway. The resulting peptides are then transported by a transporter molecule (TAP, for transporter associated with antigen processing) into the endoplasmic reticulum, where they assemble with class I MHC molecules to form a stable trimeric complex, which is then exported, via the Golgi complex, to the cell surface for presentation to Tc cells. Both LMP and TAP proteins are coded for within the MHC gene complex.

FIGURE 8.3.

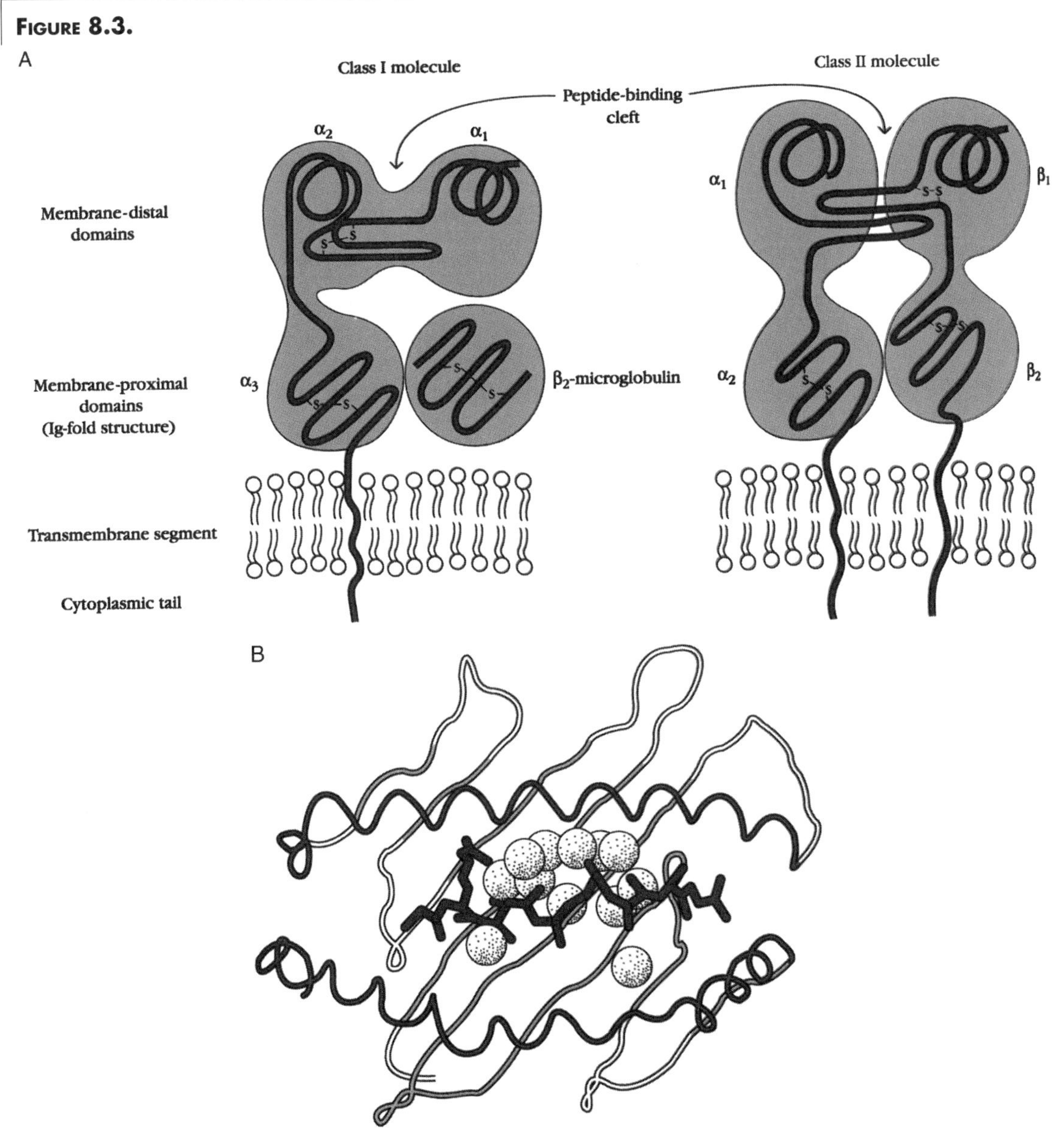

(A) Schematic diagram of MHC class I and MHC class II molecules showing the external domains, transmembrane domains, and cytoplasmic tail. The peptide-binding clefts are formed by the distal domains. (B) Viral peptide (stick model) lying in the cleft of an MHC class I molecule. The peptide arches up away from the β strands that form the floor of the binding cleft and interacts with 12 water molecules (spheres). (Adapted from J. Kuby, "Immunology," 3rd ed. Freeman, New York, 1997.)

Figure 8.4.

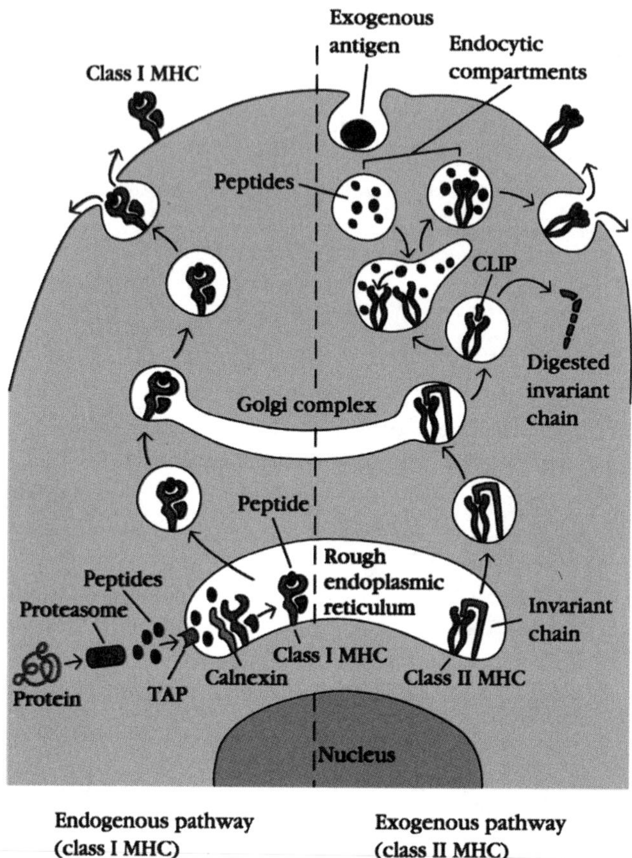

The endogenous and exogenous pathways of antigen processing and presentation. The mode of antigen entry into cells and the site of antigen processing appear to determine whether antigenic peptides associate with MHC class I molecules in the rough endoplasmic reticulum (left of dotted line) or with MHC class II molecules in endocytic compartments (right of dotted line). (From J. Kuby, "Immunology," 3rd ed. Freeman, New York, 1997.)

Cytokines

Cytokines are low molecular weight hormone-like proteins that stimulate or inhibit the proliferation, differentiation, and/or maturation of immune cells (Table 8.1; Figure 8.5). They differ from true hormones in a number of ways, including being produced by nonspecialized cells. Many are produced by T lymphocytes (lymphokines) or monocytes/macrophages (monokines) and serve to regulate the immune response by coordinating the activities of the various cell types involved. Thus, while cytokines are not antigen specific, their production and actions are often antigen driven.

Cytokines may act on the cell that produced them (autocrine) or on cells in the immediate vicinity (paracrine), particularly at cell–cell interfaces, where directional secretion may occur and very low concentrations may be effective, or they may act on cells at more distant locations (endocrine). Responsive target cells carry receptors for the particular cytokines. A single cytokine may exert a multiplicity of biological effects, often acting on more than one type of cell. Moreover, different cytokines may exert similar effects, although perhaps via distinct postreceptor signal transduction pathways, resulting in synergism (Figure 8.6). There is much redundancy in the actions of cytokines, presumably linked to the need to provide fail-safe defense mechanisms; it is frequently the case that the use of *knockout* mice characterized by the deletion of a single cytokine gene fail to succumb to particular virus challenges.

Cytokines up-regulate or down-regulate the target cell, and different cytokines can antagonize one another. Typically, a cytokine secreted by a particular type of cell activates another type of cell to secrete a different cytokine or to express receptors for a particular cytokine, and so on in a sort of chain reaction (Figure 8.1). Because of the intricacy of the cytokine cascade, it is rarely possi-

Table 8.1
Cytokines: Sources, Targets, and Effects[a,b,c]

Cytokine	Principal source	Principal target/effects
IL-1α, β	Monocytes/macrophages, B cells, dendritic cells	Proliferation of T cells, IL-2 receptor expression, antibody, fever
IL-2	Th1 cells	Proliferation and differentiation of T cells
IL-3	T cells, NK cells, mast cells	Stem cells and mast cells; hematopoiesis, histamine release
IL-4	Th2 cells, mast cells, NK cells	Proliferation and differentiation of B cells, T cells, and macrophages; switch from IgM to IgG1 and IgE; up-regulates MHC class II expression
IL-5	Th2 cells, mast cells	Proliferation and differentiation of B cells and eosinophils; class switch to IgA
IL-6	Th2 cells, macrophages, other cells	Proliferating B cells, plasma cells hepatocytes; promotes differentiation to plasma cells; synthesis of acute-phase proteins (fever)
IL-7	Bone marrow and thymic stromal cells	Proliferation of pre-B and pre-T cells; increases expression of IL-2 and its receptor
IL-8	Macrophages, endothelial cells	Chemotaxis, adhesion, and diapedesis of neutrophils
IL-9	Th cells	Some Th cells; acts as a mitogen supporting proliferation in the absence of antigen
IL-10	Th2 cells	Inhibits cytokine production by macrophages and hence indirectly reduces cytokine production by T cells
IL-11	Bone marrow stromal cells	Pre-B cells, plasmocytoma cells, megakaryocytes, hepatocytes; growth and differentiation
IL-12	Macrophages, B cells	Acts synergistically with IL-2 to promote differentiation of Tc cells; proliferation of NK cells
IL-13	Th cells	Macrophages; inhibits activation and release of inflammatory cytokines
IL-15	T cells, intestinal epithelium, NK, and activated B cells	Growth and proliferation of intestinal epithelium and T cells; comitogen
IL-16	T cells (primarily Tc cells), macrophages, eosinophils	Th cells, chemotaxis, MHC class II expression, suppression of antigen-induced proliferation
TNF-α, β	Macrophages, Th1, Tc, and mast cells	Antiviral; proliferation and differentiation of T cells, B cells, macrophages, NK cells and fibroblasts; fever; cytotoxic, induces cachexia
TGF-β	Platelets, macrophages, lymphocytes, mast cells	Inhibits proliferation of T cells, B cells, and stem cells and induces increased IL-1 production, thereby inhibiting inflammation and promoting wound healing; induces class switch to IgA
IFN-α, β	Leukocytes, other cells	Antiviral; fever
IFN-γ	Th1, Tc, and NK cells	Antiviral; activation of Th2 cells, macrophages, and NK cells; IgM to Ig2a switch; blocks IL-4-induced class switch to IgE and IgG1; up-regulates MHC and Fc receptors
GM-CSF	T cells, macrophages, endothelium	Hematopoiesis, granulocytes, monocytes

[a]Cytokines are pleiotropic, i.e., single molecules have several distinct and seemingly unrelated phenotypic effects.
[b]Only certain major activities of the best-studied cytokines are listed in this condensed summary.
[c]IL, Interleukin; TNF, tumor necrosis factor; TGF, transforming growth factor; IFN, interferon; CSF, colony-stimulating factor.

ble to attribute a given biological event *in vivo* to a single cytokine.

Cytokines can influence viral pathogenesis in a number of ways: (1) augmentation of the immune response, e.g., of cytotoxic T cells by tumor necrosis factor α or by interferon γ, which up-regulates MHC expression; (2) regulation of the immune response, e.g., antibody isotype switching by interleukin 4, 5, 6, or interferon γ; (3) suppression of the immune response, e.g., interleukin 10 inhibits the synthesis of interferon γ; (4)

FIGURE 8.5.

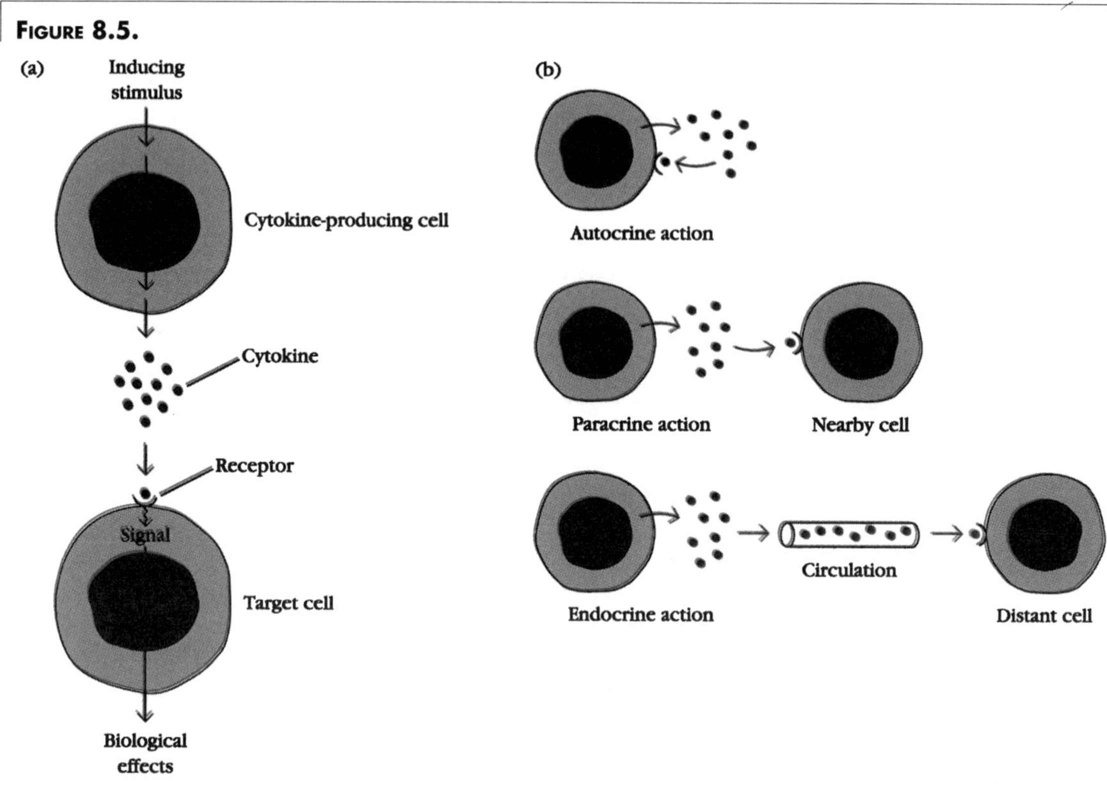

(A) General overview of the induction and function of cytokines. (B) Most cytokines have autocrine and/or paracrine actions; some also have endocrine actions. (From J. Kuby, "Immunology," 3rd ed. Freeman, New York, 1997.)

inhibition of viral replication by interferons; and (5) upregulation of viral gene expression.

Antibodies

The end result of activation and maturation of B cells is the production of antibodies, which react specifically with the epitope identified initially by their receptors. Antibodies fall into four main classes: two monomers, IgG and IgE, and two polymers, IgM and IgA. All immunoglobulins of a particular class have a similar structure, but they vary widely in the amino acid sequences comprising the antigen-binding site, which determines their specificity for a given antigenic determinant. The commonest immunoglobulin found in serum, IgG, consists of two H and two L chains, and each chain consists of a *constant* and a *variable* domain. The chains are held together by disulfide bonds. Papain cleavage separates the molecules into two identical *Fab fragments,* which contain the antigen-binding sites, and an *Fc fragment,* which carries the sites for various effector functions such as complement fixation, attachment to phagocytic cells, and placental or colostrum transfer (Figure 8.7).

The immunologic specificity of an antibody molecule is determined by its ability to bind specifically to a particular epitope. The binding site, i.e., the *antibody-binding groove,* is located at the amino-terminal end of the molecule. The variable regions of both L and H chains comprise about 107 amino acids within which there are three hypervariable domains termed *complementary determining regions* interspersed between four conserved regions called *framework regions.* When the peptides fold to form the three-dimensional functional Ig structure, the six complementary determining regions (three each from L and H chains) are located in the antigen-binding groove. It is the variability of the complementary determining regions that accounts for the limitless range of different epitopes recognized by these molecules. (Similar principles underlie the generation of antigenic diversity found in T cell receptor variable regions.)

Antibodies directed against certain epitopes on the surface of virions neutralize infectivity; they may also act as opsonins, facilitating the uptake and destruction of virions by macrophages. In addition, antibody may attach to viral antigens on the surface of infected cells, leading to their destruction following activation of the

Figure 8.6.

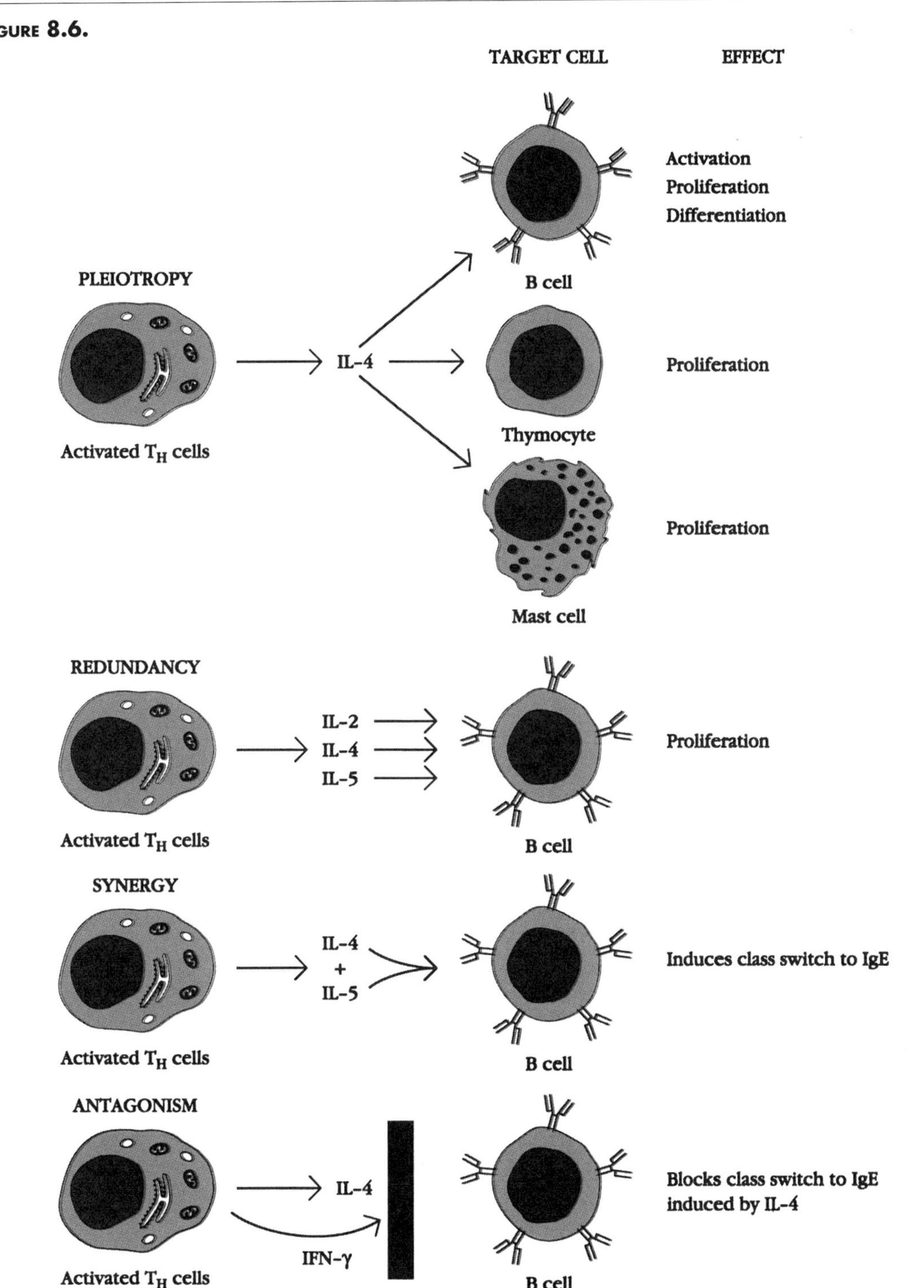

Examples of cytokine pleiotropy, redundancy, synergy, and antagonism. (From J. Kuby, "Immunology," 3rd ed. Freeman, New York, 1997.)

FIGURE 8.7.

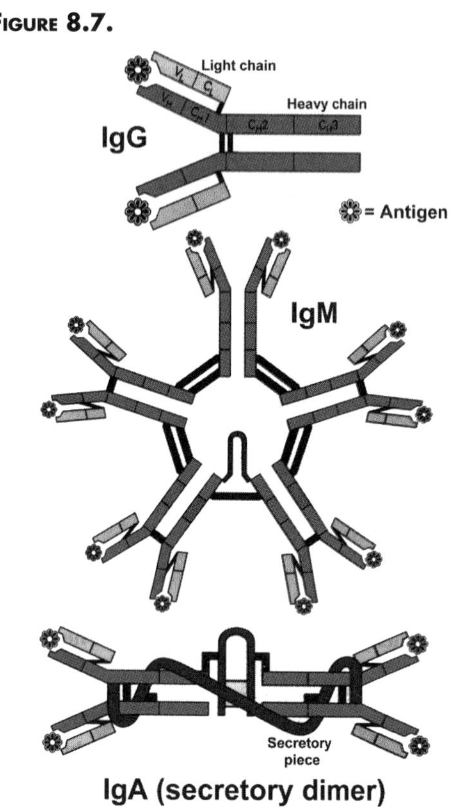

The basic structure of the immunoglobulins. The antigen-binding end of each class of immunoglobulin molecule consists of two identical light polypeptide chains and two identical heavy chains linked together by disulfide bonds. Each chain is made up of individual globular domains. Different antibodies have different V_L and V_H domains, which are highly variable, whereas the remaining domains (C_L, and C_H 1, 2, etc.) are relatively constant in amino acid sequence and structure. IgG occurs as four subclasses—IgG1,2,3, and 4—each with somewhat different properties (e.g., IgG1 is secreted in very large amounts in bovine colostrum). IgM molecules are pentameric, with five antigen-binding sites—IgM binds antigens most avidly. IgA, in its soluble form as found in the circulation, resembles IgG; in its secretory form, as found in mucus and other secretions, it is a dimer, formed by the binding of a J chain (secretory piece), which facilitates its movement across mammary epithelium and into mucus secretions.

classical or alternative complement pathways or by arming and activating Fc receptor-bearing cells such as NK cells, polymorphonuclear leukocytes, and macrophages (antibody-dependent cell-mediated cytotoxicity).

Immunoglobulin G

The major class of antibody in the blood is immunoglobulin G (IgG), which occurs as IgG1, IgG2, IgG3, and IgG4 subclasses. Following systemic viral infections, IgG continues to be synthesized for many years and is the principal mediator of protection against reinfection. The subclasses of IgG differ in the constant region of their heavy chains and consequently in biological properties such as complement fixation and binding to phagocytes.

Immunoglobulin M

Immunoglobulin M (IgM) is a particularly avid class of antibody, being a pentamer of five IgG equivalents, with 10 Fab fragments and therefore 10 antigen-binding sites. Because IgM is formed early in the immune response and is later replaced by IgG, specific antibodies of the IgM class are diagnostic of recent (or chronic) infection. Low levels of IgM may be found in the fetus as it develops immunologic competence in the second half of pregnancy. In fact, because IgM does not cross the placenta from dam to fetus in any species, the presence of IgM antibodies against a particular virus in a newborn animal may be indicative of intrauterine viral infection.

Immunoglobulin A

Immunoglobulin A (IgA) is a dimer, with four Fab fragments. Passing through epithelial cells, IgA acquires a J fragment (J, for joining, also called the secretory piece) to become *secretory IgA,* which is secreted through the epithelium into the respiratory, intestinal, and urogenital tracts. Secretory IgA is more resistant to proteases than other immunoglobulins and is the principal immunoglobulin on mucosal surfaces and, in some species of animals, in milk and colostrum. For this reason IgA antibodies are important in resistance to infection of the respiratory, intestinal, and urogenital tracts, and IgA antibody responses are much more effectively elicited by oral or respiratory than by systemic administration of antigen, a matter of importance in the design and route of delivery of some vaccines (see Chapter 13).

Immunoglobulins D and E

IgD and IgE are minor immunoglobulin species, accounting for less than 1% of total immunoglobulin levels: (1) most IgD is bound to the surface of B lymphocytes but its function there is not clear; (2) IgE, which is produced by subepithelial plasma cells in the respiratory and intestinal tracts, binds strongly to mast cells where it reacts with certain kinds of antigens (allergens). It stimulates the release of mediators of anaphylaxis such as serotonin and histamine.

Complement

The *complement system* consists of about 30 serum proteins, which can be activated to "complement" the immune response (Figure 8.8). As well as the classical complement activation pathway, which is dependent on the presence of antibody–antigen complexes, there is also

Figure 8.8.

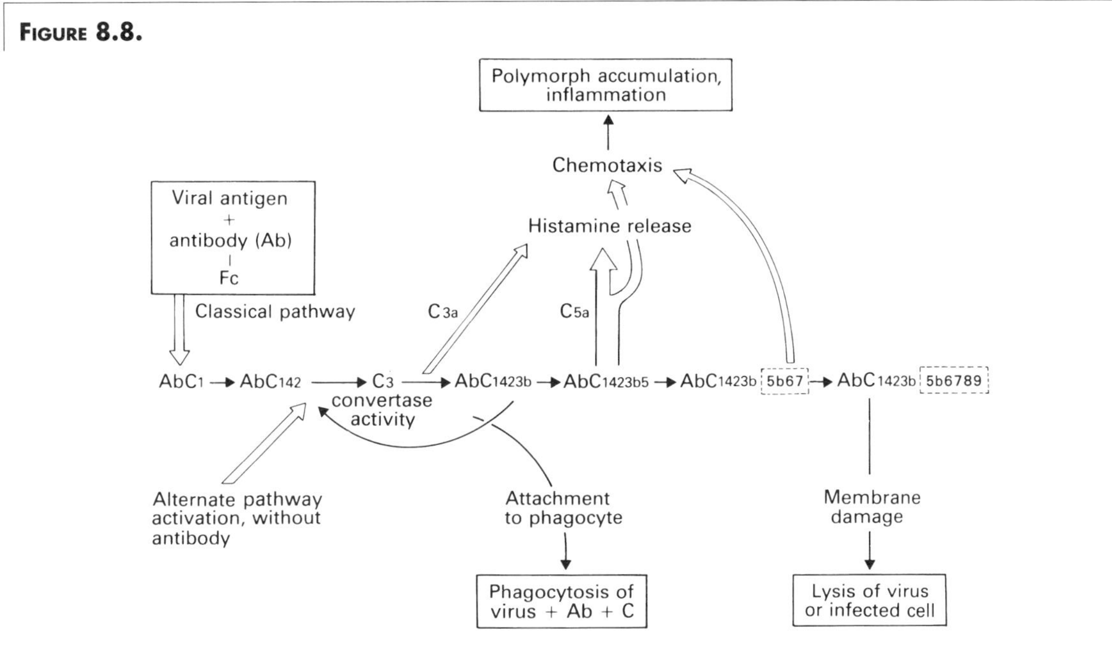

Diagram of the complement activation sequence by the classical and alternate pathways and the antiviral action of complement. The numbers of the complement components are not sequential because they were assigned before the sequence of action was elucidated. (Courtesy of C. A. Mims and D. O. White.)

an alternative antibody-independent pathway. Both are important in viral infections.

Activation of complement by the classical pathway may lead to the destruction of virions or virus-infected cells, as well as to inflammation. Virions are destroyed as a result of opsonization, enhancement of neutralization, or lysis of the viral envelope. Complement activation following interaction of antibody with viral antigens in tissues leads to inflammation and the accumulation of leukocytes. Activation of complement via the alternative pathway appears to occur mainly after infections with enveloped viruses that mature by budding through the plasma membrane; because it does not require antibody, the alternate pathway can occur immediately after viral invasion of the body.

Immunologic Memory

Following priming by antigen and clonal expansion of lymphocytes, a population of long-lived *memory cells* arises that persists indefinitely. Memory T cells are characterized by particular surface markers (notably CD45RO) and homing molecules (*adhesins*) that are associated with distinct recirculation pathways. When reexposed to the same antigen, even many years later, they respond more rapidly and more vigorously than in the primary encounter. Memory B cells, on reexposure to antigen, also display an *anamnestic (secondary) response,* with the production of larger amounts of specific antibody.

Little is known about the mechanism of the longevity of immunologic memory in T or B lymphocytes in the absence of demonstrable chronic infection. The cells may be restimulated periodically by the original antigenic peptide retained for long periods as peptide–MHC complexes on follicular dendritic cells in lymphoid follicles or by surrogate antigen in the form of either fortuitously cross-reactive antigens or anti-idiotypic antibodies. Memory T and B lymphocytes may survive for years without dividing, until restimulated following reinfection.

Immune Responses to Viral Infection

An overview of the major features of the immune response to a typical acute viral infection is illustrated in Figure 8.1. As shown, at least three phenomena contribute to recovery from infection: (1) destruction of infected cells, (2) production of interferons, and (3) neutralization of the infectivity of virions. Shortly after infection, some virus particles are phagocytosed by macrophages. Except in the case of certain viruses that are capable of growing in macrophages, the engulfed virions are destroyed. Their proteins are cleaved into short peptides that are presented on the surface of the macrophage in association with class II MHC protein. This combination is recognized by the appropriate clones of $CD4^+$ lymphocytes. Th1 lymphocytes respond by clonal proliferation and release of lymphokines, which attract blood monocytes to the site and induce them to proliferate and differentiate into activated macrophages, the basis of the inflammatory response. Th2 lymphocytes respond by secreting a different set of lymphokines that assist the appropriate clones of B cells, following binding of viral antigen, to divide and differentiate into plasma cells. Tc cells are activated following the recognition of viral peptides in association with MHC class I on the surface of infected cells. The Tc response usually peaks at about 1 week after infection, compared with the antibody response that peaks later (2 to 3 weeks). NK cell activity is maximal by 2 days, and interferon activity peaks in concert with the peak titer of virus.

Antibody synthesis takes place principally in the spleen, lymph nodes, gut-associated lymphoid tissues (GALT), and bronchus-associated lymphoid tissues (BALT). The spleen and lymph nodes receive viral antigens via the blood or lymphatics and synthesize antibodies mainly restricted to the IgM class early in the response and IgG subclasses subsequently. However, the submucosal lymphoid tissues of the respiratory and digestive tracts, such as the tonsils and Peyer's patches, receive antigens directly from overlying epithelial cells and make antibodies mainly of the IgA class.

Immune Cytolysis of Virus-Infected Cells

Destruction of infected cells is an essential feature of recovery from viral infections and it results from any of four different processes, involving cytotoxic T cells, antibody complement-mediated cytotoxicity, antibody-dependent cell-mediated cytotoxicity, or NK cells. Because some viral proteins, or peptides derived therefrom, appear in the plasma membrane before any virions have been produced, lysis of the cell at this stage brings viral replication to a halt before significant numbers of progeny virions are released.

Antibody-complement-mediated cytotoxicity is demonstrable readily *in vitro* even at very low concentrations of antibody. The alternative complement activation pathway (Figure 8.8) appears to be particularly important in this phenomenon. *Antibody-dependent cell-mediated cytotoxicity (ADCC)* is mediated by leukocytes that carry Fc receptors: macrophages, polymorphonuclear leukocytes, and other kinds of killer cells. NK cells, however, are activated by interferon or directly by viral glycoproteins. They demonstrate no immunologic specificity, but preferentially lyse virus-infected cells. In addition, in the presence of antibody, macrophages can phagocytose and digest virus-infected cells.

Neutralization of Viral Infectivity

In contrast to T cells, B cells and antibody generally recognize epitopes that are *conformational,* i.e., critical residues that make contact with the antigen-binding site of the antibody molecule are not necessarily contiguous in the primary amino acid sequence but are brought into close apposition as a result of the folding of the polypeptide chain(s) to produce the native conformation. Such B cell epitopes are generally located on the surface of the protein, often on prominent protuberances or loops, and generally represent relatively variable regions of the molecule, differing between strains of that species of virus.

While a specific antibody of any class can bind to any accessible epitope on a surface protein of a virion, only those antibodies that bind with reasonably high affinity to particular epitopes on a particular protein of the outer capsid or envelope of the virion are capable of neutralizing viral infectivity. The key protein is usually the one containing the ligand by which the virion attaches to receptors on the host cell. Mutations in critical epitopes on such a protein allow the virus to escape from neutralization by antibody, and the gradual emergence of mutations in a majority of these epitopes leads to the emergence of a novel strain (genetic/antigenic drift; see Chapter 4).

Neutralization is not simply a matter of coating the virion with antibody nor indeed of blocking attachment to the host cell. Except in the presence of such high concentrations of antibody that most or all accessible antigenic sites on the surface of the virion are saturated, neutralized virions may still attach to susceptible cells. In such cases the neutralizing block occurs at some point following adsorption and entry. One hypothesis is that whereas the virion is normally uncoated intracellularly in a controlled way that preserves its infectivity, a virion–antibody complex may be destroyed by lysosomal enzymes. For example, in the case of picornaviruses, the neutralizing antibody appears to distort the capsid, leading to loss of a particular capsid protein, which renders the virion vulnerable to enzymatic attack. With influenza virus, more subtle conformational changes in the hemagglutinin molecule may prevent the fusion event that precedes the release of the nucleocapsid from the viral envelope.

Recovery from Viral Infection

Cell-mediated immunity, antibody, complement, phagocytes, interferons, and other cytokines are all involved in recovery from viral infections—in most cases several of these arms of the immune system act in concert, again depending on the particular host–virus combination.

Role of T Lymphocytes

Lymphocytes and macrophages normally predominate in the cellular infiltration of virus-infected tissues; in contrast to bacterial infections, polymorphonuclear leukocytes are not at all plentiful. T cell depletion by neonatal thymectomy or antilymphocyte serum treatment increases the susceptibility of experimental animals to most viral infections; for example, T cell-depleted mice infected with ectromelia virus fail to show the usual inflammatory mononuclear cell infiltration in the liver, develop extensive liver necrosis, and die, despite the production of antiviral antibodies and interferon. Virus titers in the liver and spleen of infected mice can be reduced greatly by the adoptive transfer of immune T cells taken from recovered donors; this process is class I MHC restricted, implicating Tc cells, and is lifesaving.

Another approach used to "dissect" the immune response of experimentally infected inbred mice is to ablate completely all immune potential (using X-irradiation, cytotoxic drugs, etc.), then to separately add back individual components. In a now classic model, virus-primed cytotoxic T lymphocytes of defined function and specificity, cloned in culture and then transferred to infected animals, saved the lives of mice infected with lymphocytic choriomeningitis virus, influenza virus, and several other viruses. Generally, greater protection is conferred by $CD8^+$ T cells than by $CD4^+$ T cells. Moreover, transgenic mice lacking $CD8^+$ T cells suffer higher morbidity and mortality than normal mice following virus challenge. Nevertheless, $CD4^+$ T cells have been shown to play a significant role in recovery, as do the cytokines they secrete, notably interferon γ and IL-2.

Although T cell determinants and B cell epitopes on surface proteins of viruses sometimes overlap, the immunodominant Tc determinants are often situated on the relatively conserved proteins located in the interior of the virion or on nonstructural virus-coded proteins that occur only in virus-infected cells. Hence T cell responses are generally of broader specificity than neutralizing antibody responses and display cross-reactivity between strains and serotypes. When the gene encoding a protein that fails to elicit any neutralizing antibody (e.g., the NP, M, or NS protein of influenza virus) is incorporated into the genome of vaccinia virus, the T cells elicited following infection with this construct can adoptively transfer complete protection to naive mice against challenge with influenza virus.

Role of Antibody

In generalized diseases characterized by a viremia in which virions circulate free in the plasma, circulating antibody plays a significant role in recovery. Data are not available for veterinary and zoonotic diseases, but there are good data from human diseases: human infants with severe primary agammaglobulinemia recover normally from measles virus infection, but are about 10,000 times more likely than normal infants to develop paralytic disease after vaccination with attenuated poliovirus vaccine. These infants have normal cell-mediated immune and interferon responses, normal phagocytic cells, and a normal complement system, but cannot produce antibody, which is essential if poliovirus spread to the central nervous system via the bloodstream is to be prevented.

Although there is reasonably good evidence that antibody plays a key role in recovery from picornavirus, togavirus, flavivirus, and parvovirus infections in animals, it does not necessarily follow that antibody is acting solely by neutralizing virions. Indeed it has been shown that certain nonneutralizing monoclonal antibodies can save the lives of mice inoculated with various viruses, presumably by antibody-dependent cell-mediated cytotoxicity, antibody complement-mediated lysis of infected cells, or by opsonization of virions for macrophages.

Lessons from Experimental and Natural Congenital Immunodeficiencies

One approach to understanding the mechanisms involved in recovery from viral infection that is not subject to laboratory artifact is simple clinical observation of viral infections in animals or children suffering from primary immunodeficiencies. For example, athymic (*nude*) mice, which are congenitally deficient in T cells, are highly susceptible to many viral infections. In certain families of Arabian horses there is a total or near total absence of both B and T lymphocytes. Characteristic findings are lymphopenia and hypogammaglobulinemia, which render foals unusually susceptible to infections, especially equine adenovirus 1 infection. There are also several types of B lymphocyte deficiency that predispose newborn animals to very severe infections. Among these are a primary agammaglobulinemia of thoroughbred horses, a selective deficiency in foals of IgM-producing

B cells, a deficiency of IgG2-synthesizing cells in some breeds of cattle, and dysgammaglobulinemia in certain lines of White Leghorn chickens. Furthermore, there are conditions characterized by a T cell deficiency due to thymic hypoplasia. Of different origin and significance, but of great practical importance, are secondary agammaglobulinemias and hypogammaglobulinemias in foals, piglets, lambs, and especially calves, associated with the failure of antibody transfer via colostrum (see later).

Immunity to Reinfection

Whereas a large number of interacting phenomena contribute to recovery from viral infection, the mechanism of acquired immunity to reinfection with the same virus appears to be much simpler. The first line of defense is antibody, which, if acquired by active infection with a virus that causes systemic infections, continues to be synthesized for many years, providing solid protection against reinfection. The degree of acquired immunity generally correlates well with the titer of antibody in the serum. Further, transfer of antibody alone, whether by artificial passive immunization or by maternal antibody transfer from dam to fetus or newborn, provides excellent protection in the case of many viral infections. Thus it is reasonable to conclude that antibody is the most influential factor in immunity acquired by natural infection or by vaccination. If the antibody defenses are inadequate, the mechanisms that contribute to recovery are called into play again, the principal differences on this occasion being that the dose of infecting virus is reduced by antibody and that primed memory T and B lymphocytes generate a more rapid secondary response.

As a general rule, the secretory IgA response is short lived compared to the serum IgG response. Accordingly, resistance to reinfection with respiratory viruses and some enteric viruses tends to be of limited duration. For example, reinfection with the same serotype of parainfluenza virus or respiratory syncytial virus is not uncommon. Moreover, reinfection at a time of waning immunity favors the selection of neutralization-escape mutants, resulting in the emergence of new strains of viruses such as influenza virus by antigenic drift. Because there is little or no cross-protection between antigenically distinct strains of virus, repeated attacks of respiratory infections occur throughout life.

The immune response to the first infection with a virus can have a dominating influence on subsequent immune responses to antigenically related viruses, in that the second virus often induces a response that is directed mainly against the antigens of the original viral strain. For example, the antibody response to sequential infections with different strains of influenza A virus is largely directed to antigenic determinants of the particular strain of virus with which that individual was first infected. This phenomenon, irreverently called "original antigenic sin," is also seen in infections with enteroviruses, reoviruses, paramyxoviruses and togaviruses. Original antigenic sin has important implications for the interpretation of seroepidemiologic data, for understanding immunopathologic phenomena, and particularly for the development of efficacious vaccination strategies.

Passive Immunity

There is abundant evidence for the efficacy of antibody in preventing infection. For example, artificial *passive immunization* (injection of antibodies) temporarily protects against infection with canine distemper, feline panleukopenia, hog cholera, and many other viral infections (see Chapter 13). Furthermore, natural passive immunization, i.e., the transfer of maternal antibody from dam to fetus or newborn, protects the newborn for the first few months of life against most of the infections that the dam has experienced.

Natural Passive Immunity

Natural passive immunity is important for two major reasons: (1) it is essential for the protection of young animals, during the first weeks or months of life, from the myriad of microorganisms, including viruses, that are present in the environment into which animals are born and (2) maternally derived antibody interferes with active immunization of the newborn and must therefore be taken into account when designing vaccination schedules (see Chapter 13).

Transfer of Maternal Antibodies

Maternal antibodies may be transmitted in the egg yolk in birds, across the placenta in primates or via colostrum and/or milk in other mammals. Different species of mammals differ strikingly in the predominant route of transfer of maternal antibodies, depending on the structure of the placenta of the species (Table 8.2). In those species in which the maternal and fetal circulations are separated by relatively few (one to three) placental layers, antibody of the IgG (but not IgM) class is able to cross the placenta, and maternal immunity is transmitted mainly by this route. However, the placenta of most domestic animals is more complex (five to six layers) and, it is hypothesized, acts as a barrier even to IgG; in these species,

Table 8.2
Transfer of Natural Passive Immunity in Mammals

Species	Type of Placentation	Number of Placental Layers: Maternal	Number of Placental Layers: Fetal	Prenatal Transfer (via Placenta)	Postnatal Transfer (via Gut)	Translocation Cut-off Time (Days)
Cattle, swine, horses	Epitheliochorial	3	3	0	+++	2
Sheep, goats	Syndesmochorial	2 or 3	3	0	+++	2
Dogs, cats	Endotheliochorial	1	2 or 3	±	+++	2
Mice, rats	Hemochorial	0	3	++	+	16–20

maternal immunity is transmitted to the newborn via colostrum and, to a much lesser extent, via milk.

Different species differ in regard to the particular class or subclass of immunoglobulin that is transferred preferentially to the newborn in colostrum (Table 8.3), but in most domestic animals it is mainly IgG. In cattle and sheep there is a selective transfer of IgG1 from the serum across the alveolar epithelium of the mammary gland during the last few weeks of pregnancy, such that the level of IgG1 in colostrum may reach 40 to 70 g/liter, compared with about 1.0 to 1.8 g/liter in milk and 13 g/liter in serum. Antibodies of the IgG1 class are important in protection against enteric infections as long as suckling continues.

The selective transfer of IgG from the maternal circulation across the mammary alveolar epithelium is a function of the Fc fragment of the molecule. The very large amounts of IgG present in colostrum are ingested and *translocated* in large intracytoplasmic vesicles by specialized cells present in the upper part of small intestine to reach the circulation of the newborn in an undergraded form. Small amounts of other antibodies (IgM, IgA) present in colostrum or milk may, in some species, also be translocated across the gut, but disappear quickly from the circulation of the young animal. The period after birth during which antibody, ingested as colostrum, is translocated (called the *translocation cutoff* time) is sharply defined and very brief (about 48 hours) in most domestic animals (Table 8.2).

In birds there is a selective transfer of IgG from the maternal circulation; the level of IgG in chicken egg yolk is 25 g/liter compared to 6 g/liter in the maternal circulation. A laying hen produces about 100 g of IgG per year for transfer to yolk, which is about as much as she synthesizes for her own needs. IgG enters the vitelline circulation and hence that of the chick from day 12 of incubation. Some IgG is also transferred to the amniotic fluid and is swallowed by the chick. Close to the time of hatching, the yolk sac with the remaining maternal immunoglobulin is completely taken into the abdominal

Table 8.3
Concentrations of Immunoglobulin Classes IgG, IgA, and IgM in Colostrum and Milk of Some Mammalian Species[a]

	Immunoglobulin concentration (grams/liter)					
	Colostrum			Milk		
Species	IgG	IgA	IgM	IgG	IgA	IgM
Cattle	36–77	4–5	3.2–4.9	1.0–1.8	0.2	0.04
Swine	62	10	3.2	1.4	3.0	1.9
Horse	80	9	4	0.35	0.8	0.04
Dog	2.0	13.5	0.3	0.01	3.6	0.06
Human	0.3	120	1.2	0.1	1.5	0.01

[a]An underbar indicates major components.

cavity and incorporated into the wall of the small intestine of the chick.

Maternal antibody in the bloodstream of the newborn mammal or newly hatched chick is destroyed quite rapidly, with first-order kinetics. The half-life, which is somewhat longer than in adult animals, ranges from about 21 days in the cow and horse through 8 to 9 days in the dog and cat to only 2 days in the mouse. Of course, the newborn animal will be protected against infection with any particular virus only if the dam's IgG contains specific antibodies, and protection may last much longer than one IgG half-life if the initial titer against that virus is high.

Although the levels of IgA transferred via colostrum to the gut of the newborn animal are considerably lower than those of IgG, it helps to protect the neonate against enteric viruses against which the dam has developed immunity. Moreover, there is evidence that after translocation cutoff immunoglobulins present in ordinary milk, principally IgA but also IgG and IgM, may continue to provide some protective immunity against gut infections. Often the newborn encounters viruses while still partially protected. Under these circumstances the virus replicates, but only to a limited extent, stimulating an immune response without causing significant disease. The newborn thus acquires active immunity while partially protected by maternal immunity.

Failure of Maternal Antibody Transfer

The failure or partial failure of maternal antibody transfer is the most common immunodeficiency disease of domestic animals. For example, between 10 and 40% of dairy calves and up to 20% of foals fail to receive adequate levels of maternal antibody. Mortality during the neonatal period, particularly from enteric and respiratory diseases, is higher than at any other time of life and there is a strong correlation with failure of antibody transfer. Biologic reasons for failure are (1) premature birth of weak animals, (2) delay to first suckle, (3) death of the dam, (4) low colostrum production by the dam, (5) low antibody levels in maternal serum and thus in colostrum, (6) poor maternal instinct, particularly in primiparous dams, (7) premature lactation, (8) too many in the litter, and (9) domination of the weak in the litter by the strong. Of these, the most critical factors are the amount of colostrum available and the delay between birth and first suckling. Poor management also plays a major role by the imposition of unnatural conditions on parturition and early suckling. Especially in large production units, making sure that every newborn receives colostrum is a major challenge. Maternal immunization to protect newborn animals has become an important strategy in veterinary medical practice (see Chapter 13).

Further Reading

Berke, G. (1995). Unlocking the secrets of CTL and NK cells. *Immunol. Today* **16**, 343–346.

Bjorkman, P. J., and Burmeister, W. P. (1994). Structures of two classes of MHC molecules elucidated: Crucial differences and similarities. *Curr. Opin. Struct. Biol.* **4**, 852–856.

Bloom, B. R., and Zinkernagel, R. eds. (1996). Immunity to infection—overview. *Curr. Opin. Immunol.* **8**, 465–466.

Braciale, T. J., ed. (1993). Immune responses to virus infection. *Semin. Virol.* **4**(2), 81–82.

Brandtzaeg, P. (1995). Basic mechanisms of mucosal immunity: A major adaptive defense system. *Immunologist* **3**, 89–95.

Brown, J. H., Jardetzky, T. S., Gorga, J. C., Stern, L. J., Urban, R. G., Strominger, J. L., and Wiley, D. C. (1993). Three-dimensional structure of the human class II histocompatability antigen, HLA-DR1. *Nature (London)* **364**, 33–39.

Caux, C. Y., Liu, J., and Banchereau, J. (1995). Recent advances in the study of dendritic cells and follicular dendritic cells. *Immunol. Today* **16**, 2–4.

Dimmock, N. J. (1995). Update on the neutralization of animal viruses. *Rev. Med. Virol.* **5**, 165–179.

Doherty, P. C. (1993). Inflammation in virus infections. *Semin. Virol.* **4**, 117–122.

Doherty, P. C., Allan, W., Eichelberger, M., and Carding, S. R. (1992). Roles of α/β and γ/δ T cell subsets in viral immunity. *Annu. Rev. Immunol.* **10**, 123–151.

Engelhard, V. H. (1994). How cells process antigens. *Sci. Am.* **271**(2), 54–61.

Jorgensen, J. L., Reay, P. A., Ehrich, E. W., and Davis, M. M. (1992). Molecular components of T-cell recognition. *Annu. Rev. Immunol.* **10**, 835–873.

Kuby, J. (1997). "Immunology," 3rd ed. Freeman, New York.

Mims, C. A., Playfair, J. H. L., Roitt, I. M., Wakelin, D., and Williams, R. (1993). "Medical Microbiology." Mosby, London.

Notkins, A. L., and Oldstone, M. B. A., eds. (1984, 1986, 1989). "Concepts in Viral Pathogenesis," Vol. 1, 2, and 3. Springer-Verlag, New York.

Paul, W. E., ed. (1993). "Fundamental Immunology," 3rd ed. Raven, New York.

Roitt, I. M. (1997). "Essential Immunology," 9th ed. Blackwell, Oxford.

Thomas, D. B., ed. (1993). "Viruses and the Immune Response." Dekker, New York.

van Regenmortel, M. H. V., and Neurath, A. R., eds. (1985, 1991). "Immunochemistry of Viruses," Vols. 1 and 2. Elsevier, Amsterdam.

Whitton, J. L., and Oldstone, M. B. A. (1996). Immune response to viruses. *In* "Fields Virology" (B. N. Fields, D. M. Knipe, P. M. Howley, R. M. Chanock, J. L. Melnick, T. P. Monath, B. Roizman, and S. E. Straus, eds.), 3rd ed., pp. 345–374. Lippincott-Raven, Philadelphia, PA.

CHAPTER 9

Pathogenesis of Viral Diseases: Viral Strategies and Host Defense Mechanisms

In previous chapters various aspects of viral infections have been reviewed from the perspective of the host cell: this has centered on the mechanisms used by viruses to gain entry into their target cells, to replicate, and perpetuate themselves. This has also centered on the mechanisms used by host animals to counter viral infection, again primarily at the cellular level but with emphasis on the host immune response. This chapter and the next two center on the clinical and pathologic consequences of these interactions at the level of the intact host animal. This is the essence of *viral disease pathogenesis* and the essence of a concept first defined by the great pathologist, Howard Florey, as the *pathophysiologic basis of disease.* Mechanisms operating at the level of the individual host animal pertain to (1) viral strategies used to evade host defenses and host strategies used to counter them; (2) viral injury to tissues, organs, and entire animals, and again, host strategies used to overcome functional loss; and (3) viral injury to the immune system, and again, host strategies used to overcome dysfunction while avoiding immunopathological consequences. The same mechanisms that pertain to the individual infected animal, in turn, become the basis for understanding the nature of viral diseases in populations and in ecosystems.

Viral Strategies Used to Evade Host Defenses

Many strategies are employed by viruses to evade host immune and inflammatory responses *in vivo*. Their remarkable diversity is difficult to categorize, but most pertain to viral survival in the face of the onslaught of host inflammatory and immune defenses (Table 9.1). Of course, these strategies used by viruses also point to host strategies used to overcome them. The following represent only some of the many strategies presently known.

Evasion by Noncytocidal Infection

Arenaviruses and hantaviruses are examples of noncytocidal viruses that establish chronic infections in their rodent hosts without killing the cells in which they replicate. Infection causes little or no damage except rarely when certain immunopathological complications may develop later in life. Retroviruses are noncytocidal in virtually all target cells, tissues, and organs in all the various hosts that they infect.

Table 9.1
Some Viral Strategies used to Evade Host Defenses

PHENOMENON	MECHANISM	EXAMPLES
Noncytocidal infection	Failure to shut down host cell nucleic acid and protein synthesis	Arenaviruses, hantaviruses, retroviruses in natural host animals
Cell-to-cell spread	Membrane fusion	Lentiviruses (equine infectious anemia virus), morbilliviruses (canine distemper virus), herpesviruses
Infection of nonpermissive, resting, or undifferentiated cells	Failure to up-regulate viral gene expression	Herpesviruses in ganglionic neurons, papillomaviruses in basal epithelial layers, lentiviruses in lymphocytes
Little or no viral antigen on cell membrane	Infection with restricted viral gene expression	Lentiviruses in lymphocytes and macrophages, herpesviruses in ganglion neurons
	Loss of viral antigen by "stripping" and endocytosis	Marek's disease virus in T cells, canine distemper virus in neurons, cytomegaloviruses in epithelium
Destruction of immune effector cells and macrophages	Infection of lymphocytes	Infectious bursal disease virus, cytomegaloviruses, feline panleukopenia virus, feline immunodeficiency virus, human immunodeficiency virus
	Infection of macrophages	Lactate dehydrogenase elevating virus, African swine fever virus
Down-regulation of MHC antigen expression	Viral proteins inhibit production or maturation of MHC proteins	Adenoviruses, retroviruses
Evasion of cytokines	Viral proteins interfere with interferon and other cytokine actions	Adenoviruses, herpesviruses
Evasion of neutralizing antibody	Production of large amounts of soluble viral protein that "soaks up" antibody	Ebola and Marburg viruses, Lassa virus, and other arenaviruses
	Masking of viral epitopes by carbohydrates on glycoproteins	Rift Valley fever virus, arenaviruses, Ebola and Marburg viruses
Induction of nonneutralizing antibody	Production of low-affinity antibody or antibody reacting with irrelevant epitopes—an immune decoy	Aleutian disease virus of mink, African swine fever virus, lymphocytic choriomeningitis virus
Enhancing antibody	Antibody attached to virus enhances infection of macrophages	Cytomegaloviruses, lactate dehydrogenase elevating virus, feline infectious peritonitis virus, dengue viruses in humans
No antibody produced	Nonimmunogenic agent	Scrapie
Induction of immunologic tolerance	Induction of clonal anergy or specific suppressor T cells	Bovine viral diarrhea virus, hog cholera virus, arenaviruses, some retroviruses
Sequestration in immunologically privileged tissues	Viral replication in sites inaccessible to afferent or efferent limbs of immune response	Rabies virus in muscle cells, pseudorabies and rabies viruses in neurons
Integration of the viral genome into the host cell genome	Recombination-like process	Retroviruses
Genetic/antigenic drift	Mutations leading to antigenic variants	Maedi/visna virus, equine infectious anemia virus, influenza viruses

Evasion by Cell-to-Cell Spread (Membrane Fusion)

Lentiviruses (e.g., equine infectious anemia virus), morbilliviruses (e.g., canine distemper virus), and herpesviruses (e.g., cytomegaloviruses of many species) cause adjacent cells to fuse together, enabling the viral genome to spread contiguously from cell to cell without ever being exposed to the host's immune mediators. This may not help the virus in regard to host-to-host transmission, but it is important in viral spread, especially within the central nervous system.

Evasion by Infection of Nonpermissive, Resting, or Undifferentiated Cells

Viruses may undergo productive replication in one cell type but nonproductive latent infection in another. For example, many herpesviruses assume a latent state in ganglionic neurons or B lymphocytes but replicate productively and cause acute lesions in mucosal epithelial cells. Even in a given cell type, permissiveness may be determined by the state of cellular differentiation or activation. For example, papillomaviruses invade basal cells of stratified epithelium but produce infectious virions only in fully differentiated cells near the body surface.

Evasion by Infection with Restricted Viral Gene Expression

Viral latency may be maintained by restricted expression of genes that have the capacity to kill the cell. During latent infection, some viruses, such as the herpesviruses, express only a few early genes that are necessary in the maintenance of latency. During reactivation, which is often stimulated by immunosuppression and/or by the action of a cytokine or hormone, the whole viral genome is transcribed again. This strategy protects the virus during its latent state from all host immune actions.

Evasion by Destruction of Immune Effector Cells and Macrophages

Many viruses can replicate productively or abortively in cells of the lymphoid and reticuloendothelial systems and it is noteworthy that these systems are often implicated in persistent infections. Lymphocytes and monocytes/macrophages represent tempting targets for any virus, in that they move readily throughout the body and can seed virus to any organ, as well as being key players in the immune response. The extreme example of destruction of the body's immune system is provided by human immunodeficiency viruses 1 and 2 in AIDS in humans, wherein the virus replicates in $CD4^+$ T lymphocytes and cells of the monocyte/macrophage series. Virtual elimination of helper T cells from the body results in such profound depression of the immune response that patients die from opportunistic infections or from cancer.

Evasion by Down-Regulation of MHC Antigen Expression

Because $CD8^+$ T cells only recognize viral peptides bound to MHC class I antigen (and $CD4^+$ T cells only recognize them in the context of MHC class II antigen), viral persistence is favored by reduction of the concentration of MHC molecules on the cell surface. Adenoviruses encode an early protein that binds to newly synthesized MHC class I antigen, preventing its normal processing and thus reducing its cell surface expression. Betaherpesviruses, in addition to down-regulating MHC class I expression to avoid lysis of their host cells by Tc lymphocytes, synthesize MHC class I-like molecules that act as a decoy to prevent lysis by NK cells, which lyse cells that do not express a normal complement of MHC class I molecules.

Evasion of Cytokines

Interferons display a wide range of antiviral as well as immunomodulatory activities, as described in Chapter 5. However, some viruses have evolved genes that in one way or another sabotage the specific antiviral actions of effector molecules. For example, some viruses interfere with cellular proteins known as interferon-regulated proteins, which are instrumental in the up-regulation of interferon synthesis and secretion. Other viruses counter antiviral cytokines in a more direct fashion; for example, an adenovirus gene product protects infected cells against tumor necrosis factor α, thereby assuring host cell survival until viral production is complete.

Evasion of Neutralizing Antibody (Masking of Epitopes and the Immune Decoy)

Some viruses have evolved strategies for evading neutralization by the antibody they elicit. Filoviruses and arenaviruses resist neutralization by convalescent sera by still mysterious means. One notion is that the Ebola virus uses an "immune decoy" to evade neutralizing antibody: the virus produces two glycoproteins, one forming its surface peplomers, the other, a truncated version of the same protein is made in large amounts and secreted extracellularly. This protein seems to "soak up" antibody, thereby protecting the virus. Glycoproteins of filoviruses, arenaviruses, and many bunyaviruses (e.g., Rift Valley fever virus) are also glycosylated very heavily—carbohydrate may constitute one-third of the mass of their surface peplomers. It has been hypothesized that epitopes on virions and virion budding sites on the plasma membrane of infected cells may be masked by these carbohydrates. In such cases they may not present B cell or T cell recognition signals or, once sensitization has occurred, may not present optimal targets for the immune response.

Evasion by Induction of Nonneutralizing Antibody

Many persistent infections are characterized by the presence of (1) low antibody titers or (2) high antibody titers against nonneutralizing viral epitopes. In the latter case, virus–antibody and viral antigen–antibody complexes may accumulate at the basement membranes of renal glomeruli and other sites, causing a variety of immune complex or neoplastic diseases.

Nonneutralizing antibody is often directed against viral proteins or immunodominant epitopes that are not relevant in immune clearance; in fact, such antibodies, by binding to virions, may block the attachment of neutralizing antibody by steric hindrance. For example, the lethal course of Aleutian disease in mink and many retrovirus infections is a direct result of this phenomenon. Research has suggested the feasibility of refocusing the neutralizing antibody response by targeted dampening of immunodominant epitopes, using molecular and chemical means—this approach offers exciting possibilities for vaccines against viral diseases that have so far resisted all vaccine design strategies. For example, novel vaccines, expressing natural nondominant neutralizing epitopes, are being considered to protect animals against feline infectious peritonitis, bovine respiratory syncytial disease, bovine viral diarrhea, equine infectious anemia, and caprine arthritis–encephalitis.

Evasion by Induction of Immunologic Tolerance

The probability of an acute infection becoming persistent is strongly age related; congenital infections are most likely to induce immunologic tolerance and thereby persist. Bovine viral diarrhea, hog cholera, arenavirus infections, and some retrovirus infections are particular problems because of chronic viral shedding from newborns in the absence of effective immunity. In many cases, no B cell tolerance is demonstrable but there is a degree of T cell unresponsiveness to the virus. In lymphocytic choriomeningitis virus infection of mice, newborns infected from their dams while *in utero* do not mount any T cell response to the virus; the fact that this is reversible indicates that it is due, not to the deletion of virus-reactive T cell clones during embryonic life, but to clonal anergy or production of suppressor T cells.

Evasion by Sequestration in Immunologically Privileged Tissues

A striking proportion of persistent infections involve the central nervous system. The brain is insulated from the immune system to some degree by the blood–brain barrier and, further, neurons express very little MHC antigen on their surface, thereby conferring some protection against destruction by cytotoxic T lymphocytes. During their latent phase, most alphaherpesviruses avoid immune elimination by remaining within cells of the nervous system, as episomal DNA.

Certain viruses grow primarily in epithelial cells on lumenal surfaces: for example, cytomegaloviruses replicate in the kidney, salivary glands, and mammary glands and are shed more or less continuously in the corresponding secretions, even when there are abundant neutralizing antibodies and cytotoxic T cells in surrounding tissues. The anatomic barrier (basement membranes, connective tissue, etc.) surrounding glandular epithelia is a major contributor to this sequestration.

Evasion by Integration of Viral Genome into Host Cell Genome

The integration of retroviral proviral DNA into the genome of the host germ line cells assures indefinite maintenance from one generation to the next; such proviral DNA is implicated in oncogenesis (see Chapter 11). The proviral DNA of lentiviruses, however, becomes integrated only in somatic cells during the viral replication cycle—it is not transmitted to offspring except across the placenta or at birth. Viruses of the acquired immunodeficiency disease subgroup of the lentiviruses destroy lymphocytes and/or macrophages, permitting the unchecked proliferation of a variety of opportunistic infectious agents.

FIGURE 9.1.

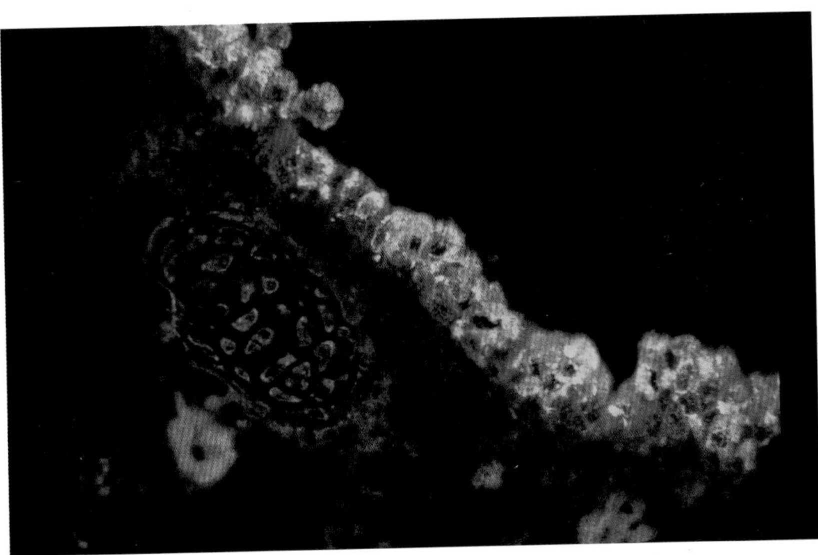

Tracheal epithelium of a mouse infected with parainfluenza virus 1 (Sendai virus) at 60 hours postinfection. In this experimental model, virtually every epithelial cell in the trachea, bronchi, and bronchioles is infected at this stage; later, these cells become necrotic and slough, filling the airways with debris and contributing to respiratory distress. Paraffin section (rapid formalin fixation, paraffin embedment, and deparaffinization); immunofluorescence using fluorescein isothiocyanate-conjugated goat anti-parainfluenza virus 1 globulin. Magnification: ×500.

Evasion by Genetic/Antigenic Drift

Maedi/visna and equine infectious anemia viruses avoid the host immune response by antigenic drift. During persistent infection, sequential antigenic variants are produced, with each successive variant different enough to evade the immune response raised against the preceding variant. In equine infectious anemia, clinical signs occur in cycles, with each cycle being initiated by a new variant. In addition to providing a mechanism for escape from immune elimination, each new variant may be more virulent than its predecessor and this may directly affect the severity and progression of the disease.

Viral Damage to Tissues and Organs

The severity of a disease is not necessarily correlated with the degree of cytopathology produced by the virus in cells in culture. Many viruses that are cytocidal in cultured cells do not produce clinical signs (e.g., many enteroviruses), whereas some that are noncytocidal *in vitro* cause lethal disease in animals (e.g., retroviruses and rabies virus). Further, depending on the organ affected, cell and tissue damage can occur without producing clinical signs of disease, e.g., a large number of liver cells may be destroyed in Rift Valley fever in sheep without significant clinical signs. When damage to cells does impair the function of an organ or tissue, this may be of minor importance in one part of the body, such as muscle or subcutaneous tissue, but of great importance in another part of the body, such as the heart or the brain. Likewise, inflammation and edema may be unimportant in many sites in the body but may have serious consequences in particular tissues and organs, such as the brain. In this case it is the host's response to infection that results in increased intracranial pressure and disease. In the same way, the host's response to viral infection in the lungs may interfere with gaseous exchange and infection in the heart may interfere with conduction.

Direct Tissue and Organ Damage

Sometimes all clinical signs and all pathologic changes in an animal may be explained by the direct damage to cells caused by a highly cytocidal virus. Mice inoculated intravenously with a large dose of Rift Valley fever virus, for example, develop hepatic necrosis within 4 hours; virions pass quickly through the Kupffer cells and infect hepatocytes, which are lysed rapidly. In this experimental model, all defense mechanisms of the host are overwhelmed and the destruction of cells in the target organ, the liver, is lethal.

Damage to the Epithelium of the Respiratory Tract

Respiratory viruses initially invade and destroy just a few epithelial cells, but such microscopic lesions progressively damage the protective layer of mucus and lay bare more and more epithelial cells. As viral replication progresses, large numbers of progeny virions are released into the lumen of the airway. Early in infection, the beating of cilia, the primary function of which is to cleanse the respiratory tract of inhaled particles, may actually help to move released progeny virus along the airway, thereby spreading the infection. As secretions become more profuse and viscous, the cilial beating becomes less effective and ceases as epithelial cells are destroyed.

In respiratory virus infections the spread of infection via contiguous expansion from initial foci may progress until virtually every columnar epithelial cell at many airway levels is infected (Figures 9.1, 9.2, and 9.3). This can result in complete denuding of large areas of epithelial surface and the accumulation of large amounts of transudates, exudates containing inflammatory cells, and necrotic epithelial cell debris in the airways. Where infection of the epithelium of the nasal passages, trachea, and bronchi proceeds to a fatal outcome, there are usually one or more complications: bacterial superinfection (nurtured by the accumulation of fluid and necrotic debris in the airways), infection and destruction of the lung parenchyma and the alveolar epithelium, and/or blockage of airways that are so small in diameter that mucous plugs cannot be dislodged by forced air movements. Blockage of the airways is of most significance in newborn animals. In all of these complications there is hypoxia and a pathophysiologic cascade that leads to acidosis and uncontrollable fluid exudation into airways.

Degeneration of respiratory tract epithelial surfaces may be extremely rapid, but so is regeneration. In studies of influenza in ferrets, for example, it has been shown that the development of a complete new columnar epithelial surface via hyperplasia of remaining transitional cells may be complete in a few days. The transitional epithelium and the newly differentiated columnar epithelium that arises from it are resistant to infection, probably by virtue of interferon production and a lack of virus receptors. The role of other host defenses, including soluble factors such as mannose-binding lectins and lung surfactants, as well as macrophages, NK cells, IgA and IgG antibodies, and T cell-mediated immune mecha-

Figure 9.2.

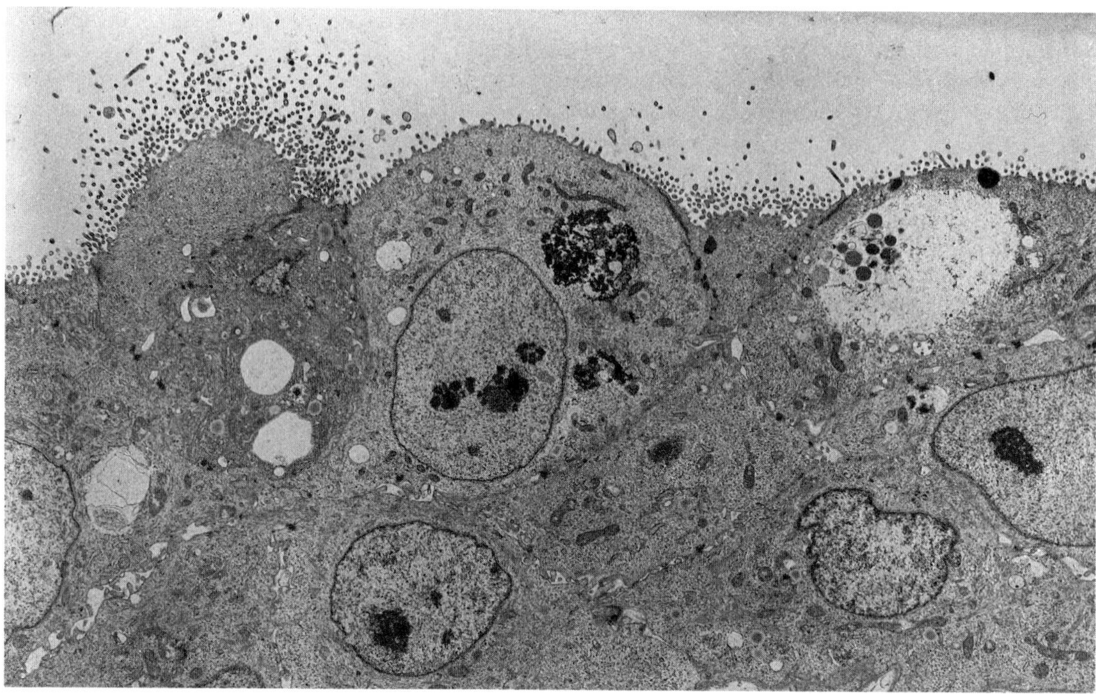

Avian influenza virus infection in the respiratory tract of a chicken. The normal side-by-side position of columnar epithelial cells has been replaced by cuboidal cells without cilia, several of which exhibit massive viral budding from their apical surface. Thin section electron microscopy. Magnification: ×10,000.

Figure 9.3.

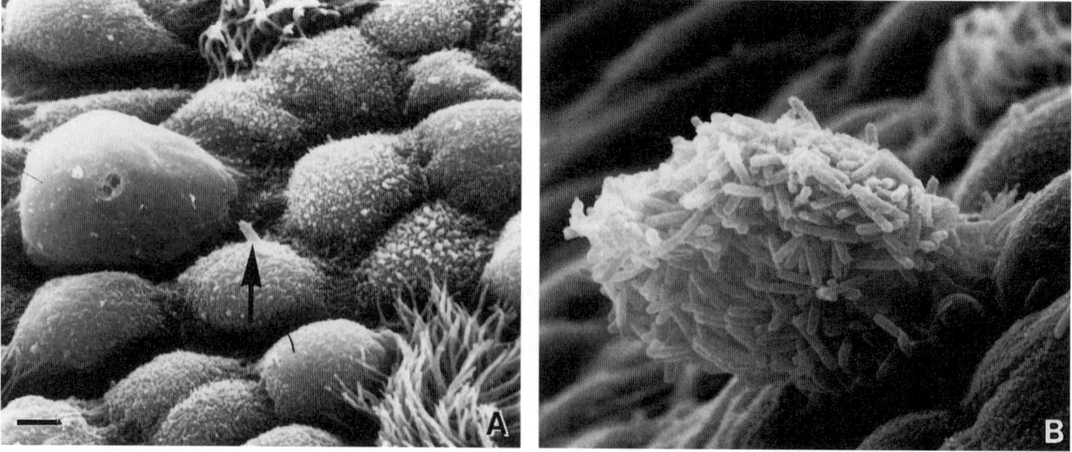

Scanning electron micrographs showing desquamating cells in an influenza virus-infected mouse trachea and the adherence of *Pseudomonas aeruginosa*. Bar: 2 μm. (A) Normal mouse trachea showing a single bacterium (arrow) on a serous cell. (B) Microcolony of *P. aeruginosa* adhering to a residual epithelial cell on an otherwise denuded surface. (Courtesy of P. A. Small, Jr.)

nisms in terminating infection, is covered in Chapters 7 and 8.

Damage to the Epithelium of the Intestinal Tract

Nearly all enteric infections occur following virus entry by ingestion; in most cases the incubation period is very short and the onset of disease is without any prodromal signs. The principal agents causing viral diarrhea in animals are the rotaviruses; other viruses that produce diarrhea include coronaviruses, toroviruses, caliciviruses, astroviruses, and certain adenoviruses and parvoviruses. Rotaviruses infect cells at the tip of villi and cause marked shortening and occasional fusion of adjacent villi (Figures 9.4 and 9.5) so that the absorptive surface of the intestine is reduced. This results in fluid accumulation in the lumen of the gut and diarrhea. In contrast, parvoviruses infect and destroy dividing crypt epithelium, thereby removing the source of the short-lived villus epithelial cells.

FIGURE 9.4.

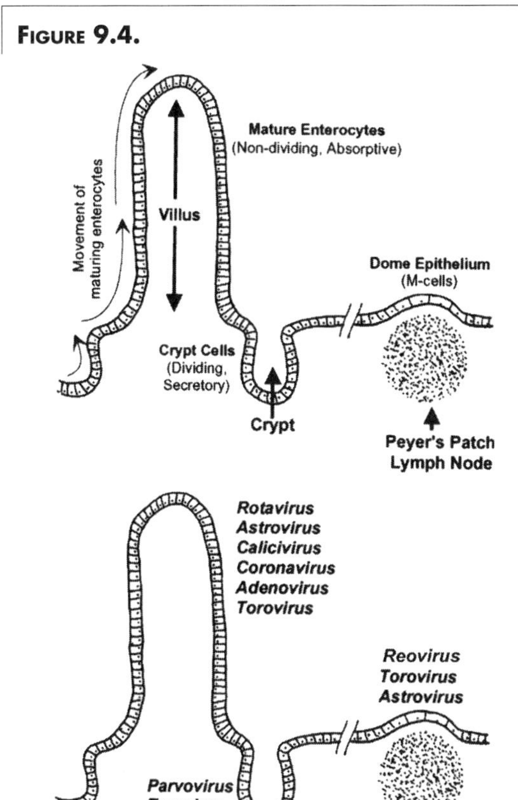

Structure of the villus epithelium of the small intestine with locations targeted by certain viruses. (Top) Cross section through a villus and crypt showing the movement and maturation of dividing crypt cells to form nondividing mature enterocytes. (Bottom) Cells infected by various enteric viral pathogens. [From M. E. Conner, and R. E. Ramig. Viral enteric diseases. *In* "Viral Pathogenesis" N. Nathanson, R. Ahmed, F. Gonzalez-Scarano, D. E. Griffin, K. V. Holmes, F. A. Murphy, and H. L. Robinson, eds.), pp. 713–743. Lippincott-Raven, Philadelphia, PA. 1997.]

Infection generally begins in the proximal part of the small intestine and spreads progressively to the jejunum and ileum and sometimes to the colon. The extent of such spread depends on the amount of virus ingested, the virulence of the virus, and the host's immunologic status. As the infection progresses, the absorptive cells are replaced by immature cuboidal epithelial cells whose absorptive capacity and enzymatic activity are greatly reduced. Because these cells are relatively resistant to viral infection, the disease is often self-limiting if dehydration is not so severe as to be lethal. The rate of recovery is rapid, especially when infection does not involve the crypt epithelium.

Fluid loss in viral infections from the intestinal tract is mainly a loss of extracellular fluid due to impaired absorption and osmotic loss due primarily to the presence of undigested lactose in the lumen (in newborn animals) rather than active secretion. As virus destroys the absorptive cells there is a loss of those enzymes responsible for the digestion of disaccharides, and the loss of differentiated cells diminishes glucose carrier, sodium carrier, and Na^+, K^+, and -ATPase activities. This leads to a loss of sodium, potassium, chloride, bicarbonate, and water and to the development of acidosis. Another cause of acidosis is increased microbial activity associated with the fermentation of undigested milk. Acidosis can create a K^+ ion exchange across the cellular membrane, affecting cellular functions that maintain the normal potassium concentration. Dehydration, as noted earlier, and hypoglycemia, due to decreased intestinal absorption, reduced glyconeogenesis, and increased glycolysis follow, completing a complex of pathophysiologic changes that, if not corrected promptly by fluid and electrolyte therapy, results in death.

Pathophysiologic Changes without Tissue and Organ Damage

In some viral infections damage may not be obvious, but infected cells may carry out their functions less effectively and clinical signs may reflect this. The virus may cause a loss in specialized functions of cells required not so much for their own survival but for systemic homeostasis. In mice infected with lymphocytic choriomeningitis virus there is a reduction in normal levels of growth and thyroid hormones due to infection of the cells that produce them. The mRNA levels for these hormones are reduced significantly in infected mice. Reduced growth hormone synthesis is associated with a runting syndrome in young infected mice, and reduced thyroid hormone synthesis is associated with myxedema and a subnormal

Figure 9.5.

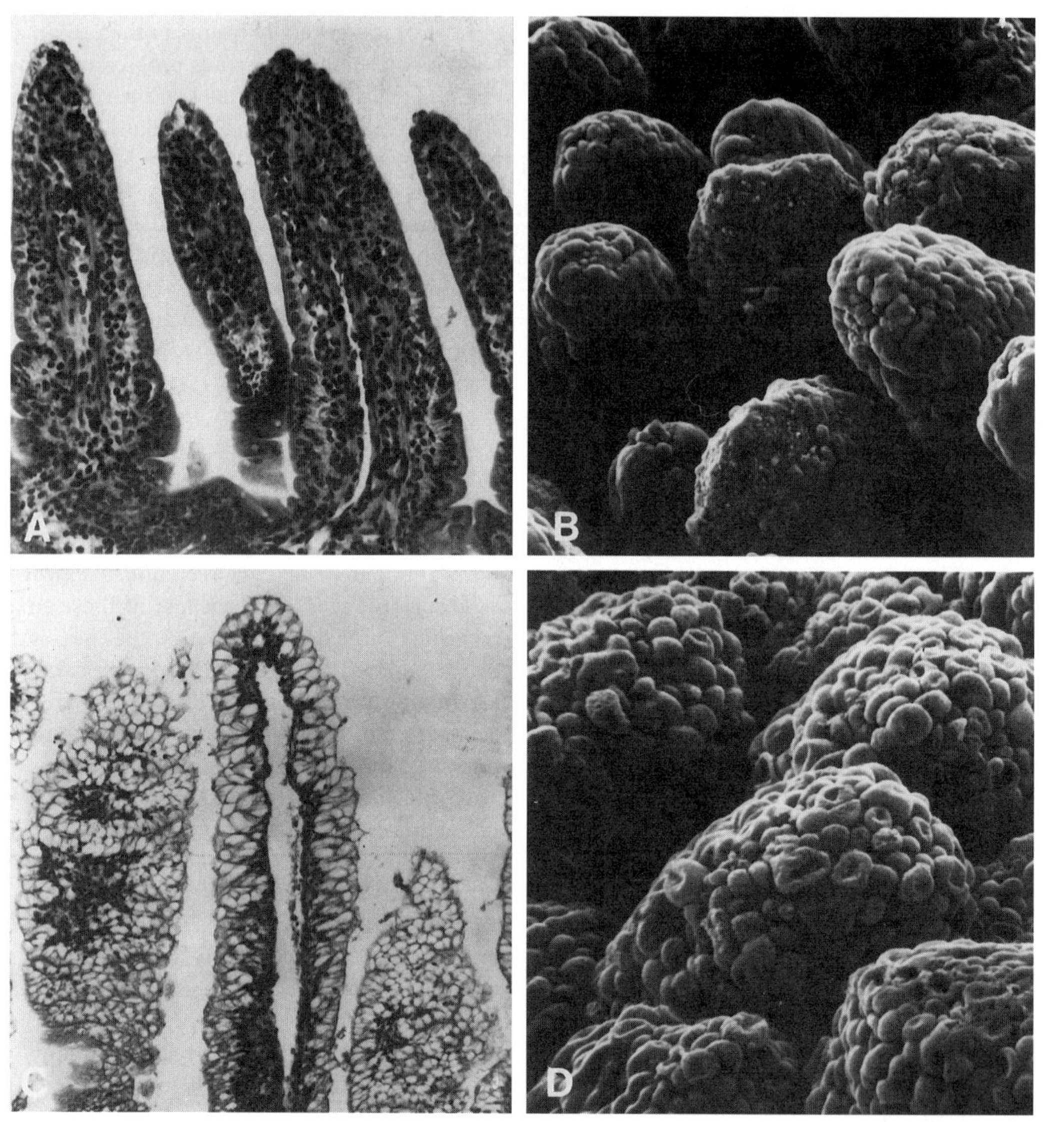

Scanning electron and light micrographs of intestinal tissues from a gnotobiotic calf sacrificed 30 minutes after onset of rotavirus diarrhea. (A) Proximal small intestine with shortened villi and denuded villus tips. (Hematoxylin and eosin. Magnification: ×120). (B) Same level of intestine as in (A), depicting denuded villi by scanning electron microscopy. Magnification: ×180). (C) Distal small intestine with normal vacuolated epithelial cells and normal villi. (Hematoxylin and eosin. Magnification: ×120). (D) Same area as in (C) by scanning electron microscopy; epithelial cells appear round and protruding. Magnification: ×210. (From C. A. Mebus, R. G. Wyatt, and A. Z. Kapikian. Intestinal lesions induced in gnotobiotic calves by the virus of human infantile gastroenteritis. *Vet. Pathol.* **14,** 273–282. (1977).)

basal metabolic rate. Persistent lymphocytic choriomeningitis virus or encephalomyocarditis virus (a picornavirus) infection of pancreatic islet cells may result in a lifelong reduction of insulin and elevation of blood glucose levels (diabetes). Viruses may also alter the expression of cell surface molecules, such as class II MHC markers, by indirect mechanisms, which may be the basis for clinical signs.

Tissue and Organ Damage Predisposing to Secondary Bacterial Infection

As well as having direct adverse effects, viral infections of the respiratory and digestive tracts often predispose animals to secondary infections with bacteria, even those that may belong to the normal flora in the nose and throat. In cattle, parainfluenza virus 3 and other respiratory viruses may destroy the ciliated epithelium and cause fluid exudation into the lumen of airways, thereby allowing *Pasteurella hemolytica* and other bacteria to invade the lungs and cause secondary bacterial pneumonia (shipping fever). In equine influenza the virus destroys large patches of ciliated epithelium in the airways and causes exudation, thereby allowing streptococci and other bacteria to invade the lungs and cause pneumonia. Conversely, proteases secreted by bacteria help activate influenza virus infectivity by proteolytic cleavage of the viral hemagglutinin (see Chapter 30).

Similarly, in the intestinal tract, rotavirus and coronavirus infections may lead to an increase in susceptibility to enteropathogenic *Escherichia coli* and this synergistic effect may lead to more severe diarrhea than if the bacterium or the virus were acting separately. In veterinary and zoonotic diseases there is a particular concern for the potentiating effect of viral infections on intercurrent infestations with parasites. Because domestic animals are almost universally infested with protozoa and helminths, and it is known that such infestations generally lower resistance to viruses and bacteria, individual animal and herd health management systems must accommodate all aspects of such multifactorial infectious disease problems.

Persistent Infection and Chronic Damage to Tissues and Organs

Persistent infections of one type or another are produced by a wide range of viruses; indeed in veterinary medicine acute self-limiting infections seem to be the exception rather than the rule. Apart from most viral diarrheas and respiratory infections, most other categories of viral infections have more or less important chronic manifestations. For example, in some cases of canine distemper the virus is not eliminated with the termination of the acute disease, instead the virus persists for months or years, causing late pathologic manifestations in several organs. In other instances, persistent viruses have been found to be responsible for subtle chronic diseases even when the acute manifestations of infection have been trivial or subclinical.

Persistent viral infections are important for several reasons: (1) they may be reactivated and cause recrudescent episodes of disease in the individual host, (2) they may lead to immunopathologic disease, (3) they may be associated with neoplasia, (4) they may allow viral survival in individual vaccinated animals and herds, and (5) they may be of epidemiologic importance, the source of contagion in long-distance viral transport and in reintroduction after viral elimination from a given herd, flock, region, or country.

For convenience, persistent viral infections may be subdivided into several categories.

Persistent infections, per se, in which infectious virus is demonstrable continuously, whether or not there is ongoing disease. Disease may develop late, often with an immunopathologic or neoplastic basis. For example, in the deer mouse (*Peromyscus maniculatus*), the reservoir rodent host of Sin Nombre virus and the etiologic agent of hantavirus pulmonary syndrome in humans, virus is shed in urine, saliva, and feces probably for the life of the animal, even in the face of neutralizing antibody.

Latent infections, in which infectious virus is not demonstrable except when reactivation occurs. For example, in infectious pustular vulvovaginitis, the sexually transmitted disease caused in cattle by bovine herpesvirus 1, virus usually cannot be isolated from the latently infected carrier cow except when there are recrudescent lesions.

Slow infections, in which infectious virus gradually increases during a very long preclinical phase, leading to a slowly progressive lethal disease. For example, in scrapie the infectious agent, the scrapie prion, only becomes detectable in target tissues years after infection but by the time of death it has reached very high titers in the brain.

Acute infections with late clinical manifestations, in which continuing replication of the causative virus is not involved in the progression of the disease. For example, in the cerebellar syndrome that occurs in young cats as a result of fetal infection with feline panleukopenia virus, virus cannot be isolated at the time neurologic damage is diagnosed. In fact, because of this the cerebellar syndrome was for many years considered to be an inherited malformation.

It may be noted that these categories are defined primarily in terms of the extent and continuity of viral replication during the long period of persistence. The presence or absence of shedding and disease are secondary issues as far as this categorization is concerned. Further, some persistent infections possess features of more than one of these categories. For example, all retrovirus infections are persistent and most exhibit features of latency, but the diseases they cause may be subacute with late clinical manifestations or only manifest as slowly progressive diseases. The variety of patterns of persistent viral infections is shown diagrammatically in Figure 9.6; further examples are given in Table 9.2.

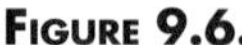

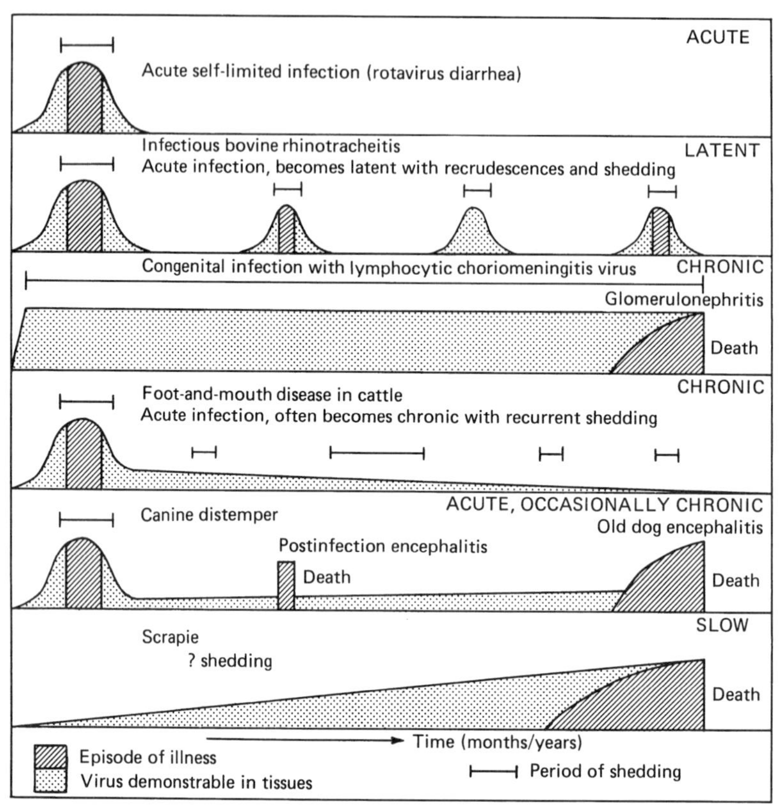

The shedding of virus and the occurrence of clinical signs in acute self-limited infections and various kinds of persistent infection, as exemplified by the diseases indicated. The time scale is notional and the duration of various events approximate.

Infection-Induced Damage to the Immune System

Because the immune system plays a key role in protection against infections, viral damage to its components can exacerbate the severity of disease or predispose to superinfection with other infectious agents. In addition, both specific acquired immunodeficiency and generalized immunosuppression can occur in viral infections.

Infection of the bursa of Fabricius in chickens (the site of B cell differentiation) with infectious bursal disease virus leads to atrophy of the bursa and a severe deficiency of B lymphocytes, with an increase in susceptibility to bacteria, particularly *Salmonella* spp. and *E. coli,* and Marek's disease, Newcastle disease, infectious bronchitis, and infectious laryngotracheitis viruses. Similarly, B cell-based immune deficiency caused by feline leukemia and feline immunodeficiency viruses predisposes to a wide range of secondary infections.

Since the discovery in 1981 of acquired immunodeficiency syndrome (AIDS) in humans and the discovery in 1983 of its etiologic agents, human immunodeficiency viruses (HIV 1 and 2), similar viruses have been discovered in monkeys [simian immunodeficiency viruses (SIVs)], cattle [bovine immunodeficiency virus (BIV)], and cats [feline immunodeficiency virus (FIV)]. In susceptible animals, each of these viruses acts in a similar way, destroying specific but different cells of the immune system, thereby causing immunosuppression. Immunosuppression may be inconspicuous (as in SIV infection of some monkey species and in virtually all BIV infections) or may lead to death from opportunistic infections after a prolonged clinical course (as in feline AIDS).

Infections with certain other viruses (e.g., hog cholera, bovine viral diarrhea, canine distemper viruses, feline and canine parvoviruses) may temporarily suppress humoral and/or cell-mediated immune responses. The immune response to unrelated antigens is reduced or abrogated in such animals, and the situation is thus distinct from suppression of the immune response to a specific virus by immune tolerance after intrauterine infection. The mechanisms involved in such general immunosuppression are not fully understood, but may result from the replication of virus in lymphocytes and/

Table 9.2
Slow Infections: Long Preclinical Phase, Slowly Progressive Fatal Disease

Virus	Host	Site of infection	Antibodies	Disease
Maedi/visna virus	Sheep	Macrophages	+ (nonneutralizing)	Slowly progressive neurological and pulmonary disease
Ovine progressive pneumonia virus	Sheep	Brain, lung	+	Slowly progressive pulmonary and neurological disease
Caprine arthritis–encephalitis virus	Goats	Macrophages, brain, joints	+ (nonneutralizing)	Slowly progressive arthritis, encephalitis
Feline immunodeficiency virus	Cats	? Helper T cells	+ (nonneutralizing)	Feline acquired immunodeficiency syndrome
Scrapie prion	Sheep	Central nervous system and lymphoid tissue	None	Slowly progressive neurological disease
Bovine spongiform encephalopathy prion	Cattle	Central nervous system and lymphoid tissue	None	Slowly progressive neurological disease
Chronic wasting disease prion	Deer, elk	Central nervous system and lymphoid tissue	None	Slowly progressive neurological disease

or macrophages. Many viruses are capable of replication in macrophages and several have been shown to grow in T cells, especially activated T cells. Some herpesviruses replicate nonproductively in B cells, transforming them and altering their function.

Virus-induced immunosuppression may in turn lead to enhanced viral replication. When the immune system is suppressed by endogenous or exogenous factors, latent herpesvirus, adenovirus, or papovavirus infections can be reactivated. Such situations are encountered frequently following the use of cytotoxic drugs or irradiation for organ transplantation in humans and are a feature of AIDS as well. Immunosuppression, usually of unknown origin, is probably responsible, at least in part, for the reactivation of herpesviruses in animals.

Immunopathology in Viral Disease

The immune response plays a two-edged role in the pathogenesis of most viral diseases. Infiltration of affected tissues by lymphocytes and macrophages, release of cytokines, and the resultant inflammation are regular features of viral infections, but have both protective and destructive effects. Fever, erythema, edema, and enlargement of lymph nodes also have an immunologic basis and have both protective and destructive effects. There are viral infections in which such manifestations of the immune response are the cardinal factors in the onset and progression of the disease (Table 9.3).

Autoimmune Disease

One traditional hypothesis proposed to explain autoimmune diseases in animals and humans has been that they are manifestations of subtle viral infections. Many variations on this hypothesis have been elaborated: (1) viral infection causes polyclonal T and B cell activation, which becomes directed indiscriminately at normal host antigens; (2) viral infection evokes altered self- or neoantigens, the new determinants becoming targets of an immune response; (3) viral infection induces an anti-idiotypic response, i.e., a response to structural domains on the oligoclonal antibody molecules synthesized in response to the infection; and (4) viral infection of lymphoid cells causes aberrant unregulated expansion of immune effector cells.

Autoimmune Damage Caused by Molecular Mimicry

The presence of structural homologies, linear or conformational, between host and viral proteins is known as *molecular mimicry*. If viral and host determinants are similar enough to cross-react, yet different enough to break normal immunologic tolerance, mimicry may in-

Table 9.3
Chronic Infections with Late Immunopathologic or Neoplastic Consequences

Virus (family/genus)	Host	Site of persistent infection	Late disease
Aleutian disease virus (*Parvoviridae/Parvovirus*)	Mink	Macrophages	Hypergammaglobulinemia, arteritis, glomerulonephritis
Avian leukosis viruses (*Retroviridae/Alpharetrovirus*)	Chickens	Widespread	Leukosis, leukemia
Equine infectious anemia virus (*Retroviridae/Lentivirus*)	Horses	Macrophages	Anemia, vasculitis, glomerulonephritis
Feline immunodeficiency virus (*Retroviridae/Lentivirus*)	Cats	Macrophages, lymphocytes	Opportunistic infections due to profound immunodeficiency
Human immunodeficiency virus (*Retroviridae/Lentivirus*)	Humans	Macrophages, lymphocytes	Opportunistic infections due to profound immunodeficiency
Lymphocytic choriomeningitis virus (*Arenaviridae/Arenavirus*)	Mice	Widespread	Glomerulonephritis

duce autoimmune disease. The concept of molecular mimicry has been verified with the aid of monoclonal antibodies, and indeed common immunological determinants on viruses and host proteins are quite common: about 4% of antiviral monoclonal antibodies react with host cell components. The molecular basis for these common determinants has been established by sequencing—in turn, peptides synthesized to match common determinants, when injected into experimental animals, have evoked antiviral and anti-self immune responses.

For example, a monoclonal antibody recognizing a neutralizing epitope on coxsackie B4 virus also reacts against heart muscle; coxsackie B4 virus is known to target muscle, including myocardial muscle of mice and humans, and to cause myocarditis in humans. Sequence homologies have also been found between normal myelin basic protein and proteins of hepatitis B virus, adenoviruses, Epstein–Barr virus, papillomaviruses, and human herpesvirus 6. At one time or another these viruses have been implicated as triggers (along with measles, canine distemper, and human coronaviruses) of multiple sclerosis, the debilitating autoimmune neurologic disease of humans.

This triggering concept, however, has never been proven; however, autoimmune encephalomyelitis has been considered pathogenetically similar to multiple sclerosis and it can be induced experimentally by immunization of animals with peptides common to some of these viruses and myelin basic protein. These peptides, which have worked as molecular mimics of epitopes on myelin, have a similar stereochemical fit into the HLA DR groove of the MHC complex. It has been hypothesized that sensitization of host T cells by viral antigens in infection target sites delivers activated T cells in the bloodstream from where they cross the blood–brain barrier and attack self-antigens in the brain. In a similar fashion, molecular mimicry may be involved in the neurologic disorders associated with maedi/visna and caprine arthritis–encephalitis virus infections, and rarely in post-vaccinial encephalitis.

Hypersensitivity Reactions in Viral Infections

Immunopathologic (hypersensitivity) reactions are traditionally classified into types I, II, III, and IV (Table 9.4). Although advances in cellular immunology have now blurred some of the distinctions, the classification is still convenient. For most viral infections it is not known whether immunopathology makes a significant contribution to disease and, if so, which of the four classical hypersensitivity reactions is implicated. Nevertheless, it is instructive to discuss the possible involvement of different kinds of hypersensitivity reactions in viral diseases.

Type I Hypersensitivity Reaction (Anaphylactic Reaction)

Type I hypersensitivity reactions depend on the interaction of antigens with IgE bound to the surface of mast cells via an Fc receptor, resulting in the release of histamine and heparin and the activation of serotonin and plasma kinins. Except for its contribution to erythema

TABLE 9.4
Hypersensitivity Reactions in Viral Infections

CHARACTERISTIC	TYPE I (ANAPHYLACTIC)	TYPE II (ANTIBODY-DEPENDENT CYTOTOXIC)	TYPE III (IMMUNE COMPLEX)	TYPE IV (DELAYED, CELL-MEDIATED)
Time course				
Initiation	Minutes	Minutes	3–6 hours	18–24 hours
Persistence	Minutes	Dependent on antigen and antibody	Dependent on antigen and antibody	Weeks
Transfer with	IgE	IgM, IgG	IgG	T lymphocytes
Complement required	No	Usually	Yes	No
Histamine dependent	Yes	No	Yes	No
Histology	Edema, congestion, eosinophils	Cell destruction, phagocytosis	Necrosis, neutrophils, later plasma cells	Lymphocytes, macrophages, necrosis
Viral immunopathology	Minor, some erythema	Minor, some erythema	Major acute: fever Chronic: immune complex disease	Major in brain, lung

and in some acute respiratory infections, anaphylaxis is probably not important in viral immunopathology; it is responsible, however, for adverse reactions to some viral vaccines.

Type II Hypersensitivity Reaction (Antibody-Dependent Cytotoxic Reaction)

Originally identified in cytotoxic reactions attributable to antibodies to autologous antigens, as in blood transfusion reactions, type II cytolytic reactions also occur when antigen–antibody complexes at the cell surface activate the complement system, leading to cell lysis. Alternatively, antibodies can sensitize virus-infected cells to destruction by cytotoxic T lymphocytes, natural killer cells, polymorphonuclear leukocytes, or macrophages via antibody-dependent cell-mediated cytotoxicity. While it has been demonstrated that virus-infected cells are lysed by these mechanisms *in vitro,* their role in viral diseases is unclear. They may be operative in certain herpesvirus infections, but definitive proof of this is lacking. Uninfected cells can be targets for type II reactions as when complement-mediated lysis occurs after equine infectious anemia virus binds to equine erythrocytes and contributes to the anemia seen in this disease.

Type III Hypersensitivity Reaction (Immune Complex-Mediated Cytotoxic Reaction)

Antigen–antibody reactions cause inflammation and tissue damage by various mechanisms. If the reaction occurs in extravascular tissues, there is edema, inflammation, and infiltration of polymorphonuclear leukocytes, which later may be replaced by mononuclear cells. This is a common course of mild inflammatory reactions. This type of immune complex reaction constitutes the classical Arthus response, which is especially important in persistent viral infections.

If antigen–antibody reactions occur in the blood, they produce circulating immune complexes, which are found in most viral infections. The fate of the immune complexes depends on the ratio of antibody to antigen. If there is a large excess of antibody, each antigenic moiety (e.g., each virion) becomes covered with antibody and is removed by macrophages that have receptors for the Fc component of the antibody molecule. If the amounts of antigen and antibody are about equal, lattice structures, which develop into large aggregates, are formed and removed rapidly by the reticuloendothelial system.

In some persistent infections, viral antigens or virions themselves are released continuously into the blood but the antibody response is weak and antibodies are of low avidity. Complexes continue to be deposited in glomeruli over periods of weeks, months, or even years, leading to the impairment of glomerular filtration and eventually to chronic glomerulonephritis. A classic example is lymphocytic choriomeningitis infection in mice infected *in utero* or as neonates. Viral antigens are present in the blood and small amounts of nonneutralizing antibody are formed, giving rise to immune complexes that are deposited progressively on renal glomerular membranes. Depending on the strain of mouse, the end result may be glomerulonephritis, uremia, and death. Circulating immune complexes may also be deposited in the walls of the small blood vessels in the skin, joints, and choroid plexus, where they attract macrophages and activate complement. In addition to these local effects, by mobilizing soluble mediators, antigen–antibody complexes contribute to systemic reactions, such as fever and malaise.

Systemic immune complex reactions may activate the enzymes of the coagulation cascade, leading to histamine release and increased vascular permeability. In such cases, fibrin may be deposited in the kidneys, lungs, adrenals, and pituitary gland, causing multiple thromboses, infarcts, and scattered hemorrhages—this is known as disseminated intravascular coagulation. This is seen in viral hemorrhagic fevers in humans, all of which are zoonoses caused by arenaviruses, bunyaviruses, filoviruses, and flaviviruses. Kittens infected with feline infectious peritonitis virus exhibit disseminated intravascular coagulation and it also occurs in fowl plague, hog cholera, and rabbit hemorrhagic disease.

Type IV Hypersensitivity Reaction (Cell-Mediated or Delayed Hypersensitivity Reaction)

Unlike the other reactions, type IV reactions, also called delayed hypersensitivity reactions, are mediated by cells—T lymphocytes—and are manifested as inflammation, lymphocytic infiltration, and macrophage infiltration and activation. They are important, for example, in the pathogenesis of Borna disease and may also contribute to consolidation of the lung in various severe lower respiratory tract diseases.

Once again, the classic virological model is lymphocytic choriomeningitis virus infection—this time primary infection of adult mice. After intracerebral inoculation the virus replicates harmlessly in the meninges, ependyma, and choroid plexus epithelium until about the seventh day, when $CD8^+$ class I MHC-restricted cytotoxic T cells invade and damage the infected cells. This causes a massive breakdown of the blood–brain barrier, producing meningitis, cerebral edema, convulsions, and death. Elsewhere than in the central nervous system, cytotoxic T cells help control the infection (by destroying infected cells); within the rigid confines of the skull this host response is fatal. The death of mice infected in this way can be prevented by chemical immunosuppression, by X-irradiation, or by antilymphocyte serum.

Although occasionally the cause of immunopathology, cell-mediated immune responses are generally an important component of the process of recovery from viral infections (see Chapter 8), as becomes evident if they are abrogated by cytotoxic drugs or are absent, as in some immunodeficiency diseases. Elimination of cells supporting the growth of a lytic virus is essential if the individual is to survive. Whether this process results in a crisis depends on the extent of the infection and how vital the infected cells are to the survival of the host. Perhaps this is the evolutionary reason why neurons, which cannot be replaced, do not express MHC antigens on their plasma membranes.

Nonspecific Pathophysiologic Changes in Viral Diseases

Some pathologic changes found in viral infections cannot be attributed to direct cell destruction by the virus, to inflammation, or to immunopathology. Perhaps the most important of these effects relates to alterations in the function of the adrenal glands in response to the stress of the infection. Most examples of this kind of indirect damaging effect come from well-studied experimental animal models; similar changes probably occur in natural infections but they have not yet been documented.

Most viral diseases are accompanied by a number of vague general clinical signs, such as fever, malaise, anorexia, and lassitude. Little is known about the causes of these clinical signs, which collectively can significantly reduce the animal's performance and impede recovery. Fever can be attributed to interleukin 1 and possibly to interferons. These and other soluble mediators produced by responding leukocytes or released from virus-infected cells may be responsible for other vague clinical signs as well.

Further Reading

Ada, G. L. (1998). Immune response. *In* "Encyclopedia of Virology" (R. G. Webster and A. Granoff, eds.), 2nd ed. (CD-ROM). Academic Press, London.

Babiuk, L. A., Lawman, M. P. J., and Bielefeldt, O. H. (1988). Viral-bacterial synergistic interaction in respiratory disease. *Adv. Virus Res.* **35**, 219–250.

Connor, D. H., Chandler, F. W., Schwartz, D. A., Manz, H. J., and Lack, E. E. (1997). "Pathology of Infectious Diseases." Appleton & Lange, Stamford, CT.

Jubb, K. V. F., Kennedy, P. C., and Palmer, N., eds. (1993). "Pathology of Domestic Animals," 4th ed. Academic Press, San Diego, CA.

Lawman, M. J. I., Campos, M., Ohmann, H. B., Griebel, P., and Babiuk, L. A. (1989). Recombinant cytokines and their therapeutic value in veterinary medicine. *In* "Animal Biotechnology" (L. A. Babiuk and J. P. Phillips, eds.), Comprehensive Biotechnology Series. pp. 1–260. Pergamon, Oxford.

Mason, P. W., Rieder, E., and Baxt, B. (1994). RGD sequence of foot-and-mouth disease virus is essential for infecting cells via the natural receptor but can be bypassed by an antibody-dependent enhancement pathway. *Proc. Natl. Acad. Sci. U.S.A.* **91**, 1932–1936.

McFadden, G., ed. (1995). "Viroceptors, Virokines and Related Immune Modulators Encoded by DNA Viruses." R. G. Landes, Austin, TX.

Mims, C. A., and White, D. O. (1984). "Viral Pathogenesis and Immunology." Blackwell, Oxford.

Mims, C. A., Dimmock, N., Nash, A., and Stephen, J. (1995). "Mims' Pathogenesis of Infectious Diseases," 4th ed. Academic Press, London.

Notkins, A. L., and Oldstone, M. B. A., eds. (1984, 1986, 1989). "Concepts in Viral Pathogenesis," Vols. 1, 2, and 3. Springer-Verlag, New York.

Oldstone, M. B. A., ed. (1989). Molecular mimicry. Cross-reactivity between microbes and host proteins as a cause of autoimmunity. *Curr. Top. Microbiol. Immunol.* **145**, 1–150.

Oldstone, M. B. A. (1996). Principles of viral pathogenesis. *Cell* **87**, 799–801.

Oldstone, M. B. A. (1997). How viruses escape from cytotoxic T lymphocytes: Molecular parameters and players. *Virology* **234**, 179–185.

Smith, G. L. (1994). Virus strategies for evasion of the host response to infection. *Trends Microbiol.* **2**, 81–88.

von Herrath, M. G., and Oldstone, M. B. A. (1996). Virus-induced autoimmune disease. *Curr. Opin. Immunol.* **8**, 878–885.

CHAPTER 10

Pathogenesis of Viral Diseases: Representative Model Diseases

To this point the pathogenesis of viral infections has been dissected in several ways, seeking understanding of the bases for disease in a piecemeal fashion. Driven by sophisticated experimental methods, this kind of reductionistic, mechanistic approach is at the heart of much of modern pathogenetic research. However, this approach often leads to too many generalizations and too much oversimplification in explaining viral diseases as they occur in nature. There is merit in considering the pathogenesis of representative model viral diseases as they occur in domestic and wild animals, if only to provide a "reality check," a reminder of how many viral and host factors come to influence the clinical course of disease and how little is known about their interrelationships. This constitutes the intersection between virology and pathology and clinical veterinary medicine.

Viral Respiratory Disease

Equine Influenza

Influenza viruses are maintained among horses by sporadic clinical cases and by inapparent infections. In outbreaks, virus is spread to susceptible horses introduced into the herd by birth, transport for show, sale, training, or racing and to horses with waning immunity. The clinical outcome following exposure depends on the nature of the virus and the immunological status of the horses in the population at risk. Infection of horses in a nonimmune population may be severe, even fatal, especially in the young, old, or debilitated. More commonly, infection results in fever up to 42°C, a cough that may last for weeks, and often secondary bacterial (usually streptococcal) bronchitis and pneumonia. Full recovery may take months.

The pathogenesis of this syndrome is the same as in influenza in other mammalian species, and as in other species interrupting the pathogenetic progression has proven difficult. Influenza virus virions in aerosolized droplets are inhaled and alight on the film of mucus that covers the epithelium of the upper respiratory tract. Alternatively, virions contained on fomites may gain entry into the nares, the conjunctiva, or the oral cavity and from there move to the respiratory tract. Aerosolized droplets of different sizes alight at different levels of the respiratory tree and infection may accordingly be initiated at different levels, but in general the upper respiratory tract is the site of initial infection, and the trachea and bronchi are the sites of infection that cause the most common clinical signs. Immediately upon alighting, the virus is met by host defense mechanisms—if the horse has previously been infected or vaccinated with the same or a very similar strain of virus, antibody (mainly IgA) present in the mucus may neutralize it. Mucus also contains glycoproteins similar to the receptor molecules on respiratory epithelial cells, which may combine with virions and prevent them from attaching to epithelial cells.

In turn, the viral neuraminidase may destroy enough of this host glycoprotein to allow virions to attach to and infect epithelial cells.

Very small virus-containing aerosolized droplets carried deeper into the airways face another physiologic barrier, namely the cleansing action of beating cilia. Inhaled particles are normally carried in the flow of mucus generated by cilial beating to the pharynx where they are swallowed. However, initial invasion and destruction of just a few epithelial cells by influenza viruses can initiate lesions that progressively damage the mucus layer, thereby baring more and more epithelial cells. Viral replication progresses, and large numbers of progeny virions are budded into the lumen of the airways. Early in infection, cilial beating helps to move released progeny virus along the airways, thereby spreading the infection. As the secretions become more profuse and viscous, cilial beating becomes less effective and ceases as epithelial cells are destroyed.

The spread of the infection via contiguous expansion from initial foci often does not stop until virtually every columnar epithelial cell at the particular airway level is infected. The result is complete denuding of large areas of epithelial surface and the accumulation in the airways of transudates and exudates containing inflammatory cells and necrotic epithelial cell debris. In the process of infecting and destroying epithelial cells, the virus induces cytokine production; these cytokines are the cause of many of the clinical signs. These cytokines also have a central role in the induction of the immune response and in the exacerbation of the inflammatory response.

Respiratory distress follows, which is made worse when animals are forced to move. There may be one or more complications: (1) secondary bacterial infection (again usually streptococcal infection), nurtured by the accumulation of fluid and necrotic debris in the airways; (2) infection and destruction of the lung parenchyma and alveolar epithelium (interstitial pneumonia); and/or (3) blockage of airways that are so small in diameter that mucous plugs cannot be dislodged by forced air movements. In all of these complications there is hypoxia and a pathophysiologic cascade that leads to acidosis and uncontrollable fluid exudation into airways.

Degeneration of respiratory tract epithelial surfaces during influenza infection is extremely rapid, but so is regeneration—development of a complete new columnar epithelial surface via hyperplasia of remaining transitional cells may be complete in a few days. The transitional epithelium and the newly differentiated columnar epithelium that arises from it are resistant to infection, probably by virtue of interferon production. Other host defenses, including antibody and cell-mediated immune effector mechanisms, also play a part in terminating the infection.

Immunity is fleeting, whether evoked by natural infection or vaccination, and reinfection is common. Unlike the situation with human influenza where the individual's immune status is often rendered moot by antigenic drift of viruses circulating in the population, equine influenza viruses have shown only modest drift. It is the failure to stimulate a strong enough, long-lasting enough, mucosal immune response in the airways that makes equine influenza such a problem. As an indication of the problem, the "Guidelines for Vaccination of Horses of the American Association of Equine Practitioners" includes the following protocol: primary vaccination, two to three doses, 3 to 4 weeks apart, and booster vaccinations at intervals of 2 to 12 months, depending on the level of exposure. If the immunogenicity of equine vaccines was better, certainly fewer doses would be needed. Clearly, the localization of the infection in the respiratory tract without systemic spread and the rather sequestered location of viral budding from apical plasma membranes of airway epithelial cells (and perhaps characteristics of the key viral glycoproteins themselves) combine to favor the virus over the host. Better vaccines and better vaccination protocols are required.

Bovine Pneumonia (Shipping Fever)

In cattle there is a seasonal incidence of bronchopneumonia in fall and early winter that corresponds with the extra stress of harsh climatic conditions and husbandry practices as well as the extra activity of respiratory viruses and mycoplasmas. This syndrome of bronchopneumonia, often extending to a true fibrinous pleuropneumonia, is called shipping fever in many countries. In the United States and Canada the syndrome represents the most economically important health problem in cattle, especially feedlot cattle—it is estimated that this syndrome costs the North American cattle industry more than $1 billion per year. Despite having diverse initial causes, the syndrome has a common terminal pathway and etiology, with terminal manifestations being caused by overwhelming infection by *Pasteurella hemolytica* and, to a lesser extent, *P. multocida*. Respiratory virus infections (e.g., bovine herpesvirus 1, parainfluenza virus 3, bovine respiratory syncytial virus) contribute to the susceptibility of cattle to the bacteria that are always present in the respiratory tract. Respiratory epithelial damage and fluid exudation, as described earlier for influenza, are major factors favoring bacterial growth. Viral infections can also alter bovine host defense mechanisms in other ways: (1) they can be directly immunosuppressive or can damage macrophage and neutrophil function in the lungs and airways; (2) they may induce such an exuberant inflammatory response that the delicate epithelial surfaces of the alveoli are destroyed; and (3) they can alter the surface properties of respiratory epithelial cells, thereby favoring bacterial adherence and growth.

In these circumstances, bacterial microcolonies resist phagocytosis and the effects of antibodies and antibiotics, and bacteria can therefore enter the lower respiratory tract more readily. Another effect of viral damage is the release of iron, which also enhances bacterial growth and colonization. Interactions between various factors during the development of bovine pneumonia are summarized in Figure 10.1.

It is more important to control the viral infections that initiate shipping fever than the bacterial superinfections that produce the pneumonia. The *Pasteurella* species that are always present in the bovine respiratory tract are unlikely to be eliminated by any means. Antibiotic therapy may yield positive results, but in many cases extensive damage has already occurred by the time the diagnosis is made. If microcolonies have been established and infection has progressed to the formation of abscesses, it is impossible to obtain effective antibiotic levels at target sites. If infected cattle survive, they are often unthrifty and are prone to further debilitating diseases. Viral vaccine programs aimed at preventing the pathogenetic cascade must be assessed and justified by their overall effect on the prevalence of the multifactorial pneumonia. So far such vaccine programs, especially those involving the use of *Pasteurella* spp. vaccines, have not proven their worth—there has always been anecdotal evidence of positive effects, but in controlled trials efficacy and economic benefit are never confirmed. As in the case of equine influenza, better vaccines and better strategies for their delivery are required.

Viral Intestinal Disease

Rotavirus, Coronavirus, and Torovirus Enteritis

Enteritis in animals is often multifactorial and interactions of infectious agents with immunologic, environmental, and nutritional factors can often exacerbate the disease. The entry into the body of viruses destined to infect the gastrointestinal tract usually starts with the ingestion of contaminated food, water, or fomites. The virus must survive the acidic conditions of the stomach and then the alkaline conditions and the presence of enzymes and bile salts in the small intestine before reaching intestinal epithelial cells, which are invaded directly. The harsh environmental conditions in the digestive system must destroy large numbers of virions continuously, but in nature, there are physiologic circumstances when pH extremes are buffered (e.g., in newborn animals by milk and in adult animals by normal intermittent gastric alkalosis) so that enough virus is protected and can go on to cause infection. In fact, the old generalization that viral enteric pathogens must be stable, i.e., acid and bile salt resistant, as are the enteroviruses, reoviruses, rotaviruses, parvoviruses, and adenoviruses, is now known to be faulted. Important pathogens that are sensitive to low pH and intestinal enzymes and bile salts include enteric coronaviruses, pestiviruses, toroviruses, and paramyxoviruses (the latter particularly in birds) (Table 10.1).

In the intestinal tract, entry and shedding involve the same cells, i.e., epithelial cells that are infected by invading virus and are also the source of the virus, which is shed and continues the transmission chain. Most viruses that infect intestinal epithelium exhibit common pathogenetic characteristics, such as rapid

Figure 10.1.

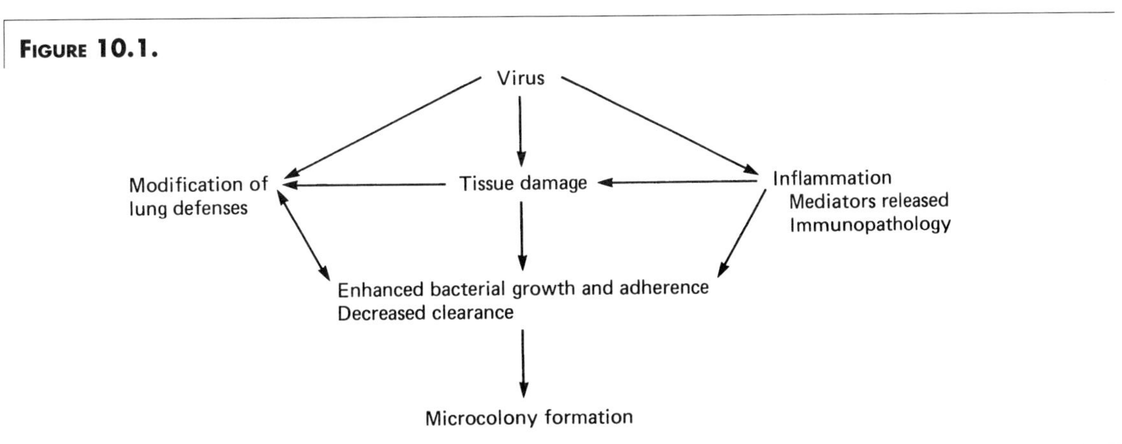

Interactions between events associated with viral and bacterial infections in the development of bovine pneumonia (shipping fever). (Courtesy of L. A. Babiuk.)

Table 10.1
Viruses Causing Diarrhea[a]

Family/Genus	Cell type infected	Distribution of virus-induced injury
Parvoviridae	Dividing cells of the crypt	Small intestine
Adenoviridae	Mature enterocytes	Apices of villi, small intestine
Caliciviridae	Mature enterocytes	Sides of villi, proximal small intestine
Astroviridae	Mature enterocytes, M cells covering Peyer's patches	Apices of villi, small intestine (ovine) Peyer's patches, proximal small intestine (bovine)
Reoviridae/ Rotavirus	Mature enterocytes	Apices of villi in proximal or distal small intestine, depending on host
Coronaviridae/ Coronavirus	Mature enterocytes Surface and crypt cells	Small intestine Large intestine
Coronaviridae/ Torovirus	Villus enterocytes M cells covering Peyer's patches and crypt cells	Distal small intestine Peyer's patches Large intestine

[a]From M. E. Conner, and R. F. Ramig, Viral enteric diseases. *In* "Viral Pathogenesis" (N. Nathanson, R. Ahmed, F. Gonzalez-Scarano, D. E. Griffin, K. V. Holmes, F. A. Murphy, and H. L. Robinson, eds.), pp. 713–744. Lippincott-Raven, Philadelphia, PA, 1997.

growth and high yield, all aimed at completing the fecal–oral transmission cycle before host immune defenses intervene.

The incubation period of these infections is usually very short—as short as 12 hours in some cases of rotavirus enteritis. Clinical signs include watery diarrhea, anorexia, depression, dehydration, and, in some species, vomiting. Repeated bouts of diarrhea often cause a failure to thrive. Deaths attributed to viral enteritis result from severe dehydration secondary to loss of water from diarrhea; newborn animals and small species with less fluid reserve are more vulnerable. Because very high concentrations of virus are shed by infected animals and because the infectious dose is small in most enteric viral infections, minimal environmental contamination is enough to cause widespread disease.

The severity of the enteritis caused by the various enteric viruses varies according to the immune status, age, and general condition of the animal at the time of infection. In enteritis caused by rotaviruses, coronaviruses, and toroviruses, there is epithelial cell destruction, with marked shortening and occasional fusion of adjacent villi (see Chapter 9). Because absorptive cells are concentrated at the tips and secretory cells at the base of villi, there is a change in the ratio of absorptive and secretory capacities. This results in fluid accumulation in the lumen of the gut and diarrhea. Infection generally begins in the proximal part of the small intestine and spreads progressively to the jejunum and ileum and sometimes to the colon. The extent of such spread depends on the initial dose, the virulence of the virus, and the host's immunologic and physiologic status. In piglets and lambs, viral enteritis is most often centered in the jejunum and ileum and in calves in the duodenum and jejunum. In mice, where rotavirus enteritis is a major problem in laboratory colonies, infection is most often centered in the duodenum and jejunum. Infection does not usually cause much inflammatory response; little is seen macroscopically and microscopically there is usually only a mild mononuclear cell infiltration into the lamina propria of the small intestine. Perpetuation of enteropathogenic viruses is favored by an explosive infection causing diarrhea and a burst of virus shedding rather than a smoldering infection. Nearly all such infections are localized. The failure to penetrate into deeper tissues and cause systemic disease may represent an evolutionary progression that maximizes shedding capacity and transmissibility without destroying the host population.

In many cases of diarrhea more than one virus is active; if two viruses have different sites of replication, their combined effect may be more severe than either alone. Furthermore, many bacterial infections (e.g., enterotoxic *Escherichia coli* infection) are more severe if combined with a viral infection.

Viral enteritis is essentially a problem in the first few weeks or months of life and susceptibility decreases rapidly with increasing age. To prevent infection of newborn animals, antibody must be present continuously in the lumen of the gut. This does not occur

FIGURE 10.2.

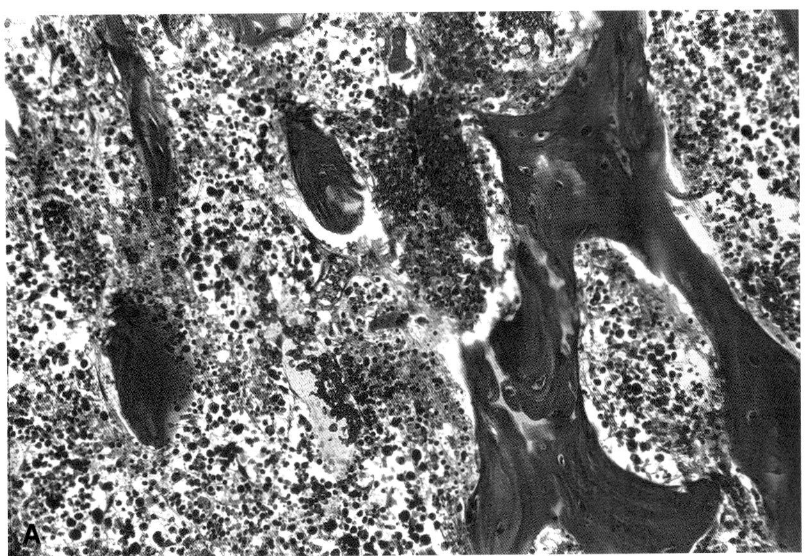

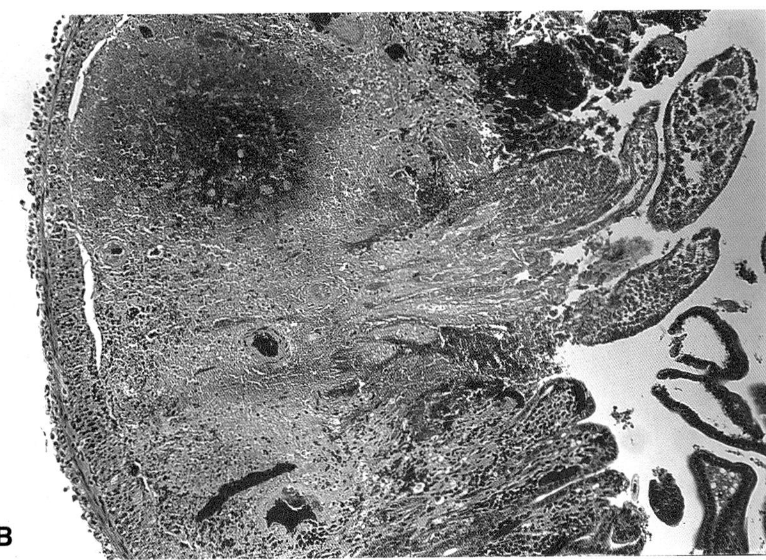

(A) Femoral bone marrow of a hamster inoculated with Venezuelan equine encephalitis virus at 3 days postinfection. Seemingly, every cell is undergoing necrosis. The progression of this infection in the hamster is rapid, extremely destructive, and dependent on the sensitivity to infection of reticuloendothelial, lymphoid, and hematopoietic cells. This model reflects only a modest exaggeration in magnitude of what occurs in horses infected with epidemic strains (types IAB and IC) of this virus. (B) Peyer's patch at 4 days postinfection (at which time the hamster was moribund); the germinal centers of this Peyer's patch are totally necrotic and the local integrity of the intestinal wall is breaking down—this could be the basis for sepsis as is seen in some horses.

for more than about 7 days unless the dam is hyperimmunized against the common enteric viruses. Because vaccination of newborns is often not practical, maternal vaccination is gaining widespread support. More and more specific protocols are being introduced—in controlled trials, many of these are proving that this strategy is efficacious and economically sound in many settings (see Chapter 13).

Viral Lymphoreticular and Hematopoietic Disease

Venezuelan Equine Encephalitis

Every cell in the lymphoreticular and hematopoietic systems could be used to illustrate an important effect of virus infection in these organ systems. The lessons from pathogenetic studies in these systems are complex and intertwined with the immune response and other crucial host functions. In most instances, these interactions are not fully understood. Many encounters between viruses and cells of the reticuloendothelial and lymphoid systems are subtle and have been studied most thoroughly by nonmorphological means using isolated cells. However, such studies usually turn our attention to the host immune response to these encounters rather than to the infection per se. When the pathology and pathogenesis of these encounters are studied *in vivo*, however, it becomes clear that they can be devastating.

Venezuelan equine encephalitis virus infection stands out as a representative model because there is a precise chronological and topographical progression of infection and destruction of lymphoreticular and hematopoietic tissues. In hamsters, in the thymus, spleen, lymph nodes, bone marrow, and Peyer's patches, there is early productive infection of reticular cells (dendritic macrophages and less differentiated reticular cells) and later infection and severe cytonecrosis of lymphoid and myeloid cells that leads to the acute death of all infected animals (Figure 10.2).

The phagocytosis of virus by macrophages is expected to trigger the afferent limb of the immune response—viral peptides should be presented to lymphocytes that have virus-specific receptors on their surface and the immune response initiated. However, when the initiation of this cascade is prevented by acute cytonecrosis of macrophages, subsequent immunologically specific events are obviated. When this kind of destruction occurs in Peyer's patches in the small intestine, the local integrity of the intestinal wall breaks down—this is thought to be the basis for the sepsis seen in some infected animals. All in all, this precise progression in the pathogenesis of Venezuelan equine encephalitis virus infection in the hamster is rapid, efficient, and extremely destructive.

Although quantitative virologic data are not available, studies of infected horses using histopathology and frozen-section immunofluroescence of tissues have indicated that the pathogenetic pattern is similar to that in hamsters. Infection of lymphoreticular and hematopoietic tissues leads to the death of most horses before the virus gains entry into the central nervous system. Infection induces the secretion of many soluble mediators (cytokines, clotting factors, complement factors, etc.), which likely contribute to the severity of the disease. Finally, in some horses that survive long enough there is an acute necrotizing encephalitis, resembling that seen in eastern and western equine encephalitis. In the case of Venezuelan equine encephalitis, it is the virus produced in lymphoreticular and hematopoietic tissues that seeds the viremia that brings the virus to the central nervous system.

Viral Central Nervous System Disease

Rabies

Infection by the bite of a rabid animal usually results in the deposition of rabies-infected saliva deep in striated muscles, but rabies can also occur, albeit with less certainty, after superficial abrasion of the skin or mucous membranes. Initially, the virus replicates in muscle cells until it has reached a sufficient concentration to reach nearby sensory or motor nerve endings. Here the virus binds specifically to the acetylcholine receptor or to other receptors expressed at sensory end organs or motor end plates. The virus enters these distal reaches of the nervous system and begins its second stage of infection, in which there is neuronal infection and centripetal passive movement of the viral genome within axons.

The incubation period, i.e., the time between the infective bite and the development of signs of central nervous system involvement, is usually between 14 and 90 days, but may occassionally be as long as several years, possibly because virus remains sequestered in striated muscle cells before entering peripheral nerves and ascending to the brain. Movement of the viral genome within axons eventually delivers virus to the central nervous system, usually initially to the spinal cord. An ascending wave of neuronal infection and neuronal dysfunction then occurs. Virus reaches the limbic system of the brain, where it replicates extensively and causes the release of cortical control of behavior—this is the basis for the aberrant behavior that we call "furious rabies." Spread within the central nervous system continues, and when replication occurs in the neocortex, the clinical picture changes to that of "dumb rabies." Depression, coma, and death from respiratory arrest follow. On histopathologic examination there is little evidence of brain damage, yet electron microscopic or fluorescent antibody studies show that almost all neurons are infected—there is minimal cellular destruction to match the extensive neurologic dysfunction seen in this disease.

Coincidentally with its replication in the limbic system of the brain, rabies virus moves centrifugally from the central nervous system, down peripheral nerves to a variety of organs: the adrenal cortex, pancreas, and, most importantly, the salivary glands (Figure 10.3). In the nervous system, most virus is assembled on intracytoplasmic membranes. In the salivary gland, however, virions bud almost exclusively from plasma membranes at the lumenal surface of mucous cells and are released in high concentrations into the saliva. In reservoir hosts, such as the fox, virus titers in saliva may reach 10^6 infectious units per milliliter. Diabolically, at the time when viral replication within the central nervous system causes the infected animal to become furious and bite indiscriminately, its saliva is maximally infectious. Virus shedding from salivary gland epithelium into saliva offers certain advantages to the virus. Shedding may continue for a longer time than is the case with shedding from airway or intestinal epithelium. Shedding may continue after the immune response is initiated because of the immunologically sequestered status of the salivary gland epithelium and the directional shedding of virus only on apical plasma membranes directly into salivary duct lumens. This is the pattern of shedding not only of

FIGURE 10.3.

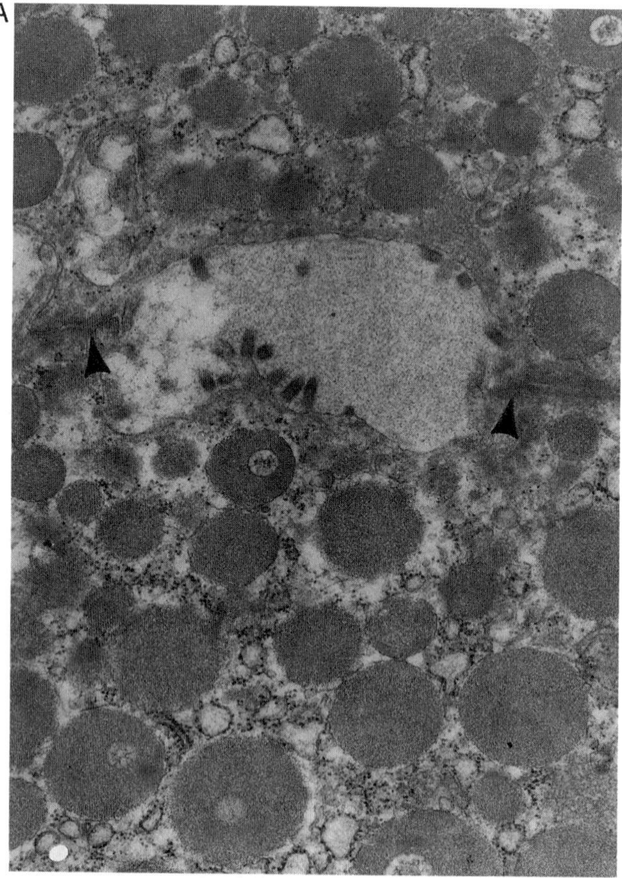

Rabies virus infection in the submandibular salivary gland and brain of a rabid fox. (A) Virions budding from the lateral plasma membrane of two mucogenic epithelial cells (tight junctions between cells defining an intercellular canaliculus are marked with arrowheads). This site of budding is delivering virus into saliva into the furthest "upstream" channel of the salivary duct system.

FIGURE 10.3. (continued)

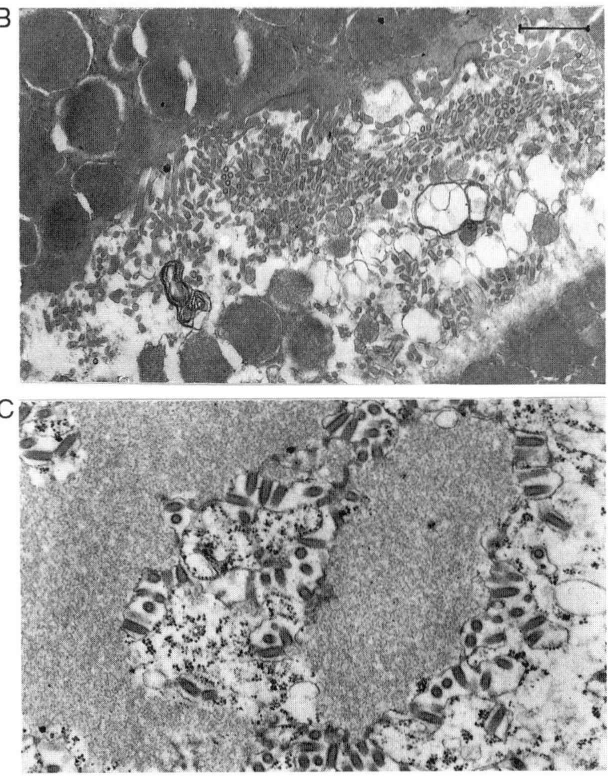

(B) Massive accumulation of virions "downstream" in the major salivary duct of the same fox. (C) Infection in the brain of the same fox. Bullet-shaped virions are budding on internal cellular membranes; the granular material is excess viral nucleocapsids forming an inclusion body, which by light microscopy is seen as a Negri body. In both the salivary glands and the brain the infection is noncytopathic, but in the brain nearly all virus is formed by budding on internal membranes of neurons and so is trapped, whereas in the salivary gland nearly all virus is formed by budding on the apical plasma membranes where it is free to enter the saliva. Some reservoir host species can have 10^6 ID_{50} of rabies virus per milliliter of saliva at the time of peak transmissibility. Thin-section electron microscopy. Magnification A, ×70,000; B, ×25,000; C ×55,000.

rabies virus, but other viruses that are shed in saliva, such as cytomegaloviruses, hantaviruses, and arenaviruses.

The pathogenesis of rabies is remarkable in that infection, spread to the central nervous system, and the development of clinical signs occur with minimal immunologic response. Although rabies proteins are highly immunogenic, neither humoral nor cell-mediated responses can be detected during the stage of movement of virus from the site of the bite to the central nervous system. The basis for this seems to be that very little antigen is presented to the immune system. Most viral antigen is sequestered within muscle cells or within neurons. However, this early stage of infection would be affected by antibodies if they were produced. The proof of this is the efficacy of classical Pasteurian postexposure vaccination, especially when vaccine is used in combination with hyperimmune immunoglobulin. Immunologic intervention is effective during the long incubation period because of the delay in most cases between the initial viral replication in muscle cells and the entry of virus into the protected environment of the nervous system. When the bite of a rabid animal occurs on the head or when the virus is introduced directly into peripheral nerves, the incubation period is often short and in some cases postexposure treatment fails.

Viral Multisystem Disease

Canine Distemper

Canine distemper has for many years been a prototypic multisystem viral disease model, largely because of the pioneering pathogenetic research of Max Appel of Cornell University. Canine distemper is typically an acute/-subacute disease, but its variable clinical presentations and variable clinical course make it quite complex (Fig-

FIGURE 10.4.

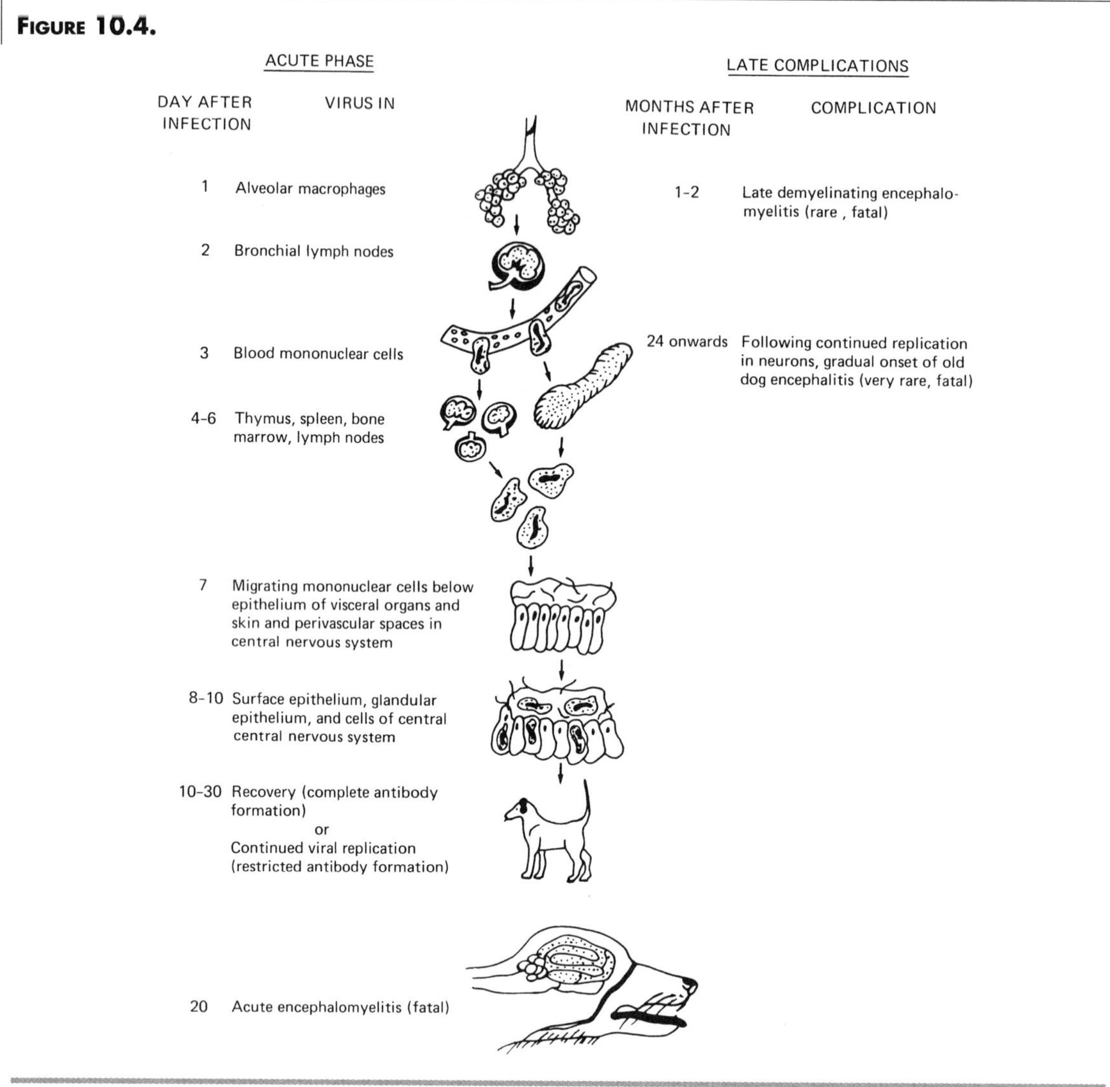

ACUTE PHASE
DAY AFTER INFECTION
VIRUS IN
1 Alveolar macrophages
2 Bronchial lymph nodes
3 Blood mononuclear cells
4-6 Thymus, spleen, bone marrow, lymph nodes
7 Migrating mononuclear cells below epithelium of visceral organs and skin and perivascular spaces in central nervous system
8-10 Surface epithelium, glandular epithelium, and cells of central central nervous system
10-30 Recovery (complete antibody formation)
or
Continued viral replication (restricted antibody formation)
20 Acute encephalomyelitis (fatal)
LATE COMPLICATIONS
MONTHS AFTER INFECTION
COMPLICATION
1-2 Late demyelinating encephalo-myelitis (rare , fatal)
24 onwards Following continued replication in neurons, gradual onset of old dog encephalitis (very rare, fatal)

The pathogenesis of canine distemper. (Courtesy of M. J. G. Appel.)

ure 10.4). Infection occurs via virus inhalation into the respiratory tract. Following initial infection of the respiratory epithelium and alveolar macrophages, the virus is transferred within 2 days to mononuclear cells in the bronchial lymph nodes and tonsils. During the first week following exposure, before the onset of clinical signs, cell-associated virus spreads via the bloodstream to the bone marrow, spleen, thymus, cervical and mesenteric lymph nodes, and macrophages in the lamina propria of the stomach and small intestine.

The rate of spread and distribution of virus after days 8 and 9 varies and appears to depend on the rate of development of neutralizing antibody, although the role of cell-mediated immunity has not been studied adequately. No neutralizing antibody is found on day 7, but in some dogs the titer reaches 100 or higher by days 8 or 9. In such dogs the virus disappears rapidly from the lymphatic tissues and the infection remains subclinical. If measurable antibody is not present by day 9 or a titer of 100 has not been attained by day 14, the virus spreads throughout the body. Extensive infection of the epithelium in the intestinal, respiratory, and urogenital tracts, skin, and exocrine and endocrine glands occurs, as well as continued infection of mononuclear cells in the lymphoreticular system. Infection of the gastrointestinal tract causes vomiting and diarrhea, infection of the respiratory tract causes bronchitis and sometimes pneumonia, and infection of the skin is associated with dermatitis.

When the brain is infected, usually after the virus has replicated in visceral organs, it appears in meningeal macrophages and mononuclear cells in the perivascular adventitia and later in ependymal and glial cells and neurons. Neuronal infection is associated with behavioral changes, myoclonia, tonic–clonic spasms, and paresis, which often persist after recovery. Forty to 60 days after apparent recovery, encephalitis with characteristic demyelination develops in some dogs, often leading to death. In these dogs, high titers of neutralizing antibody are found in both blood and cerebrospinal fluid. Recovery is followed by prolonged immunity, probably lifelong, but even in the face of high titers of neutralizing antibody, a second type of encephalitis, called *old dog encephalitis* may, in rare cases, occur years later (see later).

Canine Parvovirus Disease

The remarkable *host-range mutation* (species-jumping mutation) that transformed a feline parvovirus into canine parvovirus 2 and led to its rapid dissemination around the world is dealt with in Chapter 21. A second remarkable aspect of the emergence of canine parvovirus 2 involves its pathogenicity and the pathogenesis of the disease it causes in dogs—it is clear that the canine virus has retained characteristics from its progenitors. The central characteristic that underpins the pathogenesis of canine parvovirus disease is the requirement of the virus for cells in the S phase of the cell division cycle for its replication. In the fetus or neonatal dog, where cell division goes on at a high level in a wide variety of tissues, many tissues are infected and damaged. In older animals the virus replicates primarily in lymphoid tissues, hematopoietic tissues, and the intestinal epithelium, sites of continuing cell division. In its target cells the virus causes an acute lytic infection, ending in cell death without residual evidences of the infection. In keeping with the localized sites of high level cell division, two syndromes are seen in dogs.

1. Puppies may develop a multifocal necrosis of the myocardium and die of acute heart failure days to weeks after infection, usually in ventricular fibrillation. Many clinical signs seen in puppies, such as lethargy, dyspnea, and pulmonary edema, are consequences of this myocarditis.

2. Dogs older than about 5 weeks at the time of infection develop a leukopenia (with relative lymphopenia) and about 20% of animals develop severe hemorrhagic enteritis, seen as diarrhea and sometimes vomiting. Dogs may die as a result of dehydration and possibly endotoxemia. In these animals, characteristic lesions are seen in lymphoid organs and the intestine—in the former there is necrosis and in the latter there is a shortening and blunting of the villi with an intense inflammatory infiltration into the lamina propria.

The pathogenetic events leading to these syndromes have been studied in depth, starting with benchmark work by L. E. Carmichael, M. J. G. Appel, R. V. H. Pollock, and colleagues at Cornell University. Such studies have involved serial sampling of experimentally infected puppies and older dogs and examination of appropriate specimens by (1) hematological and serological methods, (2) virus titration in cell culture, (3) histopathology, and (4) immunohistochemistry and frozen-section immunofluorescence.

Following viral entry via the oropharynx, initial viral replication has been found to occur in the tonsils and regional lymph nodes and immediately thereafter in the thymus, spleen, and bone marrow. In these tissues, it is lymphoid cells that are infected first (lymphocytes in the cortex of the thymus, germinal centers in the tonsils, lymph nodes and Peyer's patches and white pulp of the spleen). Viral replication in lymphocytes in these tissues has been detected as early as 24 hours after oral infection. Virus produced in these initial sites of infection seed nearby cells and very quickly there is necrosis and a generalized decrease in cellularity in these sites. This infection produces the plasma viremia that by day 2 brings virus to other target tissues. In the bone marrow, cells of the myeloid, erythroid, and megakaryocytic series are destroyed—it is not known whether all damage is a direct result of infection or whether some may be due to "bystander effects" and the release of cytotoxic lymphokines. In puppies, cardiac muscle cells are destroyed (cardiac muscle cell division ceases at about 15 days of age—puppies infected after this time do not develop myocarditis). Virus infects the rapidly dividing crypt epithelial cells mainly in the ileum and jejunum and by day 3 postinfection high titers of virus are shed in the feces (up to 10^9 ID_{50}/gram of feces). Damage to crypt epithelium is most severe adjacent to Peyer's patches. The loss of crypt epithelial cells interferes with replacement of the normal high rate of cellular loss from the tips of villi and results in a flattened (attenuated) epithelium with shortened villi. These changes affect the balance between secretory and absorptive functions of villous epithelium and lead to an osmotic dysregulation and diarrhea. It has also been suggested that some clinical signs are a result of endotoxemia, perhaps related to the damage to the integrity of the epithelium over Peyer's patches.

In dogs that survive these peracute events, recovery is rapid: (1) antibody is detected from day 5, rising to high levels by day 7 postinfection; (2) the regeneration of lymphoid, hematopoietic, and intestinal epithelial cells is exuberant—lymphoid hyperplasia is seen by day 7 postinfection; (3) the amount of virus in blood and tissues declines rapidly and in most instances by day 6 to 8 virus is no longer detectable in tissues; and (4) the amount of virus in feces declines at the same time, although in rare instances it has been detected for as long as 22 days. If it were not for the destruction of cells that are not replaced, such as cardiac muscle cells (and in kittens infected with feline panleukopenia virus, cells of the cerebellum), there would be no late traces of the infection. These pathogenetic events point to the difficulty in attributing any late or continuing clinical signs in dogs to an earlier canine parvovirus infection—even at necropsy there is no confirming evidence that myocardial damage may have been caused by an earlier acute parvovirus infection.

Ebola Hemorrhagic Fever

A number of severe diseases of humans are described clinically as viral hemorrhagic fevers; the viruses that cause these diseases are all zoonotic and generally occur in life cycles in nature that only rarely involve humans (see Table 15-4). The pathogenesis and pathophysiology of these infections are poorly understood; clearly there are more differences than similarities but all are pathogenetically intriguing. One representative model disease stands out: Ebola hemorrhagic fever (caused by Ebola virus subtypes Zaire, Sudan, and Côte d'Ivoire), one of the most severe hemorrhagic fevers in humans. It has been said that "the evolution of the disease often seems inexorable and invariable." Following an incubation period of usually 4 to 10 days there is an abrupt onset of illness with initial nonspecific signs and symptoms, including fever, severe headache, malaise, myalgia, bradycardia, and conjunctivitis. Deterioration over the following 2 to 3 days is marked by pharyngitis, nausea and vomiting, hematemeses, and melena. There is prostration and bleeding, which is manifested as petechiae, ecchymoses, uncontrolled bleeding from venipuncture sites, and visceral hemorrhagic effusions. Death usually occurs 6 to 9 days after the onset of disease. Abortion is a common consequence of infection, and infants born to sick mothers are infected fatally. Convalescence is slow and marked by prostration, weight loss, and often by amnesia.

There is considerable similarity in the way Ebola virus attacks humans and certain species of monkeys. In rhesus (*Macaca mulatta*), cynomolgus (*Macaca fascicularis*), and African green (*Cercopithecus aethiops*) monkeys and baboons (*Papio* spp.) the incubation period is 4 to 6 days. With the onset of clinical disease there is interstitial hemorrhage, which is most evident in the gastrointestinal tract, profound prostration, and shock. Infection nearly always ends in death.

The pathogenesis of Ebola virus infection in humans and monkeys centers on the reticuloendothelial system (including macrophages in lymph nodes and spleen), endothelium throughout the body, and the parenchyma of multiple organs, especially the liver (Figure 10.5). The infection of these tissues is devastating, with swelling, hemorrhage, and focal necrosis. The rapid destruction of lymphoreticular tissues may be partially responsible for the common absence of an effective immune response, although the virus may also use an "immune decoy" to evade the traces of neutralizing antibody that may be produced (see Chapter 9). Disseminated intravascular coagulation is an important end event. Virus is shed from all body surfaces and orifices, including the skin and mucous membranes, and especially from hemorrhagic diatheses.

In common with other successful pathogens, Ebola virus is thus effective in humans and monkeys in gaining entry, escaping innate resistance factors and the host immune response, finding receptors on specific cells in several organs, finding cellular substrates for systemic infection, and assuring itself of shedding and continuation of its life cycle. Despite the complexity of the multiorgan systemic infection, the virus outmaneuvers host defenses by (1) its speed—animals often die before it might be expected that they could mount an effective primary inflammatory/immune response, and (2) its tropism(s)—the early reticuloendothelial and lymphoid tropisms likely minimize the response that might be elicited otherwise. There is no evidence for latency or persistence in the infection in humans or animals that have been studied. Neither is there evidence that subclinical or silent productive infections play any important role in animals or humans. Until the natural reservoir host of Ebola virus is found, there is no way to say how the pattern of infection seen in humans and monkeys might contribute to the survival of the virus in nature—infection in the reservoir hosts(s) is likely to be quite different and infection of humans is certainly so incidental as to not play an essential role in the natural history of the virus.

Chronic Viral Disease

Feline Infectious Peritonitis

Most domestic cats are persistently infected with coronaviruses. Many antigenically similar strains have been isolated that vary in their spectrum of infectivity and virulence. Feline coronavirus strains of low virulence that are not systemically invasive and replicate only in mature intestinal epithelial cells are called *feline enteric coronaviruses*. These strains usually cause only mild,

FIGURE 10.5.

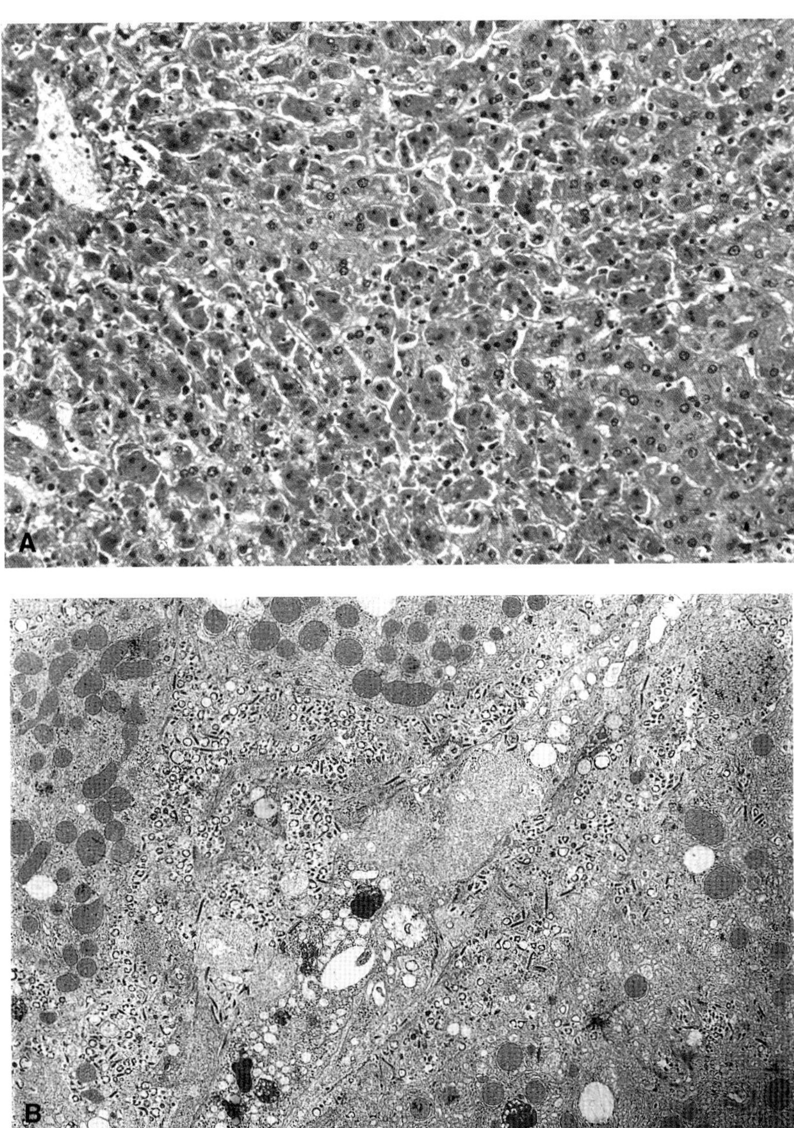

(A) Histopathologic changes in Ebola hemorrhagic fever in monkeys include massive necrosis of liver, lymphatic organs, lungs, kidneys, testes, and ovaries. Most dramatic, as seen in this section of liver from a rhesus monkey (*Macaca mulatta*) at 5 days postinfection, are focal necrotic lesions in the liver—hepatocytes exhibit eosinophilic hyaline change, but there is very little inflammatory infiltration, probably because the disease develops so rapidly. (B) Liver from a rhesus monkey infected with Ebola virus at 5 days postinfection; incredible numbers of virions are present in association with debris from necrotic hepatocytes and Kupffer cells. A, hematoxylin and eosin, magnification ×200; B, thin-section electron microscopy; magnification ×15,000.

self-limiting diarrheal illness in kittens; in adult cats these strains usually cause only subclinical infection. As these virus strains replicate, however, mutants appear at the periphery of their quasispecies swarm (see Chapter 4). Sequence analyses have shown that every cat harbors its own unique quasispecies swarm, its own variant population, which evolves continuously during low-level virus replication in the intestine.

There is considerable evidence, but no absolute proof, that enteric coronaviruses mutate and thereby develop the pathologic and invasive characteristics that are associated with *feline infectious peritonitis virus*. Virulence varies markedly among strains—some isolates consistently produce severe disease whereas others rarely do so. Sequence analysis of multiple isolates from the same cat confirm the existence of very closely related pairs of virulent/endemic viruses, indicating that the former arise from the latter. The genomes of such pairs are >98% identical, whereas any two virus strains collected from different cats show <90% sequence identity. From studies in experimentally infected cats, it has been shown that the outcome of infection depends not only on the virus strain, but also on the infecting dose and route of entry, the age of the cat, and on conditions of housing and husbandry. Genetic predisposition may be another contributing factor; this has not been proven in domestic cats, but the lack of genetic diversity in the cheetah and its exquisite susceptibility to feline infectious peritonitis virus infection are likely related.

The variance in virulence among virus strains is related to their ability to infect and replicate in macrophages. This tropism seems to stem from mutations in the gene encoding the virion S glycoprotein, the peplomer protein responsible for viral attachment and membrane fusion, and the usual target of virus-neutralizing antibodies (see Chapter 33). Endogenous mutations are the likely cause of disease in cats living in isolated environments that develop disease late in life. Stress, crowding, poor sanitation, parasites, and intercurrent diseases, particularly immunosuppressive diseases, such as feline leukemia and feline immunodeficiency virus disease, may exacerbate the impact of feline infectious peritonitis virus infection in these settings.

The endemic presence of virus in catteries is supported by chronic asymptomatic carriers/shedders. Infected cats are immune to superinfection—active immunity, although unable to clear the infection, prevents infection by antigenically related variants. This explains why littermates, which most likely are infected at the same time and from the same source, harbor genetically related but slightly different variants (quasispecies) long after weaning. The incidence of feline infectious peritonitis is age related and biphasic: cats 6 to 12 months of age have the highest incidence of disease, cats between 5 and 10 years of age have a lower incidence, but then incidence increases again in cats over 13 years of age, the latter probably because of a decline in the capacity of the cell-mediated immune system.

Clinically, there are two major forms of feline infectious peritonitis: an effusive form ("wet form"), characterized by high protein fluid accumulation in body cavities, and a noneffusive form ("dry form"), characterized by multiple pyogranulomatous lesions. In the effusive form of the disease, damage is caused by the deposition of immune complexes in small blood vessels; this leads to leakage of serum proteins and fluids into body cavities. Cats with the effusive form of the disease usually develop progressive abdominal distention due to peritoneal fluid accumulations. There may also be pleural and pericardial fluid accumulations. In the noneffusive form of the disease, the cell-mediated immune response of the cat results in localized perivascular infiltrations of inflammatory cells (lymphocytes, macrophages, neutrophils, and plasma cells) in the parenchyma of many organs, especially the eyes, central nervous system, and abdominal organs. These cellular infiltrates cause local tissue necrosis and functional disruptions.

The course of feline infectious peritonitis virus infection is established quickly following infection, with the dynamics of the development of cell-mediated and antibody responses determining the outcome. Cats that produce antibody but fail to generate a cell-mediated immune response develop effusive disease, which in fact is an immune complex-mediated immediate hypersensitivity reaction. Antibodies to feline infectious peritonitis virus are not only nonprotective—there is evidence of antibody-dependent enhancement of infection. That is, when antibody is present, the uptake of infectious antibody–virus complexes by monocytes and macrophages is facilitated; the virus then replicates in these cells and the progress of disease is accelerated. Noneffusive disease is believed to result from a partially protective cell-mediated immune response.

Cats that mount a rapid cell-mediated immune response apparently do not develop disease, although they harbor virus latently and persistently. This persistent infection seems to provide the antigenic stimulus to maintain their immune status. In these cats, infection may be reactivated by intercurrent infections that are immunosuppressive, such as feline leukemia or feline immunodeficiency virus disease. If latently infected cats clear their infection they may lose their cell-mediated immune reactivity; if this happens while they continue to produce antibody they may be hypersensitive if reexposed to virulent virus.

Understanding the pathogenesis of feline infectious peritonitis helps explain its refractoriness in regard to vaccine development. A vaccine based on a temperature-sensitive virus strain has been licensed in the United States; however, its efficacy has been questioned and, moreover, it has been said to evoke the same kind of antibody-dependent enhancement seen in natural infection.

Latency, Lifelong Carrier Status, and Recurrent Herpesvirus Diseases

Several alphaherpesviruses of animals and herpes simplex viruses 1 and 2 of humans have similar pathogenic patterns in which primary infection is followed by lifelong, latent infection that results in intermittent episodes of recurrent disease and virus shedding. The mechanisms involved have been described in greatest detail for infectious bovine rhinotracheitis (bovine herpesvirus 1 infection), pseudorabies in swine, and herpes simplex virus infections in humans.

Following initial invasion via the nasopharynx, virus infects mucocutaneous epithelial cells, causing necrosis that is seen as vesicles and ulcerative lesions (rhinotracheitis). In many cases these lesions are too small to be recognized, but they are the source of progeny virus, some of which enters nearby nerve endings and is transported in the axoplasm of sensory nerve fibers to sensory cranial (particularly the trigeminal) and/or spinal ganglia. In the case of invasion via the genital tract during sexual contact, virus causes similar epithelial lesions (vulvovaginitis and balanoposthitis), again with lesions often too small to be recognized, and then enters nerve endings and is transported to spinal ganglia. The precise details of how the virus, viral nucleocapsid, or viral genome alone is transported along nerve pathways to the ganglion cells is not known but transit occurs in the face of a vigorous immune response that eliminates all nonneuronal infected cells and all cell-free virus.

The establishment of latency is a key element in alphaherpesvirus pathogenesis. Whereas all viral synthetic processes proceed rapidly in infected epithelial cells (see Chapters 3 and 18), in ganglionic neurons the replication of the virus is restricted greatly. When these neurons are first infected, replicative processes, including messenger RNA synthesis, occur to some extent but do not result in cell lysis. After a few days the level of transcription from the circularized, episomal form of the viral genome becomes restricted to a few transcripts known as *latency associated transcripts* (and perhaps several other viral gene products, including thymidine kinase, ribonucleotide reductase, and immediate early protein IE110).

Latency associated transcripts are the only viral products synthesized in large amounts in latently infected cells; there is, however, conflicting evidence of their role: some mutant viruses that do not synthesize these transcripts can still become latent; these transcripts do not appear to be translated into proteins and there is no understanding of the mechanism by which they may maintain the latent state or their role in reactivation of the virus.

The maintenance of latency is of crucial value to the virus. There is no advantage to the virus in eliminating its site of latency—to the contrary, because neurons do not divide there is no need for continuing viral replication that might damage the host cell. In latent herpes simplex infection in humans it is estimated that from 1 to 30% of trigeminal ganglionic neurons may contain viral DNA, with 20–100 copies per cell.

Periodically, the latent viral infection in ganglionic neurons is reactivated. In most cases, reactivation leads to the transit of virus (or more likely viral nucleocapsids) down the sensory nerves back to the same neuroepidermal junctions in the nasopharyngeal or genital epithelium where the primary infection occurred. Here, there is infection of epithelial cells, vesicle formation and necrosis, and a burst of virus shedding just as in primary infection. The nature of recurrent lesions is influenced by the amount of virus reactivated and the swiftness of the host's immune response—usually lesions are less pronounced, more restricted in their distribution and in many instances inapparent. It is not clear whether there is any host cell damage during the latent state—if there is it is minimal. However, during reactivation there is substantial inflammatory cell infiltration and destruction of neurons and surrounding ganglionic tissues. In some cases during reactivation virus is transported through axons to the brain where it causes a necrotizing encephalitis—this is not uncommon when pseudorabies virus infects cattle, but is rare in bovine herpesvirus 1 infections of cattle.

Every element in this pathogenic pattern contributes to the survival and spread of the alphaherpesviruses among their host animal populations—transmission from acutely involved primary infection sites is important, but so is the "back-up" provided by reactivation, recurrent disease, and further virus shedding. Throughout the life of latently infected animals there are continuing intermittent rounds of viral shedding and transmission. Reactivation is usually associated with stress, intercurrent disease, trauma, hormonal irregularities, immunosuppression, and/or waning immunity. It so happens that these contributing factors are most pronounced when uninfected animals in the population are most vulnerable, e.g., as when cattle are shipped to feedlots.

Cytomegaloviruses (betaherpesviruses) establish latent infections in salivary gland and bladder epithelia as well as in blood mononuclear cells. The viruses are shed, intermittently or continuously, in saliva and urine. Murine cytomegaloviruses may become a problem in mouse and rat colonies when they are transmitted in this way. Human cytomegalovirus infections may be reactivated after organ transplantation, even when the donor was demonstrably free of infectious virus or viral antigen. In fact, cytomegalovirus infection is the most common cause of death in organ transplant recipients. This matter gains in importance as xenotransplantation gains momentum—the risk to recipients and to the population from "species jumping" cytomegaloviruses of donor species (swine, nonhuman primates) is a matter of scientific and public debate.

The gammaherpesviruses typified by equine herpesvirus 2 and Epstein–Barr virus of humans infect and lyse epithelial cells and become latent in B lymphocytes, which do not permit full cycle replication. Epstein–Barr virus causes glandular fever/infectious mononucleosis (a misnomer because the cells are in fact B lymphocytes undergoing blastogenesis). There is lifelong carrier status and intermittent shedding, ensuring that the viruses are reliably passed from one generation to the next. The diseases produced are described as low grade: mild fever, inflammation of the oropharynx, lymph node swelling, loss of appetite, and malaise with a prolonged recovery time. In the case of the equine herpesvirus 2, antigenically different viruses occur and horses are infected with different viruses throughout life so that recurrent disease associated with reactivation of latent virus as well as reinfection with different stains of virus are recognized. Epstein–Barr virus is associated with the production of B cell lymphomas (Burkitt's lymphoma) and nasopharyngeal carcinoma.

Foot-and-Mouth Disease

Although convalescence after foot-and-mouth disease in cattle is often protracted, for many years it was thought that recovery was complete, with elimination of the virus. However, it is now known that foot-and-mouth disease viruses can cause persistent infection of the pharynx in cattle, sheep, goats, and other ruminants. Not all infected animals become carriers nor is there any correlation between antibody levels and the carrier state. Cattle vaccinated with inactivated vaccine may become carriers if subsequently infected. The recovery of virus from pharyngeal fluids is often intermittent, possibly because of variability in sampling techniques, but isolations have been made from cattle and Cape buffalo for up to 2 years after infection. The mechanism of persistence is unknown and its epidemiologic significance has been difficult to assess. Pharyngeal fluids may contain large amounts of virus, which may be aerosolized by cattle when they cough, but attempts to demonstrate transmission from carriers to susceptible cattle have given equivocal results. Epidemiological data, however, indicate that in Africa transmission from persistently infected Cape buffalo to cattle occurs often enough to be a factor in eradication programs.

Old Dog Encephalitis

Some dogs that have recovered from canine distemper continue to harbor the virus in neurons, where slow, continuous replication eventually produces old dog encephalitis. The situation is analogous to subacute sclerosing panencephalitis in humans, caused by persistent neuronal infection by measles virus. In subacute sclerosing panencephalitis, at the time of death, some neurons contain large masses of viral nucleocapsids but complete virions are not made, apparently because a mutant virus is selected that is defective in the production of matrix protein and other envelope components. Nevertheless, the complete viral genome is present, as measles virus can be isolated by cocultivation of brain cells with permissive cells. In old dog encephalitis, the situation is similar, but virus can be cultivated directly from the brain of affected dogs if tissue samples are washed to remove neutralizing antibody. Old dog encephalitis, like acute/subacute canine distemper, has virtually disappeared in countries where vaccination has become widespread.

Lymphocytic Choriomeningitis

Lymphocytic choriomeningitis has been the preeminent representative model viral disease, the ultimate model for understanding the complexities of viral immunology and immunopathology. Lymphocytic choriomeningitis virus is maintained in nature by lifelong persistent infection of mice (*Mus musculus*). The virus is usually transmitted *in utero* and horizontally to newborns, such that every individual in a wild cohort or a laboratory colony may become infected. Infected mice are normal at birth and appear normal for most of their lives, although careful study may reveal certain functional impairments. Almost every cell in infected mice may become infected and remain so throughout life; infected mice also have persistent viremia and viruria. Some circulating free antibody can be detected, but most circulates as virion–IgG–complement complexes, which are infectious. Late in life some inbred mouse strains exhibit a "late disease," which is due to the deposition of these complexes in tissues. This may be manifested as glomerulonephritis, arteritis, and/or chronic inflammatory lesions in virtually any organ. In contrast, when laboratory mice become infected as adults they either clear the virus with lasting immunity or, if infected via intracranial injection, they die of a fulminant immunopathological meningoencephalitis.

The basis for these seemingly paradoxical patterns of infection has been made clear through the work of many virologists and immunologists over many years. In all of these patterns the infection, per se, is without pathogenic consequence—infection is noncytopathic and cellular functions essential for the life of the cell are mostly unimpaired. However, persistently infected mice exhibit a split tolerance to the virus, i.e., although they mount an antibody response, they do not generate virus-specific cytotoxic T lymphocytes ($CD8^+$ T lymphocytes), which are needed to clear the infection. In the acute infection in adult mice, both the clearance of the virus and the lethal meningoencephalitis are due to this virus-specific cytotoxic T lymphocyte response.

Antiviral cytotoxic T lymphocytes were first demonstrated in the lymphocytic choriomeningitis virus model: Doherty and Zinkernagel, in their Nobel Prize-winning work, used this model to demonstrate the important concept of MHC class I restriction in cytotoxic T lymphocyte recognition. Acutely infected adult mice usually succumb between 6 and 9 days postinfection at which time their meninges, choroid plexuses, and ependyma are infiltrated by large numbers of T lymphocytes and monocytes/macrophages (Figure 10.6). Tissue damage is mediated by the secretion by cytotoxic T cells and infiltrating macrophages of tumor necrosis factor α, IL-1α and -1β, IL-6 and interferon γ. In the absence of virus-specific cytotoxic T cells the animal survives and a persistent infection is established. Abrogation of the usual cytotoxic T cell response may be produced experimentally by antilymphocyte serum, γ-irradiation, or immunosuppressive drugs (e.g., cyclophosphamide).

When mice are infected *in utero* or are inoculated with virus within a day of birth they fail to mount a virus-specific cytotoxic T lymphocyte response. These mice may appear runted, but survive. They are not generally immunosuppressed—their unresponsiveness is highly specific. They can reject skin grafts, elicit usual immune responses, and do not succumb to opportunistic infections. The basis for this phenomenon is that virus-specific T cells are deleted in a manner identical to the deletion of self-reactive T cells—virus-specific T cells do not leave the thymus. Therefore, the virus is not recognized as non-self and is not attacked. If virus-specific cytotoxic T lymphocytes (spleen cells or lymph node cells) from immune mice are infused into these mice the infection is terminated. Infusion of B cells or $CD4^+$ T cells does not achieve this end—only $CD8^+$ cytotoxic T lymphocytes can terminate the infection.

The patterns of lymphocytic choriomeningitis virus infection can also vary according to the virus strain: lymphotropic or macrophage-tropic variants may fail to kill adult mice even when inoculated intracerebrally, whereas neurotropic variants do. Further, a virus strain may appear less virulent in one strain of mice while appearing more virulent in another strain. Another basis for the varying virulence of particular strains of virus pertains to their immunosuppressive nature, particularly when inoculated into mice at a high dose—lethal meningoencephalitis does not occur when the cytotoxic T cell response is severely compromised in this way. Immunosuppressive variants tend to replicate to very high levels in lymphoid organs and may mediate immunosuppression by replicating in $CD4^+$ T cells and macrophages or by inducing a high antigen dose tolerance.

One interesting pathogenic feature of lymphocytic choriomeningitis virus is its ability to cause a loss in specialized cellular functions required not for cell survival but for homeostasis of the whole mouse. For example, persistent infection results in reduced levels of growth and thyroid hormones in mice. Infection of pituitary and thyroid epithelia causes significant reductions in levels of mRNA encoding these hormones. Reduced growth hormone synthesis is associated with a runting syndrome in young mice.

Slowly Progressive Viral Disease

The term "slow virus disease" was coined by the Icelandic veterinarian Sigurdsson to describe the slowly progressive lentivirus diseases, maedi and visna, found in sheep in Iceland. The term is now used in a general sense to categorize viral infections with a very long preclinical phase followed by a slowly progressive clinically patent phase that is invariably fatal. There are two groups of slow diseases, one caused by prions, the agents of the spongiform encephalopathies (see Chapter 40), the other by lentiviruses. Maedi/visna disease is the prototypic lentivirus disease, providing insight into the diseases caused by equine infectious anemia virus, caprine arthritis–encephalitis virus, feline immunodeficiency virus, bovine immunodeficiency virus, simian immunodeficiency viruses (African green monkey, sooty mangabey, stump-tailed macaque, pig-tailed macaque, Rhesus, chimpanzee, and mandrill viruses), and of course human immunodeficiency viruses 1 and 2 (see Chapter 23). Our understanding of the pathogenesis of maedi/visna virus infection in sheep has been advanced over years, espe-

FIGURE 10.6.

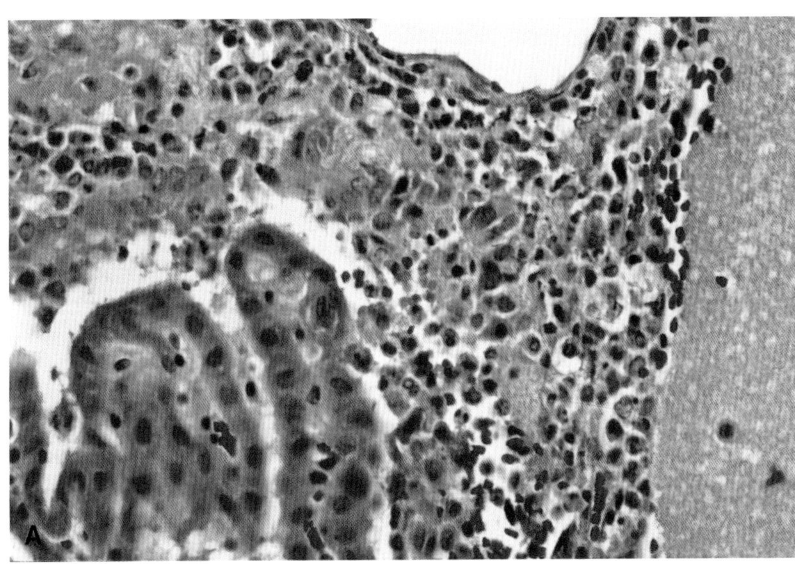

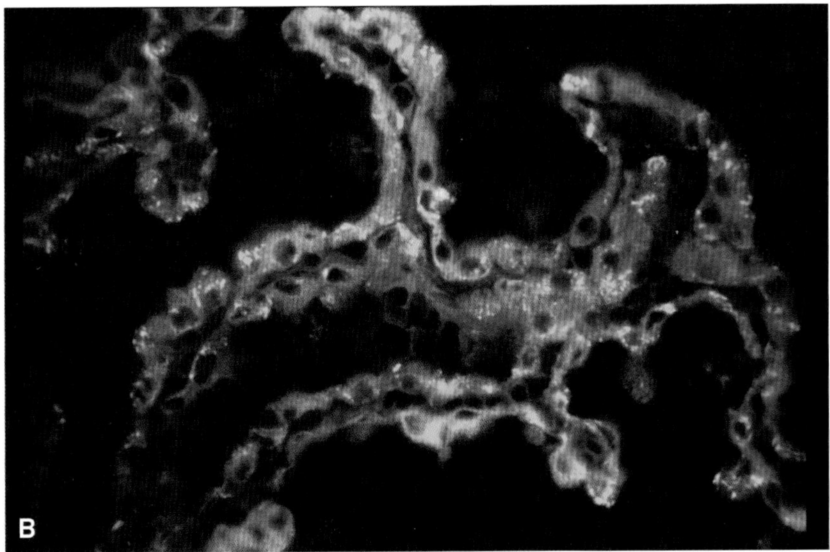

(A) Choroid plexus in the brain of an adult mouse inoculated intracerebrally with lymphocytic choriomeningitis virus at 6 days postinfection. Adult mice usually succumb to this infection between 6 and 9 days postinfection at which time their choroid plexuses, meninges, and ependyma are infiltrated by large numbers of cytotoxic T lymphocytes ($CD8^+$ T lymphocytes) and monocytes/macrophages. Tissue damage is mediated by the secretion by these cells of tumor necrosis factor α, IL-1α and 1β, IL-6, and interferon γ. (B) Immunofluorescent staining of the choroid plexus from a similarly infected mouse showing that the virus has infected every cell, presenting a massive target for the cell-mediated immunopathological attack. (A) Hematoxylin and eosin. Magnification: ×500; (B) Polyethylene glycol embedment—frozen section—direct immunofluorescence technique using fluorescein isothiocyanate-conjugated mouse anti-lymphocytic choriomeningitis virus globulin. Magnification: ×500.

cially through the work of the Icelandic scientists who followed Sigurdsson and by the work of the veterinarian Narayan and colleagues.

Maedi/Visna Disease (Ovine Progressive Pneumonia)

The pathogenesis of maedi/visna virus infection in sheep, like that of other lentivirus infections of animals, involves many features that favor the virus over host defenses. The result is persistent, lifelong infection, late manifestations of disease, and inevitably death. These pathogenetic features may be categorized, as follows.

Pathogenetic features pertaining to the nature of the virus. Like other lentiviruses, maedi/visna virus is an exogenous, nononcogenic retrovirus, which, in the course of its replication, inserts its genome into that of the host cell chromosomal DNA, thereby persisting indefinitely in the individual infected animal (but not in the population as is the case with endogenous retroviruses). The virus has a high mutation rate—it exists as a quasispecies, a swarm of mutant viruses constantly selected for fit. Mutants that escape host immunity have selective advantage—many of these mutants are more virulent than parental genotypes.

Pathogenetic features pertaining to the nature of the infection of host cells. Unlike many viruses, maedi/visna and other lentiviruses are able to replicate in nondividing, terminally differentiated cells. In these cells infection may be activated by host factors (see Chapter 23). In effect, the infection is rather indifferent to many nonspecific host defenses and is at the same time activated by changes associated with stress and physiological disturbances.

Pathogenetic features pertaining to the nature of the infection of host tissues and organs. Maedi/visna virus, like other lentiviruses of ungulates, infects cells of the macrophage lineage. Infection does not involve lymphocytes, such as is the case in human immunodeficiency virus infection in humans. This tropism results in the activation of macrophages and the consequent massive inflammatory infiltrations seen in infected tissues and organs. In turn, this inflammatory response causes massive cytokine release and secondary tissue damage. The variation that is seen in the sites of these lesions relates to the targets presented by variant viruses: in visna the result is meningoencephalomyelitis, choroiditis, and demyelination; in maedi the result is classic interstitial pneumonia. This is immunopathologic disease in its clearest manifestations, varying in target sites, not in character of lesions.

Pathogenetic features pertaining to the infection in the individual sheep. Maedi/visna virus infection in sheep progresses through specific phases. Like human immunodeficiency virus infection in humans, the early phase involves very high levels of production and a wide dissemination of virus throughout the body (high viral load). This phase is followed by some immune dampening of viral load and a long prodromal status. This phase is followed by a resurgence of virus production caused by the emergence of immune escape mutants, viral-induced immunosuppression, and secondary immunosuppressive effects. This leads to the insidious onset of disease, seen as either cachexia, dyspnea, and progressive respiratory distress (maedi) or incoordination, neurogenic weakness, and progressive neurologic deficit (visna). The long prodromal (not latent) state and late onset of disease ensure virus transmission as new generations of susceptible lambs are born into the flock.

Pathogenetic features pertaining to the nature of the host response. By replicating in macrophages the virus causes a dysregulation of the immune response. The response is exuberant, yet rather ineffective in clearing virus and virus-infected cells. Most importantly, there is a specific and progressive immune escape phenomenon (which has been best studied in equine infectious anemia). The infected animal produces neutralizing antibody but it is not effective in eliminating virus. Instead, it selects certain variants from among the quasispecies swarm—variants that represent mostly point deletions and single base substitutions that are nonneutralizable and proliferate. Curiously, the parental virus does not disappear—another evidence of the ineffectiveness of the immune response. In equine infectious anemia, sequential episodes of fever and hemolytic crisis are associated with each round of emergence of a new immune escape variant. In maedi/visna infections, such episodes are not seen clinically. As virus replication continues in this way the inflammatory response continues to build and damage to organs and tissues accelerates. There is also a host genetic predisposition involved: fatal maedi and visna were most pronounced in the highly inbred and isolated sheep of Iceland. Much milder disease is seen in sheep in the United States—visna is not seen and maedi-like disease (called ovine progressive pneumonia) is usually so indolent that death is not commonly seen.

All these features serve to illustrate the complexities of lentivirus disease pathogenesis and the shortcomings of the immune system when faced with this kind of infection. Nevertheless, in some countries, prevention and control must be considered. As might be expected from the ineffectiveness of infection immunity, vaccine development for lentivirus infections, including maedi/visna virus infection, has been disappointing—in fact no lentivirus vaccine candidates have been successful. It might be imagined that any vaccine would just provoke the emergence of further immune escape variants, some of which might be even more virulent than those that emerge naturally. The one Achilles' heel in the pathogenesis and natural history of the lentiviruses of animals is their rather inefficient transmission: the viruses are only transmitted by body fluids (mucus, milk, etc.—and insects such as horseflies in the case of equine infectious anemia). In The Netherlands, a rather successful control program is based on removal of clinically affected sheep and their lambs from flocks. Over time this reduces the exposure of new generations of lambs to the virus and may even lead to elimination if the chain of transmission is interrupted. Development of this kind of control strategy in other parts of the world where maedi is a problem, such as Peru, will require further investigation and proof of concept in the field.

Further Reading

Ahmed, R., Morrison, L. A., and Knipe, D. M. (1996). Persistence of viruses. *In* "Fields Virology" (B. N. Fields, D. M. Knipe, P. M. Howley, R. M. Chanock, J. L. Melnick, T. P. Monath, B. Roizman, and S. E. Straus, eds.), 3rd ed., pp. 219–250. Lippincott-Raven, Philadelphia, PA.

Appel, M. J. G., and Gillespie, J. H. (1972). Canine distemper virus. *Virol. Monogr.* **11**, 1–153.

Babiuk, L. A., Lawman, M. P. J., and Bielefeldt, O. H. (1988). Viral-bacterial synergistic interaction in respiratory disease. *Adv. Virus Res.* **35**, 219–250.

Buchmeier, M. J., and Zajac, A. J. (1998). Lymphocytic choriomeningitis virus. *In* "Persistent Virus Infections" (R. Ahmed and I. Chen, eds.) pp. 575–605. J. Wiley, Chichester, Sussex.

Conner, M. E., and Ramig, R. F. (1997). Viral enteric diseases. *In* "Viral Pathogenesis" (N. Nathanson, R. Ahmed, F. Gonzales-Scarano, D. E. Griffin, K. V. Holmes, F. A. Murphy, and H. L. Robinson, eds.), pp. 713–743. Lippincott-Raven, Philadelphia, PA.

DeMartini, J. C., Brodie, S. J., de la Concha-Bermejillo, A., Ellis, J. A., and Lairmore, M. D. (1993). Pathogenesis of lymphoid interstitial pneumonia in natural and experimental ovine lentivirus infection. *Clin. Infect. Dis. Suppl.* **1**(S), 236–242.

Gibbs, E. P. J. (1981). Persistent viral infections of food animals: Their relevance to the international movement of livestock and germplasm. *Adv. Vet. Sci. Comp. Med.* **25**, 71–95.

Harder, T. C., and Osterhaus, A. D. (1997). Canine distemper virus—a morbillivirus in search of new hosts? *Trends Microbiol.* **5**, 120–124.

Hecht, S. J., Sharp, J. M., and DeMartini, J. C. (1996). Retroviral etiology and pathogenesis of ovine pulmonary carcinoma: A critical appraisal. *Br. Vet. J.* **152**, 395–409.

Jackson, A. C. (1997). Rabies. *In* "Viral Pathogenesis" (N. Nathanson, R. Ahmed, F. Gonzalez-Scarano, D. E. Griffin, K. V. Holmes, F. A. Murphy, and H. L. Robinson, eds.), pp. 575–592. Lippincott-Raven, Philadelphia, PA.

Joag, S. V., Stephens, E. B., and Narayan, O. (1996). Lentiviruses. *In* "Fields Virology" (B. N. Fields, D. M. Knipe, P. M. Howley, R. M. Chanock, J. L. Melnick, T. P. Monath, B. Roizman, and S. E. Straus, eds.), pp. 1977–1996. Lippincott-Raven, Philadelphia, PA.

Jones, C. (1998). Alphaherpesvirus latency: Its role in disease and survival of the virus in nature. *Adv. Virus Res.* **51**, 82–133.

Macartney, L., McCandlish, I. A. P., Thompson, H., and Cornwell, H. J. C. (1984). Canine parvovirus enteritis 2: Pathogenesis. *Vet. Rec.* **115**, 453–460.

Mahy, B. W. J. (1985). Strategies of virus persistence. *Br. Med. Bull.* **41**, 50–55.

Mettenleiter, T. C. (1996). Immunobiology of pseudorabies (Aujeszky's disease). *Vet. Immunol. Immunopathol.* **54**, 221–229.

Mims, C. A., and White, D. O. (1984). "Viral Pathogenesis and Immunology." Blackwell, Oxford.

Mumford, J. A., and Hannant, D. (1996). Equine influenza. *In* "Virus Infections of Vertebrates" (M. J. Studdert, ed.), vol. 6, pp. 285–293. Elsevier, Amsterdam.

Murphy, F. A. (1977). Rabies pathogenesis. A review. *Arch. Virol.* **54**, 279–297.

Murphy, F. A., and Nathanson, N. (1997). An atlas of viral pathogenesis. *In* "Viral Pathogenesis" (N. Nathanson, R. Ahmed, F. Gonzalez-Scarano, D. E. Griffin, K. V. Holmes, F. A. Murphy, and H. L. Robinson, eds.), pp. 433–463. Lippincott-Raven, Philadelphia, PA.

Murphy, F. A., and Peters, C. J. (1998). Ebola virus: Where does it come from and where is it going? *In* "Emerging Infections" (R. Krause and A. Fauci, eds.), pp. 375–410. Academic Press, New York.

Narayan, O., Joag, S. V., Chebloune, Y., Zink, M. C., and Clements, J. E. (1997). Visna-Maedi: The Prototype Lentiviral Disease. *In* "Viral Pathogenesis" (N. Nathanson, R. Ahmed, F. Gonzalez-Scarano, D. E. Griffin, K. V. Holmes, F. A. Murphy, and H. L. Robinson, eds.), pp. 433–463. Lippincott-Raven, Philadelphia, PA.

Notkins, A. L., and Oldstone, M. B. A., eds. (1984, 1986, 1989). "Concepts in Viral Pathogenesis," Vol. 1, 2, and 3. Springer-Verlag, New York.

Parrish, C. R. (1995). Pathogenesis of feline panleukopenia virus and canine parvovirus. *Bailliere's Clin. Haematol.* **8**, 57–71.

Pedersen, N. C. (1995). An overview of feline enteric coronavirus and infectious peritonitis virus infections. *Feline Pract.* **23**, 7–20.

Pedersen, N. C., Addie, D., and Wolf, A. (1995). Recommendations from working groups of the international feline enteric coronavirus and feline infectious peritonitis workshop. *Feline Pract.* **23**, 108–111.

Pétursson, G. (1994). Experience with visna virus in Iceland. *Ann. N. Y. Acad. Sci.* **724**, 43–49.

Pollock, R. V. H. (1982). Experimental canine parvovirus infection in dogs. *Cornell Vet.* **72**, 103–119.

Wright, P. F. (1997). Respiratory diseases. *In* "Viral Pathogenesis" (N. Nathanson, R. Ahmed, F. Gonzalez-Scarano, D. E. Griffin, K. V. Holmes, F. A. Murphy, and H. L. Robinson, eds.), pp. 703–743. Lippincott-Raven, Philadelphia, PA.

CHAPTER 11

Mechanisms of Viral Oncogenesis

The revolution in molecular cell biology during the last few years has provided remarkable insights into the mechanisms of regulation of cell growth and differentiation, and these insights have, in turn, advanced our understanding of the mechanisms underpinning failures of regulatory processes that are expressed as cancer. The genetic changes seen in cancer may be caused by chemical or physical agents or viruses, but all involve certain common cellular pathways. Study of these pathways in cells and animals infected with oncogenic viruses is providing crucial information that pertains to cancers caused by nonviral agents as well.

The discoveries of the viral etiology of avian leukemia by Ellerman and Bang and of avian sarcoma by Rous in 1908 and 1911, respectively, were long regarded as curiosities unlikely to be of any fundamental significance. However, study of these avian viruses and related retroviruses of mice has increased our overall understanding of oncogenesis greatly, and since the 1950s there has been a steady stream of discoveries clearly incriminating other viruses in a variety of benign and malignant tumors of numerous species of mammals, birds, amphibians, reptiles, and fish (Table 11.1). Many avian retroviruses are major pathogens of poultry. Many other retroviruses produce tumors in domestic animals and two have been implicated as causes of human leukemia. Some herpesviruses, hepadnaviruses, and several papillomaviruses are also implicated in cancers of animals and humans. It is noteworthy that the list embraces five families of DNA viruses, but only two families of RNA viruses.

Definitions for a few commonly used terms are needed: *oncology* is the study of tumors or cancers; a *benign tumor* is a growth produced by abnormal cell proliferation that remains localized and does not invade adjacent tissue; *a malignant tumor,* in contrast, is locally *invasive* and may also be *metastatic,* i.e., spread to other parts of the body. Malignant tumors are often referred to as *cancers.* Malignant tumors of epithelial cell origin are known as *carcinomas,* whereas those that arise from cells of mesenchymal origin are known as *sarcomas.* Solid tumors arising from leukocytes are known as *lymphomas,* or if circulating cells are involved *leukemias.* Collectively, especially in veterinary medicine, lymphomas and leukemias are known as *leukoses.* The process of development of tumors is termed *oncogenesis,* synonyms for which are *tumorigenesis* and *carcinogenesis.*

Cell Transformation

The capacity to study oncogenesis at a molecular level was facilitated greatly when it became possible to induce genetic changes in cultured cells that resemble those that occur in cancer—this process is known as *cell transformation.*

Transformed cells, like cells in malignant tumors, express distinctive antigens, called *tumor-associated antigens.* Cells transformed by nondefective retroviruses also express the full range of viral proteins and antigens, and new virions bud from their membranes. In contrast, transformation by DNA viruses usually occurs in cells undergoing nonproductive infection. In this case, viral DNA is integrated into the cellular

Table 11.1
Viruses That Can Induce Tumors in Domestic or Laboratory Animals or Humans

Family/genus	Virus	Kind of tumor
DNA viruses		
Poxviridae[a]/*Leporipoxvirus*	Rabbit fibroma virus and squirrel fibroma virus	Fibromas and myxomas in rabbits and squirrels (hyperplasia rather than neoplasia)
Poxviridae[a]/*Yatapoxvirus*	Yaba monkey tumor virus	Histiocytoma in monkeys
Herpesviridae/*Alphaherpesvirinae*/unnamed genus	Marek's disease virus	T cell lymphomatosis in fowl
Herpesviridae/*Gammaherpesvirinae*/*Rhadinovirus*	Ateline herpesvirus 2 and saimirine herpesvirus 2	Nil in natural hosts, lymphomas and leukemia in certain other monkeys
Herpesviridae/*Gammaherpesvirinae*/*Lymphocryptovirus*	Epstein–Barr virus	Burkitt's lymphoma, nasopharyngeal carcinoma, and B cell carcinomas in humans and monkeys
	Baboon herpesvirus	Lymphoma in baboons
Herpesviridae/*Gammaherpesvirinae*/ungrouped	Cottontail rabbit herpesvirus	Lymphoma in rabbits
Herpesviridae/ungrouped	Lucké frog herpesvirus	Renal adenocarcinoma in frogs and tadpoles
Adenoviridae/*Mastadenovirus*	Many adenoviruses	Solid tumors in newborn rodents, no tumors in natural hosts
Papovaviridae/*Papillomavirus*	Cottontail rabbit papillomavirus	Papillomas, skin cancers in rabbits
	Bovine papillomavirus 4	Papillomas, carcinoma of intestine, bladder
	Bovine papillomavirus 7	Papillomas, carcinoma of eye
	Human papillomaviruses 5, 8	Squamous cell carcinoma
	Human papillomaviruses 16, 18	Genital carcinomas
Papovaviridae/*Polyomavirus*	Murine polyomavirus and simian virus 40	Solid tumors in newborn rodents
Reverse transcribing Viruses		
Hepadnaviridae/*Orthohepadnavirus*	Human, woodchuck hepatitis viruses	Hepatocellular carcinomas in humans and woodchucks
Hepadnaviridae/*Avihepadnavirus*	Duck hepatitis virus	Hepatocellular carcinomas in ducks
Retroviridae/*Alpharetrovirus*	Avian leukosis viruses	Leukosis (lymphoma, leukemia), osteopetrosis, nephroblastoma in fowl
	Rous sarcoma virus	Sarcoma in fowl
	Avian erythroblastosis virus	Erythroblastosis in fowl
	Avian myeloblastosis virus	Myeloblastosis in fowl
Retroviridae/*Betaretrovirus*	Mouse mammary carcinoma virus	Mammary carcinoma in mice
	Mason–Pfizer monkey virus	Sarcoma and immunodeficiency disease in monkeys
Retroviridae/*Gammaretrovirus*	Feline leukemia virus	Leukemia in cats
	Feline sarcoma virus	Sarcoma in cats
	Murine leukemia and sarcoma viruses	Leukemia, lymphoma, and sarcoma in mice
	Avian reticuloendotheliosis virus	Reticuloendotheliosis in fowl

Table 11.1—Continued

Family/Genus	Virus	Kind of Tumor
Retroviridae/Deltaretrovirus	Bovine leukemia virus	Leukemia (B cell lymphoma) in cattle
	Ovine pulmonary adenocarcinoma virus (Jaagsiekte virus)	Pulmonary adenocarcinoma in sheep
	HTLV 1 and 2 viruses and simian HTLV viruses	Adult T cell leukemia and hairy cell leukemia in humans, leukemia in monkeys
RNA viruses		
Flaviviridae/Hepacivirus	Hepatitis C virus	Hepatocellular carcinoma in humans

[a]Not true oncogenic viruses. They differ from all other viruses listed in that poxviruses replicate in cytoplasm and do not affect the cellular genome.

DNA of the transformed cells, except in the case of papillomaviruses and herpesviruses where the viral DNA remains episomal.

Certain virus-specific antigens are demonstrable in transformed cells. Some tumor-associated antigens are expressed on the plasma membrane where, *in vivo,* they constitute potential targets for immunologic attack. One view of cancer is that it represents a failure of immunologic surveillance mechanisms, a failure to eliminate cells expressing tumor-associated antigens on their surfaces.

Transformed cells differ in many ways from normal cells (Table 11.2). One major difference is a loss of regulation of cell growth (Figure 11.1); transformed cells may continue to divide in an uncontrolled fashion. This can be demonstrated in a variety of ways, including the production by such cells of tumors in athymic mice, which have defective T cell immunity but do not support the growth of normal foreign cells. Similarly, this can be demonstrated in transgenic (knockout) mice lacking certain immune response genes.

Oncogenes and Oncoproteins

An important element in our present understanding of oncogenesis has come from the discovery of *oncogenes* by Harold Varmus and J. Michael Bishop. Oncogenes were originally found in retroviruses, where they are collectively referred to as v-*onc* genes. For each of the more than 60 v-*onc* genes identified so far there is a corresponding normal cellular gene, which is referred to as a c-*onc* gene, or as a *proto-oncogene,* a term that suggests the origin of v-*onc* genes of retroviruses. The term oncogene is now applied broadly to any genetic element associated with cancer induction, including some cellular genes not known to have viral homologueues and some DNA virus genes not known to have cellular homologues.

In normal cells, c-*onc* genes are involved in the regulation of cell growth, division, and differentiation. The proteins they encode, called *oncoproteins,* act in five major ways—they serve as (1) growth factors, (2) growth factor receptors, (3) intracellular signal transducers, (4) nuclear transcription factors, and (5) cell cycle control proteins.

Table 11.2
Characteristics of Cells Transformed by Viruses

- Viral DNA sequences present, integrated into cellular DNA or as episomes
- Greater growth potential *in vitro*
  - Formation of three-dimensional colonies of randomly oriented cells in monolayer culture, usually due to loss of contact inhibition
  - Capacity to divide indefinitely in serial culture
  - Higher efficiency of cloning
  - Capacity to grow in suspension or in semisolid agar (anchorage independence)
  - Reduced serum requirement for growth
- Altered cell morphology
- Altered cell metabolism and membrane changes
- Chromosomal abnormalities
- Virus-specified tumor-associated antigens
  - Some at the cell surface behave as tumor-specific transplantation antigens
  - New intracellular antigens (e.g., T antigens)
- Capacity to produce malignant neoplasms when inoculated into isologous or severely immunosuppressed animals

FIGURE 11.1.

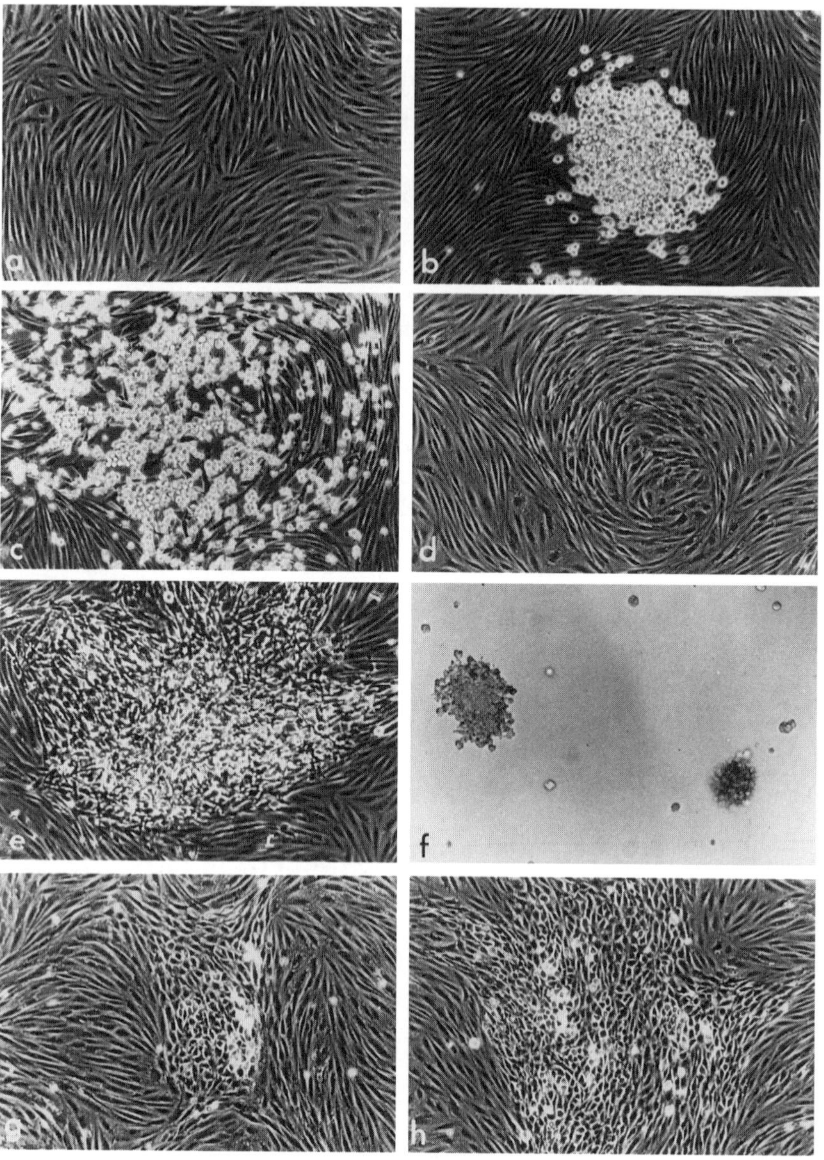

Transformation of a rat fibroblast cell line by different viruses. (A) Normal F111 cells. (B) Cells transformed by Rous sarcoma virus. (C) Cells transformed by Harvey murine sarcoma virus. (D) Cells transformed by Abelson leukemia virus. (E) Cells transformed by mouse polyomavirus. (F) Polyomavirus-transformed cells in soft agar. (G) Cells transformed by SV40. (H) Cells transformed by simian adenovirus 7. [From J. R. Nevins, and P. K. Vogt. Cell transformation by viruses. *In* "Fields Virology" (B. N. Fields, D. M. Knipe, P. M. Howley, R. M., Chanock, J. L. Melnick, T. P. Monath, B. Roizman, and S. E. Straus, eds.), 3rd ed., pp. 301–344. Lippincott-Raven, Philadelphia PA, 1996. With permission.]

Tumor Suppressor Genes and Cell Cycle Control Proteins

Cell cycle control proteins are encoded by a completely different class of cellular genes from the genes encoding other proteins involved in oncogenesis—these are called *tumor suppressor genes*—they play essential regulatory roles in normal cell division. Their protein products are involved in negative regulation of the cell cycle in that they hold the cell at the G1 phase (Figure 11.2). This regulatory role may be ablated by mutations in tumor suppressor genes or by the binding of other oncoproteins to these genes. It is estimated that at least half of all cancers, including those caused by viruses, may be associated with altered tumor suppressor genes.

Retinoblastoma (Rb) and p53 tumor suppressor proteins each block the progression of the cell cycle at

FIGURE 11.2.

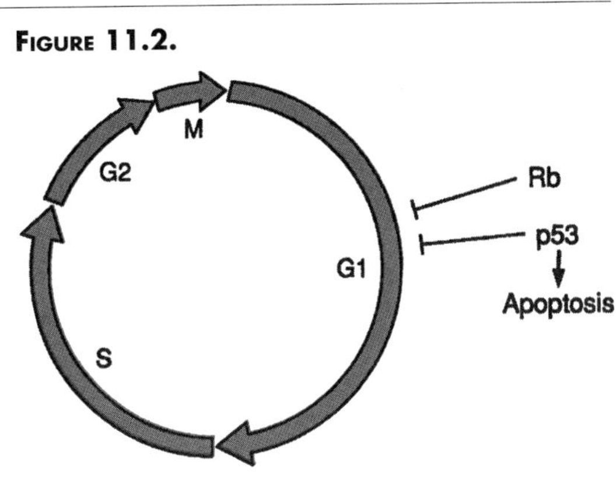

Cell cycle targets of viral oncoproteins. Cell cycle may be held in G1 because of disruption of the normal action of p53 or Rb tumor suppressor proteins. Various DNA tumor virus oncoproteins act to disrupt normal control by Rb and p53, allowing uncontrolled cell division. [From J. R. Nevins, and P. K. Vogt. Cell transformation by viruses. *In* "Fields Virology" (B. N. Fields, D. M. Knipe, P. M. Howley, R. M., Chanock, J. L. Melnick, T. P. Monath, B. Roizman, and S. E. Straus, eds.), 3rd ed., pp. 301–344. Lippincott-Raven, Philadelphia, PA, 1996. With permission.]

G1. The p53 protein, in response to various signals, also plays a role in triggering programmed cell death (apoptosis). Adenovirus E1B oncoprotein inhibits the action of these two key tumor suppressor proteins and thereby drives an otherwise resting (in G1) cell to enter S phase. The expression of the viral E1B gene in a cell is the equivalent of a mutation in the p53 gene—it renders p53 protein inactive, leading to uncontrolled cell growth.

Retrovirus Oncogenes and Oncoproteins

Retrovirus v-*onc*[1] genes are not essential for viral replication; rather, these genes have been acquired over time by the viruses and have been selected for, most likely because they cause cellular transformation, which in turn favors viral growth and perpetuation in nature. Many retroviruses carrying a v-*onc* gene are replication defective and are always found in the company of a replication-competent helper virus that supplies missing functions, such as an environmentally stable envelope. The advantage to both viruses is presumably that when they are together they can infect more cells and produce more progeny of both viruses.

[1] By convention, v-*onc* genes, such as *src*, are designated in lowercase and in italics; the oncoproteins they encode, such as Src protein, are designated in Roman script, with the first letter capitalized.

The oncoprotein products of the various retroviral oncogenes act in many different ways to affect cell growth, division, differentiation, and homeostasis. A remarkable amount of information is available about the mechanism of action of the oncoproteins of the major retrovirus pathogens of animals. It is clear that v-*onc* genes differ from c-*onc* genes in several significant ways:

- v-*onc* genes usually contain only that part of their corresponding c-*onc* gene that is transcribed into messenger RNA—in most instances they lack the introns that are so characteristic of eukaryotic genes.
- v-*onc* genes are separated from the cellular context that normally controls gene expression, including the normal promoters and other sequences that regulate c-*onc* gene expression.
- v-*onc* genes are under the control of the viral *long terminal repeats (LTRs)*, which are not only strong promoters but are also influenced by cellular regulatory factors. For some retrovirus v-*onc* genes, such as *myc* and *mos*, the presence of viral LTRs is all that is needed for tumor induction.
- v-*onc* genes may undergo mutations (deletions and rearrangements) that alter the structure of their protein products; such changes can interfere with normal protein–protein interactions leading to escape from normal regulation.
- v-*onc* genes may be joined to other viral genes in such a way that their functions are modified. For example, in Abelson murine leukemia virus the v-*abl* gene is expressed as a fusion protein with a gag protein; this arrangement directs the fusion protein to the plasma membrane where the Abl protein functions. In feline leukemia virus the v-*onc* gene *fms* is also expressed as a fusion protein with a gag protein, thus allowing the insertion of the Fms oncoprotein in the plasma membrane.

As with c-*onc* genes and gene products in normal cells, the mechanisms of action of the various v-*onc* genes and the proteins they encode are assigned to major classes: (1) growth factors, (2) growth factor receptors and hormone receptors, (3) intracellular signal transducers, and (4) nuclear transcription factors (Table 11.3 and Figure 11.3).

Retroviral Oncoproteins That Act as Growth Factors

Only one example of an oncogene encoding a growth factor analogue is known, v-*sis*, which codes for one of the two polypeptide chains of platelet-derived growth factor (PDGF). This oncogene, under the control of the

Table 11.3
Retroviral Oncogenes and Functions of Oncoproteins They Encode[a]

Viral oncogene	Virus	Subcellular location of oncogene product	Nature of oncoprotein/ associated tumors
Retroviral oncogenes that encode growth factors			
v-*sis*	Feline leukemia virus Simian sarcoma virus	Secreted and cytoplasm	Platelet-derived growth factor/ leukemia, sarcoma
Retroviral oncogenes that encode growth factor receptors and hormone receptors			
v-*erb*B	Avian leukosis viruses[b]	Plasma membrane	Truncated epidermal growth factor receptor/erythroblastosis
v-*erb*A	Avian leukosis viruses[b]	Nucleus	Thyroxine receptor; activated form prevents differentiation/erythroblastosis
v-*fms*	Feline sarcoma virus	Plasma membrane	Mutated CSF-1 receptor/sarcoma
Retroviral oncogenes that encode intracellular signal transducers (plasma membrane-associated tyrosine kinases)			
v-*src*	Rous sarcoma virus	Cytoplasm	Tyrosine phosphokinase/sarcoma
v-*fps* and v-*fes*[c]	Avian sarcoma viruses Feline leukemia and sarcoma viruses	Cytoplasm	Tyrosine phosphokinase/leukemia and sarcoma
v-*abl*	Feline leukemia virus and murine leukemia viruses	Cytoplasm	Tyrosine phosphokinase/leukemia and sarcoma
Retroviral oncogenes that encode intracellular signal transducers (cytoplasmic serine/threonine kinases)			
v-*mos*	Murine leukemia viruses	Cytoplasm	Serine/threonine kinase (cytostatic factor)/leukemia and sarcoma
Retroviral oncogenes that encode intracellular signal transducers (membrane-associated GTP-binding proteins)			
v-Ha-*ras*	Murine sarcoma viruses	Plasma membrane	GTP-binding protein/sarcoma
Retroviral oncogenes that encode intracellular signal transducers (cytoplasmic regulatory proteins)			
v-*crk*	Avian leukemia viruses	Cytoplasm	Signaling protein/sarcoma
Retroviral oncogenes that encode nuclear transcription factors			
v-*myc*	Feline leukemia virus and avian leukemia viruses	Nucleus	Binds to DNA; regulates transcription/ lymphoma and myeloblastosis

[a]Oncogenes are designated by three letters in lowercase and italics.
[b]Transducing retrovirus with two oncogenes.
[c]*fps* and *fes* are the same oncogene derived from avian and feline genomes, respectively.

powerful enhancer/promoter complex in the viral LTR, induces fibroblasts to synthesize a growth factor that they do not normally express. This leads, in cell culture, to immortalization of fibroblasts and, *in vivo,* possibly to the induction of malignant tumors.

Retroviral Oncoproteins That Act as Growth Factor Receptors and Hormone Receptors

In normal cells, growth factor receptors bind particular growth factors, thereby sending a growth signal to the cell nucleus. For example, the v-*erbB* oncogene product is a modified epidermal growth factor (EGF) receptor that retains tyrosine kinase activity. In normal cells this kinase becomes activated only after the binding of circulating epidermal growth factor to the receptor. However, in the presence of the v-*erbB* gene product, ErbB, the enzyme is activated permanently, phosphorylating any intracytoplasmic protein in its vicinity, thereby initiating a cascade of events culminating in the transmission of conflicting signals to the nucleus. In some cells this results in uncontrolled growth.

The product of the v-*erbA* gene mimics the intracellular receptor for thyroid hormone. This oncoprotein, ErbA, competes with the natural receptor for the hor-

FIGURE 11.3.

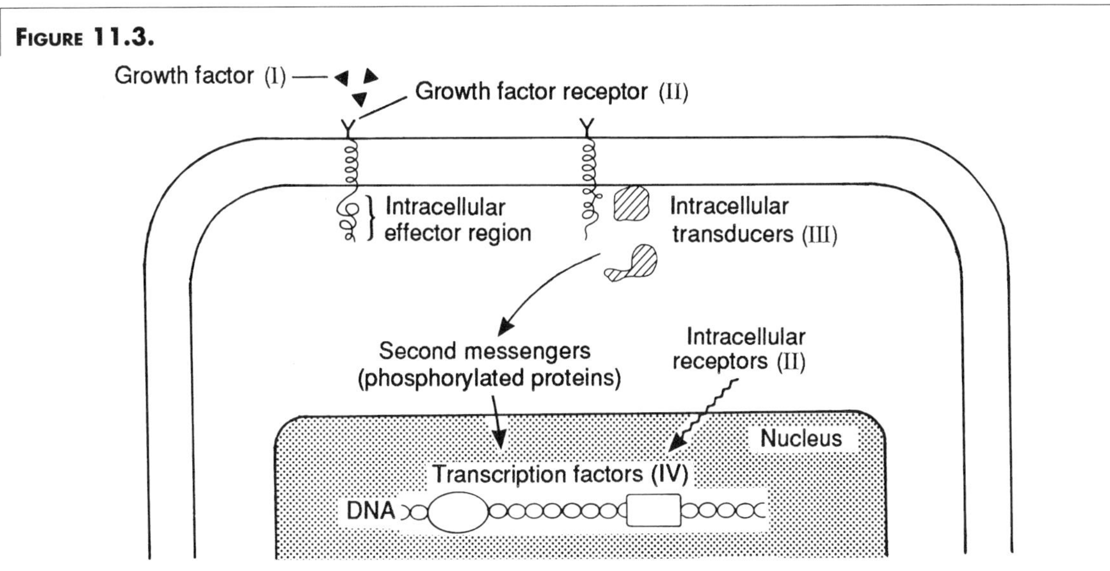

Cellular growth control involves several different types of proteins, the genes for which can give rise to oncogenes. They include (I) growth factors, (II) growth factor receptors and hormone receptors (III) intracellular signal transducers, and (IV) nuclear transcription factors. (Adapted from H. Lodish, D. Baltimore, and A. Berk, "Molecular Cell Biology," 3rd ed. with CD ROM. Scientific American Books/Freeman, New York, 1995.)

mone, causing uncontrolled growth. In avian erythroblastosis virus, v-*erbA* and v-*erbB* oncogenes act synergistically to cause uncontrolled cell growth.

Retroviral Oncoproteins That Act as Intracellular Signal Transducers

Most retrovirus v-*onc* genes mediate their oncogenic effects by altering signal transduction pathways (Figure 11.4). Signal transduction pathways link the cell surface to synthetic and regulatory functions in the nucleus. Taken together, the various v-*onc* genes encode proteins that interfere at virtually every step along these pathways.

A typical growth signal arrives at the surface of the cell in the form of a polypeptide growth factor (ligand) that binds to its specific receptor. The receptor, often an integral membrane protein with tyrosine kinase activity, is activated by binding the ligand; i.e., its kinase activity is switched on, resulting in autophosphorylation of specific residues in the tail of the molecule that protrudes into the cytoplasm. The signal is propagated further by specific sequential protein/protein interactions involving numerous different intracytoplasmic proteins and eventually the signal reaches the nucleus. The ultimate recipients of the propagated signal are transcription factors that up-regulate specific sets of genes and start a cascade of synthesis that leads to cell growth.

The best understood of the v-*onc* genes that act as signal transducers are Ha-*ras* and Ki-*ras*; their cellular equivalents were the first nonviral oncogenes to be discovered. Most Ras protein molecules exist in an inactive state in the resting cell, where they bind guanosine diphosphate. When they receive a physiologic stimulus from a transmembrane receptor they are temporarily activated, leading to the synthesis of guanosine triphosphate, one of the key ingredients in DNA synthesis. *ras* genes acquire transforming properties by mutational changes, mostly point mutations at specific sites, which stabilize Ras proteins in their active state. This causes a continuous flow of signal, leading to malignant transformation.

Retroviral Oncoproteins That Act as Nuclear Transcription Factors

By one mechanism or another, the activity of oncogenes eventually results in a change in gene expression in the cell nucleus. In most cases this effect is indirect, as noted earlier; however, some oncogenes encode proteins that bind to DNA or directly affect transcription. The v-*jun* gene product is homologous to AP-1, an important transcription factor, which can bind tightly to another nuclear oncoprotein, Fos. The oncoproteins that switch on v-*jun* so that it begins to direct the synthesis of Jun protein are components of mitotic signal chains—v-*jun* induces cancer through its role as a transcriptional regulator.

FIGURE 11.4.

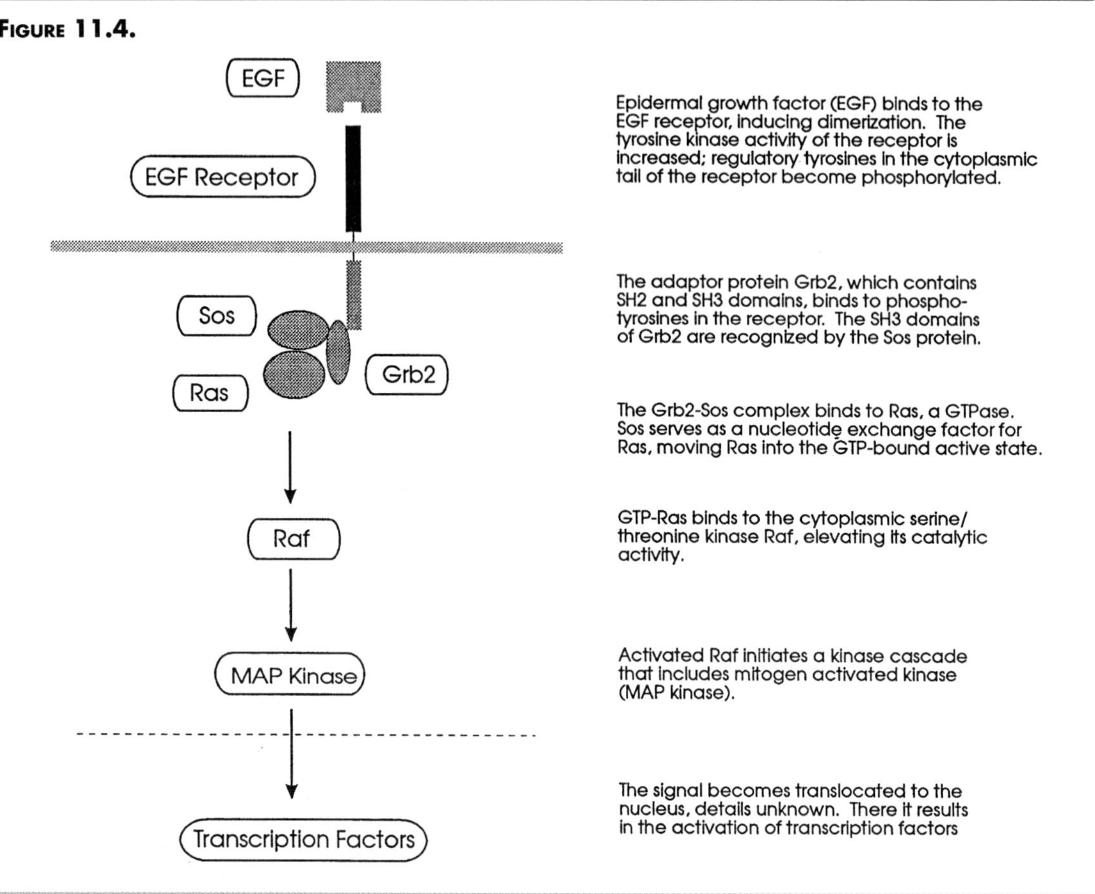

EGF
EGF Receptor
Sos
Ras
Grb2
Raf
MAP Kinase
Transcription Factors
Epidermal growth factor (EGF) binds to the EGF receptor, inducing dimerization. The tyrosine kinase activity of the receptor is increased; regulatory tyrosines in the cytoplasmic tail of the receptor become phosphorylated.
The adaptor protein Grb2, which contains SH2 and SH3 domains, binds to phosphotyrosines in the receptor. The SH3 domains of Grb2 are recognized by the Sos protein.
The Grb2-Sos complex binds to Ras, a GTPase. Sos serves as a nucleotide exchange factor for Ras, moving Ras into the GTP-bound active state.
GTP-Ras binds to the cytoplasmic serine/threonine kinase Raf, elevating its catalytic activity.
Activated Raf initiates a kinase cascade that includes mitogen activated kinase (MAP kinase).
The signal becomes translocated to the nucleus, details unknown. There it results in the activation of transcription factors

An example of a multistep signal transduction pathway. The epidermal growth factor(EGF) receptor forms the first link in a chain connecting the cell surface and synthetic and regulatory functions in the nucleus. The signal is propagated by specific sequential protein/protein interactions involving numerous different intracytoplasmic proteins. Eventually the signal reaches the nucleus where sets of genes are up-regulated. In this example, various v-*onc* gene products, such as Raf, Ras, Sos, and Grb2, affect this pathway, leading to uncontrolled cell growth and division. [From J. R. Nevins, and P. K. Vogt. Cell transformation by viruses. *In* "Fields Virology" (B. N. Fields, D. M. Knipe, P. M. Howley, R. M., Chanock, J. L. Melnick, T. P. Monath, B. Roizman, and S. E. Straus, eds.), 3rd ed., pp. 301–344. Lippincott-Raven, Philadelphia, PA, 1996.]

Activation of Cellular Oncogenes

There is evidence that c-*onc* genes may themselves be responsible for some oncogenic transformations. It is not difficult to imagine a tumor arising from overexpression or inappropriate expression of a c-*onc* gene, e.g., in the wrong cell or at the wrong time. Such abnormal c-*onc* gene expression may occur in a variety of ways.

Oncogene Activation via Insertional Mutagenesis

The presence upstream from a c-*onc* gene of an integrated provirus, with its strong promoter and enhancer elements, may amplify the expression of the c-*onc* gene greatly. This is the likely mechanism whereby the weakly oncogenic avian leukosis viruses, which lack a v-*onc* gene, produce tumors. When avian leukosis viruses cause malignant tumors, the viral genome is generally found to be integrated at a particular location, immediately upstream from a c-*onc* gene. Integrated avian leukosis provirus increases the synthesis of the normal c-*myc* oncogene product 30- to 100-fold. Experimentally, only the LTR need be integrated to cause this effect; furthermore, by this mechanism c-*myc* may be expressed in cells in which it is not normally expressed or is normally expressed at much lower levels.

Oncogene Activation via Transposition

Transposition of c-*onc* genes may result in their enhanced expression by bringing them under the control of strong promoter and enhancer elements. For instance, the 8:14 chromosomal translocation that characterizes

Burkitt's lymphoma (a tumor of African children associated with Epstein–Barr herpesvirus infection) brings the c-*myc* gene into position just downstream of a strong immunoglobulin promoter. v-*onc* genes may be transposed from their initial site of integration in a similar way.

Oncogene Activation via Gene Amplification

Amplification of oncogenes is a feature of many tumors; for example, a 30-fold increase in the number of c-*ras* gene copies is found in a cell line derived from a human cancer and the c-*myc* gene is amplified in several human tumors. The increase in gene copy number leads to a corresponding increase in the amount of oncogene product, thus producing cancer.

Oncogene Activation via Mutation

Mutation in a c-*onc* gene, e.g., c-*ras*, may alter the function of the corresponding oncoprotein. Such mutations can occur either *in situ* as a result of chemical or physical mutagenesis or in the course of recombination with integrated retroviral DNA. Given the high error rate of reverse transcription, v-*onc* gene homologues of c-*onc* genes will always carry mutations and the strongly promoted production of the viral oncoprotein will readily exceed that of the normal cellular oncoprotein. The result can be uncontrolled cell growth.

Tumor Induction by Retroviruses

Retroviruses are the major cause of leukemias and lymphomas in many species of animals, including cattle, cats, nonhuman primates, mice, and chickens. They are also the cause of certain rare forms of leukemia in humans. Oncogenic retroviruses are subdivided in two ways; according to whether they are replication competent or replication-defective and according to whether they are endogenous or exogenous.

Replication-Competent and Replication-Defective Retroviruses

The genome of a typical replication-competent retrovirus (Figure 11.5 A) consists of two identical copies of a positive sense, single-stranded RNA molecule, each of which has three genes: *gag*, encoding core proteins; *pol*, encoding the reverse transcriptase; and *env*, encoding envelope glycoproteins. A second kind of rapidly onco-

FIGURE 11.5.

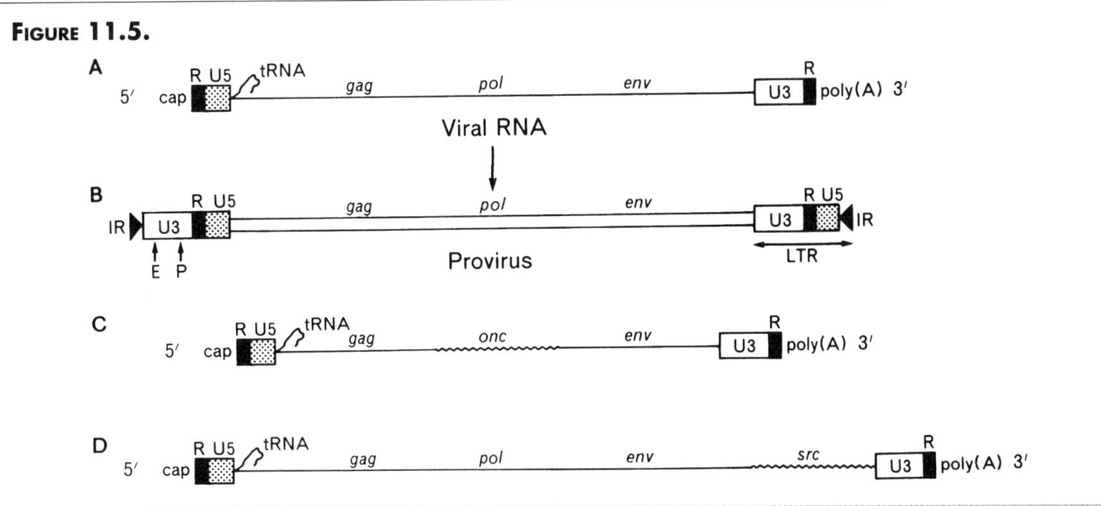

Simplified diagrams of the structure of retrovirus genomes and integrated provirus; in A, C, and D only one of the two identical RNA molecules is shown. (A) The genome of a replication-competent slowly transforming retrovirus. The major coding regions *gag, pol,* and *env* encode the viral proteins. The 5′ terminus is capped and the 3′ terminus is polyadenylated. A short sequence, R, is repeated at both ends of the molecule, whereas unique sequences, U5 and U3, are located near the 5′ and 3′ termini, immediately proximal to R. There is a 16–18 nucleotide sequence adjacent to U5, the primer binding site which is complementary to the 3′ terminus of a tRNA, which binds to it and acts as a primer for reverse transcriptase. (B) Provirus, a double-stranded DNA, is integrated into cellular DNA. The genome is flanked at each terminus by additional sequences to form the long terminal repeat (LTR). Each long terminal repeat comprises U3, R, and U5 plus short inverted repeat sequences (IR) at the distal end. U3 contains the promoter (P) and enhancer (E) sequences, as well as several other sequences with important functions. (C) The genome of a replication-defective rapidly transforming retrovirus. A v-*onc* gene (wavy line) has replaced all of the *pol* and part of the *gag* and *env* genes. (D) The genome of a Rous sarcoma virus, a replication-competent, rapidly transforming retrovirus. A v-*onc* gene (v-*src*) is present in addition to complete *gag, pol,* and *env* genes.

genic exogenous retrovirus carries an additional gene, a v-*onc,* that is responsible for the rapid malignant change in infected cells. Because the oncogene is usually incorporated into the viral RNA in place of part of one or more normal viral genes (Figure 11.5 C), such viruses are usually defective, i.e., they are dependent on nondefective helper retroviruses for their replication. However, Rous sarcoma virus is atypical in that its genome contains a viral oncogene (v-*src*) in addition to complete functioning *gag, pol,* and *env* genes (Figure 11.5 D)—Rous sarcoma virus is replication competent and rapidly oncogenic.

In evolutionary terms, retroviral oncogenes have very recently been derived from the host, most likely from the species from which the virus was isolated. There is little evidence that the defective rapidly transforming viruses are transmitted efficiently. Retroviruses, in general, are transmitted horizontally very inefficiently, and because rapidly transforming viruses kill their hosts quickly there is even less chance of transmission. Although the virus/host recombination events that give rise to new oncogene-carrying viruses are probably very rare, Darwinian selection of such viruses is very efficient—such viruses are amplified in rapidly growing tumors and preferentially transmitted in certain circumstances, such as between chickens in usual commercial husbandry systems.

Endogenous and Exogenous Retroviruses

A complete DNA copy of the genome (known as the *provirus*) of one, or sometimes more than one, retrovirus may be transmitted in the germ line DNA from parent to progeny (i.e., via ova or sperm) and may thus be perpetuated in every cell of every individual of certain vertebrate species. Such proviral genomes are under the control of cellular regulatory genes and are normally completely silent in normal animals. Such retroviruses are said to be *endogenous* (Table 11.4). Expression of such proviruses can be induced by various factors such as irradiation and exposure to mutagenic or carcinogenic chemicals or hormonal or immunological stimuli, so that virions may be produced in some circumstances with some viruses.

In contrast, other retroviruses behave as more typical infectious agents, spreading horizontally to contacts—they are said to be *exogenous.*

Most endogenous retroviruses never produce disease, cannot transform cultured cells, and contain no oncogene in their genome. Most exogenous retroviruses, however, are oncogenic; some characteristically induce leukemias or lymphomas, others sarcomas, and yet others carcinomas, usually displaying a predilection for a particular target cell (Table 11.5).

Exogenous retroviruses can be subdivided further into rapidly oncogenic and slowly oncogenic viruses. The rapidly oncogenic sarcoma viruses, like Rous sarcoma virus, are the most rapidly acting carcinogens known, transforming cultured cells in a day or so and causing death in chickens in as little as 2 weeks after infection. These properties are attributable to the v-*onc* gene, which they carry as part of their genome. Most exogenous retroviruses carry only one particular v-*onc* gene, e.g., v-*src* in the case of Rous sarcoma virus. The genomes of slowly transforming viruses contain no v-*onc* gene, but can induce B cell, T cell, or myeloid leukemia with

Table 11.4
Comparison of Endogenous and Exogenous Retroviruses

		Exogenous retroviruses	
Characteristic	Endogenous retroviruses	Slowly transforming or *cis*-acting retrovirus	Rapidly transforming or transducing retrovirus
Transmission	Vertical (germ line)	Horizontal	Horizontal
Expression	Usually not, but inducible	Yes	Yes
Genome	Complete	Complete	Defective[a]
Replication	Independent	Independent	Requires helper[a]
Oncogene	Absent	Absent	Present
Tumorigenicity	Nil, or rarely leukemia	Leukemia after long incubation period	Sarcoma, leukemia, or carcinoma, after short incubation period
In vitro transformation	No	No	Yes

[a]Except for Rous sarcoma virus.

Table 11.5
Mechanisms of Oncogenicity of Retroviruses[a]

Virus category	Tumor latency period	Efficiency of tumor formation	Oncogenic effector	State of viral genome	Ability to transform cultured cells
Transducing retroviruses	Short (days)	High (can involve 100% of animals)	Cell-derived oncogene carried in viral genome	Viral–cellular chimera, replication defective	Yes
cis-activating retroviruses	Intermediate (weeks to months)	High to intermediate	Cellular oncogene activated *in situ* by provirus	Intact, replication-competent genome	No
trans-activating retroviruses	Long (months to years)	Very low ($<1\%$)	Virus-coded regulatory protein controlling transcription	Intact, replication-competent genome	No

[a]From J. R. Nevins and P. K. Vogt, Cell transformation by viruses. *In* "Fields Virology" (B. N. Fields, D. M. Knipe, P. M. Howley, R. M., Chanock, J. L. Melnick, T. P. Monath, B. Roizman, and S. E. Straus, eds.), 3rd ed., pp. 301–344. Lippincott-Raven, Philadelphia, PA, 1996.

low efficiency and after a much longer incubation period. For example, avian leukosis viruses, which are endemic in many chicken flocks, produce lifelong viremia, which usually causes no disease. However, a small percentage of birds late in life develop a wide variety of tumors involving the hematopoietic system and even fewer birds develop solid tumors—sarcomas, carcinomas, and endotheliomas—as c-*onc* genes are activated (see Chapter 23).

Mechanisms of Tumor Induction by Retroviruses

The replication cycle of retroviruses is described in Chapter 23, but certain aspects associated with the integration of the DNA copy of the RNA genome into the cellular DNA need to be described here in order to explain retroviral oncogenesis. When released in the cytoplasm, the single-stranded RNA genome is converted to double-stranded DNA, which is integrated into the chromosomal DNA as provirus (Figure 11.5B). The expression of mRNA from the provirus is under the control of the viral transcriptional regulatory sequences, which include promoter and enhancer elements that are located in the long terminal repeats. In some ways, the proviral DNA behaves like other chromosomal genes, segregating during mitosis and in some cases gaining access to the germ line of the animal.

Retroviruses produce tumors in one of three ways: (1) *transducing retroviruses* introduce a v-*onc* gene into the chromosome of the cell; (2) *cis-activating retroviruses,* which lack a v-*onc* gene, transform cells by becoming integrated in the host cell DNA close to a c-*onc* gene and thus usurping normal cellular regulation of this gene; and (3) *trans-activating retroviruses* contain a gene that codes for a regulatory protein that may either increase transcription from the viral long terminal repeat or interfere with the transcriptional control of specific cellular genes.

Because most transducing retroviruses have lost part of their genome in the course of the original recombination event that led to the acquisition of a c-*onc* gene (now a v-*onc* gene), they are replication defective and rely on a helper retrovirus for their replication that is always found with them in the host animal. Transducing retroviruses transform cells rapidly both *in vitro* and *in vivo*. Whereas *cis*-activating retroviruses are replication competent, induce tumors more slowly, and do not transform cells in culture, *trans*-activating retroviruses either have no oncogenic activity or induce tumors very late by affecting cellular transcription.

Tumor Induction by DNA Viruses

Although retroviruses are the most important oncogenic viruses in animals, certain DNA viruses are also important as known causes of cancers (Table 11.1). DNA tumor viruses interact with cells in one of two ways: (1) productive infection, in which the virus completes its replication cycle, resulting in cell lysis, or (2) nonproductive infection, in which the virus transforms the cell without completing its replication cycle. During such nonproductive infection, the viral genome or a truncated version of it is integrated into the cellular

DNA or, alternatively, the complete genome persists as an autonomously replicating plasmid (episome). The genome continues to express early gene functions. The molecular basis of oncogenesis by DNA viruses is best understood for polyomaviruses, papillomaviruses, and adenoviruses, all of which contain genes that behave as oncogenes, including tumor suppressor genes (Table 11.6).

These oncogenes appear to act by mechanisms similar to those described for retrovirus oncogenes: they act primarily in the nucleus, where they alter patterns of gene expression and regulation of cell growth. In every case the relevant genes encode early proteins having a dual role in viral replication and cell transformation. With a few possible exceptions, the oncogenes of DNA viruses have no homologue or direct ancestors (c-*onc* genes) among cellular genes of the host.

The protein products of DNA virus oncogenes are multifunctional, with particular functions that mimic functions of normal cellular proteins related to particular domains of the folded protein molecule. They interact with host cell proteins at the plasma membrane or within the cytoplasm or nucleus. Polyoma middle T protein (Py-mT), for example, interacts with c-*src*, resulting in increased levels of the protein kinase activity of Src protein.

Tumors Induced by Polyomaviruses and Adenoviruses

During the 1960s and 1970s two members of the family *Papovaviridae,* genus *Polyomavirus,* murine polyomavirus and simian virus 40 (SV40), as well as certain human adenoviruses (types 12, 18, and 31), were found to induce malignant tumors following inoculation into baby hamsters and other rodents. With the exception of murine polyomavirus, none of these viruses induces cancer under natural conditions in its natural host, they transform cultured cells of certain other species (Figure 11.1) and provide good experimental models for analysis of the molecular events in cell transformation.

Polyomavirus- or adenovirus-transformed cells do not produce virus. Viral DNA is integrated at multiple sites in the chromosomes of the cell. Most of the integrated viral genomes are complete in the case of the polyomaviruses, but defective in the case of the adenoviruses. Only certain early viral genes are transcribed, albeit at an unusually high rate. By analogy with retrovirus genes, they are now called oncogenes. Their products, demonstrable by immunofluorescence, used to be known as *tumor (T) antigens.* A great deal is now known about the role of these proteins in transformation. For example,

Table 11.6
Oncogenes of Adenoviruses and Papovaviruses and Their Products

		Oncogene product	
Virus	Oncogene	Function	Location
Adenoviruses			
	E1A	Regulates transcription	Nucleus
	E1B	?	Nucleus, membranes
Papillomaviruses			
	E5	Signaling	Nuclear membrane
	E6	Transcription/replication	Nucleus, cytoplasm
	E7	Transcription/replication	Nucleus, cytoplasm
Polyomaviruses (murine polyoma virus)			
	Py-t	Regulates phosphatase activity	Cytoplasm, (nucleus)
	Py-mT	Binds and regulates product of *c-src* and related kinases	Plasma membrane
	Py-T	Transcription/replication	Nucleus
Polymaviruses (simian virus 40)			
	SV-t	Regulates phosphatase activity	Cytoplasm, nucleus
	SV-T	Initiates DNA synthesis, regulates transcription	Plasma membrane, nucleus

Py-mT of polyomavirus (like the product of the v-*ras* gene of retroviruses) seems to bring about the change in cell morphology and enables the cells to grow in suspension in semisolid agar medium as well as on solid substrates (anchorage independence), whereas Py-T, like the product of the v-*myc* gene of retroviruses, is responsible for the reduction in dependence of the cells on serum and enhances their life span in culture.

Virus can be rescued from polyomavirus-transformed cells, i.e., virus can be induced to replicate, by irradiation, treatment with certain mutagenic chemicals, or cocultivation with certain types of permissive cells. This cannot be done with adenovirus-transformed cells, as the integrated adenovirus DNA contains substantial deletions.

It should be stressed that the integration of viral DNA does not necessarily lead to transformation. Many or most episodes of integration of papovavirus or adenovirus DNA have no recognized biological consequence. Transformation by these viruses in experimental systems is a rare event, requiring that the viral transforming genes be integrated in the location and orientation needed for their expression. Even then, many transformed cells revert (*abortive transformation*). Furthermore, cells displaying the characteristics of transformation do not necessarily produce tumors.

Tumors Induced by Papillomaviruses

Papillomaviruses produce papillomas (warts) on the skin and mucous membranes of most animal species. These benign tumors are hyperplastic outgrowths that generally regress spontaneously. Occasionally, however, they may progress to malignancy. There is evidence that cofactors may be required.

One of the most instructive models is bovine papillomavirus, of which seven types are recognized (see Chapter 20). Different bovine papillomaviruses are associated with the development of tumors in different sites. In the Scottish Highlands, multiple benign papillomas are common but only cattle that consume bracken fern develop carcinoma of the alimentary tract or bladder. Mature virions are demonstrable readily in papillomas but are absent from carcinomas. However, *in situ* hybridization with a labeled bovine papillomavirus 4 DNA probe reveals that the cells of carcinomas contain the viral genome, not integrated but free, in the form of a closed circular molecule of double-stranded DNA. Viral DNA is also found in distant metastatic tumors, ruling out the possibility that it represents contamination from papillomas. The fact that it is all episomal indicates that integration of viral DNA is not required for the induction of malignancy.

Bovine papillomavirus 4 does not have an open reading frame E6, which is present in most other papillomaviruses; the E6 gene product binds to p53 and it is this interaction that is linked to cell proliferation. In the case of the bovine virus, transformation has been mapped to E7 and E8 genes. The E7 protein possesses conserved motifs required for interaction with Rb (retinoblastoma) protein, a potent tumor suppressor gene. Cattle vaccinated with E7 protein undergo early regression of papillomas, pointing to the role of E7 as a tumor rejection antigen and as a candidate therapeutic vaccine. The viral E8 protein, which localizes in the cell membrane, confers the capacity for anchorage-independent growth to *in vitro*-transformed cells and mutations of E8 abrogate this property.

In hot, sunny climates, such as in northern Australia and Texas, viral papillomas around the eye and on hairless or nonpigmented patches of skin, particularly of polled Hereford cattle, may become malignant; ultraviolet light is considered a cofactor for the virus in the progression of these papillomas to malignant carcinomas.

Certain human papillomaviruses initiate changes that lead to malignant carcinomas. Papillomaviruses 16 and 18 induce cervical dysplasia that may progress to invasive carcinoma. The viral genome, in the form of an unintegrated, autonomously replicating episome, is found regularly in the nuclei of premalignant cells in cervical dysplasia. In contrast, cells in invasive cervical carcinomas contain chromosomally integrated DNA of human papillomaviruses 16 or 18. Each cell carries at least one, and some up to hundreds, of incomplete copies of the viral genome. Integration disrupts one of the early genes, E2, and other genes may be deleted, but the viral oncogenes E6 and E7 remain intact and are expressed efficiently and cause the malignant transformation.

Tumors Induced by Hepadnaviruses

Mammalian and avian hepadnaviruses are associated strongly with naturally occurring hepatocellular carcinomas in their native hosts. Chronically infected woodchucks almost inevitably develop carcinoma even in the absence of other carcinogenic factors. Duck hepatitis virus is probably not oncogenic by itself, but its integrated DNA has been found in mycotoxin-associated hepatocellular carcinomas in Pekin ducks. Oncogenesis by mammalian hepadnaviruses is a multifactorial process. These viruses contain a protein, HBx, which stimulates transcription of many growth-activating host cell genes (e.g., c-*myc* and c-*fos*) and possibly inhibits cellular growth suppressor proteins. HBx protein can complement E1A-defective adenoviruses. Deregulated overexpression of HBx and viral surface proteins is often found in the early stages of hepatocellular carcinoma. In carcinoma cells, the viral genome is integrated at five to seven sites scattered through the genome. Insertional activation of positive growth factors, such as N-Myc in woodchucks, has been described. Furthermore, host cell DNA seems to be destabilized by hepadnavirus DNA, leading to gene rearrangements, deletions, and even chromosomal translocations. The hepatocellular regeneration accompanying cirrhosis of the liver also promotes the development of tumors. The likelihood of hepadnavirus-associated carcinoma is greatest in animals (and humans) infected at birth.

Tumors Induced by Herpesviruses

Tumors Induced by Members of the Subfamily *Alphaherpesvirinae*

Marek's disease virus of chickens transforms T lymphocytes, causing them to proliferate to produce a generalized polyclonal T lymphocyte tumor (lymphomatosis). The disease is preventable by vaccination with live-attenuated virus vaccines. Marek's disease virus, but not the related vaccine strains, contains retrovirus v-*onc* genes. One of the v-*onc* genes codes for a protein called bZip, a member of a family of transcription factors called leucine zippers, which include the oncogenes *jun, fos,* and *maf.*

Tumors Induced by Members of the Subfamily *Gammaherpesvirinae*

Herpesviruses of the subfamily *Gammaherpesvirinae* are lymphotropic and the etiologic agents of lymphomas and carcinomas in hosts ranging from amphibians, to primates, including humans.

Epstein–Barr virus in otherwise healthy young human adults causes infectious mononucleosis (glandular fever), in which there is B lymphocyte proliferation which resolves. The mechanism by which the virus goes on to produce malignancy in some subjects has been best studied in Burkitt's lymphoma, a malignant B cell lymphoma found in children in East Africa and less frequently in children in other parts of the world. The Epstein–Barr virus genomic DNA is present in multiple copies in each cell of most African Burkitt's lymphomas. It is generally in the form of closed circles of complete genomic DNA, which occur as autonomously replicating episomes. The tumor cells express EB virus nuclear antigen, but do not produce virus. These cells also contain a characteristic 8:14 chromosomal translocation. Burkitt's lymphoma may develop as a consequence of c-*myc* deregulation due to this translocation, which in turn causes an arrest of normal cellular maturation and differentiation processes. In parallel, host defense mechanisms may be weakened by suppression of Epstein–Barr virus membrane antigen expression and by blocking programmed cell death mediated by tumor necrosis factor. Some Burkitt's lymphomas also have mutations in the cellular tumor suppressor gene p53. It has been proposed that Burkitt's lymphoma develops in three stages: (1) Epstein–Barr virus infection arrests B cell differentiation and stimulates cell division, thereby enhancing the probability of chromosomal damage; (2) an environmental cofactor, postulated to be infection with the malaria parasite *Plasmodium falciparum,* impairs the capacity of Tc cells to control this proliferation of Epstein–Barr virus-immortalized B cells; and (3) chromosomal translocation leads to constitutive activation of the c-*myc* oncogene, resulting in Burkitt's lymphoma. It has been postulated that similar events occur in B cell lymphomas seen in immunocompromised patients, particularly AIDS patients.

The genus *Rhadinovirus* includes viruses that cause lymphomas in heterologous primate hosts (e.g., herpesvirus siamiri), human herpesvirus 8, associated with Kaposi sarcoma mostly in HIV-infected humans, and bovine malignant catarrhal fever virus, an acute fatal lymphoproliferative disease (see Chapter 18). These viruses are lymphotropic and contain at least 20 unspliced genes that seem to have been captured over considerable evolutionary time from the host during viral replication. These captured genes typically encode proteins that (1) regulate cell growth, (2) are immunosuppressive, or (3) are enzymes involved in nucleic acid metabolism—they include genes for interleukin 6 (originally called B cell growth factor), interleukin 10, an interleukin 8, receptor and bcl2, among others. Interleukin 6 and bcl2 can block apoptosis and some of the other proteins have functions that are consistent with the lymphotropic and transforming properties of these viruses.

Epstein–Barr nuclear antigens and latent membrane proteins that are required for the maintenance of viral latency and for lymphocyte transformation are not present in oncogenic rhadinoviruses. However, there is a striking correlation between the putative functions of some of the cellular homologue genes found in rhadinoviruses and the cellular genes induced by Epstein–Barr virus. Thus, these herpesviruses seem to have evolved/acquired different strategies to overcome cell cycle arrest, apoptosis, and activation of cellular immunity, all to favor viral replication and survival, all also causing lymphocyte proliferation and transformation.

Tumors Induced by Poxviruses

Although some poxviruses are regularly associated with the development of benign tumor-like lesions, there is no evidence that these ever become malignant, nor is there evidence that poxvirus DNA is ever integrated into cellular DNA. A very early viral protein produced in poxvirus-infected cells displays homology with epidermal growth factor and is probably responsible for the epithelial hyperplasia characteristic of many poxvirus infections. For some poxviruses (e.g., fowlpox, orf, and rabbit fibroma viruses), epithelial hyperplasia is a dominant clinical manifestation and may be a consequence of a more potent form of the poxvirus epidermal growth factor.

Multistep Oncogenesis

The development of malignancy requires multiple steps. A potentially neoplastic clone of cells must bypass apoptosis (programmed death), circumvent the need for growth signals from other cells, escape from immunologic surveillance, organize its own blood supply, and possibly metastasize. Thus, tumors other than those induced by rapidly transforming retroviruses like Rous sarcoma virus generally do not arise as the result of a single event, but by a series of steps leading to progressively greater loss of regulation of cell division. Significantly, the genome of some retroviruses (e.g., avian erythroblastosis virus) carries two different oncogenes (and that of murine polyomavirus, three), whereas two or more distinct oncogenes are activated in certain human tumors (e.g., Burkitt's lymphoma). Cotransfection of normal rat embryo fibroblasts with a mutated c-*ras* gene plus the polyomavirus large PyT gene, with c-*ras* plus the *E1A* early gene of oncogenic adenoviruses, or with v-*ras* plus v-*myc* converts them into tumor cells. Whereas v-*ras* and v-*myc* are typical v-*onc* genes, originally of c-*onc* origin, the other two had been assumed to be typical viral genes. Furthermore, a chemical carcinogen can substitute for one of the two v-*onc* genes; following immortalization of cells *in vitro* by treatment with a carcinogen, transfection of a cloned oncogene can convert the cloned continuous cell line into a tumor cell line. To achieve full malignancy, mutations in tumor suppressor genes may also be needed.

These points resurrect earlier unifying theories of cancer causation that viewed viruses as analogous to other mutagenic carcinogens, any one of which is capable of initiating a chain of two or more events leading eventually to malignancy. If viruses or oncogenes are considered as cocarcinogens in a chain of events culminating in the formation of a tumor, it may be important to determine whether their role is that of initiator, promoter, or both. The most plausible hypothesis is that (1) c-*onc* genes represent targets for carcinogens, including chemicals, irradiation, and other tumor viruses, and (2) the full expression of malignancy may generally require the mutation or enhanced expression of more than one class of oncogene, and perhaps also mutations in both copies of critical tumor suppressor genes.

Further Reading

Aaronson, S. A. (1991). Growth factors and cancer. *Science* **254,** 1146–1148.

Bishop, J. M. (1991). Molecular themes in oncogenesis. *Cell* **64,** 235–245.

Coffin, J. M. (1996). Retroviridae: the viruses and their replication. *In* "Fields Virology" (B. N. Fields, D. M. Knipe, P. M. Howley, R. M. Chanock, J. L. Melnick, T. P. Monath, B. Roizman, and S. E. Straus, eds.), 3rd ed., pp. 1767–1848. Lippincott-Raven, Philadelphia, PA.

Coffin, J. M., Hughes, A. H., and Varmus, H. E., eds. (1997). "Retroviruses." Cold Spring Harbor Laboratory Press, Cold Spring Harbor, NY.

Dulbecco, R. (1990). Oncogenic viruses II: RNA-containing viruses (retroviruses). *In* "Microbiology" (B. D. Davis, R. Dulbecco, H. N. Eisen and H. S. Ginsberg, eds.), 4th eds., pp. 1123–1130. Lippincott, Philadelphia, PA.

Hunter, T. (1997). Oncoprotein networks. *Cell* **88,** 333–346.

Levine, A. J. (1997). p53, the cellular gatekeeper for growth and division. *Cell* **88,** 323–331.

Lodish, H., Baltimore, D., and Berk, A. (1995). "Molecular Cell Biology," 3rd ed. with CD ROM. Scientific American Books Freeman, New York.

Nevins, J. R., and Vogt, P. K. (1996). Cell transformation by viruses. *In* "Fields Virology" (B. N. Fields, D. M. Knipe, P. M. Howley, R. M. Chanock, J. L. Melnick, T. P. Monath, B. Roizman, and S. E. Straus, eds.), 3rd ed., pp. 301–344. Lippincott-Raven, Philadelphia, PA.

Teich, N., ed. (1991). "Viral oncogenes. Parts I and II. *Semin. Virol.* **2,** 305–330.

Varmus, H., and Weinberg, R. A. (1993). "Genes and the Biology of Cancer." Scientific American Library, New York.

CHAPTER 12

Laboratory Diagnosis of Viral Diseases

Tests for the specific diagnosis of a viral infection are of two general types: (1) those that demonstrate the presence of infectious virus, viral antigen, or viral nucleic acid and (2) those that demonstrate the presence of viral antibody. While many traditional methods are still widely used, most are too slow to have any direct influence on clinical management of a particular case, providing results after several days. A major thrust of the developments in diagnostic virology has been toward rapid methods that provide a definitive answer in less than 24 hours or even during the course of the initial examination of the animal. The best of these methods fulfill five prerequisites: speed, simplicity, sensitivity, specificity, and low cost. For many viruses, (1) standardized diagnostic tests and reagents of good quality are available commercially, (2) assays have been miniaturized to conserve reagents and lower costs, (3) instruments have been developed to automate tests, again often lowering costs, and (4) computerized analyses and printouts make interpretation of results as objective as possible as well as facilitating reporting, record keeping, and billing.

Although less spectacular in veterinary medicine in comparison with human medicine (for reasons of economic return on investment and range of tests required across each species), there has been a rapid expansion in the number of commercially available rapid diagnostic kits. These tests detect viral antigens, allowing a diagnosis from a single specimen taken directly from the animal during the acute phase of the illness, or they test for antibody. Solid-phase *enzyme immunoassays,* (EIAs), in particular, have revolutionized diagnostic virology for both antigen and antibody detection and are now methods of choice in many situations. For laboratory-based diagnosis, the *polymerase chain reaction (PCR)* is being widely exploited to detect viral nucleic acids in clinical specimens as a very rapid alternative to other virus detection methods.

The provision, by a single laboratory, of a comprehensive service for the diagnosis of viral infections of domestic animals is a formidable undertaking. Over 200 individual viruses, belonging to some 25 viral families, cause infections of veterinary significance in the eight major domestic animal species (cattle, sheep, goat, swine, horse, dog, cat, and chicken). If viral subtypes, strains, and variants are considered and if the number of animal species is broadened to include turkey, duck, laboratory animals, and wildlife species, then the number of known viruses becomes very large indeed. It is estimated that international reference centers and culture collections track over 30,000 viral variants. It is therefore not surprising that no single laboratory can have the necessary specific reagents available or the skills and experience for the identification of all viruses. For this reason, veterinary diagnostic laboratories tend to specialize [e.g., in diseases of food animals, companion animals, poultry or laboratory species, or in diseases caused by exotic viruses (foreign animal diseases)]. Within these specialized laboratories there is considerable scope for the development of rapid diagnostic methods that short circuit the need for virus isolation and traditional means of identification, all of which are expensive, time-consuming, and, in some cases, insensitive. Table 12.1 provides a guide to the principles and interrelationship

Table 12.1
Principles and Objectives of Diagnostic Methods

Principle	Method	Specimens/findings	Characteristics
Visual information leading to a presumptive diagnosis			
	Review of the disease history, clinical examination, chemistry, hematology, etc.	Subject animal and its body fluids/abnormal values	Essence of differential and rule out diagnosis; presumptive diagnosis determines the specimens and methods for further testing
	Pathology, histopathology, ultrastructural pathology	Animals, organs, tissues, cells/characteristic lesions, inclusion bodies	Although slow and expensive, still important in veterinary diagnostics
	Detection of viruses by electron microscopy	Tissues, cells, secretions, excretions, vesicular contents/particles of uniform, characteristic morphology	Rapid; sensitive enough with many diseases, especially diarrheas; expensive; technically demanding, expertise unavailable in many settings
Detection and identification of viral antigens			
	Enzyme immunoassay methods (e.g., antigen-capture enzyme immunoassay)	Tissues, cells, secretions, excretions/reaction of viral antigen with antibody of known specificity	Rapid; sensitive and specific. Most common methods in use today, especially methods based on antigen capture
	Immunochromatography, immunogold-binding assays (the equivalent of the home pregnancy test)	Blood, secretions, excretions/viral antigen identified by reaction with antibody of known specificity	Rapid, sensitive, specific. Very expensive, but suitable for testing of individual specimens in the clinical setting
	Immunofluorescence	Tissues, cells, secretions, excretions/viral antigen identified *in situ* by reaction with antibody of known specificity	Rapid; sensitive and specific. Localization of antigen in specific cells adds to surety of diagnosis; technically demanding
	Immunohistochemistry (immunoperoxidase staining)	Tissues, cells, secretions, excretions/viral antigen identified *in situ* by reaction with antibody of known specificity	Slow, but sensitive and specific. Localization of antigen in specific cells adds to surety of diagnosis; the technical expertise involved is more like an extension of histopathology
	Immunoelectron microscopy	Tissues, cells, secretions, excretions/character and aggregation of virus by specific antibody of known specificity	Extension of diagnostic electron microscopy. Rapid; sensitive and specific. Expensive and technically demanding; expertise unavailable in many settings
	Radioimmunoassay	Tissues, cells, secretions, excretions/viral antigen identified by reaction with antibody of known specificity	Very elaborate equipment and reagents needed; rarely used in veterinary diagnostics

Table 12.1—Continued

Principle	Method	Specimens/Findings	Characteristics
	Latex particle agglutination	Extracts from tissues, cells, secretions, excretions/viral antigen identified by reaction with antibody of known specificity	Most simple method of all; modeled after the brucellosis slide agglutination test where +/− results are obtained quickly; insensitive and subject to nonspecific reactions
	Immunodiffusion	Extracts from tissues, cells, secretions, excretions/viral antigen identified by reaction with antibody of known specificity	Another very simple method; insensitive and subject to nonspecific reactions
Direct detection and identification of viral nucleic acids			
	Hybridization methods, including *in situ* hybridization, Southern blot hybridization and dot blot filter hybridization methods	Extracts from tissues, cells, secretions, excretions/viral nucleic acid identified by reaction with specific DNA probe	Dot blot methods are rapid, simple to carry out, very sensitive, and with suitable reagents very specific. There will be more use of these methods in the future
	Polymerase chain reaction (PCR) and amplification by isothermal amplification	Extracts from tissues, cells, secretions, excretions/viral nucleic acid specifically amplified using primer sets and then identified by various methods such as fragment size analysis, labeled DNA probes, probe hydrolysis, and partial sequencing	Subject to contamination causing false-positive results. Nevertheless, because of incredible sensitivity and specificity becoming used very widely in circumstances where the "state of the art" is required. Automation and new methods for identifying amplified products are leading to quicker, more reliable, and less expensive tests
	Viral genomic sequencing and partial sequencing	Extracts from tissues, cells, secretions, excretions/viral nucleic acid specifically amplified, usually via the PCR and then subjected to automated sequencing, usually of only 100–300 bases in selected genomic regions	Slow and expensive, but when automated, combined with automated genome amplification methods and computer-based analyses of results, this becomes the new "gold standard" in identifying a virus. Partial sequencing is used exclusively to precisely identify polioviruses and dengue viruses for public health purposes
	Oligonucleotide fingerprinting and restriction endonuclease mapping	Extracts from tissues, cells, secretions, excretions/viral nucleic acid amplified, usually via the PCR or growing the virus in cell culture, then restriction enzyme digestion and gel electrophoresis to determine characteristic banding patterns ("viral bar coding")	Very slow, expensive, difficult to automate, and complex to analyze. However, method is well suited for identifying isolates of viruses with large genomes (e.g., herpesviruses) at the level needed for molecular epidemiological studies
Virus isolation and identification			
	Virus isolation in cultured cells	Tissues, cells, secretions, excretions/specimens inoculated into suitable cell cultures and presence of virus detected by various methods, usually immunological methods	Very slow, expensive, and technically demanding. However, this is the only method that provides a viral isolate for further testing (e.g., strain typing) and is therefore widely used in reference centers
	Virus isolation in animals and chick embryos	Tissues, cells, secretions, excretions/specimens inoculated into animals, usually newborn or 3-week-old mice, usually by the intracerebral or intraperitoneal routes or	Even slower, more expensive, and technically demanding than virus isolation in cell culture. However, for viruses that do not grow well in cell culture this is the only method

Table 12.1—Continued

Principle	Method	Specimens/findings	Characteristics
		chick embryos, by various routes, with sickness or death as indication of viral growth. Identification of virus by various methods, usually immunological methods	that provides a viral isolate for further testing (e.g., strain typing) and is therefore still used in reference centers in special circumstances. The method of choice for some viruses (e.g., influenza viruses)
	Virus quantitation, especially plaque assay	Tissues, cells, secretions, excretions, and products of virus isolation in cell culture or animals/specimens inoculated into animals or cell culture. Assays in animals: usually newborn or 3-week-old mice, usually by intracerebral or intraperitoneal routes, with sickness or death as indication of viral growth, identification of virus by various immunological methods	Special addition to virus isolation methods used to determine key biological properties of viral isolates. Very slow, expensive, cumbersome, and technically demanding. However, in certain circumstances it is crucial to know virulence properties and potential for emergence of variants, etc.
Detection and quantitation of antiviral antibodies (serologic diagnosis)			
	Enzyme immunoassay (EIA)—enzyme-linked immunosorbent assay (ELISA)	Serum/specimens tested for presence of specific antibodies indicating recent or past infection	Rapid, sensitive, and specific; the pillar of retrospective diagnosis for many clinical and epidemiological purposes. All serological diagnoses suffer from the need to wait until antibodies are produced, in some cases a few days but in others weeks after infection. In many cases paired sera are needed
	IgM class-specific antibody EIA—ELISA	Serum/specimens tested for presence of specific IgM antibodies indicating recent infection	Rapid, sensitive, and specific; becoming the pillar of serologic diagnosis of recent infection. In most cases a single serum suffices
	Serum neutralization assay	Serum/specimens tested for presence of specific antibodies indicating recent or past infection	Cell culture-based method; slow, expensive, and technically demanding. However, this is the "gold standard" of serology as neutralizing antibodies correlate best with immune protection
	Immunoblotting (western blotting)	Serum/specimens tested for presence of specific antibodies indicating recent or past infection	Slow, expensive, and technically demanding. However, this is another "gold standard" because of its capacity to identify antibodies to specific viral proteins
	Indirect immunofluorescence assay	Serum/specimens tested for presence of specific antibodies indicating recent or past infection	Rapid, sensitive, but subject to major problems because of uncontrollable nonspecific reactions
	Hemagglutination–inhibition assay	Serum/specimens tested for presence of specific antibodies indicating recent or past infection	Rapid, sensitive, and specific; widely used for retrospective diagnosis for epidemiological and regulatory purposes. Still a pillar in avian viral diagnostics and for many mammalian viral diseases
	Immunodiffusion	Serum/specimens tested for presence of specific antibodies indicating recent or past infection	Rapid but insensitive and subject to specificity problems

of those rapid diagnostic tests in current veterinary use that do not rely on virus isolation or cytopathology.

Rationale for Specific Diagnosis

Why bother to establish a definitive laboratory diagnosis? Many viral diseases can be diagnosed clinically and others with the assistance of the pathologist, but there are several circumstances under which laboratory confirmation of the specific virus involved is desirable or, indeed, essential.

At the Individual Animal or Individual Herd Level

Diseases in which the management of the animal or its prognosis is influenced by the diagnosis. Respiratory diseases (e.g., in a broiler facility, kennel cough in a boarding kennel, shipping fever in a feedlot), diarrheal diseases (e.g., rotavirus, coronavirus, torovirus, calicivirus infections in calves), and some skin diseases may be caused by a variety of agents, viral and bacterial. Proper management of individual cases or infected herds or flocks is often improved by specific differential diagnoses.

Certification of freedom from specific infections. For diseases in which there is lifelong infection, such as bovine and feline leukemia, equine infectious anemia, and herpesvirus infections, a negative test certificate is often required as a condition of sale, particularly export sale, for exhibition at a state fair or show, or for competition, as at race meetings.

Artificial insemination, embryo transfer, and blood transfusion. Males used for semen collection and females used in embryo transfer programs, especially in cattle, and blood donors of all species are usually screened for a range of viruses to minimize the risk of viral transmission to recipient animals.

Zoonoses. Several viral diseases such as rabies, Rift Valley fever, and eastern, western, and Venezuelan equine encephalitis are zoonotic and are of sufficient public health significance as to require the maintenance of specialized diagnostic laboratories. Early warning of a potential equine encephalitis virus epidemic through diagnosis of disease on an individual farm allows the implementation of mosquito control and other measures, such as restriction of the movement of horses. Confirmation of the diagnosis of rabies in a skunk that has bitten a child provides the basis for postexposure treatment decisions.

Xenotransplantation for humans. It has been proposed that animal organs and tissues obtained from animals, notably pigs, that have been "humanized" by transgenic insertion of human major histocompatibility genes be used as an alternative to scarce human cadaver material for transplantation programs. An overriding concern is the exclusion of passenger viruses and prions from such donor animals.

At the State, Country, and International Level

Epidemiologic and economic awareness. Provision of a sound veterinary service in any state or country depends on a knowledge of prevailing viral diseases, hence epidemiologic studies to determine the prevalence and distribution of particular viral infections are frequently undertaken, usually based on the detection of a specific antibody. Such programs are also directed against zoonotic, food-borne, water-borne, rodent-borne, and arthropod-borne viruses.

Test and removal programs. For retrovirus infections, Marek's disease, infectious bovine rhinotracheitis, pseudorabies, bovine viral diarrhea, and certain other diseases, it is possible to reduce substantially the incidence of disease or eliminate the causative virus from the herd or flock by test and removal programs. The elimination of pseudorabies from several countries in Europe and states in the United States is an example. Laboratory diagnosis is essential for the implementation of such programs; it is particularly effective when differential tests (tests that discriminate between naturally infected and vaccinated animals) are linked to the use of modern vaccines (see Chapter 13).

Surveillance programs in support of endemic disease research and control activities. Surveillance of viral infections, based on laboratory diagnostics, is the key in all epidemiologic research, whether to determine the significance of a particular virus in a new setting, to unravel the natural history and ecology of a virus in a particular host animal population, to establish priorities and means of control, or to monitor and evaluate immunization programs.

Surveillance programs in support of exotic disease research and control activities. The developed countries of Europe, North America, Australia, and Japan are free of many devastating diseases of livestock that are still endemic in other parts of the world, such as foot-and-mouth disease, African swine fever, rinderpest, and fowl plague. Clearly it is of the utmost importance that the clinical diagnosis of a suspected exotic virus be confirmed quickly and accurately (see Chapter 15). All developed countries maintain or share the use of specialized biocontainment laboratories devoted to diagnosis and research on exotic viruses that cause "foreign animal diseases."

Prevention of new, emerging, and reemerging viral diseases of animals. Continuous surveillance of animal populations for evidence of new viruses, new diseases, and new epidemics is essential if new threats are to be dealt with rapidly and comprehensively. New viruses and new virus–disease associations continue to be discovered virtually every year. We need only make the point that over 90% of all the pathogenic viruses known today were completely unknown at the end of World War II. Vigilance by astute veterinary clinicians as well as by diagnostic virologists and epidemiologists is essential for early recognition of such occurrences.

Collection, Packaging, and Transport of Specimens

The chance of isolating a virus depends critically on the attention given by the attending veterinarian to the collection of the specimen. Clearly, such specimens must be taken from the right place at the right time. The right time is as soon as possible after the animal first develops clinical signs because virus is usually present in maximum amount at about this time then falls away, often rapidly, during the ensuing days. Specimens taken as a last resort when days or weeks of empirical therapy have failed are almost invariably useless and will usually consume more laboratory time than an early well-collected specimen.

The site from which the specimen is collected will be influenced by the clinical signs, together with a knowledge of the pathogenesis of the suspected disease. As a general rule the epithelial surface that constitutes the portal of entry and the primary site of viral replication should be sampled (Table 12.2). The most important specimen, routine in respiratory infections as well as in many generalized infections, is a nasal or throat swab or a nasopharyngeal aspirate in which mucus is sucked from the back of the nose and throat. The second important specimen, routine in enteric and many generalized infections, is feces. Swabs may be taken from the genital tract, from the eye, or from vesicular skin lesions. Skin scrapings may be obtained with a scalpel blade from pock-like skin lesions. Some viruses responsible for systemic infections can be isolated from blood leukocytes (buffy coat). Biopsy or necropsy specimens may be taken from any appropriate part of the body—obviously, tissue taken for the purpose of virus isolation must not be placed in formalin or other fixative.

Because of the lability of many viruses, specimens intended for virus isolation must always be kept cold and moist. Immediately after collection a plain cotton or dacron swab should be swirled around in a small screw-capped container containing virus transport medium. This medium consists of a buffered salt solution, to which has been added protein (e.g., gelatin, albumin, or fetal calf serum) to protect the virus against inactivation, and antibiotics to prevent the multiplication of bacteria and fungi. If it is at all probable that the specimen will also be used for attempted isolation of bacteria, rickettsiae, chlamydiae, or mycoplasmas, the collection medium must not contain antibiotics—the portion used for virus isolation can be treated with antibiotics later or a completely separate set of often specially impregnated swabs should be obtained for the isolation of these organisms. The swab stick is then broken or cut off aseptically into the fluid, the cap is fastened tightly and secured with adhesive tape to prevent leakage, the bottle is labeled with the identity of the animal/owner, date of collection, and nature of specimen, and is then dispatched immediately to the laboratory. The specimen is accompanied by a properly completed laboratory submission form (seal in a plastic sleeve to prevent it getting wet) that includes all necessary details, including an informative clinical history, a provisional diagnosis, and a request for a particular test(s). The specimens should be protected from breaking in transit and should be sent refrigerated (but not frozen), with "cold packs" (4°C) or ice in a thermos flask or Styrofoam box (Figure 12.1). International or transcontinental transport generally requires that specimens be packed in dry ice (solid CO_2). Governmental and IATA regulations relating to the transport of such specimens require precautions such as double-walled containers with absorbent padding in case of breakage. Permits must be obtained from the appropriate authorities for interstate and international transportation.

Table 12.2
Specimens Appropriate for Laboratory Diagnosis of Various Clinical Syndromes

Syndrome	Specimen
Respiratory	Nasal or throat swab; nasopharyngeal aspirate
Enteric	Feces
Genital	Genital swab
Eye	Conjunctival swab
Skin	Vesicle swab or scraping; biopsy of solid lesion
Central nervous system	Cerebrospinal fluid, feces, nasal swab
Generalized	Nasal swab[a], feces[a], blood leukocytes[a]
Autopsy/biopsy	Relevant organ
Any disease	Blood for serology[b]

[a]Depending on presumed pathogenesis.
[b]Blood allowed to clot, serum kept for assay of antibody.

Figure 12.1.

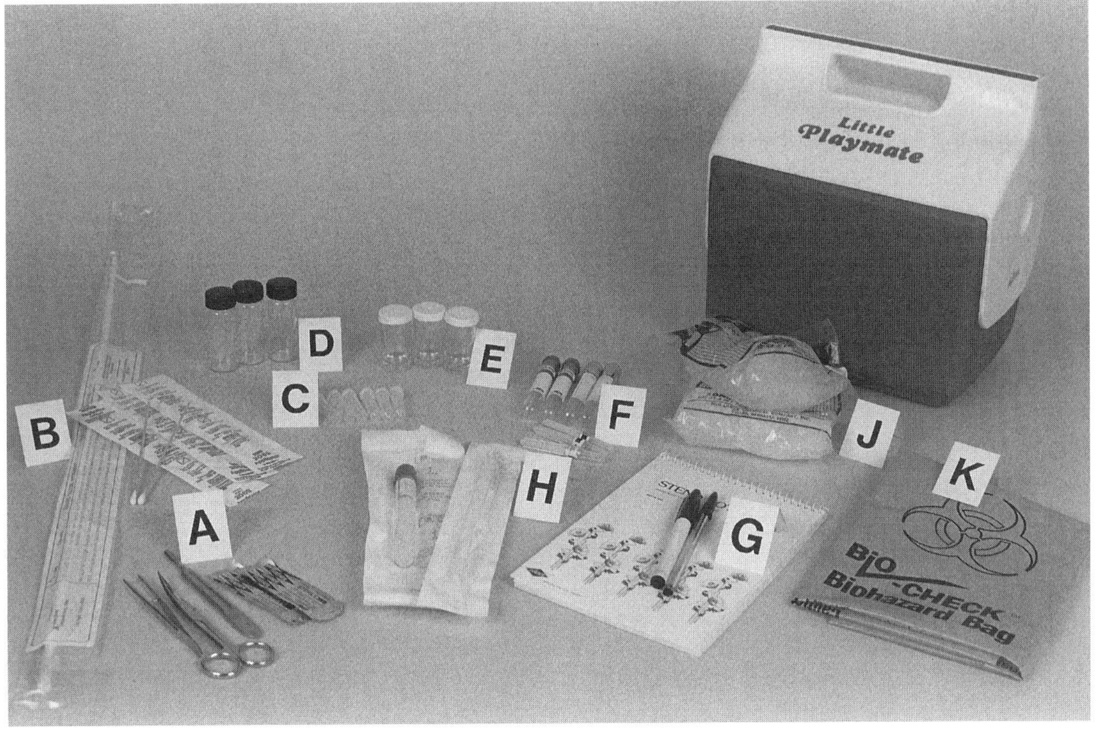

Equipment required for collection of virus samples. (A) Sterile forceps, scissors, and scalpels. (B) Selection of sterile swabs. (C) Vials containing virus transport medium (with antibiotics) for collection of samples for virus isolation or identification. (D) Bottles for collection of feces, blood, and other samples that do not require virus transport medium. (E) Bottles containing formalin or Bouin's fixative for tissues to be examined by histology. (F) Blood collection equipment—without additive for serum, with anticoagulant for virus isolation. (G) Notebook and equipment for labeling specimens. (H) Swabs and transport medium for bacteriological investigation. (J) Cool box. (K) Heavy-duty plastic bags for postmortem material.

Initial Processing in the Laboratory

On arrival in the laboratory the specimen is processed immediately or refrigerated when this is not practical. For inoculation into cell culture, swabs are shaken in fluid medium, feces are dispersed in fluid medium, and tissue specimens are homogenized in a high-speed blender. Cell debris and bacteria are deposited by low-speed centrifugation, after which the supernatant is usually passed through a 0.45-μm syringe-top membrane filter to remove remaining nonviral contaminating organisms. Some of the original sample and of the filtrate is retained at 4°C or frozen at −70°C, at least until virus isolation attempts are completed. The filtrate is inoculated into cell cultures and/or sometimes into chick embryos or newborn mice. Clinical specimens processed in this way are generally suitable for detection of viral antigens/DNA/RNA by *in vitro* tests.

In this chapter, the titer of a virus, the concentration of antigen, or gene copy number is usually expressed per milliliter of the virus transport material into which the specimen was collected and processed within the laboratory; the dilution factor relative to the high concentrations in which viruses and antigens can occur in secretions/excretions and tissues is generally of minor significance; further the weight/volume of clinical material collected is seldom known, making the correction difficult. For critical studies on pathogenesis, the dilution factor is acknowledged and the titer adjusted to reflect concentration per measured/weighed milliliter of secretion/excretion or gram of tissue collected.

Diagnosis of Viral Infections by Histopathology

If biopsy/necropsy samples are collected for possible histopathological diagnosis, then appropriate tissue specimens in appropriate fixative, routinely formalin or Bouin's fixative, are required. If special procedures such as frozen sections, histochemistry, or thin section electron microscopy are to be requested, the receiving laboratory should be consulted for procedural and material details.

Direct Identification of Viruses

Detection of Viruses by Electron Microscopy

Perhaps the most obvious method of virus identification is direct visualization of the virus itself (Figure 12.2). The morphology of most viruses is sufficiently characteristic to assign an unknown virus to the correct family and, in the context of the particular case (e.g., detection of parapoxvirus in a scraping from a pock-like lesion on a cow's teat), the method may provide an immediate definitive diagnosis. Noncultivable viruses may also be detectable by electron microscopy. Beginning in the late 1960s, electron microscopy was the means to the discovery in feces of several new groups of previously noncultivable viruses, notably rotaviruses, caliciviruses, astroviruses, and previously unknown adenoviruses and coronaviruses.

Low sensitivity is the biggest limitation of electron microscopy as a diagnostic tool. Quite a bit of time is required (15 minutes or more) for a skilled microscopist, using a very expensive machine, to scan the grid adequately and detect viruses when the specimen contains fewer than 10^7 virions per milliliter. Such levels are often surpassed in feces and vesicle fluid, but not in respiratory mucus. Feces are first clarified by low-speed centrifugation; the supernatant is then subjected to ultracentrifugation, often through a sucrose cushion, to deposit the virions. Alternatively, salts and water can be removed from a drop of virus suspension hanging from a carbon-coated plastic support film by

FIGURE 12.2.

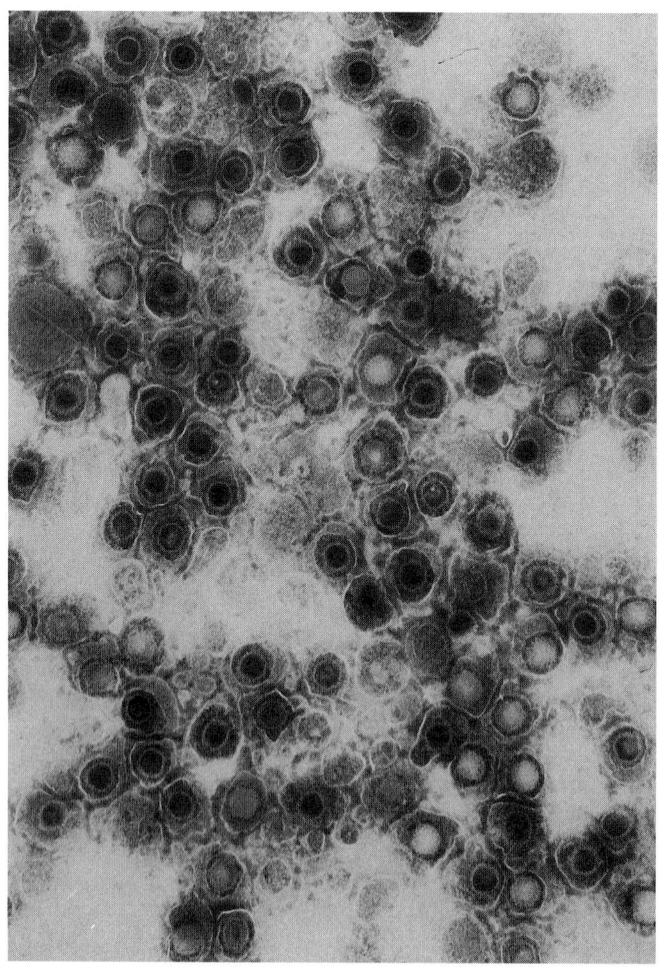

Diagnostic electron microscopy. The morphology of most viruses is sufficiently characteristic to assign an unknown virus to the correct family. In this case, direct negative staining of vesicular fluid revealed large numbers of herpesvirus particles, allowing a presumptive diagnosis of infectious bovine rhinotracheitis. Magnification: ×10,000.

diffusion into agar, leaving the concentrated virions on the film. Specimens are then stained negatively with phosphotungstate, or sometimes uranyl acetate, and scanned by electron microscopy.

Identification of Viruses by Immunoelectron Microscopy

Definitive identification (and further concentration) of virions may be achieved by adding specific antibody to the specimen before depositing the virus–antibody complexes onto the electron microscopic grid by centrifugation. Negative staining reveals the virions as aggregates (Figure 12.3).

To improve detection, the antibody may be labeled with gold. Solid-phase immunoelectron microscopy techniques have been developed in which virus-specific antibody is first bound to the plastic supporting film on the copper grid. Sensitivity can also be enhanced by a double layering procedure, whereby staphylococcal protein A (which binds the Fc fragment of IgG) is first bound to the film, to which virus-specific antibody and the unknown sample are added sequentially.

Direct Identification of Viral Antigens

Immunofluorescence

If antibody is labeled with a fluorochrome, often fluorescein isothiocyanate, the antigen–antibody complex, when excited by light of short wavelength, emits light of a particular longer wavelength, which can be visualized as fluorescence in an optical microscope when light of all other wavelengths is filtered out. The sensitivity of the method is generally too low to detect complexes of fluorescent antibody with virions or soluble antigen, hence, the antigen in the test typically takes the form of virus-infected cells. There are two main variants of the technique, direct immunofluorescence and indirect immunofluorescence:

Direct immunofluorescence involves the visualization of viral antigens in the specimen of interest by "staining" with a specific fluorescein-tagged antiviral antibody. A frozen tissue section, a cell smear, or a cell monolayer on a coverslip is fixed, usually with methanol or acetone, and flooded with fluorescein isothiocyanate conjugated to antiviral antibody (Figure 12.4, left). Unbound antibody is then washed away and the tissue or cells are

FIGURE 12.3.

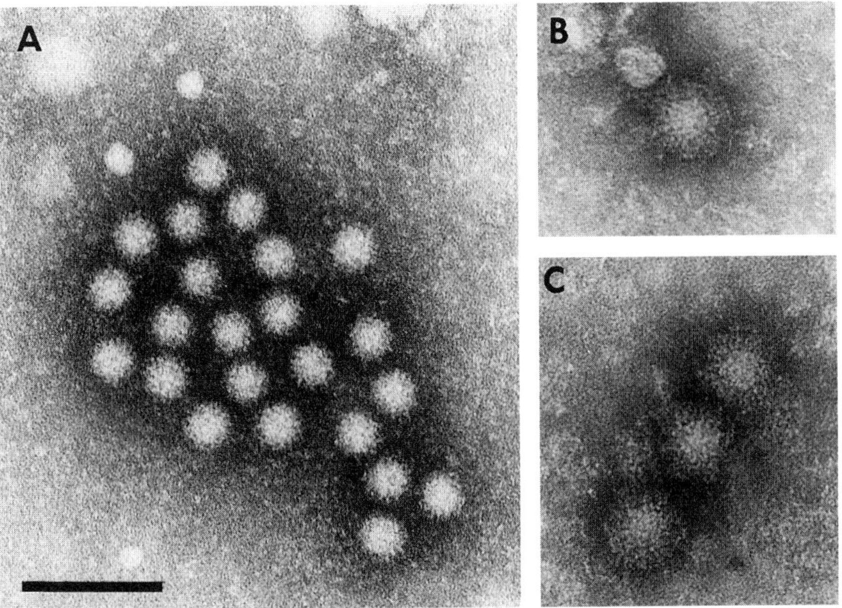

Immunoelectron microscopy. An enteric calici virus was seen by direct negative staining of a fecal specimen. An aliquot of the specimen was then treated with an antiserum of known specificity. The virus was aggregated by the reference antiserum and by convalescent serum from the same animal, but not by antisera to different viruses. Aggregation patterns are different according to the amount of antibody present: (A) high dilutions of the antiserum cause clumping of the virus; (B and C) low dilutions of the antiserum cause fuzzy halos around individual virions or small clumps of virions. Bar: 100 nm. (Courtesy of A. Z. Kapikian.)

Figure 12.4.

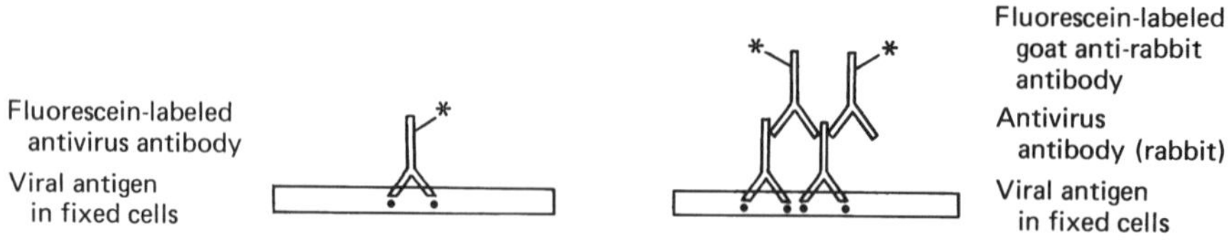

Immunofluorescence. (Left) Direct method. (Right) Indirect method.

examined by light microscopy using a powerful ultraviolet/blue light source. The apple-green light emitted from the specimen is revealed (against a black background) by incorporating filters in the eyepieces that absorb all the blue and ultraviolet incident light (Figure 12.5).

Indirect immunofluorescence differs in that the antiviral antibody is untagged. It binds to antigen and is itself recognized by fluorescein-conjugated anti-immunoglobulin or a second antibody (Figure 12.4, right). The high affinity of avidin for biotin can also be exploited in immunofluorescence, by coupling biotin to antibody and fluorescein to avidin.

Although technically demanding, immunofluorescence has proved to be of great value in the early identification of viral antigens in infected cells taken from animals with diseases known to have a relatively small number of possible etiological agents. There is no difficulty in removing partly detached infected cells from the mucous membrane of the upper respiratory tract, genital tract, eye, or skin, simply by swabbing or scraping the infected area with reasonable firmness. Cells are also present in mucus aspirated from the nasopharynx or in fluids from other sites, including tracheal and bronchial lavages, or pleural, abdominal, or cerebrospinal fluids; cells must be washed, extensively in the case of mucus, by low-speed centrifugation before fixation and staining. Respiratory infections with paramyxoviruses, orthomyxoviruses, adenoviruses, and herpesviruses are particularly amenable to rapid diagnosis by immunofluorescence. The method can also be applied to tissue, e.g., biopsies for the diagnosis of herpesvirus diseases, or at necropsy, for the verification of rabies infection of the brain of animals euthanized after biting humans (Figure 12.5).

Immunohistochemistry (Immunoperoxidase Staining)

An alternative method of locating and identifying viral antigen in tissues is to use antibody coupled to horseradish peroxidase. Subsequent addition of hydrogen peroxide together with a benzidine derivative forms a colored insoluble precipitate. Advantages of the method are that the preparations are permanent and it requires less expensive equipment than immunofluorescence—an ordinary light microscope is used. A disadvantage is that endogenous peroxidase is present in the cells of many tissues, particularly leukocytes. This may produce false positives, but this problem can be circumvented by meticulous technique and adequate controls (Figure 12.6).

Enzyme Immunoassay—Enzyme-Linked Immunosorbent Assay

Enzyme immunoassays, often referred to as enzyme-linked immunosorbent assays (ELISAs), have revolutionized diagnostic virology. Assays can be designed to detect viral antigens or antibodies. The exquisite sensitivity of the method enables less than 1 ng of viral antigen per milliliter to be detected in specimens taken directly from the animal. A wide variety of different assay procedures are used, including direct, indirect, and competitive assays and assays may be conducted on a single sample in the veterinarian's clinic or on many hundreds at a time using automated systems in centralized laboratories. Most enzyme immunoassays are solid-phase enzyme immunoassays; the "capture" antibody is attached by adsorption at pH 9.3 to a solid substrate, typically the wells of polystyrene or polyvinyl microtiter plates. The simplest format is a direct enzyme immunoassay (Figure 12.7, left). Enzyme immunoassays have replaced the complement fixation test for most applications, including those for the differentiation of the serotypes of foot-and-mouth disease.

Virus and soluble viral antigens from the specimen are allowed to bind to the capture antibody. After unbound components are washed away, an enzyme-labeled antiviral antibody (the "detector" antibody) is added. (Various enzymes can be linked to antibody; horseradish peroxidase and alkaline phosphatase are the most commonly used.) After a washing step, an appropriate organic substrate for the particular enzyme is added and

Figure 12.5.

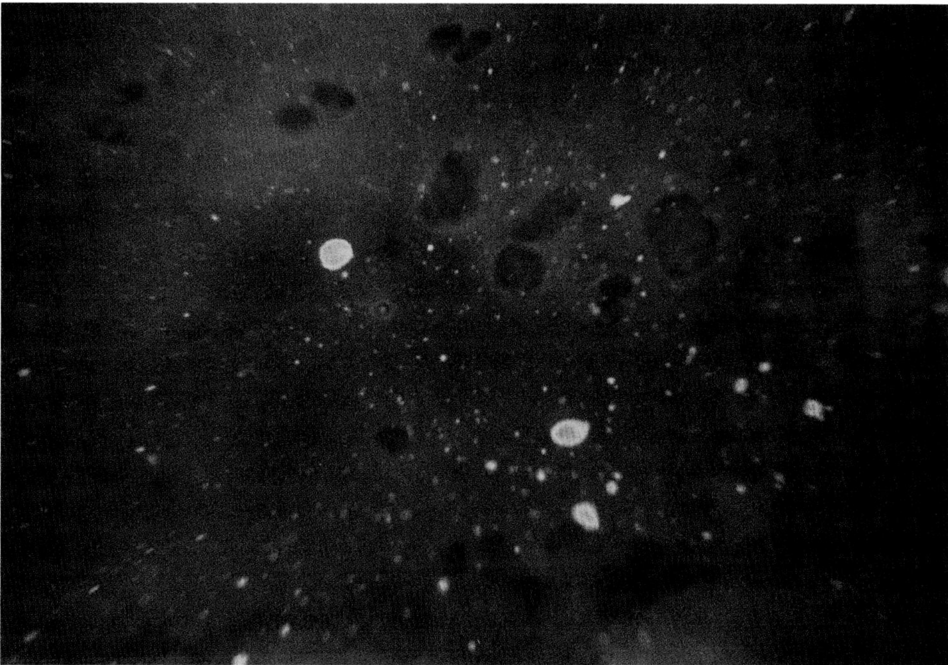

Direct immunofluorescence for the diagnosis of rabies. Tissue impressions are made from medulla, cerebellum, and hippocampus of the suspect animal by lightly touching tissues to a microscope slide. Following air-drying and acetone fixation the tissue impressions are stained with fluorescein-conjugated antirabies virus globulin; they are then washed, mounted, and examined by ultraviolet/blue light microscopy. Identified by its specific apple-green fluorescence against a black background, rabies virus antigen appears as dust-like particles or as large masses, equivalent to Negri bodies in histologic sections. Direct immunofluorescence has a 97–98% correlation with virus isolation techniques, which are very slow and cumbersome. Magnification: ×400.

Figure 12.6.

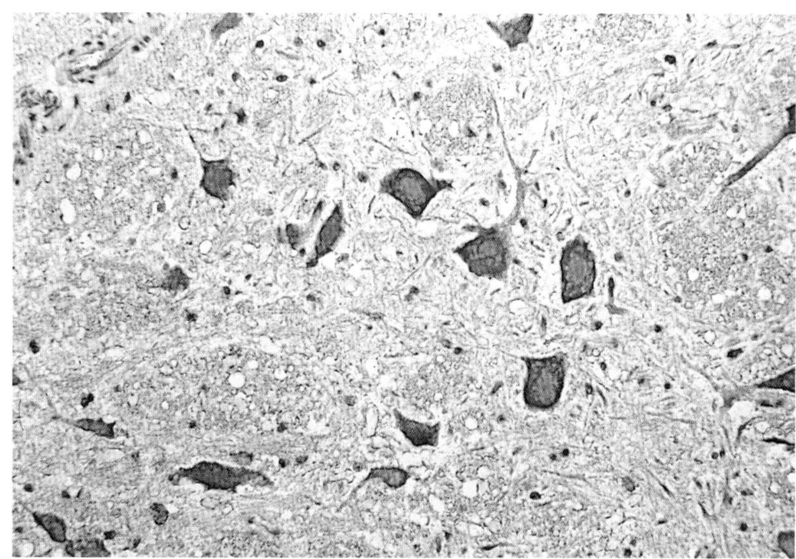

Immunohistochemistry. Rabies virus infection in the brain of a dog. Paraffin section, avidin–biotin–immunoperoxidase method, using mouse monoclonal antirabies virus globulin and counterstain. Viral antigen stands out as brick-colored masses in the cytoplasm of infected cells. Magnification: ×300. (Courtesy of M. Fekadu.)

readout is based on the color change that follows. The colored product of the action of the enzyme on the substrate is recognizable by eye. The test can be made quantitative by serially diluting the antigen to obtain an end point or by spectrophotometry to measure the amount of enzyme-conjugated antibody bound to the captured antigen.

A further refinement takes advantage of the extraordinarily high binding affinity of avidin for biotin. The antibody is conjugated to biotin, a reagent that gives reproducible labeling and does not alter the antigen-binding capacity of antibody. The antigen–antibody complex is recognized with high sensitivity simply by adding avidin-labeled enzyme, then substrate (Figure 12.7, right). Other modifications of enzyme immunoassays, such as high-energy substrates that release fluorescent, chemiluminescence, or radioactive products, further increase the sensitivity.

Indirect enzyme immunoassays are widely used because of their greater sensitivity and avoidance of the need to label each specific antiviral antibody in the repertoire of the laboratory. Here, the detector antibody is unlabeled and a second labeled (species-specific) anti-immunoglobulin is added as the "indicator" antibody; of course, the antiviral antibodies constituting the capture and detector antibodies, respectively, must be raised in different animal species (Figure 12.7, right). Alternatively, labeled staphylococcal protein A, which binds to the Fc moiety of IgG of most mammalian species, can be used as the indicator in indirect immunoassays.

Monoclonal antiviral antibodies may be used as capture and/or detector antibodies in enzyme immunoassays. Their obvious advantages are that they represent well-characterized, highly pure, monospecific antibody of a defined class, recognizing only a single epitope, are free of "natural" and other extraneous antibodies against host antigens or adventitious agents concurrently infecting the animal, and can be made available in large amounts as reference reagents. It is important to select monoclonal antibodies of high affinity, but not of such high specificity that some strains of the virus sought might be missed in the assay. Indeed, the specificity of the assay can be predetermined by selecting a monoclonal antibody directed at an epitope that is either confined to a particular viral serotype or common to all serotypes within a given species or genus.

Enzyme immunoassays have also been adapted to formats suitable for use in veterinary clinics on single animal specimens (Figure 12.8).

Immunochromatography

Immunochromatography tests are modeled after the home pregnancy tests now used by women in many countries; they differ from usual systems for measuring antigen–antibody reactions in that the specimen from the subject animal is made to flow through a filter after which it is immobilized in a membrane at a site where antigen (or antibody) in the specimen comes

Figure 12.7.

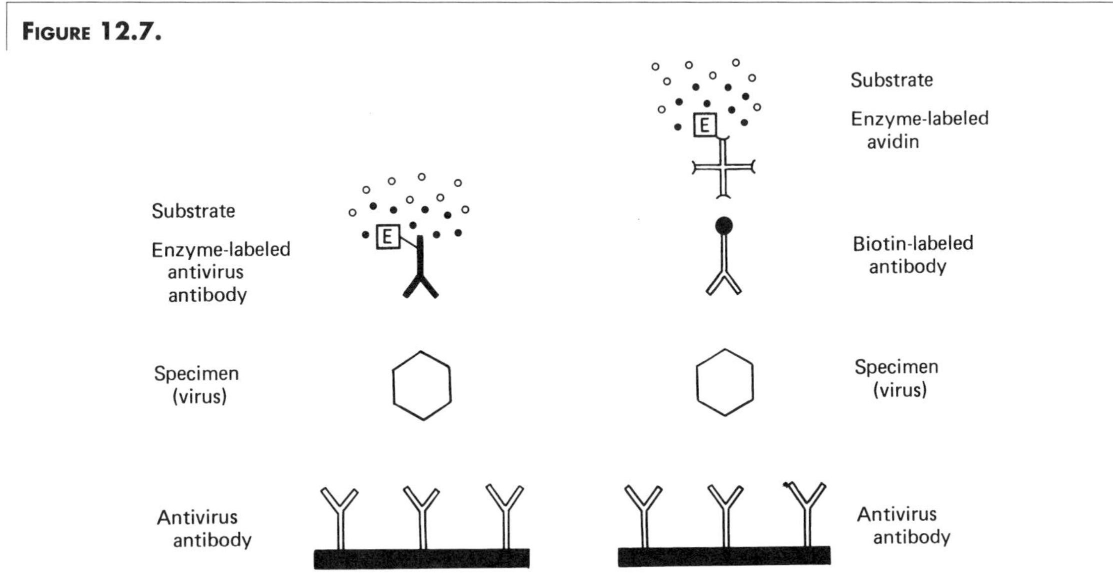

Enzyme immunoassay (EIA, also called enzyme-linked immunosorbent assay, ELISA) for the detection of virus and/or viral antigen. (Left) Direct method. (Right) Indirect method using biotinylated antibody, enzyme (e.g., peroxidase)-labeled avidin, and an enzyme substrate and chromogen for color reaction.

FIGURE 12.8.

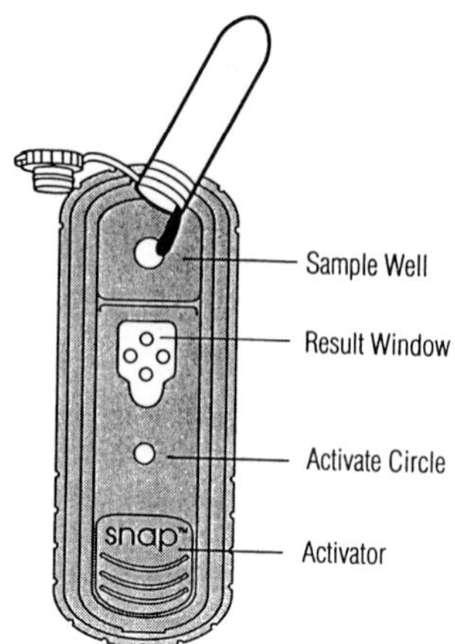

Interpreting Test Result

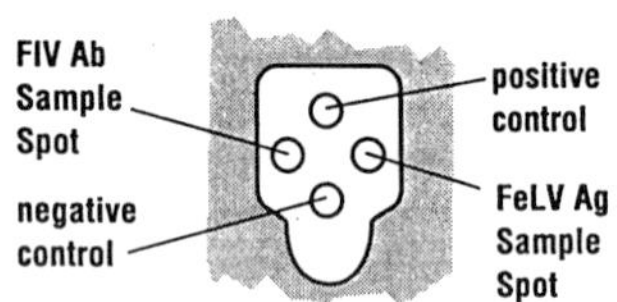

To determine test results, read the reaction spots in the Result Window. Color development in sample spots is proportional to the concentration of FeLV antigen or FIV antibody in the sample. If no color develops in the positive control spot, repeat the test.

Negative Result

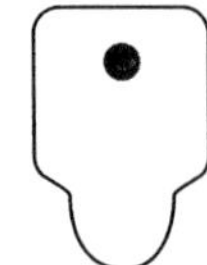

Only positive control spot develops color.

Positive Result

FeLV Antigen

1) 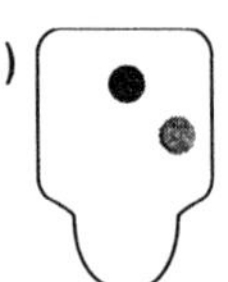

Positive control spot and FeLV Ag sample spot develop color.

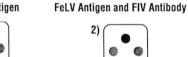

FeLV Antigen and FIV Antibody

2) 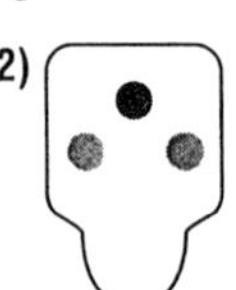

Positive control spot and both sample spots develop color.

FIV Antibody

3) 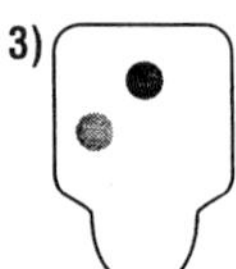

Positive control spot and FIV Ab sample spot develop color.

Reaction with Negative Control

The negative control spot serves as a safeguard against false positives.

1) 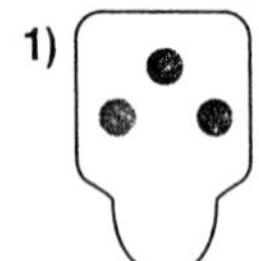

Positive Result
If color in the FIV Ab or FeLV Ag sample spot is darker than negative control spot, result is positive for that spot.

2) 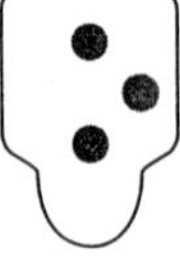

Invalid Result
If color in the negative control spot is equal to or darker than FIV Ab or FeLV Ag sample spot, the test is invalid for that sample spot.

Invalid Results

1. **Background**
   If the sample is allowed to flow past the activate circle, background color may result. Some background color is normal. However, if colored background obscures test result, repeat the test.
2. **No Color Development**
   If positive control does not develop color, repeat the test.

(A) Commercial enzyme immunoassay device for clinical use on a single animal. This kit is for the simultaneous detection of feline leukemia virus (FeLV) antigen and feline immunodeficiency virus (FIV) antibody in feline serum, plasma, or whole blood. The detection of FeLV group-specific

FIGURE 12.8. (continued)

B

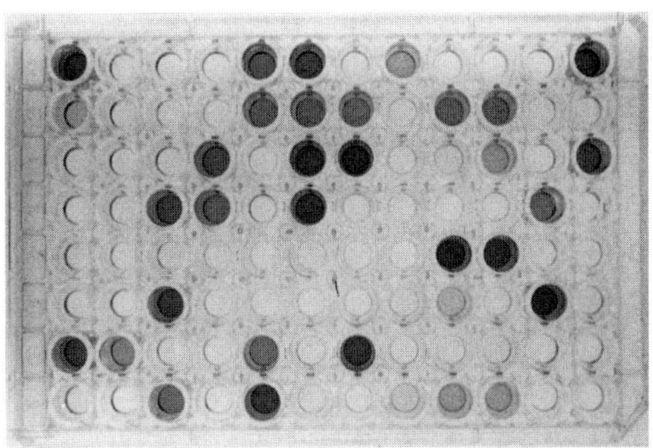

antigen (p27) is diagnostic of FeLV infection, and the detection of specific antibody to FIV is indicative of infection. The test utilizes a monoclonal antibody to FeLV p27, inactivated FIV antigen, and positive and negative controls. A conjugate mixture contains enzyme-conjugated antibody to p27 and enzyme-conjugated FIV antigen. Upon mixing the conjugate and the test sample, conjugated monoclonal antibody will bind p27 antigen (if present) and the conjugated FIV antigen will bind to FIV antibody (if present). The sample/conjugate mixture is then added to the "Snap" device and flows across the spotted matrix. The matrix-bound p27 antibody (FeLV spot) will capture the p27-conjugated antibody complex, whereas the matrix-bound FIV antigen (FIV spot) will capture the FIV antibody-conjugated antigen complex. The device is then activated (snapped), releasing wash, and substrate reagents stored within the device. Color development in the FeLV antigen sample spot indicates the presence of FeLV antigen, whereas color development in the FIV antibody sample spot indicates the presence of FIV antibody. (Courtesy of Idexx Laboratories, Inc.) (B) FIV antibody detection by enzyme immunoassay in a 96-well microtiter plate. The three wells in the first vertical row at the top left corner are controls—they represent a strong positive serum (first well), a medium positive serum (second well), and a negative serum (third well). The remaining 93 wells contain various feline serum samples. By visual inspection of this black and white rendition of the plate, a spectrum of positive reactions can be seen as varying shades of gray/black. The enzyme used actually produces a blue reaction product; the density of the blue color is measured spectrophotometrically and the results are printed out automatically. Cats whose serum produces an indeterminant result are retested some weeks later. In the example shown, the wells contain a single dilution of serum from individual cats; this is a qualitative test (the results are read as positive, negative, or indeterminant). For screening purposes, this is usually sufficient; it is inexpensive and can be fully automated. The test can be made quantitative by serially diluting the sera.

into contact with a test antibody (or antigen) already present in the membrane. All controls are included in the membrane as well and results are seen as colored spots or bands, as one of the test reagents is conjugated to colloidal gold or a chromogenic substance. Because all this is done in a plastic device, often with only one step required to activate the reaction, tests are quite simple to do and seemingly foolproof. Of course, the latter depends on the quality of the reagents and the conditions of the test. In any case, these tests are usually quite expensive.

Radioimmunoassay

Radioimmunoassay predates enzyme immunoassay but is progressively being superseded by it. The only significant difference is that the label is not an enzyme but a radioactive isotope such as ^{125}I and the bound antibody or antigen is measured in a gamma counter (Figure 12.9). It is a highly sensitive and reliable assay that lends itself well to automation, but the cost of the equipment and the health hazard of working with radioisotopes argue against its use in small laboratories.

Latex Particle Agglutination

Perhaps the simplest of all immunoassays is the agglutination by antigen of small latex beads previously coated with antiviral antibody. The test can be read by eye within a minute or so. Not surprisingly, diagnostic kits based on this method have become popular with small laboratories and with some veterinary practitioners. However, current tests suffer from low sensitivity and low specificity. Thus, false negatives occur unless large numbers of virions are present, therefore this assay for antigen tends to be restricted to examination of feces. False positives, however, occur quite commonly with fecal specimens. If these problems can be overcome, latex agglutination may develop a better reputation for reliability.

Immunodiffusion

In agar gel diffusion, also called immunodiffusion assays, a sample suspected to contain viral antigen is placed in a well cut in agar opposite a similar well containing antibody; the reactants diffuse toward each other and

FIGURE 12.9.

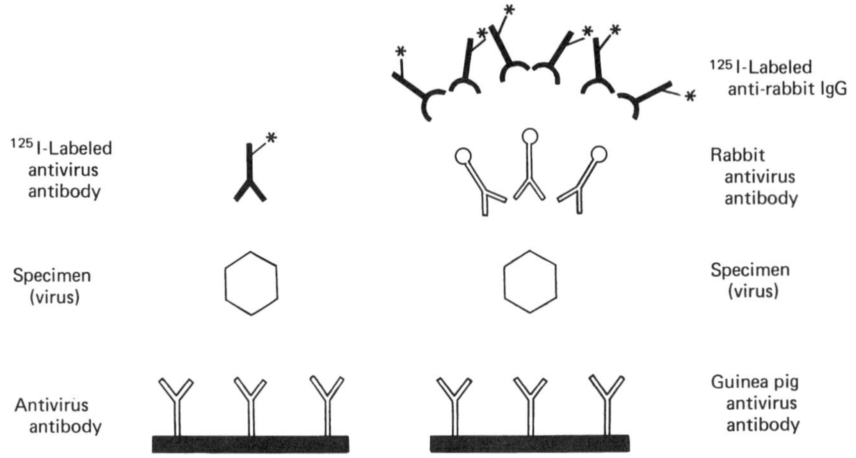

Radioimmunoassay for the detection of virus and/or viral antigen. (Left) Direct method. (Right) Indirect method.

form a visible line of precipitation if antigen is present. Such assays are seldom used, although a few examples where the antibody is the unknown are still used.

Direct Identification of Viral Nucleic Acids

The sensitivity and versatility of nucleic acid hybridization techniques have been expanded rapidly such that probing for the viral genome has overtaken probing for antigen as the diagnostic method of choice in many laboratories. More dramatic still has been the extraordinary adoption of PCR as an amplification step for enhancing the detection of viral nucleic acid in clinical specimens. It is now theoretically possible for a single laboratory with access to a complete panel of oligonucleotide primers to use the polymerase chain reaction to provide a comprehensive diagnostic service within 24 hours from specimen submission. However, the added sensitivity provided by amplification of viral nucleic acid can actually create new problems. Unlike the situation with bacterial pathogens, it has usually been the case that just detecting a pathogenic virus in a lesion, or from a clinically ill animal, has been enough evidence of its etiologic role. As detection methods have become increasingly sensitive, questions of viral "passengers" and noninfectious degraded viral genomes become more pertinent.

Nucleic acid detection methods are invaluable when dealing with (1) viruses that cannot be cultured satisfactorily, (2) specimens that contain predominantly inactivated virus, as a result of prolonged storage or transport, or (3) latent infections in which the viral genome lies dormant and infectious virus is absent.

For most routine diagnostic purposes it is often not necessary to "type" the virus of interest down to the level of strain, variant or local vs exotic variety. However, there are certain situations when important epidemiologic information can be obtained by viral nucleic acid characterization. There are several methods for deriving valuable information from the detection of viral nucleic acids.

Hybridization Methods

The detection of specific viral nucleic acid by hybridization using labeled viral DNA and RNA probes to detect nucleic acid has been widely used for rapid diagnosis, although the methods have been superseded in many instances by the polymerase chain reaction.

The principle of nucleic acid hybridization is that single-stranded DNA will hybridize by hydrogen-bonded base pairing to another single strand of DNA (or RNA) of complementary base sequence. Thus the two strands of the target DNA molecule are first separated by heating, then following cooling, allowed to hybridize with a labeled single-stranded DNA or RNA probe present in excess. The reaction can be accomplished in solution, which is useful for determining the kinetics of annealing or the stoichiometry of the reaction, from which can be calculated the percentage identity between the two sequences calculated from the kinetics of annealing. The conditions set for annealing, especially temperature and ionic strength, determine the degree of discrimination (stringency) of the test. Under conditions of low stringency, a number of mismatched base pairs are tolerated, whereas at high stringency such a heteroduplex is unstable.

The other major factor determining the specificity of the test is, of course, the nature of the probe itself. This may correspond in length to the whole viral genome or a single gene or a much shorter nucleotide sequence deliberately chosen to represent either a variable or a conserved region of the genome, depending on whether it is intended that the probe be type specific or more versatile. The oligonucleotide sequence intended as a probe is produced by chemical synthesis or by cloning in a bacterial plasmid or bacteriophage.

Traditionally, radioactive isotopes such as ^{32}P and ^{35}S were used to label nucleic acids or oligonucleotides intended as probes for hybridization tests, with the signal being read by counting in a spectrometer or by autoradiography. The trend is now toward nonradioactive labels. Some of these (e.g., fluorescein or peroxidase) produce a signal directly, whereas others (e.g., biotin or digoxigenin) act indirectly by binding to another labeled compound, which then emits the signal. Biotinylated probes can be combined with various types of readout, e.g., an avidin-based enzyme immunoassay. Chemiluminescent substrates, such as luminol, are also being widely exploited. Indeed, we are witnessing a proliferation of diagnostic kits for various diseases, many of them based on novel labels and/or methods of readout.

Dot Blot (Filter Hybridization) Methods

The most popular hybridization methods are two-phase systems, generically known as filter hybridization. In its simplest format, dot (blot) hybridization, DNA or RNA extracted from virus or infected cells, is denatured and then spotted directly onto a charged nylon or nitrocellulose membrane to which it binds tightly on baking. The single-stranded DNA or RNA probe is then hybridized to the target nucleic acid *in situ* on the membrane, and unbound probe is washed away. The signal generated by the bound probe is measured by autoradiography if the probe is radioactive or by the formation of a colored precipitate if an enzyme-labeled probe is used. By choosing RNA as a probe, sensitivity can be improved and the incidence of false positives reduced by treating the filters with RNase before counting.

In Situ Hybridization Methods

In situ hybridization has been widely used by pathologists to screen animals with persistent infections or viral-induced cancers for evidence of integrated or nonintegrated copies of the viral genome. Frozen sections on slides are probed, much as described earlier, and the intracellular location of viral nucleic acid sequences is revealed by autoradiography or immunoperoxidase cytochemistry.

Southern Blot Hybridization Methods

The introduction of Southern blotting (Figure 12.10) has been of great significance and wide application. Restriction endonucleases are used to cleave the DNA into fragments of various size and number, depending on the

Figure 12.10.

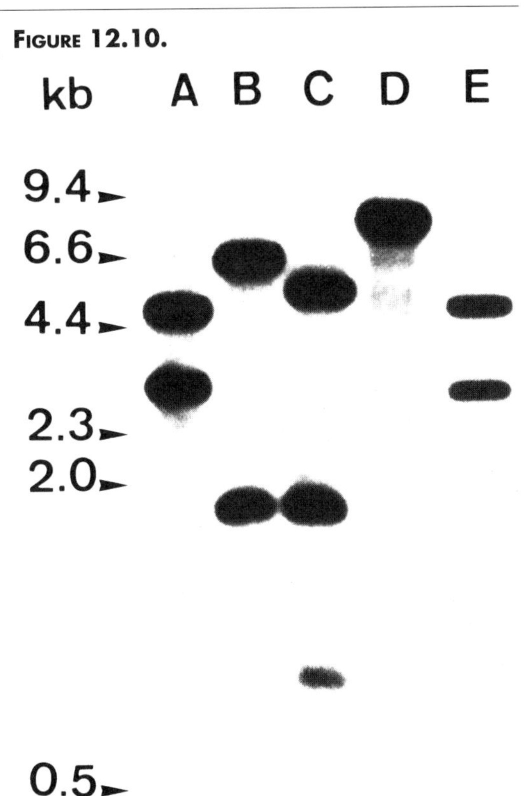

Southern blot hybridization of DNA extracted from a wart-like skin lesion. The DNA was first digested with restriction enzymes *Bgl* II (lane A), *Eco*RI (lane B), *Pst*I (lane C), *Pvu*II (lane D), and *Bam*HI (lane E). The fragments were then separated on the basis of size by agarose gel electrophoresis. After transfer to a nylon membrane, the blot was hybridized at high stringency to a probe consisting of ^{32}P-labeled type-specific papillomavirus DNA, washed, and used to expose X-ray film. The pattern of restriction fragments is used to identify the virus. The genome of papillomaviruses is normally found in cells as a circular plasmid of about 8 kbp, but it is easier to estimate DNA size by gel electrophoresis when it is linear (i.e., after digestion of the plasmid with restriction enzymes). In lane D (*Pvu*II digest), the plasmid is cut only once (to produce the full-length linear form), whereas the other enzymes cut two or more times. (Courtesy of H. E. Trowell and M. L. Dyall-Smith.)

location and number of restriction sites. The fragments are then separated by electrophoresis on an agarose or polyacrylamide gel. After staining with ethidium bromide to reveal the position of the fragments, the gel is treated successively with acidic and basic solutions to depurinate and denature the DNA, which is then transferred by electrophoresis, diffusion, or other means ("blotting") onto a nylon or nitrocellulose membrane. Individual bands (fragments) are revealed by hybridization of a labeled DNA or RNA probe followed by autoradiography or a color development process. Northern blotting for the detection of RNA follows similar principles.

FIGURE 12.11.

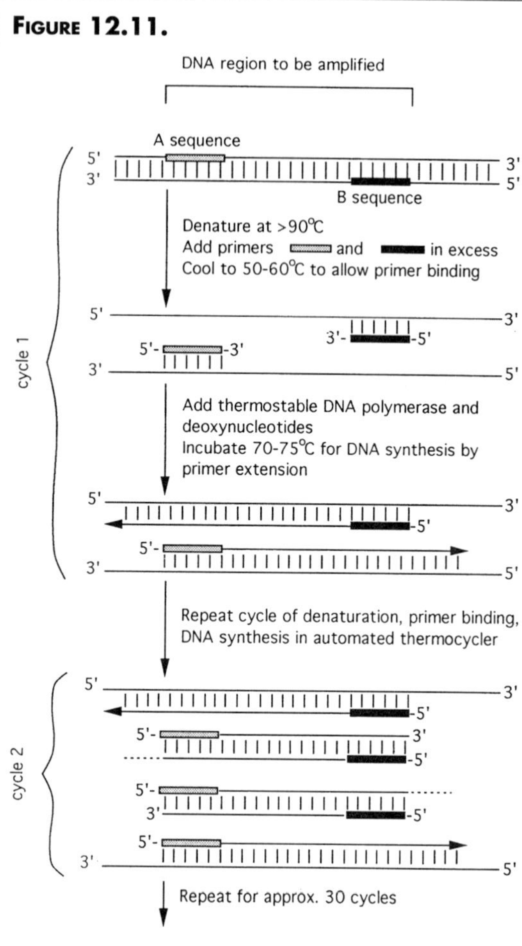

Amplification of part of a DNA sequence by the polymerase chain reaction. Oligonucleotide primers must first be made according to the sequences at either end of the portion of DNA to be amplified. After the DNA has been denatured by heating, the primers can hybridize to the complementary sequences on the opposite strand. In the presence of heat-resistant DNA polymerase and deoxynucleotide triphosphates, two new copies of the desired region are produced. The cycles of melting, annealing, and extension are repeated rapidly; each time, the amount of target DNA sequence doubles. After the first few cycles, virtually all the templates consist of just the short region chosen for amplification. After 30 cycles, taking about 3 hours, this region bounded by the chosen primers has been amplified many millionfold. (Courtesy of I. H. Holmes and R. Strugnell.)

Polymerase Chain Reaction

In 1983 Kary Mullis envisioned a method for the *in vitro* amplification of DNA, which became known as the polymerase chain reaction, and for which Mullis received the Nobel prize. As for other major advances in molecular biology, the polymerase chain reaction has been applied in many areas, including genetics, evolutionary biology, forensic medicine, parentage determination, and the diagnosis of infectious diseases. In 1997 over 20,000 entries in the Current Contents reference database were obtained from a search for the keyword "PCR." The immense potential of the polymerase chain reaction to specifically amplify minimal amounts of target DNA was particularly appealing for the diagnosis of viral diseases. It is said that "the polymerase chain reaction detects a needle in a haystack and makes a haystack out of the needle." It must not be forgotten that polymerase chain reaction technology amplifies the target gene sequence, in itself it is not a diagnostic test; specific detection of the amplified product is by one of the techniques described later.

Principles of the Polymerase Chain Reaction

The polymerase chain reaction is an *in vitro* method for the enzymatic synthesis of specific DNA sequences using two oligonucleotide primers, usually of about 20 residues (20-mers), that hybridize to opposite strands and flank the region of interest in the target DNA; the primer pairs are sometimes referred to as forward and reverse primers (Figure 12.11). Computer programs are used for the design of optimum primer sets and to predict the parameters (time/temperature) for the reactions. Depending on the degree of conservation of the putative target sequence, primers may be chosen to be strain, genus, or family specific. Where there are either knowingly or unknowingly mismatched bases between the primer and target sequences, the primers are said to be degenerate. Reactions are carried out under carefully controlled conditions of ionic strength, temperature, primer concentration, and nucleotide concentration. Reaction mixtures include the template (clinical specimen), the primers, polymerase, and single nucleotides. In a programmable instrument known as a thermocycler, repetitive cycles involving template denaturation by heating, primer annealing, and extension of the annealed primers by DNA polymerase at a lower temperature result in the exponential accumulation of a specific DNA fragment whose termini are defined by the 5′ ends of the primers. The primer extension products synthesized in one cycle serve as templates in the next, hence the number of target DNA copies approximately doubles every cycle; 20 cycles yields about a millionfold amplification.

The specificity of the reaction is *de facto* indicated by obtaining a reaction product of the expected size; base pair size markers are always included in the gels used to visualize the amplified products. The identity of the reaction products may be confirmed more specifically as target virus by restriction enzyme digestion, Southern blotting and use of a specific probe, or direct sequencing of the fragment (Figure 12.12).

Modifications of Original Polymerase Chain Reaction

Originally, the polymerase chain reaction used the Klenow fragment of *Escherichia coli* DNA polymerase I for primer extension, which was inactivated in the denaturation step and therefore had to be replenished in each cycle. The introduction of a thermostable polymerase derived from the thermophilic bacterium *Thermus aquaticus* termed *Taq* polymerase improved and simplified polymerase chain reaction assays considerably. It also increased the specificity of the reaction because the annealed primers could be extended at considerably higher temperatures, which reduced secondary structure formation.

Among other modifications most relevant to viral diagnosis are nested polymerase chain reaction methods, multiplex polymerase chain reaction methods, reverse transcriptase polymerase chain reaction methods for the detection of RNA viruses, quantitative polymerase chain reaction methods, and improved methods for the visualization of amplified products by colorimetric reactions.

Nested polymerase chain reaction methods. This method uses two sets of primers in two sequential amplification reactions. The first primer pair amplifies through 20 or so cycles, a DNA fragment which is then used as template in the second reaction. The primers for the second round of amplification are either both different from the first set, i.e., both are located within the first amplified DNA region (nested PCR), or one is the same and one, located within the amplified region, is different (seminested PCR). Nested amplification is highly sensitive. The second set of primers serves to verify the specificity of the first round product, and the transfer of the first round product into a new reaction mixture has the useful effect of diluting possible inhibitors that may be present in the original sample. However, nested polymerase chain reaction increases the risk of template contaminations.

Multiplex polymerase chain reaction methods. In this method, two or more primer pairs specific for different target sequences are included in the same amplification reaction. Coamplification of several targets is more cost effective where multiple pathogens are possible etiologic agents. Coamplification of internal controls may also be included in multiplex reactions.

Reverse transcriptase polymerase chain reaction methods. The development of reverse transcriptase polymerase chain reaction (RT-PCR) methods to assist in the detection of RNA viruses has been a major advance in viral diagnostics and research. The RNA template is first transcribed into cDNA using reverse transcriptase originally derived from retroviruses. The virus-derived

FIGURE 12.12.

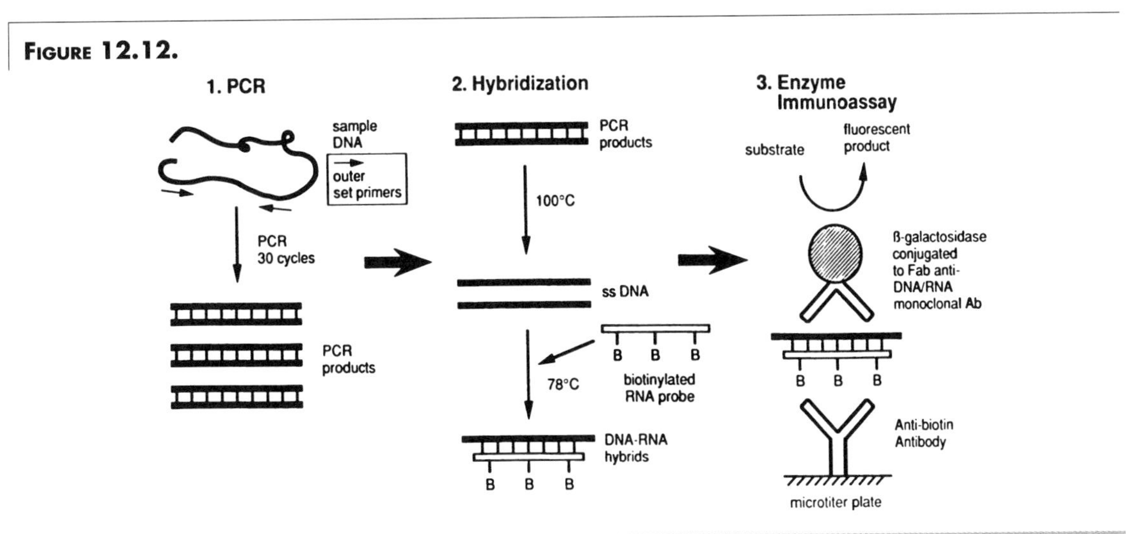

Detection of polymerase chain reaction products using a biotinylated RNA probe and an enzyme immunoassay readout based on capture of labeled DNA–RNA hybrid molecules by antibiotin antibody. (Courtesy of R. H. Yolken.)

enzymes cannot tolerate temperatures above 42°C, which is a nonstringent hybridization temperature for most primers. Furthermore, at low temperatures, single-stranded RNA templates tend to form stable secondary structures. The combination of low stringency of template binding and secondary structure reduced the efficiency of cDNA synthesis. The introduction of a recombinant DNA polymerase derived from the thermophilic bacterium *T. thermophilus* that also had efficient reverse transcriptase activity allowed reactions to be performed at 70°C. This allowed high stringency of primer–template binding and the elimination or marked reduction of secondary structure formation and thus improved specificity and sensitivity.

Quantitative polymerase chain reaction methods. To quantify the amount of template DNA or RNA in clinical samples, quantitative polymerase chain reaction assays have been developed. One approach uses a competitive template that is amplified by the same primer set and can be discriminated (e.g., by size difference) from the target sequence. A known quantity of the competitive template is mixed with the sample. When the amounts of target sequence and competitor template are equivalent, equal amounts of the respective polymerase chain reaction products are produced. The amount of target sequence present in the sample is determined by interpolation of the equivalence point of both products.

Methods for Detection of Amplified Products

The products of polymerase chain reaction amplification are usually detected by agarose gel electrophoresis analysis and ethidium bromide staining. To circumvent this time-consuming step, colorimetric and chemiluminescence methods have been developed. Although the approaches to visualize DNA products are diverse, most are based on enzyme-linked assays. Some procedures use biotinylated or digoxigeninated primers to label the polymerase chain reaction products, whereas others detect the unlabeled amplified DNA by anti-DNA monoclonal antibodies or biotinylated and fluoresceinated DNA probes. The enzyme-linked oligonucleotide sorbent assay (ELOSA) for the detection of bluetongue virus, for example, relies on annealing of separate biotinylated and fluoresceinated probes to the amplified viral nucleic acid; these complexes are captured on streptavidin-coated microtitration wells and detected using a horseradish peroxidase-labeled antifluorescein antibody conjugate.

Advantages and Limitations of the Polymerase Chain Reaction

There are few limits to the use of the polymerase chain reaction in assisting the diagnosis of virus diseases of veterinary importance as long as some viral sequence is available. The polymerase chain reaction is the method of choice to detect viral template directly in clinical specimens. However, molecular diagnostic procedures employing the polymerase chain reaction are unnecessary if the diagnostic procedures currently in use are cost effective, rapid, sensitive, reliable, and meet national and/or international legislative requirements.

The polymerase chain reaction is useful in the diagnosis of virus infections where viral antigens or virus-specific antibodies cannot be detected and where the presence of viral nucleic acid may be the only evidence of infection. This is particularly true for latent virus infections, including herpesvirus, retrovirus, or papillomavirus infections. The polymerase chain reaction is most useful for the detection of viruses such as certain enteric adenoviruses, papillomaviruses, astroviruses, or rotaviruses that are either noncultivable or difficult to cultivate and for viruses that grow without a visible cytopathic effect such as respiratory syncytial virus, bovine viral diarrhea virus, coronaviruses, or certain gammaherpesviruses. For the study of viruses that cause zoonotic infections, including rabies virus, poxviruses, or influenza viruses, the polymerase chain reaction may be the preferred method to minimize the risk of exposure for laboratory personnel.

The polymerase chain reaction may be superior to conventional virus detection methods in the differentiation of vaccine virus from wild-type virus. The use of attenuated virus vaccines that have nucleotide deletions in so-called marker genes has gained considerable importance in veterinary medicine (e.g., in the vaccination of pigs against pseudorabies). Detection of marker genes is important for herd health, regulatory, eradication, and forensic purposes and for studies of latency and epidemiology. Although deletions in marker genes can be monitored serologically, the detection of virus and differentiation by the polymerase chain reaction is a fast and sensitive alternative.

The immense potential is also considered the greatest hazard of the polymerase chain reaction. As for any procedure, inconclusive or indeterminate results are obtained with the polymerase chain reaction. It is argued that the risk of cross-contamination between specimens may outweigh the advantage. This is particularly the case for polymerase chain reaction assays based on nested amplification, which can detect as little as a single copy of viral nucleic acid. Strict precautions to avoid cross-contamination between specimens and adequate quality controls must be adopted as for any other technique used in diagnostic clinical virology.

Current procedures are labor intensive and expensive, which limits their use to large laboratories or research-oriented diagnostic laboratories at universities.

The ability to automate polymerase chain reaction procedures is therefore considered a key factor in determining how large a role the polymerase chain reaction will play in the future. For some viruses, commercially available polymerase chain reaction kits have been introduced. Particular kits are designed for clusters of pathogens that may be involved in say respiratory, enteric, or genital infections and could be developed for exotic viral disease clusters of a particular species such as vesicular disease of ruminants and pigs. These multiplex polymerase chain reaction kits are designed for amplification in conventional thermocyclers with colorimetric detection of the biotinylated polymerase chain reaction products. Second generation kits for use in automated workstations are being tested and appear to be extremely accurate, sensitive, fast, and versatile. Real time computerized analysis of polymerase chain reaction results allows for sequential testing and/or simultaneous detection of different pathogens in the same specimen. Minimization of cross-contaminations between samples is considered a major advantage of the automated polymerase chain reaction system.

There has been an extraordinary large number of what may be considered initial reports of the use of the polymerase chain reaction for viral diagnosis. Development of diagnostic polymerase chain reaction to a stage where it will become even more widely adopted and for many viruses the procedure of first choice, will require time, knowledge, money, and rigorous validation.

Gene Amplification by Isothermal Amplification

Isothermal amplification is a technique that does not require the temperature cycling and accompanying equipment used in the polymerase chain reaction. Three enzymes involved in the replication of retroviruses are simply mixed with either a DNA or a RNA template and DNA primers at a constant temperature and millionfold amplification is achieved rapidly.

Viral Genomic Sequencing

Direct viral genomic sequencing has become a major factor in viral diagnostics, particularly in protocols based on viral nucleic acid amplification via the polymerase chain reaction. Sequencing methods in viral diagnostics are the same as in the rest of the world of molecular biology; in the diagnostic setting, where large numbers of specimens are of interest and where diagnostically unique sequences must, for practical reasons, be detected quickly, critical primers for the polymerase chain reaction, automated sequencers, and computer analysis of partial sequence information is the key to overall value.

Today, all human polioviruses of interest are subjected to partial sequencing immediately upon isolation—epidemiologically important information stemming from such sequencing includes identification of wild vs vaccine strains, local or imported strains, and, in the latter case, often the geographic source of the virus. The same is being done with dengue and measles virus isolates. In veterinary medicine, partial sequencing is being used to detect further mutations in canine parvovirus that might predict the need for another reformulation of the vaccine.

Two noncultivable putative herpesviruses, ovine herpesvirus 2, the cause of sheep-associated bovine malignant catarrhal fever, and the herpesvirus associated with Kaposi sarcoma in humans, were discovered by methods that were based on strategies that required large amounts of sequencing. The ovine herpesvirus was detected by use of the polymerase chain reaction and progressive sequencing of amplified products. Human herpesvirus 8 was discovered by representational difference analysis (RDA), a very complex method based on amplifying differences in DNA sequences in tissue specimens of interest and control specimens thought not to contain the putative virus. This method employs the polymerase chain reaction (or reverse transcriptase polymerase chain reaction), cloning, subtractive hybridization, sequencing, and computer technology to eliminate unique nonviral DNA sequences.

Oligonucleotide Fingerprinting and Restriction Endonuclease Mapping

For most routine diagnostic purposes it is usually not necessary to "type" the isolate. Sometimes, however, important epidemiologic information can be obtained by going even further, to identify differences between subtypes within a given type. This may be accomplished using the polymerase chain reaction and partial sequencing, oligonucleotide fingerprinting of viral RNA, or the determination of restriction endonuclease fragment patterns (fingerprints) of viral DNA. For example, in 1981 the origin and spread of foot-and-mouth disease virus in an epidemic that spread between countries in Europe were accomplished by the use of oligonucleotide fingerprinting of viral RNA obtained from isolates from key sites.

Viral DNA prepared from virions or infected cells can be cut with appropriately chosen restriction endonucleases and the fragments separated by agarose gel electrophoresis. When stained with ethidium bromide or silver, restriction endonuclease fingerprints are obtained. The method has found application in all DNA virus families, particularly in epidemiologic studies. Depending on the viral family, the resolution of these methods is such that different isolates of the same virus are distinguishable. Minor degrees of genetic drift, often not reflected in serologic differences, can sometimes be detected in this way.

Virus Isolation in Cultured Cells

Despite the explosion of new techniques for "same-day diagnosis" of viral disease by demonstration of virus, viral antigen, or viral nucleic acid in specimens taken directly from the animal, it is still true to say that few of them achieve quite the sensitivity of virus isolation in cell culture. Theoretically at least, a single viable virion present in a specimen can be grown in cultured cells, thus expanding it many millionfold to produce enough material to be characterized antigenically. Virus isolation remains the "gold standard" against which newer methods must be compared. There is an excitement in isolating viruses. Moreover, it is the only technique that can detect the unexpected, i.e., identify a totally unforeseen virus, or even discover an entirely new agent. Accordingly, even those laboratories well equipped for rapid diagnosis sometimes also inoculate cell cultures in an attempt to isolate the virus. Culture is the only method of producing a supply of live virus for further examination, such as antigenic variation. Research and reference laboratories, in particular, are always on the lookout for new viruses within the context of emerging diseases; such viruses require comprehensive characterization. Moreover, large quantities of virus must be grown up in cultured cells to produce diagnostic antigens and monoclonal antibodies for distribution to other laboratories. Vaccine development is currently dependent, in nearly all cases, on the availability of viruses grown in culture, even though the production of the vaccine may not be dependent on culturing because of recombinant DNA technology, as discussed in Chapter 13.

Cell Culture Methods

The choice of the optimal cell culture for the primary isolation of a virus of unknown nature from clinical specimens is largely empirical. Primary cells derived from fetal tissues of the same species usually provide the most sensitive cell culture substrates for virus isolation. Continuous cell lines derived from the homologous species are, in most cases, almost as good. Often the nature of the disease from which the material was obtained will suggest what virus may be found, and in such cases the optimum cell culture for that virus can be chosen, often in parallel with a second type of culture with a wide spectrum. Cell lines offer some advantages and are available for most domestic mammals.

Special types of cell and organ culture are utilized for particular viruses. For example, betaherpesviruses and gammaherpesviruses may be recovered from monolayer cultures propagated directly from tissues taken from the diseased animal, whereas inoculation of established monolayer cell cultures with cell-free material may be negative. For some coronaviruses and rhinoviruses that do not grow well in monolayer cultures, growth may occur in explant cultures (e.g., small cubes of tissue with intact epithelium taken from the trachea or gut). Cocultivation of explant tissues with cell monolayers can be used to enhance the isolation of viruses associated with latency (e.g., herpesviruses from the trigeminal nerve ganglia). Arthropod cell cultures are used frequently as a parallel system for isolating arboviruses.

Inoculation and Maintenance of Cell Cultures

Monolayer cultures for viral diagnostic purposes are generally grown in screw-capped plastic flasks. Multiwell plates are very convenient for serum neutralization tests, where large numbers of cultures are required and economy of medium, equipment, and space is important, but the risk of cross-contamination argues against them for virus isolation. The inoculated cultures are usually incubated at 37°C, even though the normal body temperature of various domestic animal species varies somewhat above and below 37°C. In the case of viruses of the upper respiratory tract such as influenza viruses, rhinoviruses, and coronaviruses (which grow best at 33°C, the temperature encountered in the nasal mucosa), incubators may be set at 33°C. Cultures are usually inspected daily for the development of cytopathic effects.

Recognition of Viral Growth in Cell Cultures

Although rapidly growing viruses such as most picornaviruses or most alphaherpesviruses can be relied upon to produce detectable cytopathic effect within a day or two, other viruses such as some beta- and gammaherpesviruses are notoriously slow and may not produce an obvious cytopathic effect for 1–4 weeks or not at all on first passage. By this time, the uninoculated control cultures will usually start to show nonspecific degeneration, which may resemble a cytopathic effect. In such cases the cells and supernatant fluid, usually after freezing and thawing several times, from the infected culture are inoculated into fresh monolayers (blind passage), after which the cytopathic effect usually appears.

When changes indicative of viral replication become evident, a number of courses are open. The cytopathic effect is often sufficiently characteristic, even in the living unstained culture viewed *in situ* (see Chapter 5), for a provisional diagnosis to be made. Some viruses that are relatively noncytopathic for cultured cells may be recognized by means of hemadsorption. Most viruses that hemagglutinate will be amenable to test by hemadsorption; the growth of paramyxoviruses, for example, is routinely recognized in this way. Alternatively, it is usually instructive to fix and stain the infected monolayer that has been grown on coverslips or in special cell culture slide chambers to more closely examine the cells showing a cytopathic effect. Inclusion bodies, multinucleate giant cells (syncytia), and other findings can be identified after staining with hematoxylin and eosin; if present, these changes are usually sufficiently characteristic to enable the isolate to at least be assigned to a family. Such cultures can also be stained with fluorescent antibody for positive identification. It is usually most advantageous to submit some of the cell culture-grown virus for negative stain electron microscopic examination.

One of the key goals in a busy diagnostic laboratory is to reach a point at which sufficient information has been obtained to confirm the diagnosis. An isolate can be characterized further if necessary; the decision as to which tests to do is the mark of a knowledgeable and skillful laboratory diagnostician; there is art as well as science in diagnostic virology!

Identification of Viral Isolates: Antigenic Characterization

A newly isolated virus can usually be allocated provisionally to a particular family, and sometimes to a genus or species, on the basis of the clinical findings, the particular type of cell culture yielding the isolate, and the visible result of viral growth (cytopathic effect, hemadsorption, inclusion body formation, etc.). Definitive identification, however, rests on antigenic characterization. By using the new isolate as antigen against a panel of antisera, for example, in an enzyme immunoassay, the virus can first be placed into its correct family or genus (e.g., *Adenoviridae*). If it is considered important to do so, one can then go on to identify the species (e.g., canine hepatitis virus) or serotype by moving to monoclonal antibodies or to one of the more discriminating serologic procedures, such as neutralization or hemagglutination inhibition. This sequential approach is applicable only to families that share a common family antigen. The choice of available immunologic techniques is very wide. Some are best suited to particular families of viruses. Each laboratory makes its own choice of favored procedures based on considerations of sensitivity, specificity, reproducibility, speed, convenience, and cost. For virus diseases important in national or international commerce, it is usual that the identification conform to a defined panel of tests for a particular virus.

One of the simplest ways of identifying a newly isolated virus is by fluorescent antibody staining of the infected cell monolayer itself. This can provide a definitive answer within an hour or so of recognizing the earliest indication of a cytopathic effect. Immunofluorescence is best suited to the identification of viruses with no close relatives or in epidemic situations when a particular virus is suspected; otherwise replicate cultures must be screened with a range of antisera.

Most other immunologic approaches are applied to the identification of virions and soluble antigen present in the cell culture supernatant. Enzyme immunoassays are now probably the most commonly used, although virus neutralization remains the gold standard for defining and distinguishing serotypes (Figure 12.13). Monoclonal antibodies with defined specificity have become the standard for identifying many viruses. These make it possible to proceed quickly to very specific diagnosis, even to the level of subtypes, strains, or variants (e.g., rabies viruses from different geographic areas). Family-, genus-, and type-specific monoclonal antibodies are also available in some instances (e.g., influenza virus antibodies). As they become available commercially, we can expect monoclonal antibodies to be more widely used.

Identification of Viral Isolates: Hemadsorption and Hemagglutination

Cells infected with member viruses of several families bind red blood cells on their plasma membranes at the sites of virion budding—this is called hemadsorption. It may be used to determine specific viruses via a hemadsorption–inhibition assay in which antibodies of known specificities are used. Hemagglutination–inhibition assays are somewhat similar: many viruses bind to red blood cells of various species of mammals and birds, forming bridges between cells and agglutination of large clumps of cells. When specific antibody and virus are mixed prior to the addition of red blood cells, hemagglutination is inhibited—therefore, the specificity of the antibody used serves to identify the virus isolated in cell culture. The hemagglutination–inhibition reaction is highly sensitive and specific. Moreover, it is simple, inexpensive, and rapid and has been historically the serologic procedure of choice for identifying isolates of hemagglutinating viruses.

Figure 12.13.

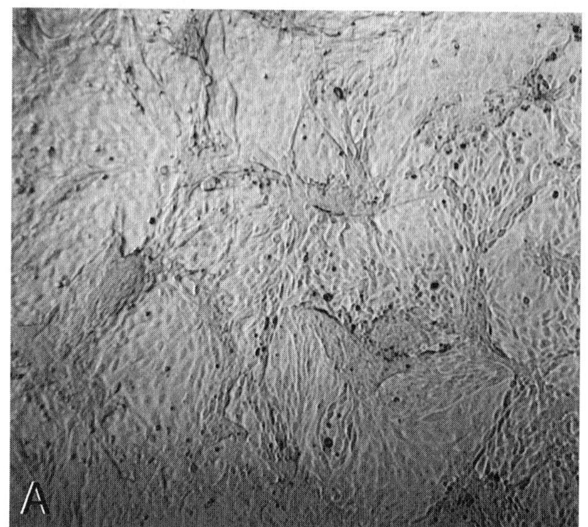

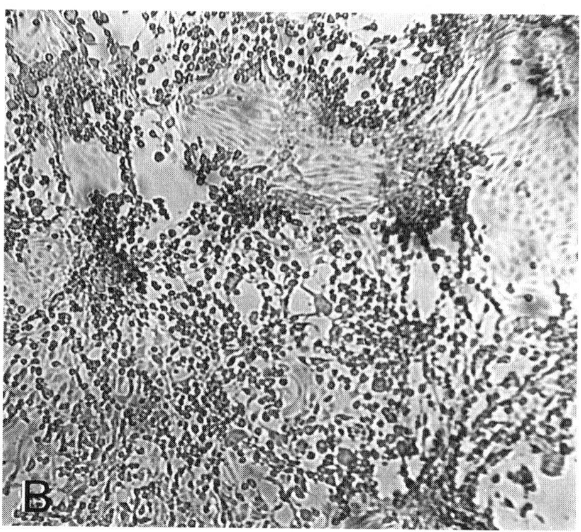

Virus neutralization. A pig developed encephalitis during an epidemic of porcine enterovirus 1 infection. An enterovirus was isolated from the feces. One hundred tissue culture infectious doses ($TCID_{50}$) of this virus were incubated at 37°C for 60 minutes with a suitable dilution of "inactivated" (56°C, 30 minutes) porcine enterovirus 1 antiserum (a reference serum raised in a rabbit). (A) Mixtures were inoculated onto monolayers of swine kidney cells in wells of a microculture tray. (B) Virus was similarly incubated with normal rabbit serum and inoculated onto identical cells. The cultures were incubated at 37°C for several days and inspected daily for cytopathic effect. The infectivity of the virus isolate has been neutralized by this antiserum, thereby identifying the isolate as porcine enterovirus 1; the control culture (B) shows the typical cytopathic effect caused by this virus. Unstained. Magnification: ×25. (Courtesy of I. Jack.)

Virus Isolation in Animals and Chick Embryos

Many viruses will grow satisfactorily in chick embryos or newborn mice but neither is now commonly used because cell culture is generally the simpler option. Mice can be used to isolate arboviruses and rabies virus; suckling mice less than 24 hours old are injected intracerebrally and/or intraperitoneally, then observed for up to 2 weeks for the development of pathognomonic signs before euthanizing them for examination by various means such as histopathology, immunofluorescence, immunohistochemistry, or serology.

Where all other methods have failed, it is also an option in veterinary medicine to use the putative natural host animal to "isolate" viruses. Natural host animals are also used for other purposes such as pathogenesis and immunity research.

Embryonated hens' eggs are used for the isolation of influenza A viruses and for many avian viruses. Indeed, there are several important pathogens that replicate much better in eggs than in cell cultures derived from chick embryo tissues. According to the virus of interest, the diagnostic specimen is inoculated in the amniotic cavity, the allantoic cavity, the yolk sac, or on the chorioallantoic membrane. Evidences of viral growth may be seen on the chorioallantoic membrane (e.g., characteristic pocks caused by poxviruses) but otherwise other means are used to detect virus growth (e.g., hemagglutination, immunofluorescence).

Virus Quantitation

Many viral identification procedures cannot be performed until the quantity or "dose" of the virus has been determined. Quantitation is accomplished by preparing serial, 10-fold dilutions of the virus-infected material; an aliquot from each dilution serves as inoculum for susceptible hosts (a cell culture is also a "host" in this context). Ideally, replicate numbers of hosts are inoculated with each virus dilution. Most commonly five or six replicates for each dilution are used. This approach, although best scientifically, is impractical in clinical virology; the cost of large numbers of animals or cell cultures is too high. Most laboratories utilize modified titration methods to gauge the viral dose within acceptable accuracy limits.

Most virus titration procedures are quantal rather than truly quantitative in that results do not really indicate the number of infectious virions in the specimen, but instead provide an approximation. Estimation of viral dose by quantal techniques is satisfactory for most purposes. These assays provide a result defined in terms of the highest virus dilution in which the virus affects 50% of the hosts. When the titration is done in animals (e.g., mice) or embryonated eggs and the end point is death, the unit is expressed as the 50% lethal dose (LD_{50}). When the end point measured is some parameter other than death (e.g., paralysis, presence of skin lesions) the unit is expressed as the 50% infective dose (ID_{50}). When the titration is done in replicate cell cultures (tube cultures, microtiter well cultures, etc.) and the end point is cytopathology, the presence of inclusion bodies, antigen, immunofluorescent antigen, and so on, the unit is expressed as the 50% tissue culture infective doses ($TCID_{50}$). In all of these kinds of quantal assays, raw end point data are analyzed by standard statistical methods, with the result being the best approximation of the dilution of the specimen that has enough virus in it to affect 50% of the mice, eggs, or cell cultures inoculated. Two statistical methods have been used in virology laboratories for many years: the Reed-Muench method and the Kärber method—they are described in any diagnostic laboratory methods manual. When a virus present in a clinical specimen has been quantitated in these ways, the results are expressed as a $\log_{10}$ value: for example, "$10^{7.95}$ TCID/ml," which is to say that there are 89,125,093 infectious units of virus in 1 ml of the original undiluted specimen (an unrealistic degree of precision, of course).

Plaque Assays

The most common methods of virus quantitation, representing adaptations of the previously described methods, are plaque assays. Plaque assays, first described by Renato Dulbecco in 1952, involve adsorption of 10-fold serial dilutions of the virus-containing specimen onto monolayer cell cultures. The monolayers are overlaid with agar containing nutrient medium, which prevents free virus spread throughout the culture but allows cell-to-cell spread. A circular plaque of infected cells is formed around each infectious unit. The cultures are stained with a vital dye, and plaques are counted to determine the titration end point. The unit is expressed as plaque-forming units (PFU) per unit volume of specimen. Again, statistical methods are used to convert raw plaque counts into precise units. Plaque assays are the standard for quantitating many viruses, e.g., many animal herpesviruses, togaviruses, picornaviruses, and vesiculoviruses.

Other Methods for Virus Quantitation

Physical methods for virus quantitation include counting virus particles by electron microscopy, a method that is quite complex and not often used, and many innovative methods based on molecular biologic technologies. For example, the quantitative polymerase chain reaction is used in human medicine to quantitate HIV virus load in patients as the basis for prescribing various antiviral drug regimens. Quantitative enzyme immunoassays and various other immunologic procedures in which titration end point determinations are based on measuring the presence of viral antigens in each dilution are also widely used, partly because they lend themselves to automated dilution, addition of reagents, and colorimetric readout. Statistical methods are used to convert raw readout data into precise units, indicating the number of infectious units per unit volume of the original clinical specimen.

Interpretation of Virologic Laboratory Findings

The isolation, identification, and quantitation of a particular virus from an animal with a given disease is not necessarily meaningful in itself. The name *diagnostic laboratory* is in fact a misnomer; the laboratory provides data upon which the submitting veterinarian can base his/her diagnosis within the context of the clinical history. The laboratory does not provide a definitive diagnosis. For example, concurrent subclinical infection with a virus unrelated to the causative agent of the disease in question is not uncommon. Koch's postulates or Evans' criteria for disease causation (see Chapter 2) are as relevant here as in any other microbiological context, but are not always easy to fulfill. When attempting to interpret the significance of the detection of a virus from a clinical specimen, one must be guided by the following considerations.

The site from which the virus was isolated. For example, one would be quite confident about the etiological significance of equine herpesvirus 1 isolated from the tissues of a 9-month-old aborted equine fetus with typical gross and microscopic lesions. However, recovery of an enterovirus from the feces of a young pig may not necessarily be significant because such viruses are often associated with inapparent infections.

The epidemiologic circumstances under which the virus was isolated. Interpretation of the significance of a virus isolation may be much more meaningful if the same virus is isolated from several cases of the same illness in the same place and time.

The pathogenetic character of the virus isolated. Knowledge that the virus isolated is nearly always etiologically associated with frank disease, i.e., rarely is found as a "passenger," engenders confidence that the isolate is significant.

Detection and Quantitation of Antiviral Antibodies (Serologic Diagnosis)

Innovative assay strategies based on increasing knowledge of the nature of the immune response to viral infection, miniaturization of assay systems affecting the cost of reagents (e.g., multiwell plates), automated equipment, and integrated communication systems for rapid reporting of diagnostic laboratory data have all contributed to a revolution in clinical veterinary and zoonotic virology. In particular, innovative enzyme immunoassays, often based on monoclonal antibodies or viral antigens produced by recombinant DNA technologies, have led to the widespread development of diagnostic kits by commercial vendors. Thus, assays that are extremely complex in design, engineering, materials, and readout are reduced to the most straightforward, simple procedures in the clinical setting. These same assays, of proven sensitivity and specificity, are now also incorporated into epidemiologic surveys, disease control programs, and even regional eradication programs (see Chapters 14 and 15). Nowhere has this revolution had more impact than in laboratory methods based on serology, i.e., the measurement of the host's immune response to viral infection.

For the serologic diagnosis of a viral disease in an individual animal, the classic approach has been to test paired sera, i.e., an acute and convalescent serum from the same animal, for the presence of a specific antibody. The acute-phase serum sample is taken as early as possible in the illness, the convalescent-phase sample usually at least 2 weeks later. Given this time line, diagnosis based on this approach is said to be "retrospective." In recent years this approach has, in many cases, been complemented by serologic methods for detecting specific IgM antibodies—in many viral diseases a presumptive diagnosis may be made on the basis of detecting IgM antibody in a single acute-phase serum specimen.

Serum Specimens for Serologic Assays

Blood, collected in plain tubes, is allowed to clot and the serum is separated. Paired acute and convalescent sera are tested simultaneously. For certain tests that measure inhibition of some biologic function of the virus, e.g., virus neutralization or hemagglutination inhibition, sera must first be "inactivated" by heating at 56°C for 30 minutes. Sometimes sera must also be treated additionally, e.g., by absorption with kaolin or treatment with neuraminidase, to remove nonspecific inhibitors. Prior treatment of the serum is not generally required for assays that simply measure antigen–antibody binding, such as enzyme immunoassays, immunofluorescence, or immunodiffusion. Paired sera are then titrated for antibodies using any of a wide range of available serologic techniques. The basic principles of the most widely used tests are set out in Table 12.1.

Enzyme Immunoassay—Enzyme-Linked Immunosorbent Assay

Enzyme immunoassays (EIAs), also called enzyme-linked immunosorbent assays (ELISAs), are the serologic assays of choice for the qualitative (positive or negative) or quantitative determination of viral antibodies. Enzyme immunoassays offer the advantage that quantitative assays can be based on a single dilution of serum—the colorimetric (optical density) end point being interpolated by the spectrophotometric instrument and attached computer ("the reader" in the usual vernacular usage). In the most common formats for serologic enzyme immunoassays, the wells of 96-well microtiter plates are coated with purified antigen so as to reduce nonspecific binding of antibody. Positive and negative serums are included in every run and cutoff limits are adjusted by the reactivity of these controls in the given run. Kits have been designed for in-clinic testing of single serum samples in which only three wells are used for each case: the test sample and a positive and negative control serum (Figure 12.8).

In a more widely used format, the test serum flows through a membrane filter that has three circular areas impregnated with antigen, two of which have already interacted with a positive and a negative serum, respectively (Figure 12.8). After the test serum flows through the membrane and a washing step is completed, a second antispecies antibody with an enzyme linked to it is added and the membrane is again rinsed before the addition of the enzyme substrate. The result is read as a color change in the test sample circle, which is compared to the color change in the positive control and no change in the negative control. Such single patient tests are relatively expensive compared to the economies of testing hundreds of sera in a single run in a fully automated laboratory, but the great savings in time and effort to send samples to the laboratory, as well as the fact that decisions can be made while both client and patient are still in the consulting room, make single tests attractive and useful in the immediate clinical management of sometimes critically ill animals.

Serum Neutralization Assay

As virus isolation is considered the gold standard for the detection of virus against which other assays must be compared, so it has been that serum neutralization has been the gold standard, when available, for the detection and quantitation of antiviral antibodies. Neutralizing antibody also attracts great interest because it is considered a direct correlate of protective antibody *in vivo*. For the assay of neutralizing antibody, two general procedures are available: the alpha or *constant serum-variable virus* method and the beta or *constant virus variable serum* method.

In the alpha procedure, two 10-fold dilution series of virus are set up, usually in a 96-well microtiter plate. To one of the series a constant amount of the test serum, usually diluted 1 : 10 or 1 : 100, is added and to the other series a negative or perhaps an acute-phase serum from the test animal is added. The assay is based on the difference in virus titer between the two titrations. The amount to which the virus titer is reduced by the test (or convalescent) serum compared to the normal or acute-phase serum is a measure of the amount of antibody in the test serum.

In the beta procedure, a constant amount of virus, usually 100 $TCID_{50}$, obtained by previous titration and dilution of a stock virus, is mixed with serial, usually twofold dilutions, of the test serum. The highest dilution of serum that neutralizes the test dose of virus is the titer of the serum. In both the alpha and the beta versions of the test, end points may be indicated by cytopathology, immunofluorescence, or even by enzyme immunoassay.

In both alpha and beta systems the serum–virus mixtures are inoculated into disposable, nontoxic, sterile, plastic plates with 96 flat-bottomed wells in each of which a cell monolayer has been established. Plates are then incubated until the wells containing the "virus only" controls develop evidence of infection (Figure 12.13). By neutralizing the infectivity of the virus, antibody protects the cells against viral destruction—the highest dilution of antibody that protects cells from the virus represents the titer of neutralizing antibody contained in the serum specimen. Again, statistical methods are used to convert raw end point data into precise units of neutralizing antibody.

Immunoblotting (Western Blotting)

Western blotting tests simultaneously but independently measure antibodies against all of the proteins present in a particular virus. There are four key steps to Western blotting (Figure 12.14). First, purified virus is solubilized with the anionic detergent sodium dodecyl sulfate and the constituent proteins are separated into discrete bands according to their molecular mass (M_r) by sodium dodecyl sulfate–polyacrylamide gel electrophoresis (SDS-PAGE). Second, the separated proteins are transferred electrophoretically ("blotted") onto nitrocellulose to immobilize them. Third, the test serum is allowed to bind to the viral proteins on the membrane. Fourth, their presence is demonstrated using a radiolabeled or, most

FIGURE 12.14.

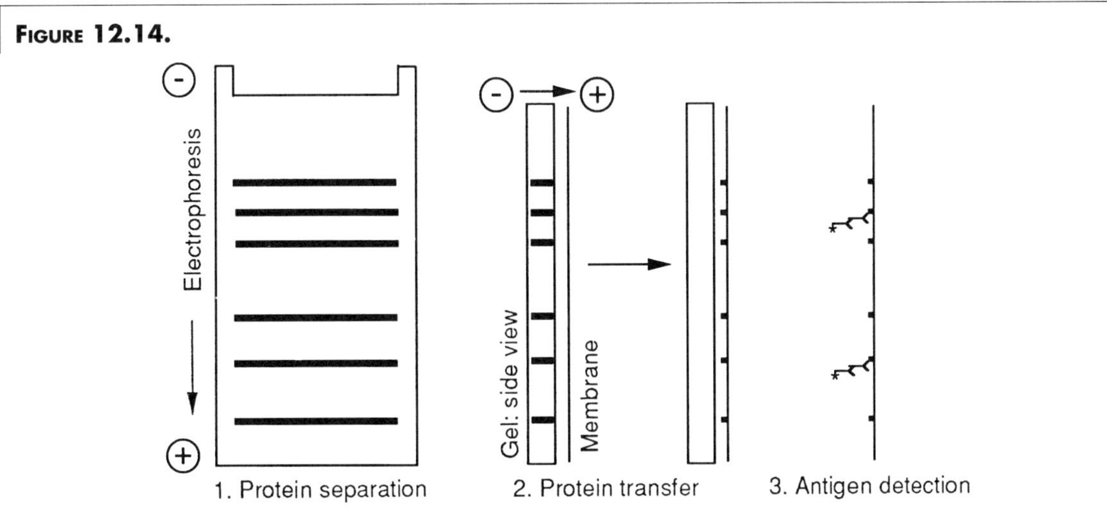

Immunoblotting (Western blotting) for the identification of antibodies. (1) Purified virus is disrupted with the anionic detergent SDS and is subjected to electrophoresis in a polyacrylamide gel (PAGE), which separates the different viral proteins according to their molecular mass (M_r). (2) These bands of viral protein are then transferred ("blotted") onto a nitrocellulose membrane and immobilized. (3) The unoccupied areas of the nitrocellulose membrane are then blocked ("quenched") by saturation with a suitable protein, washed, dried, and cut into strips that can be used to test individual animal sera. Each strip is incubated with an individual test serum to enable antibodies to bind to the individual viral proteins. Following rinsing, bound antibody is detected by the addition of enzyme-labeled antispecies immunoglobulin. Following another wash, the bands are revealed by the addition of a substrate for the enzyme and a chromogen chosen to produce an insoluble colored product. (Courtesy of I. H. Holmes and R. Strugnell.)

commonly, an enzyme-labeled antispecies antibody. Thus, immunoblotting permits demonstration of antibodies to some or all of the proteins of any given virus and can be used not only to discriminate between infection with closely related viruses sharing certain antigens, but also to monitor the presence of antibodies to different antigens at different stages of infection. Dip stick versions of these assays in which membrane strips containing the separated viral proteins are exposed to the serum and the strips are "developed" are designed for consulting room use.

Indirect Immunofluorescence Assay

Indirect immunofluorescence assays for the detection and quantitation of antibody have been widely used in many clinical and research laboratories for many years. The assay, which is similar in principle to enzyme immunoassays and radioimmunoassays, involves two steps: first the serum of interest is layered over the substrate containing the virus (usually virus-infected cells fixed on glass microscope slides); following incubation of the slide to allow binding of antibodies in the serum to the viral substrate and washing to remove unbound antibody, fluorescein isothiocyanate-conjugated antiglobulin (matched to the species from which the serum specimen was obtained) is added. Slides are examined in a microscope equipped with an ultraviolet light source and filters that transmit only light emitted from the fluorescent label. A positive reaction is seen, as apple-green color localized where viral antigen is present in the infected cell substrate, only when the serum specimen contains antibodies to the virus in question. Although the method is rapid and may be useful in detecting antibodies that are difficult or even impossible to demonstrate by any other means, nonspecific fluorescence frequently confuses interpretation of results.

Hemagglutination–Inhibition Assay

For those viruses that hemagglutinate red blood cells of one or another species, such as many of the arthropod-borne viruses and influenza and parainfluenza viruses, hemagglutination–inhibition assays are widely used. For detecting and quantitating antibodies in the serum of animals, the methods are sensitive, specific, simple, reliable, and quite inexpensive. Assays are conducted in 96-well microtiter plates in a procedure similar to that of a constant virus-variable serum dilution neutralization assay. Serum is diluted serially in the wells of the microtiter plate, usually in twofold steps, and to each well a constant amount of virus, usually four or eight hemagglutinating units, is added. The highest dilution of serum that inhibits the agglutination of the red blood cells by the standardized amount of virus represents the hemagglutination–inhibition titer of the serum (Figure 12.15).

Immunodiffusion

Historically, agar gel diffusion assays were used for the specific diagnosis of a number of diseases, including hog cholera, equine infectious anemia (Coggins test), and bovine leukemia. This was because the assays require only very simple, readily available materials. A further advantage of the assays was that the antigen used could be a relatively crude preparation (e.g., spleen pulp from an infected animal). In a commonly used format, six peripheral wells and a single central well, all 3 mm in diameter, were cut in agar with a punch. Antigen was placed in the central well, a known positive serum was placed in every other peripheral well, and three sera from animals of interest were placed in the remaining wells. Precipitin lines were formed by antibodies diffusing from the wells containing the positive control sera and antigen diffusing from the central well. Precipitin lines produced by any of the test sera and the antigen indicated that they contained antibody; precipitin lines from test sera that fused with lines produced by the positive control sera were considered as a confirmed indication of the presence of specific antibody.

IgM Class-Specific Antibody Assay

A rapid antibody-based diagnosis of a disease can be made on the basis of a single acute-phase serum by demonstrating virus-specific antibody of the IgM class. Because IgM antibodies appear early after infection but drop to low levels within 1 to 2 months and generally disappear altogether within 3 months, they are usually indicative of recent (or chronic) infection. Moreover, if found in a newborn animal, they are diagnostic of intrauterine infection, because maternal IgM does not cross the placenta.

The most common method used is the IgM antibody capture assay, in which the viral antigen is bound on a solid-phase substrate, say a microtiter well. The test serum is allowed to react with this substrate and then specific IgM antibodies "captured" by the antigen are detected with labeled anti-IgM antibody matched to the species from which the specimen was obtained. All of the immunoassays described earlier can readily be rendered IgM class-specific—enzyme immunoassays, radioimmunoassays, and indirect immunofluorescence

FIGURE 12.15.

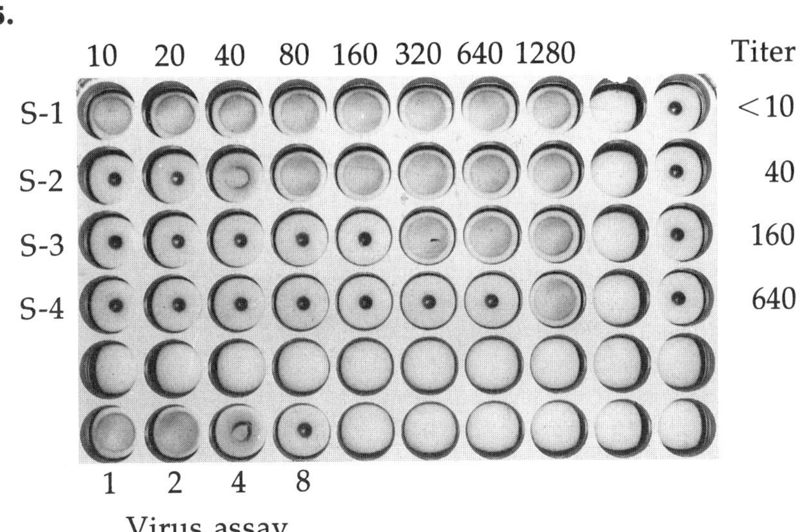

Hemagglutination–inhibition test used for titrating antibodies to the influenza virus hemagglutinin. In the example illustrated, a horse was immunized against the prevalent strain of influenza virus. Serum samples—S-1, S-2, S-3, and S-4—were taken, respectively, before immunization, 1 and 4 weeks after the first vaccine dose, and 4 weeks after the second. Sera were treated with periodate and heated at 56°C for 30 minutes to inactivate nonspecific inhibitors of hemagglutination and then diluted in wells of a microtiter plate in twofold steps from 1 : 10 to 1 : 1280 (dilutions indicated across top of figure.) Each well then received four hemagglutinating (HA) units of the relevant strain of influenza virus. After incubation at room temperature for 30 minutes, 0.05 ml of a 0.5% suspension of red blood cells was added to each well. Where enough antibody is present to complex the virions, hemagglutination is inhibited, hence the erythrocytes settle to form a button on the bottom of the well. Where insufficient antibody is present, erythrocytes are agglutinated by virus and form a mat. The virus titration (bottom row) indicates that the dilution of virus used gave partial agglutination (the end point) when diluted 1:4, i.e., that about four hemagglutinating units of virus were used in the assay. The horse originally had no hemagglutinin-inhibiting antibodies against this particular strain of influenza virus (top row). One dose of vaccine produced an antibody (titer 20); the second injection boosted the response to a titer of 640. (Courtesy of I. Jack.)

assays have proven generally useful. Typical indirect immunoassays for virus-specific IgM are depicted in Figure 12.16. Class-specific immunoassays can also be designed to measure IgG subclasses (useful in measuring colostral antibodies in cattle and sheep), IgA (useful in measuring mucosal immunity), and IgE (useful in measuring IgE-mediated hypersensitivity states). Such immunoglobulin class-specific antibody capture assays have an increasingly important place in the armamentarium of diagnostic laboratories.

FIGURE 12.16.

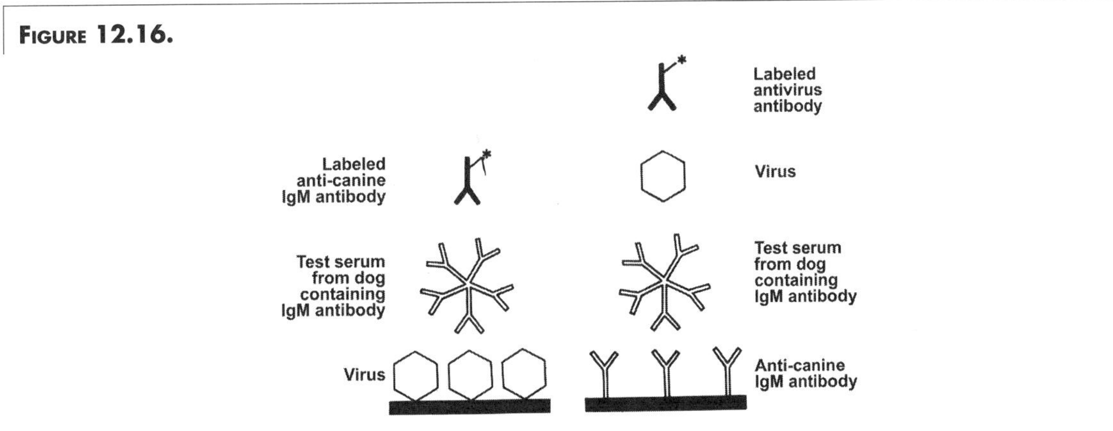

Immunoassays for the detection of specific antiviral antibodies of the IgM class using canine serum as an example and immunological reagents suitable for testing for canine IgM antibodies to a given virus. (Left) Indirect method. (Right) IgM antibody-capture method.

Interpretation of Serologic Laboratory Findings

A rise in antibody titer between acute and convalescent samples is a basis, albeit in retrospect, for a specific viral diagnosis; in some diseases, such as eastern equine encephalitis, a significant rise can occur within 48 hours of the onset of clinical signs. Sometimes the demonstration of antibody in a single serum sample is diagnostic of current infection (e.g., with retroviruses and herpesviruses, because these viruses establish lifelong infections). However, in such circumstances there is no assurance that the persistent virus was responsible for the disease under consideration. Assays designed to detect IgM antibody provide evidence of recent or current infection. A summary of the major strengths and limitations of the several alternative approaches to the serological diagnosis of viral infections is given in Table 12.1.

Detection of antiviral antibody in presuckle newborn cord or venous blood provides a basis for specific diagnosis of *in utero* infections. This approach was used, for example, to show that Akabane virus was the cause of arthrogryposis-hydranencephaly in calves (see Chapter 31). Because transplacental transfer of immunoglobulins does not occur in most domestic animals, the presence of either IgG or IgM antibodies in presuckle blood is indicative of infection of the fetus.

Sensitivity and Specificity

The interpretation and value of a particular serologic test is critically dependent on an understanding of two key parameters: sensitivity and specificity. The *sensitivity* of a given test is expressed as a percentage and is the number of animals with the disease (or infection) in question that are identified as positive by that test, divided by the total number that have the disease. For example, a particular enzyme immunoassay used to screen a population for bovine leukemia virus antibody may have a sensitivity of 98%, i.e., of every 100 infected cattle tested, 98 will be diagnosed correctly and 2 will be missed (the false-negative rate = 2%). In contrast, the *specificity* of a test is a measure of the percentage of those without the disease (or infection) who yield a negative result. For example, the same enzyme immunoassay for bovine leukemia virus antibody may have a specificity of 97%, i.e., of every 100 uninfected cattle, 97 will be diagnosed correctly as negative but 3 will be diagnosed incorrectly as infected (the false-positive rate = 3%). Whereas sensitivity and specificity are fixed percentages intrinsic to the particular diagnostic assay, the *predictive value* of an assay is affected greatly by the prevalence of the disease (or infection) involved. Thus, if the same enzyme immunoassay is used to screen a high-risk population with a known bovine leukemia prevalence of 50%, the predictive value of the assay will be high, but if it is used to screen a population with a known prevalence of 0.1%, the great majority of the 3.1% of animals that test positive will in fact be false positives and will require follow-up with a confirmatory test of much higher specificity. This striking illustration draws attention to the importance of selecting diagnostic assays with a particular objective in mind. An assay with high sensitivity is required when the aim is to screen for a serious infection or where eradication of the disease is the aim, in which case positive cases must not be missed. An assay, usually based on an independent technology, with very high specificity is required for confirmation that the diagnosis is correct.

The sensitivity of a given immunoassay is also a measure of its ability to detect small amounts of antibody (or antigen). For instance, enzyme immunoassays, radioimmunoassays, and neutralization assays generally display substantially higher sensitivity than immunodiffusion. Improvements in sensitivity may be obtained by the use of purified reagents and sensitive instrumentation. However, the specificity of an immunoassay is a measure of its capacity to discriminate the presence of antibody directed against one virus versus another. This quality is influenced mainly by the purity of the key reagents, especially the antigen when testing for antibody and the antibody when testing for antigen.

Quite apart from the problem of spurious cross-reactions caused by impure reagents or mysterious substances in specimens that bind to antigens or antibodies, it is crucial to understand that the specificity of any assay can be manipulated to match one's particular objective. For example, because of the presence of antigenic determinants common to many or all related viruses, say all the viruses within a given genus, the serum of an animal infected with just one of these viruses may contain antibodies that cross-react broadly. To render the assay more specific it is often necessary to use absolutely pure antigens, e.g., antigens produced by recombinant DNA technologies or peptides produced by organic synthesis. Alternatively, one can select an immunoassay that registers only those particular antibodies that bind to type-specific epitopes on the virus; virus neutralization and hemagglutination–inhibition assays are very specific because they measure only antibodies directed against epitopes involved in virus binding and attachment to cells that are usually extremely type specific.

Applications of Serology

A significant (conventionally, fourfold or greater) rise in antibody titer to a given virus between acute and convalescent serum samples is indicative of recent infection. Because of the necessary interval between the two specimens, a diagnosis is provided only in retrospect. Nevertheless, there are several circumstances wherein serology may still be the diagnostic method of choice.

There are circumstances when it is not practicable to attempt virus isolation or when the virus in question is one that is notoriously difficult to isolate from clinical specimens. For example, some togaviruses and bunyaviruses disappear so rapidly from the blood and tissues of infected animals that only serological diagnoses are practicable.

There are circumstances when the management of the case or the question of risk of transmission to uninfected animals is not an urgent matter. For example, when a cat returns to its home cattery from a show where there have been a number of cases of suspected feline herpesvirus 1 disease the first question might be whether the virus is present in the cattery or not. If the home cattery is virus free and if the exposed cat can be quarantined, it may be prudent to wait for as long as it takes to obtain laboratory results before allowing the cat to reenter the cattery.

There are circumstances when the presence of persistently infected animals in a herd pose a continuing threat. For example, the presence of pseudorabies virus in a herd may be determined serologically and an eradication program initiated.

There are circumstances when it is important to assay the dynamics of immunity to a given virus. For example, assessment of vaccine coverage, i.e., the prevalence of animals with antibody through vaccination may be in question if vaccine use has not resulted in expected reductions in disease incidence. Large poultry and swine operations include serological assessments as part of their preventive medicine programs. Decisions to retain and, if necessary, boost vaccination when the incidence of disease has fallen dramatically are often related to the percentage of the herd presumed to be protected. Continued suppression of rinderpest in cattle in some countries of West Africa in the 1970s was based on this approach. When the herd immunity fell because of civil strife interfering with vaccination programs, rinderpest reemerged.

Laboratory Safety

Many cases of serious illness and several hundred deaths from laboratory-acquired infection have been recorded over the years, particularly from togaviruses, flaviviruses, bunyaviruses, arenaviruses, filoviruses, and other Biosafety level 3 and 4 pathogens. Precautions to avoid laboratory hazards consist essentially of good laboratory practices and adequate facilities and equipment (Tables 12.3, 12.4 and Figure 12.17). Safe practices include:

1. Rigorous aseptic technique must be used. The practice veterinarians have in aseptic surgery provides a valuable base upon which similar laboratory techniques may be learned. For example, the proper way to put on gown and gloves for surgery is similar to the proper

Figure 12.17.

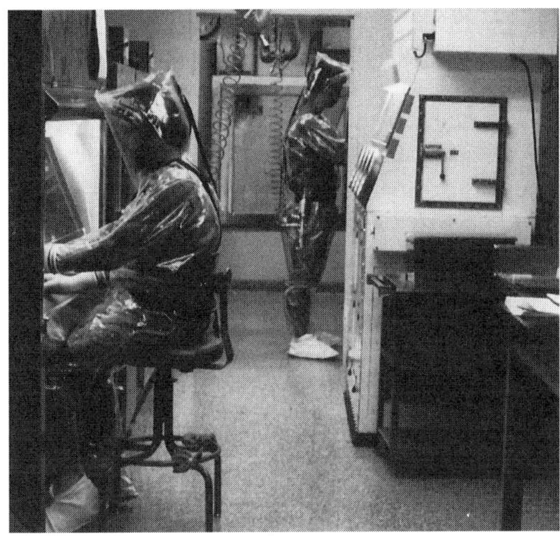

Maximum containment laboratory, Centers for Disease Control, Atlanta, Georgia. Workers are protected by positive-pressure suits with an independent remote source of breathing air. Primary containment of aerosols is achieved by use of filtered vertical laminar-flow workstations. The ultracentrifuge is contained in an explosion-proof laminar-flow hood. A full range of equipment is available, and animals as large as monkeys can be used for experiments. (Courtesy of K. M. Johnson.)

Table 12.3
Recommended Biosafety Levels for Infectious Agents[a]

Biosafety level	Agents	Practice	Safety equipment (primary barriers)	Facility (secondary barriers)
BSL 1	Not known to cause human disease	Standard microbiological practices	None required	Open bench
BSL 2	Associated with human disease, hazard of autoinoculation, ingestion, mucous membrane exposure	BSL 1 practices plus limited access, biohazard warning signs, "sharps" precautions, protocol for medical surveillance, waste decontamination	Primary barriers: Class I or II BSCs[b] for all manipulations that cause splashes or aerosols, laboratory coats, gloves, face protection as needed	BSL 1 plus autoclave available
BSL 3	Indigenous or exotic agents with potential for aerosol transmission; disease may have serious or lethal consequences	BSL 2 practice plus controlled access, decontamination of all waste, baseline serum, decontamination of lab clothing before laundering	Primary barriers: Class I or II BSCs used for all manipulations, protective lab clothing, gloves; respiratory protection as needed	BSL 2 plus physical separation from access corridors self-closing, double door access, exhaust air not recirculated, negative air flow into laboratory
BSL 4	Dangerous/exotic agents that pose high risk of life-threatening disease, aerosol-transmitted lab infections, or related agents with unknown risk of transmission	BSL 3 practices plus clothing change before entering, shower on exit, all material decontaminated before exit from facility	Primary barriers: Class III BSCs or Class I or II BSCs *in combination with* positive pressure full-body suit with contained air supply, for all procedures	BSL 3 plus separate building or isolated zone with dedicated air supply and exhaust, vacuum, and decontamination systems, other requirements as well

[a]From Centers for Disease Control and National Institutes for Health, "Biosafety in Microbiological and Biomedical Laboratories," 3rd Ed. U.S. Government Printing Office, Washington, DC, 1993. There are additional guidelines for practices, safety equipment, and facilities for working with experimental animals infected with pathogens.
[b]Biological safety cabinet.

way of removing gown and gloves after working with a dangerous virus in the laboratory.

2. Laboratory clothing, gloves, and even masks or respirators are chosen to match the virus or clinical material being worked with. Laboratory clothing is decontaminated before being sent to the laundry.

3. Various classes of biological safety cabinets providing increasing levels of containment are available for procedures of various degrees of biohazard; their use is summarized in Table 12.4. Biosafety level 4 viruses, such as Ebola, Marburg, Lassa, and equine morbillivirus, are handled only in maximum-containment laboratories.

4. Careful attention must be given to the autoclaving of all potentially infectious waste.

5. Mouth pipetting is banned; instead mechanical pipetting devices are used.

6. Particular care is taken when centrifuging material containing or possibly containing a dangerous virus.

7. Where possible, particularly dangerous viruses employed in various laboratory tests are inacti-

Table 12.4
Laboratory Hazards

Hazard	Cause
Aerosol	Homogenization (e.g., of tissue in blender) Centrifugation Ultrasonic vibration Broken glassware Pipetting
Ingestion	Mouth pipetting Eating or smoking in laboratory Inadequate washing/disinfection of hands
Skin penetration	Needle-stick Hand cut by broken glassware Leaking container contaminating hands Handling infected organs at necropsy Splash into eye Animal bite

Table 12.5
Restricted Animal Viruses[a]

Virus	Family/genus
African horse sickness viruses	*Reoviridae/Orbivirus*
African swine fever virus	*Asfarviridae/Asfivirus*
Avian influenza viruses (certain viruses such as those H5 and H7 viruses that cause severe disease with high mortality—previously called fowl plague)	*Orthomyxoviridae/ Influenzavirus A*
Borna disease virus	*Bornaviridae/Bornavirus*
Bovine ephemeral fever virus	*Rhabdoviridae/ Ephemerovirus*
Camelpox virus	*Poxviridae/Orthopoxvirus*
Foot-and-mouth disease viruses	*Picornaviridae/Aphthovirus*
Lumpy skin disease virus	*Poxviridae/Capripoxvirus*
Nairobi sheep disease virus	*Bunyaviridae/Nairovirus*
Newcastle disease virus (velogenic strains)	*Paramyxoviridae/ Rubulavirus*
Porcine polioencephalomyelitis virus	*Picornaviridae/Enterovirus*
Rift Valley fever virus	*Bunyaviridae/Phlebovirus*
Rinderpest virus	*Paramyxoviridae/ Morbillivirus*
Swine vesicular disease virus	*Picornaviridae/Enterovirus*
Vesicular exanthema virus	*Caliciviridae/Vesivirus*
Wesselsbron virus	*Flaviviridae/Flavivirus*

[a]For the United States. In other developed countries there are similar listings; some are even longer, e.g., the Australian list includes exotic bluetongue viruses, epidemic hemorrhagic disease of deer virus, hog cholera virus, malignant catarrhal fever virus, ovine progressive pneumonia virus, pseudorabies virus, rabies virus, sheeppox virus, vesicular stomatitis viruses, and the scrapie and bovine spongiform encephalopathy prions, but excludes bovine ephemeral fever virus, which is endemic in Australia. Additionally, certain viruses of fish and mollusks are notifiable to the Office International des Épizooties, in Paris: epizootic hematopoietic necrosis virus, infectious hematopoietic necrosis virus, spring viremia of carp virus, viral hemorrhagic septicemia virus, channel catfish herpesvirus, viral encephalopathy and retinopathy virus, and infectious pancreatic necrosis virus.

vated (e.g., filoviruses, arenaviruses and certain togaviruses, bunyaviruses, and flaviviruses). This can be done, without destroying viral antigenicity, by γ-irradiation or by photodynamic inactivation with ultraviolet light in the presence of psoralen. Increasingly, viral proteins produced by recombinant DNA technologies are being employed instead of whole virus as safe antigens for serologic tests.

8. Spills are cleaned up with an appropriate chemical disinfectant.
9. Where zoonotic or human or primate tissues are handled, personnel are immunized against such pathogens as hepatitis B virus, polioviruses, and rabies virus, as well as against exotic agents such as Rift Valley fever virus in the special laboratories handling them.
10. Limitations are placed on the type of work undertaken by pregnant women or immunosuppressed employees.

The United States Centers for Disease Control and Prevention, in conjunction with the United States Department of Agriculture and similar bodies in other countries, including the Office International des Épizooties, provide guidelines for appropriate laboratory practices, procedures, containment facilities, and equipment for working with dangerous viruses (and other microorganisms).

Security for National Livestock Industries

In addition to personal hazard, exotic animal viruses pose special community risks such that major industrialized countries with large livestock industries support special laboratories for their investigation and for reference diagnosis. These laboratories are popularly designated by their location: for example, *Plum Island* in the United States, *Pirbright* in the United Kingdom, *Geelong* in Australia, *Ondestepoort* in South Africa, and so on. Animal viruses that are restricted to these laboratories in the United States are listed in Table 12.5. The importation, possession, or use of these viruses is prohibited or restricted by law or regulation. The importation of some is totally prohibited (e.g., foot-and-mouth disease viruses and vesicular stomatitis viruses into Australia); more often their importation and study are restricted to national maximum containment laboratories.

Further Reading

Arnheim, N., and Erlich, H. (1992). Polymerase chain reaction strategy. *Annu. Rev. Biochem.* **61,** 131–162.

Centers for Disease Control/National Institutes for Health. (1993). "Biosafety in Microbiological and Biomedical Laboratories," 3rd ed., Publ. NIH 88-8395. U.S. Government Printing Office, Washington, DC.

Fleming, D. O., Richardson, J. H., Tullis, J. J., and Vesley, D. (1995). "Laboratory Safety. Principles and Practices," 2nd ed., American Society for Microbiology Press, Washington, DC.

Freshney, R. I. (1988). "Culture of Animal Cells: A Manual of Basic Techniques," 2nd ed. Liss/Wiley, New York.

Hierholzer, J. C. (1991). Rapid diagnosis of viral infection. *In* "Rapid Methods and Automation in Microbiology and Immunology" (A. Vaheri and A. Balows, eds.), pp. 556–590. Springer-Verlag, New York.

Innis, M. A., Gelfand, D. H., Sninsky, J. J., and White, T. J., eds. (1990). "Polymerase Chain Reaction Protocols: A Guide to Methods and Applications." Academic Press, San Diego, CA.

James, K. (1990). Immunoserology of infectious diseases. *Clin. Microbiol. Rev.* **3**, 132–155.

Johnson, F. B. (1990). Transport of viral specimens. *Clin. Microbiol. Rev.* **3**, 120–139.

Katz, J. B., Alstad, A. D., Gustafson, G. A., and Moser, K. M. (1993). Sensitive identification of bluetongue virus serogroup by a colorimetric dual oligonucleotide sorbent assay of amplified viral nucleic acid. *J. Clin. Microbiol.* **31**, 3028–3030.

Lennette, E. H., Halonen, P., and Murphy, F. A., eds. (1988). "Laboratory Diagnosis of Infectious Diseases. Principles and Practice," Vol. 2. Springer-Verlag, New York.

Murray, P. R., Baron, E. J., Pfaller, M. A., and Tenover, F. C., (1995). "Manual of Clinical Microbiology," 6th ed. American Society for Microbiology Press, Washington, DC.

Palmer, E. L., and Martin, M. L. (1988). "Electron Microscopy in Viral Diagnosis." CRC Press, Boca Raton, FL.

Reubel, G. H. and Studdert, M. J. (1998). Benefits and limitations of polymerase chain reaction in veterinary diagnostic virology. *Vet. Bull.* **68**, 505–516.

Rose, N. R., de Macario, E. C., Folds, J. D., Lane, H. C., and Nakamura, R. M., eds. (1997). "Manual of Clinical Laboratory Immunology," 5 ed. American Society of Microbiology Press, Washington, DC.

CHAPTER 13

Vaccination against Viral Diseases

Vaccination is the most effective way of preventing viral diseases. The control of so many viral (and other infectious) diseases of animals by vaccination is probably the single most outstanding achievement of veterinary medicine. The history of vaccination is a fascinating one; vaccines were introduced by Edward Jenner in 1798 to protect humans against smallpox, then, nearly a century later, the concept was shown by Louis Pasteur to have wider applications and, most notably, could be used to prevent rabies. With the advent of cell culture techniques in the 1950s, a second era of vaccination was introduced and many attenuated virus and inactivated virus vaccines were developed. Today, the field of vaccinology has entered a third era through the application, in many different ways, of recombinant DNA technologies. While the attenuated virus and inactivated virus vaccines of the second era are still the "work horses" of veterinary practice, third generation vaccines are now complementing and, in some cases, replacing them.

There are some important differences between vaccination practices in humans and animals. Except in developing countries, economic constraints are of less importance in human medicine than in veterinary practice. There is greater agreement about the safety and efficacy of vaccines in use in human medicine than there is with animal vaccines. At the international level, the World Health Organization (WHO) exerts persuasive leadership for human vaccine usage and maintains a number of programs such as the Global Program for Vaccines and Immunization, a program that is unmatched for animal vaccine usage by its sister agencies, the Food and Agriculture Organization and the Office International des Épizooties. Further, within countries, greater latitude is allowed in the manufacture and use of vaccines for veterinary and zoonotic diseases than is allowed by national regulatory authorities for human vaccines. As may be seen in the tables in Chapter 42, there are many viral vaccines available for use in domestic animals, whereas, currently, only about 13 are available for use in humans. Finally, even a very small number of vaccine-associated illnesses or deaths constitutes a major objection to the use of a vaccine in humans. If a vaccine is effective and the potential cost of failure to control the disease is sufficiently high, mild disease (and even, in the past, occasional death) is tolerated in veterinary medicine.

Traditionally, until the advent of the third generation vaccines, there were two major strategies for the production of viral vaccines; one employing attenuated virus and the other employing chemically inactivated virus. Today, the situation is far more complex; while most of the vaccines in wide-scale production contain either attenuated or inactivated virus, new vaccines are being developed through recombinant DNA technologies that promise significant improvements in safety, efficacy, and cost (Table 13.1). The excitement of the prospect of "DNA vaccines" is conspicuous in this regard.

Live virus vaccines replicate in the vaccine recipient and, in so doing, amplify the amount of antigen presented to the host's immune system. There are important benefits in this because the replication of vaccine virus mimics infection to the extent that the host immune response is more similar to that occurring after natural infection than is the case with inactivated or subunit vaccines. When inactivated virus vaccines are produced, the chemical or physical treatment used to eliminate infectivity may be damaging enough to modify immunogenicity, especially cell-mediated immunogenicity, usually resulting in an immune response that is shorter in duration, narrower in antigenic spectrum, weaker in cell-mediated and mucosal immune responses, and possibly less effective in totally preventing viral entry. Nonetheless, very serviceable and safe inactivated vaccines are available and widely used.

Live-Virus Vaccines

Attenuated virus vaccines, when they have been proven to be safe, have been the best of all vaccines. Several of them have been dramatically successful in reducing the incidence of important diseases of animals and humans. Most live-virus vaccines are injected subcutaneously or intramuscularly, but some are delivered orally and a few by aerosol or to poultry in their drinking water. For these vaccines to be successful the vaccine virus must replicate in the recipient, thereby eliciting a lasting immune response, while causing little or no disease. In effect, a live-virus vaccine mimics a subclinical infection. Live-virus vaccines are derived from several sources.

Vaccines Produced from Naturally Occurring Attenuated Viruses

The original vaccine (*vacca* = cow), introduced by Jenner in 1798 for the control of human smallpox, utilized cowpox virus, a natural pathogen of the cow. This virus produced only a mild lesion in humans, but, because it

Table 13.1
Approaches to the Design of Viral Vaccines

Live-virus vaccines
- Vaccines produced from naturally occurring attenuated viruses
- Vaccines produced by serial passage in cultured cells
- Vaccines produced by serial passage in a heterologous host animal
- Vaccines produced by selection of cold-adapted mutants and reassortants

Nonreplicating native antigen vaccines
- Vaccines produced from inactivated whole virions
- Vaccines produced from native viral subunits
- Vaccines produced from purified native viral proteins

Vaccines produced by recombinant DNA and other innovative technologies
- Vaccines produced by recombinant DNA technology by the attenuation of viruses by gene deletion or site-directed mutagenesis
- Vaccines produced by recombinant DNA technology by the expression of viral proteins in eukaryotic (yeast, mammalian, insect) or bacterial cells
- Vaccines produced by recombinant DNA technology by the expression of viral proteins that self-assemble into virus-like particles
- Vaccines produced by recombinant DNA technology by the expression of viral antigens in viral vectors.
- Vaccines produced by recombinant DNA technology by the expression of viral antigens in bacterial vectors
- Vaccines produced by recombinant DNA technology by the formation of viral chimeras (viruses with the replicative machinery of one virus and the protective antigens of another)
- Vaccines produced by recombinant DNA technology by the organic synthesis of viral peptides
- Vaccines produced by recombinant DNA technology by the production and administration of anti-idiotypic antibodies
- DNA vaccines

is antigenically related to smallpox virus, it conferred protection against the severe human disease. The same principle has been applied to other diseases (e.g., the protection of chickens against Marek's disease using a vaccine derived from a related herpesvirus of turkeys and the protection of piglets against porcine rotavirus infection using a vaccine derived from a bovine rotavirus).

Virulent viruses given by an unnatural route have historically been used as vaccines in veterinary practice (e.g., wild-type avian infectious laryngotracheitis virus).

Vaccines Produced by Attenuation of Viruses by Serial Passage in Cultured Cells

Most of the live-virus vaccines in common use today have been derived empirically by serial passage in cultured cells. The cells may be of homologous or, more commonly, heterologous host origin. Adaptation of virus to more vigorous growth in cultured cells is fortuitously accompanied by progressive loss of virulence for the natural host. Loss of virulence may be demonstrated initially in a convenient laboratory model, often a mouse, before being confirmed by clinical trials in the species of interest. Because of the practical requirement that the vaccine must not be so attenuated that it fails to replicate satisfactorily *in vivo*, it is sometimes necessary to compromise by using a strain that may induce mild clinical signs in a few of the recipient animals.

During multiple passages in cultured cells, vaccine seed viruses may accumulate numerous point mutations in the genome, which lead to attenuation. In recent years, genomic sequencing has brought considerable understanding of attenuation, allowing better predictions of vaccine efficacy and safety. It has been shown that for most viruses, several genes contribute to virulence and tropism and do so in several different ways. For example, in contrast to the systemic infection associated with the wild-type virus, it has been found that some vaccine viruses, administered by the respiratory route, replicate only in the upper respiratory tract; in other cases, vaccine viruses, administered orally, replicate only in specific intestinal epithelial cells.

Despite the outstanding success of empirically derived attenuated virus vaccines, extensive research is currently aimed at replacing what some veterinarians see as "genetic roulette" with "rationally designed, engineered" vaccines. In these engineered vaccines, the mutations associated with the attenuation are known, stable, and predictable. This approach has already yielded several promising vaccines, as discussed later.

Vaccines Produced by Attenuation of Viruses by Serial Passage in Heterologous Host

Serial passage in a heterologous host was a classic means of empirically attenuating viruses for use as vaccines. For example, rinderpest and hog cholera viruses were each adapted to grow in rabbits and in serial passage became sufficiently attenuated to be used in earlier vaccines. Many viruses were passaged in embryonated hen's eggs in similar fashion.

Vaccines Produced by Attenuation of Viruses by Selection of Cold-Adapted Mutants and Reassortants

The observation that *temperature-sensitive (ts) mutants* (unable to replicate satisfactorily at temperatures much higher than normal body temperature) generally display reduced virulence suggested that they might make satisfactory live vaccines. Unfortunately, even vaccines containing more than one ts mutation have displayed a disturbing tendency to revert toward virulence during replication in vaccinated animals. Attention accordingly moved to *cold-adapted (ca) mutants,* derived by adaptation of virus to grow at suboptimal temperatures. The rationale is that such mutant viruses might comprise safer vaccines for intranasal administration in that they would replicate well at the lower temperature of the nasal cavity (about 33°C in most mammalian species), but not at the temperature of the more vulnerable lower respiratory tree and lungs. Cold-adapted influenza vaccines containing mutations in almost every gene do not revert to virulence. In 1997, influenza vaccines based on such mutations were licensed for human use in the United States—the same approach is currently under study for the development of improved vaccines against equine influenza.

Nonreplicating Native Antigen Vaccines

Vaccines Produced from Inactivated Whole Virions

Inactivated virus vaccines are usually made from virulent virus; chemical or physical agents are used to destroy infectivity while maintaining immunogenicity. When prepared properly, such vaccines are safe, but they need to contain large amounts of antigen to elicit an antibody response commensurate with that attainable by a much smaller dose of attenuated virus vaccines. Normally the primary vaccination course comprises two or three injections; further ("booster") doses may be required at intervals to maintain immunity.

The most commonly used inactivating agents are formaldehyde, β-propiolactone, and ethylenimine. One of the advantages of β-propiolactone, which is used in the manufacture of rabies vaccines, and ethylenimine, which is used in the manufacture of foot-and-mouth disease vaccines, is that they are completely hydrolyzed within hours to nontoxic products. Because virions in the center of aggregates may be protected from inactivation, it is important that aggregates be broken up before inactivation. In the past, failure to do this occasionally resulted in vaccine-associated disease outbreaks—several foot-and-mouth disease outbreaks have been traced to this problem (see Chapter 15).

Vaccines Produced from Purified Native Viral Proteins

Lipid solvents such as sodium deoxycholate are used in the case of enveloped viruses to solubilize the virion and release the components, including the glycoprotein spikes of the envelope. Differential centrifugation is used to semipurify these glycoproteins, which are then formulated for use as so-called "split" vaccines. Examples include vaccines against herpesviruses, influenza viruses, and coronaviruses.

Vaccines Produced from Purified Naturally Occurring Viral Proteins

The earliest vaccine for human hepatitis B virus was unusual in that it was prepared as purified hepatitis B surface antigen (HBsAg) from human blood of chronically infected carriers of the virus. There are no commonly used veterinary vaccines of this kind.

Vaccines Produced by Recombinant DNA and Other Innovative Technologies

Vaccines Produced by Attenuation of Viruses by Gene Deletion or Site-Directed Mutagenesis

The problem of back mutation (i.e., a mutation by which the vaccine virus regains virulence) may be largely circumvented by completely deleting nonessential genes that contribute to virulence. The large DNA viruses, in particular, carry a significant number of genes that are not essential for replication, at least for replication in cultured cells. "Genetic surgery" is used to construct deletion mutants that are stable over many passages. Several herpesvirus vaccines have been constructed using this strategy; one of these, pseudorabies vaccine for swine, produced by recombinant DNA technology with a deletion of the thymidine kinase (TK) gene of the virus, is in wide use in veterinary practice in many countries. Other pseudorabies virus vaccines have been constructed that are TK^- and also have deletions in one or more glycoprotein gene(s) (gE, gB, or gG). The deleted glycoprotein may be used as capture antigen in an ELISA, so that vaccinated, uninfected pigs, which would test negative, can be distinguished from naturally infected pigs, enabling eradication programs to be conducted in parallel with continued vaccination.

Site-directed mutagenesis permits the introduction of prescribed nucleotide substitutions into viral genomes at will. As more becomes known about particular genes that are influential in virulence and immunogenicity, these genes may be modified. Further, other meaningful insertions or changes in the viral nucleotide sequence may be tested easily. Indeed, the day is coming when licensing authorities may demand that new vaccines be fully defined genetically, i.e., that the complete nucleotide sequence of the vaccine virus be known and perhaps stipulated in the license application.

Vaccines Produced by Expression of Viral Proteins in Eukaryotic (Yeast, Mammalian, Insect) or Bacterial Cells

Recombinant DNA technology provides a means of producing large amounts of viral proteins that can be purified readily and formulated into vaccines. Once the critical viral protein conferring protection has been identified, its gene (or, in the case of an RNA virus, a cDNA copy of the gene) may be cloned into one of a wide choice of expression plasmids and expressed in any of several cell systems. If the immunogenic viral protein of interest is glycosylated, eukaryotic expression systems must be used so that the expressed protein is glycosylated and produced ideally in its proper conformation.

Useful eukaryotic expression systems include yeast cells (*Saccharomyces cerevisiae*), insect cells (*Spodoptera frugiperda*), and various mammalian cells. Yeast offers the advantage that there is extensive experience with scaleup for industrial production; the first vaccine produced by expression of a cloned gene, human hepatitis B vaccine, was produced in yeast. Insect cells offer the advantage of simple technology derived from the silk industry: moth cell cultures (or caterpillars!) may be made to express very large amounts of viral proteins through infection with baculoviruses carrying the gene(s) of the virus of interest. The promoter for the gene encoding the baculovirus polyhedrin protein is so strong that the product of a viral gene of interest inserted within the baculovirus polyhedrin gene may comprise up to half of all the protein the infected moth cells or caterpillars make.

Mammalian cells offer the advantage over cells from lower eukaryotes in that they are more likely to possess the machinery for correct posttranslational processing, including glycosylation and secretion, of viral proteins. The relative advantages of these systems are presented in Table 13.2.

Vaccines Produced by Expression of Viral Proteins That Self-Assemble into Virus-like Particles

When the genes coding for the production and cleavage of capsid proteins of viruses within certain families of nonenveloped icosahedral viruses are cloned into plasmids and expressed, the resulting individual capsid proteins assemble into virus-like particles (VLPs). These VLPs may be used as a vaccine. Examples of viruses for which VLPs have been made and shown to be immunogenic include picornaviruses, caliciviruses, rotaviruses, and orbiviruses. Virus-like particles may be equated to so-called "empty virus particles" (which are not always empty) in that they are totally devoid of nucleic acid and therefore are safe. They may also be equated to an inactivated whole virus vaccine but without the potentially epitope-damaging step of chemical inactivation. Surprisingly, no virus-like, particle-based vaccines are in commercial use. Possible reasons for this include cost of production, low yields, and less effective immunity compared to existing vaccines, even when these are whole-virus inactivated vaccines.

Vaccines Utilizing Bacteria as Vectors for Expression of Viral Antigens

Rather than proceed to formulate a vaccine using the protein derived from the systems described previously, recombinant DNA technology allows the expression of viral epitopes on the surface of bacteria that infect the host directly. The general approach is to insert the DNA encoding a protective viral antigen or epitope into a region of the genome of a bacterium, or one of its plasmids, that encodes a prominent surface protein. Provided that the added viral protein structures do not seriously interfere with the transport, stability, or function of the

Table 13.2
Advantages and Limitations of Attenuated, Inactivated, and DNA Vaccines

Property	Attenuated virus vaccine	Inactivated virus vaccine	DNA vaccine
Route of administration	Injection, inhalation or oral	Injection	Injection
Amount of virus in vaccine dose	Low	High	Nil
Number of doses	Single, generally	Multiple	Single, generally
Need for adjuvant	No	Yes	No
Duration of immunity	Many years	Generally 1 year or less	Many years
Antibody response	IgG, IgA (if via mucosal route)	IgG	IgG
Cell-mediated response	Good	Generally modest	Good
Heat lability	Yes, for most viruses	No	No
Interference by prior antibody	Yes	Usually no	Apparently no
Side effects	Occasional, local, or systemic	Occasional, local	Uncertain
Use in pregnant animals	Often not advised, but commonly done	Yes	Yes
Reversion to virulence	Rarely	No	No
Cost	Low	High	High

bacterial protein, the bacterium can multiply and present the viral epitope to the immune system of the host. Enteric bacteria that multiply naturally in the gut would seem to be ideal expression vectors for presenting protective epitopes of virulent enteric viruses to the gut-associated lymphoid tissue. The main vaccines under development employ attenuated strains of *Escherichia coli*, *Salmonella* spp., and *Mycobacteria* spp. for immunization against enteric organisms and/or for the preferential stimulation of mucosal immunity.

Vaccines Utilizing Viruses as Vectors for Expression of Viral Antigens

DNA Viruses as Vectors

Recombinant DNA techniques allow any foreign gene to be introduced into the viral genome, and the product of the foreign gene is then carried into and expressed in the cell. The method is in use in veterinary medicine and involves the use of viruses as vectors to carry the genes for the protective antigens of other viruses. The same technology is being explored seriously in other contexts, including the correction of defective genes, anticancer therapy, and the correction of some degenerative diseases associated with aging in humans. The concept for vaccines against disease involves inserting the gene coding for the antigen (against which protective responses are generated in the host) of the virus causing the disease of interest into the genome of an avirulent virus. This modified avirulent virus is then administered as a live-virus vector. Cells in which the vector virus replicates *in vivo* will express the foreign protein and the animal will mount both a humoral and a cell-mediated immune response to it. In the original proof test of this concept, the human hepatitis B surface antigen (HBsAg) gene, flanked by the nonessential vaccinia gene for thymidine kinase and its promoter, was inserted into a bacterial plasmid (Figure 13.1). Mammalian cells infected with vaccinia virus were then transfected with this chimeric plasmid, which by homologous recombination produced vaccinia virus carrying the HBsAg. The recombinant virus was then used as a hepatitis B vaccine. Genes for many antigens from a variety of viruses have been incor-

FIGURE 13.1.

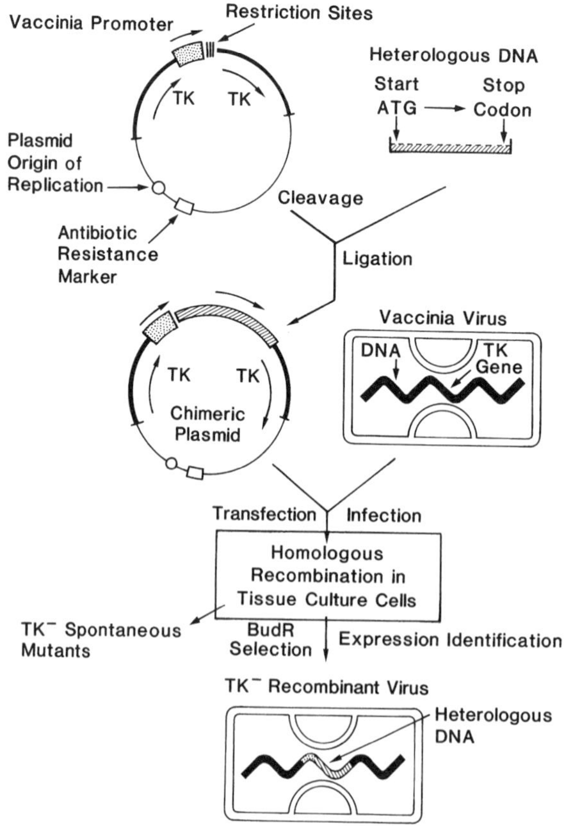

Method of constructing a vaccinia virus vector carrying a selected gene from another virus. TK, thymidine kinase gene of vaccinia virus; BudR, bromodeoxyuridine; TK, thymidine kinase. (Courtesy of B. Moss and J. Esposito.)

porated into the genome of vaccinia virus, and vaccination of animals with these recombinant-vectored vaccines has, in nearly every case, produced a good antibody response. For example, vaccinia virus-vectored rabies vaccines have been shown to protect foxes and raccoons when incorporated into baits administered orally. Because the large vaccinia genome can accommodate at least a dozen foreign genes and still be packaged satisfactorily within the virion, it is theoretically possible to construct, as a vector, a single recombinant virus capable of protecting against several different viral diseases. Fowlpox virus is a logical choice as a vector for avian vaccines. Most surprisingly, fowlpox virus has also been shown to be a useful vector in mammals. Even though this virus and the closely related canarypox virus do not replicate to produce infectious virus in mammals (including humans), the inserted genes are expressed and induce an antibody response.

So far, the only vectored vaccines to be used in the field are vaccinia–rabies constructs used for the vaccination of foxes in Europe and raccoons in the United States and rinderpest vaccines (based on vaccinia and capripox viruses) in Africa. Recent research suggests that adenoviruses, herpesviruses, and parvoviruses will also have value as vectors and may have advantages in terms of long-term antigen expression.

RNA Viruses as Vectors

Several RNA viruses, such as Sindbis virus and several picornaviruses, are also being developed as vectors. This approach opens up the possibility of designing vaccines for the range of viral and bacterial and perhaps parasitic infections common in each species of domestic animal in any particular country.

Viral Chimeras (Viruses with Replicative Machinery of One Virus and Protective Antigens of Another) as Vaccines

Conceptually, this is a subtle form of vectored vaccine. When a particular virus strain has very well tested and useful properties, such as safety and high yield, it is possible to add or substitute gene segments from a less well-characterized virus of the same species into the genome of the former for use as a vaccine. A hypothetical example might be a recently isolated variant of avian encephalomyelitis virus that grows poorly in cultured cells and embryonated hen eggs. A cDNA of the capsid-coding region of the virus of interest is used to replace the corresponding region of a high-yielding existing vaccine strain. The chimeric virus is then used as vaccine for the newly isolated virus strain.

For influenza viruses and other viruses with segmented genomes, the principle of chimeric viruses was well established before the advent of recombinant DNA technology. Reassortant viruses were produced by homologueous reassortment (segment swapping) by cocultivation of an existing vaccine strain virus with the new isolate. Viruses with the desirable growth properties of the vaccine virus but with the immunogenic properties of the recent isolate were selected, cloned, and used as vaccine.

Synthetic Peptide Vaccines

Techniques have been developed for locating and defining epitopes on viral proteins and it is possible to synthesize peptides chemically corresponding to these antigenic determinants (Table 13.3). Such synthetic peptides have been shown to elicit neutralizing antibodies against foot-and-mouth disease virus, rabies virus, and certain other animal pathogens, but in general this approach has been disappointing. While the approach merits further research, one limitation is that most epitopes that elicit humoral immunity are conformational. Epitopes are not composed of linear arrays of contiguous amino acids, but rather are assembled from amino acids that, while separated in the primary sequence, are brought into close apposition by the folding of the polypeptide chain(s). An effective antigenic stimulus requires that the three-dimensional shape that an epitope has in the native protein molecule or virus particle be maintained in a vaccine. Because short synthetic peptides lack any tertiary or qua-

Table 13.3
Synthetic Peptides as Potential Vaccines

Advantages

- Short defined amino acid sequence representing protective epitope
- Safe, nontoxic, stable
- T cell epitopes are naturally presented in the form of linear peptides so they can be included easily in the vaccine
- May be engineered to contain B cell and T cell epitopes or several epitopes of one or more proteins
- May be engineered to lack immunosuppressive domains present in naive proteins

Disadvantages

- Poorly immunogenic; adjuvant, liposome, ISCOM, or polymerization needed
- Most B cell epitopes are nonlinear (discontinuous) and therefore not reproduced by peptides
- May be too narrowly specific, not protecting against natural variants
- Single-epitope vaccine may readily select mutants in the field
- No response in animals lacking appropriate MHC class II antigen

ternary conformation, most antibodies raised against them are incapable of binding to virions, hence neutralizing antibody titers may be orders of magnitude lower than those induced by inactivated whole virus vaccines or purified intact proteins.

In contrast, the epitopes recognized by T lymphocytes are short linear peptides (bound to MHC protein). Some of these T cell epitopes are conserved between strains of virus and therefore elicit a cross-reactive T cell response. Thus, attention is moving toward the construction of artificial heteropolymers of T cell epitopes and B cell epitopes, perhaps coupled to a peptide facilitating fusion with cell membranes to enhance uptake. Such constructs might prime T cells to respond more vigorously when boosted with an inactivated whole-virus vaccine or on natural challenge. This approach may have merit for developing vaccines effective in thoroughbred horses in which the MHC diversity is restricted. Peptide-based vaccines have shown promise in eliciting protection against canine parvovirus, mink parvovirus and foot-and-mouth disease virus infections.

Vaccines Utilizing Anti-idiotypic Antibodies

The antigen-binding site of the antibody produced by each B cell contains a unique amino acid sequence known as its *idiotype* or *idiotypic determinant.* Because anti-idiotypic antibody is capable of binding to the same idiotype as binds the combining epitope on the original antigen, the anti-idiotypic antibody mimics the conformation of that epitope so that anti-idiotypic antibody raised against a neutralizing monoclonal antibody to a particular virus can conceivably be used as a vaccine. Anti-idiotypic antibodies raised against antibodies to the reovirus S1 capsid antigen elicit an antiviral antibody response upon injection into animals, and an anti-idiotypic antibody generated against a T cell receptor for parainfluenza virus 1 (Sendai virus) has been shown to induce both humoral and cell-mediated immune responses in mice. It is still uncertain whether this points the way to a practical vaccine strategy, but there are situations, probably in human rather than veterinary medicine, where such vaccines, if efficacious, would be have advantages over orthodox vaccines, primarily because of their safety.

Vaccines Utilizing Viral DNA ("DNA Vaccines")

Perhaps the most revolutionary new approach to vaccination to emerge from the onward rush of recombinant DNA technology stems from the discovery that viral DNA itself can be used as a vaccine. In the early 1990s, it was observed that a plasmid construct that included the β-galactosidase gene, when inoculated into mouse skeletal muscle, expressed the enzyme for up to 60 days postinoculation. From this early observation, there has been an explosion of interest in the development of DNA vaccines. Experimental vaccines exist for a wide range of applications, including bacterial, viral (Table 13-1), parasitic, antitumor, and antiallergic therapies. Experimentally, the methodology can be applied to screening for protective antigens.

With hindsight, such a discovery may not be that surprising. In 1960, it was shown that cutaneous inoculation of a phenol extract of DNA from Shope papillomavirus induced papilloma in rabbit skin at the site of inoculation. Subsequently, it was shown for many viruses that whole viral DNA, RNA, or cDNA of viral RNA, when transfected into cells, could undergo full cycle viral replication. In principle, the technique is relatively simple; most notably, it cuts out the step of constructing an infectious viral or bacterial vector. Recombinant plasmids are constructed to contain genes capable of expressing viral antigens. The DNA insert in the plasmid, on injection, transfects cells. The expressed protein elicits an immune response that simulates, for the particular antigen of interest, the response elicited by the viral infection. Both humoral and cellular immune responses are detectable. Most importantly, for a growing number of viruses the immune response has been shown to be protective.

DNA vaccines usually consist of an *E. coli* plasmid with a strong promoter, the gene of interest being cloned into a polycloning site, with a polyadenylation/transcriptional termination sequence and a selectable marker (ampicillin resistance). Because it is a strong promoter with broad cell specificity the human cytomegalovirus immediate early promoter is commonly used. The plasmid is amplified, commonly in *E. coli,* purified, suspended in buffered saline, and then simply injected into the host. Cells, initially at least, at the site of injection are transfected by the plasmid; the DNA is transported to the nucleus where the protein of interest is translated. Intramuscular immunization is most effective. It was initially believed that myocytes were transfected and were responsible for sustained antigen production and acted as antigen-presenting cells. It is now believed that "professional" antigen-presenting cells of bone marrow origin are required; these cells infiltrate the site, take up the antigen, and carry them to regional lymph nodes. Direct transfection of antigen-presenting cells, particularly Langerhans cells of the skin, may also occur.

A significant improvement in response to vaccination has been achieved by coating the plasmid DNA onto microparticles, commonly 1- to 3-μm-diameter gold particles, and injecting them by "bombardment" using a helium gas-driven gun-like apparatus (the *gene gun*); less than 1 μg DNA delivered by a gene gun is adequate. As is possible with other recombinant vaccines, the incorporation of genes encoding immunostimulatory proteins, including interleukin 2, interleukin 12, and interferon γ, has been used.

Advantages of DNA vaccines include purity, physiochemical stability, simplicity, a relatively low cost of production, distribution, and delivery, inclusion of multiple antigens in a single plasmid, and expression of antigens in their native form (thereby facilitating processing and presentation to the immune system). Repeated injection may be given without interference and both Th and Tc as well as antibody responses are elicited. One interesting aspect of DNA immunization is that it induces immunity in the presence of maternal antibodies.

Among disadvantages of DNA vaccines is an overriding concern about the fate of the foreign, genetically engineered DNA. Concerns relate to possible integration into chromosomal DNA, leading to insertional mutagenesis or oncogenicity, induction of autoimmune disease including anti-DNA antibodies, and induction of tolerance or breaking of self-tolerance due to sustained expression of antigen. These concerns are being addressed. The plasmids used lack an origin of replication and therefore are not themselves replicated. Plasmids are also designed without sequences that would knowingly enable them to integrate into the chromosomal DNA. For animals that will enter the human food chain, the costs of proving safety will be significant. Table 13.2 summarizes the advantages and limitations of live, inactivated, and DNA vaccines.

Methods for Enhancing Immunogenicity

The immunogenicity of inactivated vaccines, especially that of purified protein vaccines and synthetic peptides, usually needs to be enhanced; this may be achieved by mixing the antigen with an *adjuvant,* incorporation of the antigen in *liposomes,* or incorporation of the antigen in an immunostimulating complex (ISCOM).

Adjuvants

Adjuvants are formulations that, when mixed with vaccines, potentiate the immune response, both humoral and/or cellular, so that a lesser quantity of antigen and/or fewer doses will suffice. Adjuvants differ greatly in their chemistry and in their modes of action, which may include (1) prolongation of release of antigen; (2) activation of macrophages, leading to secretion of lymphokines and attraction of lymphocytes; and (3) mitogenicity for lymphocytes. The adjuvants used most widely in animal vaccines are alum and mineral oils. One of the most promising new adjuvants being developed is muramyl dipeptide, which can be coupled to synthetic antigens or incorporated into liposomes.

Liposomes and Immunostimulating Complexes

Liposomes consist of artificial lipid membrane spheres into which viral proteins can be incorporated. When purified viral envelope proteins are used, the resulting "virosomes" (or "immunosomes") resemble somewhat the original envelope of the virion. This enables not only a reconstitution of virus envelope-like structures lacking nucleic acid and other viral components, but also allows the incorporation of nonpyrogenic lipids with adjuvant activity.

When viral envelope glycoproteins or synthetic peptides are mixed with cholesterol plus a glycoside known as Quil A, spherical cage-like structures 40 nm in diameter are formed. Several veterinary vaccines based on ISCOM technology have reached the market.

Factors Affecting Vaccine Efficacy and Safety

Attenuated virus vaccines delivered by mouth or nose depend critically for their efficacy on replication in the intestinal or respiratory tract, respectively. Interference can occur between the vaccine virus and enteric or respiratory viruses incidentally infecting the animal at the time of vaccination. In the past, interference occurred between different attenuated viruses contained in certain vaccine formulations (e.g., bluetongue vaccines). Canine parvovirus infection may be immunosuppressive to such an extent that it interferes with the response of dogs to vaccination against canine distemper.

In much of the world, vaccines are made under a broad set of guidelines, termed *Good Manufacturing Practices (GMP).* Properly prepared and tested, all vaccines should be safe in immunocompetent animals. As a minimum standard, licensing authorities insist on rigorous safety tests for residual infectious virus in inactivated virus vaccines. There are other safety problems that are unique to attenuated virus vaccines.

Immunologic Considerations

The objective of vaccination is to protect against disease and ideally to prevent infection and virus transmission within the population at risk. If infection with wild-type virus occurs as immunity wanes following vaccination, the infection is likely to be subclinical, but it will boost immunity. For endemic viruses, this is a frequent occurrence in farm animals and birds in crowded pens.

IgA is the most important class of immunoglobulin relevant to the prevention of infection of mucosal surfaces, such as those of the intestinal, respiratory, genitourinary, and ocular epithelia.

One of the advantages of an oral attenuated virus vaccine, such as Newcastle disease vaccine, is that by virtue of its replication in the intestinal tract, it leads to prolonged synthesis of local IgA antibody. By preventing infection, such a vaccine regimen may make feasible the prospect of eradication of the virus from the local population.

Immunity to reinfection is virtually lifelong following infection with most viruses that reach their target organ(s) via systemic (viremic) spread. This solid immunity is attributable to antibody of the IgG class, which successfully neutralizes any virus to which an animal is reexposed. Immunity to those respiratory and enteric viruses whose pathogenic effects are manifested mainly at the site of entry is attributable mainly to antibodies of the IgA class and tends to be of shorter duration. Thus the principal objective of vaccination is to mimic natural infection, i.e., to elicit a high titer of neutralizing antibodies of the appropriate class, IgG and/or IgA, directed against the relevant epitopes on the virion in the hope of preventing infection.

Special difficulties also attend vaccination against viruses known to establish persistent infections, such as herpesviruses and retroviruses; a vaccine must be outstandingly effective if it is to prevent not only the primary disease, but also the establishment of lifelong latency. Attenuated virus vaccines are generally found to be much more effective in eliciting cell-mediated immunity than inactivated viruses. Further, cell-mediated immunity is the most effective arm of the immune system in modulating, if not eliminating, latent/persistent infections.

Underattenuation

Some attenuated virus vaccines in routine use produce some clinical signs in some animals—in effect, a very mild case of the disease. For example, some early canine parvovirus vaccines that had undergone few cell culture passages were used in an attempt to overcome residual maternal immunity, but were found to produce an unacceptably high incidence of disease. Attempts to attenuate virulence further by additional passages in cultured cells have been accompanied by a decline in the capacity of the virus to replicate in the vaccinated animal, with a corresponding loss of immunogenicity.

Such side effects, as occur with current animal virus vaccines, are minimal and do not constitute a significant disincentive to vaccination. However, it is important that attenuated virus vaccines are used only in the species for which they were produced; for example, canine distemper vaccines cause fatalities in some members of the family *Mustelidae,* such as the black footed ferret, where an inactivated whole virus vaccine must be used.

Genetic Instability

Some vaccine strains may revert toward virulence during replication in the recipient or in contact animals to which the vaccine virus has spread. Most vaccine viruses are incapable of such spread, but in those that do there may be an accumulation of back mutations that gradually leads to a restoration of virulence. The principal example of this phenomenon is the very rare reversion to virulence of Sabin poliovirus type 3 oral vaccine in humans, but temperature-sensitive mutants of bovine viral diarrhea virus have also proven to be genetically unstable.

Heat Lability

Live-virus vaccines are vulnerable to inactivation by high ambient temperatures, a particular problem in the tropics. Because most tropical countries also have underdeveloped veterinary services, formidable problems are encountered in maintaining the "cold chain" from manufacturer to the point of administration to animals in remote, hot, rural areas. To some extent the problem has been alleviated by the addition of stabilizing agents to the vaccines, selection of vaccine strains that are inherently more heat stable, and by packaging them in freeze-dried form for reconstitution immediately before administration. Simple portable refrigerators for use in vehicles and temporary field laboratories are invaluable. The control of rinderpest in West Africa is a classical case study of this approach.

Contaminating Viruses

Because vaccine virsuses are grown in animals or cells derived from them, there is always a possibility that a vaccine will be contaminated with another virus from that animal or from the medium used for culturing its cells. An early example, which led to restrictions on international trade in vaccines and sera that are still in effect, was the introduction into the United States in 1908 of foot-and-mouth disease virus as a contaminant of smallpox vaccine produced in calves. The use of embryonated eggs to produce vaccines for use in chickens may pose problems (e.g., the contamination of Marek's disease vaccine with reticuloendotheliosis virus). Another important source of viral contaminants is bovine fetal calf serum, used universally in cell cultures; all batches must be screened for contamination with bovine viral diarrhea virus. Likewise, porcine parvovirus is a common contaminant of crude preparations of trypsin prepared from pig pancreases, which is used commonly in the preparation of animal cell cultures. The risk of contaminating viruses is greatest with live-virus vaccines, but may also occur with inactivated whole virus vaccines, as some viruses are more resistant to inactivation than others.

Adverse Effects in Pregnant Animals

Attenuated virus vaccines are not generally recommended for use in pregnant animals because they may be abortigenic or teratogenic. For example, many infectious bovine rhinotracheitis vaccines are abortigenic, and feline panleukopenia, hog cholera, bovine viral diarrhea, Rift Valley fever, and bluetongue vaccines are teratogenic. These adverse effects are usually due to primary immunization of a nonimmune pregnant animal. Proprietors of large dog and cat breeding establishments often wish to boost antibody titers in pregnant animals, especially to parvovirus, so as to provide high antibody levels for maternal transfer, but it is better to immunize the dam just before mating or use inactivated virus vaccine. Contaminating viruses in vaccines sometimes go unnoticed until used in pregnant animals. The discovery that bluetongue virus contamination of canine vaccines caused abortion and death in pregnant bitches was unexpected.

Adverse Effects from Nonreplicating Vaccines

Some inactivated whole virus vaccines have been found to potentiate disease. The earliest observations were made with inactivated vaccines for measles and human respiratory syncytial virus. In veterinary medicine, attempts to produce a vectored vaccine for the coronavirus that causes feline infectious peritonitis illustrate the problem. A recombinant vaccinia virus that expressed the coronavirus E2 protein was used to immunize kittens. Despite the production of neutralizing antibodies, the kittens were not protected; when challenged, they died quickly of feline infectious peritonitis, probably because of antibody-dependent enhancement of the disease. While not studied in such detail, eastern equine encephalitis in young horses, previously vaccinated with formalin-inactivated virus, has many similarities to the earlier problems seen with human respiratory syncytial vaccines.

Vaccination Frequency and Inoculation Site Reactions

In veterinary medicine, beyond the primary vaccination schedule, there is no general consensus on how often animals need to be revaccinated. For most vaccines, there is comparatively little information available on the duration of immunity. For example, it is well recognized that immunity following attenuated canine distemper vaccine is of long duration, perhaps lifelong. However, the duration of immunity to other viruses or components in a combined vaccine may not be of such long duration. In companion animal practice the cost of vaccination, relative to other costs, is small when clients visit their veterinarian, so it has been argued that if revaccination does no harm it may be considered a justified component of the routine annual "checkup" in which a wide spectrum of health care needs may be addressed. In many countries, annual revaccination has become a cornerstone of broad-based companion animal preventive health-care programs.

This rationale was disturbed in the mid-1990s by reports of subcutaneous fibrosarcomas in cats at sites (often behind the shoulder) corresponding to actual or possible vaccination sites—more than 3000 instances have been reported. These occurrences have not been fully explained: there are still several epidemiological questions that need to be answered, including true incidence (the fibrosarcomas are relatively infrequent), type of vaccines involved (inactivated, alum-adjuvanted vaccines, mainly feline leukemia and rabies vaccines have been incriminated), frequency of vaccination, and other possible cofactor correlations. In any case, however, these occurrences have reopened the issue of revaccination. In the United States, for many companion animal vaccines there have been new recommendations on the preferred vaccination site, vaccination interval (extended from 1 to 3 years for some vaccines), and systems for reporting adverse responses. In general, vaccine manufactures have supported these recommendations. It remains to be seen whether other issues pertaining to the safety of revaccination when it is not necessary to maintain the immune status of the recipient animal will emerge.

Passive Immunization

Instead of actively immunizing with viral vaccines it is possible to confer short-term protection by the subcutaneous administration of antibody, as immune serum or immunoglobulin. Homologous immunoglobulin is preferred because heterologous protein may provoke a hypersensitivity response. Pooled normal immunoglobulin contains sufficient high concentrations of antibody against all the common viruses that cause systemic disease in the respective species. Higher titers occur in convalescent serum from donor animals that have recovered from infection or have been hyperimmunized by repeated vaccinations; such hyperimmune globulin is the preferred product if available commercially (e.g., for canine distemper and canine parvovirus infection). Passive immunization by subcutaneous injection of antibody is not used routinely in practice.

A more common practice is to vaccinate (preferably using an inactivated virus vaccine) the pregnant dam or female bird approximately 3 weeks before anticipated parturition or egg laying. This provides the offspring with passive (maternal) immunity via antibodies present in the egg (in birds) or in colostrum and milk (in mammals). This is particularly important for diseases in which the major impact occurs during the first few weeks of life, when active immunization of the newborn cannot be accomplished early enough. With avian encephalomyelitis, this strategy is employed for the further reason that the attenuated virus vaccines themselves are pathogenic in young chicks.

Vaccination Policy

Design of Vaccination Programs

Epidemiologic theory is applied less widely in the study of animal diseases than in human diseases. Two possible reasons have been suggested; data on animal disease incidence are more difficult to obtain and theoretical analysis is not promoted so widely.

The optimal design of a veterinary vaccination program depends on both the characteristics of the vaccine and the epidemiology of the virus. Relevant vaccine characteristics are the proportion of those vaccinated that are protected initially, the duration of protection, and the coverage achieved by the vaccination program. The most important epidemiological parameter is the *reproduction number,* R_0; this is defined as the number of secondary cases arising from a single primary case in the absence of any constraints on the spread of infection. Mathematical theory can integrate this information to address such questions as to whether it is possible to eliminate an infection; what proportion of hosts must be vaccinated to achieve this; what age should hosts first be vaccinated; and at what interval, if at all, should hosts be revaccinated. Rabies in foxes and foot-and-mouth disease in cattle have been used as guides to the design of vaccination programs and the general usefulness of the models. The models indicate, as one might expect for diseases that are transmitted directly between animals of the same species, that vaccination has advantages not only for the vaccinated hosts, which are directly protected, but also for unvaccinated hosts. The latter are protected indirectly because opportunities for the transmission of the virus in the population as a whole are reduced.

There is an important threshold defined by the condition $R_0 = 1$. If $R_0 > 1$, each primary case will, on average, produce more than one secondary case and the infection will spread through the host population, leading to an epidemic. Conversely, if $R_0 < 1$, each primary case will, on average, produce less than one secondary case and, although some secondary cases may occur, the infection will tend to die out without a major epidemic. An epidemic is possible only if R_0 is greater than or equal to one.

The value of R_0 for a given virus in a given host population is determined by a number of different factors, including the transmissibility of the virus, the period over which an infected host is infectious, the population density of hosts, and, where appropriate, the density of arthropod vectors and the capacity of the vectors to transmit the virus. The details of these relationships depend on the mode of transmission (e.g., direct contact, venereal, vector-borne transmission). Equations have been developed to take account of the impact of host life expectancy, duration of protection due to maternal antibody, and the duration of protection afforded by a vaccine.

The predictive value of the equations is based on certain assumptions; hosts are considered homogeneous with respect to the epidemiology of infection and the consequences of vaccination. All hosts are considered to be equally exposed and equally susceptible (unless vaccinated) to infection, the assumption being that the populations of infectious and susceptible hosts are perfectly mixed. While these assumptions are rarely satisfied in practice, the approach appears to work well. Other factors that have an impact on the basic R_0 number are stocking density and management practices and variation between host breeds and between virus types. The influences of climate and other environmental factors are difficult to assess. In the case of rabies in foxes in two areas of Belgium, estimates for R_0 were between 2 and 5 and vaccine had a major impact in reducing the incidence of disease with vaccine takes above 90% and a duration of protection of at least 1.5 years compared with a fox mean life expectancy of 2.0 years. The objective was to achieve coverage sufficient to eliminate endemic infection. According to mathematical predictions, the requirement was for 50 to 80% of the foxes to be vaccinated successfully. This was achieved in both areas using vaccine containing baits, and endemic rabies infection was eliminated successfully.

In a second study, outbreaks of foot-and-mouth disease on cattle farms in Saudi Arabia were analyzed. The R_0 was as high as 70 and the vaccine take was in excess of 95%, but the duration of immunity was less than 0.5 years compared with a mean cattle life expectancy of 5.0 years, giving a low vaccine impact (which was lower still with virus antigenically different from the vaccine strain). In these circumstances the mathematical formula predicted that the critical interval between vaccinations to provide herd immunity would be extremely short, perhaps as low as a few days, which was clearly impractical. Although vaccinations were given on some farms at intervals as little as 3 months, the disease was not controlled.

These contrasting examples illustrate the potential for epidemiological theory to provide helpful insights into the predicted consequences of vaccination at the population level, to the interpretation of the results of vaccine trials, and as an aid in the design of optimal vaccination programs.

Economic Considerations

Cost–benefit factors are critical in determining the usage of veterinary vaccines. For example, good vaccines are available for the control of many diseases of swine and poultry, but their costs limit their use to large producers, and the diseases remain endemic elsewhere. Economic constraints are most evident in developing countries. For example, in the 1970s, economic constraints led to the abandonment of vaccination against rinderpest in sub-Saharan Africa, despite the fact that a concerted vaccination program could well have led to regional elimination and eventually to global eradication of this virus.

Because of large markets (economy of scale of production), together with somewhat less stringent licensing requirements, veterinary vaccines are generally less expensive than those used in humans. Some avian viral vaccines cost less than 1 cent per dose; many human (and some veterinary) viral vaccines cost many dollars per dose. The pattern of vaccine usage differs strikingly from country to country, with many of the principal diseases against which vaccines are employed in South Africa, for example, being exotic to the United States.

The decision to use a vaccine is governed by a complex equation, balancing expected extra profit against costs and risks. If the disease is lethal or causes major economic losses, the need for vaccination is clear; both the owners and the vaccine-licensing authorities will accept a risk of occasional quite serious side effects. If, however, the disease is perceived as trivial or economically unimportant, no vaccine would be used. Where equally satisfactory vaccines are available against a particular disease, considerations of cost and ease of administration usually tip the balance (e.g., toward vaccines administered via drinking water in poultry).

Once a disease has been controlled in an area to the point where it is of low incidence, continued vaccination is often difficult to sustain because of fading awareness of the risk. Yet it is essential because a reduction in circulation of wild-type virus leaves nonvaccinated animals highly susceptible by removing the protective effect of repeated subclinical infections. Legislation for compulsory vaccination against particular diseases is perhaps the most effective single measure for maintaining protection in the apparent absence of disease.

Vaccination Schedules

The available range of vaccines, often in multivalent formulations and with somewhat different recommendations from each manufacturer regarding vaccination schedules, means that the practicing veterinarian needs to constantly educate her/himself about vaccine choice and usage. Multivalent vaccine formulations, such as those available for canine distemper/hepatitis/parvovirus/coronavirus/parainfluenza virus/bordetella/leptospirosis for dogs, confer major practical advantages by reducing the number of visits the owner must make to the veterinarian. Also, multivalent vaccines allow more extensive use of vaccines against agents of secondary importance. Unlike the situation in human medicine, however, where there is general agreement on vaccine formulations and schedules for vaccination against all the common viral diseases of childhood, there is no such consensus in veterinary medicine. Furthermore, unlike the situation in human medicine, where there are few vaccine manufacturers, there are many veterinary vaccine manufacturers, each promoting their own products. Some of the principles underlying decisions on vaccination schedules are outlined and tables of schedules for the vaccination of various domestic animals are provided in this chapter.

Optimal Age for Vaccination

The risk of most viral diseases is greatest in young animals. Most vaccines are therefore given during the first 6 months of life. Maternal antibody, whether transferred transplacentally or, as in domestic animals, in the colostrum or via the yolk sac, inhibits the immune response of the newborn or newly hatched to vaccines. Optimally, vaccination should be delayed until the titer of maternal antibody in the young animal has declined to near zero. However, waiting may leave the animal defenseless during the resulting "window of susceptibility." This is life-threatening in crowded, highly contaminated environments or where there is intense activity of arthropod vectors. There are a number of approaches to handling this problem in different animal species, but none is fully satisfactory. The problem is complicated further because young animals do not necessarily respond to vaccines in the same way as older animals do. In horses, for example, antibody responses to inactivated influenza vaccines are poor until recipients become yearlings.

Because the titer of passively acquired antibody in the circulation of newborn animals after receiving colostrum is proportional to that in the dam's blood and because the rate of its subsequent clearance in different animal species is known, it is possible to estimate, for any given maternal antibody titer, the age at which no measurable antibody remains in the offspring. This can be plotted as a nomograph, from which the optimal age of vaccination against any particular disease can be read (Figure 13.2). The method is seldom used, but should be considered for exceptionally valuable animals.

In practice, relatively few vaccine failures are encountered if one simply follows the instructions from the vaccine manufacturers, who have used averaged data on maternal antibody levels and rate of IgG decay in that animal species to estimate an optimal age for vaccination. It is recommended commonly, even in the case of live-virus vaccines, that a number of doses of vaccine be administered, say at monthly intervals, to cover the window of susceptibility in animals with particularly high maternal antibody titers. This precaution is even more relevant to multivalent vaccine formulations because of the differences in maternal antibody levels against each virus.

Dam Vaccination

The aim of vaccination is generally thought of as the protection of the vaccinee. This is usually so, but in the case of certain vaccines (e.g., those for equine abortion virus, rotavirus infection in cattle, parvovirus infection in swine, infectious bursal disease of chickens) the objective is to protect the vaccinee's offspring either *in utero* (e.g., equine abortion) or as a neonate/hatchling. This is achieved by vaccination of the dam. For neonates/hatchlings, the level of maternal antibody transferred in the colostrum and milk or in the egg ensures that the offspring have a protective level of antibody during the critical early days. Since many attenuated virus vaccines are abortigenic or teratogenic, inactivated vaccines are recommended for dam vaccination.

FIGURE 13.2.

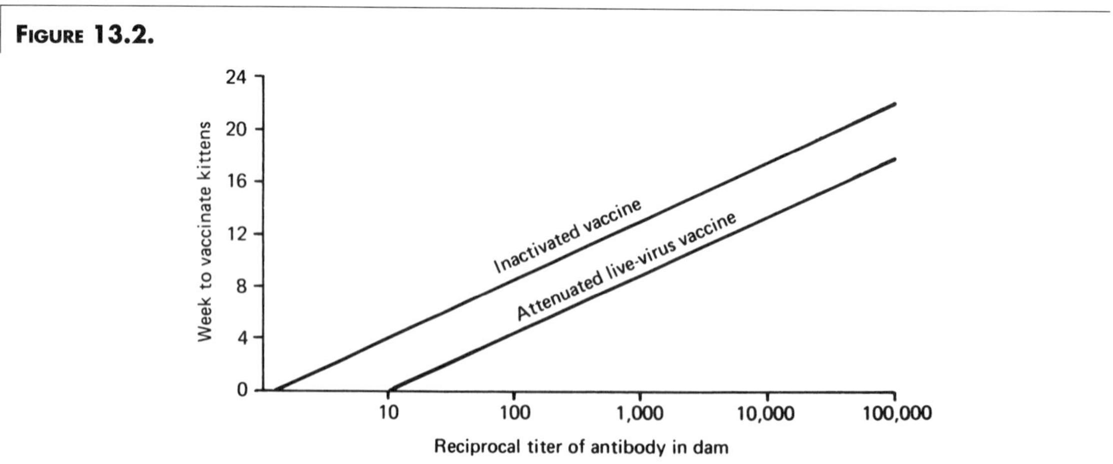

Nomograph indicating optimum times for vaccinating kittens with feline panleukopenia vaccines, based on the antibody titer of the dam and a half-life of IgG in the kitten of 9.5 days. (Courtesy of F. W. Scott.)

TABLE 13.4
Schedule for Vaccination against Viral Diseases of Cattle

VACCINE	BASIC COURSE	REVACCINATION
Attenuated virus vaccines		
Bovine viral diarrhea virus	4–9 months of age (single dose)[a,b]	Annual
Infectious bovine rhinotracheitis virus	3–4 months of age (single dose)	Annual
Rinderpest virus[c]	6–8 months of age (single dose)	None
Respiratory syncytial virus	4–6 months of age (two doses with a 4-week interval)	Annual
Parainfluenza virus 3	4–6 months of age (two doses with a 4-week interval)	Annual
Inactivated virus vaccines		
Foot-and-mouth disease viruses[d]	4 weeks of age (single dose)	4–12 months
Infectious bovine rhinotracheitis virus	3–4 months of age (two doses at a 4-week interval)	6–12 months
Rotaviruses	6–8 weeks and 2 weeks before end of gestation	Each pregnancy
Coronavirus[e]	6–8 weeks and 2 weeks before end of gestation	Each pregnancy
Parainfluenza virus 3, reovirus, various adenoviruses	6 weeks, 3 months, 7 months of age	Annual

[a]When vaccination is carried out at early age, a second dose is recommended because of possible interference with maternal antibodies.
[b]Emergency vaccination: all cattle older than 2 weeks of age except animals during the first trimester of pregnancy.
[c]Only in countries where the disease occurs.
[d]Compulsory in some countries; multivalent vaccine.
[e]Dam vaccination.

In Ovo and Other Vaccination Methods for Chickens

In the United States alone, the annual production of poultry birds exceeds $8 billion. All commercially produced birds are vaccinated against as many as eight different viral diseases. The cost of each dose is usually a fraction of a cent; much of this economy of scale is linked to low-cost delivery systems (aerosol and drinking water). Further economies have been achieved

TABLE 13.5
Schedule for Vaccination against Viral Diseases of Sheep and Goats

VACCINE	BASIC COURSE	REVACCINATION
Attenuated virus vaccines		
Bluetongue viruses[a] (polyvalent vaccines; up to 15 types)	3–6 months of age (two doses with a 3-week interval)	Annual
Sheeppox virus[a]	3 months of age (single dose)	2 years
Rinderpest virus[a] (and peste des petits ruminants virus)	3 months of age (single dose)	None
Wild-type virus vaccines		
Orf virus[b]	2–3 months of age (single dose)	None
Inactivated virus vaccines		
Foot-and-mouth disease viruses[a]	3–4 months of age (single dose)	Annual

[a]Only in countries where the disease occurs.
[b]In some countries; only on properties where scabby mouth is a problem.

Table 13.6
Schedule for Vaccination against Viral Diseases of Swine

Vaccine	Basic course	Revaccination
Attenuated virus vaccines		
Hog cholera virus[a]	8 weeks of age (single dose)	None
Pseudorabies virus[a]	All ages (two doses with a 4-week interval)	4–6 months
Inactivated virus vaccines		
Pseudorabies virus[a]	4 weeks of age (two doses with a 4-week interval)	5–6 months
Porcine polioencephalitis virus[a]	8–12 weeks of age (two doses with a 4-week interval)	None
Porcine parvovirus	Before mating (two doses with a 4-week interval)	Annual
Influenza viruses	Any age (two doses with a 4-week interval)	Annual

[a]Depends on current policy in particular countries.

by the introduction of *in ovo* immunization of 18-day-old embryonated eggs; an instrument (called an Inovoject) capable of immunizing 40,000 eggs per hour, is been used. Thus far, only Marek's disease vaccine, which was formerly inoculated individually into 1-day-old chicks, is delivered in this way, but others vaccines are being explored. In 1997, over 80% of birds in the United States were vaccinated by this method. In rural economies with village chickens, methods have been developed for the delivery of Newcastle disease virus vaccine in feed pellets.

Available and Recommended Vaccines

The types of vaccines available for each viral disease (or the lack of any satisfactory vaccine) are discussed in each chapter of Part II of this book and in the tables in Chapter 42. There are obvious geographic variations in the requirements for particular vaccines (e.g., between some countries in South America where vaccination against foot-and-mouth disease is practiced and the United States where it is not). There are also different requirements

Table 13.7
Schedule for Vaccination against Viral Diseases of Horses

Vaccine	Basic course	Revaccination
Attenuated virus vaccines		
Equine abortion virus (equine herpesvirus 1)	3 months of age (three doses with 2- and 6-month intervals)	9–12 months
Equine arteritis virus[a]	3 months of age (two doses with a 4-week interval)	1–2 years
African horse sickness viruses[a] (polyvalent vaccine)	6–8 months of age (single dose)	2–3 years
Inactivated virus vaccines		
Influenza viruses (bivalent vaccine)	3–5 months of age (three doses with 2- and 6-month intervals)	Every 3–6 months
Eastern, western, and Venezuelan encephalitis viruses	3 months of age (two doses with a 3-week interval)	Annual
Equine abortion virus[b] (equine herpesvirus 1) and equine rhinopneumonitis virus (equine herpesvirus 4)	10 weeks of age (three doses with 1- and 6-month intervals)	6–12 months

[a]Only recommended in areas where the disease occurs.
[b]Also in combination with influenza and reovirus types 1 and 3. Mares should be vaccinated additionally at 5, 7, and 9 months of pregnancy.

TABLE 13.8
Schedule for Vaccination against Viral Diseases of Dogs

VACCINE	BASIC COURSE	REVACCINATION
Attenuated virus vaccines		
Canine distemper virus	6–8 weeks of age (three doses with 3 week intervals)	Every 2 years
Canine hepatitis virus	6–8 weeks of age (three doses with 3 week intervals)	Every 2 years
Canine parvovirus 2[a]	6 weeks of age (three doses with 3 week intervals)	Annual
Inactivated virus vaccines		
Rabies virus	12 weeks of age (single dose)	Annual or every 3 years
Canine parvovirus 2[a]	6–8 weeks of age (three doses with 3 week intervals)	Annual
Canine coronavirus	9–16 weeks of age (three doses with 3 week intervals)	Annual
Parainfluenza viruses	6–8 weeks of age (three doses with 3 week intervals)	Annual

[a]See Chapter 21.

appropriate to various types of husbandry (e.g., for dairy cattle, beef cows, and their calves on range or cattle in feedlots and in poultry for breeders, commercial egg layers, and broilers) (see Tables 13.4 to 13.10).

Chemotherapy of Viral Diseases

If this had been a book about bacterial diseases of domestic animals, there would have been a large section on antimicrobial chemotherapy. However, the antibiotics that have been so effective against bacterial diseases have few counterparts in our armamentarium against viral diseases. The reason is that viruses are intimately dependent on the metabolic pathways of their host cell for their replication, hence most agents that interfere with viral replication are toxic to the cell. In recent years, however, increased knowledge of the biochemistry of viral replication has led to a more rational approach in the search for antiviral chemotherapeutic agents, and a small number of such compounds have now become a standard part of the armamentarium against particular human viruses. As yet there are no specifically antiviral chemotherapeutic

TABLE 13.9
Schedule for Vaccination against Viral Diseases of Cats

VACCINE	BASIC COURSE	REVACCINATION
Attenuated virus vaccines		
Feline panleukopenia virus[a]	6–12 weeks of age (three doses with 3 week intervals)[b]	Annual or every 3 years
Feline calicivirus	6–12 weeks of age (three doses with 3 week intervals)[b]	Annual
Feline herpesvirus	6–12 weeks of age (three doses with 3 week intervals)[b]	Annual
Inactivated virus vaccines		
Feline panleukopenia virus	6–12 weeks of age (three doses with 3 week intervals)	Annual
Rabies virus	12 weeks of age (single dose)	Annual or every 3 years
Feline calicivirus	6–12 weeks of age (three doses with 3 week intervals)	Annual
Feline herpesvirus	6–12 weeks of age (three doses with 3 week intervals)	Annual
Feline leukemia virus (subunit)	9 weeks of age (two doses with 3- to 15-week intervals)	Annual
Feline leukemia virus (whole virus)	10 weeks of age (two doses with a 1-month interval)	Annual

[a]Attenuated panleukopenia virus vaccines should not be used in pregnant cats because of the risk of placental passage of the vaccine virus.
[b]If first vaccination is given at more than 9 weeks of age, only one additional dose is needed.

Table 13.10
Schedule Vaccination against Viral Diseases of Poultry[a]

Age	Vaccine	Route
Broilers		
1 day	Infectious bronchitis virus	Spray
	Newcastle disease virus	Spray (if required)
18 days	Infectious bronchitis virus	Drinking water or spray
	Newcastle disease virus	Drinking water or spray (if required)
Chickens: Broilers, layers, breeders		
3 days before hatching or	Marek's disease virus	*In ovo*
1 day or		Intramuscular injection
3 weeks	Newcastle disease virus	Drinking water
	Infectious bronchitis virus	Drinking water
	Marek's disease virus	Intramuscular injection
8 weeks	Infectious bronchitis virus	Drinking water or spray
	Newcastle disease virus	Drinking water or spray
10 weeks	Infectious bursal disease virus	Drinking water
14 weeks	Avian encephalomyelitis virus	Drinking water
16 weeks	Newcastle disease virus	Intramuscular injection
	Infectious bronchitis virus	Intramuscular injection
	Infectious bursal disease virus	Intramuscular injection
Chickens: Layers		
3 days before hatching or	Marek's disease virus	*In ovo*
1 day or		Intramuscular injection
3 weeks	Newcastle disease virus	Drinking water or spray
	Infectious bronchitis virus	Drinking water or spray
7 weeks	Infectious bronchitis virus	Drinking water or spray
	Newcastle disease virus	Drinking water or spray
10 weeks	Avian encephalomyelitis virus	Drinking water
14 weeks	Newcastle disease virus	Intramuscular injection
	Infectious bronchitis virus	Intramuscular injection
	Egg drop syndrome virus	Intramuscular injection
Turkeys: Breeders		
3 weeks	Newcastle disease virus	Spray
6 weeks	Newcastle disease virus	Spray
12 weeks	Newcastle disease virus	Intramuscular injection
	Paramyxovirus 3 virus	Intramuscular injection
24 weeks	Newcastle disease virus	Intramuscular injection
	Paramyxovirus 3 virus	Intramuscular injection

[a]All are attenuated live-virus vaccines except those for egg drop syndrome and infectious bursal disease virus used at 16 weeks for broiler or layer breeders.

agents in common use in veterinary practice, partly because of the very high cost. Several antiviral drugs are now in use in human medicine and the day is sure to come when they are cost effective for veterinary medicine. Accordingly it is appropriate to outline briefly some potential developments in this field.

Strategy for Development of Antiviral Agents

Several steps in the viral replication cycle (see Chapter 3) represent potential targets for selective antiviral drug attack. Theoretically, all virus-coded enzymes are vulnerable, as are all processes (enzymatic or nonenzymatic) that are more essential to the replication of the virus than to the survival of the cell. Table 13.11 sets out the most vulnerable steps and provides examples of antiviral drugs that display activity, indicating those that have already been licensed for use in humans.

A logical approach to the development of new antiviral drugs is to isolate or synthesize substances that might be predicted to serve as inhibitors of a known virus-coded enzyme such as a transcriptase, replicase, or protease. Analogs of this prototype drug are then synthesized with a view to enhancing activity and/or selectivity. A further refinement of this approach is well illustrated by the nucleoside analog acycloguanosine (Acyclovir), an inhibitor of herpesvirus DNA polymerase. Acyclovir is in fact an inactive *prodrug* that requires another herpesvirus-coded enzyme, thymidine kinase, to phosphorylate it to its active form. Because this viral enzyme occurs only in infected cells, Acyclovir is nontoxic for uninfected cells, but very effective in herpesvirus-infected cells. So far, such drugs have found only limited use in veterinary medicine (e.g., for treatment of feline herpesvirus 1 corneal ulcers), but again this will surely change.

Table 13.11
Possible Targets for Antiviral Chemotherapy in Veterinary Medicine

Target	Prototype drug
Attachment of virion to cell receptor	Receptor analogs
Uncoating	Rimantadine[a]
Primary transcription from viral genome	Transcriptase inhibitors
Reverse transcription	Zidovudine—AZT[a]
Regulation of transcription	Lentivirus tat inhibitors
Processing of RNA transcripts	Ribavirin[a]
Translation of viral mRNA into protein	Interferons[a]
Posttranslational cleavage of proteins	Protease inhibitors
Replication of viral DNA genome	Acycloguanosine (Acyclovir[a])
Replication of viral RNA genome	Replicase inhibitors

[a]Licensed for human use.

X-ray crystallography has opened a major new approach in the search for antiviral drugs. Now that the three-dimensional structure of many icosahedral virions, such as those of picornaviruses, is known, it has been possible to characterize receptor-binding sites on capsid proteins at the atomic level of resolution. Complexes of viral proteins with bound cellular receptors can be crystallized and examined directly. For example, for some rhinoviruses, receptor-binding sites on virions are in "canyons," i.e., clefts in the capsid surface. Drugs have been found that fit into these clefts, thereby preventing viral attachment to the host cell. Further information is provided by mapping the position of the particular amino acid residues that form these clefts, thereby allowing the design of drugs that better fit and better interfere with the viral infection process. This approach also lends itself to the development of drugs that block viral penetration of the host cell or uncoating once inside. Of course, the close similarity between human rhinoviruses and important animal pathogens, such as foot-and-mouth disease viruses and equine rhinoviruses, means that as human drugs come closer to licensing, adaptation to veterinary usage may follow.

Further Reading

Ada, G. L. (1998). Vaccines. *In* "Encyclopedia of Virology," (R. G. Webster and A. Granoff, eds.), 2nd ed. (CD-ROM). Academic Press, London.

American Veterinary Medical Association. (1985). Guidelines for vaccination of horses. *J. Am. Vet. Med. Assoc.* **185**, 32–36.

American Veterinary Medical Association. (1989). Canine and feline immunization guidelines. *J. Am. Vet. Med. Assoc.* **195**, 314–316.

Anderson, R. M., and May, R. M. (1991). "Infectious Diseases of Humans: Dynamics and Control." Oxford University Press, New York.

Anonymous. (1992). "International Symposium on the First Steps Towards an International Harmonization of Veterinary Biologicals." International Association of Biological Standardization and Office International des Epizooties. Karger, Basel.

Babiuk, L. A., van Drunen Little-van den Hurk, S., Tikoo, S. K., Lewis, P. J., and Liang, X. (1996). Novel viral vaccines for livestock. *Vet. Immunol. Immunopathol.* **54**, 355–363.

Bittle, J. L., and Muir, S. (1989). Vaccines produced by conventional means to control major infectious diseases of man and animals. *Adv. Vet. Sci. Comp. Med.* **33**, 1–64.

Bittle, J. L., and Murphy, F. A. eds. (1989). Vaccine biotechnology. *Adv. Vet. Sci. Comp. Med.* **33**, 1–444.

Brown, F., ed. (1985–1998). "Vaccines '85–'98: Molecular Approaches to the Control of Infectious Diseases (published annually)." Cold Spring Harbor Laboratory Press, Cold Spring Harbor, NY.

Brown, F. ed. (1991). Impact of biotechnology on protection against infectious diseases. *World J. Microbiol. Biotechnol.* **7**, 105–109.

Coyne, M. J., Reeves, N. C. P., and Rosen, D. K. (1997). Estimated prevalence of injection-site sarcomas in cats during 1992. *J. Am. Vet. Med. Assoc.* **210**, 249–251.

De Clercq, E. (1993). Antiviral agents: Characteristic activity spectrum depending on the molecular target with which they interact. *Adv. Virus Res.* **42**, 1–56.

Donnelly, J. J., Ulmer, J. B., Shiver, J. W., and Liu, M. A. (1997). DNA vaccines. *Annu. Rev. Immunol.* **15**, 617–648.

Green, C. E. (1998). "Infectious Diseases of the Dog and Cat, 2nd Edition," W. B. Saunders, Philadelphia, PA.

Morein, B., Villacres-Erikisson, M., Sjoülander, A., and Bengtsson, K. L. (1996). Novel adjuvants and vaccine delivery systems. *Vet. Immunol. Immunopathol.* **54**, 373–384.

Mowat, N., and Rweyemamu, M. (1997). "Vaccine Manual: The Production and Quality Control of Veterinary Vaccines for Use in Developing Countries." Food and Agriculture Organization of the United Nations, Rome.

Murphy, B. R., and Chanock, R. M. (1996). Immunization against virus disease. *In* "Fields Virology," (B. N. Fields, D. M. Knipe, P. M. Howley, R. M. Chanock, J. L. Melnick, T. P. Monath, B. Roizman, and S. E. Straus, eds.), 3rd ed., pp. 467–498. Lippincott-Raven, Philadelphia, PA.

Ogra, P. L., and Garofalo, R. (1990). Secretory antibody response to viral vaccines. *Prog. Med. Virol.* **37**, 156–179.

Paoletti, E. (1996). Applications of pox virus vectors to vaccination: An update. *Proc. Nat. Acad. Sci. U.S.A.* **93**, 11349–11353.

Peters, A. R., ed. (1993). "Vaccines for Veterinary Applications." Butterworth-Heinemann, Oxford.

Powell, D. G. (1996). Epidemiology and control of equine viral disease. *In* "Virus Infections of Vertebrates" (M. J. Studdert, ed.), Vol. 6. Chapter 22. Elsevier, Amsterdam.

van Regenmortel, M. H. V., and Neurath, A. R., eds. (1985, 1991). "The Basis for Serodiagnosis and Vaccines. Immunochemistry of Viruses," Vol. 1 and 2. Elsevier, Amsterdam.

White, D. O., and Fenner, F. (1993). Chemotherapy of viral diseases. *In* "Medical Virology," 4 ed. Academic Press, Orlando, FL.

Woodhouse, M. E. J., Haydon, D. T., and Bundy, A. P. (1997). The design of veterinary vaccination programmes. *Vet. J.* **153**, 41–47.

CHAPTER 14

Epidemiology of Viral Diseases

Epidemiology is the study of the determinants, dynamics, and distribution of diseases in populations. The risk of infection and/or disease in an animal or animal population is determined by characteristics of the virus (e.g., antigenic variation), the host and host population (e.g., innate and acquired resistance), and behavioral, environmental, and ecological factors that affect virus transmission from one host to another. Epidemiology, which is part of the science of population biology, attempts to meld these factors into a unified whole.

Although originally derived from the root term *demos,* meaning people, the word epidemiology is widely used now no matter what host is concerned, and the words endemic, epidemic, and pandemic are used to characterize disease states in populations, whether of humans or other animals. By introducing quantitative measurements of disease trends, epidemiology has come to have a major role in advancing our understanding of the nature of diseases and in alerting and directing disease control activities. Epidemiologic study is also effective in clarifying the role of viruses in the etiology of diseases, in understanding the interaction of viruses with environmental determinants of disease, in determining factors affecting host susceptibility, in unraveling modes of transmission, and in large-scale testing of vaccines and drugs.

Computations and Databases

Calculations of Rates

The comparison of disease experience in different populations is expressed in the form of rates. Multipliers (e.g., rates per 10^n) are used to provide rates that are manageable whole numbers—the most common rate multiplier used is 100,000, i.e., the given rate is expressed per 100,000 of the given population. Four rates are most widely used: the *incidence rate,* the *prevalence rate,* the *morbidity rate,* and the *mortality rate.* In all four rates the denominator (total number of animals at risk) may be as general as the total population in a state or country or as specific as the population known to be susceptible or at risk (e.g., the number of animals in a specified population that lack antibodies to the virus of interest). In each situation it is imperative that the nature of the denominator is made clear—indeed, epidemiology has been called "the science of the denominator." Each of these rates may be affected by various attributes that distinguish one individual animal from another: age, sex, genetic constitution, immune status, nutrition, pregnancy, and various behavioral parameters. The most widely applicable attribute is age, which may encompass, and can therefore be confounded by, the animal's immune status as well as by various physiologic variables.

Incidence Rate

Incidence rate

$$= \frac{\text{number of cases} \times 10^n}{\text{population at risk}} \text{ in a specified period of time}$$

The incidence rate, or *attack rate,* is a measure of the occurrence of infection or disease in a population over time, e.g., a month or a year, and is especially useful for describing acute diseases of short duration. For acute infections, three parameters determine the incidence of infection or disease in a population: the percentage of susceptible animals, the percentage of susceptible animals that are infected, and the percentage of infected animals that suffer disease. The percentage of animals susceptible to a specific virus reflects their past history of exposure to that virus and the duration of their immunity. The percentage infected during a year or a season may vary considerably, depending on factors such as animal numbers and density, season, and, for arbovirus infections, the vector population. Of those infected, only some may develop overt disease. The ratio of clinical to subclinical (inapparent) infections varies greatly with different viruses. The *secondary attack rate,* when applied to comparable, relatively closed groups such as herds or flocks, is a useful measure of the "infectiousness" of viruses transmitted by aerosols or droplets. It is defined as the number of animals in contact with the primary or *index case(s)* that become infected or sick within the maximum incubation period as a percentage of the total number of susceptible animals exposed to the virus.

Prevalence Rate

Prevalence rate

$$= \frac{\text{number of cases} \times 10^n}{\text{population at risk}} \text{ at a particular time}$$

It is difficult to measure the incidence of chronic diseases, especially where the onset is insidious, and for such diseases it is customary to determine the prevalence rate, i.e., the ratio, at a particular point in time of the number of cases currently present in the population divided by the number of animals in the population; it is a snapshot of the occurrence of infection or disease at a given time.

The prevalence rate is thus a function of both the incidence rate and the duration of the disease. *Seroprevalence* relates to the occurrence of antibody to a particular virus in a population. Because neutralizing antibodies often last for many years, or even for life, seroprevalence rates usually represent the cumulative experience of a population with a given virus.

Morbidity Rate

The morbidity rate is the percentage of animals in a population that develop disease attributable to a particular virus over a defined period of time (commonly the duration of an outbreak).

Mortality Rate

Mortality from a disease can be categorized in two ways: the *cause-specific mortality rate* (the number of deaths from the disease in a given year, divided by the total population at midyear), usually expressed per 100,000 population, or the *case-fatality rate* (the percentage of animals with a particular disease that die from the disease).

Other Terms and Concepts Used in Epidemiology

Endemic disease refers to the presence of multiple or continuous chains of transmission resulting in the continuous occurrence of disease in a population over a period of time.

Epidemic disease refers to peaks in disease incidence that exceed the endemic baseline or expected incidence of disease. The size of the peak required to constitute an epidemic is arbitrary and is influenced by the background infection rate, the morbidity rate, and the anxiety that the disease arouses because of its clinical severity or potential economic impact. Thus, a few cases of velogenic Newcastle disease in a poultry flock might be regarded as an epidemic, whereas a few cases of infectious bronchitis would not be.

Pandemic disease refers to worldwide epidemics, such as the canine parvovirus pandemic that swept around the world in the early 1980s.

Note: the terms *enzootic, epizootic,* and *panzootic* have often been used for diseases of animals, but, in this book, in keeping with modern usage, the general terms *endemic, epidemic,* and *pandemic* are used when referring to diseases of both animals and humans.

Incubation period refers to the interval between infection and the onset of clinical signs. In many diseases there is a period of a day or so during which animals are infectious before they become sick.

Period of contagiousness refers to the time during which an infected animal sheds virus. This period varies depending on the disease concerned. For example, in lentivirus infections such as feline immunodeficiency virus infection, animals shed virus for a very long period before showing clinical signs. In such infections the amount of virus shed may be very small, but because the period of infectivity is so long, the virus is maintained readily in the population.

Seroepidemiology simply denotes the use of serological data as the basis of epidemiological investigation. Serological techniques employed are outlined in Chapter 12. Seroepidemiology is extremely useful in veterinary disease control operations and in veterinary research. Because of the expense of collecting and storing sera properly, advantage is often taken of a wide range of sources of representative serum samples, such as abattoirs, culling operations (especially useful for assessment of wildlife populations), and vaccination programs. Such sera can be used to determine the prevalence or incidence of particular infections, to evaluate eradication and immunization programs, and to assess the impact, dynamics, and geographic distribution of new, emerging, and reemerging viruses. By detecting antibodies to selected viruses in various age groups of the population, it is possible to determine how effectively viruses have spread or how long it has been since the last appearance of a particular virus in the population. Correlation of serologic data with clinical observations makes it possible to determine the ratio of clinical to subclinical infections.

Molecular epidemiology denotes the use of molecular biological data as the basis of epidemiological investigation. Many of the molecular diagnostic techniques described in Chapter 12 are used. For example, with DNA viruses (e.g., pseudorabies virus and equine herpesvirus 1), restriction endonuclease fingerprinting, nucleic acid hybridization, and other approaches to genome mapping are used for the identification of field isolates with a precision that surpasses serologic methods. With viruses that have segmented double-stranded RNA genomes, such as orbiviruses and rotaviruses, polyacrylamide gel electrophoresis of genomic RNA is used to characterize isolates as to genotype—this level of specificity is valuable in tracking the introduction and relative prevalence of different viral genotypes in livestock populations. Other techniques, such as partial sequencing, the polymerase chain reaction (with identification of amplified products), and oligonucleotide fingerprinting, are also used to characterize viral variants among large numbers of isolates that might be considered homogeneous by serology. For example, the 1981 outbreak of foot-and-mouth disease in the United Kingdom was traced by oligonucleotide fingerprinting to the presence of a residual infectious virus in a vaccine being used in France.

Determining the occurrence of a particular disease in a given animal population is more difficult than the computation of the rates just described. The denominator, i.e., the number of animals in the population at risk, is often impossible to calculate or estimate accurately. Determining the number of cases of the disease may also prove impossible. Where such information is regarded as essential, government regulations may declare a disease to be *notifiable,* requiring veterinarians to report all cases to authorities. For example, suspicion of the presence of foot-and-mouth disease is notifiable in virtually all developed countries.

Types of Epidemiologic Investigation

Conceptual Framework

The *case-control study,* the *cohort study,* the *cross-sectional study,* and the *long-term herd study* provide the conceptual framework upon which can be determined the relationships between cause and effect, the incidence and prevalence of disease, the evaluation of risk factors of disease, the safety and efficacy of vaccines, and the therapeutic value of vaccines and drugs.

Case-Control Studies

Case-control studies are *retrospective,* i.e., investigation starts after the disease episode has occurred. In human disease epidemiology, this is the most common type of study, often used to identify the cause of a disease outbreak. Advantages of retrospective studies are that they make use of existing data and are relatively inexpensive to carry out. In many instances they are the only practicable method of investigating rare occurrences. Although case-control studies do not require the creation of new data or records, they do require careful selection of the control group, carefully matched to the subject group, so as to avoid bias. Because necessary records are generally not available in most animal disease outbreaks, this can present irresolvable difficulties in veterinary medicine.

Cohort Studies

Cohort studies are *prospective* or *longitudinal,* i.e., investigation starts with a presumed disease episode, say a suspected viral disease outbreak, and with a population exposed to the suspected causative virus. The population is monitored for evidence of the disease. This type of study requires the creation of new data and records. It also requires careful selection of the control group, designing it to be as similar as possible to the exposed group except for the absence of contact with the presumed causative virus. Cohort studies do not lend themselves to quick analysis as groups must be followed until disease is observed, often for long periods of time. This makes such studies expensive. However, when cohort studies are successful, proof of cause–effect relationships is usually incontrovertible.

Once the causal agent is identified, and serological and other diagnostic tests have been developed, case-control and cohort studies can progress to cross-sectional and long-term herd studies.

Cross-Sectional Studies

When the cause of a specific disease is known, a cross-sectional study can be carried out relatively quickly using serology and/or virus identification. This provides data on the prevalence of the particular disease/infection in a population in a specific area.

Long-Term Herd Studies

Long-term herd studies are another kind of epidemiologic investigation that can provide unique information about the presence and continued activity (or lack of activity) of a given virus in an area. They can be regarded as a series of cross-sectional studies. They can also be designed to provide information on the value of vaccines or therapeutic drugs. Despite automation of diagnostic methods and computerization of data files, such studies are still very expensive and require long-term dedication of both personnel and funds. When used for evaluating vaccines or therapeutic agents, long-term herd studies have the advantage that they include all of the variables attributable to the entire husbandry system.

When used to determine the introduction of a particular virus into a population in a given area, such investigations are referred to as *sentinel studies.* For example, such studies are widely used for determining the initial introduction of arboviruses into high-risk areas—sentinel animals, usually chickens, are bled at weekly intervals and sera are tested serologically for the first evidence of viral activity. The first seroconversions often presage infection of horses, other animals, and humans by several weeks, enough time to initiate vector control actions.

Examples of How Various Kinds of Epidemiological Investigations Are Used in Prevention and Control of Viral Diseases

Investigating Causation of Disease

The original investigations of the production of congenital defects in cattle by Akabane virus provide examples of both case-control and cohort studies. Case-control studies of epidemics of congenital defects in calves, characterized by deformed limbs and abnormal brain development [referred to as congenital arthrogryposis-hydranencephaly (see Chapter 31)], were carried out in Australia in the 1950s and 1960s, but the cause of the disease was not identified. During the summer and early winter months from 1972 to 1975, approximately 42,000 calves were born with these congenital defects in central and western Japan, causing significant economic loss. Japanese scientists postulated that the disease was infectious, but were unable to isolate a virus from affected calves. However, when precolostral sera from such calves were tested for antibody to a number of viruses, antibody to Akabane virus, a bunyavirus, which was first isolated from mosquitoes in Akabane Prefecture in Japan in 1959, was found in almost all sera. A retrospective serologic survey indicated a very high correlation between the geographic distribution of the disease and the presence of antibody to the virus, suggesting that Akabane virus was the etiologic agent of the congenital arthrogryposis-hydranencephaly in cattle. Cohort (prospective) studies were then organized. Sentinel herds were established in Japan and Australia, and it was soon found that the virus could be isolated from fetuses obtained by slaughter or cesarean section for only a short period after infection, thus explaining earlier failures in attempts to isolate virus after calves were born. Experimental inoculation of pregnant cows with Akabane virus during the first two trimesters resulted in congenital abnormalities in calves similar to those seen in natural cases of the disease; clinical signs were not seen in the cows. Following these studies and estimates of the economic impact of the disease, a vaccine was developed and control programs were set in place, which are still being used.

Investigating Geographical Distribution and Genetic Variation of Viruses

The concerted investigations of veterinary scientists in many countries interested in understanding the global epidemiology of bluetongue virus (an orbivirus; Chapter 24) illustrate the use of cross-sectional and long-term herd studies and the application of both seroepidemiology and molecular epidemiology. Bluetongue of sheep was considered an emerging disease of great international importance from the late-1950s to the mid-1980s; evidence of the presence of the virus in a country was used as a *nontariff trade barrier,* i.e., a means to curtail unwanted international trade in animal products, breeding animals, and germ plasm. For example, bluetongue virus 20 was isolated from collections of *Culicoides* spp. in Australia in 1977 and bluetongue virus 2 from similar collections in Florida in 1983, in each case without any disease being recognized. Serologic surveys were used to determine the geographic distribution of both viruses; stored sera were used to estimate how long the viruses had been present. Using long-term herd studies, which relied heavily on sentinel animals and extended respectively into countries to the north of Australia and into the Caribbean region from Florida, it was discovered that there were several additional serotypes of bluetongue virus present in each region. Further, these studies confirmed that clinical signs were rarely, if ever, seen and established that different species of *Culicoides* spp. vectors were able to transmit the virus in different regions of the world. Molecular techniques were used to monitor the evolution of the viruses within each region; from data generated, it was concluded that bluetongue had been present in these ecosystems for a considerable time and that the presence of the virus did not constitute an "emerging disease" threat. Import regulations were changed by some countries and international trade expanded in some instances on the basis of these discoveries.

Vaccine Trials

The immunogenicity, potency, safety, and efficacy of vaccines are first studied in laboratory animals, followed by small-scale closed trials in the target animal species, and finally by large-scale open field trials. In the latter, epidemiologic methods like those employed in cohort studies are used. There is no alternative way to evaluate new vaccines, and the design of field trials has now been developed so that they yield maximum information with minimum risk and cost. Even with this system, however, a serious problem may be recognized only after a vaccine has been licensed for commercial use. This occurred after the introduction of attenuated virus vaccines for infectious bovine rhinotracheitis (caused by bovine herpesvirus 1) in the United States in the 1950s. Surprisingly, the vaccines had been in use for 5 years before it was recognized that abortion was a common sequel to vaccination. Case-control and cohort studies confirmed the causal relationship.

Mathematical Modeling

From the time of William Farr, who studied both medical and veterinary problems in the 1840s, mathematicians have been interested in "epidemic curves" and secular trends in the incidence of infectious diseases. With the development of mathematical modeling using the computer there has been a resurgence of interest in the dynamics of infectious diseases within populations. Because modeling involves predictions about future occurrences of diseases, models carry a degree of uncertainty; skeptics have said that "for every model there is an equal and opposite model," but in recent years models have played an increasing role in directing disease control activities.

Mathematical models have been developed to predict various epidemiologic parameters, such as (1) critical population sizes required to support the continuous transmission of animal viruses with short and long incubation periods; (2) the dynamics of endemicity of viruses that establish persistent infection; and (3) the important variables in age-dependent viral pathogenicity. Computer modeling also provides insights into the effectiveness of disease control programs. In this regard, most attention has been given to the potential national and international spread of exotic virus diseases. Figure 14.1 illustrates the modeling of an outbreak of foot-and-mouth disease in the United States, commencing with the introduction of the virus and progressing through discovery of its presence to the stage where the disease becomes well established and traditional control measures (quarantine, slaughter, and disinfection) become ineffective. The model suggests that in the so-called "worst-case scenario," 60% of the cattle herds in the United States could become infected within a 30-week period. In this model, if it were decided not to vaccinate or if sufficient vaccine of the correct antigenic type were not available, the disease would increase again in incidence after 60 weeks and begin a series of endemic cycles.

Such models bring a number of issues into focus. The results are often unexpected, pointing to the need for better data and different strategies for disease control. They are also dependent on detailed information on the mechanisms of virus transmission and virus survival in nature as is now discussed.

Virus Transmission

Viruses survive in nature only if they can be transmitted from one host to another, whether of the same or another species (Table 14.1). Transmission cycles require virus entry into the body, replication, and shedding with subsequent spread to another host. These basic aspects of viral activity are described in relation to individual animal hosts in Chapters 3 and 6; aspects relevant to the spread of viruses in populations are covered here.

Virus transmission may be *horizontal* or *vertical.* Vertical transmission describes transmission from dam to offspring. However, most transmission is horizontal, i.e., between animals within the population at risk, and can occur via direct contact, indirect contact, or a common vehicle or may be airborne, vector-borne, or iatrogenic. Some viruses are transmitted in nature via several modes, others exclusively via one mode.

Horizontal Transmission

Direct Contact Transmission

Direct contact transmission involves actual physical contact between an infected animal and a susceptible animal (e.g., licking, rubbing, biting). This category also includes sexual contact, which, for example, is important in the transmission of some herpesviruses.

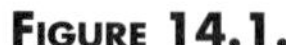

FIGURE 14.1.

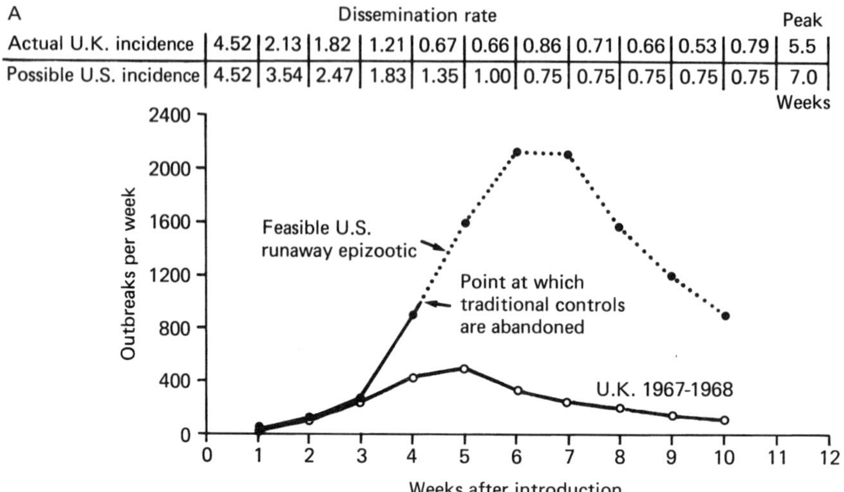

A Dissemination rate

											Peak
Actual U.K. incidence	4.52	2.13	1.82	1.21	0.67	0.66	0.86	0.71	0.66	0.53	0.79	5.5
Possible U.S. incidence	4.52	3.54	2.47	1.83	1.35	1.00	0.75	0.75	0.75	0.75	0.75	7.0

Weeks

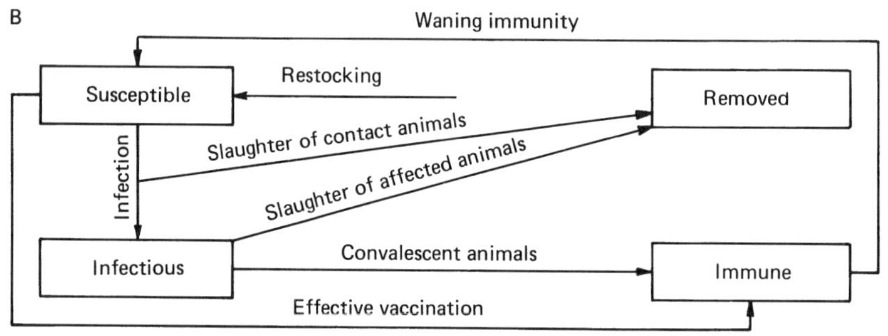

(A) A state-transition model of a major epidemic of foot-and-mouth disease in the United States from the point of virus introduction, through the time of discovery of its presence, to the stage where the disease is well established and traditional control measures (quarantine, slaughter, and disinfection) are no longer effective. The model is based on data from a 1967–68 epidemic in the United Kingdom, during which outbreaks were recorded on 2364 farms. The model permits a variety of disease-control strategies to be examined. It illustrates several key characteristics of a useful model: (1) its pathways are intuitively acceptable, (2) it behaves in a biologically and mathematically logical way (i.e., it is sensitive to appropriate variables), (3) it mimics real-life situations, and (4) it is simple enough to be tested rigorously, but is not naively simplistic. (Courtesy of M. W. Miller.) (B) In the model the basic unit is the herd. Each herd is considered to be in one of four mutually exclusive categories: "susceptible," "infectious," "immune," or "removed/dead." For each week the probability of transition from one category to another and the number of herds expected to be in each category during the next week are calculated. A key factor in determining the probability of a susceptible herd becoming infected in a particular week is the *dissemination rate,* which is the average number of herds to which the virus spreads from each infected herd. This depends on a number of factors, such as topography, weather, husbandry, animal movement, and quarantine effectiveness. The dissemination rate used in the model is based on that calculated for the 1967–1968 epidemic in the United Kingdom. With this dissemination rate, a situation wherein traditional control methods fail is reached 4–5 weeks after introduction of the virus.

Indirect Contact Transmission

Indirect contact transmission occurs via *fomites,* such as shared eating containers, bedding, dander, restraint devices, vehicles, clothing, improperly sterilized surgical equipment, or improperly sterilized syringes or needles (the later also comes under the heading iatrogenic transmission).

Common Vehicle Transmission

Common vehicle transmission includes fecal contamination of food and water supplies (fecal–oral transmission) and virus-contaminated meat or bone products (e.g., for the transmission of vesicular exanthema of swine, hog cholera, pseudorabies, and bovine spongiform encephalopathy).

Airborne Transmission

Airborne transmission, resulting in infection of the respiratory tract, occurs via droplets and droplet nuclei (aerosols) emitted from infected animals during coughing or sneezing (e.g., influenza) or from environmental sources such as dander or dust from bedding (e.g., Marek's dis-

Table 14.1
Common Modes of Transmission of Viruses of Animals

Virus family	Mode of transmission
Poxviridae	Contact (e.g., orf, cowpox viruses)
	Arthropod (mechanical, e.g., myxoma virus, fowlpox virus)
	Respiratory, contact (e.g., sheeppox virus)
Asfarviridae	Respiratory, arthropod (ticks), ingestion of garbage (infected meat)
Herpesviridae	Sexual (e.g., equine coital exanthema virus)
	Respiratory (e.g., infectious bovine rhinotracheitis virus)
	Transplacental (e.g., pseudorabies virus)
Adenoviridae	Respiratory, fecal–oral
Papovaviridae	Direct contact, skin abrasions (e.g., papillomaviruses)
Parvoviridae	Fecal–oral, respiratory, contact, transplacental (e.g., feline panleukopenia virus)
Circoviridae	Fecal–oral, respiratory, contact
Retroviridae	Contact, *in ovo* (germ line), ingestion, mechanically by arthropods
Reoviridae	Fecal–oral (e.g., calf rotavirus)
	Arthropod (e.g., bluetongue viruses)
Birnaviridae	Fecal–oral, water
Paramyxoviridae	Respiratory, contact
Rhabdoviridae	Animal bite (e.g., rabies virus)
	Arthropod and contact (e.g., vesicular stomatitis viruses)
Filoviridae	Unknown in nature; human-to-human spread is by direct contact
Bornaviridae	Unknown in nature; animal-to-animal spread is by direct contact
Orthomyxoviridae	Respiratory
Bunyaviridae	Arthropod (e.g., Rift Valley fever virus)
Arenaviridae	Contact with contaminated urine, respiratory
Coronaviridae	Fecal–oral, respiratory, contact
Arteriviridae	Direct contact, fomites
Picornaviridae	Fecal–oral (e.g., swine enteroviruses)
	Respiratory (e.g., equine rhinoviruses)
	Ingestion of garbage (infected meat) (e.g., foot-and-mouth disease viruses in swine)
Caliciviridae	Respiratory, fecal–oral, contact
Togaviridae	Arthropod (e.g., Venezuelan equine encephalitis virus)
Flaviviridae	Arthropod (e.g., Japanese encephalitis virus)
	Respiratory, fecal–oral, transplacental (e.g., bovine viral diarrhea virus)
Prions	Contaminated pastures (scrapie); contaminated feedstuff (e.g., bovine spongiform encephalopathy); unknown (e.g., chronic wasting disease of deer and elk)

ease). Large droplets settle quickly, but microdroplets evaporate, forming droplet nuclei (less than 5 μm in diameter) that remain suspended in the air for extended periods. Droplets may travel only a meter or so, but droplet nuclei may travel long distances—many kilometers if wind and other weather conditions are favorable.

Arthropod-Borne Transmission

Arthropod-borne transmission involves the bites of arthropod vectors (e.g., mosquitoes transmit equine encephalitis viruses, ticks transmit African swine fever virus, *Culicoides* spp. transmit bluetongue viruses) (see section on Arthropod-Borne Virus Transmission Pattern later in this chapter and Table 14.2).

Table 14.2
Major Arthropod-Borne Viral Zoonoses

Family	Genus	Virus	Reservoir Host	Arthropod Vector
Togaviridae	*Alphavirus*[a]	Eastern equine encephalitis virus[a]	Birds	Mosquitoes
		Western equine encephalitis virus	Birds	Mosquitoes
		Venezuelan equine encephalitis virus[a]	Mammals, horses	Mosquitoes
		Ross River virus[a]	Mammals	Mosquitoes
Flaviviridae	*Flavivirus*	Japanese encephalitis virus	Birds, pigs	Mosquitoes
		St. Louis encephalitis virus	Birds	Mosquitoes
		West Nile virus	Birds	Mosquitoes
		Murray Valley encephalitis virus	Birds	Mosquitoes
		Yellow fever virus[b]	Monkeys, humans	Mosquitoes
		Dengue viruses[b]	Humans, monkeys	Mosquitoes
		Kyasanur Forest disease virus	Mammals	Ticks
		Tick-borne encephalitis viruses	Mammals, birds	Ticks
Bunyaviridae	*Phlebovirus*	Rift Valley fever virus	Mammals	Mosquitoes
		Sandfly fever viruses[a]	Mammals	Sandflies
	Nairovirus	Crimean-Congo hemorrhagic fever virus	Mammals	Ticks
	Bunyavirus	California encephalitis virus	Mammals	Mosquitoes
		La Crosse encephalitis virus	Mammals	Mosquitoes
		Tahyna virus	Mammals	Mosquitoes
		Oropouche virus	? Mammals	Mosquitoes, midges
Reoviridae	*Coltivirus*	Colorado tick fever virus	Mammals	Ticks

[a] In certain episodes, virus is transmitted by insects from human to human.
[b] Usually transmitted by mosquitoes from human to human.

Other terms are used to describe transmission by mechanisms that embrace more than one of the just-described routes.

Iatrogenic Transmission

Iatrogenic ("caused by the doctor") transmission occurs as a direct result of some activity of the attending veterinarian, veterinary technologist, or other person in the course of caring for animals, usually via nonsterile equipment, multiple-use syringes, or inadequate handwashing. Iatrogenic transmission has been important in the spread of equine infectious anemia virus via multiple-use syringes and needles. Similarly, chickens have been infected with reticuloendotheliosis virus via contaminated Marek's disease vaccine.

Nosocomial Transmission

Nosocomial transmission occurs while an animal is in a veterinary hospital or clinic. During the peak of the canine parvovirus epidemic in the 1980s, many puppies became infected in veterinary hospitals and clinics. In some hospitals, the disinfectants in routine use were found to be ineffective against the virus. Feline respiratory infections are also acquired nosocomially. In human medicine, the Ebola virus episodes in Zaire (now Democratic Republic of Congo) in 1976 and 1995 were classic examples of iatrogenic nosocomial epidemics.

Zoonotic Transmission

Because most viruses are host restricted, the majority of viral infections are maintained in nature within populations of the same or closely related species. However, a number of viruses are spread naturally between several different species of animals, e.g., rabies and the arboviral encephalitides. The term *zoonosis* is used to describe infections that are transmissible from animals to humans (Table 14.3). Zoonoses, whether involving domestic or wild animal reservoirs, usually occur only under conditions where humans are engaged in activities involving close contact with animals or where viruses are transmitted by arthropods (Table 14.2).

Vertical Transmission

Vertical transmission is usually used to describe infection that is transferred from dam to embryo or fetus or newborn prior to, during, or shortly after parturition, although some authorities prefer to restrict the term to situations where infection occurs before birth. Certain retroviruses are transmitted vertically via the integration of proviral DNA directly into the DNA of the germ line of the fertilized egg. Cytomegaloviruses are often transmitted to the fetus via the placenta, whereas other herpesviruses are transmitted during passage through the birth canal. Yet other viruses are transmitted via colostrum and milk (e.g., caprine arthritis–encephalitis virus and maedi/visna virus of sheep). Vertical transmission of a virus may cause early embryonic death or abortion (e.g., several lentiviruses) or may be associated with congenital disease (e.g., bovine viral diarrhea virus), or the infection may be the cause of congenital defects (e.g., Akabane virus). Herpesviruses of many species and parvoviruses of several species are important causes of congenital diseases.

Mechanisms of Survival of Viruses in Nature

Perpetuation of a virus in nature depends on the maintenance of serial infections, i.e., a chain of transmission; the occurrence of disease is neither required nor necessarily advantageous (Table 14.4). Indeed, although clinical cases may be somewhat more productive sources of virus than inapparent infections, the latter are generally more numerous and more important because they do not restrict the movement of infectious individuals and thus provide a better opportunity for viral dissemination. As our knowledge of the different features of the pathogenesis, species susceptibility, routes of transmission, and environmental stability of various viruses has increased,

Table 14.3
Major Nonarthropod-Borne Viral Zoonoses

Family	Virus	Reservoir host	Mode of transmission to humans
Poxviridae	Cowpox virus	Rodents, cats, cattle	Contact, abrasions
	Monkeypox virus	Squirrels, monkeys	Contact, abrasions
	Pseudocowpox virus	Cattle	Contact, abrasions
	Orf virus	Sheep, goats	Contact, abrasions
Herpesviridae	B virus	Monkey	Animal bite
Paramyxoviridae	Equine morbillivirus	Fruit-eating bats	Uncertain
Rhabdoviridae	Rabies virus	Various mammals	Animal bite, scratch, respiratory
	Vesicular stomatitis viruses	Cattle	Contact with secretions[a]
Filoviridae	Ebola, Marburg viruses	Monkeys	Contact; iatrogenic (injection)[b]
Orthomyxoviridae	Influenza A viruses[c]	Birds, pigs	Respiratory
Bunyaviridae	Hantaviruses	Rodents	Contact with rodent urine
Arenaviridae	Lymphocytic choriomeningitis, Junin, Machupo, Lassa, Guanarito viruses	Rodents	Contact with rodent urine

[a] May be arthropod-borne.
[b] Also human-to-human spread.
[c] Usually maintained by human-to-human spread; zoonotic infections occur only rarely, but reassortants between human and avian influenza viruses (perhaps arising during coinfection of pigs) may result in human pandemics due to antigenic shift.

Table 14.4
Modes of Survival of Viruses in Nature

Family	Example	Mode of survival
Poxviridae	Orf virus	Virus stable in environment
Asfarviridae	African swine fever virus	Acute self-limiting infection; persistent infection in soft ticks
Herpesviridae	Bovine herpesvirus 1	Persistent infection, intermittant shedding
Adenoviridae	Canine adenovirus 1	Persistent infection; virus stable in environment
Papovaviridae	Papillomaviruses	Persistent in lesions; virus stable in environment
Parvoviridae	Canine parvovirus	Virus stable in environment
Circoviridae	Psittacine beak and feather disease virus	Virus stable in environment
Retroviridae	Avian leukosis viruses	Persistent infection; vertical transmission
Reoviridae	Calf rotaviruses	Acute self-limiting infection; very high yield of virus from infected animals
	Bluetongue viruses	Arthropod-borne
Birnaviridae	Infectious bursal disease virus	Acute self-limiting infection
Paramyxoviridae	Newcastle disease virus	Acute self-limiting infection; vertical with velogenic strains
Rhabdoviridae	Rabies virus	Long incubation period
	Vesicular stomatitis viruses	Virus stable, arthropod-borne
Filoviridae	Ebola virus	Unknown
Bornaviridae	Borna disease virus	Persistent infection
Orthomyxoviridae	Influenza viruses	Acute self-limiting infection
Bunyaviridae	Rift Valley fever virus	Arthropod-borne; vertical transmission in flood-water mosquitoes
Arenaviridae	Lassa virus	Persistent infection
Coronaviridae	Feline infectious peritonitis virus	Persistent infection with enteric virus
Arteriviridae	Equine arteritis virus	Persistent infection
Picornaviridae	Foot-and-mouth disease viruses	Acute self-limiting infection; sometimes persistent infection
Caliciviridae	Feline calicivirus	Persistent infection with continuous shedding
Togaviridae	Equine encephalitis viruses	Arthropod-borne
Flaviviridae	Japanese encephalitis virus	Arthropod-borne
	Bovine viral diarrhea virus	Acute self-limiting infection; persistent after congenital infection
Prions	Scrapie prion	Prion stable in environment

epidemiologists have been able to recognize four major patterns by which viruses maintain serial transmission in their host(s): (1) the acute self-limiting infection pattern, in which transmission is always affected by host population size, (2) the persistent infection pattern, (3) the vertical transmission pattern, and (4) the arthropod-borne virus transmission pattern.

The physical stability of a virus affects its survival in the environment; in general, viruses that are transmitted by the respiratory route have low environmental stability whereas those transmitted by the fecal–oral route have a higher stability. Thus, stability of the virus in water, fomites, or on the mouthparts of mechanical arthropod vectors favors transmission—this is particularly important in small or dispersed animal communities. For example, the parapox virus that causes orf in sheep survives for months in pastures. During the winter, myxoma virus, which causes myxomatosis in rabbits, can survive for several weeks on the mouthparts of mosquitoes.

Most viruses have a principal mechanism for survival, but if this mechanism is interrupted, e.g., by a sudden decline in the population of the host species, a second or even a third mechanism may exist as a "backup." For example, in bovine viral diarrhea there is a primary fecal–oral transmission cycle that is backed up by the less common persistent shedding of virus by congenitally infected calves. An appreciation of these mechanisms for viral perpetuation is valuable in designing and implementing control programs.

Acute Self-Limiting Infection Pattern

The most precise data on the importance of population size in acute, self-limiting infections come from studies of measles, which is a cosmopolitan human disease. Measles has long been a favorite disease for modeling epidemics because it is one of the few common human diseases in which subclinical infections are rare, clinical diagnosis is easy, and postinfection immunity is lifelong. Measles virus is related closely to rinderpest and canine distemper viruses, and many aspects of the model apply equally well to these two viruses and the diseases they cause. Survival of measles virus in a population requires a large continuous supply of susceptible hosts. Analyses of the incidence of measles in large cities and in island communities have shown that a population of about half a million persons is needed to ensure a large enough annual input of new susceptible hosts, by birth or immigration, to maintain the virus in the population. Because infection depends on respiratory transmission, the duration of epidemics of measles is correlated inversely with population density. If a population is dispersed over a large area, the rate of spread is reduced and the epidemic will last longer so that the number of susceptible persons needed to maintain the transmission chain is reduced. However, in such a situation a break in the transmission chain is much more likely. When a large percentage of the population is susceptible initially, the intensity of the epidemic builds up very quickly and attack rates are almost 100% (*virgin-soil epidemic*). There are many examples of similar transmission patterns among viruses of domestic animals, but quantitative data are not as complete as those for measles. *Exotic viruses,* i.e., those that are not present in a particular country or region, represent the most important group of viruses with a potential for causing virgin-soil epidemics.

The history of rinderpest in cattle in Africa in the early 20th century shows many parallels with measles in isolated human populations. When it was first introduced into cattle populations the initial impact was devastating. Cattle and wild ruminants of all ages were susceptible, and the mortality was so high that in Tanzania the ground was so littered with the carcasses of cattle that a Masai tribesman commented that "the vultures had forgotten how to fly." The development of vaccines beginning in the 1920s changed the epidemiology of rinderpest, leading to a period in the 1960s when its global eradication was anticipated. Unfortunately, in the 1970s, vaccination programs in West Africa were maintained poorly and by the 1980s the disease had once again become rampant and the cause of major losses in many parts of Africa. This prompted renewed vaccination campaigns in African and the Indian subcontinents; once again the prospect of global eradication of rinderpest is being considered.

The cyclical nature of the occurrence of such diseases is determined by several variables, including the rate of buildup of susceptible animals, introduction of the virus, and environmental conditions that promote viral spread.

Persistent Infection Pattern

Persistent viral infections, whether they are associated with acute initial disease or with recurrent episodes of clinical disease, play an important role in the perpetuation of many viruses. For example, recurrent virus shedding by a persistently infected animal can reintroduce virus into a population of susceptible animals, all of which have been born since the last clinically apparent episode of infection. This transmission pattern is important for the survival of bovine viral diarrhea virus, hog cholera virus, equine arteritis virus, and herpesviruses, and such viruses have a much smaller critical population size than occurs in acute self-limited infections; indeed the sustaining population for some herpesviruses may be as small as a single farm, kennel, cattery, or breeding unit.

Sometimes the persistence of infection, the production of disease, and the transmission of virus are dissociated; for example, togavirus and arenavirus infections have little adverse effect on their reservoir hosts (arthropods, birds, and rodents) but transmission is very efficient. However, the persistence of infection in the central nervous system, as with canine distemper virus, is of no epidemiologic significance, as no infectious virus is shed from this site; infections of the central nervous system may have a severe effect on the dog, but is of no consequence for survival of the virus.

Vertical Transmission Pattern

Transmission of virus from the dam to the embryo, fetus, or newborn, as described earlier, can be important in virus survival in nature: all arenaviruses, several herpesviruses, parvoviruses, and retroviruses, some orbiviruses and togaviruses, and a few bunyaviruses and coronaviruses may be transmitted in this way. Indeed, if the consequence of vertical transmission is lifelong persistent infection, as in the case of arenaviruses and retroviruses, the long-term survival of the virus is assured. Virus transmission in the immediate perinatal period, by contact or via colostrum and milk, is also important.

Arthropod-Borne Virus Transmission Pattern

Several arthropod-borne diseases are discussed in appropriate chapters of Part II of this book; this chapter considers some common features that will be useful in understanding their epidemiology and control. Over 500 arboviruses are known, of which some 40 cause disease in domestic animals and many of the same cause zoonotic diseases (Table 14.2). Sometimes arthropod transmission may be mechanical, as in myxomatosis and fowlpox, in which mosquitoes act as "flying needles." More commonly, transmission involves replication of the virus in the arthropod vector, which may be a tick, a mosquito, a sandfly (*Phlebotomus* spp.), or a midge (*Culicoides* spp.).

The arthropod vector acquires virus by feeding on the blood of a viremic animal. Replication of the ingested virus, initially in the insect gut, and its spread to the salivary gland take several days (the *extrinsic incubation period*); the interval varies with different viruses and is influenced by ambient temperature. Virions in the salivary secretions of the vector are injected into new animal hosts during blood meals. Arthropod transmission provides a way for a virus to cross species barriers, as the same arthropod may bite birds, reptiles, and mammals that rarely or never come into close contact in nature.

Most arboviruses have localized natural habitats in which specific receptive arthropod and vertebrate hosts are involved in the viral life cycle. Vertebrate reservoir hosts are usually wild mammals or birds; domestic animals and humans are rarely involved in primary transmission cycles, although the exceptions to this generalization are important (e.g., Venezuelan equine encephalitis virus in horses, yellow fever, and dengue viruses in humans). Domestic animal species are, in most cases, infected incidentally, e.g., by the geographic extension of a reservoir vertebrate host and/or a vector arthropod.

Most arboviruses that cause periodic epidemics have ecologically complex endemic cycles, which often involve different arthropod as well as different vertebrate hosts from those involved in epidemic cycles. Endemic cycles, which are generally poorly understood and inaccessible to effective control measures, provide for the amplification of virus and therefore are critical in dictating the magnitude of epidemics.

When arthropods are active, arboviruses replicate alternately in vertebrate and invertebrate hosts. A puzzle that has concerned many investigators has been to understand what happens to these viruses during the winter months in temperate climates when the arthropod vectors are inactive. One important mechanism for "overwintering" is *transovarial* and *transstadial transmission.* Transovarial transmission occurs with the tick-borne flaviviruses and has been shown to occur with some mosquito-borne bunyaviruses and flaviviruses. Some bunyaviruses are found in high northern latitudes where the mosquito breeding season is too short to allow virus survival by horizontal transmission cycles alone; many of the first mosquitoes to emerge each summer carry virus as a result of transovarial and transstadial transmission and the pool of virus is amplified rapidly by horizontal transmission in mosquito–vertebrate–mosquito cycles.

Vertical transmission in arthropods may not explain overwintering of all arboviruses, but other possibilities are still unproven or speculative. For example, hibernating vertebrates have been thought to play a role in overwintering. In cold climates, bats and some small rodents, as well as snakes and frogs, hibernate during the winter months. Their low body temperature has been thought to favor persistent infection, with recrudescent viremia occurring when the temperature rises in the spring. Although demonstrated in the laboratory, this mechanism has never been proven to occur in nature.

Many human activities disturb the natural ecology and hence the natural arbovirus life cycles and have been incriminated in the geographic spread or increased prevalence of the diseases caused by these viruses:

1. Population movements and the intrusion of humans and domestic animals into new arthropod habitats have resulted in dramatic epidemics. Some have had historic impact: the Louisiana Purchase came about because of the losses Napoleon's army experienced from yellow fever in the Caribbean. Several decades later the same disease affected the building of the Panama canal. Ecologic factors pertaining to unique environments and geographic factors have contributed to many new, emergent disease episodes. Remote econiches, such as islands, free of particular species of reservoir hosts and vectors, are often particularly vulnerable to an introduced virus.

2. Deforestation has been the key to the exposure of farmers and domestic animals to new arthropods—there are many contemporary examples of the importance of this kind of ecological disruption.

3. Increased long-distance travel facilitates the carriage of exotic arthropod vectors around the world. The carriage of the eggs of the Asian mosquito, *Aedes*

albopictus, to the United States in used tires represents an unsolved problem of this kind.

4. Increased long-distance livestock transportation facilitates the carriage of viruses and arthropods (especially ticks) around the world. Ecologic factors pertaining to water usage, i.e., increasing irrigation and the expanding reuse of water, are becoming very important factors in virus disease emergence. The problem with primitive water and irrigation systems, which are developed without attention to arthropod control, is exemplified in the emergence of Japanese encephalitis in new areas of southeast Asia.

5. New routings of long-distance bird migrations brought about by new man-made water impoundments represent an important yet still untested new risk of introduction of arboviruses into new areas. The extension of the geographical range of Japanese encephalitis virus into new areas of Asia has likely involved virus carriage by birds.

6. Ecologic factors pertaining to environmental pollution and uncontrolled urbanization are contributing to many new, emergent disease episodes. Arthropod vectors breeding in accumulations of water (tin cans, old tires, etc.) and sewage-laden water are a worldwide problem. Environmental chemical toxicants (herbicides, pesticides, residues) can also affect vector–virus relationships directly or indirectly. For example, mosquito resistance to all licensed insecticides in parts of California is a known direct effect of unsound mosquito abatement programs; this resistance may also have been augmented indirectly by uncontrolled pesticide usage against crop pests.

7. Global warming, affecting sea level, estuarine wetlands, fresh water swamps, and human habitation patterns, may be affecting vector–virus relationships throughout the tropics; however, data are scarce and many programs to study the effect of global warming have not included the participation of infectious disease experts.

The history of the European colonization of Africa is replete with examples of new arbovirus diseases resulting from the introduction of susceptible European livestock into that continent, e.g., African swine fever, African horse sickness, Rift valley fever, Nairobi sheep disease, and bluetongue. The viruses that cause these diseases are now feared in the industrialized countries as exotic threats that may devastate their livestock. Another example of the importance of ecologic factors is the infection of horses in the eastern part of North America with eastern equine encephalitis virus when their pasturage is made to overlap the natural swamp-based mosquito–bird–mosquito cycle of this virus. Similarly, in Japan and southeastern Asian countries, swine may become infected with Japanese encephalitis virus and become important amplifying hosts when they are bitten by mosquitoes that breed in rice fields.

Tick-borne flaviviruses illustrate two features of epidemiologic importance. First, transovarial infection in ticks is often sufficient to ensure survival of the virus independently of a cycle in vertebrates; vertebrate infection amplifies the population of infected ticks. Second, for some of these viruses, transmission from one vertebrate host to another, once initiated by the bite of an infected tick, can also occur by mechanisms not involving an arthropod. Thus, in central Europe and the eastern part of Russia, a variety of small rodents may be infected with tick-borne encephalitis viruses. Goats, cows, and sheep are incidental hosts and sustain inapparent infections, but they excrete virus in their milk. Adult and juvenile ungulates may acquire virus during grazing on tick-infested pastures, and newborn animals may be infected by drinking infected milk. Humans may be infected by being bitten by a tick or by drinking milk from an infected goat.

Variations in Disease Incidence Associated with Seasons and Animal Management Practices

Many viral infections show pronounced seasonal variations in incidence. In temperate climates, arbovirus infections transmitted by mosquitoes or sandflies occur mainly during the summer months, when vectors are most numerous and active. Infections transmitted by ticks occur most commonly during the spring and early summer months. Other biologic reasons for seasonal disease include both virus and host factors. Influenza viruses and poxviruses survive better in air at low rather than at high humidity, and all viruses survive better at lower temperatures in aerosols. It has also been suggested, without much supporting evidence, that there may be seasonal changes in the susceptibility of the host, perhaps associated with changes in the physiological status of nasal and oropharyngeal mucous membranes.

More important in veterinary medicine than any natural seasonal effects are the changes in housing and management practices that occur in different seasons. Housing animals such as cattle and sheep for the winter often increases the incidence of respiratory and enteric diseases. These diseases often have obscure primary etiologies, usually viral, followed by secondary infections caused by opportunistic pathogens (see Chapter 9). In such cases, infectious disease diagnosis, prevention, and treatment must be integrated into an overall system for the management of facilities as well as husbandry practices. In areas where animals are moved, e.g., to feedlots or seasonally to distant pasturage, there are two major problems: animals are subjected to the stress of transportation and they are brought into contact with new populations carrying and shedding different infectious agents. Often summer pasturage is at high altitude, adding the stress of pulmonary vascular dysfunction and pulmonary edema to the insult of respiratory virus infections. Secondary *Pasteurella* pneumonia is not limited to animals subjected to the stress of transportation to feedlots.

In areas of the world where cattle are moved hundreds of miles each year, such as in the Sahel zone of Africa, viral diseases such as rinderpest are associated with the contact between previously separate populations brought about by this traditional husbandry practice. In southern Africa, the communal use of waterholes during the dry season promotes the exchange of viruses such as foot-and-mouth disease virus between different species of wildlife and, in certain circumstances, between wildlife and domestic animals.

Epidemiologic Aspects of Immunity

Immunity acquired from prior infection or from vaccination plays a vital role in the epidemiology of viral diseases; in fact, vaccination (see Chapter 13) is the single most effective method of controlling viral diseases. Canine distemper, caused by a single, antigenically stable virus, is associated with a very effective immune response. In industrialized countries, the widespread vaccination of puppies with attenuated virus canine distemper vaccine has sharply decreased the incidence of both canine distemper and its complications, old dog encephalitis, and hard pad disease.

For some viruses, immunity is relatively ineffective because of the absence of antibodies at the site of infection (e.g., the respiratory or intestinal tract). Respiratory syncytial viruses cause mild to severe respiratory tract disease in cattle and sheep. Infections usually occur during the winter months when the animals are housed in confined conditions. The virus spreads rapidly by aerosol infection and reinfection of the respiratory tract is not uncommon. Preexisting antibody, whether derived passively by maternal transfer or actively by prior infection, does not prevent viral replication and excretion, although clinical signs are usually mild where the antibody titer is high. Not surprisingly, vaccination is not very effective.

Further Reading

Anderson, R. M. (1998). Analytic theory of epidemics. *In* "Emerging Infections" (R. Krause and A. Fauci, eds.), pp. 23–50. Academic Press, New York.

Anderson, R. M., and May, R. M. (1985). Herd immunity. *Nature (London)* **318,** 323–325.

Berg, E. (1987). "Methods of Recovering Viruses from the Environment." CRC Press, Boca Raton, FL.

Black, F. L., and Singer, B. (1987). Elaboration versus simplification in refining mathematical models of infectious disease. *Annu. Rev. Microbiol.* **41,** 677–698.

Coyne, M. J., Smith, G., and McAllister, F. E. (1989). Mathematical model for the population biology of rabies in raccoons in the mid-Atlantic states. *Am. J. Vet. Res.* **50,** 2148–2153.

Gibbs, E. P. J., ed. (1981). "Virus Diseases of Food Animals. A World Geography of Epidemiology and Control," Vols. 1 and 2. Academic Press, London.

Gloster, J. (1983). Forecasting the airborne spread of foot-and-mouth disease and Newcastle disease. *Philos. Trans. R. Soc. London. Ser. B.* **302,** 535–545.

James, A. D. and Rossiter, P. B. (1989). An epidemiological model of rinderpest. I. Description of the model. *Trop. Anim. Health Prod.* **21,** 59–68.

Kramer, M. S. (1988). "Clinical Epidemiology and Biostatistics." Springer-Verlag, New York.

Miller, W. M. (1979). A state-transition model of epidemic foot-and-mouth disease. *In* "A study of the Potential Economic Impact of Foot-and-Mouth Disease in the United States" (E. H. McCauley, N. A. Aulaqi, J. C. New, W. Sundquist, and W. M. Miller, eds.). U. S. Government Printing Office, Washington, DC.

Mims, C. A. (1981). Vertical transmission of viruses. *Microbiol. Rev.* **41,** 267–275.

Pech, R. E., and Hone, J. (1988). A model of the dynamics and control of an outbreak of foot-and-mouth disease in feral pigs in Australia. *J. Appl. Biol.* **25,** 63–67.

Rossiter, P. B. and James, A. D. (1989). An epidemiological model of rinderpest. II. Simulations of the behavior of rinderpest in populations. *Trop. Anim. Health Prod.* **21,** 69–78.

Smith, G., and Grenfell, B. T. (1990). Population biology of pseudorabies in swine. *Am. J. Vet. Res.* **51,** 148–156.

CHAPTER 15

Surveillance, Prevention, Control, and Eradication of Viral Diseases

Principles of Disease Prevention, Control, and Eradication

A new political and economic paradigm is emerging with the turn of the century that is affecting the prevention, control, and eradication of veterinary and zoonotic diseases. Ever more complex and intertwined global political systems are exemplified by the European Union. Ever more complex and intertwined trading patterns are exemplified by the North American Free Trade Agreement and other similar agreements. Ever more complex and intertwined food production, processing, and distribution systems are exemplified by international trade in meat and poultry, dairy products, and seafood and shellfish. These trends are leading to increased public awareness of disease risks and to a rising public expectation of the veterinary medical profession as the global steward of animal health and the related areas of environmental quality, food safety, animal welfare, and zoonotic disease control. All these responsibilities will require the application of the principles of preventive medicine: surveillance, particularly on the international scene, and time-honored investigative and disease prevention and control actions must expand in scope and scale.

Good preventive medicine starts with the local practitioner, on the farm, ranch, feedlot, or poultry house and in the veterinary clinic. In this respect, little has changed: the basic principles of good husbandry, knowledge of the prevalence of specific diseases and how they are transmitted, and the best methods for disinfection and vaccination and vector control still apply. With the turn of the century, however, it seems clear that *knowledge-based practice,* whether private practice with producers as clients or public practice with the public as constituent, will become more demanding. Depth of knowledge of the scientific base underpinning preventive medicine practice will advance rapidly—in many instances it will be the prevention and control of viral diseases that will lead the way for other veterinary medical risk assessment and risk management activities.

Prevention Strategies

Nowhere in veterinary medicine is the adage "an ounce of prevention is better than a pound of cure" more appropriate than in viral diseases. Apart from therapeutic regimes for ameliorating clinical signs of disease, such as the administration of fluids in viral diarrhea or using antibiotics to prevent secondary bacterial infections after viral respiratory diseases, there are no effective and practical treatments for most viral diseases of domestic animals. Nevertheless, there are many well-proven approaches to the prevention, control, and even the regional eradication of many important viral diseases of animals. Progress indicates that some viral diseases of animals will be eradicated globally in the next century.

Viral disease prevention and control is based on diverse strategies, each chosen in keeping with the characteristics of the virus, its transmission pattern(s) and environmental stability, and its pathogenesis and threat (to animal health, productivity, and profitability, zoonotic risk, etc.). When available, the most valuable preventive measure is the comprehensive use of vaccines, not solely for the protection of the individual animal, but to build up a level of population immunity sufficient to break chains of transmission (see Chapter 13). Hygiene and sanitation measures are important methods of controlling fecal–oral infections in kennels and catteries, on farms and ranches, and in commercial aquaculture facilities. Arthropod vector control is the key to regional prevention of several arthropod-borne viral diseases. Test-and-removal programs continue to be used on regional and country-wide bases to eradicate several viral diseases of livestock and poultry. The importation of exotic diseases (the term *foreign animal diseases* is used officially in some countries) into countries or regions is prevented by surveillance and quarantine programs. Finally, following the lead taken in human medicine to globally eradicate smallpox (accomplished in 1977) and polio (expected to be accomplished in 2002), the global eradication of rinderpest is now considered attainable.

Disease Surveillance

The implementation of disease control programs and regulatory policy is critically dependent on accurate intelligence on disease incidence, prevalence, transmission, endemic presence, epidemic spread, and so on. *Surveillance* of viral diseases provides this basic information; it is the systematic and regular collection, collation, and analysis of data on disease occurrence. Its main purpose is to detect trends—changes in the distribution of diseases.

The need for data on the occurrence of infectious diseases has led to the concept of "notifiable" diseases, whereby veterinary practitioners are required to report to central authorities such as state or national veterinary authorities. In turn, through regional or international agreement, national authorities may elect, or be obliged, to inform other countries immediately of even the suspicion, let alone confirmation of disease in their country. Clearly the list of "notifiable" diseases must not be too large; if so, notification will be ignored. However, data provided by a system of notification influence decisions on resource allocation for the control of diseases and the intensity of follow-up.

Many countries collect data on diseases that are not notifiable. Such data provide useful information on strategies of prevention, especially by allowing calculations of cost–benefit equations and indices of vaccine efficacy. Dependent on the characteristics of the disease, the availability of effective vaccines, and sensitivity and specificity of the diagnostic tests, progressive eradication programs can be planned and implemented over a time period of several years through access to this information. The ongoing eradication of pseudorabies in the United States and several European countries is an excellent example of this approach.

Sources of Surveillance Data

The methods of surveillance used commonly for animal diseases are (1) notifiable disease reporting, (2) laboratory-based surveillance, and (3) population-based surveillance. The key to surveillance is the veterinary practitioner. Although any one practitioner may see only a few cases of a particular disease, data from many practitioners can be accumulated and analyzed to reveal trends in the occurrence of diseases. One key to effective surveillance, especially for exotic or unusual animal diseases, is a sense of heightened awareness among veterinary practitioners—"when you hear hoofbeats, think horses, not zebras" may be good diagnostic advice to clinicians in general, but heightened awareness means that one should not totally dismiss the possibility that the hoofbeats may be, indeed, zebras.

Each country has its own system for collecting and collating data. International agencies such as the Food and Agricultural Organization of the United Nations and the Office International des Épizooties coordinate information exchange between countries. For example, the United States Department of Agriculture has its Centers for Epidemiology and Animal Health, with three units: (1) the Center for Animal Disease Information and Analysis, which collects, manages, analyzes, and disseminates epidemiological information; (2) the Center for Animal Health Monitoring, which operates the National Animal Health Monitoring System (NAHMS) and DxMonitor, an animal health report covering ongoing monitoring and surveillance; and (3) the Center for Emerging Issues, which identifies emerging issues and provides risk assessment studies.

There are several sources of information on disease incidence that are used by veterinary authorities in most developed countries, not all of which are pertinent in any particular disease:

1. Morbidity and mortality data assessed through information submitted to national, state, and local diagnostic laboratories and made available, with varying degrees of access, through national, regional, and international agencies. Some of these data are published through annual reports, scientific journals and so on.
2. Information from case and outbreak investigations, again often linked to diagnostic laboratories and state and national veterinary investigations units.
3. Monitoring of virus activity by clinical, pathologic, serologic, and virologic examination of animals presented for slaughter at abattoirs, tested for legal movement, examined in pathology laboratories, or exposed as sentinels to detect virus activity.
4. Monitoring of arthropod populations and virus infection rates and sentinel animal monitoring to detect arbovirus activity.
5. Specific serologic and virologic surveys.
6. Analyses of vaccine manufacture and use.
7. Reviews of local media reports of disease.
8. List servers, special interest group communications, and other Internet resources.

Having collected data, it is important that they should be analyzed quickly enough to influence necessary follow-up measures. If action is intended, the accuracy of the information needs to be evaluated carefully. For example, data available from national databases are likely to be reliable and annotated but often reflect information collected several weeks or even several months earlier. In contrast, information gleaned from reviews of local media and from individual reports of unconfirmed disease on the WorldWide Web, may represent the earliest warning of an impending epidemic. However, such sources may provide well-intended, but false, information. Quick action when necessary and dissemination of information, particularly to local veterinary practitioners, is a vital component of effective surveillance systems. Caution must be exercised, however, to avoid unnecessary public alarm. Having to retract false information undermines credibility severely.

Investigation and Action in Disease Outbreaks

When there is a disease outbreak, it must first be recognized, hopefully at the level of primary veterinary care. This is not always easy when a new disease occurs or a disease occurs in a new setting. Investigation and actions may be described in the form of a *discovery-to-control continuum*. The continuum involves three major phases, each with several elements.

Early Phase

Initial investigation at the first sign of an unusual disease episode must focus on practical characteristics such as mortality, severity of disease, transmissibility, and remote spread, all of which are important predictors of epidemic potential and risk to animal populations. Clinical and pathologic observations often provide key early clues.

Discovery. The precise recognition of a new disease in its host population is the starting point. For diseases that are identified as endemic or present sporadically in a given animal population, outbreaks are usually handled by veterinary practitioners working directly with producers and owners. For diseases that are identified as exotic or as having epidemic potential, most further investigation and action depends on specialized expertise and resources.

Epidemiologic field investigation. Many of the early investigative activities surrounding a disease episode must be carried out in the field, not in the laboratory. This is the world of "shoe-leather epidemiology."

Etiologic investigation. Identification of the etiologic virus is crucial—it is not enough to find a virus, its causative role in the episode must be established.

Diagnostic development. It is often difficult to move from identifying a causative virus to adapting it to sensitive, specific, and practical diagnostic tests (tests for the presence of virus, viral nucleic acids, antigens, and antibodies) that can be used in epidemiologic investigations. Here, there is need for controlled sensitivity, specificity, reproducibility, rapidity, simplicity, and economy. There is also a need for proof-testing of the diagnostics system in the field in the setting of the disease episode at hand.

Intermediate Phase

The continuum progresses to the general area of risk management, the area represented not by the question, "What's going on here?," but by the question, "What are we going to do about it?" This phase may include expansion of many elements.

Focused research. The importance of focused research, aimed at determining more about the etiologic virus, the pathogenesis and pathophysiology of the infection, and related immunologic, ecologic (including vector biology, zoonotic host biology, etc.), and epidemiologic sciences, plays a major role in disease control programs.

Training, outreach, continuing education and public education. Each of these elements requires professional expertise and adaptation to the special circumstances of the disease locale.

Communications. Risk communications must be of an appropriate scope and scale, employing the technologies of the day, including newspapers, radio, television, and the Internet.

Technology transfer. Diagnostics development, vaccine development, sanitation and vector control, and many veterinary care activities require the transfer of information and specialized knowledge to those in need. This is especially true regarding transfer from national centers to local disease control units.

Commercialization or governmental production. Where appropriate, the wherewithal for the production of diagnostics, vaccines, and so on must be moved from research-scale sites to production-scale sites. This differs in different countries and with different viral diseases.

Late Phase

As one goes further and further along the continuum, actions become more and more complex. More and more expensive, specialized expertise and resources come into play.

Animal health systems development. This includes rapid case/herd reporting systems, ongoing surveillance systems, and records and disease registers. This also includes staffing and staff support and logistical support such as facilities, equipment, supplies, and transport. This often requires the development of legislation and regulation. The systems needed to control a foot-and-mouth disease epidemic in an otherwise disease-free country or region is exemplary of these elements.

Special clinical systems. In some cases, isolation of cases by quarantine (usually requiring legal authorization and enforcement) and special clinical care and herd/flock management are necessary.

Public infrastructure systems. In some cases, new or additional sanitation and sewage systems, clean water supplies, environmental control, and reservoir host and vector control are needed on a long-term basis. These elements usually require new or modified government organizational structures. The largest epidemics may require incredible resources, e.g., limiting the movement of animals on a national or regional scale, test-and-slaughter programs, and similar actions often require special new funding and the involvement of international agencies such as the Office International des Épizooties (OIE), the Food and Agriculture Organization, and/or the World Health Organization. The public infrastructure systems developed in the United Kingdom to control the epidemic of bovine spongiform encephalopathy is exemplary in this regard. The systems developed in Hong Kong and elsewhere in China to deal with H5N1 avian influenza provide further lessons.

Of course not all of these elements are appropriate in every viral disease episode—decisions must be made and priorities must be set—"we must do this, but we need not do that"—"what is the minimum that must be done to deal with this viral disease outbreak in this given circumstance?"

Disease Control through Hygiene and Sanitation

Intensive animal husbandry leads to a buildup in the local environment of feces, urine, hair, feathers, and so on that may be contaminated with viruses. For viruses that are thermostable, the buildup of such contamination provides a ready source of virus for infecting newly introduced animals. To avoid this, many pork, veal, and poultry farmers operate an "all in, all out" management system, by which the animal houses are emptied, cleaned, and disinfected between cohorts of animals.

Hygiene and disinfection are most effective in the control of fecal–oral infections; they have much less effect on the incidence of respiratory infections. In general, attempts to achieve "air sanitation" have failed and respiratory viral infections constitute the single most important group of diseases in intensive animal production systems. Respiratory viral infections are probably more common now than they have ever been because of growing animal populations and increasing population densities in many settings. For example, the typical poultry broiler facility, operating as a single ecosystem, exposes thousands to tens-of-thousands of birds equally when avian influenza virus is introduced by a wild bird.

Nosocomial Infections

Nosocomial infections are less common in large animal veterinary practices, as animals are usually treated on the farm, than in companion animal practices. The use of appointment systems in veterinary practices reduces the risk of disease transmission in the waiting room; further, the preference of many clients to wait in their cars so that their animals become less excited also cuts down the risk of disease transmission. Veterinary clinics should require that all inpatients have current immunization records or receive booster immunization. Clinics should be designed for easy disinfection, with wash-down walls and flooring and as few permanent fixtures as possible. They should also have efficient ventilation and air conditioning, not only to minimize odors, but also to reduce the aerosol transmission of viruses. Frequent hand washing and decontamination of contaminated equipment are essential.

Disinfection and Disinfectants

Disinfectants are chemical germicides formulated for use on inanimate surfaces, in contrast to *antiseptics,* which are chemical germicides designed for use on the skin or mucous membranes. Disinfection of contaminated premises and equipment plays an important role in the control of diseases of livestock.

Viruses of different families vary greatly in their resistance to disinfectants, with enveloped viruses usually being much more sensitive than nonenveloped viruses. However, most modern disinfectants inactivate most viruses rapidly. Their effective action is influenced by access; viruses trapped in heavy layers of mucus or fecal material are not inactivated easily. Standard requirements by the United States Environmental Protection Agency specify that test viruses must be suspended in 5% serum and dried on a hard surface before testing the efficacy of a disinfectant. There are special problems when surfaces cannot be cleaned thoroughly or where cracks and crevices are relatively inaccessible, as in old timber buildings or the fence posts and railings of cattle and sheep yards.

Table 15.1 sets out some common disinfectants and their potential uses. The first five compounds listed

Table 15.1
Commercially Available Disinfectants Used to Inactivate Viruses

Disinfectant	Uses	Remarks
Sodium hypochlorite (Chlorox, Chlorize)	Drinking water, food and utensils, dairies, spot disinfection	Highly effective, but high protein concentrations interfere; inexpensive nontoxic, rapid action
Detergent iodophores (Betadine, Wescodyne, Redene)	Same as sodium hypochlorite	Action based on slow release of iodine and detergent action; less affected by high protein concentrations than sodium hypochlorite; expensive
Formaldehyde (formalin)	Laundry, bedding surfaces, and as vapor for surface sterilization	Low power of penetration except as vapor, but useful for terminal disinfection; irritating, hypersensitivity develops
Phenol derivatives (Lysol, Dettol, Staphene, Sudol)	2.5% aqueous solution for hands, examination tables, cages, hospital surfaces	Efficacy depends on concentration and temperature; high protein concentrations interfere
Chlorohexidine (Hibitane, Nolvasan)	Wide range, examination tables, cages, hospital surfaces	Little affected by body fluids, soap, organic compounds; expensive
Ethylene dioxide	For heat-sensitive medical supplies, plastic isolators	Toxic and explosive except as mixture, 10% with 90% CO_2, which is available commercially as compressed gas
Glutaraldehyde (Cidex)	Cold sterilization of instruments with lenses	2% solution buffered with sodium bicarbonate is virucidal in 10 minutes at pH 7.5–8.5; expensive
Alcohol (ethanol and 2-propanol)	Hands, thermometers	Moderately virucidal only in high concentrations (70–80%); ethanol preferable to methanol or 2-propanol; nontoxic
Quaternary ammonium compounds (Zephiran, Roccal, Savlon)	Zephiran (benzalkonium chloride) used for cleansing wounds	Not very effective against many viruses; high protein concentrations interfere

[a]Based on data supplied by J. Storz.

can be used in animal quarters, although some are too expensive for large-scale use. The last four are of use primarily in the consulting room, hospital, or laboratory. Lye (2% NaOH) is inexpensive and has been the traditional disinfectant for large-scale disinfection of farm premises following outbreaks of foot-and-mouth disease and other exotic viral diseases. Hot water containing detergent and steam sterilization are also useful for the decontamination of livestock premises.

Disease Control through Eliminating Arthropod Vectors

Control of arbovirus infections relies, where possible, on the use of vaccines because the large areas and extended periods over which vectors may be active make vector control difficult. However, surveillance of vector populations (e.g., mosquito larval counts) and/or the climatic conditions conducive to vector transmissions over wider geographical areas (e.g., remote sensing by satellite imagery for Rift Valley fever in East Africa; see Chapter 30) provide the justification for local vector control both as a preventive and as control strategy. For example, aerial spraying with ultra-low-volume insecticides has been used to prevent the establishment of mosquito populations carrying eastern and western equine encephalitis and St. Louis encephalitis viruses in some parts of North America. The widespread use of insecticides is a controversial issue: (1) mosquito resistance is increasing and (2) there are mounting environmental objections. Policy on insecticide use should be decided on a basis of a risk–benefit analysis on a situation-by-situation basis. Some countries have based their emergency arbovirus control program plans on aerial insecticide spraying. This strategy is aimed at rapid reduction of the adult female mosquito population in a defined area for a very short time.

Organophosphorus insecticides such as malathion or fenitrothion are delivered as an ultra-low-volume (short-acting) aerosol generated by spray machines mounted on backpacks, trucks, or low-flying aircraft. Spraying of the luggage bays and passenger cabins of aircraft with insecticides reduces the chances of intercontinental transfer of exotic arthropods, whether infected or noninfected.

Elimination of cracks and crevices in pig pens (in which soft ticks can hide) has been important in the control of African swine fever in Spain (see Chapter 17). A similar approach has been found to be successful in South Africa, where swine are often double-fenced to avoid contact with wart hogs. In the case of many other arbovirus infections, vector arthropods breed over too wide an area to make vector control feasible.

Disease Control through Quarantine

Movement of domestic animals across international and even state borders can be regulated, at least in the industrialized countries, where there are appropriate veterinary services and regulatory infrastructure. Quarantine remains a cornerstone in many animal disease control programs. A period of quarantine, with or without specific etiologic or serologic testing, is usually a requirement for the importation of animals from another country and similar requirements may be enforced within a country or local area to assist in the control or eradication of specific infectious agents.

As international movement of live animals for breeding purposes and exhibition has increased, so has the risk of introducing disease. Before the advent of air transport, the duration of shipment usually exceeded the incubation period of most diseases, but this is no longer the case. With the ever-increasing value of livestock, national veterinary authorities have tended to adopt stricter quarantine regulations to protect their livestock industries. Complete embargoes on importation are imposed for some animals by some countries. The concept of quarantine (Italian, *quarantina:* originally 40 days during which, in medieval times, ships arriving in port were forbidden to land freight or passengers if there was a suspicion of a contagious disease), where animals were simply isolated and observed for disease for a given period of time, is now augmented by extensive laboratory testing designed to detect previous exposure to selected viruses or a carrier state. Laboratory testing requirements are set down in detailed protocols and are supported by national legislation.

While historically the quarantine of dogs and cats has been a successful method for preventing the introduction of many diseases, such as rabies into Australia, New Zealand, and Great Britain (and only now, in light of the development of effective vaccines and diagnostic technology, is being reviewed), other diseases may be introduced in animal products (e.g., foot-and-mouth disease in meat products) or by virus-infected arthropods (e.g., bluetongue). It must also be recognized that most countries have land boundaries with their neighbors and cannot control human and wildlife movement easily (e.g., the movement of fox rabies in Europe). For countries with long land borders, quarantine is difficult to enforce. To help overcome this problem, most countries have agreed to notify each other through the Office International des Épizooties in Paris, France, of the disease status of their livestock. Although the recognition of internationally acceptable criteria for reporting the presence of specific disease remains a problem, the system usually provides countries with an opportunity to take appropriate action, such as increased vigilance along a national boundary and maintenance of vaccine stocks. However, there is still a long way to go in developing standards for testing animals and controlling animal movement. The problems are often social, economic, and political rather than scientific e.g., smuggling of exotic birds may play a significant role in the introduction of Newcastle disease and fowl plague viruses.

Disease Control through Vaccination

Each of the foregoing methods of control of viral diseases is focused on reducing the chances of infection. The most generally effective method of control, vaccination, is directed primarily at making animals exposed to particular viruses resistant to infection and unable to participate in the transmission and perpetuation of such viruses in the population at risk.

As outlined in Chapter 13 and discussed at length in the chapters of Part II of this book, there are now effective vaccines for many common viral diseases of animals. They are especially effective in diseases with a necessary viremic phase, such as canine distemper and feline panleukopenia. It has proved much more difficult to immunize effectively against infections that localize only in the alimentary or respiratory tracts. The effect of vaccination programs in reducing the incidence of foot-and-mouth disease in northern European livestock was dramatic from 1960 to 1990 (Figure 15.1). The penalty for prematurely discontinuing herd vaccination against foot-and-mouth disease, before disease is truly under control, is illustrated by events in southern Europe and Turkey over the last 10 years. To understand recent events, the history of foot-and-mouth disease must first be reviewed. A vaccination belt (buffer zone) was established in adjoining border areas of Turkish Thrace (Europe), Greece, and Bulgaria in 1962–1964 in response to the threat of foot-and-mouth disease (South African Territories type 1) virus from the Middle East. The Tripartite Group (European Commission for the Control of Foot-and-Mouth Disease, together with the Food and Agricultural Organization of the United Nations and the Office International des Épizooties) took responsibility for overseeing the program of annual vaccination in the zone. Vaccine was obtained from Western European

FIGURE 15.1.

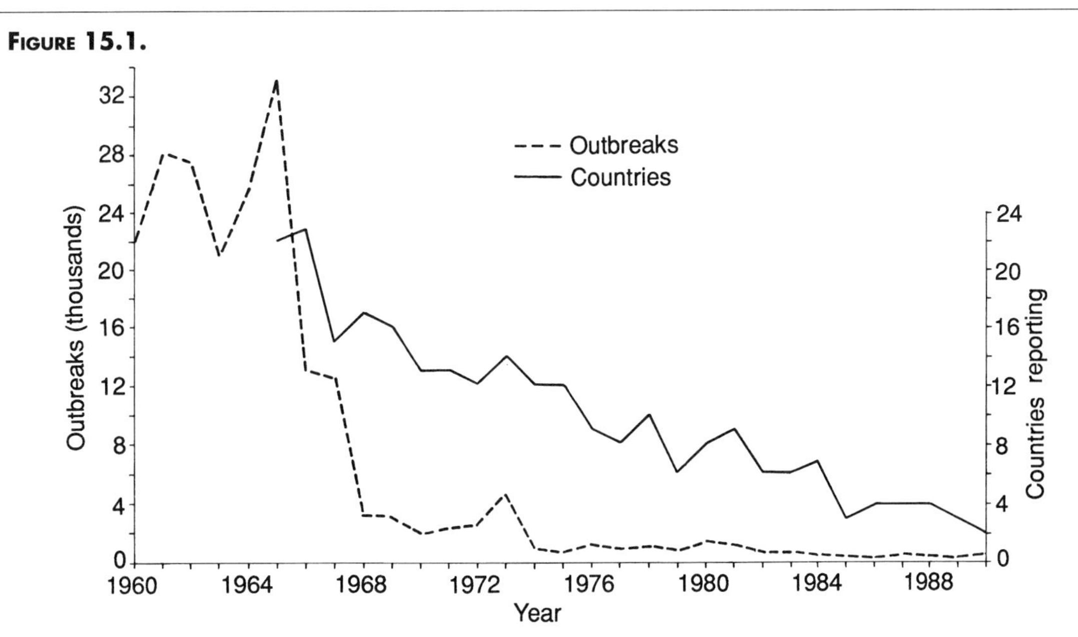

Foot-and-mouth disease in Europe, 1960–1990, showing numbers of outbreaks and numbers of countries reporting cases each year. The reduction since the mid-1960s is due to the effective use of trivalent inactivated vaccines (types A, O, and C). Since 1977 (with the exception of an epidemic in Italy in 1986–87) over two-thirds of the outbreaks each year have occurred in the Anatolian (Asian) region of Turkey. In 1990, only Turkey and Russia reported foot-and-mouth disease; of the 547 outbreaks, 542 were in Anatolian Turkey. (Data from the European Commission for the Control of Foot-and-Mouth Disease, *in* Animal Health Yearbook. FAO, Rome, 1990.)

manufacturers. During the following 25 years there were a few occasions when Middle Eastern strains of virus penetrated the buffer zone and caused outbreaks within it; however, disease did not spread further and so the zone was effective in protecting the southeastern part of Europe.

In the late 1980s, the European Union, followed by the countries of the former Eastern Bloc, decided that they would cease vaccination against foot-and-mouth disease. A consequence was that vaccination ceased in the Greek and Bulgarian parts of the buffer zone. The Tripartite Group considered what should be done about vaccination in Turkish Thrace and decided, in 1989, that vaccination should be discontinued forthwith and that a new strategic vaccination zone corresponding to approximately 12 provinces in the Marmara area of Asiatic Turkey be established. The modified strategy proved to be a failure. Foot-and-mouth disease has remained widespread in Asiatic Turkey with several hundred outbreaks being reported most years (predominantly type O1 Middle East and occasionally A22). Outbreaks have also occurred every year in the strategic vaccination zone. Of concern to Europe is that since 1989 there have been several occasions when strains of type O1 virus (with nucleotide sequences typical of Middle Eastern strains) have caused outbreaks in Bulgaria and Greece. In Bulgaria, single type O1 outbreaks occurred in 1991 and in 1993 near the border with European Turkey. In Greece, an epidemic with 95 outbreaks occurred in 1994 due to type O1 virus (closely related to the Bulgaria 1991 and 1993 strains, and to those from Anatolia).

In 1996 an epidemic due to type O1 occurred in Greece and Bulgaria. In light of this experience, the European Commission for the Control of Foot-and-Mouth Disease at its general session in Rome in April 1997 recommended that a vaccination zone should be reestablished in Turkish Thrace. This was accepted by the Turkish veterinary services and the policy has been implemented using vaccine produced at the national laboratory in Ankara. It is of interest that Europe was free of foot-and-mouth disease during 1997, but obviously it is too soon to conclude that the reestablished buffer zone has been successful in reducing the threat from the Middle East and Turkey.

Another example of the consequences of ineffective vaccines and failure to maintain herd vaccination was demonstrated by an epidemic of canine distemper in dogs in Finland in 1994–1995. Canine distemper reappeared in 1990 in Finland after a 16-year absence; initially the disease was of low incidence, but in 1994 and 1995 it is estimated that over 5000 cases occurred in areas with high densities of dogs. Analysis of vaccine sales indicated that fewer than 50% of dogs were being vaccinated annually prior to the epidemic; the epidemiological picture was further complicated by the conclusion that a disproportionate number of cases occurred in dogs vaccinated with the vaccine having the largest market share at the beginning of the outbreak. As a result of the epidemic, this vaccine was withdrawn from sale in Finland. For comparison, it is considered that 95% of children need to be vaccinated against the related virus, measles virus, to provide adequate herd immunity.

The introduction of recombinant DNA vaccines, designed in many very innovative ways, has opened up a new arena whereby vaccination and elimination programs may be conducted concurrently (see Chapter 13). For example, recombinant DNA-based, live-virus pseudorabies vaccines containing genomic deletions and thereby rendered nonpathogenic have become the basis for regional and national virus elimination programs. These vaccines, together with corresponding enzyme immunoassay test kits for differentiating vaccinated from naturally infected swine, are available commercially and are in use in Europe, New Zealand, and the United States. They are being used in very successful virus elimination programs. Similarly, recombinant DNA-based vaccinia virus-vectored rabies vaccines are currently being used in Europe, Canada, the United States, and some countries in Africa to control rabies in wildlife species.

Influence of Changing Patterns of Animal Production on Disease Control

During the latter part of the present century there has been a revolution in systems of food animal management and production, and these changes have had profound effects on disease patterns and control. Throughout some of the industrialized and nearly all of the developing world, systems of animal production for food and fiber are traditional or extensive, typified by the grazing of sheep and cattle across vast areas, as in the Americas and Australia, or by the movement of small herds of cattle or goats across the Sahel by nomadic tribes in Africa. Chickens and swine were penned and housed centuries ago, but intensive animal production systems, particularly for chickens and swine and, to a lesser extent, for cattle and sheep, were established in the middle of this century. In the industrialized world since World War II, they have been almost the only economically viable method of production for these species, but current concerns over the welfare of animals in these intensive units is promoting the reintroduction of more traditional husbandry. For example, the rural landscape of

England now features large numbers of pigs being reared in fields and so-called free-range chickens and eggs are preferred by some consumers.

Infectious diseases, particularly viral diseases, have often been the rate- and profit-limiting step in the development of intensive systems. Significant aspects of intensive animal production include the following:

1. The bringing together of large numbers of animals, often from diverse backgrounds, and confining them to limited spaces, at high density.
2. Asynchronous turnoff of animals for sale and the introduction of new animals.
3. The care of large numbers of animals by few, sometimes inadequately trained, personnel.
4. Elaborate housing systems with complex mechanical services for ventilation, feeding, waste disposal, and cleaning.
5. Limitation of the husbandry system to one species.
6. Manipulation of natural biologic rhythms (artificial daylight, estrus synchronization, etc.).
7. Use of very large batches of premixed, easily digestible foodstuffs.
8. Improved hygienic conditions.
9. Isolation of animal populations.

Some figures from North America illustrate the scale of operations of intensive animal production units. A large cattle feedlot operation in Alberta may have at any one time 100,000 cattle held in 1-acre pens of 400 animals each, with 2.5 cohort groups processed each year. A single farrowing facility in Iowa may house 5000 sows; using a fully integrated "farrow-to-finish" system there may at any one time be 50,000 swine in such a facility, of which 45,000 are sold and replaced 2.2 times a year. A dairy farm in California may milk 8000 cows, using dry lot technology for feed and waste management. A single broiler house in Georgia may house 50,000 birds, and a single farm may comprise many such houses. Further, many such farms are often located in close proximity. The growing time for a broiler is 9 weeks, so that several million birds may be produced on a single farm each year. There are also intensive systems for producing veal calves and lambs. Three consequences follow upon these situations:

1. The conditions favor the emergence and spread of endemic infectious diseases, as well as opportunistic infections.
2. The introduction of nonendemic viruses poses a great risk to such populations; although many farms are designed to provide reliable barriers against such introductions, many others are not.
3. These conditions favor multiple infections working synergistically, further complicating diagnosis, prevention, and therapy.

Disease is a component of the current concerns over welfare in intensive systems, but none of the basic characteristics of intensive livestock production systems are going to change because of disease constraints per se—the economics of these systems is such that losses due to diseases are generally small relative to gains, due mainly to feed and labor efficiency. Nevertheless, there is great merit in improving these production systems by minimizing disease losses, thereby increasing yields and lowering costs. The chief constraint is management, with the solution requiring the introduction of modern epidemiologic methods into the training and experience of veterinarians and other animal scientists concerned with livestock production.

Traditional extensive farming methods continue for all species in most developing countries, but particularly sub-Saharan Africa. In the latter, husbandry is often primitive, but requirements for animal products have increased greatly because of the continually expanding human populations. For example, in the Sahel, installation of watering points has led to a build-up of herds in good seasons, with disastrous results when droughts occur or when epidemic diseases enter the region.

More frequent and extensive movement of domestic livestock, wildlife species, and people exacerbates the spread of infectious diseases, especially in Africa, where the large populations of wildlife harbor several viruses that affect domestic livestock (e.g., malignant catarrhal fever). These are matters of national and international concern, not only for humanitarian reasons, but because of the risk of the international transfer of exotic viruses of livestock and the disastrous consequences such importations could have on animal production industries in industrialized countries.

The situation with companion animals is very different, but the risk of infectious diseases varies greatly between the single, mature-age household dog, cat, or pony and the large, sometimes disreputable, breeding establishments for these species ("puppy farms," for example) in which several hundred animals, of all ages, are kept and bred.

Biocontrol of Pest Species Using Viruses

The use of recombinant DNA "vaccines" expressing genes to control the reproduction of wildlife and feral species is technically feasible. These products have been proposed as an adjunct to disease eradication programs. One example in support of the national program for the eradication of pseudorabies from the domestic swine population in the United States features the possible use of a swinepox vector expressing genes affecting the development of the reproductive system of feral swine. The prevalence of antibody to pseudorabies virus in feral swine populations in the southern states often exceeds 30% and is considered by some to be a major impediment to the national eradication program. This approach can be justified ecologically. Feral swine are an introduced species to North America; they are not indigenous and trace their ancestry to the early European voyages of discovery.

In contrast to the proposed use of recombinant products to reduce populations through reproductive control, the use of viruses as pathogens, such as myxomatosis virus and rabbit calicivirus to control pest populations of rabbits in Australia, has already been established. The use of these viruses can be justified ecologically as the rabbit is an introduced species to the continent (see Chapter 36). While rabbits are not considered to be a reservoir of any diseases of importance to Australian wildlife or agriculture, they are an important component in endangering the long-term survival of several indigenous species of marsupials and rare plant species on the Australian continent through competitive grazing.

Eradication of Viral Diseases

Disease control, whether by vaccination alone or by vaccination plus the various other methods described earlier, is an ongoing process that must be maintained as long as the disease is of economic importance. If a disease can be eradicated within a country so that the virus is no longer present anywhere except in microbiologically secure laboratories, control measures within that country are no longer required and costs are lowered permanently. Surveillance to prevent the reintroduction of the disease into the country is still necessary. Eradication of a disease that is endemic demands major financial commitments for a long period, often decades, if success is to be achieved. Close cooperation between veterinary services and agricultural industries is essential. To achieve such cooperation, disease eradication programs must be justified by cost–benefit analyses and risk–benefit analyses. They must also be justified politically. As programs proceed, they must ensure feedback of information on progress (or problems) directly to those involved and to the public via the media.

Foot-and-mouth disease has now been eradicated from a number of countries in which it was once important: Japan, United Kingdom, United States, Mexico, and the countries of Central America. An outbreak in Taiwan in March 1997 has illustrated vividly the impact of this disease on the agricultural exports of a small country and is a salient reminder of the importance of this disease. Capitalizing on its geographical advantage of being an island, Taiwan had been free of foot-and-mouth disease since 1929, while most neighboring countries of continental Asia remained infected with the disease. Prior to March 1997, Taiwan had a robust export market of pork to Japan (6 million pigs per year). This represented 70% of its pork exports, approximately 60% of its pig production, and approximately 10% of its entire agricultural production. The presence of the disease on the island went unnoticed initially, as the virus was pathogenic only for pigs and not for cattle or other ruminants. Only when the authorities observed increasing mortality in piglets was the true nature of the problem suspected. By time the disease was confirmed as foot-and-mouth disease, the epidemic had spread widely throughout the island. Records indicate that on March 29, 1997, 1106 farms were affected, by April 22, a total of 4394, and by May 17, over 6100. When confronted with the extent of the epidemic, the Taiwanese government had little option but to ban all exports of pork. Fortunately, Taiwan has a broad-based export trade beyond agriculture and, while such a ban causes substantial economic hardship, it is not likely to have long-term adverse effects on the economy of Taiwan.

With hindsight, various factors contributed to the extremely rapid spread of the virus. Most important were a high density of pigs and ineffective control of animal and product movement until the epidemic was well into its course. There was no legislation against the feeding of waste food and several outbreaks probably originated from infected pig products. The procedures used for the disposal of pigs were chaotic and probably resulted in the dissemination of virus. The rate of spread during the first 100 days of the epidemic was at a rate of around 60 reported outbreaks per day—quite a challenge for any veterinary service!

The eradication of a specific disease from a region, through the combined efforts of several countries, brings with it incremental advantages. The experience of the United States with Canada, Mexico, and the countries of Central America in eradicating foot-and-mouth disease is a good example. So far, *global* eradication has been achieved for only one disease, and that a disease of humans. The last endemic case of smallpox occurred in Somalia in October 1977. Global eradication was achieved by an intensified effort led by the World Health Organization that involved a high level of international cooperation and made use of a potent, inexpensive and very stable vaccine. However, mass vaccination alone could not have achieved eradication of the disease from the densely populated tropical countries where it remained endemic in the 1970s because it was impossible to achieve the necessary very high level of vaccine coverage in many remote settings. A revised strategy was implemented in the last years of the eradication campaign involving *surveillance and containment.* That is, cases and niches where transmission was ongoing were actively sought out and "ring vaccination" (vaccination of everyone in the area, first in the household and then at increasing distances from the index case). The global smallpox eradication campaign was a highly cost-effective operation. The expenditure by the World Health Organization for the campaign between 1967 and 1979 was $81 million, to which could be added about $32 million in bilateral aid contributions and some $200 million in services provided by the endemic countries involved in the campaign. Against this expenditure of about $313 million over the 11 years of the campaign may be set an *annual* global expenditure of about $1 billion for vaccination, airport inspections, and so on made necessary by the existence of smallpox. This equation takes no account of the deaths, misery, and costs of smallpox itself or of the complications of vaccination.

More recently, the World Health Organization has organized a campaign to globally eradicate the three polioviruses. Massive vaccination campaigns and laboratory-based surveillance for the presence of the viruses in sewage have eliminated wild-type polioviruses from the western hemisphere and all the developed countries of the eastern hemisphere. Global eradication is expected in about the year 2002. Many lessons have been learned from these programs, which are applicable in veterinary medicine. For example, rabies was eliminated from the United Kingdom in 1901 and again in 1922 after reintroduction of the disease during World War I. The cost savings following upon this success have been very large indeed—the usual four-pronged rabies control infrastructure required in countries where rabies is endemic, i.e., surveillance, diagnostics, animals control and quarantine, and vaccination, has been replaced by an infrastructure focused on control over the importation of

Table 15.2
Biological Characteristics of Viruses That Might Enhance Their Vulnerability to Eradication

Characteristic	Variola (smallpox) virus	Canine distemper virus	Newcastle disease virus	Rinderpest virus	Foot-and-mouth disease viruses
Host species	Humans	Dogs	Chickens	Cattle	Cattle
Reservior host in wildlife	No	No	Yes	Not self perpetuating	Yes, in Africa
Persistent infection occurs	No	No	No	No	Yes, especially in African buffalo (*Syncerus caffer*)
Subclinical cases occur	No	No	Yes	Unusual	Yes
Number of serotypes	One	One	One	One	Many
Infectivity during prodromal stage	No	Yes	Yes	Yes	Yes, very infectious
Vaccine					
Effective	Yes	Yes	Yes	Yes	Usually but type-specific polyvalent formulation used
Heat stable	Yes	Moderately	Moderately	No[a]	Yes
Number of doses	One	One	Two	One	Two, then annually or more often
Early containment of outbreak possible	Yes	No	Sometimes	Yes	Difficult
High level of public concern	Yes	No	Yes	Yes	Yes

[a]Vaccina and capripox virus recombinant vaccines are available that overcome this problem but neither is in commercial use.

unvaccinated animals. The same kind of cost–benefit value has been obtained in several European countries, including Switzerland and France, and regionally in southern Germany and Belgium. Nevertheless, rabies is not a candidate for global eradication—its entrenchment in wildlife species in many countries makes this impossible.

The first animal disease that should be a target for global eradication is rinderpest. Rinderpest was a devastating disease of cattle in Europe before it was finally eliminated in 1949. It has been a scourge in sub-Saharan Africa ever since livestock farming was introduced in the late 1800s; remarkably, it was very nearly eliminated from Africa in the 1980s by massive cattle vaccination programs, but regional wars and violence interceded, programs were stopped, and the disease made a rapid comeback in many areas. The lessons learned from these vaccination programs, additional lessons from the success in eradicating smallpox and polio, the availability of very good vaccines and the technology to maintain a cold chain for assuring vaccine potency, and an improving sense of "public will" have all been used in the last decade to bring us to the point where rinderpest may well be eradicated globally. Success in eliminating rinderpest from India has been remarkable in recent years, but war-torn areas, such as southern Sudan, Afghanistan, Somalia, and northern Iraq, still present nidi of infection.

Conventional veterinary vaccination campaigns, through central government, are often impossible to implement in such areas, which has led to community-based approaches (supported by nongovernmental orga-

Table 15.3
Some Important New, Emerging, and Reemerging Animal Viruses

African horse sickness viruses (mosquito-borne; a historic problem in southern Africa; now entrenched in the Iberian peninsula; a major threat to horses worldwide)

African swine fever virus (tick borne and also spread by contact; an extremely pathogenic virus; recently present in Europe and South America; a potential threat to commercial swine industries)

Avian influenza viruses (spread by wild birds; epidemics in the United States in 1983 and Mexico in the 1990s; a major threat to commercial poultry industries of all countries)

Bluetongue viruses (*Culicoides* spp.-borne; the isolation of several strains in Australia led to an important nontariff trade barrier issue)

Bovine spongiform encephalopathy prion (the cause of a major epidemic in cattle in the United Kingdom, resulting in major economic loss and trade embargo)

Canine parvovirus (a new virus, having mutated from feline panleukopenia virus; the virus has swept around the world rapidly, causing a pandemic of severe disease in dogs)

Chronic wasting disease of deer and elk prion (a spongiform encephalopathy agent of unknown source, discovered in captive breeding herds in the United States and recently in feral animals in the United States and Canada)

Equine morbillivirus (recognized in Queensland, Australia, in 1994; the cause of fatal acute respiratory distress syndrome in horses and humans; bats serve as reservoir host)

Feline immunodeficiency virus (a rather newly recognized major cause of morbidity and mortality in cats globally)

Foot-and-mouth-disease viruses (still considered the most dangerous exotic viruses of animals in the world because of their capacity for rapid transmission and great economic loss; still entrenched in Africa, the middle East, and Asia; still capable of emergence in any commercial cattle industry)

Malignant catarrhal fever virus (the African form is an exotic, lethal herpesvirus of cattle; its presence is an important nontariff trade barrier issue)

Marine mammal morbilliviruses (epidemic disease first identified in 1988 in European seals; now realized as several important emerging viruses, endangering several species of marine mammals)

Porcine reproductive and respiratory syndrome virus (also called Lelystad virus—rather recently recognized as an important cause of disease in swine in Europe and the United States)

Rabbit hemorrhagic disease virus (rabbit biocontrol agent, newly released in Australia and New Zealand; emergent in the sense that purposeful release mimics a virgin-soil epidemic)

Rinderpest virus (potential for causing substantial economic loss; entrenched in one region of Africa; capable of reemergence, requiring wide-area surveillance)

Simian immunodeficiency virus (significance of these viruses increasingly recognized as important models in AIDS research)

nizations) sometimes linked to parallel vaccination programs for children against measles, polio, etc. This can reduce the cost of the infrastructure significantly, particularly that of maintaining the cold chain. Interestingly, in southern Sudan, some pastoral groups have been more enthusiastic to have their cattle vaccinated than their children, a feature that has led to increased childhood vaccination. In eastern Africa, there is an additional problem: recent isolates from game animals in Kenyan wildlife parks are virulent for eland, kudu, and buffalo, but not for cattle, thus unrecognized spread has probably occurred among domestic livestock.

Successful regional/country eradication of velogenic Newcastle disease, fowl plague, hog cholera, foot-and-mouth disease, scrapie, infectious bovine rhinotracheitis, pseudorabies, and bovine leukemia raises the question of whether there are other animal diseases that might one day be eradicated globally. The biologic characteristics of the viruses and diseases that have been eradicated from individual countries, and in some cases regions, are set out in Table 15-2.

The viruses that cause these diseases share several essential characteristics: (1) they have no uncontrollable reservoirs, (2) they do not cause persistent infection and chronic or recrudescent disease where long-term or intermittent viral shedding would occur, (3) they exist as one or few stable serotypes, and (4) they have been amenable to efficacious vaccine development. In addition to the biologic properties of smallpox virus being particularly favorable, there were strong financial incentives for the

Table 15.4
Some Important New, Emerging, and Reemerging Zoonotic Viruses

Bovine spongiform encephalopathy prion (recognized in 1986; the cause of a major epidemic in cattle in the United Kingdom, resulting in major economic loss and trade embargo; identified as the cause of human central nervous system disease: new-variant Creutzfeldt–Jakob disease)

Crimean-Congo hemorrhagic fever virus[a] (tick borne; reservoir in sheep; severe human disease with 10% mortality; widespread across Africa, the Middle East, and Asia)

Ebola[a] and Marburg[a] viruses (natural animal reservoirs unknown; Ebola and Marburg viruses are the causes of the most lethal hemorrhagic fevers known)

Equine morbillivirus (recognized in Queensland, Australia, in 1994; the cause of fatal acute respiratory distress syndrome in horses; spread to humans causing similar also fatal disease; bats serve as reservoir host)

Guanarito virus[a] (rodent borne; the newly discovered cause of Venezuelan hemorrhagic fever)

Hantaviruses[a] (rodent borne; the cause of important rodent-borne hemorrhagic fever in Asia and Europe; Sin Nombre virus and related viruses are the cause of hantavirus pulmonary syndrome in the Americas)

Influenza viruses (reservoir in birds, especially sea birds, with intermediate evolution in swine, and viral species jumping bringing new viruses to human populations each year; the cause of the single most deadly human epidemic ever recorded—the pandemic of 1918 in which 25–40 million people died; the cause of panic in Hong Kong in 1997 as an H5N1 avian influenza virus for the first time appeared in humans, causing severe disease and several deaths; the cause of thousands of deaths every winter in the elderly)

Japanese encephalitis virus (mosquito borne; swine serve as amplifying reservoir hosts; very severe, lethal encephalitis in humans; now spreading across southeast Asia; great epidemic potential)

Junin virus[a] (rodent borne; the cause of Argentine hemorrhagic fever)

Lassa virus[a] (rodent borne; a very important, severe disease in West Africa)

Machupo virus[a] (rodent borne; the cause of Bolivian hemorrhagic fever, recent outbreaks after many years of quiescence)

Rabies virus (transmitted by the bite of rabid animals; raccoon epidemic still spreading across the northeastern United States; coyote/dog epidemic in south Texas; thousands of deaths every year in India, Sri Lanka, the Philippines, and elsewhere)

Rift Valley fever virus[a] (mosquito borne; sheep, cattle, and wild mammals serve as amplifying hosts; the cause of one of the most explosive epidemics ever seen when the virus first appeared in 1977 in Egypt)

Ross River virus (mosquito borne; cause of human epidemic arthritis; has moved across the Pacific region several times)

Sabiá virus (rodent borne; newly discovered cause of severe, even fatal hemorrhagic fever in Brazil; two recent laboratory-acquired cases)

Yellow fever virus[a] (mosquito borne; monkeys serve as reservoir hosts; one of the most deadly diseases in history, great potential for urban reemergence)

[a]Viruses that cause hemorrhagic fevers in humans.

industrialized countries to promote the global eradication of smallpox because of the costs associated with vaccination of international travelers, port inspections, etc.

Emerging Viral Diseases

The term *emerging diseases* was used with remarkable prescience as a book title by the Food and Agricultural Organization in 1966 to describe several viral diseases of veterinary importance, such as African swine fever, that appeared to have the potential to spread beyond their known geographical distribution. In 1992, the Institute of Medicine, a branch of the National Academy of Sciences of the United States, in response to the recognition of the emergence of AIDS and nosocomial virus diseases such as Ebola hemorrhagic fever, but also to the reemergence of several bacterial diseases such as tuberculosis, issued a report in which emerging infectious

Table 15.5
New, Emerging, and Reemerging Viruses in Endangered/Threatened Species (and Species Involved in Captive Breeding and Translocation Programs)

Avian influenza viruses, velogenic Newcastle disease virus, and other avian paramyxoviruses in endangered psittacine species (threat of quarrantine and slaughter to control risk of importation of exotic viruses that are a threat to poultry industries)
Avian poxviruses in endangered avian species in Hawaii (threat of fatal disease in highly susceptible species)
Callitrichid arenavirus in golden lion tamarins in Brazil and in captive breeding/release programs (the virus is indistinguishable from lymphocytic choriomeningitis virus; a universally lethal disease; a major problem in many endangered tamarin species)
Canine distemper virus in lions and leopards in the Serengeti and elsewhere in Kenya and Tanzania (threat of fatal disease in highly susceptible species; very large numbers of lions have suffered fatal infection in the past 10 years)
Canine distemper virus in the red panda in zoos (threat of fatal disease in highly susceptible species; attenuated virus canine vaccine causes disease and immunosuppression—inactivated vaccine used)
Canine distemper virus in the black-footed ferret (lethal disease; its control remains crucial to the survival of this endangered North American species; canine attenuated virus vaccine causes disease and immunosuppression—inactivated vaccine used)
Canine parvovirus in the red wolf in captive breeding/release programs in southeastern United States (threat of fatal disease in highly susceptible species—pups now recaptured each year and vaccinated with canine vaccine)
Eastern equine encephalitis virus in the whooping crane (lethal disease; its control is crucial to the survival of this endangered North American species—chicks now captured and vaccinated with human vaccine)
Ebola virus in chimpanzees in Côte d'Ivoire and Gabon and gorillas in Gabon (threat of fatal disease in susceptible endangered species)
Encephalomyocarditis virus in elephants in the Kruger Park, South Africa (threat of fatal disease in susceptible signature species that is important in the rising tourist industry, which in turn is the funding base for most African wildlife conservation programs)
Equine morbillivirus and Australian bat lyssavirus in bats (flying foxes) in Australia (threatened bat species, the reservoir hosts of these viruses, face unwarranted killing to remove the threat of these zoonotic viruses)
Feline infectious peritonitis virus in the cheetah, the snow leopard, and small spotted felids (lethal disease; its control is crucial to the survival of these endangered species)
Marine mammal morbilliviruses (epidemic disease first identified in 1988 in European seals; a complex of lethal diseases in several species of seals, sea lions, dolphins, porpoises, and whales caused by related morbilliviruses; control is crucial to the survival of several endangered species such as the monk seal)
Psitticine beak and feather disease virus—(in captive and free-living parrots, in Australia and South America, a progressive, ultimately fatal disease in threatened and endangered species)
Rabies in endangered free-living wild canid species (lethal disease; its control is crucial to the survival of several endangered African wild canid species)
Rinderpest virus in endangered free-living ungulate species in Africa (several wild African ungulate species, such as buffalo in Tsavo West National Park, Kenya, are considered by farmers as reservoir hosts of this virus, the source of epidemics in cattle; control is crucial to the acceptance of cohabitation of domestic and wild animals by farmers)
Simian hemorrhagic fever virus in captive macaques (silent infection in several simian species serves as the reservoir of virus that cause lethal disease in macaques; a problem in macaque breeding programs)

diseases were defined as diseases whose incidence has increased within the past two decades or threaten to increase in the near future. It was this 1992 report that drew the public's attention to infectious diseases and the concept of emergence. Because of their rapidity of spread, viral diseases feature prominently in any listing of emerging disease. Their prominence has been highlighted further by recognition of epidemics throughout the 1990s of Ebola hemorrhagic fever in central Africa (Chapter 28), by an outbreak in 1994 of a new paramyxovirus disease in horses and humans in Australia (Chapter 26), and by identification in 1997 of a zoonotic outbreak of H5N1 avian influenza in Hong Kong (Chapter 30).

If the definition used by the Institute of Medicine is applied to veterinary medicine, numerous viral diseases in this book currently qualify as emerging diseases. Tables 15.3, 15.4, and 15.5 list some of these diseases and the viruses that cause them.

It hardly needs to be added that the principles outlined in this and preceding chapters of Part I of this book are key to any study of emerging diseases. Further information about these diseases and viruses may be found in the relevant chapters in Part II of this book. Several have already been referred to when illustrating specific points in this and previous chapters.

Bioterrorism and Emergence of Viral Diseases

The new world order has led to revised attitudes to biological warfare. In comparison to nuclear weapons and, to a lesser extent, chemical agents of mass destruction, biological agents combine relatively easy availability with maximum potential for destruction and terror. Many governments anticipate greater use of infectious agents by terrorists in the future with the focus on inflicting human casualties. Economic and/or ecological catastrophes in animal populations are possible as well through the orchestrated use of several viruses discussed in this book. While it would be possible to provide examples of several scenarios where viruses of veterinary importance might be used by terrorists, the authors will leave further consideration of this subject to the reader.

Further Reading

Block, S., ed. (1991). "Disinfection, Sterilization, and Preservation," 4 ed. Lea & Febiger, Philadelphia, PA.

Fenner, F., Henderson, D. A., Arita, I., Jezek, Z., and Ladnyi, I. D. (1988). "Smallpox and its Eradication." World Health Organization, Geneva.

Food and Agriculture Organization of the United Nations. (published annually). "FAO-WHO-OIE Animal Health Yearbook." Food and Agriculture Organization, Rome.

Hanson, R. P., and Hanson, M. G. (1983). "Animal Disease Control. Regional Programs." Iowa State University Press, Ames.

Lederberg, J., Shope, R. E., and Oaks, S. C., eds. (1992). "Emerging Infections: Microbial Threats to Health in the United States. Institute of Medicine, National Academy of Sciences of the United States of America, National Academy Press, Washington, DC.

Morris, R. S., ed. (1991). "Epidemiological Information Systems." Rev. Sci. Technol., vol. 10, No. 7. Office International des Épizooties, Paris.

Murphy, F. A., and Nathanson, N., eds. (1994). New and emerging viral diseases. *Semin. Virol.* 5, 85–187.

Office International des Épizooties (1995). "Disinfectants: Actions and Applications," OIE Sci. Tech. Rev. 14 (1) and 14 (2). Office International Épizooties, Paris.

Office International des Épizooties. (1998). "Disease Information (information and articles available by country and by disease)." Office International des Épizooties, Paris. Available also at: http://www.oie.org/info/info_a.htm

Office International des Épizooties." International Animal Health Code for Mammals, Birds and Bees and International Aquatic Animal Health Code." (published annually) Office International des Épizooties, Paris. Available also at: http://www.oie.org/a_code.htm

Office International des Épizooties. "World Animal Health." (published annually) Office International des Épizooties, Paris.

Quinn, P. J. (1991). Disinfection and disease prevention in veterinary medicine. *In* "Disinfection, Sterilization and Preservation," (S. S. Block, ed.), 4th ed., pp. 846–855. Lea & Febiger, Philadelphia, PA.

Radostits, O. M., and Blood, D. C. (1985). "Herd Health. A Textbook of Health and Production Management of Agricultural Animals." Saunders, Philadelphia, PA.

Russell, A. D., Hugo, W. B., and Ayliffe, G., A. J. eds. (1992). "Principles and Practice of Disinfection, Preservation, and Sterilization," 2nd ed. Blackwell, Oxford.

Schnurrenberger, P. R., Sharman, R. S., and Wise, G. H. (1987). "Attacking Animal Diseases: Concepts and Strategies for Control and Eradication." Iowa State University Press, Ames.

Truyen, U., Parrish, C. R., Harder, T. C., and Kaaden, O. R. (1995). There is nothing permanent except change. The emergence of new virus diseases. *Vet. Microbiol.* **43**, 103–122.

Watson, W. A., and Brown, A. C. L. (1981). Legislation and control of virus diseases. *In* "Virus Diseases of Food Animals" (E. P. J. Gibbs, ed.), vol. 1, pp. 265–306. Academic Press, London.

World Health Organization. (1991). "Safe Use of Pesticides. Fourteenth Report of the WHO Expert Committee on Vector Biology and Control," WHO Tech. Rep. Ser. 813. World Health Organization, Geneva.

PART II

Veterinary and Zoonotic Viral Diseases

CHAPTER 16

Poxviridae

The family *Poxviridae* includes several viruses of veterinary and medical importance. Poxvirus diseases occur in most animal species and are of considerable economic importance in some regions of the world. Diseases such as sheeppox have been eradicated in developed countries, but are still a cause of major losses in some developing countries.

The history of poxviruses has been dominated by smallpox. This disease, once a worldwide and greatly feared disease of humans, has now been eradicated by use of the vaccine that traces its ancestry to Edward Jenner and the cowsheds of Gloucestershire in England. Although Jenner's first vaccines probably came from cattle, the origins of modern vaccinia virus, the smallpox vaccine virus, are unknown. In his *Inquiry* published in 1798, Jenner described the clinical signs of cowpox in cattle and humans and how human infection provided protection against smallpox. At the time smallpox was responsible for more than 10% of all deaths in children. Jenner's discovery soon led to the establishment of vaccination programs around the world. However, it was not until Pasteur's work nearly 100 years later that the principle was used again—in fact it was Pasteur who suggested the general terms *vaccine* and *vaccination* (from *vacca,* Latin for cow) in honor of Jenner. Other landmark discoveries came from early work on poxviruses: myxoma virus, an important cause of disease in domestic rabbits, described first by Sanarelli in 1896, was the first viral pathogen of a laboratory animal. Rabbit fibroma virus, described in 1932 by Shope, was the first virus proven to cause tissue hyperplasia (which was at the time considered to be related to tumor formation).

With the eradication of smallpox, use of the smallpox vaccine was discontinued throughout the world, but it is possible that it may be widely used again, as recombinant DNA vaccines using vaccinia virus as a vector for delivering a wide range of viral and microbial antigens are the subject of intensive research (see Chapter 13). The use of other poxviruses as vaccine vectors is also being investigated vigorously.

Properties of Poxviruses

Classification

The family *Poxviridae* is subdivided into two subfamilies: *Chordopoxvirinae* (poxviruses of vertebrates) and *Entomopoxvirinae* (poxviruses of insects). The subfamily *Chordopoxvirinae* is subdivided into eight genera (Table 16.1). Each of the genera, except *Molluscipoxvirus,* includes species that cause diseases in domestic or laboratory animals. There are other poxviruses that have not yet been classified; indeed new poxviruses are being discovered constantly, including viruses isolated from lizards, frogs, deer, and kangaroos, among others. Further, because of the large size and distinctive structure of poxvirus virions, negative stain electron microscopic examination of lesion material is used in many veterinary and zoonotic virology laboratories for diagnosis—this method allows rapid visualization of poxviruses in various specimens, but it does not allow specific verification of viral species or variants. Hence, many specimens are left with a diagnosis of "poxvirus," "orthopoxvirus," or "parapoxvirus," with further identification only pertaining to the species of origin. If further characterization, including molecular methods, was used to follow up on such diagnoses, it is presumed that many more poxvirus species would be recognized as animal pathogens. For example, entomopox-like virions, previously only associated with insects, have been found in lesions in fish raised commercially.

Virion Properties

Most poxvirus virions are brick shaped, about 250 × 200 × 200 nm in size; in contrast, virions of the members of the genus *Parapoxvirus* are cocoon shaped and 260 × 160 nm in size (Figures 16.1A, 16.1B, 16.1C, and 16.1D). There is no isometric nucleocapsid conforming to either icosahedral or helical symmetry found in most other viruses (see Chapter 1); hence poxviruses are said to have a "complex" structure.

Virions of most poxviruses are composed of an outer layer of tubular structures, arranged rather irregularly, giving them a characteristic appearance; in contrast, virions of the members of the genus *Parapoxvirus* are covered with long thread-like surface tubules, which because of the superimposition of features on the tops and bottoms of virions appear to be arranged in crisscross fashion resembling a ball of yarn. Virions of some ungrouped viruses from reptiles are brick shaped but have a surface structure similar to that of parapoxviruses (Figure 16.1B). Interestingly, recent cryoelectron microscopic studies have suggested that all these virion surface structures, which have been used to identify poxviruses ever since the development of negative-contrast electron microscopy, may actually represent dehydration (shrinkage) artifacts. The outer layer encloses a dumbbell-shaped core and two lateral bodies of unknown nature. The core contains the viral DNA together with several proteins. Virions that are released from cells by budding, rather than by cellular disruption, have an extra envelope that contains cellular lipids and several virus-specified proteins.

The genome consists of a single molecule of linear double-stranded DNA varying in size from 130 kbp (parapoxviruses), 280 kbp (fowlpox virus), up to 375 kbp (entomopoxviruses). The genomes of vaccinia virus (191,636 bp) and several other poxviruses have been sequenced completely. Poxvirus genomes have cross-links that join the two DNA strands at both ends; the ends of each DNA strand have long inverted tandemly repeated nucleotide sequences that form single-stranded loops (Figure 16.2).

Poxvirus genomes have the capacity to encode about 200 proteins, as many as 100 of which are contained in virions. Only relatively few viral proteins have been assigned functions; the majority with known functions are enzymes involved in nucleic acid synthesis and virion structural components. Examples of the former are DNA polymerase, DNA ligase, RNA polymerase, enzymes involved in capping and polyadenylation of messenger RNAs, and thymidine kinase. Several poxvirus genes encode proteins that are secreted from infected cells and affect the response of the host to infection. Among these virokines is a homologue of epidermal growth factor, a protein that down-regulates complement, virokines conferring resistance to interferon, and yet others suppressing the immune response by inhibiting certain host cytokines.

Poxviruses are transmitted between animals by several routes: by introduction of virus into small skin

Table 16.1
Poxviruses: Host Range and Geographic Distribution

Genus	Virus	Major hosts	Host range	Geographic distribution
Orthopoxvirus				
	Variola (smallpox) virus	Humans	Narrow	Eradicated globally
	Vaccinia virus	Numerous: humans, cattle,[a] buffalo,[a] swine,[a] rabbits[a]	Broad	Worldwide
	Cowpox virus	Numerous: cattle, humans, rats, cats, gerbils, large felids, elephants, rhinoceros, okapi	Broad	Europe, Asia
	Camelpox virus	Camels	Narrow	Asia, Africa
	Ectromelia virus	Mice, voles	Narrow	Europe
	Monkeypox virus	Numerous: squirrels, monkeys, anteaters, great apes, humans	Broad	Western and central Africa
	Uasin Gishu disease virus	Horses	Broad	Eastern Africa
	Tatera poxvirus	Gerbils (*Tatera kempi*)	?	Western Africa
	Raccoon poxvirus	Raccoons	Broad	North America
	Vole poxvirus	Voles (*Microtus californicus*)	?	California
	Seal poxvirus	Grey seals (*Halichoerus grypus*)	?	North Sea
Capripoxvirus				
	Sheeppox virus	Sheep, goats	Narrow	Africa, Asia
	Goatpox virus	Goats, sheep	Narrow	Africa, Asia
	Lumpyskin disease virus	Cattle, Cape buffalo	Narrow	Africa
Suipoxvirus				
	Swinepox virus	Swine	Narrow	Worldwide
Leporipoxvirus				
	Myxoma virus	Rabbits (*Oryctolagus* and *Sylvilagus* spp.)	Narrow	Americas, Europe, Australia
Molluscipoxvirus				
	Molluscum contagiosum virus	Humans	Narrow	Worldwide
Yatapoxvirus				
	Yabapox virus and tanapox virus	Monkeys, humans	Narrow	West Africa
Avipoxvirus				
	Fowlpox virus	Chickens, turkeys, other birds	Narrow	Worldwide
Parapoxvirus				
	Orf virus	Sheep, goats, humans	Narrow	Worldwide
	Pseudocowpox virus	Cattle, humans	Narrow	Worldwide
	Bovine papular stomatitis virus	Cattle, humans	Narrow	Worldwide
	Ausdyk virus	Camels	Narrow	Africa, Asia
	Seal parapoxvirus	Seals, humans	Narrow	Worldwide

[a] Infected from humans; now that smallpox vaccination has been discontinued for the civilian populations of all countries, such infections are unlikely to be seen.

FIGURE 16.1.

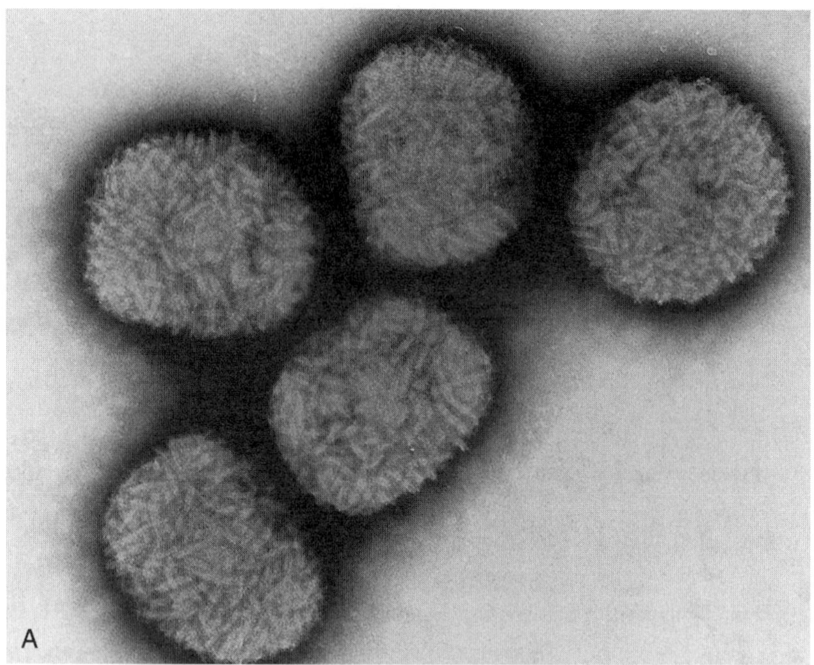

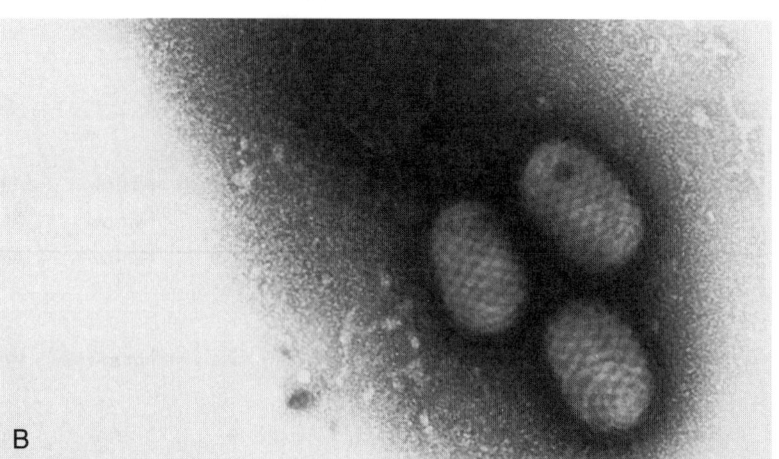

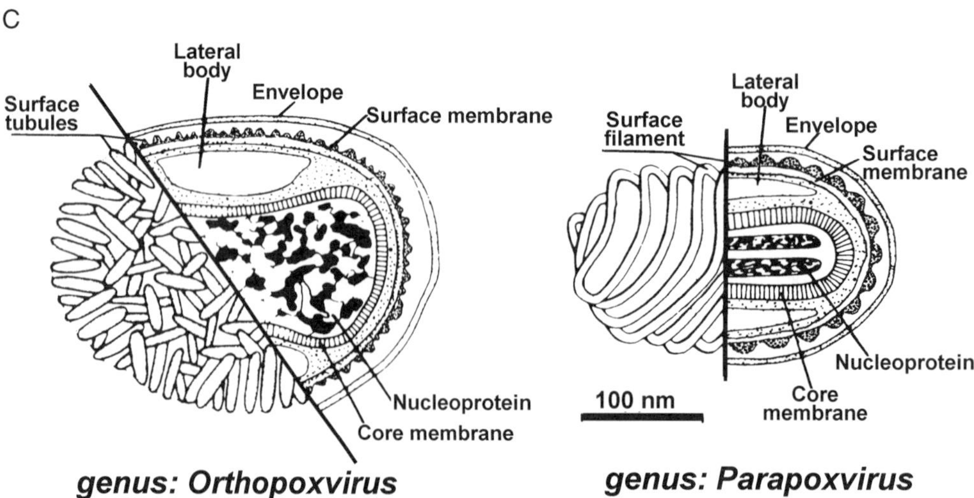

Poxviridae (bar = 100 nm). (A) Negatively stained vaccinia virus virions showing surface tubules characteristic of member viruses of all genera except the genus *Parapoxvirus*. (B) Negatively stained orf virus virions showing characteristic surface tubules of the member viruses of the genus *Parapoxvirus*. (C, left) Schematic diagram, genus *Orthopoxvirus* (and all other vertebrate poxvirus genera except the genus *Parapoxvirus*). (C, right) Schematic diagram, genus *Parapoxvirus*. Part of the two diagrams shows the surface structure of an unenveloped virion, whereas the other part shows a cross section through the center of an enveloped virion.

FIGURE 16.2.

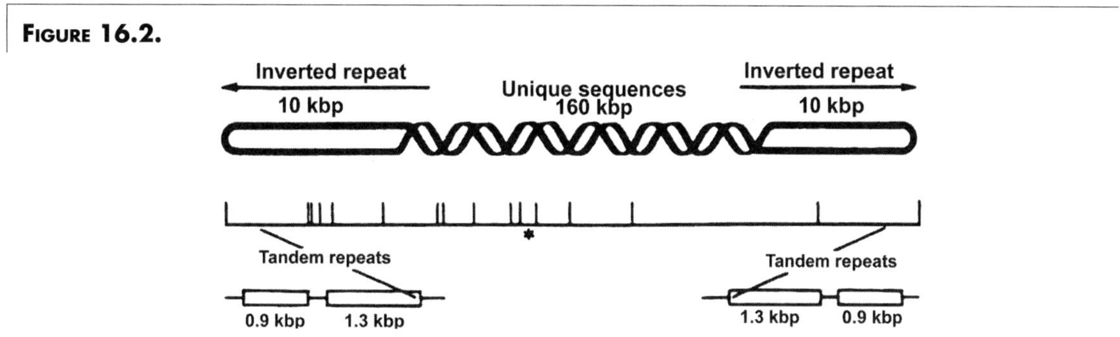

Schematic representation of the DNA of vaccinia virus. (Top) Linear double-stranded DNA molecule with terminal hairpins and inverted repeats (not to scale). Denatured DNA forms a single-stranded circular molecule. (Center) Vaccinia virus genome *Hin*dIII cleavage sites, the asterisk indicates the fragment that contains the thymidine kinase gene. (Bottom) Each 10-kbp terminal region contains two groups of tandem repeats composed of short sequences rich in AT. (From F. Fenner, R. Wittek, and K. R. Dumbell, "The Orthopoxviruses." Academic Press, New York, 1989.)

abrasions or directly or indirectly from a contaminated environment. For example, orf virus is transmitted by the respiratory route via droplets from infected animals. Sheeppox, swinepox, fowlpox, and myxomatosis are transmitted mechanically by biting arthropods. The viruses generally have narrow host ranges. Poxviruses are resistant in the environment under ambient temperatures and may survive for many years in dried scabs or other virus-laden material.

Viral Replication

Most poxviruses, except for parapoxviruses, swinepox virus, and molluscum contagiosum virus, grow readily in cell culture. They also produce pocks on the chorioallantoic membrane of embryonated hen's eggs, the appearance of which has been used to differentiate orthopoxviruses from each other. Replication of poxviruses occurs in the cytoplasm. To achieve this total independence from the cell nucleus, poxviruses, unlike other DNA viruses, have evolved to encode all of the enzymes required for transcription and replication of the viral genome, several of which must be carried in the virion itself. After fusion of the virion with the plasma membrane or after endocytosis, the viral core is released into the cytoplasm (Figure 16.3).

Transcription is characterized by a cascade in which the transcription of each temporal class of genes ("early," "intermediate," and "late" genes) requires the presence of specific transcription factors that are made by the preceding temporal class of genes. Intermediate gene transcription factors are encoded by early genes, whereas late transcription factors are encoded by intermediate genes. Transcription is initiated by the viral transcriptase and other factors carried in the core of the virion that enable the production of mRNAs within minutes after infection. Proteins produced by translation of

FIGURE 16.3.

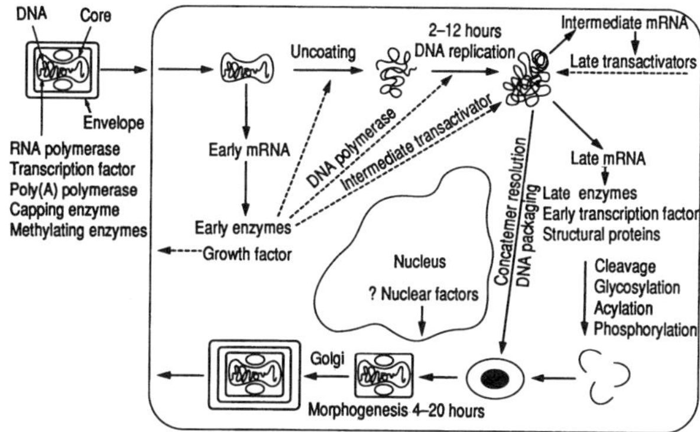

Diagram illustrating the replication cycle of vaccinia virus. (Courtesy of B. Moss.)

these mRNAs complete the uncoating of the core and transcription of about 100 early genes; all this occurs before viral DNA synthesis begins. Early proteins include DNA polymerase, thymidine kinase, and several other enzymes required for replication of the genome.

Poxvirus DNA replication involves the synthesis of long concatemeric intermediates, which are subsequently cut into unit-length genomes—the details of this process remain unknown. With the onset of DNA replication there is a dramatic shift in gene expression. Transcription of "intermediate" and "late" genes is controlled by binding of specific viral proteins to promoter sequences in the viral genome. Some early gene transcription factors are made late in infection, packaged in virions, and used in the subsequent round of infection.

Because poxviruses are composed of a very large number of proteins, it is not surprising that viral assembly is a complex process, which is still poorly understood and which requires several hours to be completed. Virion formation involves coalescence of DNA within crescent-shaped immature core structures, which then mature by the addition of outer coat layers. Replication and assembly occur in discrete sites within the cytoplasm (called *viroplasm* or viral factories), and virions are released by budding (enveloped virions) or by exocytosis, or cell lysis (nonenveloped virions). Most virions are not enveloped and are released by cell lysis. Both enveloped and nonenveloped virions are infectious, but enveloped virions are taken up by cells more readily and appear to be more important in the spread of virions through the body of the animal (Table 16.2).

Table 16.2
Properties of Poxviruses

Virions in most genera are brick-shaped, 250 × 200 × 200 nm, with an irregular arrangement of surface tubules. Virions of members of the genus *Parapoxvirus* are ovoid, 260 × 160 nm, with regular spiral arrangement of surface tubules

Virions have a complex structure with a core, lateral bodies, outer membrane, and sometimes an envelope

Gernome is composed of a single molecule of linear double-stranded DNA, 165–210 kbp (genus *Orthopoxvirus*), 280 kbp (genus *Avipoxvirus*), or 130 kbp (genus *Parapoxvirus*) in size

Genomes have the capacity to encode about 200 proteins, as many as 100 of which are contained in virions. Unlike other DNA viruses, poxviruses encode all of the enzymes required for transcription and replication, many of which are carried in the virion

Cytoplasmic replication, enveloped virions released by exocytosis; nonenveloped virions released by cell lysis

Diseases Caused by Members of the Genus *Orthopoxvirus*

Vaccinia Virus Disease (and Buffalopox)

Because of its widespread use and its wide host range, vaccinia virus sometimes has caused naturally spreading diseases in domestic animals (e.g., teat infections of cattle) and also in laboratory rabbits ("rabbitpox"). In the Netherlands in 1963, before human vaccination against smallpox had been discontinued, 8 out of 36 outbreaks of disease first thought to be cowpox were found to be caused by vaccinia virus and the rest by authentic cowpox virus.

Outbreaks of buffalopox have occurred in water buffalo (*Bubalis bubalis*) in Egypt, the Indian subcontinent, and Indonesia, where buffalo are used for milk production. The disease is caused by an orthopoxvirus that is related so closely to the vaccinia virus that is it not clear whether it should be considered a separate virus on not. By restriction endonuclease mapping, the causative virus is indistinguishable from vaccinia virus, although it is slightly different from laboratory strains of vaccinia virus and strains that had been used for smallpox vaccination in the same regions. The disease is characterized by pustular lesions on the teats and udders of milking buffalo; occasionally, especially in calves, a generalized disease is seen. Outbreaks still occur in India (even though vaccinia virus is not used for any type of vaccination in the country), sometimes producing lesions on the hands and face of milkers who are no longer protected by vaccination against smallpox.

Cowpox

Despite the name, the reservoir hosts of cowpox virus are rodents, from which the virus occasionally spreads to domestic cats, cows, humans, and zoo animals, including large felids (especially cheetahs, ocelots, panthers, lynx, lions, pumas, and jaguars) and anteaters, rhinoceroses, okapis, and elephants. During an outbreak at the Moscow zoo the virus was also isolated from laboratory rats used to feed the big cats, and a subsequent survey demonstrated infection in wild susliks (*Spermophilus citellus* and *S. suslicus*) and gerbils (*Rhombomys opimus*) in Russia. In the United Kingdom, the reservoir species are bank voles (*Clethrionomys glareolus*), field voles (*Microtus agrestis*), and wood mice (*Apodemus sylvaticus*).

Cowpox virus has been found only in Europe and adjacent regions of Russia. The virus produces lesions on the teats and the contiguous parts of the udder of cows and is spread through herds by the process of milking. Currently, infection with cowpox virus is more commonly seen among domestic cats, from which it is occasionally transmitted to humans. Lesions in humans usually appear as single maculopapular eruptions on the hands or the face; infection is accompanied by systemic signs such as nausea, fever, and lymphadenopathy. Children are often hospitalized but while human death is rare, it has occurred.

Cowpox virus infection in domestic cats is often a more severe disease than in cattle or humans. There is often a history of a single primary lesion, generally on the head or a forelimb, but by the time the cat is presented for veterinary attention, widespread skin lesions have usually developed. The primary lesions vary in character, and secondary bacterial infection is common. The widespread secondary lesions first appear as small red macular eruptions, which develop into papules and ulcers over several days. These scab over, and the cat usually recovers within 6 to 8 weeks. More severe disease with large nonhealing lesions or pneumonia usually, but not always, results from secondary bacterial infection or immunosuppression (e.g., by concurrent feline leukemia virus or feline immunodeficiency virus infection). In cheetahs, pneumonia is common, and cowpox virus infection in cheetahs has a high mortality rate.

Camelpox

Camelpox causes a severe generalized disease in camels, with extensive skin lesions. It is an important disease, especially in countries of Africa, the Middle East, and southwestern Asia where the camel is used as a beast of burden and for milk. The more severe cases usually occur in young animals, and in epidemics the case-fatality rate may be as high as 25%. The causative virus is a distinctive orthopoxvirus species and its restriction endonuclease map differentiates it from other viruses. It has a narrow host range, and despite the frequent exposure of unvaccinated humans to florid cases of camelpox, human infection has not been seen. A parapoxvirus also infect camels producing a disease that can be confused with camelpox (Ausdyk virus; Table 16.1).

Ectromelia (Mousepox)

Ectromelia virus has been spread around the world inadvertently in shipments of laboratory mice and mouse products and has been repeatedly reported from laboratories in several countries of Europe and from Japan and China. Mousepox has never been endemic for prolonged periods in mouse colonies in the United States, but accidental importations have occurred from European laboratories, e.g., via mouse tumor material, with devastating consequences. In recent years, stringent steps have been taken to prevent its entry into modern laboratory colonies.

Clinically, there are two forms of mousepox: (1) a rapidly fatal form in which there is extensive necrosis of the liver and spleen with death occurring within a few hours of the first signs of illness and (2) a chronic form characterized by ulcerating lesions of the feet, tail, and snout. Frank Fenner studied the natural history and epidemiology of mousepox during an epidemic in the colonies at the National Institutes of Health in Bethesda, Maryland. He found that when the virus is first introduced into a colony, most mice develop a primary lesion, usually on the snout, feet, or belly. Subsequently, the virus multiplies to high titer in the liver and spleen. Some mice die at this stage, but if they survive they almost invariably develop a generalized rash. There is higher mortality in suckling mice than in adults. Only after this form of disease has been established in a colony for some time, with widespread partial active and passive immunity prevailing, does the chronic form become dominant.

The consequences of the introduction of ectromelia virus into a mouse colony are so serious that definitive diagnosis is an urgent matter. Mousepox can be diagnosed by the histopathologic examination of tissues of suspected cases, its diagnostic features being distinctive eosinophilic cytoplasmic inclusion bodies, especially at the edges of skin lesions. Electron microscopy is also a valuable diagnostic adjunct: distinctive virions may be seen in any infected tissue. Virus may be isolated in mouse embryo cell cultures and identified by immunological means.

The usual mode of transmission of the virus in mouse colonies is via minor abrasions of the skin, which become contaminated from bedding or during manipulations by animal handlers. Infection may also occur by the respiratory route, but probably only between mice in close proximity to each other. Because mice are infected readily by inoculation, virus-contaminated mouse serum, ascites fluid, tumors, or tissues constitute a risk to laboratory colonies previously free of infection. Analysis of epidemics in mouse colonies has shown that C56BL/6 and AKR mice are highly resistant to mousepox and that BALB/c, DBA, and C3H mice are highly susceptible. Although there is no disease in C57BL/6 mice, serial transmission occurs and these mice may serve as silent sources of contagion for susceptible mouse strains.

Prevention and control are based on quarantine and regulation of the importation and distribution of ectromelia virus, mice, and materials that may be carrying the virus. However, because such regulations offer no protection against unsuspected sources of infection, regular serologic testing is done in many colonies housing valuable animals.

Monkeypox

Human infections with monkeypox virus are seen in villages in the tropical rain forests of west and central Africa, especially in the Democratic Republic of Congo. The disease was discovered in the early 1970s, after smallpox had been eradicated from the region. The signs and symptoms are very like those of smallpox, with a generalized pustular rash, fever, and toxemia. Monkeypox virus is a zoonotic agent; it is acquired by humans by direct contact with wild animals killed for food, especially squirrels and monkeys. There is some evidence that squirrels are the true reservoir host of the virus. A few cases of person-to-person transmission have been reported, but the secondary attack rate seems too low for the disease to become established as an endemic human infection.

The human disease had been rather rare, with only 400 or so cases diagnosed in the 1980s; however, in the 1990s there have been simmering outbreaks involving more and more people. More than 500 human cases were reported in the Congo in 1996–1997, the largest outbreak ever of the disease. Vaccination with smallpox vaccine (vaccinia virus) immunizes against monkeypox, and vaccination may be reintroduced in some villages in Africa to deal with zoonotic monkeypox infections.

Diseases Caused by Members of the Genus *Capripoxvirus*

Sheeppox and Goatpox

Sheeppox and goatpox are the most important of all pox diseases of domestic animals, causing high mortality in young animals and significant economic loss. They occur as endemic infections in southwestern Asia, the Indian subcontinent, and most parts of Africa, except southern Africa.

Although the geographic distribution of sheeppox, goatpox, and lumpyskin disease is different, suggesting that they are distinct viruses, they are indistinguishable by conventional serology and only barely distinguishable by restriction endonuclease DNA analysis. The African strains of sheeppox and lumpyskin disease viruses are related more closely to each other than sheeppox virus is to goatpox virus. However, whereas sheeppox and goatpox are considered to be host specific, in parts of Africa where sheep and goats are herded together both animal species may show clinical signs during an outbreak, indicating that some strains may affect both sheep and goats.

Clinical signs vary in different hosts and in different geographical areas. Sheep and goats of all ages may be affected, but the disease is generally more severe in young animals. An epidemic in a susceptible flock of sheep can affect over 75% of the animals, with mortality as high as 50%; case-fatality rates in young sheep may approach 100%. After an incubation period of 4 to 8 days, there is a rise in temperature, an increase in respiratory rate, edema of the eyelids, and a mucous discharge from the nose. Affected sheep may lose their appetite and stand with an arched back. One to 2 days later, cutaneous nodules about 1 cm in diameter develop, which may be distributed widely over the body. These lesions are most obvious in the areas of skin where the wool/hair is shortest, such as the head, neck, ears, axillae, and under the tail (Figure 16.4A). These lesions usually scab and persist for 3–4 weeks, healing to leave a permanent depressed scar. Lesions within the mouth affect the tongue and gums and ulcerate. Such lesions constitute an important source of virus for infection of other animals. In some sheep, lesions develop in the lungs, as multisite consolidation. Goatpox is similar clinically to sheeppox (Figure 16.4B).

Sheeppox and goatpox are notifiable diseases in most countries of the world, with any clinical suspicion of disease requiring disclosure to appropriate authorities. Apart from occasional outbreaks in partly immune flocks—where the disease may be mild—or when the presence of orf complicates the diagnosis, sheeppox and goatpox present little difficulty in clinical diagnosis. For presumptive laboratory diagnosis, negative-contrast electron microscopy can be used to demonstrate virions in clinical material, as the virions are indistinguishable from those of vaccinia virus. The viruses can be isolated in various cell cultures derived from sheep, cattle, or goats; the presence of virus is indicated by cytopathology and cytoplasmic inclusion bodies.

In common with most poxviruses, environmental contamination can lead to the introduction of virus into small skin wounds. Scabs that have been shed by infected sheep remain infective for several months. The common practice of herding sheep and goats into enclosures at night in countries where the disease occurs provides adequate exposure to maintain endemic infection. During an outbreak, the virus is probably transmitted between

Figure 16.4.

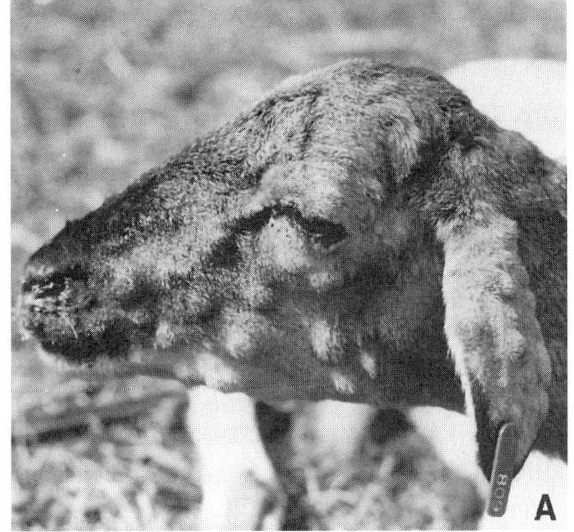

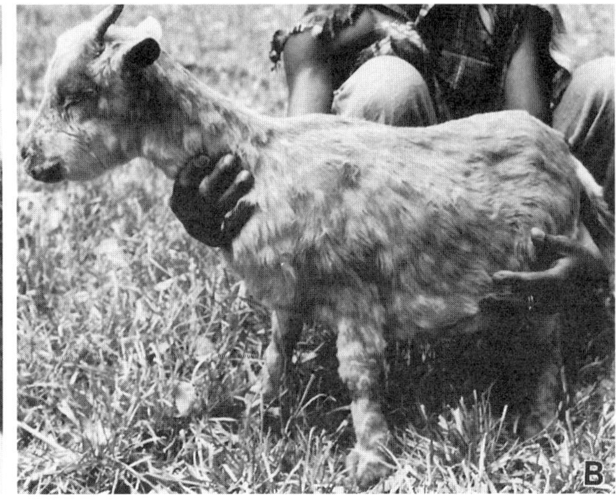

(A) Sheeppox and (B) goatpox in native breeds in Ghana. (Courtesy of M. Bonniwell.)

sheep by respiratory droplets; there is also evidence that mechanical transmission by biting arthropods, such as stable flies, may be important.

In countries where the diseases are endemic, attenuated virus and inactivated virus vaccines are used. Recombinant vaccines, with these viruses as vectors, are under development for the control of rinderpest.

Lumpyskin Disease of Cattle

Lumpyskin disease affects cattle breeds derived from both *Bos taurus* and *Bos indicus* and was first recognized in an extensive epidemic in Zambia in 1929. An epidemic in 1943–44, which involved other countries, including South Africa, emphasized the importance of this disease, which remained restricted to southern Africa until 1956, when it spread to central and eastern Africa. Since the 1950s, it has continued to spread progressively throughout Africa, first north to the Sudan and subsequently westward, to appear by the mid-1970s in most countries of western Africa. In 1988, the disease was confirmed in Egypt, and in 1989 a single outbreak occurred in Israel, the first report outside the African continent.

Lumpyskin disease is characterized by fever, followed shortly by the development of nodular lesions in the skin that subsequently undergo necrosis. Generalized lymphadenitis and edema of the limbs are common. During the early stages of the disease, affected cattle show lacrimation, nasal discharge, and loss of appetite. The skin nodules involve the dermis and epidermis; they are raised and later ulcerate and may become infected secondarily. Ulcerated lesions may be present in the mouth and nares; postmortem, circumscribed nodules may be found in lungs and the alimentary tract. Healing is slow and affected cattle often remain debilitated for several months.

Morbidity in susceptible herds can be as high as 100%, but mortality is rarely more than 1–2%. The economic importance of the disease relates to the prolonged convalescence and, in this respect, lumphyskin disease is similar to foot-and-mouth disease; indeed, in South Africa, it is regarded as economically more important.

The clinical diagnosis presents few problems to clinicians familiar with it, although the early skin lesions can be confused with generalized skin infections of pseudo-lumpyskin disease, caused by bovine herpesvirus 2.

It is likely that the virus is transmitted mechanically between cattle by biting insects, with the virus being perpetuated in a wildlife reservoir host, possibly the African Cape buffalo. Control is by vaccination. Two vaccines are currently available: in South Africa an attenuated virus vaccine (Neethling) is used and in Kenya a strain of sheep/goatpox virus propagated in tissue culture has been used.

Lumpyskin disease has shown the potential to spread outside continental Africa. Because it is transmitted principally by insect vectors, the importation of wild ruminants to zoos could establish new foci of infection, if suitable vectors were available.

Diseases Caused by Members of the Genus *Suipoxvirus*

Swinepox

Swinepox is seen sporadically in swine-raising areas throughout the world. Many outbreaks of poxvirus disease in swine have been caused by vaccinia virus, but swinepox virus, which belongs to a different genus, is now the primary cause of the disease. Swinepox is usually a mild disease with lesions restricted to the skin (Figure 16.5). Lesions may occur anywhere, but are most obvious on the abdomen. A transient low-grade fever may precede the development of papules which, within 1 to 2 days, become vesicles and then umbilicated pustules, 1–2 cm in diameter. The pocks crust over and scab by 7 days; healing is usually complete by 3 weeks. The clinical picture is characteristic; it is seldom necessary to seek laboratory confirmation of the clinical diagnosis.

Swinepox is transmitted most commonly between swine by the bite of the pig louse, *Hematopinus suis,* which is common in many herds; the virus does not replicate in the louse. No vaccines are available for swinepox, which is controlled most easily by elimination of the louse from the affected herd and by improved hygiene. As with other poxviruses of livestock, swinepox virus is being developed as a vaccine vector.

Diseases Caused by Members of the Genus *Leporipoxvirus*

Myxomatosis

Myxoma virus causes only a localized benign fibroma in wild rabbits in the Americas (*Sylvilagus* spp.); in contrast, it causes a severe generalized disease in the European rabbit (*Oryctolagus cuniculus*), with a very high mortality rate (Figure 16.6). The characteristic early signs of myxomatosis in the European rabbit are blepharoconjunctivitis and swelling of the muzzle and anogenital region, giving animals a leonine appearance. Infected rabbits become febrile and listless and often die within 48 hours of onset of clinical signs. This rapid progression and fatal outcome are seen especially with the California strain of myxoma virus. In rabbits that survive longer, subcutaneous gelatinous swellings (hence the name myxomatosis) appear all over the body within 2 to 3 days. The vast majority of rabbits (over 99%) infected from

Figure 16.5.

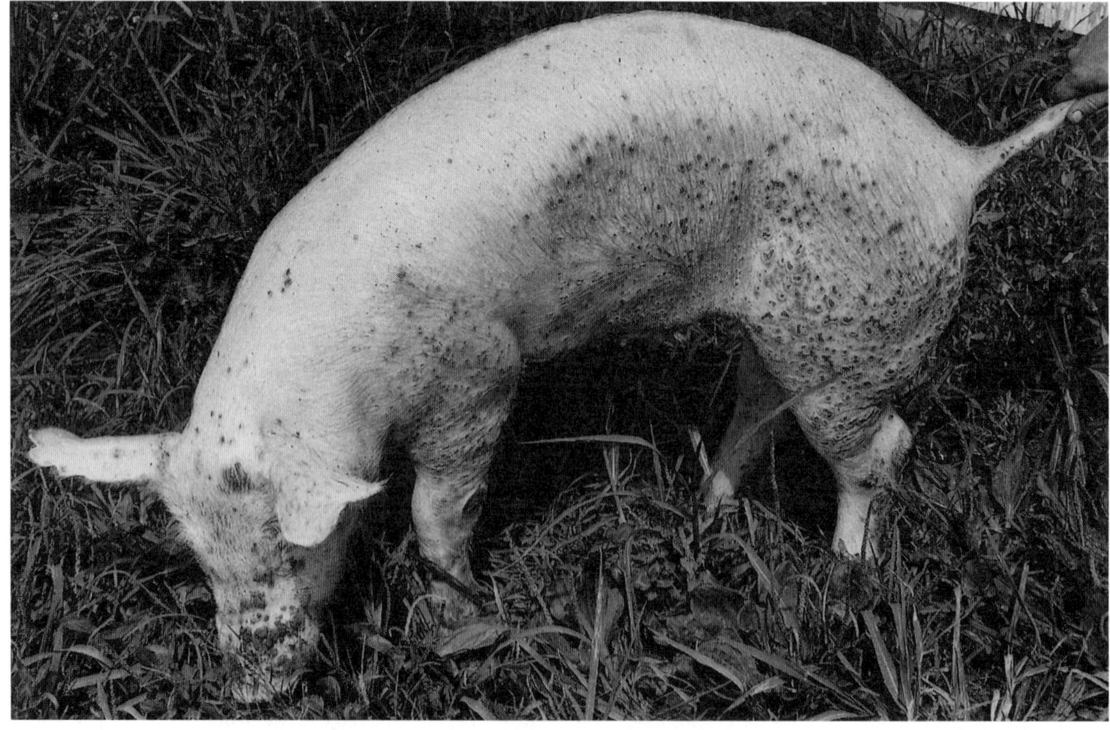

Swinepox. (Courtesy of R. Miller.)

FIGURE 16.6.

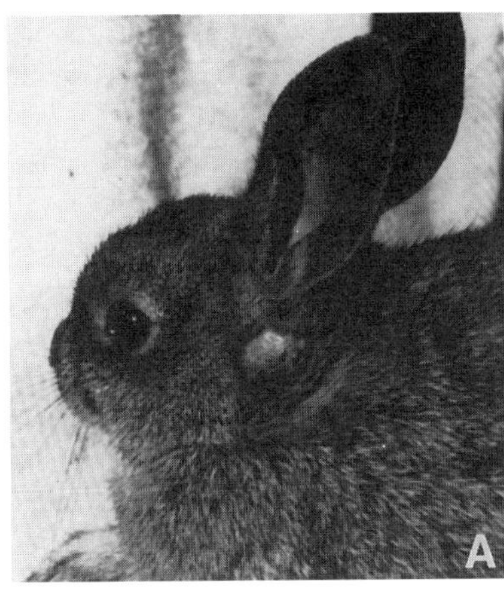

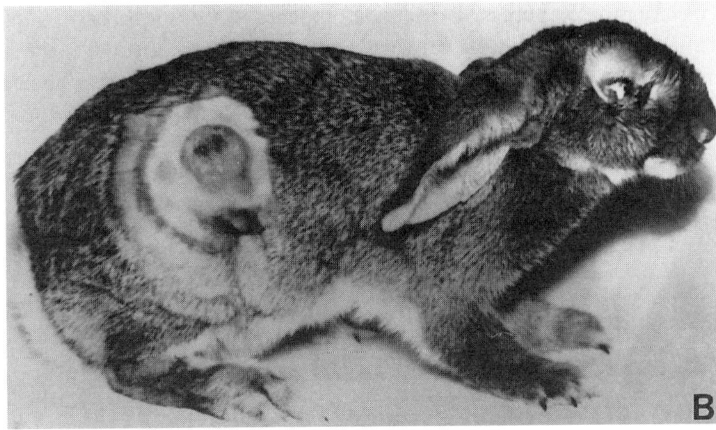

Myxomatosis. (A) Localized fibroma in *Sylvilagus bachmani*. (B) Severe generalized disease in *Oryctolagus cuniculus* showing a large tumor at the site of intradermal inoculation on the flank, generalized lesions, and blepharoconjunctivitis. (A, courtesy of D. Regnery.)

a wild (*Sylvilagus* spp.) source of myxoma virus die within 12 days of infection. Transmission can occur via respiratory droplets, but more often via mechanical transmission by arthropods (mosquitoes, fleas, black flies, ticks, lice, mites).

Diagnosis of myxomatosis in European rabbits can be made by the clinical appearance, or virus isolation in rabbits, on the chorioallantoic membrane of embryonated hen's eggs or in cultured rabbit or chicken cells. Electron microscopy of exudates or smear preparations from lesions reveal virions morphologically indistinguishable from those of vaccinia virus.

Laboratory or hutch rabbits can be protected against myxomatosis by inoculation with the related rabbit fibroma virus or with attenuated myxoma virus vaccines developed in California and France.

Myxoma virus was the first virus ever introduced into the wild for the purpose of eradicating a vertebrate pest, namely the feral European rabbit in Australia in 1950 and in Europe 2 years later (see Chapter 4).

Diseases Caused by Members of the Genus *Molluscipoxvirus*

Molluscum Contagiosum

Molluscum contagiosum is specifically a human disease, but it is often confused with zoonotic poxviruses. Infection is characterized by multiple discrete nodules 2 to 5 mm in diameter, limited to the epidermis, and occurring anywhere on the body except on the soles and palms. The nodules are pearly white or pink in color and painless. The disease may last for several months before recovery occurs. Cells in the nodule are hypertrophied greatly and contain large hyaline acidophilic cytoplasmic masses called molluscum bodies. These consist of a spongy matrix divided into cavities, in each of which are clustered masses of viral particles that have the same general structure as those of vaccinia virus. The disease is seen most commonly in children and occurs worldwide, but is much more common in some localities, e.g., parts of the Democratic Republic of Congo and Papua New Guinea. The virus is transmitted by direct contact, perhaps through minor abrasions and sexually in adults. In developed countries, communal swimming pools and gymnasiums have been sources of contagion.

Diseases Caused by Members of the Genus *Yatapoxvirus*

Yabapox and Tanapox

Yabapox and tanapox occur naturally only in tropical Africa. The yabapox virus was discovered because it produced large benign tumors on the hairless areas of the face, on the palms and interdigital areas, and on the mucosal surfaces of the nostrils, sinuses, lips, and palate of Asian monkeys (*Cercopithecus aethiops*) kept in a laboratory in Nigeria. Subsequent cases occurred in primate colonies in California, Oregon, and Texas. Yabapox is believed to be epidemic in scope in African and Asian monkeys. The virus is zoonotic, spreading to humans in contact with diseased monkeys and causing similar lesions as in affected monkeys.

Tanapox is a relatively common skin infection of humans in parts of Africa, extending from eastern Kenya to the Democratic Republic of Congo. It appears to be spread mechanically by insect bites from an unknown wild animal reservoir, probably a species of monkey. In humans, skin lesions start as papules and progress to vesicles but pustules do not occur. There is usually a febrile illness lasting 3 to 4 days, sometimes with severe headache, backache, and prostration.

Diseases Caused by Members of the Genus *Avipoxvirus*

Fowlpox and Other Avian Poxvirus Diseases

Poxviruses that are related serologically to each other and specifically infect birds have been recovered from lesions found in all species of poultry and many species of wild birds. Viruses recovered from various species of birds are given names related to their hosts, such as fowlpox, canarypox, turkeypox, pigeonpox, and magpiepox. As judged by their pathogenicity in various avian hosts, there seems to be a number of different species of avian poxviruses, but no systematic analysis of their DNAs has yet been made. Mechanical transmission by arthropods, especially mosquitoes, provides a mechanism for transfer of the viruses between a variety of different species of birds.

Fowlpox is a serious disease of poultry that has occurred worldwide for centuries. The fowlpox virus is highly infectious for chickens and turkeys, rarely so for pigeons, and not at all for ducks and canaries, but turkeypox virus is virulent for ducks.

There are two forms of fowlpox, probably associated with different routes of infection. The most common, which probably results from infection by biting arthropods, is characterized by small papules on the comb, wattles, and around the beak (Figure 16.7); lesions occasionally develop on the legs and feet and around the cloaca. The nodules become yellowish and progress to a thick dark scab. Multiple lesions often coalesce. Involvement of the skin around the nares may cause nasal discharge, and lesions on the eyelids can cause excessive lacrimation and predispose poultry to secondary bacterial infections. In uncomplicated cases, healing occurs within 3 weeks.

The second form of fowlpox is probably due to droplet infection and involves infection of the mucous membranes of the mouth, pharynx, larynx, and some-

Figure 16.7.

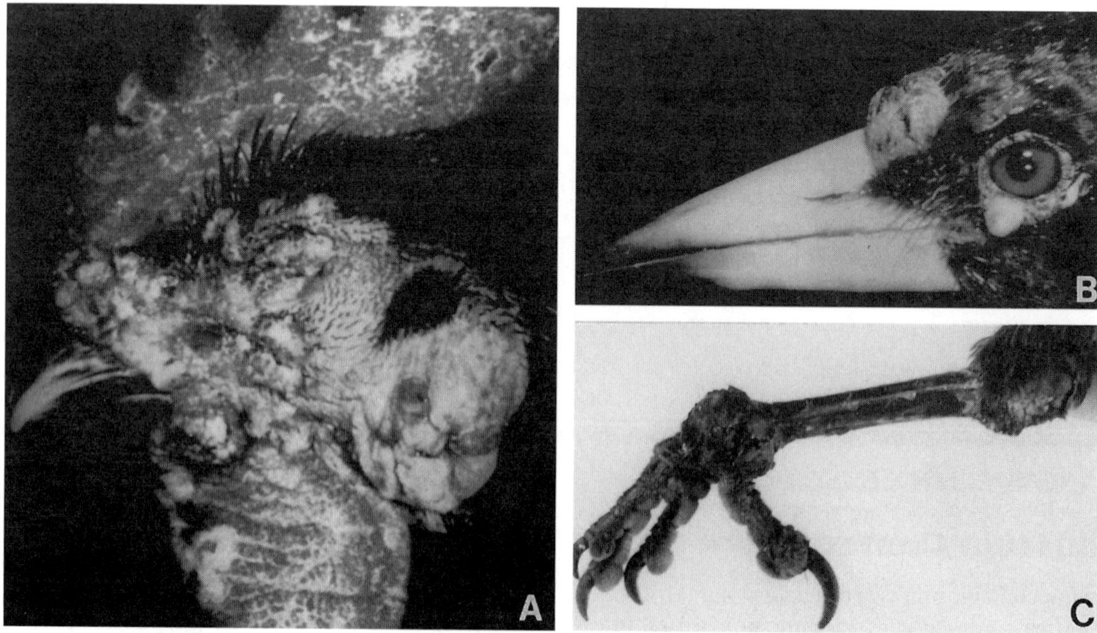

Avian poxvirus diseases. (A) Fowlpox. (B and C) Poxvirus infection in an Australian magpie. (B) Lesions at the base of the beak and under the eye. (C) Lesions on the foot. (B and C, courtesy of K. E. Harrigan.)

times the trachea. This is often referred to as the *diphtheritic form* of fowlpox because the lesions, as they coalesce, result in a necrotic pseudo-membrane, which can cause death by asphyxiation. The prognosis for this form of fowlpox is poor. Extensive infection in a flock may cause a slow decline in egg production. Cutaneous infection causes little mortality and these flocks return to normal production on recovery. Recovered birds are immune.

Under natural conditions there may be breed differences in susceptibility; chickens with large combs appear to be more affected than breeds with small combs. The mortality rate is low in healthy flocks, but in laying flocks and in chickens in poor condition or under stress, the disease may assume serious proportions with a mortality rate of 50% or higher.

The cutaneous form of fowlpox seldom presents a diagnostic problem. The diphtheritic form is more difficult to diagnose because it can occur in the absence of skin lesions and may be confused with vitamin A deficiency and several other respiratory diseases caused by viruses. Histopathology and electron microscopy are used to confirm the clinical diagnosis. The virus can be isolated by the inoculation of avian cell cultures or the chorioallantoic membrane of embryonated eggs.

Fowlpox virus is extremely resistance to desiccation: it can survive for long periods under the most adverse environmental conditions in exfoliated scabs. The virus is transmitted within a flock through minor wounds and abrasions, by fighting and pecking, mechanically by mosquitoes, lice, and ticks, and possibly by aerosols.

Several types of vaccine are available. Nonattenuated fowlpox virus and pigeonpox virus vaccines prepared in embryonated hen's eggs and attenuated virus vaccines prepared in avian cell cultures are widely used for vaccination. Vaccines are applied by scarification of the skin of the thigh. One vaccine can be administered in drinking water. In flocks infected endemically, birds are vaccinated during the first few weeks of life and again 8 to 12 weeks later. Recombinant vaccines for poultry are in development using both fowlpox and canarypox viruses as vectors. As discussed in Chapter 13, these viruses may also have application in mammalian species as vaccine vectors.

Diseases Caused by Members of the Genus *Parapoxvirus*

Parapoxviruses infect a wide range of species, generally causing only localized lesions. Disease in sheep, cattle, goats, and camels can be of economic significance. Parapoxviruses also infect several species of terrestrial and marine wildlife (e.g., chamois, red deer, seals), but their clinical importance in these species is more difficult to assess. These viruses are zoonotic; farmers, sheep shearers, veterinarians, butchers, and others who handle infected livestock or their products can develop localized lesions, usually on the hand (Figure 16.8E). Lesions, which are identical irrespective of the source of the virus, begin as an inflammatory papule, then enlarge to become granulomatous before regressing. Lesions may persist for several weeks. If the infection is acquired from milking cows, the lesion is known as "milker's nodule"; if from sheep it is known as "orf."

Orf (Contagious Pustular Dermatitis)

Orf (contagious pustular dermatitis, scabby mouth) is a more important disease in sheep and goats than either pseudocowpox or bovine papular stomatitis in cattle and is common throughout the world. Orf, which is Old English for "rough," commonly involves only the muzzle and lips (Figure 16.8D), although lesions within the mouth affecting the gums and tongue can occur, especially in young lambs. The lesions can also affect the eyelids, feet, and the teats. Human infection can occur among persons exposed occupationally (Figure 16.8E).

Lesions of orf progress from papules to pustules and then to thick crusts. The scabs are often friable and mild trauma causes the lesions to bleed. Orf may prevent lambs from suckling. Severely affected animals may lose weight and be predisposed to secondary infections. Morbidity is high in young sheep, but mortality is usually low. Clinical differentiation of orf from other diseases seldom presents a problem, but electron microscopy can be used if necessary to confirm the diagnosis.

Sheep are susceptible to reinfection and chronic infections can occur. These features, and the resistance of the virus to desiccation, explain how the virus, once introduced to a flock, can be difficult to eradicate. Spread of infection can be by direct contact or through exposure to contaminated feeding troughs and similar fomites, including wheat stubble and thorny plants.

Ewes can be vaccinated several weeks before lambing, using commercial nonattenuated virus vaccines derived from infected scabs collected from sheep or from virus grown in cell culture. Vaccines are applied to scarified skin, preferably in the axilla, where a localized lesion develops. A short-lived immunity is generated; ewes are thus less likely to develop orf at lambing time, thereby minimizing the risk of an epidemic of orf in the lambs.

Figure 16.8.

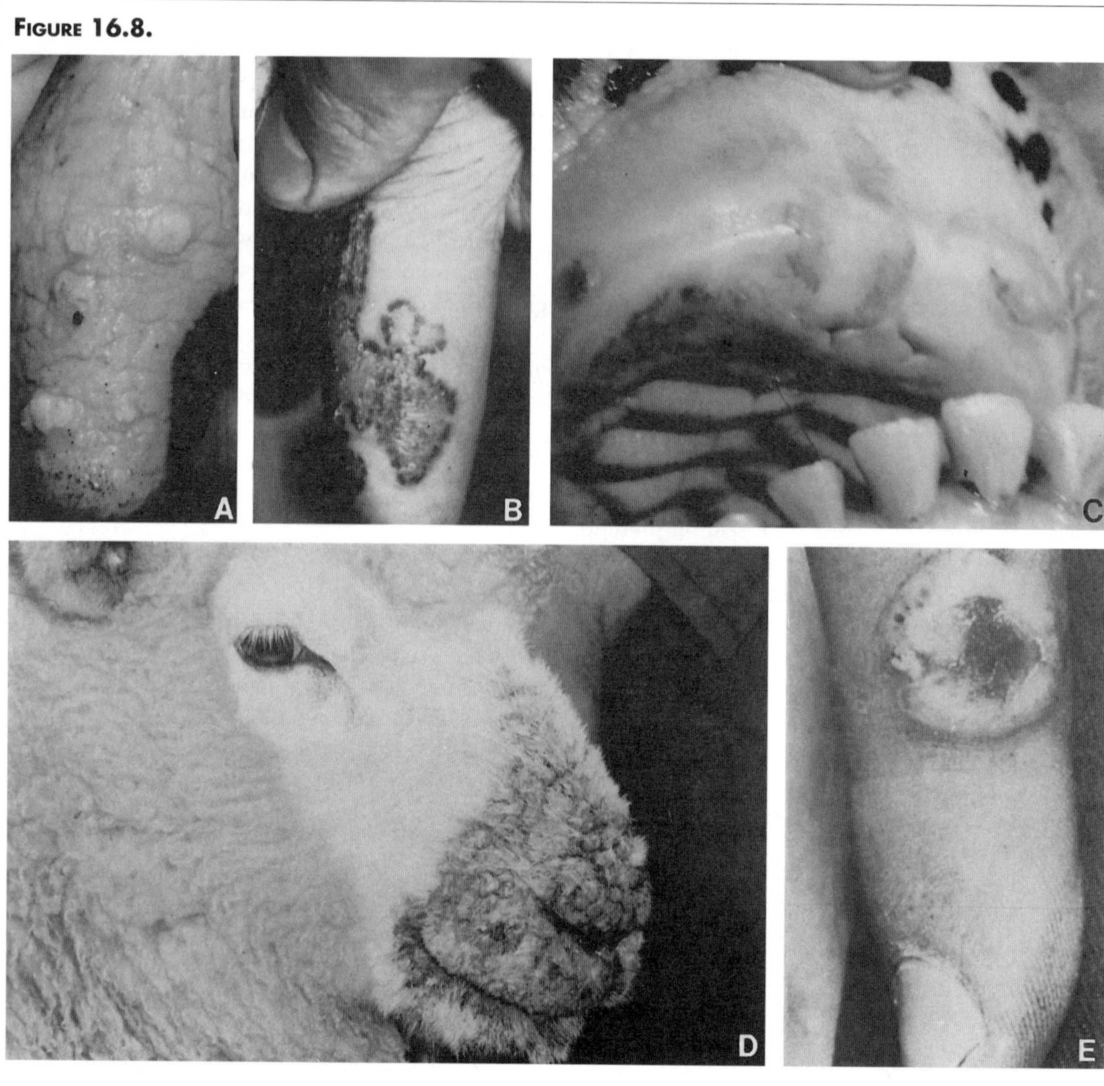

Parapoxvirus infections: pseudocowpox, bovine papular stomatitis, and orf in animals and humans. (A) and (B) Pseudocowpox lesions on teats of cow, at pustular and scab stages. (C) Bovine papular stomatitis. (D) Scabby mouth caused by orf virus in a lamb. (E) Orf lesion on the hand of a human. (A and B, courtesy of D. C. Blood; D, courtesy of A. Robinson; E, courtesy of J. Nagington.)

Orf virus is zoonotic; infections are frequent in humans, especially when they are in contact with sheep (e.g., during shearing, docking, drenching, slaughtering) or wildlife. In humans, after an incubation period of 2 to 4 days, the following stages may be observed: (1) macular lesions, (2) papular lesions, and (3) rather large nodules, becoming papillomatous in some cases. Lesions are, as a rule, solitary, although multiple lesions have been described. The duration of lesions ranges from 4 to 9 weeks. Healing takes place without scarring, but secondary infections may retard healing. Severe complications, such as fever, regional adenitis, lymphangitis, or blindness when the eye is affected, are seen only rarely.

Pseudocowpox

Pseudocowpox occurs as a common endemic infection in cattle in most countries of the world. It is a chronic infection in many milking herds and occasionally occurs in beef herds. The lesions of pseudocowpox are characterized by "ring" or "horseshoe" scabs, the latter being pathognomonic for the disease (Figure 16.8B). Similar lesions can occur on the muzzles and within the mouths of nursing calves. Infection is transmitted by cross-suckling of calves, improperly disinfected teat clusters of milking machines, and probably by the mechanical transfer of virus by flies. Attention to hygiene in the milking shed and the use of teat dips reduce the risk of transmission.

Bovine Papular Stomatitis

Bovine papular stomatitis is usually of little clinical importance, but occurs worldwide, affecting cattle of all ages, although the incidence is higher in animals less than 2 years of age. The development of lesions on the muzzle, margins of the lips, and the buccal mucosa is similar to that of pseudocowpox (Figure 16.8C). Immunity is of short duration and cattle can become reinfected. Demonstration by electron microscopy of the characteristic parapoxvirus virions in lesion scrapings is used for diagnosis.

Further Reading

Buller, R. M. L., and Palumbo, G. J. (1991). Poxvirus pathogenesis. *Microbiol. Rev.* **55,** 80–122.

Dumbell, K., and Richardson, M. (1993). Virological investigations of specimens from buffaloes affected by buffalopox in Maharashtra State, India between 1985 and 1987. *Arch. Virol.* **128,** 257–267.

Fenner, F. (1993). Poxviral zoonoses. *In* "Handbook Series in Zoonoses: Viral Zoonoses" (G. W. Beran and J. H. Steele, eds.), 2nd ed. Vol. 2, pp. 485–503. CRC Press, Boca Raton, FL.

Fenner, F. (1996). Poxviruses. *In* "Fields Virology." (B. N. Fields, D. M. Knipe, P. M. Howley, R. M. Chanock, J. L. Melnick, T. P. Monath, B. Roizman, and S. E. Straus, eds.), 3rd ed., pp. 2673–2702. Lippincott-Raven, Philadelphia, PA.

Fenner, F., and Buller, M. L. (1997). Mousepox. *In* "Viral Pathogenesis" (N. Nathanson, R. Ahmed, F. Gonzalez-Scarano, D. E. Griffin, K. V. Holmes, F. A. Murphy, and H. L. Robinson, eds.), pp. 535–554. Lippincott-Raven, Philadelphia, PA.

Fenner, F., Henderson, D. A., Arita, I., Jezek, Z., and Ladnyi, I. D. (1988). "Smallpox and its Eradication." World Health Organization, Geneva.

Moss, B. (1996). Poxviridae: The viruses and their replication. *In* "Fields Virology" (B. N. Fields, D. M. Knipe, P. M. Howley, R. M. Chanock, J. L. Melnick, T. P. Monath, B. Roizman, and S. E. Straus, eds.), 3rd ed., pp. 2637–2672. Lippincott-Raven, Philadelphia, PA.

Paoletti, E. (1996). Applications of poxvirus vectors to vaccination: An update. *Proc. Nat. Acad. Sci. U. S. A.* **93,** 11349–11353.

Chapter 17

Asfarviridae and *Iridoviridae*

Although there have been no major epidemics of African swine fever in recent years, the disease remains a serious threat to swine industries throughout the world. Since its recognition in 1921 in east Africa, the disease has emerged on several occasions, causing the death of many hundreds of thousands of domestic swine. In 1957 the disease spread for the first time outside Africa, first to Portugal, then in 1960 to Spain. In the 1960s and 1970s it occurred in France, Italy, Sardinia, and Malta and in the Americas in Cuba, Brazil, the Dominican Republic, and Haiti. In 1985 there was an outbreak in Belgium and in 1986 in The Netherlands. Today, the disease is endemic only in sub-Saharan Africa and Sardinia.

African swine fever virus had been classified for many years as a member of the family *Iridoviridae*, a family containing mostly viruses of insects, fish, and amphibians. The virus resembles iridoviruses morphologically, but there are major differences in the structure of its DNA and its mode of replication. When these properties were discovered, the virus was classified as the only member of the family *Asfarviridae* and the genus *Asfivirus*.

African swine fever virus is transmitted by soft ticks of the genus *Ornithodoros;* it is the only DNA virus that can be called an arbovirus. Interestingly, its DNA resembles linear plasmids of bacteria of the genus *Borrelia* in structure, size, and sequence. African swine fever virus and *Borrelia duttoni,* one cause of relapsing fever in Africa, share the same tick vector, *Ornithodoros moubata;* similarities between the virus and the *Borrelia* plasmid have suggested to some investigators a common ancestry or perhaps more likely some kind of horizontal genetic transfer. The genomic DNA of African swine fever virus also resembles somewhat that of poxviruses, but their evolutionary relationship is probably very distant.

The family *Iridoviridae* is large and complex and several iridoviruses have been associated with disease in fish and amphibians. This family of viruses may emerge as important pathogens in commercial fish production. Of these, lymphocystis virus is the best known. It causes tumor-like lesions on the skin of fish, which make them unmarketable. Because the virus has been reported to cause disease in more than 90 different species of marine and freshwater fish, it is an important pathogen.

Properties of Asfarviruses and Iridoviruses

Classification

As the only member of the family *Asfarviridae* and its single genus *Asfivirus,* the classification of African swine fever virus is straightforward. Restriction endonuclease analysis of the DNA of isolates of African swine fever virus from Africa, Europe, and the Americas permits classification into five groups. All European and American isolates fall within one group, whereas African isolates show greater variation. This is probably because in Africa the virus has been circulating for a long time and has diverged extensively, whereas only one or a few genotypes have been introduced into Europe and the Americas. Isolates are also categorized according to their virulence for swine, with some strains causing severe disease and near 100% mortality and others causing transient disease or even silent infection.

Virion Properties

Asfarvirus virions are enveloped, 175–215 nm in diameter, and contain a complex icosahedral capsid, 180 nm in diameter (Figure 17.1). The capsid consists of a hexagonal arrangement of structural units, each of which appears as a hexagonal prism with a central hole. Capsids have been estimated to contain between 1892 and 2172 structural units. The genome consists of a single molecule of linear double-stranded DNA, 170–190 kbp in size, depending on the isolate. The DNA has covalently closed ends with inverted terminal repeats and hairpin loops and encodes up to 200 proteins (34 structural proteins have been detected in purified virions and about 100 proteins have been detected in infected Vero cells). The entire DNA sequence of the virus has been determined.

Virions of the iridoviruses of vertebrates are morphologically rather similar to African swine fever virus virions; they are enveloped, 160–200 nm in diameter, and have an icosahedral capsid that is 120 nm in diameter (Figure 17.2). The genomes of iridoviruses range from 95 to 190 kbp in size and their termini are different from those of African swine fever virus, being circularly

Figure 17.1.

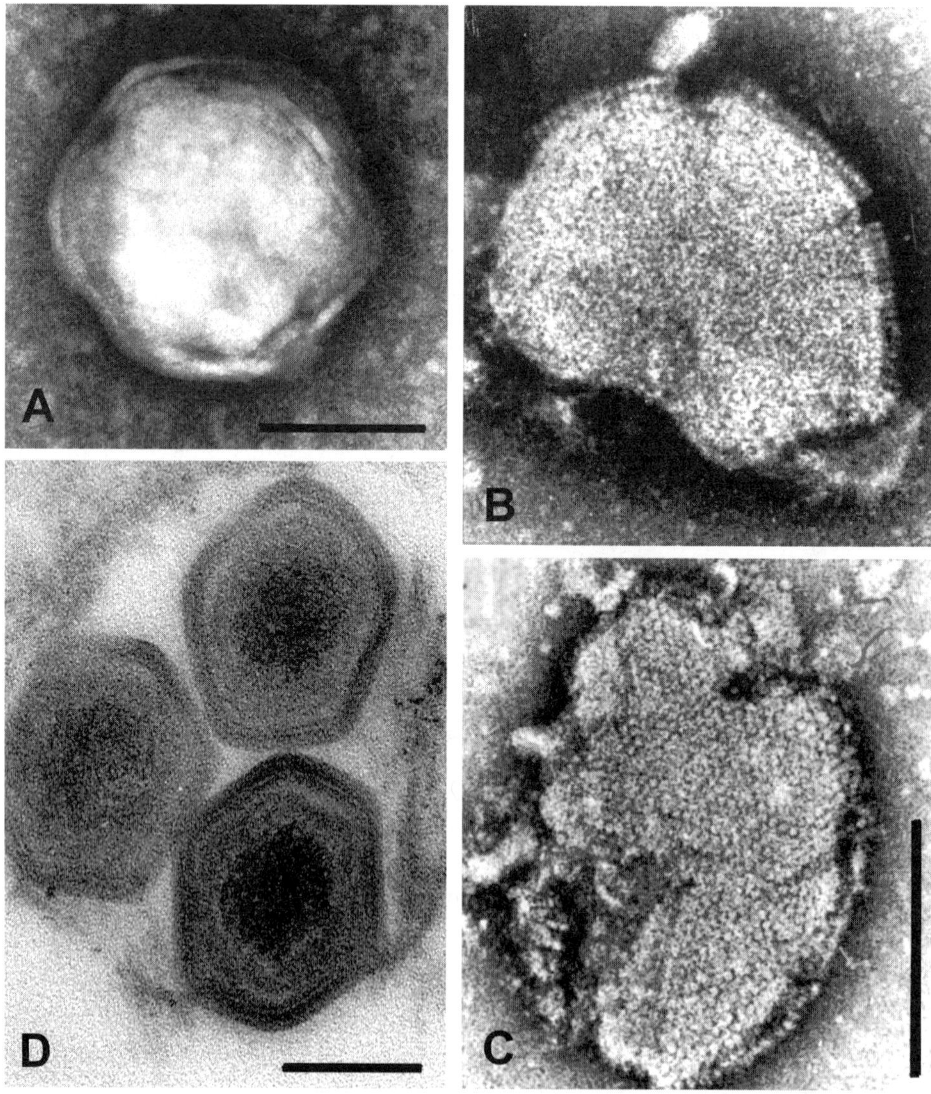

Family *Asfarviridae*, genus *Asfivirus*, African swine fever virus. (A) Negatively stained virion showing the hexagonal outline of the capsid enclosed within the envelope. (B and C) Negatively stained damaged capsids showing the ordered arrangement of the very large number of capsomers (between 1892 and 2172 structural units) that make up the capsid. (D) Thin section of three virions showing multiple layers surrounding their cores. Bars: 100 nm. (Courtesy of J. L. Carrascosa.)

FIGURE 17.2.

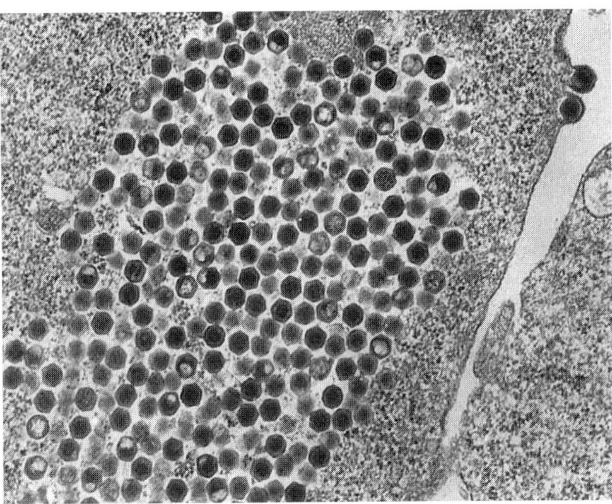

Frog virus 3, a typical member of the family *Iridoviridae*, in the cytoplasm of a frog embryo cell. Thin section electron microscopy, magnification ×18,000. (Courtesy of A. Kirn.)

permuted and terminally redundant and containing methylated bases like the DNAs of bacteria.

African swine fever virus and the iridoviruses of vertebrates are thermolabile and sensitive to lipid solvents. However, the viruses are very resistant to a wide range of pH (several hours at pH 4 or pH 13), and African swine fever virus survives for months and even years in refrigerated meat.

Viral Replication

Primary isolates of African swine fever virus replicate in swine monocytes and macrophages. After adaptation, some isolates can replicate in cultured cells such as pig kidney cells (PK 15), Vero cells, or other monkey kidney cells. Replication occurs primarily in the cytoplasm, although the nucleus is needed for viral DNA synthesis. Viral attachment is via a specific receptor and entry into host cells is via endocytosis. Like the poxviruses, virions contain genes for all the machinery necessary for transcription and replication; after entry into the cytoplasm, virions are uncoated and their DNA is transcribed by a virion-associated, DNA-dependent RNA polymerase (transcriptase). DNA replication is believed to be similar to that of poxviruses; parental genomic DNA serves as the template for the first round of DNA replication, the product of which then serves as a template for the synthesis of large replicative complexes that are cleaved to produce mature virion DNA.

The iridoviruses of vertebrates grow in a wide variety of cells of piscine, amphibian, avian, and mammalian origin at temperatures between 12 and 32°C. Their replication is similar to that of African swine fever virus, but there are two interesting differences: (1) the viruses do not encode an RNA polymerase but instead use cellular RNA polymerase II, which their structural proteins modify to favor viral mRNA synthesis; and (2) the stages of replication are compartmentalized—the first round of DNA replication takes place in the nucleus, the second, in which replicating DNA is present as large concatemers (more than 10 times genome size), takes place in the cytoplasm.

Late in infection, both African swine fever virus and vertebrate iridoviruses produce paracrystalline arrays of virions in the cytoplasm. Infected cells form many microvillus-like projections through which virions bud; however, acquisition of an envelope is not necessary for virus infectivity (Table 17.1).

DISEASES CAUSED BY MEMBERS OF THE FAMILY *ASFARVIRIDAE*

African Swine Fever

African swine fever virus infects domestic swine and other members of the family *Suidae,* including warthogs (*Potamochoerus aethiopicus*), bushpigs (*P. porcus*), and wild boar (*Sus scrofa ferus*). All efforts to infect other animals have been unsuccessful. The virus may be primarily a virus of ticks: in Africa, numerous isolates have been made from the soft tick *Ornithodoros moubata*

Table 17.1

Properties of Asfarviruses and Iridoviruses of Vertebrates

Asfarvirus virions are enveloped, 175–215 nm in diameter, and contain a complex icosahedral capsid, 180 nm in diameter

The genome of African swine fever virus is a single molecule of linear double-stranded DNA, 170–190 kbp in size. It has covalently closed ends with inverted terminal repeats and hairpin loops and encodes up to 200 proteins (at least 34 virion structural proteins)

Vertebrate iridovirus virions are similar in morphology; the genome is a single molecule of linear double-stranded DNA, 95–190 kbp in size. It is permuted circularly and has terminally redundant ends and methylated bases

The nucleus is involved in DNA replication; late functions and virion assembly occur in the cytoplasm

collected in warthog burrows. In Spain the virus has been associated with *O. erraticus*.

Clinical Features

After an incubation period of 5 to 15 days, swine develop high fever (40.5–42°C), which persists for about 4 days. Starting 1 to 2 days after the onset of fever, there is inappetence, diarrhea, incoordination, and prostration. Swine may die at this stage without other clinical signs. In some swine there is dyspnea, vomiting, nasal and conjunctival discharge, reddening or cyanosis of the ears and snout, and hemorrhages from the nose and anus. Pregnant sows often abort. In eastern and southern Africa, mortality is often 100%, with domestic swine dying within 1 to 3 days after the onset of fever. In many geographic extensions of the disease, such as that into Europe and the Americas in the 1970s and 1980s, the course of disease was usually rapid and fatal at first, but the severity of disease diminished rapidly until finally cases were predominantly subclinical and persistent. Adult warthogs do not develop any signs of disease, although virus has been found in their tissues.

Pathogenesis, Pathology, and Immunity

In acutely fatal cases in domestic swine, gross lesions are most prominent in the lymphatic and vascular systems. Hemorrhages occur widely, and the visceral lymph nodes may resemble blood clots. The spleen is often large and friable and there are petechial hemorrhages in the cortex of the kidney. The chronic disease is characterized by cutaneous ulcers, pneumonia, pericarditis, pleuritis, and arthritis.

If infection is acquired via the respiratory tract, the virus replicates first in the pharyngeal tonsils and lymph nodes draining the nasal mucosa before being disseminated rapidly throughout the body via a primary viremia in which virions are associated with both erythrocytes and leukocytes. A generalized infection follows with titers up to 10^9 ID_{50}/ml of blood or/gram of tissue. Consequently, all secretions and excretions contain large amounts of infectious virus.

Experimental studies have shown that African swine fever virus replicates in several cell types of the reticuloendothelial system and causes a severe leukopenia. Infected swine probably die through the indirect effects of viral replication on platelets and complement functions instead of by the direct cytolytic effect of the virus.

In infected macrophages, the virus effectively inhibits secretion and synthesis of antiviral immunomodulatory and pro-inflammatory cytokines, including interferons, tumor necrosis factors, IL-1, and IL-8. This inhibition is mediated by the viral gene A238L, which encodes a protein that is similar to an inhibitor of the cellular transcription factor NFκB. The viral protein has been shown to inhibit activation of NFκB and thus down-regulate the expression of all the antiviral cytokines that are controlled by NFκB. Mechanistically, the A238L protein acts as an analog of the immunosuppressive drug cyclosporin A. This seems to represent a novel viral evasion strategy; further, this protein may be the key in explaining how the virus causes a fatal hemorrhagic disease in domestic pigs while at the same time causing a temperate, persistent infection in its natural host, the African warthog.

Swine that survive may appear healthy or chronically diseased, but both groups may remain persistently infected. Indeed, swine may become persistently infected without ever showing clinical signs. The duration of the persistent infection is not known, but low levels of virus have been detected in tissues over a year after exposure. Viremia has been induced in such animals by injection of corticosteroids.

One of the most striking aspects of African swine fever virus infection is that sera from swine inoculated with the virus do not neutralize the virus. Although these animals produce virus-specific antibodies that bind to virus, the humoral immune response does not seem to have any substantial protective value. This phenomenon has been attributed to the character of the virus rather than to the host, as pigs that have recovered from infection or are chronically infected respond normally to other immunogens, producing normal levels of neutralizing antibodies. It has been suggested that the absence of neutralizing antibodies may be due to (1) the presence of a dominant epitope on the virus that suppresses the response to critical epitopes, (2) the induction of blocking antibodies that interfere with recognition of the virus by the immune system, or (3) the synthesis of very little antibody with very low avidity (actually, low-level neutralization has been obtained with high-avidity monoclonal antibodies and massive transfer of immunoglobulins from recovered pigs). Whatever the reason, efforts to produce a vaccine for African swine fever have been fruitless so far. There is, however, an extensive repertoire of both T and B cell responses to the virus in infected pigs. Accordingly, it has been considered that the best strategy for developing a vaccine might be to use nonreplicating whole virus rather than a single recombinant protein.

Laboratory Diagnosis

The clinical signs of African swine fever are similar to those of several diseases such as erysipelas and acute salmonellosis, but the major diagnostic problem is in distinguishing it from hog cholera. Any febrile disease in swine associated with hemorrhage and death should raise suspicion of African swine fever. Laboratory confirmation is essential and samples of blood, spleen, and visceral lymph nodes should be collected for virus isolation and for detection of antigen. Virus isolation is done in swine bone marrow or peripheral blood leukocyte cultures, in which hemadsorption can be demonstrated and a cytopathic effect seen within a few days after inoculation. From this point, the virus can be adapted to grow in various cell lines such as pig kidney (PK 15) and Vero cells. Antigen detection is done by immunofluorescence staining of tissue smears or frozen sections, by immunodiffusion using tissue suspensions as the source of antigen, and by enzyme immunoassay.

Epidemiology, Prevention, and Control

Two distinct epidemiologic patterns occur: a sylvatic cycle in warthogs in Africa and epidemic and endemic cycles in domestic swine.

Sylvatic Cycle

In its original ecologic niche in southern and eastern Africa, African swine fever virus is maintained in a sylvatic cycle involving asymptomatic infection in wild pigs (warthogs and, to a lesser extent, bush pigs) and argasid ticks (soft ticks, genus *Ornithodoros*), which occur in the burrows used by these animals. Ticks are biological vectors of the virus (Figure 17.3). Most tick populations in southern and eastern Africa are infected, with infection rates as high as 25%. After feeding on viremic swine, the virus replicates in the gut of the tick and subsequently infects its reproductive system, which leads to transovarial and venereal transmission of the virus. The virus is also transmitted between developmental stages of the tick—transstadial transmission—and is excreted in tick saliva, coxal fluid, and Malpighian excrement. Infected

FIGURE 17.3.

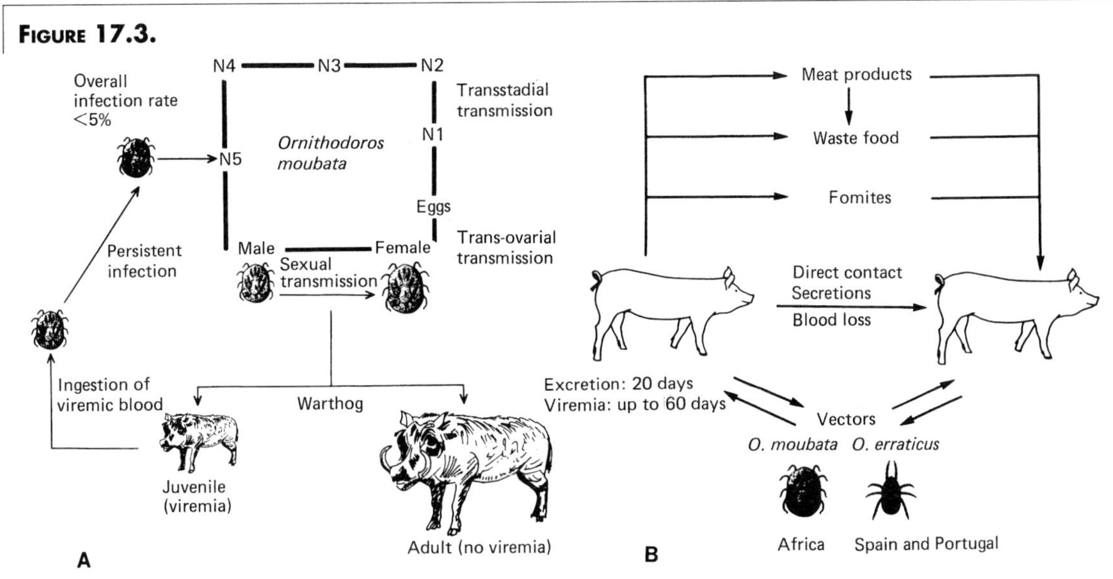

(A) Sylvatic transmission cycle of African swine fever virus between warthogs and *Ornithodoros moubata* ticks. In ticks there is transovarial (through the egg), venereal (through sex), and transstadial (through developmental stages of the tick) transmission of the virus. (B) Transmission cycle in domestic swine by direct contact, meat products and scraps, and fomites and through *Ornithodoros* spp. ticks. (Courtesy of P. J. Wilkinson.)

ticks may live for several years and are capable of transmitting disease to swine at each blood meal.

Serologic studies indicate that many warthog populations in southern and eastern Africa are infected. After primary infection, young warthogs develop viremia sufficient to infect at least some of the ticks feeding on them. Older warthogs are persistently infected but are seldom viremic. It is therefore likely that the virus is maintained in a cycle involving young warthogs and ticks.

Domestic Cycle

Primary outbreaks of African swine fever in domestic swine in Africa probably result from the bite of an infected tick, although tissues of acutely infected warthogs, if eaten by domestic swine, can also cause infection.

Introduction of the virus into a previously noninfected country may result in indigenous ticks becoming infected and acting as biological vectors and reservoirs of disease—a feature of great epidemiologic significance. Several species of soft tick found in association with domestic and feral swine in the western hemisphere (the United States and the Caribbean islands) have been shown in experimental studies to be capable of biological transmission of the virus, although there is no evidence that they have become infected naturally during the epidemics in the Caribbean islands and South America.

Once the virus has been introduced into domestic swine, either by the bite of infected ticks or through infected meat, infected animals form the most important source of virus for susceptible swine. Disease spreads rapidly by contact and within buildings by aerosol. Mechanical spread by people, vehicles, and fomites is possible because of the stability of the virus in swine blood, feces, and tissues.

The international spread of African swine fever virus has invariably been linked to feeding scraps of uncooked meat from infected swine. When the virus appeared in Portugal in 1957 and in Brazil in 1978, it was first reported in the vicinity of international airports, among swine fed on food scraps. Virus spread to the Caribbean and Mediterranean islands in 1978 may have arisen from the unloading of infected food scraps from ships.

The prevention and control of African swine fever are difficult because of several features; the lack of an effective vaccine, the transmission of virus in fresh meat and some cured pork products, the existence of persistent infection in some swine, the clinical similarity to hog cholera, and the recognition that soft ticks in some parts of the world are involved in the transmission of the disease. The presence of the virus in ticks and warthogs in many countries of sub-Saharan Africa makes it impossible to break the sylvatic cycle of the virus. However, domestic swine can be reared in Africa if the management system avoids feeding uncooked waste food scraps and prevents the access of ticks and contact with warthogs, usually by double fencing with a wire mesh perimeter fence extending beneath the ground.

Elsewhere in the world, countries that are free of African swine fever maintain their virus-free status by prohibiting the importation of live swine and swine products from infected countries and by monitoring the destruction of all waste food scraps from ships and aircraft involved in international routings.

If disease does occur in a previously noninfected country, control depends first on early recognition and rapid laboratory diagnosis. The virulent forms of African swine fever cause such dramatic mortality that episodes are brought quickly to the attention of veterinary authorities, but the disease caused by less virulent strains that has occurred outside Africa in the past can cause confusion with other diseases and therefore may not be recognized until the virus is well established in the swine population.

Once African swine fever is confirmed in a country that has hitherto been free of disease, its importance necessitates prompt action to first control and then eradicate it. All non-African countries that have become infected have elected to attempt eradication; in many cases, such countries have received financial assistance from international agencies such as the Food and Agricultural Organization of the United Nations. The strategy for eradication involves slaughter of infected swine and swine in contact with them and disposal of carcasses, preferably by burning. Movement of swine between farms is controlled and feeding of waste food prohibited. Where soft ticks are known to occur, infested buildings are sprayed with acaricides. Restocking of farms is allowed only if sentinel swine do not become infected. Using this approach, elimination has been successful, except in Sardinia.

Diseases Caused by Members of the Family *Iridoviridae*

Lymphocystis and Related Diseases of Fish

Lymphocystis Disease

Lymphocystis, caused by a typical vertebrate iridovirus, occurs worldwide, affecting a wide variety of fish—freshwater, saltwater, wild, cultured, warm water, and

FIGURE 17.4.

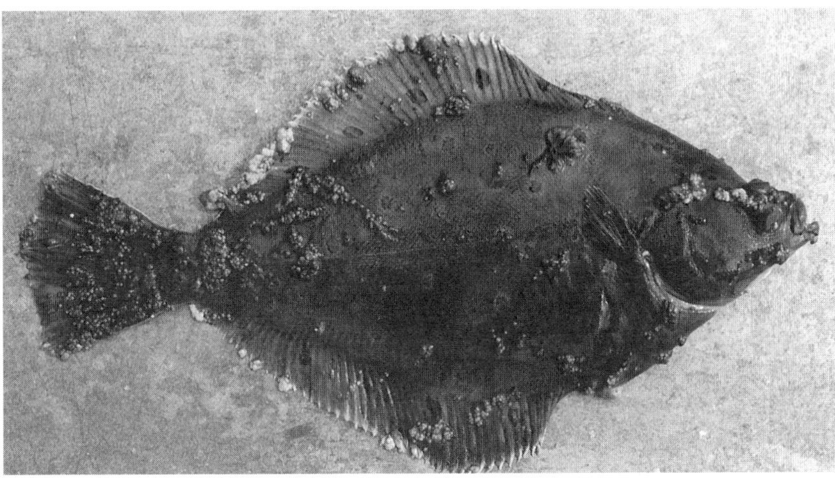

Lymphocystis in plaice. (Courtesy of P. van Banning.)

cold water species. It is a problem in aquarium fish and in commercial aquaculture, most notably in striped bass along the east coast of North America. Infection rarely, if ever, causes mortality; rather it produces unsightly external lesions that make fish unmarketable. Transmission from fish to fish is probably via contact through abrasions and therefore the disease is seen more where there is crowding. The disease is seen most commonly in brackish water or sea water with a slow circulation. Peak incidence is recorded in summer and local pollution may predispose fish to infection.

Lesions appear as raised white to gray nodules, usually on fins and skin, but internal organs and tissues may be affected as well (Figure 17.4). Histologically, lesions are remarkable: there is massive hypertrophy of fibroblasts, individual cells may reach 2 mm in diameter. Infected cells become vacuolated, necrotic, and contain basophilic cytoplasmic inclusions. Infection does not usually elicit an inflammatory response. Infection is usually self-limiting, with lesions disappearing spontaneously as infected cells are sloughed.

Viral Erythrocytic Necrosis

Viral erythrocytic necrosis (also called piscine erythrocytic necrosis) was first described in wild oceanic fish along the northeastern coast of the United States and Canada but is now recognized in a wide variety of freshwater fish as well. Wild oceanic fish may exhibit no signs of disease; however, in cultured fish, especially salmonid species raised in crowded conditions with lower oxygen levels, there may be anemia, abnormal blood clotting, increased susceptibility to bacterial diseases, a decreased tolerance to low oxygen, and a decreased osmoregulatory ability. The incidence of infection may be very high but mortality is usually low. Lesions are only seen microscopically; apparently only red blood cells are infected—these cells become distorted, exhibit karyorrhexis, and have basophilic intracytoplasmic inclusion bodies. As with the lymphocystis virus, there is some indication that there may be different strains of the virus.

Frog Virus 3 Disease

Frog virus 3 is not known to cause any disease in naturally occurring populations of frogs; however, the virus causes the death of frog embryos and causes edema of the tail in tadpoles. The significance of this virus in nature remains unknown.

Further Reading

Anonymous. (1998). "African Swine Fever Virus." Institute for Animal Health, Compton, UK. Available at: http://www.iah.bbsrc.ac.uk/reports/1996/asfv.html

Costa, J. V. (1990). African swine fever. *In* "Molecular Biology of Iridoviruses" (G. Darai, ed.), pp. 247–270. Kluwer Academic Publishers, Boston, MA.

Dixon, L. K., Wilkinson, P. J., Sumpton, K. J., and Ekue, F. (1990). Diversity of the African swine fever virus genome. *In* Molecular Biology of Iridoviruses (G. Darai, ed.), pp. 271–296. Kluwer Academic Publishers, Boston, MA.

Plowright, W., Thomson, G. R., and Neser, J. A. (1994). African swine fever. *In* "Infectious Diseases of Livestock with Special Reference to Southern Africa" (J. A. W. Coetzer, G. R. Thompson, and R. C. Tustin, eds.), Vol. 1, pp. 568–599. Oxford University Press, Cape Town.

Vinuela, E. (1985). African swine fever. *Curr. Top. Microbiol. Immunol.* **116,** 151–170.

Wilkinson, P. J. (1989). African swine fever virus. *In* "Virus Infections of Vertebrates" (M. B. Pensaert, ed.), Vol. 2, pp. 15–36. Elsevier, Amsterdam.

CHAPTER 18

Herpesviridae

Herpesviruses have been found in insects, reptiles, amphibians, and mollusks as well as in virtually every species of bird and mammal that has been investigated. At least one major disease of each domestic animal species, except sheep, is caused by a herpesvirus, including such important diseases as infectious bovine rhinotracheitis, pseudorabies, and Marek's disease. About 100 herpesviruses have been at least partially characterized and the genomes of at least 19, including equine herpesviruses 1, 2, and 4, bovine herpesvirus 1, alcelaphine herpesvirus 1, and channel catfish herpesvirus, have been sequenced completely.

Herpesvirus virions are fragile and do not survive well outside the body. In general, transmission requires close contact, particularly mucosal contact (e.g., coitus, licking and nuzzling as between mother and offspring or between foals or kittens). In large, closely confined populations, such as found in cattle feedlots, modern swine farrowing units, catteries, or broiler facilities, sneezing and short-distance droplet spread are major modes of transmission.

Herpesviruses can survive from one generation to the next via persistent, often latent, infections, from which virus is periodically reactivated and shed. In some infections, shedding may be virtually continuous. Molecular phylogenetic studies suggest that, with few exceptions, each virus is unique because it has arisen and coevolved with its host species. Latency has allowed herpesviruses to be perpetuated, even in very small isolated host groups.

Table 18.1
Herpesviruses That Cause Diseases in Animals

Virus	Disease
Subfamily *Alphaherpesvirinae*	
Bovine herpesvirus 1	Infectious bovine rhinotracheitis, infectious pustular vulvovaginitis, infectious balanoposthitis, abortion
Bovine herpesvirus 2	Bovine mammilitis, pseudo-lumpyskin disease
Bovine herpesvirus 5	Encephalitis
Caprine herpesvirus 1	Conjunctivitis, respiratory and enteric disease
Porcine herpesvirus 1	In young swine generalized disease; in older swine abortion; in secondary hosts neurologic disease (pseudorabies)
Equine herpesvirus 1	Abortion, perinatal foal mortality, respiratory disease, neurologic disease
Equine herpesvirus 3	Coital exanthema
Equine herpesvirus 4	Rhinopneumonitis
Canine herpesvirus 1	Hemorrhagic disease in pups
Felid herpesvirus 1	Feline viral rhinotracheitis
B virus (Cercopithecine herpesvirus 1)	Herpes simplex-like disease in macaques, fatal encephalitis in humans
Simian varicellavirus	Varicella-like disease in monkeys
Gallid herpesvirus 1	Infectious laryngotracheitis of chickens
Gallid herpesvirus 2	Marek's disease of chickens
Anatid herpesvirus 1	Duck plague
Subfamily *Betaherpesvirinae*	
Porcine herpesvirus 2	Inclusion body rhinitis, generalized cytomegalovirus infection
Subfamily *Gammaherpesvirinae*	
Alcelaphine herpesvirus 1	Bovine malignant catarrhal fever
Equine herpesvirus 2	Equine gammaherpesvirus infection
Equine herpesvirus 5	Equine gammaherpesvirus infection
Subfamily, unnamed, channel catfish herpesvirus-like viruses	
Ictalurid herpesvirus 1	Systemic disease in channel catfish
Unclassified herpesviruses	
Salmonid herpesviruses 1 and 2	Systemic disease

Properties of Herpesviruses

Classification

The family *Herpesviridae* is divided into four subfamilies: *Alphaherpesvirinae, Betaherpesvirinae, Gammaherpesvirinae,* and an unnamed subfamily comprising the channel catfish herpesvirus-like viruses. This division was originally based on biological properties, but in general it has accorded well with subsequent molecular characterizations, including nucleotide sequence and phylogenetic analyses (Table 18.1). The subfamilies have been divided into genera, but at this level classification is incomplete and large numbers of viruses, including many important animal pathogens, have been classified only to the subfamily level or have been left unclassified. For example, the newly established subfamily comprising the channel catfish herpesvirus-like viruses only includes one virus at this time—several other important herpesviruses of fish and mollusks have been sequenced completely and now await classification.

Antigenic relationships among the herpesviruses are complex; there are some shared antigens within the family, but different species have distinct envelope glycoproteins. A notable example of the difficulty in correlating biological and molecular properties of the herpesviruses for the purpose of completing a useful taxonomic hierarchy of the family is that of Marek's disease virus. This virus was originally classified as a gammaherpesvirus because of its tropism for T lymphocytes and its oncogenic capacity. Subsequent sequence analysis, however, indicated that the virus is an alphaherpesvirus and so it has been placed in its own genus in this subfamily. The molecular basis for the earlier confusion has come from the discovery that Marek's disease virus carries *onc* gene sequences that are similar to and probably derived from those of avian retroviruses or the cellular homologue of these *onc* genes. Also, based on sequence analysis, two equine herpesviruses, equine herpesvirus 2 and equine herpesvirus 5, formerly classified as betaherpesviruses, have been reclassified as gammaherpesviruses.

Subfamily *Alphaherpesvirinae*

The prototypic viruses of the genera of this subfamily are human herpesvirus 1 (herpes simplex virus 1; genus *Simplexvirus*) and human herpesvirus 3 (varicella-zoster virus; genus *Varicellovirus*). Gallid herpesvirus 1 (infectious laryngotracheitis virus) and Marek's disease virus are the prototypes of two new, as yet unnamed, genera in this subfamily; although having a genomic organization similar to that of the mammalian viruses of the subfamily, these viruses exhibit significant differences in their biological properties. Most alphaherpesviruses grow rapidly, lyse infected cells, and establish latent infections primarily in sensory ganglia. Some alphaherpesviruses have a broad host range.

Subfamily *Betaherpesvirinae*

This subfamily comprises the cytomegaloviruses of many species; the prototype of the subfamily is human herpesvirus 5 (human cytomegalovirus). Individual cytomegaloviruses have a restricted host range. Their replicative cycle is slow and cell lysis does not occur until several days after infection. The viruses may remain latent in secretory glands, lymphoreticular tissues, kidneys, and other tissues.

Subfamily *Gammaherpesvirinae*

This subfamily comprises the herpesviruses that are lymphotropic; the prototype is human herpesvirus 4 (Epstein–Barr virus; genus *Lymphocryptovirus*). All viruses of veterinary importance are in the genus *Rhadinovirus,* from the Greek word for fragile (prototype, ateline herpesvirus 2). Members have a narrow host range and become latent in lymphocytes; some are linked to oncogenic transformation of lymphocytes (e.g., Burkitt's lymphoma and nasopharyngeal carcinoma in humans) and some also cause cytocidal infections in epithelial and fibroblastic cells. The nonhuman primate and ungulate gammaherpesviruses are not recognized as significant causes of disease in their natural hosts where these are identified, but often cause lymphoproliferative disease in heterologous, not too distantly, related hosts.

Unnamed Subfamily Comprising Channel Catfish Herpesvirus-like Viruses

At present this subfamily comprises only channel catfish herpesvirus, but additional herpesviruses of fish and mollusks will undoubtedly be added. Channel catfish herpesvirus has been sequenced completely and found to be the most different in genomic structure of any herpesvirus yet studied.

Virion Properties

Herpesvirus virions are enveloped, about 150 nm in diameter, and contain an icosahedral nucleocapsid about 100 nm in diameter, composed of 162 hollow capsomers—150 hexamers and 12 pentamers (Figure 18.1). The DNA genome is wrapped around a fibrous spool-like core, which has the shape of a torus and appears to be suspended by fibrils that are anchored to the inner side of the surrounding capsid and pass through the hole of the torus. Surrounding the capsid is a layer of globular material, known as the tegument, which is enclosed by a typical lipoprotein envelope with numerous small glycoprotein peplomers. Because of the variable size of the

FIGURE 18.1.

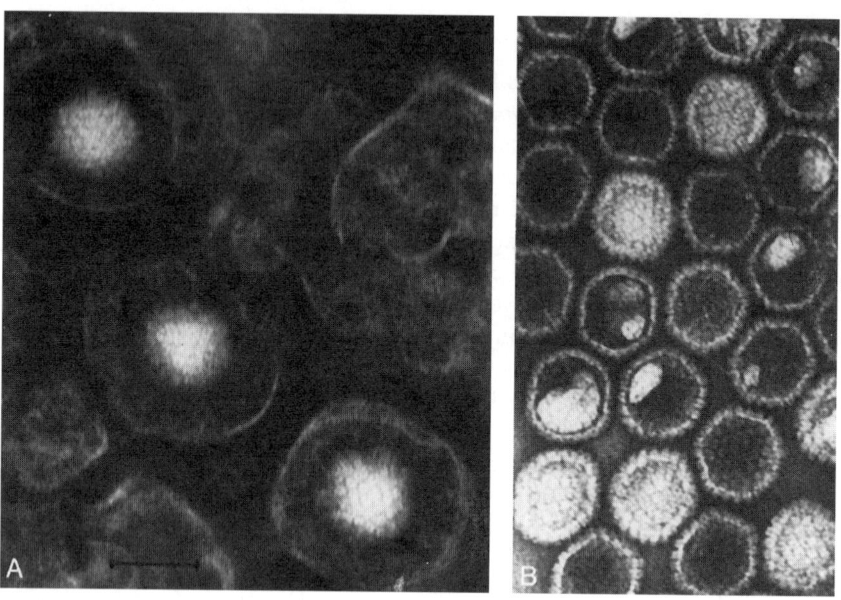

Herpesviridae. Negatively stained preparations of the prototype herpesvirus, herpes simplex virus type 1. (Left) Enveloped virions. (Right) Unenveloped capsids. Bar: 100 nm. (Courtesy of E. L. Palmer.)

envelope, virions can range in diameter from 120 to 200 nm.

The genome consists of a single linear molecule of double-stranded DNA, 125–235 kbp in size, which is infectious under appropriate experimental conditions (Figure 18.2). The complete sequences of at least 19 herpesviruses, including representatives of each of the three subfamilies, have been determined.

FIGURE 18.2.

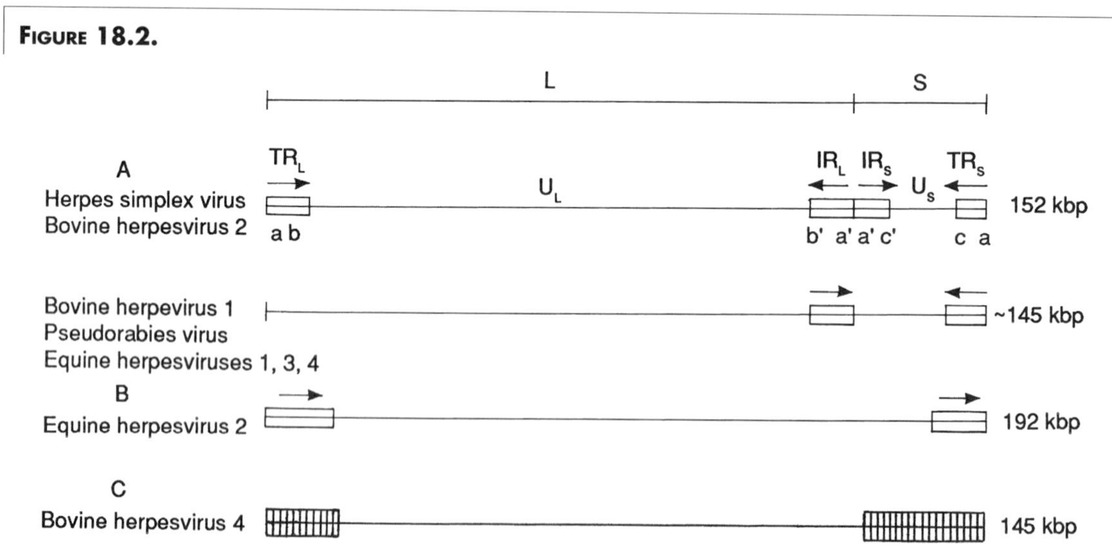

The genome structure of herpesviruses: (A) Alphaherpesvirus genomes comprise two regions designated long (L) and short (S). Terminal repeat (TR) and internal repeat (IR) sequences may bracket unique sequences (U_L, U_S) of both L and S or only S. Repeat sequences are shown as boxes and are encoded as indicated by the direction of the arrows. Repeat sequences allow the DNA they bracket to invert relative to the rest of the genome such that where both U_L and U_S are bracketed by repeat sequences, four isomers are made and packaged in equimolar amounts into virions. Where only S is bracketed by repeat sequences, two equimolar isomers are made. (B) The genome of equine herpesvirus 2, a betaherpesvirus, contains terminal direct repeat structures. (C) The genome of bovine herpesvirus 4, a gammaherpesvirus, contains multiple direct terminal repeat sequences (small boxes) in a nonequal, variable number of copies.

There is a remarkable degree of variation in the composition, size, and organization of the genomes of the herpesviruses: (1) the percentage of guanine plus cytosine (G+C ratio) varies between 32 and 74%, a range that far exceeds that found in DNAs of all eukaryotes; (2) the size of herpesvirus genomes varies between 125 and 235 kbp; and (3) the organization of genomes varies in complex fashion. Reiterated DNA sequences generally occur at both ends (and in some viruses also internally), dividing the genome into two unique sections, designated large (U_L) and small (U_s). When these reiterated sequences are inverted in their orientation, the unique L and S components can invert, relative to one another, during replication, giving rise to two or four different isomers of the genome, present in equimolar proportions. Further, intragenomic and intergenomic recombination events can alter the number of any particular reiterated sequence polymorphism.

As an example of the complex arrangement and content of a herpesvirus genome, the genome of equine herpesvirus 1 is shown in Figure 18.3 and a brief description of some of the proteins encoded by the genome is provided in Table 18.2.

In broad terms, herpesvirus genes fall into three categories: (1) those encoding proteins concerned with viral replication (immediate early and early genes), (2) those encoding structural proteins (late genes), and (3) a heterologous set of optional genes in the sense that they are not found in all herpesviruses and are not essential for replication in cultured cells. Herpesvirus virions contain over 30 structural proteins, of which 6 are present in the nucleocapsid, 2 being DNA associated. The glycoproteins, of which there are about 12, are located in the envelope, from which most project as peplomers. One of the peplomer glycoproteins (gE) possesses Fc receptor activity and binds normal IgG.

FIGURE 18.3.

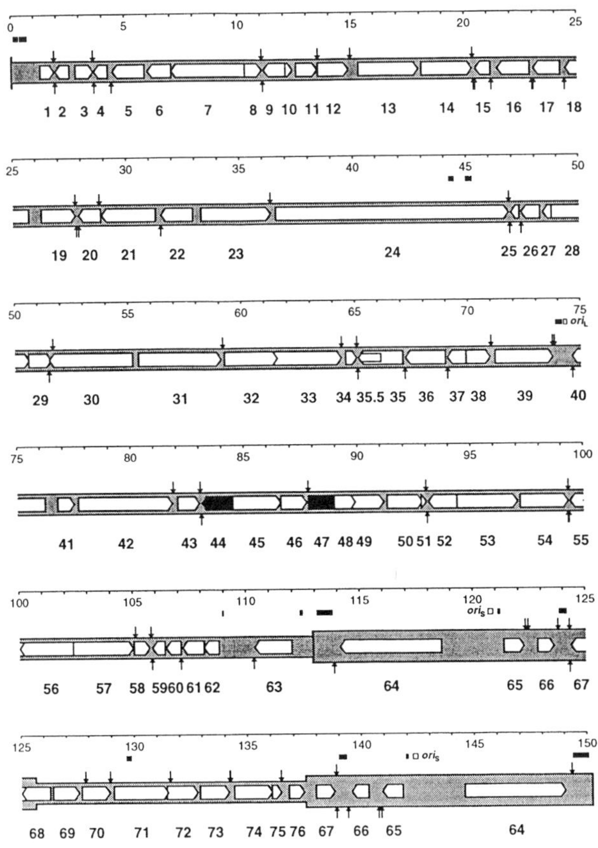

Schematic diagram of the genome of equine herpesvirus 1 as an example of the complexity of herpesvirus genomes. The 150,223-bp sequence has been determined: GenBank Data Library Accession No. M86664. The thinner and thicker bars denote the unique regions (U_L, U_S) and inverted repeats (TR_L, IR_L, TR_S, IR_S), respectively. The predicted arrangement of open reading frames (ORFs) is shown as open arrows with the head of the arrow indicating the direction of transcription. ORFs are numbered sequentially from left to right. Vertical arrows indicate candidate polyadenylation sites. The locations of reiterations and candidate origins of replication are indicated above the genome as closed and open boxes, respectively. The scale above the genome is in kbp. [From E. A. Telford, M. S., Watson, K. McBride, and A. J. Davidson. The DNA sequence of equine herpesvirus 1. *Virology* **189,** 304–316 (1992).]

Table 18.2
Some Proteins Encoded by Genome of Equine Herpesvirus 1 (an Alphaherpesvirus)[a]

Gene	Codon	Size (M_r)	Properties or functions
5	470	51,318	Transcriptional activator
7	1081	118,956	DNA helicase/primase complex
9	326	35,207	Deoxyuridine triphosphatase
11	304	33,239	Tegument protein
16	469	50,887	Membrane glycoprotein (gC)
19	497	56,540	Host shutoff factor
22	465	51,304	Capsid protein
24	3421	367,061	Tegument protein
30	1220	135,949	DNA polymerase
33	980	109,800	Membrane glycoprotein (gB)
38	352	38,748	Thymidine kinase
39	848	92,837	Membrane glycoprotein (gH)
42	1376	152,175	Major capsid protein
49	594	65,244	Virion protein kinase
50	508	56,064	Deoxyribonuclease
61	312	34,776	Uracil-DNA glycosylase
62	218	24,424	Membrane glycoprotein (gL)
65	293	32,115	*In vitro* host-range factor
69	382	42,541	Protein kinase
70	411	45,267	Membrane glycoprotein (gG)
72	452	51,097	Membrane glycoprotein (gD)
73	424	46,390	Membrane glycoprotein (gI)
74	550	61,180	Membrane glycoprotein (gE)

[a] A genome map to match these genes and proteins is shown in Figure 18.3. The functions of the proteins are inferred from homology with the proteins of herpes simplex virus of humans or non-herpesvirus protein sequences deposited in GenBank. Twenty-three of the 76 proteins identified in equine herpesvirus 1 have no known homologues. Many of the proteins not listed here have unknown functions. [From E. A. R. Telford, M. J. Studdert, C. T. Agius, M. S. Watson, H. C. Aird, and A. J. Davison. Equine herpesvirus-2 and herpesvirus-5 are gammaherpesviruses. *Virology* **195,** 492–499 (1993).]

Some of the growth-regulating and immune modulation proteins that are not necessary for viral replication and maturation in cultured cells are homologues of cellular genes that are known to be involved in growth regulation and modulation of the immune response. It is likely that these virus-coded proteins play a significant role in the pathogenesis of herpesvirus infections. Because they are clustered at the initiation site for viral DNA replication, it has been proposed that the genes for these proteins were acquired from host cells, with the viruses acting as natural cloning vectors for the capture of cellular genes. Latent herpesvirus genomes are believed to be maintained in host cells in a circular episomal (extrachromosomal) form.

Viral Replication

Herpesvirus replication has been studied most extensively with human herpesviruses 1 (herpes simplex virus 1). Betaherpesviruses and gammaherpesviruses probably follow a similar pattern, but replicate more slowly. Following attachment via the binding of virion glycoprotein peplomers to host cell receptors, one of which is heparin sulfate proteoglycan, the nucleocapsid enters the cytoplasm either by fusion of the virion envelope to the cell membrane or by endophagocytosis. The DNA–protein complex is then freed from the nucleocapsid and enters the nucleus, quickly shutting off host cell macromolecular synthesis.

Three classes of mRNA, α, β, and γ, are transcribed in sequence by cellular RNA polymerase II (Figure 18.4). Thus, α (immediate early) RNAs, when processed appropriately to become mRNAs, are translated to form α proteins, which initiate transcription of β (early) mRNAs, the translation of which produces β (early) proteins and suppresses the transcription of further α mRNAs. Viral DNA replication then commences, utilizing some of the α and β proteins as well as host cell proteins. The transcription program then switches again, and the resulting γ (late) mRNAs, which are transcribed from sequences situated throughout the genome, are translated into γ proteins. Over 70 virus-coded proteins are made during the cycle, with many of the α and β proteins being enzymes and DNA-binding proteins, whereas most of the γ proteins are structural. Intricate controls regulate expression at the level of both transcription and translation. Viral DNA is replicated in the nucleus and newly synthesized DNA is spooled into preformed immature capsids.

Maturation involves the completion of encapsidation of virion DNA into nucleocapsids and the association of nucleocapsids with altered patches of the inner layer of the nuclear envelope, followed by envelopment by budding (Figure 18.5). Mature virions accumulate within vacuoles in the cytoplasm and are released by exocytosis or cytolysis. Virus-specific proteins are also found in the plasma membrane, where they are involved in cell fusion, may act as Fc receptors, and are presumed to be targets for immune cytolysis.

Intranuclear inclusion bodies are characteristic of herpesvirus infections and can usually be found both in appropriately fixed and stained tissues from herpesvirus-infected animals and in cell cultures (Figure 18.6).

FIGURE 18.4.

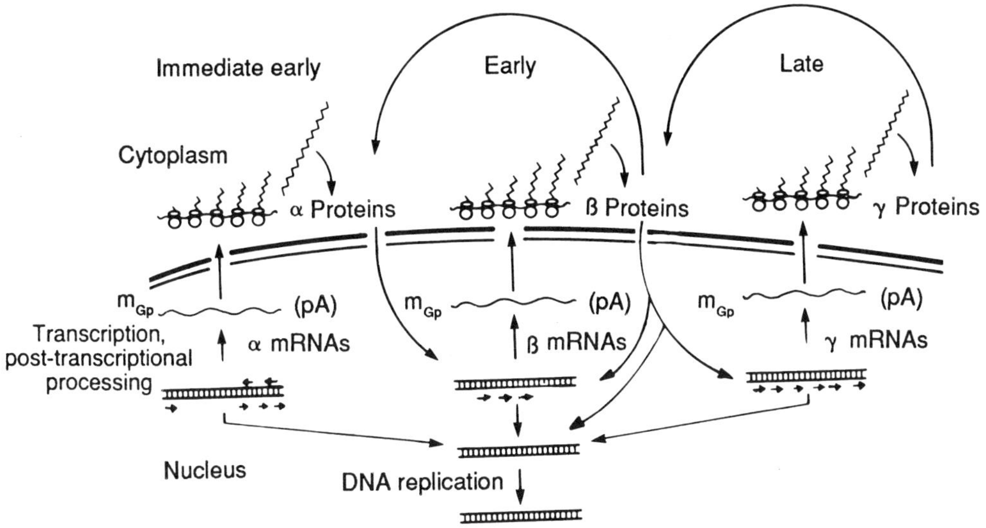

Immediate early
Early
Late
Cytoplasm
α Proteins
β Proteins
γ Proteins
m_{Gp} (pA)
m_{Gp} (pA)
m_{Gp} (pA)
Transcription, post-transcriptional processing
α mRNAs
β mRNAs
γ mRNAs
Nucleus
DNA replication

Diagram representing transcription, translation, and DNA replication of a typical herpesvirus (see text). Transcription and posttranscriptional processing occur in the nucleus, translation in the cytoplasm, and some of the α and β proteins are involved in further transcription and some β proteins in DNA replication. [From B. Roizman. Herpesviruses. *In* Microbiology (B. D. Davis, R. Dulbecco, H. N. Eisen, and H. Ginsberg, eds.) 4th ed. pp. 929–945. Lippincott-Raven, Philadelphia, PA. 1990.]

FIGURE 18.5.

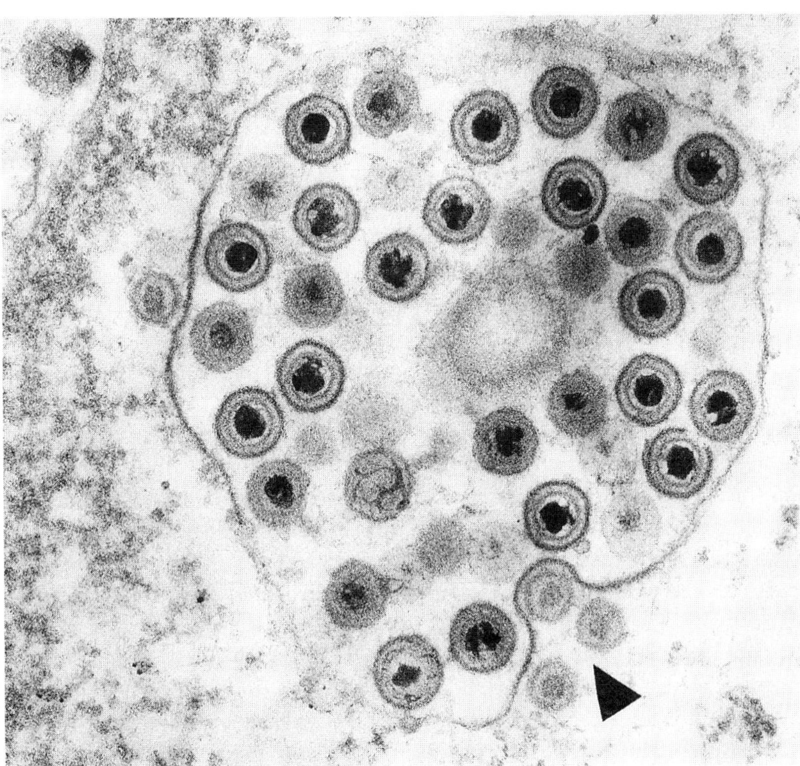

Thin section electron microscopy of a herpesvirus-infected cell showing the formation of capsids and their primary envelopment by budding through the nuclear envelope (arrow). Magnification: ×65,000.

Figure 18.6.

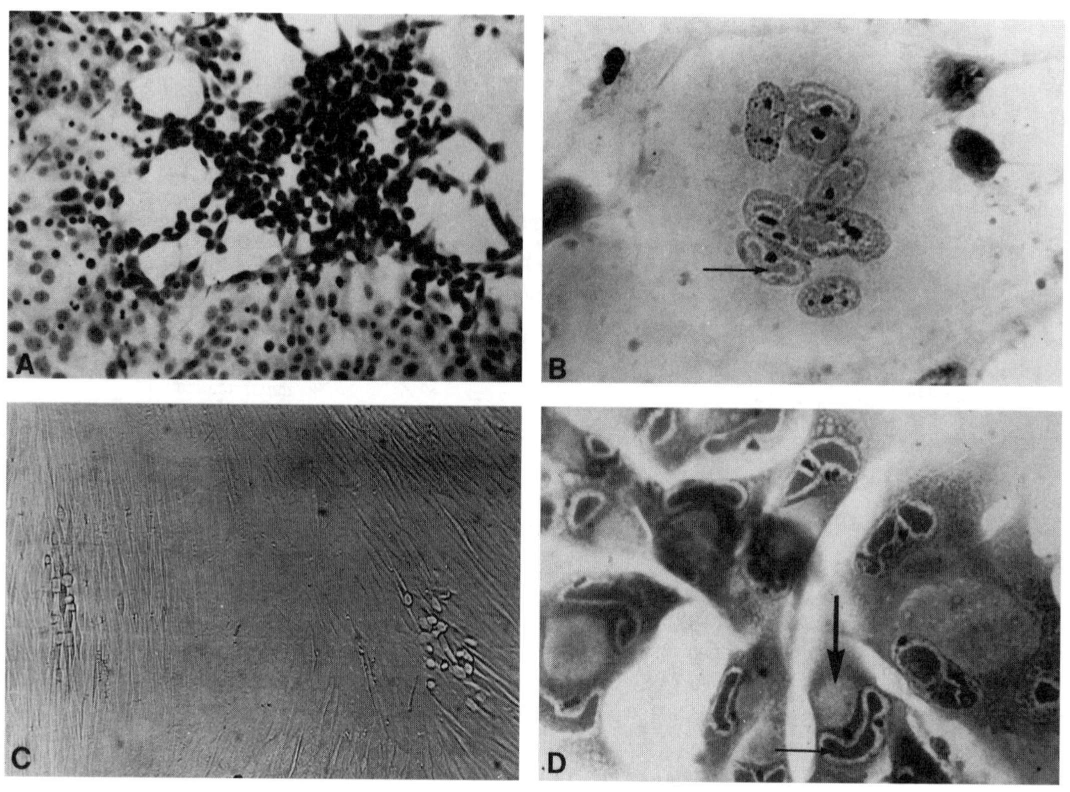

Cytopathic effects induced by herpesviruses. (A) Alphaherpesvirus in HEp-2 cells showing early focal cytopathology (hematoxylin and eosin stain; magnification: ×100). (B) Alphaherpesvirus in bovine kidney cells showing multinucleated giant cell containing acidophilic intranuclear inclusions (arrow) (hematoxylin and eosin stain, magnification ×400). (C) Cytomegalovirus in fibroblasts showing two foci of slowly developing cytopathology (unstained, magnification: ×35). (D) Cytomegalovirus in fibroblasts showing giant cells with acidophilic inclusions in the nuclei (small arrow) and cytoplasm (large arrow), the latter being characteristically large and round (hematoxylin and eosin stain, magnification: ×450). (Courtesy of I. Jack.)

Characteristics Common to Many Herpesvirus Infections

Collectively and individually the herpesviruses exhibit many extraordinary infection characteristics that make them versatile pathogens. Transmission is generally associated with mucosal contact, but droplet infection is also common. Many alphaherpesviruses produce localized lesions, particularly in the skin or on the mucosae of the respiratory and genital tracts. Generalized alphaherpesvirus infections, characterized by foci of necrosis in almost any organ or tissue, are seen when animals less than 3 months of age are infected without the protection provided by maternal antibody. In pregnant animals, a mononuclear cell-associated viremia may result in the transfer of virus across the placenta, leading to abortion, with focal necrotic lesions being found throughout the fetus. Marek's disease virus (alphaherpesvirus) causes a polyclonal T lymphocyte tumor—the genetic basis for this resides in oncogenic genes carried by the virus (see Chapter 11). Betaherpesviruses and gammaherpesviruses are not highly lytic for infected cells, they typically cause chronic infections lasting several months before clinical recovery. Some of the primate rhadinoviruses (subfamily *Gammaherpesvirinae*) produce tumors (see Chapter 11).

Persistent infection with periodic or continuous shedding occurs in all herpesvirus infections. In alphaherpesvirus infections, multiple copies of viral DNA are demonstrable either as episomes or more rarely integrated into the chromosomal DNA of latently infected neurons. The latent genome is essentially silent except for the production of a latency-associated transcript. This RNA transcript is not known to code for any protein (bovine herpesvirus 1 may be an exception); its mechanism of action in the establishment, maintenance, and reactivation of latent infection is not yet known. Reactivation is usually associated with stress, caused by intercurrent infections, shipping, cold, or

TABLE 18.3
Properties of Herpesviruses

Virions are enveloped, about 150 nm in diameter, containing an icosahedral nucleocapsid that is 100 nm in diameter and composed of 162 capsomers

Genome is linear double-stranded DNA, 125–235 kbp in size

Replication occurs in the nucleus, with sequential transcription and translation of immediate early (α), early (β), and late (γ) genes producing α, β, and γ proteins, respectively; the earlier genes and their gene products regulate the transcription of later genes

DNA replication and encapsidation occur in the nucleus; the envelope is acquired by budding through the inner layer of the nuclear envelope

Infection results in characteristic eosinophilic intranuclear inclusion bodies

Infection becomes latent, with recrudescence and intermittent or continuous viral shedding

crowding. Shedding of virus in nasal, oral, or genital secretions provides the source of infection for other animals, including transfer from dam to offspring. In domestic animals, reactivation is usually not noticed, partly because lesions on nasal or genital mucosae are not seen readily. Some betaherpesviruses and gammaherpesviruses are shed continuously from epithelial surfaces (Table 18.3).

DISEASES CAUSED BY MEMBERS OF THE SUBFAMILY *ALPHAHERPESVIRINAE*

Infectious Bovine Rhinotracheitis (Caused by Bovine Herpesvirus 1)

Bovine herpesvirus 1 (infectious bovine rhinotracheitis virus; infectious pustular vulvovaginitis virus) causes a variety of diseases in cattle, including rhinotracheitis, pustular vaginitis, balanoposthitis, conjunctivitis, abortion, enteritis, a generalized disease of newborn calves, and possibly encephalitis.

The rapid expansion of feedlots in the United States during the 1950s led to the recognition of several new disease syndromes, including rhinotracheitis, from which a herpesvirus was isolated. Comparison of the herpesvirus isolated from cases of rhinotracheitis and from cases of vulvovaginitis in dairy cattle in eastern United States indicated that the viruses were indistinguishable. Bovine herpesvirus 1 and the diseases it causes are now known to occur worldwide.

Clinical Features

Genital Disease

Infectious pustular vulvovaginitis is recognized most commonly in dairy cows. Affected cows develop fever, depression, anorexia, and stand apart, often with the tail held away from contact with the vulva; micturition is frequent and painful. The vulval labia are swollen, there is a slight vulval discharge, and the vestibular mucosa is reddened with many small pustules (Figure 18.7A). Adjacent pustules usually coalesce to form a fibrinous pseudomembrane that covers an ulcerated mucosa. The acute stage of the disease lasts 4–5 days and uncomplicated lesions usually heal by 10 to 14 days. Many cases are subclinical or go unnoticed.

Lesions of infectious balanoposthitis in bulls and the clinical course of disease are similar (Figure 18.7B). Where lesions are extensive and acute there is reluctance or complete refusal to serve. Semen from recovered bulls may be contaminated with virus as a result of periodic shedding. However, cows may conceive to the service or artificial insemination from which they acquire infectious pustular vulvovaginitis, and pregnant cows that develop the infection rarely abort. Bovine herpesvirus 1 has been isolated occasionally from cases of vaginitis and balanitis in swine, from stillborn piglets, and from aborted equine fetuses.

Respiratory Disease

Infectious bovine rhinotracheitis occurs as a subclinical, mild, or severe disease. Morbidity approaches 100% and mortality may reach 10%, particularly if complications occur. Initial signs include fever, depression, inappetence, and a profuse nasal discharge, initially serous and later mucopurulent. The nasal mucosa is hyperemic and lesions within the nasal cavity, which may be difficult to see, progress from focal pustular necrosis to large areas of shallow, hemorrhagic, ulcerated mucosa covered by a cream-colored diphtheritic membrane. The breath may be fetid. Dyspnea, mouth breathing, salivation, and a deep bronchial cough are common. Acute, uncomplicated cases last 5–10 days.

Unilateral or bilateral conjunctivitis, often with profuse lacrimation, is a common clinical sign in cattle with infectious bovine rhinotracheitis but may occur in a herd as an almost exclusive clinical sign. Gastroenteritis may occur in adult cattle and is a prominent finding in

Figure 18.7.

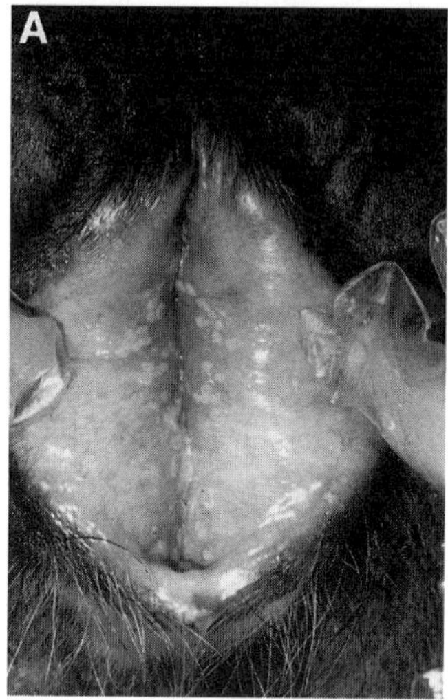

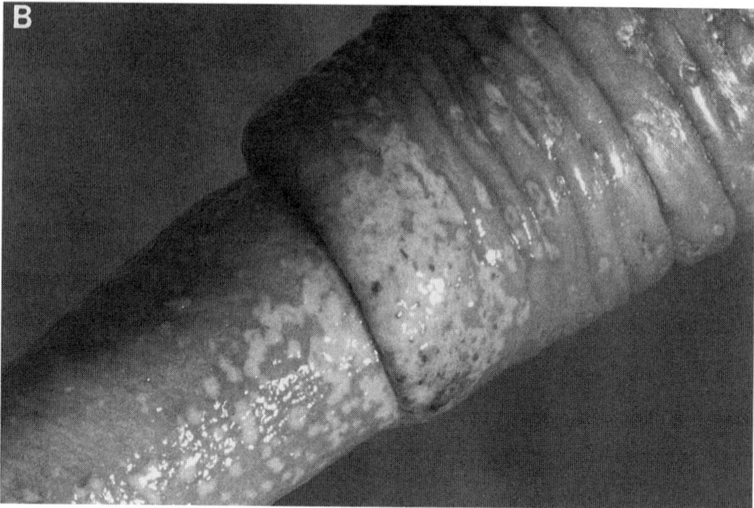

Genital disease caused by bovine herpesvirus 1. (A) Infectious pustular vulvovaginitis. (B) Infectious pustular balanoposthitis. (A, courtesy of D. F. Collings.)

the generalized disease of neonatal calves, which is often fatal. Abortion may occur at 4–7 months gestation, and the virus has also been reported to be cause mastitis.

Pathogenesis, Pathology, and Immunity

Genital disease may result from coitus or artificial insemination, although some outbreaks, particularly in dairy cows, may occur in the absence of coitus. Respiratory disease and conjunctivitis result from droplet transmission. Within the animal, dissemination of the virus from the initial focus of infection probably occurs via a cell-associated viremia.

Lifelong latent infection with periodic virus shedding occurs after bovine herpesvirus 1 infection; the sciatic and trigeminal ganglia are the sites of latency following genital and respiratory disease, respectively. The administration of corticosteroids results in reactivation of the virus and has been used as a means of detecting and eliminating carrier bulls in artificial insemination centers.

In both the genital and the respiratory forms of the disease the lesions are focal areas of epithelial cell necrosis in which there is ballooning of epithelial cells; typical herpesvirus inclusions may be present in nuclei at the periphery of necrotic foci. There is an intense inflammatory response. Gross lesions are not observed in aborted fetuses, but microscopic necrotic foci are present in most tissues and the liver is affected consistently.

Laboratory Diagnosis

Rapid diagnostic methods include electron microscopy of vesicular fluid or scrapings and immunofluorescence staining of smears or tissue sections and detection of viral nucleic acid by the polymerase chain reaction. Viral isolation and characterization provide a definitive diagnosis. Herpesviruses are grown most readily in cell cultures derived from their natural host. As with other alphaherpesviruses, there is a rapid cytopathic effect, with syncytia and characteristic eosinophilic intranuclear inclusion bodies. The polymerase chain reaction for virus detection and specific enzyme immunoassays for antibody detection have been developed and are available in reference laboratories in many countries.

Epidemiology, Prevention, and Control

Genital and respiratory disease are rarely diagnosed in the same herd at the same time. Infectious bovine rhinotracheitis is an uncommon disease in range cattle, but is of major significance in feedlots. In cattle not in feedlots, the incidence of antibody varies between 10 and 35%. Primary infection often coincides with transport and introduction to a feedlot of young, fully susceptible cattle from diverse sources. Adaptation from range to feedlot conditions and dietary changes, including the high protein diet, contribute to a stressful environment that may potentiate disease, although in well-managed operations these factors are minimized, with a corresponding reduced incidence of severe disease. The damaged necrotic mucosa provides a substrate for bacterial infection in stressed cattle and contributes to the complex syndrome called shipping fever (see Chapter 9). Transmission has occurred among bulls in artificial insemination centers when a common sponge has been used for washing the prepuce prior to semen collection. Virus may also be spread by artificial insemination.

Bovine herpesvirus 1 vaccines (mostly attenuated virus vaccines) are used extensively, alone or in multiple virus formulations. Recombinant DNA vaccines have been constructed in which the thymidine kinase and other glycoprotein "marker" genes have been deleted. Although they do not prevent infection, vaccines significantly reduce the incidence and severity of disease. Experimental vaccines produced by recombinant methods have been tested: they are based on single glycoprotein genes, particularly gD, that have been expressed in baculovirus expression systems or have been placed in plasmid vectors for delivery as DNA vaccines.

Because of the low incidence of bovine herpesvirus 1 infections in cattle in Switzerland and Denmark, successful eradication programs based on test and slaughter, combined with control of cattle movements, were initiated in the early 1980s. Vaccines were not used, so as to avoid problems of masking latently infected animals. With the probable commercial introduction of better vaccines that enable distinction between vaccinated and infected cattle in the near future, other countries in Europe are now considering eradicating the virus by an integrated program involving vaccination, movement control, and slaughter of all cattle with serologic evidence of exposure to wild type virus.

Bovine Mammillitis/Pseudo-Lumpyskin Disease (Caused by Bovine Herpesvirus 2)

Two clinical forms of bovine herpesvirus 2 infections are known: lesions localized to the teats, occasionally spreading to the udder (bovine mammillitis), and a generalized skin disease (pseudo-lumpyskin disease). Bovine herpesvirus 2 was first isolated in 1957 from cattle in South Africa with a generalized lumpyskin disease. The disease was mild and its major significance lay in the need to differentiate it from a more serious lumpyskin disease found in South Africa caused by a poxvirus (see Chapter 16). A similar herpesvirus was isolated from cattle with extensive erosions of the teats elsewhere in Africa and subsequently from similar lesions in cattle in many countries of the world.

Bovine herpesvirus 2 is related antigenically to human herpes simplex virus and the DNAs of these viruses show 15% homology, compared with less than 6% homology, between bovine herpesvirus 2 and bovine herpesvirus 1.

Clinical Features

Pseudo-lumpyskin disease has an incubation period of 5 to 9 days and is characterized by a mild fever, followed by the sudden appearance of skin nodules: a few, or many, on the face, neck, back, and perineum. The nodules have a flat surface with a slightly depressed center and involve only the superficial layers of the epidermis, which undergo necrosis. Within 7–8 days, the local swelling subsides and healing, without scar formation, is complete within a few weeks.

In many countries, the generalized skin disease is not seen and bovine herpesvirus 2 is recognized only as a cause of mammillitis, but virus isolated experimentally from cases of mammillitis can cause generalized skin disease. Lesions usually occur only on the teats, but in severe cases most of the skin of the udder may be affected. Occasionally, heifers may develop fever, coinciding with the appearance of lesions. Milk yield may be reduced by as much as 10% as a result of difficulty in milking the affected cows and intercurrent mastitis.

Pathogenesis, Pathology, and Immunity

The distribution of lesions in mammillitis suggests local spread. The generalized distribution of lesions in pseudo-lumpyskin disease suggest viremic spread, but viremia is difficult to demonstrate.

Laboratory Diagnosis

The benign nature of pseudo-lumpyskin disease, the characteristic central depression on the surface of the nodules, the superficial necrosis of the epidermis, and the shorter course of the disease are helpful in differentiating the condition from true lumpyskin disease in countries where both occur.

The clinical differentiation of the various conditions that affect the teats of cattle can be difficult; other virus diseases causing teat lesions are warts, cowpox, pseudocowpox, vesicular stomatitis, and foot-and-mouth disease. For this reason it is advisable to examine the whole herd, as a comparison of the early developmental stages helps considerably in the diagnosis. Advanced lesions are often similar, irrespective of the cause. Demonstration of virus in scrapings or vesicular fluid by electron microscopy, coupled with virus isolation, are used for confirming a diagnosis.

Epidemiology, Prevention, and Control

Pseudo-lumpyskin disease occurs most commonly in southern Africa, in moist low-lying areas, especially along rivers, and has its highest incidence in the summer months and early fall. Susceptible cattle cannot be infected by placing them in contact with diseased cattle if housed in insect-proof accommodation. It is therefore assumed that mechanical transmission of the virus occurs by arthropods but attempts to identify the vectors have failed. Buffalo, giraffe, and other African wildlife may be naturally infected with bovine herpesvirus 2.

Although milking machines were initially thought to be responsible for the transmission of mammillitis in dairy herds, there is evidence that this is rarely the case. The infection may spread rapidly through a herd, but in some outbreaks disease is confined to newly calved heifers or heavily pregnant cattle. Serologic surveys suggest that many infections are subclinical.

Bovine Herpesvirus Encephalitis (Caused by Bovine Herpesvirus 5)

Encephalitis due to bovine herpesvirus 5 has been recognized in several countries. It is believed to result from direct neural spread from the nasal cavity, pharynx, and tonsils via the maxillary and mandibular branches of the trigeminal nerve. Lesions initially occur in the midbrain and later involve the entire brain. The natural history of the causative virus, which is related to bovine herpesvirus 1, is obscure. Although frequently stated to cause encephalitis, bovine herpesvirus 1 has not been confirmed as a cause of this disease.

Caprine Herpesvirus Disease (Caused by Caprine Herpesvirus 1)

Herpesviruses have been isolated from goats in several parts of the world in association with a variety of clinical signs, including conjunctivitis and disease of the respiratory, digestive, and genital tracts, including abortion. Caprine herpesvirus 1 is related antigenically to bovine herpesvirus 1 in a one-way cross-reaction but it is not infectious for cattle or lambs and its restriction endonuclease map is quite different from that of bovine herpesvirus 1.

Pseudorabies (Caused by Porcine Herpesvirus 1)

This disease (*syn.*, Aujeszky's disease) is primarily a disease of swine, which serve as a reservoir and the principal source of natural infection for a diverse range of secondary hosts, including horses, cattle, sheep, goats, dogs, cats, and many feral species. Humans are refractory. The diverse host range is also demonstrated *in vitro;* cell cultures derived from almost any animal species support the replication of pseudorabies virus.

Pseudorabies is endemic in swine in most parts of the world. The eradication of hog cholera from the United States and the United Kingdom (see Chapter 36) has brought pseudorabies to greater prominence and is now economically the most important viral disease of swine, causing multimillion dollar losses each year in countries where it is found.

Clinical Features

Clinical Features in Swine

In herds in which the disease is endemic, reactivation of virus occurs without obvious clinical signs, but the spread of the virus within a nonimmune herd may be rapid, with the consequences of primary infection being influenced markedly by age and, in sows, by pregnancy. Pruritus, which is such a dominant feature of the disease in secondary hosts such as cattle, is rare in swine.

Pregnant Sows. In nonimmune herds, up to 50% of pregnant sows may abort over a short period of time due to rapid spread of infection from an index case or carrier. Infection of a sow before the 30th day of gestation results in death and resorption of embryos and after that time in abortion. Infection in late pregnancy may terminate with the delivery of a mixture of mummified, macerated, stillborn, weak, and normal swine, and some of these pregnancies may be prolonged for 2–3 weeks beyond the normal gestation period. Up to 20% of aborting sows are infertile on the first subsequent breeding but do eventually conceive.

Piglets. Mortality rates among piglets born to nonimmune dams depend somewhat on their age, but approaches 100%. Maternal antibody is protective, and disease in piglets born to recovered or vaccinated sows is greatly diminished in severity, with recovery the usual outcome.

Weaned, Growing, and Mature Swine. The incubation period is about 30 hours. In younger pigs the course is typically about 8 days but may be as short as 4 days. Initial signs include sneezing, coughing, and moderate fever (40°C), which increases up to 42°C in the ensuing 48 hours. There is constipation during the fever, the feces are hard and dry, and vomiting may occur. Pigs are listless, depressed, and tend to remain recumbent. By the fifth day there is incoordination and pronounced muscle spasm, circling, and intermittent convulsions accompanied by excess salivation. By the sixth day swine become moribund and die within 12 hours. In mature swine the mortality rate is low, usually less than 2%, but there may be significant weight loss and poor growth rates after recovery.

Clinical Features in Secondary Hosts

Important secondary hosts include cattle ("mad itch"), dogs ("pseudorabies"), and cats. Disease in secondary hosts is sporadic and occurs where there is direct or indirect contact with swine. Infection is usually by ingestion, less commonly inhalation, and possibly via minor wounds. In cattle the dominant clinical sign is intense pruritus. Particular sites, often on the flanks or hind limbs, are licked incessantly; there is gnawing and rubbing such that the area becomes abraded. Cattle may become frenzied. There is progressive involvement of the central nervous system; following the first signs, the course leading to death may be as short as a few hours and is never longer than 6 days.

In dogs, the frenzy associated with intense pruritus and paralysis of the jaws and pharynx accompanied by drooling of saliva and plaintive howling simulates true rabies; however, there is no tendency for dogs to attack other animals. In cats, the disease may progress so rapidly that frenzy is not observed.

Pathogenesis, Pathology and Immunity

Following primary oral or intranasal infection of swine, virus replicates in the oropharynx. There is no viremia during the first 24 hours and it is difficult to demonstrate at any time. However, within 24 hours virus can be isolated from various cranial nerve ganglia and the medulla and pons, to which virions have traveled via the axoplasm of the cranial nerves. Virus continues to spread within the central nervous system; there is ganglioneuritis at many sites, including those controlling vital functions.

The relative lack of gross lesions even in young swine is notable. Tonsillitis, pharyngitis, tracheitis, rhinitis, and esophagitis may be evident but are mild. Occasionally, small necrotic foci may be found in the liver and spleen. Microscopically the principal findings in both swine and secondary hosts are in the central nervous system. There is a diffuse nonsuppurative meningoencephalitis and ganglioneuritis, marked perivascular cuffing, and focal gliosis associated with extensive necrosis of neuronal and glial cells. There is a correlation between the site and severity of clinical signs and the histologic findings. Typical intranuclear herpesvirus inclusions are rarely found in the lesions in swine.

Some swine that have recovered from pseudorabies may shed virus continuously in their nasal secretions. Others from which virus cannot be isolated by conventional means may yield virus when explant cultures of tonsillar tissue are made. Pseudorabies virus DNA can be demonstrated in the trigeminal ganglia of recovered swine by DNA hybridization and the polymerase chain reaction, but there is debate about the relative significance of lymphoreticular cells and nerve cells as a site for latency.

Laboratory Diagnosis

The history and clinical signs often suggest the diagnosis. Enzyme immunoassay has been approved as a standard test in several countries and is used in association with vaccination and eradication programs. Fluorescent antibody staining of frozen tissue sections, virus isolation, and serum neutralization tests are used for confirmation.

Epidemiology, Prevention, and Control

Swine are the primary host and reservoir for pseudorabies virus, and the virus causes a uniformly fatal disease when transmitted to a wide variety of secondary hosts. Virus is shed in the saliva and nasal discharges of swine, so that licking, biting, and aerosols could result in transmission. Virus is not shed in the urine or feces. The contamination of livestock feed or the ingestion of infected carcasses by swine is common, and ingestion of virus-contaminated material, including pork, is probably the most common source of infection for secondary hosts. Rats may contribute to farm-to-farm transfer, and sick or dead rats and other feral animals are probably the source of infection for dogs and cats. Because of their scavenging habits, raccoons in the United States have received particular attention, but they probably play a minor role in the natural spread of pseudorabies virus.

Management practices influence epidemiologic patterns of infection and disease in swine. Losses from severe disease occur when nonimmune pregnant sows or swine less than 3 months old, born to nonimmune sows, are infected. Such a pattern is likely to be seen when the virus is newly introduced into a herd or unit within a farm. When breeding sows are immune with adequate antibody levels, overt disease in their progeny is not observed or is reduced greatly. Where breeding and growing/finishing operations are conducted separately, significant losses from pseudorabies occur when weaned swine from several sources are brought together in the growing/finishing unit, but the disease in these older swine is less severe than that in piglets. If care is taken to prevent the entry of pseudorabies, the move toward complete integration of swine husbandry, so-called "farrow-to-finish" operations, provides an ideal situation by which to produce and maintain pseudorabies-free herds and thus avoid the costs of disease losses and the problems associated with vaccination.

Vaccination of swine in areas where the virus is endemic and spreading can reduce losses. Both recombinant DNA deletion mutant and inactivated vaccines are used, but they do not prevent infection or the establishment of latent infection by the wild-type virus. A pseudorabies vaccine from which both the thymidine kinase and a glycoprotein gene have been deleted, and the E1 gene of hog cholera virus inserted, provides protection against both pseudorabies and hog cholera. Vaccination of secondary hosts is rarely undertaken because of the sporadic incidence of the disease.

Eradication programs have been established in several countries, including the United Kingdom and United States, and in 1991 the national herd in the United Kingdom was considered free of pseudorabies.

Equine Abortion (Caused by Equine Herpesvirus 1)

Following respiratory infection, usually accompanied by clinical signs similar to those caused by equine herpesvirus 4, abortion may occur as early as the fourth month of gestation, although most occur during the last 4 months. It occurs without premonitory signs and there are usually no complications. The fetus is usually born dead.

Perinatal infection may result in a fatal generalized disease in which respiratory distress due to interstitial pneumonia is the dominant clinical feature. Encephalitis occurs sporadically or as epidemics, usually in association with respiratory disease and abortion. Clinical signs vary from mild ataxia to complete recumbency with forelimb and hind limb paralysis, leading to death.

In fetuses aborted before 6 months there is diffusely scattered cell necrosis with inclusion bodies and a lack of an inflammatory cell response. Gross lesions are sometimes present in fetuses aborted after 6 months and may include small necrotic foci in the liver. Characteristic microscopic lesions include bronchiolitis, pneumonitis, severe necrosis of splenic white pulp, and focal hepatic necrosis, accompanied by a marked inflammatory cell response. Typical herpetic intranuclear inclusion bodies are demonstrated readily in these lesions.

Only certain strains of equine herpesvirus 1 cause encephalitis, which is characterized by vasculitis leading to thrombosis and hypoxic degeneration of adjacent neural tissue. In contrast to alphaherpesvirus encephalitis in other species, it is usually difficult or impossible to isolate virus from neural tissues; it is thought that the vasculitis is caused by virus–antibody complexes.

Abortion, perinatal mortality, and, less commonly, encephalitis affecting up to 70% of horses in a herd may follow the occurrence of abortion in the index case, usually a recently introduced mare. The incidence of mares that are latent carriers of equine herpesvirus 1 is lower than for equine herpesvirus 4 and hence circumstances arise where an equine herpesvirus 1 carrier mare can reactivate virus and infect a large number of nonimmune contact mares, leading to devastating "abortion storms." Vaccination with an inactivated combined equine herpesvirus vaccine can minimize losses. Management practices and adherence to well-established codes of practice will also minimize losses. While equine herpesviruses 1 and 4 share many antigens, a recombinant antigen based on a variable region at the C terminus of glycoprotein G is available to detect antibody that is specific for each virus and where vaccine is not used the test may be used as a means of separating known equine herpesvirus 1 carrier mares from noncarrier mares.

Equine Rhinopneumonitis (Caused by Equine Herpesvirus 4)

Equine herpesvirus 4 is the most important of the several viruses that cause acute respiratory disease of horses. Acute respiratory disease due to equine herpesvirus 4 occurs commonly in foals over 2 months old, weanlings, and yearlings. There is fever, anorexia, and a profuse serous nasal discharge that later becomes mucopurulent. Most affected foals recover completely and mild or subclinical infections are common. More severe disease including bronchopneumonia and death may occur when there is crowding, stress, poor hygiene, and secondary infection. The source of virus is thought to be from older horses in which inapparent virus shedding occurs, following reactivation of the latent virus. Reactivation of latent virus is probably responsible for some of the many episodes of febrile respiratory disease that occur throughout life that disrupt training and performance schedules. Combined inactivated equine herpesvirus 1 and 4 vaccines are used to control respiratory disease and abortion.

Equine Coital Exanthema (Caused by Equine Herpesvirus 3)

A disease that was probably equine coital exanthema has long been known, but its causative agent was not shown to be an alphaherpesvirus (equine herpesvirus 3) until 1968. Equine herpesvirus 3 shows no serologic cross-reactivity with other equine herpesviruses by neutralization tests, but shares antigens with equine herpesvirus 1, demonstrable by complement fixation and immunofluorescence. Equine herpesvirus 3 grows only in cells of equine origin and produces large plaques. Although rapidly cytopathic, the virus tends to remain cell associated.

Equine coital exanthema is an acute, usually mild disease characterized by the formation of pustular and ulcerative lesions on the vaginal and vestibular mucosa, on the skin of the penis, prepuce, and the perineal region, especially of the mare, and occasionally on the teats, lips, and the respiratory mucosa. The incidence of antibody in sexually active horses is much higher (about 50%) than the reported incidence of disease. The incubation period may be as short as 2 days and, in uncomplicated cases, healing is usually complete by 14 days. Where the skin of the vulva, penis, and prepuce is black, white depigmented spots mark for life the site of earlier lesions and identify potential carriers.

Although genital lesions may be extensive, there are no systemic signs and unless the affected areas are examined carefully cases are missed readily. Abortion or infertility is not associated with equine herpesvirus 3 infection; indeed mares usually conceive to the service in which they acquire the disease; although abortion occurs following experimental *in utero* inoculation.

Affected stallions show decreased libido and the presence of the disease may seriously disrupt breeding schedules. Recurrent disease is more likely to occur when stallions are in frequent use. Management of the disease consists of the removal of stallions from service until all lesions have healed and symptomatic treatment.

Equine herpesvirus 3 can cause subclinical respiratory infection in yearling horses and has been isolated from vesicular lesions on the muzzles of foals in contact with infected mares.

Canine Herpesvirus Disease (Caused by Canine Herpesvirus 1)

Canine herpesvirus 1 was first recognized in the United States in 1965 as the cause of a highly fatal, generalized hemorrhagic disease of pups under 4 weeks of age. This syndrome is rare, and the prevalence of the virus, based on antibody surveys, is low (<20%). It probably occurs worldwide. In sexually mature dogs, canine herpesvirus 1 causes genital disease, although this is rarely diagnosed clinically.

Clinical Features

The incubation period varies from 3 to 8 days and in fatal disease the course is brief, 1–2 days. Signs include painful crying, abdominal pain, anorexia, and dyspnea. In older dogs there may be vaginal or prepucial discharge and, on careful examination, a focal nodular lesion of the vaginal, penile, and prepucial epithelium may be seen. The virus may also cause respiratory disease and may be part of the kennel cough syndrome.

Pathogenesis, Pathology, and Immunity

Pups born to presumably seronegative bitches are infected oronasally either from their dam's vagina or from other infected dogs. Pups less than 4 weeks old that become hypothermic develop the generalized, often fatal disease. There is a cell-associated viremia followed by viral replication in blood vessel walls. The optimal temperature for viral replication is about 33°C, i.e., the temperature of the outer genital and upper respiratory tracts. The hypothalamic thermoregulatory centers of the pup are not fully operative until about 4 weeks of age. Accordingly, in the context of canine herpesvirus 1 infection, the pup is critically dependent on ambient temperature and maternal contact for the maintenance of its normal body temperature. The more severe the hypothermia, the more severe and rapid is the course of the disease.

Gross findings in pups are frequently dramatic. Large ecchymotic hemorrhages are particularly obvious in the kidney, adrenal, and gastrointestinal tract. Microscopically they are seen as necrotic foci, however, not all such necrotic foci are marked by gross hemorrhage, and inflammation is conspicuously absent.

Laboratory Diagnosis

This sporadic disease is rarely diagnosed during life. Gross postmortem findings, particularly the ecchymotic hemorrhages of the kidney and gastrointestinal tract, are characteristic. Inclusion bodies may be present in liver cells and the causative virus can be isolated readily in canine cell cultures.

Epidemiology, Prevention, and Control

The low incidence of severe disease in pups and the mild nature of infections in older dogs have not warranted the development of vaccines. Losses may be prevented or arrested if the ambient temperature minimizes the risk of hypothermia. Raising the body temperature by putting pups under an infrared lamp early in the course of infection may have therapeutic value.

Feline Herpesvirus Disease (Caused by Feline Herpesvirus 1)

About half of the cats presenting with respiratory disease have feline herpesvirus 1 infection, about half calicivirus infection, and a few *Chlamydia psittaci* infection. The incidence of feline herpesvirus antibody in colony cats is over 70% whereas for household cats the figure is less than 50%. All species of the family *Felidae* are believed to be susceptible.

Feline herpesvirus 1 causes acute disease of the upper respiratory tract in the first year or so of life. After an incubation period of 24–48 hours there is a sudden onset of bouts of sneezing, coughing, profuse serous nasal and ocular discharges, frothy salivation, dyspnea, anorexia, weight loss, and fever. Occasionally there may be ulcers on the tongue. Keratitis associated with punctate corneal ulcers is common. In fully susceptible kittens up to 4 weeks old the extensive rhinotracheitis and an associated bronchopneumonia may be fatal. Clinically, the acute disease is very similar to that caused by caliciviruses. Profuse frothy salivation and corneal ulcers suggest feline herpesvirus infection, whereas ulcers of the tongue, palate, and pharynx are encountered more frequently in calicivirus infections. Infection of cats over six months of age is likely to result in mild or subclinical infection. Pregnant queens may abort, although there is no evidence that the virus crosses the placenta and fatally infects fetuses, and virus has not been isolated from aborted placenta or fetuses; abortion is thought to be secondary to fever and toxemia.

There is necrosis of epithelia of the nasal cavity, pharynx, epiglottis, tonsils, larynx, and trachea and in extreme cases, in young kittens, a bronchopneumonia. Typical intranuclear inclusion bodies may be detected if death occurs within 7 to 9 days after infection.

Inactivated virus and attenuated virus vaccines are used for the control of infections due to feline herpesvirus 1; they reduce disease but do not prevent infection. An experimental genetically engineered vaccine has been developed; comprised of a gene deletion mutant of feline herpesvirus 1 into which the gene encoding the capsid protein of feline calicivirus has been inserted. This vaccine candidate has been shown to be protective against both virus infections.

B Virus Disease of Macaques (Caused by B Virus/ Cercopithecine Herpesvirus 1)

Macaques suffer from a herpesvirus infection caused by B virus (cercopithecine herpesvirus 1), the natural history of which in these animals is very like that of herpes simplex type 1 infection in humans. A number of fatal cases of ascending paralysis and encephalitis in humans have occurred, with infection being transmitted directly by monkey bite and indirectly by monkey saliva. Most cases have occurred among animal handlers and biomedical researchers who had occupational exposure to macaques, although transmission has also been documented among laboratory workers handling macaque central nervous system and kidney tissues. The risk presented to owners by pet macaques and to tourists visiting exotic wild-animal parks where there are free-ranging macaques has also been recognized.

B virus infection is common in all macaques, with rhesus, Japanese, cynomolgus, pig-tailed, and stump-tailed macaques being the species used most commonly in biomedical research. Neutralizing antibodies are found in 75 to 100% of adult macaques in captive populations. Like many herpes simplex virus infections in humans, primary B virus infection in monkeys is often minor, but is characterized by lifelong latent infection in trigeminal and lumbosacral ganglia with intermittent reactivation and shedding of the virus in saliva or genital secretions, particularly during periods of stress or immunosuppression. The virus is transmitted among free-ranging or group-housed monkeys, primarily through sexual activity and bites.

B virus disease in humans usually results from macaque bites or scratches, but a case has been reported in which exposure was via saliva contact with the eye. Incubation periods may be as short as 2 days, but more commonly are 2 to 5 weeks. In some cases, the first clinical signs are the formation of vesicles, pruritis, and hyperesthesia at the bite site. This is followed quickly by ascending paralysis, frank encephalitis, and death. In some case there are no suspect clinical symptoms prior to the onset of encephalitis. In a series of 24 cases, 19 (79%) died. Most surviving patients have had moderate to severe neurologic impairment, sometimes requiring lifelong institutionalization; however, the use of Acyclovir or Gancyclovir has prevented progression of the disease, even reversing neurologic symptoms. Rapid diagnosis and initiation of therapy are of paramount importance in preventing death or permanent disability in surviving patients.

In most developed countries, there are strict regulations regarding the importation, breeding, and handling of nonhuman primates, in many cases prohibiting their ownership as pets. Further, the American Veterinary Medical Association has issued guidelines to deal with the dangers of keeping primate species as pets. However, macaque and other primate species continue to be marketed and kept as pets.

In the United States, occupational safety guidelines are in place, based on evidence that all macaque species are inherently dangerous because of the risk of B virus transmission, as well as the likelihood of serious physical injury from bite wounds. Following occupational exposure of a human to a macaque monkey by bite, scratch, or needle-stick injury, the macaque should be evaluated for possible B virus shedding: (1) the monkey is examined, paying particular attention to any signs of ulceration of oral and genital mucosa and or neurologic abnormalities; (2) oral swab specimens are collected for viral antigen and/or nucleic acid testing and blood/serum is collected for serology at a special reference laboratory (enzyme immunoassays and immunoblot assays have replaced virus isolation and serum neutralization in these laboratories); (3) a physician specializing in such occupational risks is contacted to treat the person. Following evaluation, prophylactic Acyclovir or Gancyclovir should be started immediately.

Simian Varicella (Caused by Cercopithecine Herpesviruses 6, 7, and 9)

Simian varicella is a naturally occurring disease of Old World monkeys (superfamily *Cercopithecoidea*). The disease is characterized by varicella-like clinical signs, including fever, lethargy, and vesicular rash on the face, abdomen, and extremities. Disseminated infection often results in life-threatening pneumonia and hepatitis. Epidemics have occurred in captive African green (vervet) monkeys (*Cercopithecus aethiops*), patas monkeys (*Erythrocebus patas*), and several species of macaques (*Macaca* spp.). The causative herpesviruses isolated in several epidemics were originally given distinct names, but molecular genetic characterization has indicated that these viruses are virtually identical. Thus the names cercopithecine herpesvirus 6, 7, and 9, each with synonyms as well, should give way to a common name, the vernacular of which is simian varicella virus. Like human varicella-zoster virus, the simian virus establishes latency in sensory ganglia and is reactivated to cause recrudescent disease and shedding. Reactivation leads to transmission of the highly contagious virus to susceptible monkeys and is the basis for epidemics. In recent years there have been several rather large epidemics in primate colonies, some involving hundreds of monkeys and causing substantial morbidity.

Avian Infectious Laryngotracheitis (Caused by Gallid Herpesvirus 1)

Identified as a specific viral disease of chickens in the United States in 1926, infectious laryngotracheitis, caused by gallid herpesvirus 1, occurs among chickens worldwide. This virus rarely causes disease in other avian species. Strains of the virus vary considerably in virulence.

Clinical Features

Chickens of all ages are susceptible, but disease is most common in those aged 4–18 months. After an incubation period of 2–8 days, mild coughing and sneezing are followed by nasal and ocular discharge, dyspnea, loud gasping and coughing, and depression. In severe cases the neck is raised and the head extended during inspiration—"pump handle respiration." Head shaking with coughing is characteristic and may be associated with expectoration of bloody mucus and frank blood that appear on the beak, face, and feathers. Morbidity approaches 100% and for virulent strains the mortality may be 50–70% and for strains of low virulence, about 20%. Strains of low virulence are associated with conjunctivitis, ocular discharge, swollen infraorbital and nasal sinuses, and lowered egg production.

Pathogenesis, Pathology, and Immunity

There is severe laryngotracheitis characterized by necrosis, hemorrhage, ulceration, and the formation of diphtheritic membranes. The extensive diphtheritic membrane formation and death from asphyxia have led to the use of the term "fowl diphtheria." The virus probably persists as a latent infection and has been recovered from tracheal explant cultures over 3 months after infection.

Laboratory Diagnosis

Clinical and postmortem findings are characteristic. Fluorescent antibody staining of smears and tissues and isolation of the virus either by inoculation on the chorioallantoic membrane of embryonated eggs or cell cultures are also used. The neutralizing antibody may be detected by pock or plaque reduction assays and enzyme immunoassays have been developed.

Epidemiology, Prevention, and Control

Infectious laryngotracheitis virus is usually introduced into a flock via carrier birds and is transmitted by droplet and inhalation, less commonly by ingestion. Although it spreads rapidly through a flock, new clinical cases may occur over a period of 2 to 8 weeks; thus it spreads somewhat more slowly than Newcastle disease, influenza, and infectious bronchitis.

It is feasible to establish and maintain flocks free of infectious laryngotracheitis, and where management systems allow, this practice is increasingly adopted, particularly in the broiler industry where birds are harvested at 9 weeks of age and where "all-in-all-out" management is possible. However, for breeding and egg production flocks vaccination is still widely practiced, using attenuated virus vaccine. This protects birds against disease, but not against infection with virulent virus or the development of a latent carrier status for either the virulent or the vaccine viruses.

Marek's Disease (Caused by Gallid Herpesvirus 2)

The herpesvirus etiology of Marek's disease, which occurs worldwide, was established in 1967. Prior to the introduction of vaccination in 1970, it was the most common lymphoproliferative disease of chickens, causing annual losses in the United States of $150 million and in the United Kingdom of $40 million. Vaccination has reduced the incidence of disease dramatically, but not of infection. Because of continuing losses from disease and the costs of vaccination, it remains a most important disease of chickens. The virus is slowly cytopathic and remains highly cell associated so that cell-free infectious virus is virtually impossible to obtain, except in dander from feather follicles.

Clinical Features

Marek's disease is a progressive disease with variable signs; four overlapping syndromes are described. In its clinical presentation the disease bears several similarities and some key differences to avian leukosis (Table 18.4).

Neurolymphomatosis

Neurolymphomatosis or so-called classical Marek's disease is associated with an asymmetric paralysis of one or both legs or wings (Figure 18.8). Incoordination is a common early sign; one leg is held forward and the other backward when stationary because of unilateral paresis or paralysis. Wing dropping and lowering of the head and neck are common. If the vagus nerve is involved there may be dilation of the crop and gasping.

Acute Marek's Disease

Acute Marek's disease occurs in explosive outbreaks in which a large proportion of birds in a flock show depression followed after a few days by ataxia and paralysis of some birds. Significant mortality occurs without localizing neurologic signs.

Ocular Lymphomatosis

Ocular lymphomatosis leads to graying of the iris of one or both eyes because of lymphoblastoid cell infiltration; the pupil is irregular and eccentric and there is partial or total blindness.

Cutaneous Marek's Disease

Cutaneous Marek's disease is recognized readily after plucking, when round, nodular lesions up to 1 cm in diameter are seen, particularly at feather follicles.

Pathogenesis, Pathology, and Immunity

Enlargement of one or more peripheral nerve trunks is the most constant gross finding. In the vast majority of cases a diagnosis can be made if the celiac, cranial, intercostal, mesenteric, brachial, sciatic, and greater splanchnic nerves are examined. In a diseased bird, the

Table 18.4
Clinical and Histologic Differentiation of Marek's Disease and Avian Leukosis

Disease parameter	Marek's disease	Avian leukosis
Etiology	Herpesvirus	Retrovirus
Target cells	T lymphocytes	Various hemopoietic cells
Age of onset of signs	4 weeks	16 weeks
Paralysis	Yes	No
Gross lesions		
Liver, spleen, kidney	Yes	Yes
Gonads, lungs, heart	Yes	Rare
Nerve trunks	Yes (neural form)	Rare
Iris	Yes (ocular form)	Rare
Skin	Yes (cutaneous form)	Rare
Bursa of Fabricius	Rare	Yes (nodular)
Microscopic lesions		
Size of affected lymphoblasts	Varied	Uniform
Intranuclear inclusion bodies	Yes	No

Figure 18.8.

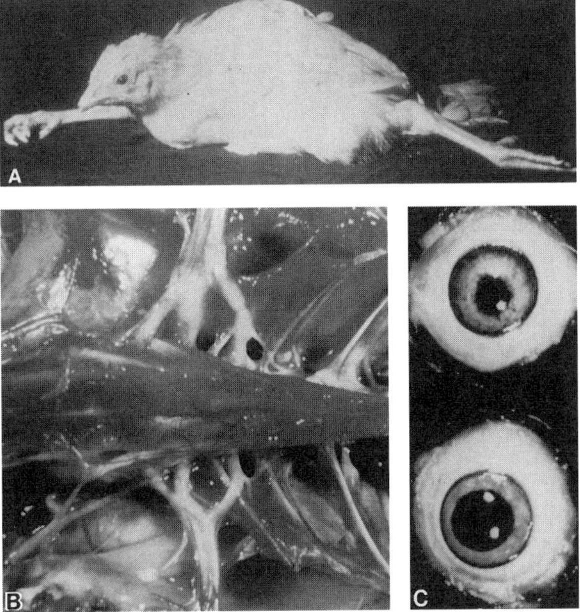

Marek's disease of chickens. (A) Paralysis. (B) Enlargement of sciatic nerves. (C) Ocular lesions. Lower eye is normal, with dilated pupil; pupil of upper eye failed to dilate and has an irregular outline due to the infiltration of transformed lymphocytes.

nerves are up to three time their normal diameter, show loss of striations, and are edematous, gray, or yellowish and somewhat translucent in appearance. Because enlargement is frequently unilateral, it is especially helpful to compare contralateral nerves.

Lymphomatous lesions, indistinguishable from those of avian leukosis, are usually small, diffuse, grayish, and translucent. They are most common in acute Marek's disease and occur in the gonads, particularly the ovary, and other tissues.

The outcome of infection of chickens by Marek's disease virus is influenced by the virus strain, dose, and route of infection and by the age, sex, immune status, and genetic susceptibility of the chickens. Subclinical infection with virus shedding is common. Infection is acquired by inhalation of dander. Epithelial cells of the respiratory tract are infected productively and contribute to a cell-associated viremia involving macrophages. By the sixth day there is productive infection of lymphoid cells in a variety of organs, including the thymus, bursa of Fabricius, bone marrow, and spleen, resulting in immune suppression. During the second week after infection there is a persistent cell-associated viremia followed by a proliferation of T lymphoblastoid cells, and a week later deaths begin to occur, although regression may also occur from this time.

The discovery that the genome of Marek's disease virus has incorporated *onc* genes that resemble those found in avian retroviruses provides a more rational basis for explaining the pathogenesis of the disease, which is considered in more detail in Chapter 11.

T lymphocytes are transformed by the virus, and up to 90 genome equivalents of Marek's disease virus DNA can be demonstrated in transformed cells in both plasmid and integrated forms.

The lesions of Marek's disease result from the infiltration and *in situ* proliferation of T lymphocytes, which may result in leukemia, but in addition there is often a significant inflammatory cell response to the lysis of nonlymphoid cells by the virus. Lesions of the feather follicle are invariably a mixture of lymphoblastoid and inflammatory cells. Epithelial cells at the base of feather follicles are exceptional in that productive infection of these cells is also associated with the release of cell-free infectious virus.

The basis for genetic resistance is not fully defined but has been correlated with birds that carry the B21 alloantigen of the B red blood cell group. Maternal antibody may persist in newly hatched chicks for up to 3 weeks, and infection of such chicks with virulent Marek's disease virus may not produce disease but may lead to an active immune response. Chickens that are bursectomized and then actively immunized also survive challenge infection.

Many apparently healthy birds are lifelong carriers and shedders of virus, but the virus is not transmitted *in ovo*. When fully susceptible 1 day-old chicks are infected with virulent virus, the minimum time for detection of microscopic lesions is 1–2 weeks, and gross lesions are present by 3 to 4 weeks. Maximal virus shedding occurs at 5–6 weeks after infection.

Laboratory Diagnosis

Where sufficient numbers of birds are examined, history, age, clinical signs, and gross postmortem findings are adequate for the diagnosis, which can be confirmed by histopathology. Detection of viral antigen by immunofluorescence is the simplest reliable laboratory diagnostic procedure. Gel diffusion, indirect immunofluorescence, or virus neutralization is used for the detection of viral antibody.

A variety of methods can be used for virus isolation: inoculation of cell cultures, the chorioallantoic membrane, or the yolk sac of 4-day-old embryonated eggs with suspensions of buffy coat or spleen cells. The presence of virus can be demonstrated by immunofluorescence or electron microscopy.

Marek's disease and avian leukosis are usually present in the same flock and both diseases may occur in the same bird. The two diseases were long confused, but can be differentiated by clinical and pathologic features or by specific tests for virus, viral antigens, or viral antibody.

Epidemiology, Prevention, and Control

Most chickens have antibody to Marek's disease virus by the time they are mature; infection persists and virus is released in dander from the feather follicles. Congenital infection does not occur and chicks are protected by maternal antibody for the first few weeks of life. They then become infected by the inhalation of virus in the dust. Epidemics of Marek's disease usually involve sexually immature birds 2 to 5 months old; a high mortality (about 80%) soon peaks and then declines sharply.

Isolates of Marek's disease virus vary considerably in virulence and in the types of lesions different strains produce. Avirulent strains are recognized and used for vaccine, although the antigenically related turkey herpesvirus is preferred as a vaccine strain, primarily because it infects cells productively. Marek's disease virus and turkey herpesvirus are about 95% homologous by DNA hybridization.

Vaccination is the principal method of control. The standard method has been to vaccinate 1-day-old chicks parenterally; however, more than 80% of the 8 billion birds vaccinated annually in the United Stated are vaccinated *in ovo* at 18 days with a robotic machine (Inovoject). The vaccine is available as either a lyophilized cell-free preparation or a cell-associated preparation. The cell-free vaccine does not take in chicks with maternal antibody whereas cell-associated vaccines do. Protective immunity develops within about 2 weeks. Vaccination decreases the incidence of disease, particularly of lymphomatous lesions in visceral organs, and has been most successful in the control of acute Marek's disease. Peripheral neurologic disease continues to occur in vaccinated flocks, but at reduced incidence.

A further level of control can be achieved if flocks are built up with birds carrying the B21 alloantigen. It is possible to establish flocks free of Marek's disease, but commercially it is extremely difficult to maintain the disease-free status. The production of chickens on the "all-in-all-out" principle, whereby they are hatched, started, raised, and dispersed as a unit, would improve the efficacy of vaccination as a control measure.

Duck Plague (Caused by Anatid Herpesvirus 1)

Duck plague occurs worldwide among domestic and wild ducks, geese, swans, and other water fowl, with migratory waterfowl contributing to spread within and between continents. Major epidemics have occurred in duck farms in the United States.

Strains of virus vary in virulence, although only a single antigenic type has been recognized. The virus grows readily on the chorioallantoic membrane of embryonated duck eggs and in duck embryo fibroblast cell cultures, but only poorly or not at all in similar substrates of chicken origin, although it may be adapted to grow in chicken cells.

Clinical Features

Attention is drawn to the disease by the occurrence of a sudden and persistent increased mortality within flocks of ducks. The incubation period is 3–7 days. There is anorexia, depression, nasal discharge, ruffled, dull feathers, adherent eyelids, photophobia, extreme thirst, ataxia leading to recumbency with outstretched wings with head extended forward, tremors, watery diarrhea, and soiled vents. Egg production drops 25 to 40%. Morbidity and mortality vary from 5 to 100%. Most ducks that develop clinical signs die. Sick wild ducks conceal themselves and die in vegetation at the water's edge.

Pathogenesis, Pathology, and Immunity

Ingested virus causes enteritis and viremic spread leads to vasculitis and widespread focal necrosis. Blood is present in the body cavities, including gizzard and intestinal lumens, and petechial hemorrhages are present in many tissues. There may be elevated crusty plaques of diphtheritic membrane in the esophagus, cecum, rectum, cloaca, and bursa. Herpesvirus inclusions are demonstrated most readily in hepatocytes, intestinal epithelium, and lymphoid tissues.

Laboratory Diagnosis

Clinical and gross postmortem findings may be confirmed by the finding of herpesvirus inclusion bodies or positive immunofluorescence. Duck plague needs to be differentiated from duck hepatitis (due to a picornavirus) and from Newcastle disease and influenza.

Epidemiology, Prevention, and Control

Ingestion of contaminated water is thought to be the major mode of transmission, although the virus may also be transmitted by contact. Virus has been isolated from wild ducks up to a year after infection. A chick embryo-adapted attenuated virus vaccine has been used in the United States. However, despite the continued threat of reintroduction from wild birds, the disease has been eliminated from the duck farms of Long Island, New York, and vaccination is not now practiced routinely.

Alphaherpesvirus Diseases of Other Species

A few species of alphaherpesviruses of other animals warrant brief mention. They have been associated with fatal diseases in hedgehogs, kangaroos, wallabies, wombats, and harbor seals. Two species of phocid herpesvirus have been isolated from pinniped species: phocid herpesvirus 1, classified in the genus *Varicellovirus,* causes significant mortalities in neonate seal pups and phocid herpesvirus 2 is a gammaherpesvirus of uncertain pathogenicity. Major epidemics of fatal illness due to alphaherpesviruses have occurred in a variety of tortoise species in captivity and are recognized as significant causes of mortality in channel catfish and salmonid species. Alphaherpesviruses related antigenically to bovine herpesvirus 1 have been isolated from several ruminant species, including red deer, reindeer, and buffalo. Equine herpesvirus 1 or viruses related very closely to it have not infrequently been the cause of abortion and/or encephalitis in ruminant species, including cattle, llama, alpaca, gazelles, and camels. A fatal herpesvirus disease of unknown origin or classification has caused the death of young elephants in zoos.

Diseases Caused by Members of Subfamily *Betaherpesvirinae*

Betaherpesviruses replicate more slowly than alphaherpesviruses and often produce greatly enlarged cells, hence the designation cytomegalovirus. Their host range is narrow, and in latent infections, viral DNA is believed to be sequestered in cells of secretory glands, lymphoreticular organs, and kidney. Rather than being subject to periodic reactivation, betaherpesviruses are often associated with continuous viral excretion. They have been associated with diseases of economic importance in swine.

Porcine Cytomegalovirus Disease (Caused by Porcine Herpesvirus 2)

First recognized in 1955, porcine herpesvirus 2 is endemic in many swine herds worldwide. In the United Kingdom, some 50% of herds are infected, while a survey in Iowa indicated infection in 12% of herds. Within a herd, up to 90% of swine may carry the virus. Often the disease is not seen in herds in which the virus is endemic; it is more likely to be associated with recent introduction of the virus or with environmental factors such as poor nutrition and intercurrent disease. Virus-free herds have been established.

Rhinitis occurs in swine up to 10 weeks of age, after which infection is subclinical, and it is most severe in swine less than 2 weeks old. There is sneezing, coughing, serous nasal and ocular discharge, and depression. The discharge becomes mucopurulent and may block the nasal passages, which interferes with suckling; such piglets lose weight rapidly and die within a few days. Survivors are stunted. A generalized disease following viremic spread is also recognized in young swine. Porcine herpesvirus 2 crosses the placenta and may cause fetal death or result in generalized disease in the first 2 weeks after birth or there may be runting and poor weight gains. Large basophilic intranuclear inclusions are found in enlarged cells of the mucous glands of the turbinate mucosa (hence the synonym "inclusion body rhinitis").

When newly introduced into a susceptible herd, virus is transmitted both transplacentally and horizontally. In herds in which the virus is endemic, transmission is predominantly horizontal but because young swine are infected when maternal antibody is present, the infection is subclinical. Disease occurs when the virus is introduced into susceptible herds or if susceptible swine are mixed with carrier swine. Virus-free swine can be produced by hysterotomy; however, because the virus crosses the placenta, swine produced in this way must be monitored carefully for antibody for at least 70 days after delivery.

Diseases Caused by Members of Subfamily *Gammaherpesvirinae*

Gammaherpesviruses are characterized by replication in lymphoblastoid cells, with different members of the subfamily being specific for either B or T lymphocytes. In lymphocytes, infection is arrested frequently at a prelytic stage, with persistence and minimum expression of the viral genome. Herpesvirus saimiri and human herpesvirus 8 (human Kaposi's sarcoma-associated herpesvirus) have viral genes that code for cyclins that regulate the cell cycle at a restriction point between G1 and S phases by phosphorylation of the retinoblastoma protein. By overriding normal cell cycle arrest, these viral-encoded proteins induce the lymphoproliferative responses characteristic of these rhadinoviruses. Gammaherpesviruses may also enter a lytic stage, causing cell death without production of virions. Latent infection can be demonstrated in lymphoid tissue.

Epstein–Barr virus causes the human disease glandular fever/infectious mononucleosis and is the prototype of the genus *Lymphocryptovirus*. Several viruses of primates, including herpesvirus saimiri, are members of the genus *Rhadinovirus*, which also includes bovine malignant catarrhal fever virus caused by alcelaphine herpesvirus 1 and bovine herpesvirus 4 and equine herpesviruses 2 and 5. Marek's disease virus has been removed from the subfamily, even though it produces lymphoblastoid tumors, because the genome architecture of virus resembles that of alphaherpesviruses.

Bovine Malignant Catarrhal Fever (Caused by Alcelaphine Herpesvirus 1)

Malignant catarrhal fever is an almost invariably fatal, generalized lymphoproliferative disease of cattle and some wild ruminants (deer, buffalo, antelope), primarily affecting lymphoid tissues and epithelial cells of the respiratory and gastrointestinal tracts. Three distinct epidemiologic patterns are recognized, from only one of which has a herpesvirus been isolated. In Africa (and zoos), epidemics of the disease occur in cattle (and captive, susceptible wild ruminants) following transmission of the virus from wildebeest (*Connochaetes gnu* and *C. taurinus*) and, to a lesser extent, from hartebeest (*Alcephus buselaphus*) and topi (*Damaliscus korrigum*), particularly at calving time. A herpesvirus (alcelaphine herpesvirus 1) has been isolated from this African form of malignant catarrhal fever and shown experimentally to reproduce the disease; it has been tentatively classified as a gammaherpesvirus.

Outside Africa and zoos, a disease described as malignant catarrhal fever in cattle and deer occurs when these species are kept in close contact with sheep, especially during lambing time. This sheep-associated form can be transmitted by inoculation of cattle or deer with blood from known carrier sheep. It has been shown that sheep have an antibody that is cross-reactive with alcelaphine herpesvirus 1. Although the virus (ovine herpesvirus 2) responsible for the ovine form of the disease has not been isolated, a DNA clone with a sequence corresponding to a gammaherpesvirus and similar to alcelaphine herpesvirus 1 has been characterized.

A third epidemiologic form of the syndrome described as malignant catarrhal fever is recognized in feedlot cattle in North America, in the absence of contact with sheep. It occurs as minor epidemics; the identity and source of virus in this third form is unknown. Both alcelaphine herpesvirus 1 and the putative sheep-associated herpesviruses produce a disease resembling malignant catarrhal fever in rabbits. The description that follows refers to the African form of the disease.

Clinical Features

After an incubation period of about 3 weeks, malignant catarrhal fever is characterized by fever, depression, leukopenia, profuse nasal and ocular discharges, bilateral ophthalmia, generalized lymphadenopathy, extensive mucosal erosions, and central nervous system signs. The ophthalmia is associated with corneal opacity, which begins peripherally and progresses centripetally, often leading to blindness. Erosions of the gastrointestinal mucosa lead to diarrhea.

Pathogenesis, Pathology, and Immunity

Postmortem findings vary according to the duration of the disease. There are usually extensive erosions, edema, and hemorrhage throughout the gastrointestinal tract. There is a generalized lymphadenopathy; all lymph nodes are enlarged, edematous, and sometimes hemorrhagic. The lymphoproliferative response involves Th and Tc cells. Frequently there are multiple raised necrotic lesions accompanied by ecchymotic hemorrhages in the kidney and erosions of the mucosa of the turbinates, larynx, and trachea. Histologically there is widespread lymphoid cell proliferation and multifocal areas of necrosis, centered on small blood vessels. Death occurs about a week after the onset of clinical signs. There is evidence that a small number of affected cattle and deer that develop clinical signs of disease survive, at least for a short time, with evidence of ocular disease, arteriosclerosis, and persistence of the virus as detected by polymerase chain reaction.

Laboratory Diagnosis

The history and clinical signs, particularly the presence of bilateral ophthalmia, suggest the diagnosis of malignant catarrhal fever. The virus can be isolated when washed peripheral blood leukocytes are inoculated in calf thyroid cells. Cell-free inocula do not yield virus. The cytopathic changes require at least 3 days to appear and several passages in cell culture are often necessary. They are characterized by syncytia and by the presence of typical herpesvirus intranuclear inclusion bodies.

Epidemiology, Prevention, and Control

The virus does not appear to be pathogenic for wildebeest and in this species it appears to be transmitted from mother to offspring in the immediate postcalving period, via nasal secretions. Cattle are believed to be infected via the relatively large amounts of virus present in the nasal secretions of wildebeest calves. The virus is not transmitted between cattle, which appear to be "dead-end" hosts. Attempts to develop a vaccine have been unsuccessful.

Bovine Herpesvirus Infection (Caused by Bovine Herpesvirus 4)

Bovine herpesvirus 4, which has a genome organization similar to that of Epstein–Barr virus, has been isolated throughout the world from cattle suffering from a variety of diseases, including conjunctivitis, respiratory disease, vaginitis, metritis, skin nodules, and lymphosarcoma.

However, there is no proven etiologic association between the diseases and the virus isolated occasionally from cases. When inoculated experimentally into susceptible cattle, these viruses produce no disease. Strains of bovine herpesvirus 4 have been isolated when cell cultures are prepared from tissues of apparently normal cattle; they have also been isolated from semen of normal bulls.

Equine Herpesvirus Infection (Caused by Equine Herpesviruses 2 and 5)

The gammaherpesvirus, equine herpesvirus 2, may be isolated from nasal swab filtrates or from buffy coat cells of up to 70% of horses, with rates of isolation increasing with age. Horses may be infected in the first weeks of life even in the presence of maternal antibody. Neutralization tests suggest that several antigenic types exist; more than one antigenic type may be recovered at different times, or at the same time, from the same horse.

Equine herpesvirus 2 has been recovered from horses with respiratory disease sometimes characterized by coughing, swollen submaxillary and parotid lymph nodes and pharyngeal ulceration, from conjunctivitis, and from the genital tract. While the role of the virus in these and other diseases is uncertain, the virus is been investigated for a causative role in these various syndromes, which are common and costly, particularly among horses in racing. A second, distinctly different, slowly growing gammaherpesvirus (equine herpesvirus 5) has been isolated from nasal swabs and from buffy coat cells; its pathologic significance is unknown.

Diseases Caused by Members of Unnamed Subfamily Comprising Channel Catfish Herpesvirus

Channel catfish herpesvirus and an oyster (mollusk) herpesvirus genomes have been sequenced completely. The striking discovery from the sequence information is that while the viruses are morphologically and biologically similar to other herpesviruses the sequences bear almost no similarity with those of mammalian and avian herpesviruses. This has led to the construction of a separate subfamily, but at present only channel catfish herpesvirus has been placed in this subfamily. The lack of sequence similarity underlines the early origin and long coevolutionary virus/host association of herpesviruses in general.

Channel Catfish Herpesvirus Disease (Caused by Ictalurid Herpesvirus 1)

Ictalurid herpesvirus 1 (channel catfish herpesvirus) was the first fish herpesvirus to be isolated. It has a greater economic impact on the commercial rearing of its host species in North America than any other virus and has been studied more extensively than other herpesviruses of fish. The virus can be remarkably virulent in susceptible populations of channel catfish. The incubation period can be as short as 3 days; signs of infection include convulsive swimming, including a "head-up" posture, lethargy exophthalmia, distended abdomen, and hemorrhages. Mortality can rise rapidly to 100%. Lesions include hemorrhage and necrosis of visceral organs, particularly the liver and digestive tract.

The lack of reported virus isolations from wild channel catfish strongly indicates that factors such as dense stocking and poor environmental conditions may predispose farmed fish stocks to outbreaks of disease. A key factor is temperature; most outbreaks occur in the summer months when water is as warm as 30°C. The acute disease occurs only in young channel catfish usually up to about 6 months of age, with the degree of mortality depending on the strain of fish. The virus is transmitted readily from fish to fish; virus shedding is probably via the urine and virus entry is probably through the gills.

Attempts to vaccinate channel catfish against channel catfish virus have shown promise. An attenuated virus vaccine prepared by serial passage in fish cells has been shown to protect recipients against lethal challenge.

Diseases Caused by Unclassified Herpesviruses

Herpesvirus Diseases of Fish and Mollusks

Herpesviruses of fish, like those of higher vertebrates, are highly species specific, suggesting that they have coevolved over all evolutionary time with their hosts. Some cause high mortalities in young fish and some cause epidermal hyperplasia or neoplasia. Some have been investigated to such a limited extent that causal links with the disease whose occurrence led to their recognition have not yet been fully established.

Herpesvirus Infections in Salmonids (Caused by Salmonid Herpesviruses 1 and 2)

Two salmonid herpesviruses have been shown to cause severe disease: salmonid herpesviruses 1 and 2. These viruses have been shown to be distinct on the basis of serological data and DNA sequence studies.

The first of these viruses was isolated on several occasions from rainbow trout (*Salmo gairdneri*) in a hatchery in the United States. The virus causes disease when inoculated into young rainbow trout maintained at 6–9°C, but not in other salmonid species.

Salmonid herpesvirus 2 has a slightly wider host range, causing disease in the young of several members of the genus *Oncorhynchus* (Pacific salmon) as well as rainbow trout. The virus causes disease when inoculated into young fish maintained at 15°C and has the interesting property of causing epithelial tumors in survivors of experimental infection.

Other Herpesvirus Infections of Fish

Three other fish herpesviruses have been described: percid herpesvirus 1 (walleye herpesvirus), which is associated with epidermal hyperplasia in the walleye (*Stizostedion vitreum*); cyprinid herpesvirus (carp pox herpesvirus), implicated as the cause of transmissible epithelial hyperplasia in the common carp (*Cyprinus carpio*); and pleuronectid herpesvirus (turbot herpesvirus), which has been found in association with episodes of substantial mortality among farmed fry.

Further Reading

Ackermann, M., Edwards, S., Keil, G., Pastoret, P.-P., van Oirschot, J. T., and Thiry, E. (1996). Infectious bovine rhinotracheitis and other ruminant herpesviruses. *Vet. Microbiol.* **53**, 1–231.

Agius, C. T., and Studdert, M. J. (1994). Equine herpesviruses 2 and 5: Comparisons with other members of the subfamily gammaherpesviruses. *Adv. Virus Res.* **44**, 357–379.

Babiuk, L. A., and Rouse, B. T. (1996). Herpesvirus vaccines. *Adv. Drug Delivery Rev.* **21**, 63–76.

Babiuk, L. A., van Drunen Little-van den Hurk, S., and Tikoo, S. K. (1996). Immunology of bovine herpesvirus 1 infection. *Vet. Microbiol.* **53**, 31–42.

Bagust, T. J., and Guy, J. S. (1997). Laryngotracheitis. *In* "Diseases of Poultry" (B. W. Calnek, ed.), 10th ed., pp. 527–531. Iowa State University Press, Ames.

Bernard, J., and Brémont, M. (1995). Molecular biology of fish viruses: A review. *Vet. Res.* **26**, 341–351.

Calnek, B. W., and Witter, R. L. (1997). Marek's disease. *In* "Diseases of Poultry" (B. W. Calnek, ed.), 10th ed., pp. 369–378. Iowa State University Press, Ames.

Carmichael, L. E., and Greene, C. E. (1990). Canine herpesvirus infection. *In* "Infectious Diseases of the Dog and Cat" (C. E. Greene, ed.), pp. 252–261. Saunders, Philadelphia, PA.

Crabb, B. S., and Studdert, M. J. (1995). Equine herpesviruses 4 (equine rhinopneumonitis virus) and 1 (equine abortion virus). *Adv. Virus Res.* **45**, 153–190.

Edington, N. (1992). Porcine cytomegalovirus. *In* "Diseases of Swine," (A. D. Leman, B. Straw, W. L. Mengeling, S. D'Allaire, and D. J. Taylor, eds.), 7th ed., pp. 250–252. Iowa State University Press, Ames.

Holmes, G. P., Chapman, L. E., Stewart, J. A., *et al.* (1995). Guidelines for the prevention of B-virus infections in exposed persons. *Clin. Infect. Dis.* **20**, 421–439.

Kit, S. (1989). Recombinant-derived modified-live herpesvirus vaccines. *Adv. Exp. Med. Biol.* **251**, 219–236.

Mettenleiter, T. C. (1997). Immunobiology of pseudorabies (Aujeszky's) disease. *Vet. Immunol. Immunopathol.* **54**, 221–229.

O'Toole, D., Li, H., Miller, D., Williams, W. R., and Crawford, T. B. (1997). Chronic and recovered cases of sheep-associated malignant catarrhal fever in cattle. *Vet. Rec.* **140**, 519–524.

Povey, R. C. (1990). Feline viral rhinotracheitis (FVR). *In* "Infectious Diseases of the Dog and Cat" (C. E. Greene, ed.), pp. 346–351. Saunders, Philadelphia, PA.

Roizman, B., and Sears, A. E. (1996). Herpes simplex viruses and their replication. *In* "Fields Virology" (B. N. Fields, D. M. Knipe, P. M. Howley, R. M. Chanock, J. L. Melnick, T. P. Monath, B. Roizman, and S. E. Straus, eds.), 3rd ed., pp. 2231–2296. Lippincott-Raven, Philadelphia, PA.

Wolf, K. (1983). Biology and properties of fish and reptilian herpesviruses. *In* "The Herpesviruses (B. Roizman, ed.), Vol. 2, pp. 319–325. Plenum, New York.

CHAPTER 19

Adenoviridae

In 1953 Wallace Rowe and colleagues, having observed that explant cultures of human adenoids degenerated spontaneously, isolated a new virus that they named *adenovirus*. The next year Cabasso and colleagues demonstrated that the etiological agent of infectious canine hepatitis was an adenovirus. Subsequently, many adenoviruses, each appearing to be highly host specific, were isolated from humans and many other mammals and birds, usually from the upper respiratory tract, but sometimes from feces. Most of these viruses produce subclinical infections, with occasional upper respiratory disease, but avian adenoviruses are associated with a variety of clinically important syndromes. Since their discovery, adenoviruses have been at the core of significant basic discoveries, including many concerning virus structure, eukaryotic gene expression and organization, RNA splicing, and apoptosis. Adenoviruses have also been used as vectors for recombinant DNA vaccines and as vectors in gene therapy.

Properties of Adenoviruses

Classification

The family *Adenoviridae* comprises two genera: the genus *Mastadenovirus* comprising viruses that infect mammalian species and the genus *Aviadenovirus* comprising viruses that infect birds. A third genus, *Atadenovirus*, has been proposed, but had not been accepted by the International Committee on Taxonomy of Viruses as of the date of publication of this book. This genus would comprise certain animal adenoviruses with distinct genomic structure, including ovine adenovirus 287, several bovine adenoviruses, and egg drop syndrome virus of chickens. The genome of the latter virus, which had been the sole member of avian adenovirus group III, has been sequenced completely and found to be exceptional—its hexon gene shows greatest similarity to that of ovine adenovirus 287, but is missing several genes found in other adenoviruses.

The number of adenoviruses known to infect each animal species is shown in Table 19.1. Some 50 different adenoviruses are recognized in humans. There is a sense that there are many more adenoviruses of animals yet to be discovered—this is just a matter of the level of activity of reference diagnostic laboratories, from where new viruses usually emerge.

Genera and complexes within the genus *Mastadenovirus* have been defined by antigenic and genome characteristics. The individual viruses assigned to each are designated by their host species and a serial number (e.g., canine adenovirus 1). Restriction endonuclease mapping and sequencing of the genomic DNA has proven useful for the precise categorization of viral strains, and in general, results have accorded well with previous categorizations based on serological cross-reactions.

After the general structuring of the family had been redone on the basis of molecular characteristics of the viruses, the bases for the immunologic relationships among the viruses became clear. For example, antigenic determinants associated with the inner part of hexons, i.e., the structural units making up the bulk of the capsid, contain the epitopes that were first used to antigenically define the two genera. Genus-specific epitopes were found to be located on pentons, i.e., structural units that are located at the vertices of capsids. Type-specific epitopes, which were first defined in neutralization and

Table 19.1
Diseases of Domestic Animals Associated with Adenoviruses

Animal species	Number of serotypes	Disease
Dogs	2	Infectious canine hepatitis (canine adenovirus 1)
		Infectious canine tracheobronchitis (canine adenovirus 2)
Horses	2	Usually asymptomatic or mild upper respiratory disease. Bronchopneumonia and generalized disease in foals with primary severe combined immunodeficiency disease
Cattle	10	Usually asymptomatic or mild upper respiratory disease
Swine	4	Usually asymptomatic or mild upper respiratory disease
Sheep	6	Usually asymptomatic or mild upper respiratory disease
Goats	2	Usually asymptomatic or mild upper respiratory disease
Deer	1	Pulmonary edema, hemorrhage, vasculitis
Rabbits	1	Diarrhea
Chickens	12	Egg drop syndrome, inclusion body hepatitis
Turkeys and pheasants	3	Hemorrhagic enteritis (turkey); marble spleen disease (pheasant); egg drop syndrome in both
Quail	1	Bronchitis
Ducks	2	Rarely, duck hepatitis
Geese	3	Isolated from liver, intestines

hemagglutination–inhibition assays, were found to be located on the outward-facing surface of the hexons. The penton fibers were found to contain other type-specific epitopes, which were also important in neutralization assays. Unexpectedly, although the distal knobs on the penton fibers contain the cell-binding ligands that are responsible for viral attachment to specific cellular receptors, antibody to these knobs or to the penton fibers was found to be only weakly neutralizing. All in all, the merits of the serological structuring of the family were based more on the relative dominance of certain epitopes in particular serological tests than on their location in the virion.

Virion Properties

Adenovirus virions are nonenveloped, precisely hexagonal in outline, with icosahedral symmetry, 80–100 nm in diameter (Figure 19.1). Virions are composed of 252 capsomers: 240 hexons that occupy the faces and edges of the 20 equilateral triangular facets of the icosahedron and 12 pentons that occupy the vertices. From each penton projects a penton fiber 20 to 50 nm in length, with a terminal knob (Figure 19.2). Avian adenovirus penton fibers are bifurcated, giving the appearance of two fibers extending from each vertex. The genome consists of a single linear molecule of double-stranded DNA, 36 to 44 kbp in size, with inverted terminal repeats. The complete sequence of the genomic DNA of several adenoviruses, including canine adenovirus 1, has been determined. Virion DNA, in association with a 55K protein linked covalently to each 5′-terminus, is infectious. About 40 proteins are coded for by the viral genome and are transcribed following complex RNA splicing. About one-third of the proteins are structural proteins. Structural proteins include those that make up the hexons, pentons, and penton fibers and others associated with the virion core.

Many adenoviruses agglutinate red blood cells, with hemagglutination occurring when the tips of penton fibers bind to cellular receptors and form bridges between cells. The optimal conditions and species of red blood cells for demonstrating this phenomenon with each adenovirus have been determined as hemagglutination–inhibition has been a major serologic diagnostic method for many years.

Adenoviruses are rather stable in the environment, but are inactivated easily by common disinfectants. All of the viruses have narrow host ranges. Many cause acute respiratory disease or gastroenteric disease and some cause persistent infections with long periods of latency that may be reactivated by immunosuppression—some viruses, such as equine adenovirus 1, cause severe disease in immunocompromised hosts. Some of the adenoviruses of humans, cattle, and chickens cause

FIGURE 19.1.

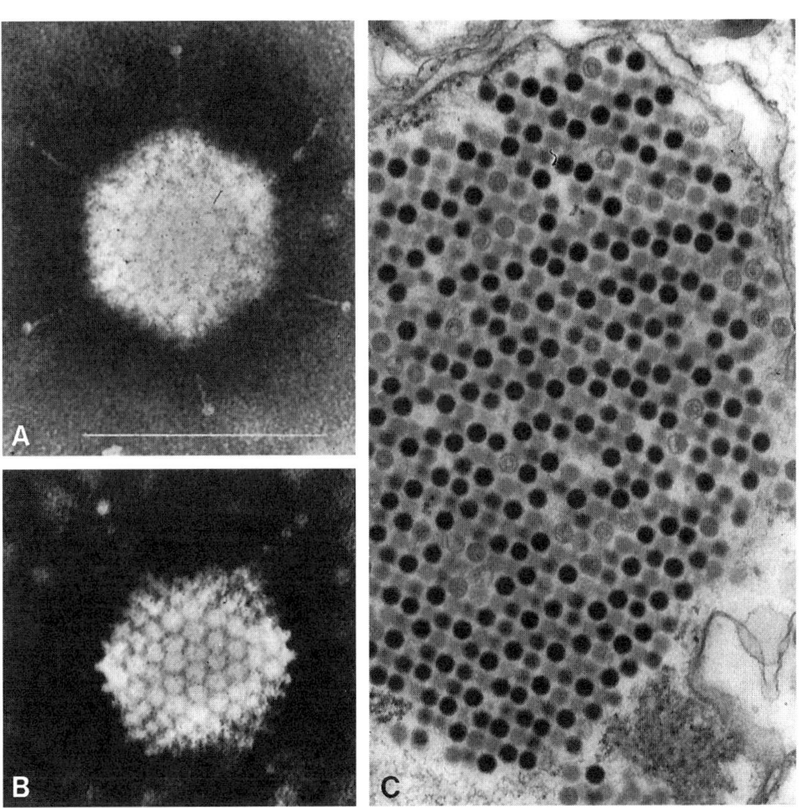

Family *Adenoviridae*, genus *Mastadenovirus*. (A) Virion showing penton fibers projecting from the vertices. (B) Virion showing the icosahedral array of capsomers—capsomers at the vertices (pentons) are surrounded by five neighbors, all the others (hexons) by six. (C) Crystalline array of virions in the nucleus of a fibroblast. A and B, negative contrast electron microscopy; C, thin section electron microscopy. [Bar: 100 nm. A and B, courtesy of R. C. Valentine and H. G. Pereira.]

tumors when inoculated into newborn hamsters and have been used in experimental oncogenesis studies, but none cause tumors in their natural hosts.

Viral Replication

Adenoviruses replicate in the nucleus and their replication is facilitated by extensive modulation of the host immune response. Viruses bind to host cell receptors via their penton fibers and enter the cell by endocytosis via clathrin-coated pits. The outer capsid is then removed and the core comprising the viral genome with its associated histones enters the nucleus where mRNA transcription, viral DNA replication, and assembly of virions occur.

In the nucleus the genome is transcribed by cellular RNA polymerase II according to a complex program involving both DNA strands (see Chapter 3). There are five early (E) transcriptional units: E1A, E1B, E2, E3 and E4, two intermediate units, IX and IVa2, and one late (L) unit from which five families of late mRNAs (L1 to L5) are transcribed. Each early region is under the control of a separate promoter whereas the late region uses a single promoter called the major late promoter. The E1A region of the viral genome encodes proteins that are essential for three main outcomes of early adenovirus transcription: (1) induction of cell cycle progression (DNA synthesis) to provide an optimal environment for viral replication; (2) protection of infected cells from host antiviral immune defenses, such as from tumor necrosis factor (TNF) activity or from apoptosis; and (3) synthesis of viral proteins necessary for viral DNA replication.

E1A and E1B gene products are also responsible for cell transformation and hence for the oncogenicity (experimental) of some adenoviruses. Both proteins interact with the cellular tumor suppresser gene p53, compromise its normal activity, and thus deregulate cell cycle progression. The E3 region is not essential for adenovirus replication in cell cultures and can be deleted or replaced without disrupting viral replication *in vitro*. It is therefore one of the insertion sites for foreign DNA when

FIGURE 19.2.

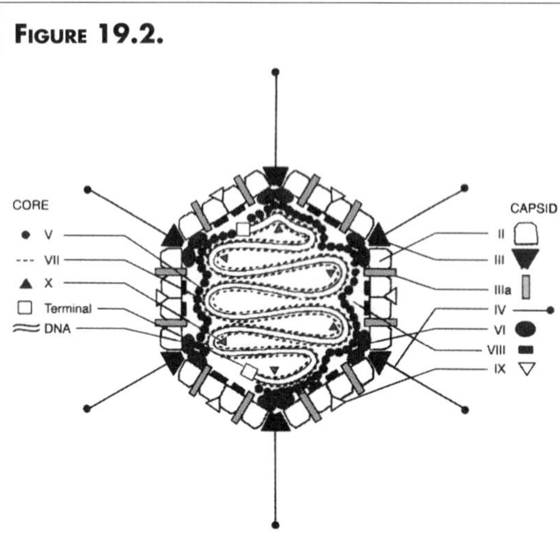

Model of an adenovirus virion showing constituents. Hexons (II) and pentons (III) are packed together to form the capsid. Penton fibers (IV) contain cell attachment ligands. Minor proteins are located between hexons (IIIa, IX), whereas others are located on the interior surface of the capsid (VI, VIII). The core consists of the genomic DNA complexed with four proteins (V, VII, X, and terminal). [From P. L. Stewart, R. M. Burnett, M. Cyrklaff, and S. D. Fuller, Image reconstruction reveals the complex molecular organization of adenovirus. *Cell* **67,** 145–154 (1991).]

constructing adenovirus vectors. E3 proteins are known to interact with host immune defense mechanisms, thus modulating the host response to adenovirus infection. Inhibition of class I major histocompatibility antigen expression by infected cells and inhibition of tumor necrosis factor are two examples of immune evasion mediated by E3-encoded proteins.

Viral DNA replication, using the 5′-linked 55K protein as primer, proceeds from both ends by a strand displacement mechanism. The repeat sequences form panhandle-like structures of single-stranded DNA that serve as origins of replication. Following DNA replication, late mRNAs are transcribed; these are translated into structural proteins, which are made in considerable excess. All adenovirus late-coding regions are transcribed from a common promoter, the major late promoter. The primary transcript is about 29 kb; at least 18 distinct mRNAs are produced by alternative splicing of the late primary transcript. Shutdown of host cell macromolecular synthesis occurs progressively during the second half of the replication cycle. Virions are assembled in the nucleus, where they form crystalline arrays (Figure 19-1C). Many adenoviruses cause severe condensation and margination of the host cell chromatin, making nuclei appear abnormal (Figure 19-3); this is the basis for the inclusion bodies seen characteristically in adenovirus-infected cells. Virions are released by cell lysis.

FIGURE 19.3.

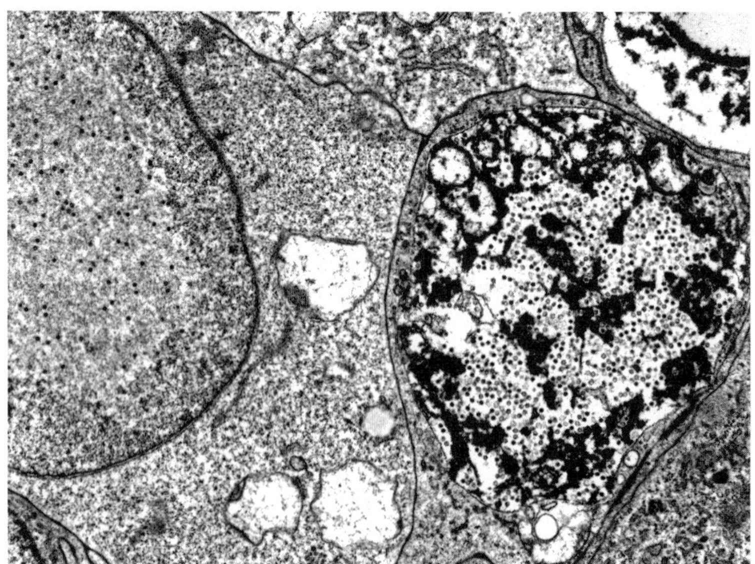

Avian adenovirus 1 infection in the spleen of a chick. The nucleus at the left contains dispersed virions and early margination of chromatin, whereas the nucleus at the right contains many virions and extremely condensed chromatin. Thin section electron microscopy, magnification ×16,000. (Courtesy of N. Cheville.)

Adenoviruses as Vectors for Delivery of Foreign DNA

Adenoviruses are being studied extensively as vectors for the delivery of foreign DNA. Examples of the expression of foreign genes in recombinant adenovirus vectors include pseudorabies virus gD protein, Epstein–Barr virus glycoprotein 340/220, vesicular stomatitis virus structural glycoprotein, rotavirus VP4, rabies virus glycoprotein, bovine parainfluenza virus 3 glycoprotein, feline immunodeficiency virus envelope glycoprotein, porcine respiratory and reproductive syndrome virus glycoprotein, human hepatitis B virus surface antigen, polyomavirus T antigen, and measles virus fusion protein (Table 19.2).

Infectious Canine Hepatitis

The two diseases caused by canine adenoviruses are the most important adenovirus infections of animals worldwide. Infectious canine hepatitis, caused by canine adenovirus 1, is also an important pathogen of foxes, wolves, coyotes, skunks, and bears. In fact, the virus was first recognized as the cause of fox encephalitis. In dogs, as well as causing acute hepatitis, the virus may cause respiratory or ocular disease, encephalopathy, chronic hepatitis, and interstitial nephritis. Canine adenovirus 2 causes respiratory disease: tonsillitis, pharyngitis, tracheitis, bronchitis, and bronchopneumonia.

Table 19.2
Properties of Adenoviruses

Two genera, *Mastadenovirus* and *Aviadenovirus*
Virions are nonenveloped, hexagonal in outline, with icosahedral symmetry, 80–100 nm in diameter, with one (genus *Mastadenovirus*) or two (genus *Aviadenovirus*) fibers (glycoprotein) projecting from each vertex of the capsid
The genome consists of a single linear molecule of double-stranded DNA, 36–44 kbp in size, with inverted terminal repeats
Replication takes place in the nucleus by a complex program of early and late transcription (before and after DNA replication); virions are released by cell lysis
Intranuclear inclusion bodies are formed, containing large numbers of virions, often in paracrystalline arrays
Viruses agglutinate red blood cells
Some viruses are oncogenic in rodents

Clinical Features

Most infections with canine adenovirus 1 are asymptomatic or are seen as undifferentiated respiratory disease. In some cases, however, the infection proceeds from the initial respiratory site to cause systemic disease. The systemic disease may be divided into three overlapping syndromes, which are usually seen in pups less than 6 months of age: (1) peracute disease in which the pup is found dead either without apparent preceding illness or after an illness lasting only 3 or 4 hours; (2) acute disease, which may be fatal, marked by fever, depression, loss of appetite, vomiting, bloody diarrhea, petechial hemorrhages of the gums, pale mucous membranes, and jaundice; and (3) mild disease, which may actually be a vaccine-modified disease, i.e., the result of partial immunity.

The incubation period of the acute disease is 4 to 9 days. Clinical signs include fever, apathy, anorexia, thirst, conjunctivitis, serous discharge from the eyes and nose, and occasionally abdominal pain and petechiae of the oral mucosa. There is tachycardia, leukopenia, prolonged clotting time, and disseminated intravascular coagulopathy. In some cases there is hemorrhage (e.g., bleeding around deciduous teeth and spontaneous hematomas). Although central nervous system involvement is not common, dogs affected severely may convulse. Upon recovery, dogs eat well but regain weight slowly. Seven to 10 days after acute signs disappear, about 25% of dogs develop bilateral corneal opacity, which usually disappears spontaneously.

In foxes, canine adenovirus 1 causes primarily central nervous system disease; infected animals may exhibit intermittent convulsions during the course of their illness and terminally may suffer paralysis of one or more limbs.

Pathogenesis, Pathology, and Immunity

The virus enters through nasopharyngeal, oral, and conjunctival routes; initial infection occurs in tonsillar crypts and Peyer's patches. There is viremia and infection of endothelial and parenchymal cells in many tissues, leading to hemorrhages and necrosis, especially in the liver, kidneys, spleen, and lungs. Canine adenovirus 1 is also one of the several causes of kennel cough, although it is probably less important than canine adenovirus 2. The syndrome that gave the disease its name, infectious canine hepatitis, involves the massive destruction of hepatocytes, resulting in peracute death. Invariably in such cases, histologic examination reveals characteristic inclusion bodies in hepatocytes (Figure 19.4A).

Figure 19.4.

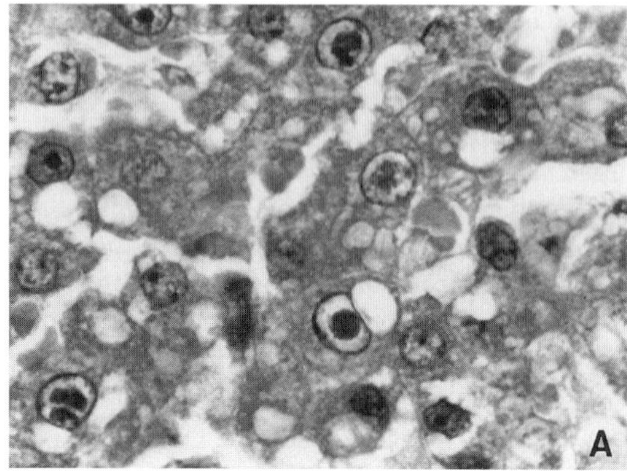

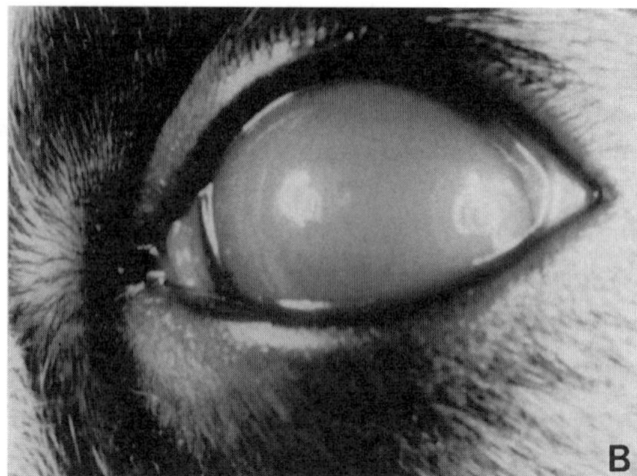

Canine adenovirus 1 (infectious canine hepatitis) infection. (A) Intranuclear inclusion bodies within hepatocytes in peracute infectious canine hepatitis (hematoxylin and eosin stain, magnification ×400). (B) "Blue eye" in a pup 9 days after vaccination with canine adenovirus 1 vaccine. (Courtesy of L. E. Carmichael.)

In the convalescent stages of natural infection and 8–12 days after vaccination with canine adenovirus 1-attenuated virus vaccine, corneal edema ("blue eye") is occasionally observed (19.4B). Although clinically dramatic and alarming, especially after vaccination, the edema usually resolves after a few days without consequence. The edema is due to virus–antibody complexes, deposited in the small blood vessels of the ciliary body, interfering with normal fluid exchange within the cornea. A similar pathogenesis underlies glomerulonephritis due to canine adenovirus 1.

Laboratory Diagnosis

Diagnosis of canine adenovirus infections is done by either virus isolation or serology using an enzyme immunoassay, hemagglutination–inhibition, or neutralization. The polymerase chain reaction is becoming a useful assay as well. Virus isolation is performed in any of several cell lines of canine origin (e.g., Madin-Darby canine kidney cells). Cytopathology occurs in most cases in 24 to 48 hours and the identification of the cause of this is determined immunologically.

Epidemiology, Prevention, and Control

Infection of the kidney is associated with viruria, which is a major mode of transmission, along with feces and saliva. Recovered dogs may shed virus in their urine for up to 6 months.

Both inactivated virus and attenuated virus canine adenovirus 1 vaccines had been in general use for many years. The antigenic relationship between canine adenoviruses 1 and 2 is sufficiently close for canine adenovirus 2 vaccine to be cross-protective; it has the advantage that it does not cause corneal edema. Annual revaccination is recommended by many manufacturers. Maternal antibody interferes with active immunization until puppies are 9 to 12 weeks of age.

One of the most remarkable phenomena in veterinary practice has been the virtual disappearance of infectious canine hepatitis from regions where vaccination had been performed for many years. This has been a result of the shedding of vaccine virus by vaccinated dogs, thereby "seeding" the environment with attenuated virus, immunizing many dogs secondarily, and building up a high level of herd immunity.

Equine Adenovirus Disease

Clinical Features

In horses, most adenovirus infections are asymptomatic or present as mild upper or lower respiratory tract disease. The latter are marked by fever, nasal discharge, and cough. Secondary bacterial infections, which produce a mucopurulent nasal discharge and exacerbate the cough, are not uncommon.

Certain Arabian foals that have primary severe combined immunodeficiency disease, an autosomal inherited defect in which there is a total absence of both

T and B cells, are particularly susceptible to equine adenovirus 1. As maternal antibody wanes, these foals become extremely susceptible to adenovirus infection. Infection is progressive and these foals invariably die within 3 months of age.

Pathogenesis, Pathology, and Immunity

Little is known about the pathology or pathogenesis of adenovirus infections in horses, primarily because infections are usually self-limited. Much research has been done on adenovirus infections in foals with primary severe combined immunodeficiency disease. Among all the potentially important opportunistic pathogens that may take advantage of the immune incompetence of these foals, the dominant role of equine adenovirus 1 in the overall pathogenesis of this syndrome is intriguing. In addition to bronchiolitis and pneumonia, the virus destroys cells in a wide range of other tissues in these foals, particularly the pancreas and salivary glands, but also renal, bladder, and gastrointestinal epithelium.

Laboratory Diagnosis

A diagnosis of adenovirus infection can, in most cases, be made by virus isolation, serology, or detection and analysis of viral nucleic acid. Adenovirus antigen detection using enzyme immunoassay and monoclonal antibodies may also be used. Virus isolation (from nasal swabs of suspect cases or tissues of foals with primary severe combined immunodeficiency disease) is performed in any of several cell lines of equine origin. Cytopathology typical of adenovirus infections (rounding and grape-like clustering of infected cells) occurs in most cases in 24 to 48 hours. Serological diagnosis is usually made by hemagglutination–inhibition or neutralization tests. DNA restriction endonuclease mapping (fingerprinting), Southern, dot-blot, and *in situ* hybridization and, most recently, polymerase chain reaction assays are also available. Of these the polymerase chain reaction is becoming the most widely applicable assay.

Epidemiology, Prevention, and Control

Like most other adenoviruses, equine viruses are most likely transmitted by oral and nasopharyngeal routes. Nothing is done to prevent or control infections, given their self-limiting nature.

Adenovirus Disease of Deer

In 1993 an epidemic of severe systemic disease in mule deer (*Odocoileus hemionus*) in California was found to be caused by an adenovirus. Since then there have been "die-offs" in other deer species, and evidence has accumulated that this may be a rather common disease. The disease is marked by pulmonary edema and erosions, ulcerations, hemorrhage, and abscesses of the intestinal tract. Histologically, there is widespread vasculitis with endothelial intranuclear inclusions. Laboratory diagnosis is based on the detection of viral antigen in tissues by immunofluorescence and by the detection of virions by electron microscopy.

Avian Adenovirus Diseases

Egg Drop Syndrome

Egg drop syndrome, first reported in 1976, is characterized by the production of soft-shelled and shell-less eggs by apparently healthy chickens. The disease has been recognized in fowl and both wild and domestic ducks and geese worldwide, except in the United States. The disease is caused by three avian adenoviruses that agglutinate avian red blood cells: one is associated with classical egg drop syndrome in many countries, another with ducks in the United Kingdom, and a third with egg drop syndrome in Australia. The viruses grow to high titers in embryonated eggs or cell cultures derived from ducks, geese, or chickens (e.g., chick kidney or chick embryo liver cells).

In chicken flocks without prior experience with these viruses the first clinical signs of infection are loss of color in pigmented eggs and soft-shelled and shell-less eggs. Because birds tend to eat the shell-less eggs, they may be missed. In flocks in which there is antibody the disease is seen as a failure to achieve production targets. There is also an endemic form of the disease, similar but more difficult to detect. Major lesions in infected birds are seen in the pouch shell gland and oviduct where epithelial cells become necrotic and contain intranuclear inclusion bodies. There is associated inflammatory infiltration. These findings are virtually pathognomonic, but diagnosis may be confirmed by virus isolation or serology (hemagglutination–inhibition or neutralization assay)

The main route of transmission is through contaminated eggs. Droppings also contain virus, and contaminated fomites such as crates or trucks can spread virus. The virus is also transmitted by needles used for vaccinations. At one time these viruses were spread by the contamination of Marek's disease vaccine, which was produced in duck embryo fibroblasts. Breeding flocks were infected and the viruses were spread widely through fertile eggs. Because infection usually remained latent until birds reached sexual maturity and because the viruses are transmitted vertically in eggs, the detection of this source of contagion was very difficult. Sporadic outbreaks have also been traced to contact of chickens with domestic ducks or geese and to water contaminated with wildfowl droppings.

This disease has been eradicated from primary breeder flocks in most countries. Its entry into layer flocks is further managed by (1) preventing contact with other birds, especially waterfowl; (2) disinfecting all equipment regularly; and (3) chlorination of water. Inactivated vaccines are available for use in chickens before they begin laying eggs, but they only reduce rather than eliminate virus transmission.

Hemorrhagic Enteritis of Turkeys and Marble Spleen Disease of Pheasants

Hemorrhagic enteritis is a common acute infection of turkeys older than 4 weeks of age; it is characterized by splenomegaly and intestinal hemorrhage. Clinically, the disease is characterized by acute onset, depression, bloody droppings, and death. Infection causes both humoral- and cell-mediated immunosuppression, so opportunistic bacterial infections are often an intercurrent problem. Flock mortality may reach 60%, although the usual mortality is 1 to 3%. The disease is caused by turkey adenovirus 2, a virus that is serologically indistinguishable from the virus that causes marble spleen disease of pheasants.

The lesions are pathognomonic: there is prominent reticuloendothelial hyperplasia and intranuclear inclusion bodies in the spleen. Diagnosis may be confirmed by virus isolation (with identification of isolates by neutralization assay) or by serology using an enzyme immunoassay.

The virus is transmitted readily by contact and fomites and is very stable in contaminated droppings, litter, etc. Control of the disease in turkeys or pheasants is based on vaccination, using an attenuated virus produced either in turkey spleen cells or in turkey B lymphoblastoid cells. Vaccine is administered via drinking water. Because maternal antibody interferes with vaccination, the optimum age for vaccination (usually 4 to 5 weeks) may vary according to the level of antibody in the flock.

Quail Bronchitis

Quail bronchitis is an important disease of wild and captive-bred bobwhite quail worldwide; in young birds it is seen as respiratory distress, coughing, sneezing, rales, lacrimation, and conjunctivitis. In older birds there is also diarrhea. Mortality may be 100% in young birds, but falls to less than 25% in birds more than 4 weeks of age when infected. The disease is marked by tracheitis, air sacculitis, and gaseous, mucoid enteritis. The etiologic agent is avian adenovirus 1, which can be isolated readily from the respiratory tract of acutely affected birds and from the intestinal tract of mildly affected birds. The virus is highly contagious and spreads rapidly through flocks. Control is based on strict isolation, quarantine of introduced birds, and regular decontamination of premises and equipment. In some instances, recovered birds are retained as breeders, as there is no long-term shedding and immunity is long lasting.

Further Reading

Horwitz, M. S. (1996). Adenoviruses. *In* "Fields Virology" (B. N. Fields, D. M. Knipe, P. M. Howley, R. M. Chanock, J. L. Melnick, T. P. Monath, B. Roizman, and S. E. Straus, eds.), 3rd ed., pp. 2149–2172. Lippincott-Raven, Philadelphia, PA.

McFerran, J. B. (1997). Adenovirus infections. *In* "Diseases of Poultry," (B. W. Calnek, ed.), 10th ed., pp. 607–610. Iowa State University Press, Ames.

McGuire, T. C., and Perryman, L. E. (1981). Combined immunodeficiency of Arabian foals. *In* "Immunologic Defects in Laboratory Animals" (M. E. Gershwin and B. Merchant, eds.), vol. 2, pp. 185–191. Plenum, New York.

Morrison, M. D., Onions, D. E., and Nicholson, L. (1997). Complete sequence of canine adenovirus 1. *J. Gen. Virol.* **78**, 873–878.

Shenk, T. (1996). Adenoviridae: The viruses and their replication. *In* "Fields Virology" (B. N. Fields, D. M. Knipe, P. M. Howley, R. M. Chanock, J. L. Melnick, T. P. Monath, B. Roizman, and S. E. Straus, eds.), 3rd ed., pp. 2111–2148. Lippincott-Raven, Philadelphia, PA.

Studdert, M. J. (1996). Equine adenovirus infections. *In* "Virus Infections of Vertebrates" (M. J. Studdert, ed.), vol. 4, pp. 65–80. Elsevier, Amsterdam.

Timoney, J. F., Gillespie, J. H., Scott, F. N., and Barlough, J. E. (1988). "Hagan and Bruner's Infectious Diseases of Domestic Animals," 8th ed. Cornell University Press, Ithaca, NY.

CHAPTER 20

Papovaviridae

Papillomas or warts have been recognized in animals for centuries; a stable master for the Caliph of Baghdad described equine warts in the 9th century. That papillomas have a viral etiology was recognized as long ago as 1907, but it was not until 1978 that it was realized that bovine papillomas and papillomas in other species are caused by several different viruses. In 1935, Peyton Rous observed that benign rabbit papillomas occasionally progressed to carcinomas; this was one of the earliest associations of viruses with cancer. Today, bovine papillomatosis, canine oral papillomatosis, and equine sarcoid may present significant clinical problems.

With few exceptions, papillomaviruses cannot be grown in cell culture; nevertheless, DNAs of many of the viruses that infect animals and about half of the many viruses that infect humans have been purified, cloned, and sequenced completely. This work was stimulated by the discovery in the 1980s that certain papillomaviruses cause cervical, anogenital, and laryngeal carcinomas in humans. This discovery, in turn, has prompted much research on the nature and mechanisms of papillomavirus oncogenesis, which is now advancing our understanding of papillomas in animals.

Polyomaviruses are also highly species specific. Except for rare neurologic and urologic diseases in immunologically incompetent humans and a disease in budgerigars, these viruses are of little concern as pathogens in nature.

Properties of Papovaviruses

Classification

The family *Papovaviridae* comprises two rather disparate genera: (1) the genus *Papillomavirus,* containing the many papillomaviruses of mammals and birds, (2) the genus *Polyomavirus,* containing a few pathogens of animals and humans. The first two syllables of the name *Papovaviridae* refer to the genera *Papillomavirus* and *Polyomavirus;* "va" alludes to "vacuolating agent," an old name for the prototype polyomavirus, simian virus 40 (SV40).

Papillomaviruses are distinguished on the basis of host range and DNA sequence relatedness. Types are designated by numbers following the chronological order of their identification. By convention, a new virus type must have less than 50% overall DNA sequence homology with other viruses from the same species (greater than 50% but less than 100% homology defines new subtypes, which are designated by serial letters). Using this system, 6 types of bovine, 2 types of equine, and more than 77 types of human papillomaviruses have been identified (Table 20.1). Papillomaviruses have also been found in chimpanzees, colobus and rhesus monkeys, deer, dogs, elephant, elk, opossum, mice, turtles, chaffinches, and parrots. There is little sequence homology between DNAs of papillomaviruses from different species.

Table 20.1
Diseases Caused by Papillomaviruses

Virus	Principal species affected	Disease
Bovine papillomaviruses 1 and 2	Cattle	Cutaneous fibropapilloma
	Horses	Sarcoid
Bovine papillomavirus 3	Cattle	Cutaneous papilloma
Bovine papillomavirus 4	Cattle	Intestinal tract papilloma (may become malignant)
Bovine papillomavirus 5	Cattle	Teat fibropapilloma ("rice grain papilloma")
Bovine papillomavirus 6	Cattle	Teat papilloma ("frond papilloma")
Ovine papillomavirus	Sheep	Cutaneous fibropapilloma
Equine papillomaviruses 1 and 2	Horses	Cutaneous papilloma
Porcine genital papillomavirus	Swine	Cutaneous papilloma
Canine oral papillomavirus	Dogs	Oral papilloma
Deer papillomavirus	Deer	Fibropapilloma, papilloma, fibroma
Cottontail rabbit papillomavirus[a] and rabbit papillomavirus	Rabbits	Cutaneous papilloma (may become malignant)
Human papillomavirus (>77 types)	Humans	Cutaneous and mucosal papillomas (may become malignant)
Fringilla (finch) papillomavirus	Finches	Papilloma
Avian papillomavirus	Parrots	Papilloma

[a]Also called Shope papillomavirus, much used in early studies of oncogenic viruses.

Bovine papillomaviruses have been divided further into two "groups": (1) bovine papillomaviruses 1, 2, and 5 are related immunologically, have the same genome size, and share nucleotide sequence homologies and (2) bovine papillomaviruses 3, 4, and 6 have smaller genomes and share DNA sequence homologies. The two groups are related only distantly.

Papillomaviruses can also be categorized according to their tissue tropism and the histologic character of the lesions they cause: group I (bovine papillomaviruses types 3 and 6 and cottontail rabbit papillomavirus) induce cutaneous neoplasia; group II (bovine papillomavirus type 4) induce hyperplasia of nonstratified squamous epithelium; group III (bovine papillomaviruses types 1, 2, and 5) induce subcutaneous fibromas in addition to cutaneous papillomas; and group IV (deer papillomavirus) induce primarily fibromas with minimal cutaneous hyperplasia.

Virion Properties

Papovavirus virions are nonenveloped, spherical in outline, with icosahedral symmetry. Virions are 55 (genus *Papillomavirus*) or 45 (genus *Polyomavirus*) nm in diameter. Virions are constructed from 72 hexavalent (six-sided) capsomers arranged most unusually in pentameric (five-sided) arrays (Figures 20.1 and 20.2). Both "empty" and "full" virus particles and tubular and other aberrant forms are seen by electron microscopy. The genome consists of a single molecule of circular double-stranded DNA, 8 (genus *Papillomavirus*) or 5 (genus *Polyomavirus*) kbp in size. The DNA has covalently closed ends, is supercoiled, and is infectious. Six polypeptides have been identified, two forming the capsid (Figure 20.3). The viruses are resistant to diverse environmental insults: infectivity survives lipid solvents and detergents, low pH, and high temperatures.

Viral Replication

Papillomavirus replication is linked tightly to the growth and differentiation of cells in stratified squamous and mucosal epithelium from their origin in basal layers to their shedding at the epidermal surface of the skin or mucous membranes. Actively dividing basal cells in the stratum germinativum are infected initially and are be-

FIGURE 20.1.

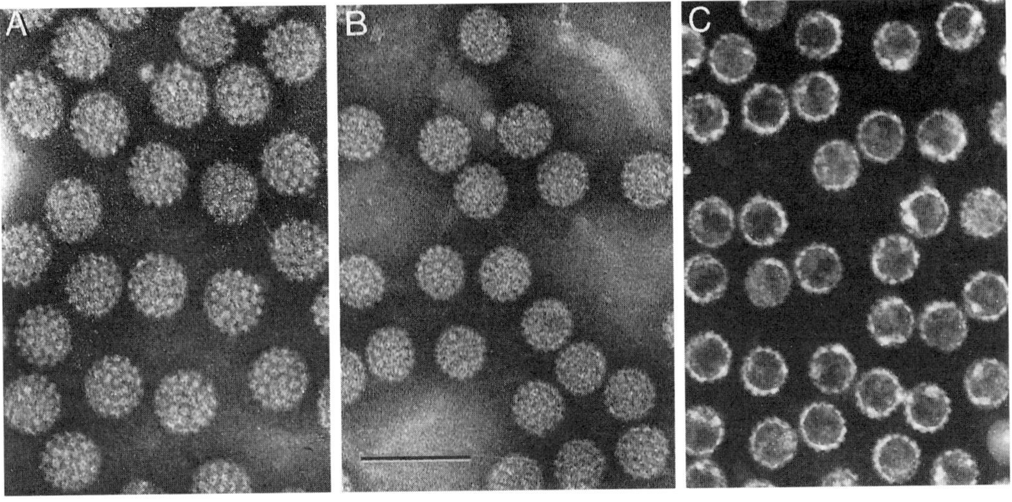

Family *Papovaviridae*. (A) Genus *Papillomavirus*, bovine papillomavirus 1. (B) Genus *Polyomavirus*, SV40 virus. (C) Genus *Polyomavirus*, empty SV40 capsids. Bar: 100 nm. (Courtesy of E. A. Follett.)

lieved to maintain the virus in a proviral, possibly latent, state throughout cellular differentiation. Virus-induced hyperplasia, induced by early viral gene products, leads to increased basal cell division and delayed maturation of cells in the stratum spinosum and stratum granulosum. These cells become massed into nascent papillomas. Late viral genes encoding capsid proteins are expressed, first in cells of the stratum spinosum. Virions are first seen at this stage of cellular differentiation. The accumulation of large numbers of virions and associated cytopathology are most pronounced in the stratum granulosum. Virions are shed with exfoliated cells of the stratum corneum of the skin or nonkeratinized cells of mucosal surfaces (Figure 20.4).

FIGURE 20.2.

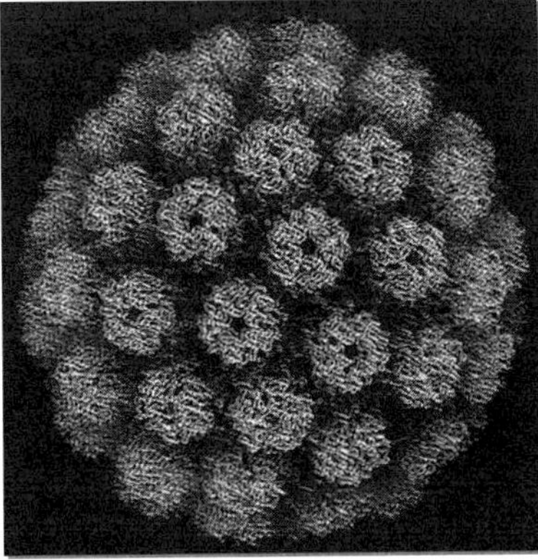

SV40 virus structure at 3.8-Å resolution, determined using X-ray crystallography. [From J. S. Butel, Papovaviruses. *In* Encyclopedia of Virology (R. G. Webster and A. Granoff, eds.), 2nd ed. (CD-ROM). Academic Press, London, 1998.]

Virions attach to cellular receptors, enter via receptor-mediated endocytosis, and are transported to the nucleus where they are uncoated, releasing their DNA. During productive infection, transcription of the viral genome is divided into early and late stages. Transcription of early and late coding regions is controlled by separate promoters and occurs on opposite DNA strands in the case of polyomaviruses and on the same strand with papillomaviruses. First, the half of the genome that contains the early genes is transcribed, forming mRNAs that direct the synthesis of enzymes involved in viral replication. Late mRNAs that direct the synthesis of virion structural proteins are transcribed from the other half of the viral genome after DNA synthesis has begun. Progeny DNA molecules serve as additional template, amplifying the production of structural proteins greatly. Several different translational strategies are employed to enhance the limited coding capacity of the viral genomes.

Papovavirus DNA replication begins at a single unique origin of replication and proceeds bidirectionally, terminating about 180° away on the circular DNA. An initiation complex binds to the origin and unwinds a region (the replication bubble and fork); nascent DNA chains are formed; one strand synthesized continuously in the direction of unwinding, the other synthesized discontinuously in the opposite direction. As replication proceeds the torsional strain created by the unwinding

Figure 20.3.

Bovine papillomavirus 1

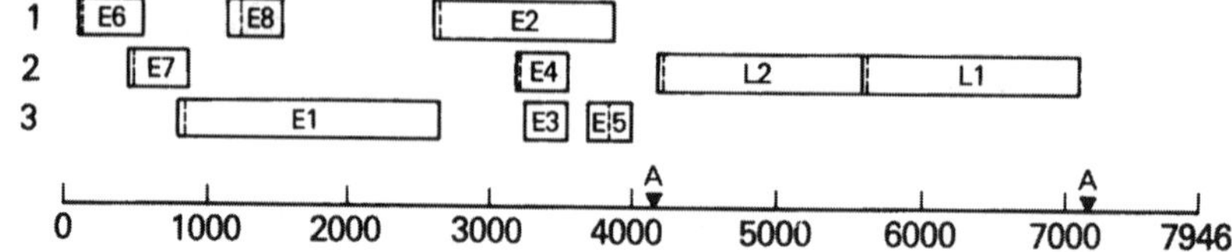

Cottontail rabbit papillomavirus

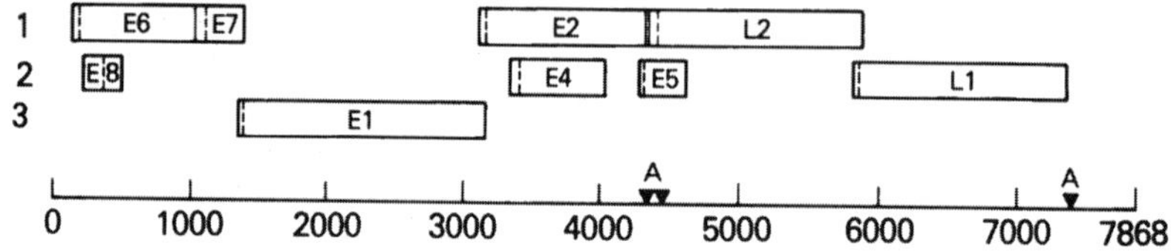

The genomic organization of two papillomaviruses, bovine papillomavirus 1 and cottontail rabbit papillomavirus (Shope papillomavirus), deduced from DNA sequence data. Although the genomes are circular, they have been linearized by cutting at a standard site. All papillomavirus open reading frames are located on one of the DNA strands and only that strand is transcribed. Transcription is complex, involving the use of seven different promoters and alternate and multiple splicing patterns and producing over 20 different mRNAs. The E (for early) genes encode mainly proteins with regulatory functions concerned with persistence, DNA replication, and activation of the lytic cycle; the L (for late) genes encode structural proteins. A, polyadenylation sites. [From P. M. Howley, Papillomaviruses: The viruses and their replication. *In* "Fields Virology" (B. N. Fields, D. M. Knipe, P. M. Howley, R. M. Chanock, J. L. Melnick, T. P. Monath, B. Roizman, and S. E. Straus, eds.), 3rd ed., pp. 2045–2076. Lippincott-Raven, Philadelphia, 1996.]

of the parental strands of DNA is released by the action of a specific viral enzyme. Bidirectional replication proceeds around the full genomic DNA circle, at which point the progeny DNA circles separate.

Virions are assembled in the nucleus and are released on cell death, often just as a consequence of cellular replacement in epithelia. Some cells exhibit a characteristic cytopathic effect, marked by cytoplasmic vacuolization. An infected cell may produce 10,000 to 100,000 virions.

Bovine papillomaviruses 1 and 2 and DNA isolated from them can transform cells *in vitro*. In contrast to other transforming DNA viruses, papillomavirus DNA remains episomal and is rarely integrated into the cellular genome. The genes expressed in such cells encode proteins concerned with replication and regulation of viral transcription as well as proteins that affect cellular transformation directly. In association with cofactors, bovine, rabbit, and human papillomaviruses may produce carcinomas *in vivo* (Table 20.2).

Figure 20.4.

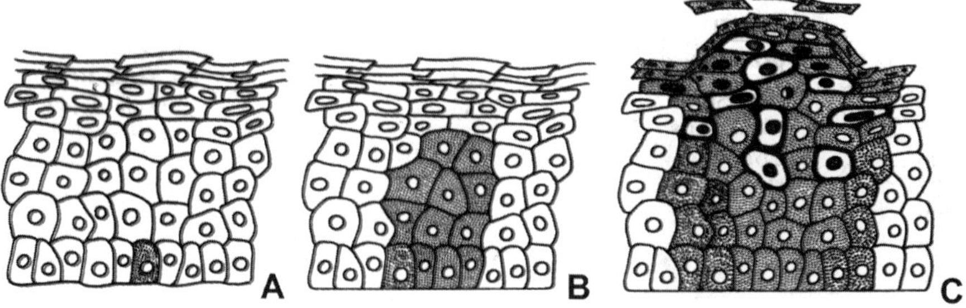

Schematic representation of the events in papillomavirus infection of keratinocytes. (A) The primary infection occurs in a cell of the stratum germinativum, with the virus gaining entry via an abrasion, etc. (B) This results in a proliferating clone of infected cells that spreads laterally in association with virus-induced delay in the maturation of infected cells. (C) Cellular differentiation occurs eventually and large numbers of virions are produced in association with the formation of a papilloma. This is most pronounced in the stratum granulosum. Virions are shed with exfoliated cells of the stratum corneum. (Courtesy of H. zur Hausen.)

Table 20.2
Properties of Papovaviruses

Two genera, *Polyomavirus* and *Papillomavirus*

Virions are nonenveloped, spherical in outline, with icosahedral symmetry. Virions are 55 (genus *Papillomavirus*) or 45 (genus *Polyomavirus*) nm in diameter

The genome consists of a single molecule of circular double-stranded DNA, 8 (genus *Papillomavirus*) or 5 (genus *Polyomavirus*) kbp in size. The DNA has covalently closed ends, is circular and supercoiled, and is infectious

Members of both genera replicate in nucleus; members of the genus *Polyomavirus* grow in cultured cells; most members of the genus *Papillomavirus* have not been grown in culture, but will transform cultured cells; infectious virions produced only in terminally differentiated epithelial cells

During replication, polyomavirus DNA is transcribed from both strands, whereas papillomavirus DNA is transcribed from one strand

Integrated (genus *Polyomavirus*) or episomal (genus *Papillomavirus*) DNA may be oncogenic

Table 20.3
Host Responses to Papillomavirus Infections

Host response	Virus
Group 1	
Neoplasia of cutaneous stratified epithelium (cutaneous papilloma)	Bovine papillomaviruses 3 and 6, equine, and cottontail rabbit papillomaviruses[a]
Group 2	
Hyperplasia of normal nonstratified squamous epithelium or metaplastic squamous epithelium	Bovine papillomavirus 4[b] and canine oral papillomaviruses
Group 3	
Cutaneous papilloma with underlying fibroma of connective tissue	Bovine papillomaviruses 1, 2, and 5

[a]May progress to squamous carcinoma.
[b]With cofactors, alimentary tract and bladder papillomas may progress to carcinomas.

Diseases Caused by Members of the Genus *Papillomavirus*

Bovine Papillomatosis

Papillomas or warts are seen more commonly in cattle than in any other domestic animal. All ages are affected, but the incidence is highest in calves and yearlings.

Bovine papillomaviruses 1 and 2 exhibit a somewhat broader host range and tissue tropism than other types, causing fibropapillomas in cattle and sarcoids in horses. Bovine papillomaviruses 3 to 6 have been shown by both natural and experimental infection to be restricted to cattle. Transmission from cattle to humans was suspected from the high incidence of cutaneous warts in butchers; however, the virus isolated from these people does not appear to be related to any known bovine virus.

Clinical Features

The various papillomaviruses recognized in cattle are associated with distinct lesions (Table 20.3); bovine papillomaviruses 1, 2, and 5 cause "teat frond" warts, common cutaneous warts, and "rice grain" fibropapillomas, respectively. These papillomas have a fibrous core covered to a variable depth with stratified squamous epithelium, the outer layers of which are hyperkeratinized. The lesions vary from small firm nodules to large cauliflower-like growths; they are grayish to black in color and rough and spiny to the touch. Large fibropapillomas are subject to abrasion and may bleed. Fibropapillomas are common on the udder and teats and on the head, neck, and shoulders; they may also occur in the omasum, vagina, vulva, penis, and anus (Figure 20.5A).

In contrast, bovine papillomaviruses 3, 4, and 6 induce epithelial and cutaneous lesions without fibroblast proliferation. Lesions caused by bovine papillomavirus 3 have a tendency to persist and are usually flat with a broad base in contrast to the more usual fibropapillomas that protrude and are often pedunculated. In upland areas of Scotland and northern England, papillomas due to bovine papillomavirus 4 occur only in the alimentary tract and in the urinary bladder and may progress to squamous cells carcinomas (Figure 20-5B) (see Chapter 11). Ingestion of bracken fern (*Pteridium aquilinum*) is a major contributing factor (both cocarcinogen and immunosuppressive agent) in the transition from benign papillomas to invasive carcinoma of the alimentary tract (type 4) or bladder (type 2), the latter leading to so-called chronic endemic hematuria.

Pathogenesis, Pathology, and Immunity

Papillomas develop after the introduction of virus through abrasions of the skin. Infection of epithelial cells results in hyperplasia with subsequent degeneration and hyperkeratinization. These changes begin usually 4 to 6 weeks after exposure. In general, fibropapillomas persist for 4 to 6 months before spontaneous regression; multiple warts usually regress simultaneously. Stages in the pattern of papilloma develop-

FIGURE 20.5.

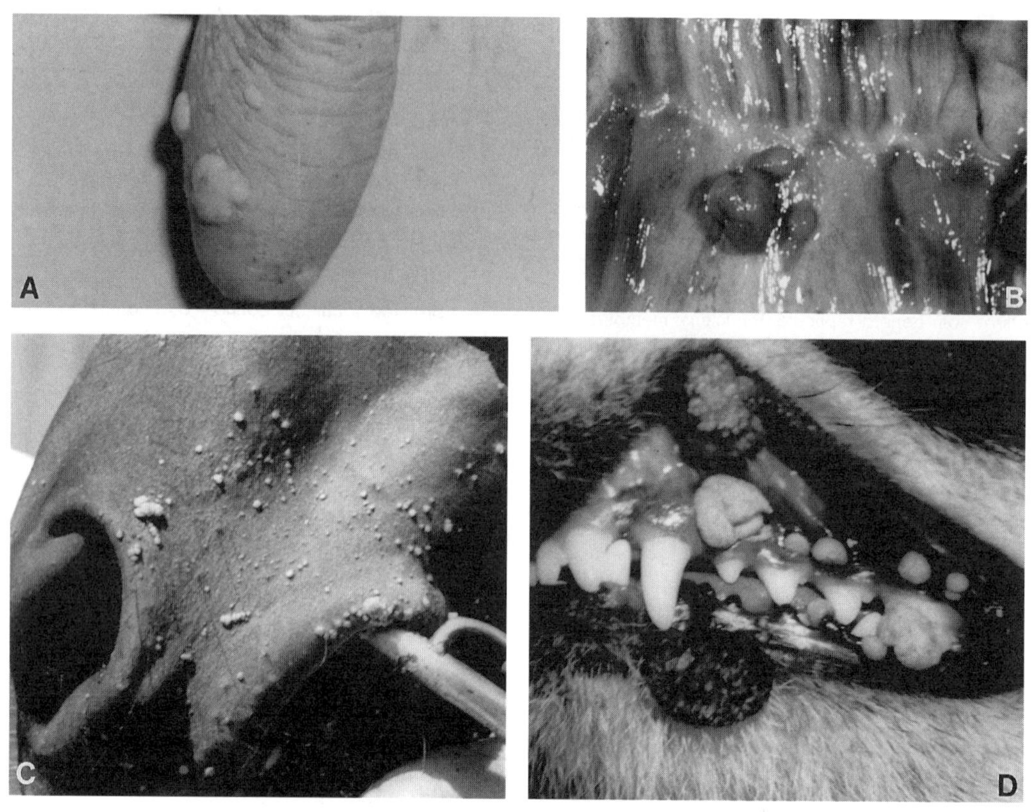

Papillomas of various host species. (A) Bovine fibropapilloma—teat warts—caused by bovine papillomavirus 5. (B) Bovine bladder papilloma caused by bovine papillomavirus 4. (C) Equine papillomatosis. (D) Canine oral papillomatosis.

ment can be discerned. Thus, stage 1 papillomas appear as slightly raised plaques, starting at about 4 weeks after exposure. Stage 2 papillomas are characterized by cytopathology, virus replication, and crystalline aggregates of virions in lesions, starting at about 8 weeks. Stage 3 papillomas are characterized by fibrotic, pedunculated bases and rough, lobate, or fungiform surfaces, starting after about 12 weeks. The level of neutralizing antibody appears to be correlated with the regression of lesions and with protection against re-infection.

Laboratory Diagnosis

The clinical appearance of papillomas is characteristic, and laboratory diagnosis is seldom necessary. Virions can be seen by electron microscopic examination. Hybridization assays and the polymerase chain reaction can be used to detect papillomavirus DNA, but these methods are seldom used for routine diagnosis in veterinary medicine.

Epidemiology, Prevention, and Control

Virus is transmitted between animals by contaminated halters, nose leads, grooming and earmarking equipment, rubbing posts, and other articles contaminated by contact with diseased cattle. Cattle that have been groomed for show may have extensive lesions. Sexual transmission of warts in cattle is likely as such lesions are rare in animals that are artificially inseminated. The disease is more common in housed cattle than in cattle on pasture. Natural bovine papillomavirus infection of horses generally occurs after housing animals in stalls that previously held cattle.

Prevention and treatment of papillomas are difficult to evaluate because the disease is self-limiting and its duration varies. Bovine interferon α has been used to treat cattle, but rarely seems indicated. Psoralen-based photodynamic therapy has been used, but again appropriate clinical circumstances are rarely encountered. Inoculation with homogenized, autologous wart tissue, treated with formalin, has been used for many years, but its efficacy has always been evaluated anecdotally.

Vaccination with viral capsid proteins produced by recombinant DNA technology has been encouraging, but vaccines must contain multiple virus types because there is no cross-protection.

Equine Papillomatosis and Sarcoids

Lesions caused by equine papillomavirus appear occasionally as small, elevated, keratinized papillomas around the lips and noses of horses (Figure 20.5C). They generally regress after 1 to 9 months. Warts that interfere with the bit or bridle can be removed surgically. Congenital equine papillomas have been recorded on several occasions.

Sarcoids are naturally occurring skin tumors of horses that have the histological appearance of fibrosarcomas. Although they do not metastasize, they persist for life and are locally invasive, often recurring after surgical removal or treatment with radioactive implants. Transmission trials with sarcoid material have usually been unsuccessful. Sarcoids have not been observed to spread from affected horses to other horses by direct contact.

On the basis of their appearance, sarcoids have been classified into type 1 (verrucous type, usually hairless and slowly growing), type 2 (fibroblastic, "proud flesh" type, comprising an intradermal fibroblastic proliferative response, often growing rapidly and ulcerating), type 3 (mixed type, showing features of types 1 and 2), and type 4 (occult type, flat with rough thickened skin and a surrounding area of alopecia). Types 1 to 3 may be either sessile or pedunculated. Subcutaneous fibrous nodules beneath apparently normal skin have been observed in association with sarcoids, particularly in the periorbital region, and may represent a fifth category.

Horses are susceptible to experimental infection with bovine papillomaviruses 1 and 2, and the tumors produced are similar to sarcoids. Bovine papillomavirus DNA sequences have been detected in high copy number by hybridization in both experimental and natural lesions. Also, bovine papillomaviruses have been shown to be able to transform equine fibroblasts *in vitro*. These data, together with the observation that sarcoids can occur in epidemic form, suggest that bovine papillomaviruses may be the cause of equine sarcoids. However, unlike their natural counterparts, the induced tumors regress spontaneously, and horses infected experimentally develop antibodies against bovine papillomaviruses, which are absent in horses with naturally occurring sarcoids.

The variable success and hazards of several attempted therapies (surgery, laser surgery, radiation, topical drugs) have led to an interest in immunotherapy. Stimulation of cell-mediated responses by the injection of immunopotentiators has been somewhat successful. Ocular sarcoids have regressed following the injection of viable Bacillus Calmette-Guerin (BCG) mycobacteria.

Canine Papillomatosis

Warts in dogs usually begin on the lips and can spread to the buccal mucosa, tongue, palate, and pharynx before regressing spontaneously (Figure 20-5D). The lesions occasionally become extensive, requiring veterinary attention.

Papillomatosis in Other Mammalian Species

Classic studies on viral oncogenesis were carried out in the late 1930s with the Shope rabbit papillomavirus. Papillomas caused by this virus often progress to carcinomas in both their natural host, the cottontail rabbit (*Sylvilagus* spp.), and in laboratory rabbits infected experimentally.

Oral papillomatosis occurs naturally in domestic rabbits (*Oryctologus cuniculus*); the tumors are small, gray-white, filiform or pedunculated nodules (5 mm in diameter) and are localized mostly on the underside of the tongue. The causative papillomavirus is distinct from the Shope rabbit papilloma virus (cottontail rabbit papillomavirus). Experimentally, oral papillomatosis has been reproduced in various rabbit species, and in nature it is widespread among domestic rabbits, particularly in older animals. Virus spread in animal rooms seems not to occur, but transmission from the mother to offspring during the suckling period is common. Oral papillomas of rabbits show no tendency to malignancy and may persist for many months.

Papillomatosis in Birds

A member of the genus *Papillomavirus* has been identified in birds: the Fringilla (finch) papillomavirus. Infection with a second papillomavirus-like virus has been described in African green parrots. Both viruses have been demonstrated in papillomatous lesions in their respective host species. In finches, papillomas occur exclusively on the legs and show stages of development from a slight node on a digit to heavy involvement of the foot and tarsometatarsus, often obscuring the individual digits and resulting in overgrowth and distortion of the claws. In severe cases the tumor may account for up to 5% of the bird's total body weight, but affected birds seem to remain in good condition otherwise.

Diseases Caused by Members of the Genus *Polyomavirus*

Polyomaviruses cause inapparent infections in most hosts; they have restricted host ranges and their oncogenic potential has often only been revealed when inoculated experimentally into heterologous hosts. Several polyomaviruses have been found in rodents and lagomorphs in addition to murine polyoma virus, the virus that gave this genus its name: K virus of mice, latent hamster virus, and rabbit kidney vacuolating virus. Polyomaviruses of interest in veterinary medicine occur in cattle and birds.

Bovine Polyomavirus Infection

About 60% of bovine sera, including fetal and neonatal calf sera, contain a bovine polyomavirus, which grows well in monkey kidney cells. A construct containing its early genes transforms rodent cells, and these cells induce tumors in immunocompromised rats. In a survey done in The Netherlands, about 60% of veterinarians were found to have antibodies to this virus. Despite this prevalence, the possible significance of this virus remains unknown.

Budgerigar Fledgling Disease

An avian polyomavirus has been identified as the cause of an acute generalized disease in fledgling budgerigars (*Melopsittacus undulatus*). The same virus may also be responsible for "French molt," which is a milder disease of budgerigars that results in chronic disorders of feather formation, and it is also widespread among chickens as a subclinical infection.

Budgerigar fledgling disease has been reported from various aviaries in the United States, with mortalities ranging between 30 and 80%. Affected birds have full crops, die acutely, and exhibit abdominal distention and reddening of the skin. Postmortem examination reveals visceral changes such as hydropericardium, enlarged heart and liver, and swollen congested kidneys. On histologic examination, cells with enlarged nuclei containing inclusions are seen along with necrotic foci in several organs. By electron microscopy, polyomavirus virions can be visualized in the nuclei of epithelial cells, e.g., in renal tubules.

The virus has been isolated in budgerigar embryo fibroblasts inoculated with tissue homogenates from affected birds and can be adapted easily to growth in chicken embryo fibroblasts. The virus is similar to polyomaviruses of mammals, having a similar genome but a smaller large T antigen and a different organization of its origin of replication. Little similarity was observed by physical mapping with restriction endonucleases.

Further Reading

Campo, M. S. (1997). Bovine papillomavirus and cancer. *Vet. J.* **154**, 175–188.

Howley, P. M. (1996). Papillomaviruses: The viruses and their replication. *In* "Fields Virology" (B. N. Fields, D. M. Knipe, P. M. Howley, R. M. Chanock, J. L. Melnick, T. P. Monath, B. Roizman, and S. E. Straus, eds.), 3rd ed., pp. 2045–2076. Lippincott-Raven, Philadelphia, PA.

Olson, C. (1987). Animal papillomas: Historical perspectives. *In* "The Papovaviridae" (N. P. Salzman and P. M. Howley, eds.), vol. 2, pp. 39–49. Plenum, New York.

Osterhaus, A. D. M. E., and Moreno-Lopez, J. (1993). Papovaviruses. *In* "Virus Infections of Vertebrates" (J. B. McFerran and M. S. McNulty, eds.), vol. 4, pp. 147–151. Elsevier, Amsterdam.

Shah, K. V. (1996). Polyomaviruses. *In* "Fields Virology" (B. N. Fields, D. M. Knipe, P. M. Howley, R. M. Chanock, J. L. Melnick, T. P. Monath, B. Roizman, and S. E. Straus, eds.), 3rd ed., pp. 2027–2044. Lippincott-Raven, Philadelphia, PA.

Shah, K. V., and Howley, P. M. (1996). Papillomaviruses. *In* "Fields Virology" (B. N. Fields, D. M. Knipe, P. M. Howley, R. M. Chanock, J. L. Melnick, T. P. Monath, B. Roizman, and S. E. Straus, eds.), 3rd ed., pp. 2077–2110. Lippincott-Raven, Philadelphia, PA.

Vanselow, B. A., and Spradbrow, P. B. (1997). Equine and bovine papillomavirus infections. *In* "Virus Infections of Vertebrates" (M. J. Studdert, ed.), vol. 6, pp. 83–94. Elsevier, Amsterdam.

CHAPTER 21

Parvoviridae

Feline panleukopenia has been recognized for about 100 years, mink enteritis was first described in 1947, and canine parvovirus disease was recognized as a new nosologic entity in 1978. The parvoviruses that cause these diseases are closely related, the mink and canine viruses seemingly having arisen as host range mutants of the feline virus. The diseases in cats, mink, and dogs are remarkably similar, particularly in causing leukopenia and enteritis. In animals infected *in utero* or in the perinatal period, there may be generalized disease and sequelae; for example, when the feline virus infects the fetus or newborn kitten it produces cerebellar hypoplasia and when the canine virus infects the newborn pup it produces myocarditis.

Porcine parvovirus infection is usually subclinical in adult swine but causes important disease in the fetus. Goose parvovirus causes a lethal disease in goslings and there is another parvovirus that causes lethal disease in muscovy ducklings. Rodent parvoviruses, particularly minute virus of mice, are used as models in studies of the pathogenesis of certain fetal abnormalities and are common contaminants of cultured rodent cells and tumors. A human parvovirus, parvovirus B19, is the cause of a common exanthematous disease of children, erythema infectiosum, also called fifth disease, and hemolytic crisis in people with sickle cell disease. Parvoviruses have been isolated from chickens, rabbits, and an equine fetus, but their roles as pathogens in these species are not clear.

Properties of Parvoviruses

Classification

The family *Parvoviridae* comprises two subfamilies: the subfamily *Parvovirinae,* which contains viruses of vertebrates, and the subfamily *Densovirinae,* which contains viruses of insects that will not be discussed further. There are three genera in the subfamily *Parvovirinae:* the genus *Parvovirus,* the members of which infect vertebrates and replicate autonomously; the genus *Erythrovirus,* which includes human parvovirus B19 and a related virus of cynomolgus monkeys (*Macaca fascicularis*), which also replicate autonomously; and the genus *Dependovirus,* the members of which are called adeno-associated viruses because they are defective and unable to replicate except in the presence of a helper virus, usually an adenovirus.

Member viruses of the genus *Parvovirus* cause important diseases in swine, cats, dogs, mink, mice, rats, hamsters, geese, and ducks (Table 21.1). The original canine virus, called canine parvovirus 1 or minute virus of canines, is taxonomically distinct. The other canine virus, called canine parvovirus 2, is related closely to feline and mink viruses: (1) the canine virus can replicate in both canine and feline cells but the feline virus replicates only in feline cells; (2) feline and mink viruses are indistinguishable antigenically by

TABLE 21.1
Manifestations of Parvovirus Diseases in Animals[a]

VIRUS	DISEASE
Feline panleukopenia virus	Generalized neonatal disease, cerebellar hypoplasia, panleukopenia, enteritis
Canine parvovirus 1 (minute virus of canines)	Mild diarrhea
Canine parvovirus 2 (subtypes 2a and 2b)	Generalized neonatal disease, enteritis, myocarditis, leukopenia
Porcine parvovirus	Stillbirth, abortion, fetal death, mummification, infertility
Mink enteritis virus	Panleukopenia, enteritis
Aleutian disease virus of mink	Chronic immune complex disease, encephalopathy
Minute virus of mice	Congenital fetal malformations
Rat virus	Congenital fetal malformations
H-1 virus of rats	Congenital fetal malformations
Goose parvovirus	Hepatitis, myocarditis
Duck parvovirus	Hepatitis, myocarditis

[a] Parvoviruses have also been recovered from cattle and from rabbits, but under natural conditions are not known to cause disease in these species.

hemagglutination–inhibition and serum neutralization tests (canine parvovirus is distinguishable by these methods); and (3) the three viruses are distinguishable by genomic DNA sequencing. When parvoviruses are compared by sequencing, their phylogenetic interrelationships are as depicted in Figure 21.1. Since its emergence in 1978, canine parvovirus 2 has undergone further mutations affecting its antigenic and genetic properties—these changes are recognized as subtypes 2a and 2b and are depicted in Figure 21.2.

FIGURE 21.1.

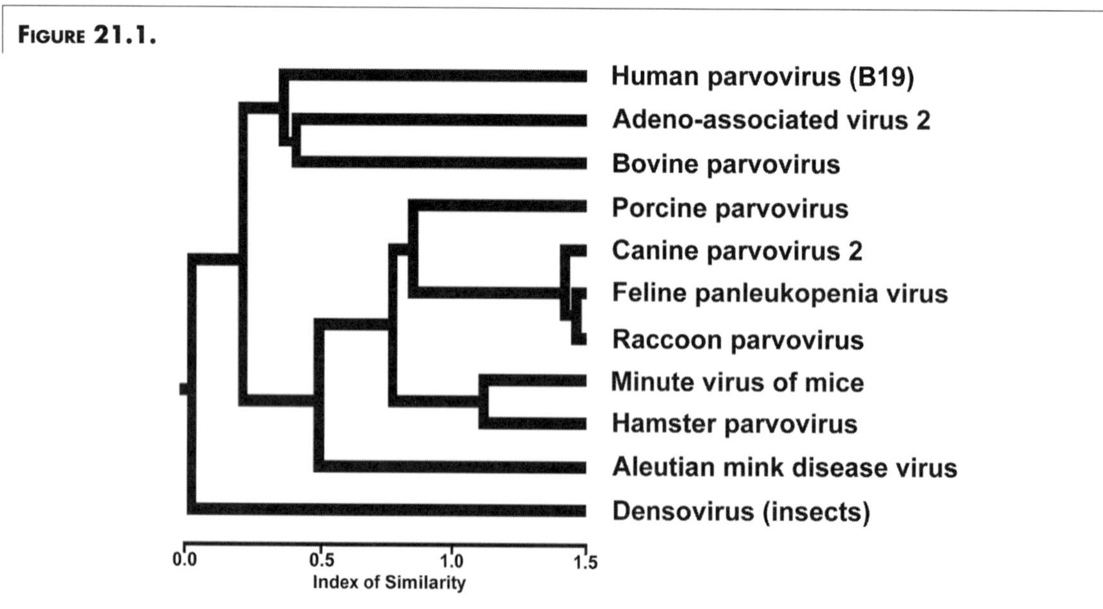

Phylogenetic interrelationships among the parvoviruses, presented as a general index of similarity of their genomic DNA sequences. (Courtesy of A. Simpson and M. G. Rossmann.)

FIGURE 21.2.

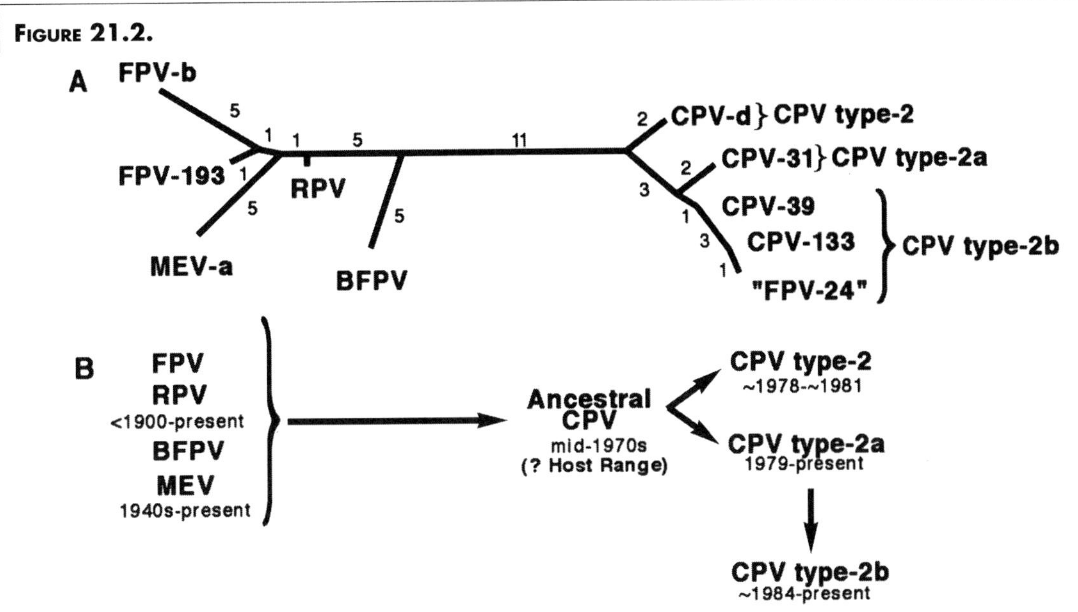

The evolution of the carnivore parvoviruses leading to the emergence of canine parvoviruses 2, 2a, and 2b. (A) Genetic diversity of the different viruses and the various variants of these viruses that are important in veterinary medicine (e.g., variants that must be covered by up-to-date vaccines) are founded in point mutations (nucleotide substitutions)—the length of the branches of the tree and the small numbers indicate the number of nucleotide differences between adjacent viruses. (B) This evolution has taken place in recent times; the latest, involving the emergence of canine parvovirus 2b from 2a, occurred around 1984. FPV, feline panleukopenia virus (numbers and letters indicate strains); MEV, mink enteritis virus; RPV, raccoon parvovirus; BFPV, blue fox parvovirus (an isolate made in Finland from an arctic fox); CPV, canine parvovirus; "FPV-24", a canine parvovirus 2b-like virus from a cat. (Courtesy of C. R. Parrish.)

Virion Properties

Parvovirus virions are nonenveloped, 25 nm in diameter, and have icosahedral symmetry (Figures 21.3). The surface features of the capsid revealed by X-ray crystallography include a hollow cylinder at each fivefold axis of symmetry that is surrounded by a circular depression (called the canyon), a prominent protrusion at each threefold axis of symmetry (called the spike), and a depression at each twofold axis of symmetry (called the dimple) (Figure 21.4). The determinants of the host range difference between feline and canine parvoviruses have been mapped to the spike, where there are just two amino acid differences between the two viruses.

The genome consists of a single molecule of linear single-stranded DNA, 5.2 kb in size (Figure 21.5). The complete nucleotide sequences of all important parvoviruses are available. Some parvoviruses encapsidate only the negative-sense DNA strand (e.g., canine parvovirus 2, minute virus of mice), whereas others encapsidate different proportions of either strand. The genome has 6 to 10 terminal palindromic sequences, enabling each end to form hairpin structures.

The capsid is composed of 60 molecules of VP2 protein (M_r 65,000), along with a few molecules of VP1 (M_r 84,000). VP1 and VP2 are formed by alternative splicing of the same mRNA, and the entire sequence of VP2 is encoded within the VP1 gene. A third structural protein, VP3, is formed only in "full" (DNA-containing) capsids by cleavage of 15–20 amino acids from the amino terminus of VP2. As determined by X-ray crystallography, the central structural motif of VP2 of canine parvovirus has an eight-stranded, antiparallel β-barrel motif as found in several other icosahedral viruses. The strands of the β-barrel are linked at each turn by four extensive loops; these loops form most of the outer surface of the virus particle and are responsible for the environmental stability of these viruses. Indeed, parvoviruses are extremely stable to environmental conditions (extremes of heat and pH); disinfection of contaminated premises using commercially available disinfectants is a major challenge.

Viral Replication

Viral replication takes place in the nucleus and requires host cell functions of late S phase or early G2 phase of the cell division cycle. This requirement for cycling cells

FIGURE 21.3.

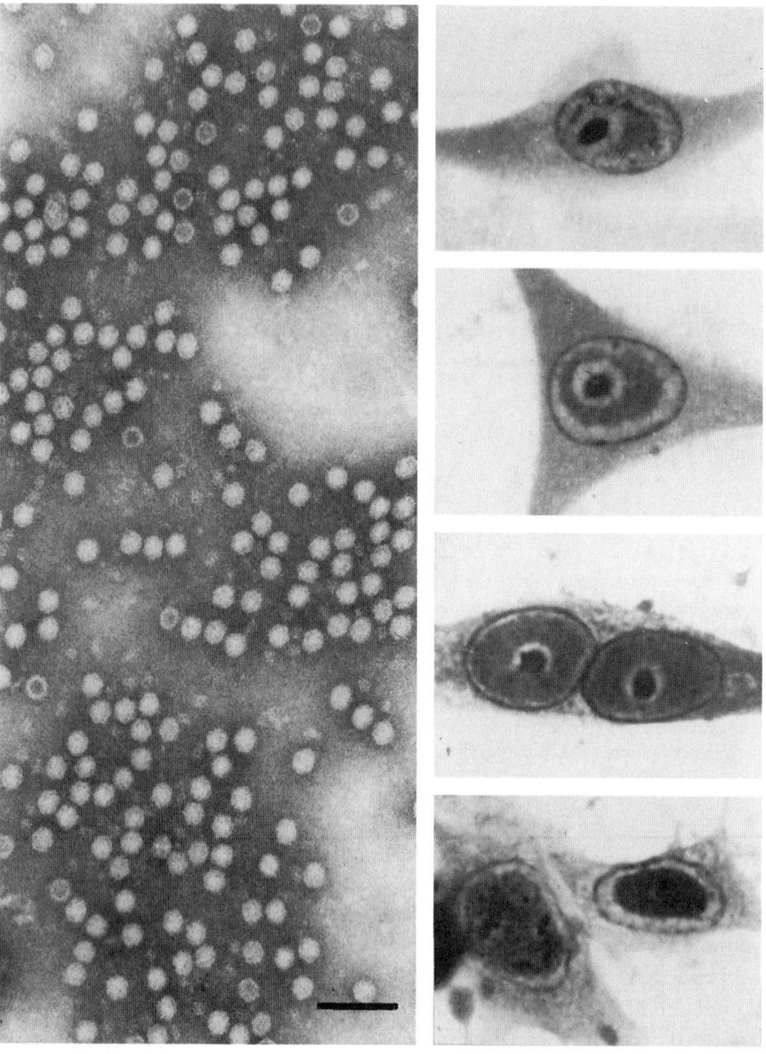

Family *Parvoviridae*, genus *Parvovirus*, canine parvovirus. (Left) Virions, negative stain electron microscopy. Bar 100 nm). (Right) Feline embryo cells infected with feline panleukopenia virus; the appearance of intranuclear inclusion bodies varies, becoming more dense as infection progresses. Hematoxylin and eosin. Magnification: ×800.

for viral replication is the basis for many aspects of the pathogenesis of parvovirus infections. In infections of the fetus (pig or cat) or newborn (dog or cat) where there is considerable cell division in many organs, the infection may be widespread; in older animals a narrower range of tissues is affected. Thus, the cerebellum is destroyed selectively in feline fetuses or kittens infected in the perinatal period, and the myocardium is damaged in pups and goslings. At all ages, the continuous division of cells in lymphoid tissues and the intestinal epithelium leads to the common occurrence of leukopenia and enteritis.

The requirement for cycling cells for viral replication indicates a viral requirement for host DNA replication machinery. Specifically, there is no polymerase enzyme in the virion itself nor does the virus encode any such enzyme. Instead, cellular DNA polymerase II is employed to transcribe viral DNA into a double-stranded DNA intermediate, which is then used as a template as other cellular enzymes catalyze the transcription of viral mRNAs. Alternative splicing patterns give rise to several mRNA species that are translated into a greater number of different proteins than the limited coding potential of the small genome might suggest. The

FIGURE 21.4.

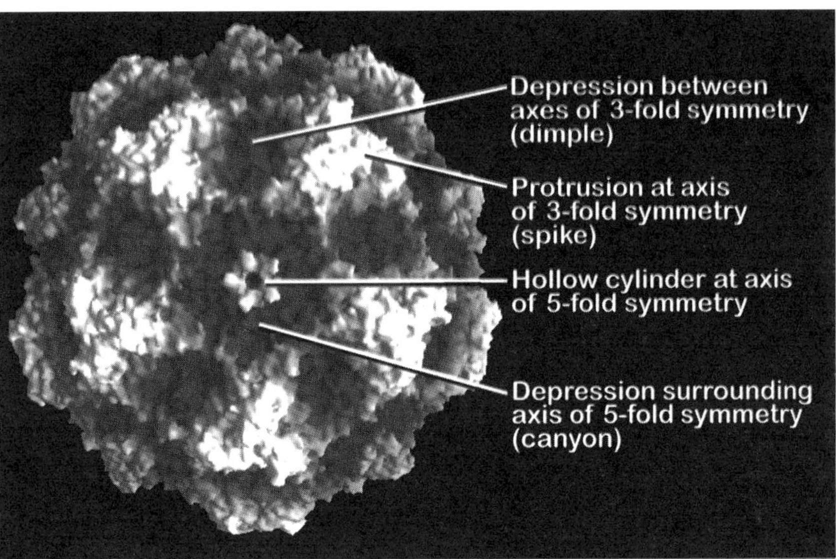

Canine parvovirus: virion model computer-generated from X-ray crystallographic data. The virion is centered on its axis of five-fold symmetry. Surface features include (1) a hollow cylinder at each axis of five-fold symmetry, (2) a depression surrounding the hollow cylinder (called the canyon), (3) a prominent protrusion at each axis of three-fold symmetry (called the spike), and (4) a depression at each axis of two-fold symmetry (called the dimple). The major host cell-binding ligand that determines the host range specificity of the virus is located on the spike (a minor determinant is located nearby). Host range differences between feline panleukopenia virus and canine parvovirus have been mapped to the spike, where there are just two amino acid differences between the two viruses. (Adapted from the work of C. R. Parrish, U. Truyen, J. S. Parker, and J.-Y. Sgro.)

most abundant mRNA, which is encoded in the 3′-half of the genome, directs the synthesis of the structural proteins. The nonstructural protein (NS1), encoded in the 5′-half of the genome, is also produced in very large amounts and serves a number of functions: (1) it binds to DNA and is required for viral DNA replication, (2) it serves as a helicase, (3) it serves as an endonuclease, and (4) it interferes with cellular DNA replication by producing nicks in cellular DNA. This latter activity leads to the arrest of the cell division cycle in S phase.

The mechanism of replication of the genome is amazingly complex (Figure 21.6). The 3′-terminal hairpins on the negative-sense DNA genome serve as a self-primer for the initiation of synthesis of a double-stranded circular DNA replicative intermediate. The detection of a dimeric form of the replicative intermediate, i.e., a concatemer of two covalently linked double-stranded forms, has led to a model in which the growing DNA strand replicates back on itself to produce a tetrameric form from which two complete positive strands and two complete negative strands are generated by a complicated series of reopening of circular forms, reinitiation of replication at transiently formed hairpins, and repeated single-strand endonuclease cleavages (Table 21.2).

TABLE 21.2
Properties of Parvoviruses

Three genera: *Parvovirus,* replication autonomous; *Dependovirus,* defective, requires helper adenovirus; and *Densovirus,* infects insects

Virions are icosahedral, 25 nm in diameter, and composed of 60 protein subunits

The genome is a single molecule of negative-sense, single-stranded DNA, 5.2 kb in size

Replication occurs in the nucleus of dividing cells; infection leads to large intranuclear inclusion bodies

Viruses are very stable, resisting 60°C for 60 minutes and pH 3 to pH 9

Most viruses hemagglutinate red blood cells

FIGURE 21.5.

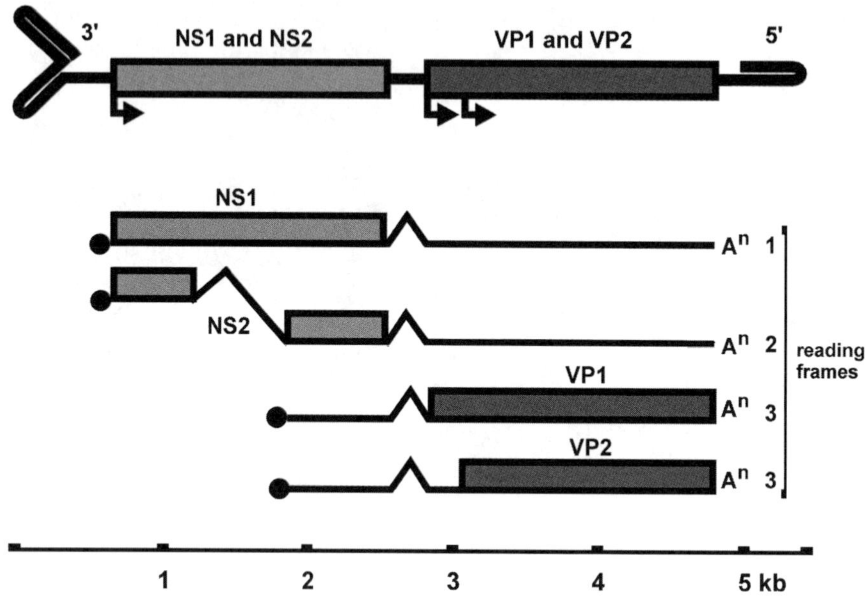

Genomic DNA of canine parvovirus and its transcription strategy. The genome has terminal palindromic sequences enabling each end to form hairpin structures; these structures serve as the origin of DNA replication and also facilitate encapsidation (packaging) of viral DNA within nascent virions. The 5′ ends of RNA transcripts are capped (black circles) and the 3′ ends are polyadenylated (A^n). VP1 and VP2, which are produced in very large amounts, are encoded in the same mRNA. They are formed by alternative initiation codons (arrowheads)—the entire sequence of VP2 is encoded within the VP1 gene. The nonstructural protein NS1, also produced in very large amounts, serves a number of functions: (1) it binds to DNA and is required for viral DNA replication, (2) it serves as a helicase, (3) it serves as an endonuclease, and (4) it interferes with cellular DNA replication, causing the arrest of the cell division cycle in the S phase. NS2, which is encoded in two open reading frames and is formed by splicing, also regulates viral gene expression. There is a remarkable diversity in transcription details (frameshifting, splicing, etc.) and products among the different parvoviruses that cannot be shown using any one virus as a model. (Courtesy of C. R. Parrish.)

Feline Panleukopenia

It is thought that all members of the family *Felidae* are susceptible to infection with feline panleukopenia virus, which occurs worldwide and is arguably the most important of all feline viral diseases.

Clinical Features

Feline panleukopenia is most common in kittens at about the time of weaning, but cats of all ages are susceptible (Table 21.3). The incubation period is about 5 days (range 2 to 10 days). At the onset of clinical signs, there is a profound leukopenia—there may be fewer than 100 white blood cells per cubic millimeter of blood. The severity of the disease and the mortality rate parallel the severity of the leukopenia—prognosis is grave if the white blood cell count falls below 1000 cells per cubic millimeter of blood. Clinical signs include fever (greater than 40°C), which persists for about 24 hours and during which, in the peracute form of the disease, death occurs. The temperature returns to normal and rises again on the third or fourth day of illness, at which time there is lassitude, inappetence, a rough coat, and repeated vomiting. A profuse, persistent, frequently bloody diarrhea develops on the third or fourth day of illness. Dehydration due to severe enteritis is a major contributing factor in the fatal outcome of the disease in many cats. Where the clinical course is more prolonged, dehydration is a major factor contributing to death, but most cats given adequate fluid therapy will recover.

Kittens that are infected from 2 weeks before to about 2 weeks after birth may develop cerebellar hypoplasia. Affected kittens are noticeably ataxic when they become ambulatory at about 3 weeks of age; they have a wide-based stance and move with exaggerated steps, tending to overshoot the mark and to pause and oscillate about an intended goal.

Figure 21.6.

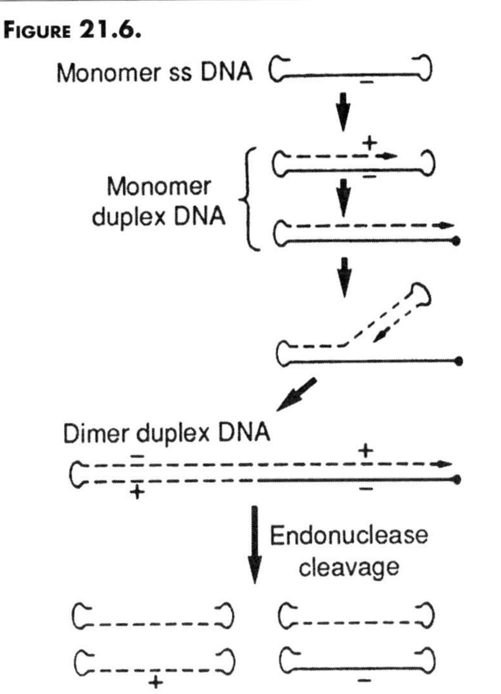

Parvovirus DNA replication—a highly simplified model. DNA replication involves a single-strand displacement mechanism. First, the 3′-terminal hairpins serve as a primer to initiate DNA synthesis; elongation leads to a double-stranded replicative intermediate (monomer duplex DNA) that is cross-linked covalently at one end by the terminal hairpin. A dimeric duplex form of the replicative intermediate, i.e., a concatemer of two covalently linked double-stranded forms, is synthesized from which two complete positive strands and two complete negative strands are generated by a complicated series of steps (reopening of circular forms, reinitiation of replication at transiently formed hairpins, repeated single-strand endonuclease cleavages, etc.). The presence of 3′-terminal hairpins on progeny negative-sense DNA strands favors their encapsidation.

Pathogenesis, Pathology, and Immunity

Following viral entry in the oropharynx, initial viral replication occurs in pharyngeal lymphoid tissue. From here the virus is distributed to other organs and tissues via the bloodstream. Cells that have appropriate receptors and are in the S phase of the cell cycle are infected and killed or prevented from entering mitosis. The characteristic profound leukopenia involves all white blood cell elements: lymphocytes, neutrophils, monocytes, and platelets. These cells are destroyed, both those present in the circulation and those in lymphoid organs, including the thymus, bone marrow, lymph nodes, spleen, and Peyer's patches. Resting peripheral leukocytes may be stimulated to proliferate, thereby becoming permissive for viral replication. Alternatively, the presence of virus bound to the surface of cells may render them targets for cytotoxic lysis.

Rapidly dividing intestinal epithelial cells in the crypts of Lieberkühn are very susceptible to infection. The loss of cells from villus tips continues in normal fashion, but the failure in replacing these cells with cells from the crypts leads to greatly shortened, nonabsorptive villi and hence to diarrhea. At necropsy, lesions in the small intestine are usually patchy in their distribution; the entire small intestine must be examined for evidence of congestion and thickening, which is visible from the serosal as well as the lumenal surface. Where enteritis has been present for several days before death the intestinal lesions are usually obvious, consisting of segmental thickening and necrosis; histologically, in addition to shortened and blunted intestinal villi, the crypts are dilated and distended with mucus and cell debris. Rarely, intranuclear inclusions may be found in cells near the base of the crypts. The lymph nodes may be enlarged and edematous and the bone marrow pale and fluid; histologically, there is evidence of widespread destruc-

Table 21.3

Relationship between Age of Host and Occurrence of Various Syndromes in Feline Panleukopenia and Canine Parvovirus Infection

Syndrome	Animal species	Age
Generalized neonatal disease	Cat and dog	2 to 12 days
Leukopenia/enteritis	Cat and dog	2 to 4 months
Enteritis	Cat and dog	4 to 12 months
Cerebellar hypoplasia	Cat	2 weeks before to 4 weeks after birth
Myocarditis	Dog	
Acute		3 to 8 weeks
Chronic		After 8 weeks

tion of lymphoid cells and massive neutrophil infiltrations into lymphoid tissues.

In fetuses infected during the last 2 weeks of pregnancy and the first 2 weeks of life, dramatic lesions are found in the external granular layer of the cerebellum—this is the basis for the cerebellar hypoplasia seen grossly at necropsy (Figure 21.7). During this period, cells of the external granular layer of the cerebellum normally undergo rapid division and migrate to form internal granular and Purkinje cell layers; this migration is arrested and affected kittens remain permanently ataxic.

Following natural infection in previously healthy cats there is a rapid immune response. Neutralizing antibody can be detected within 3 to 5 days of infection and may rise to very high levels. The presence of high titer antibody is correlated with protection, and immunity after natural infection appears to be lifelong. The titer of passively acquired antibody in kittens parallels the maternal antibody titer and is therefore quite variable, providing protection and compromising active immunization for only a few weeks or for as long as 22 weeks.

Laboratory Diagnosis

Clinical signs, hematological examination, and postmortem findings are characteristic and are used for a presumptive diagnosis. Confirmatory tests include (1) direct hemagglutination of swine or rhesus monkey red blood cells by virus present in suitably prepared fecal samples; (2) virus isolation in cell culture; (3) antigen-capture enzyme immunoassay or immunofluorescence for the detection of antigen in tissues; (4) and polymerase chain reaction assay for the detection of viral DNA in tissues. Serologic diagnosis is done by enzyme immunoassay or indirect immunofluorescence.

Epidemiology, Prevention, and Control

Feline panleukopenia virus is highly contagious. The virus may be acquired by direct contact with infected cats or via fomites (bedding, food dishes); fleas and humans may act as mechanical vectors. Virus is shed in the feces, vomitus, urine, and saliva. Recovered cats may excrete small amounts of virus for many months. Neither the exact duration of such excretion nor the underlying basis for persistent infection has been determined.

The stability of the virus and the very high rates of viral excretion (up to 10^9 ID_{50}/g of feces) result in high levels of environmental contamination, hence it may be extremely difficult to disinfect contaminated premises. The virus may be acquired from premises following the introduction of susceptible cats many months, even up to a year, after previously affected cats have been removed. The virus may also be carried a considerable distance on wind-blown fomites.

Vaccination is practiced universally with both attenuated virus and inactivated virus vaccines being used. When there are vaccine breaks, the usual problem is interference caused by maternal antibody (see section on canine parvovirus vaccination).

In large catteries, strict hygiene and quarantine of incoming cats are essential if the virus is to be excluded; cats should be held in isolation for several weeks before entry and sick cats should be removed

FIGURE 21.7.

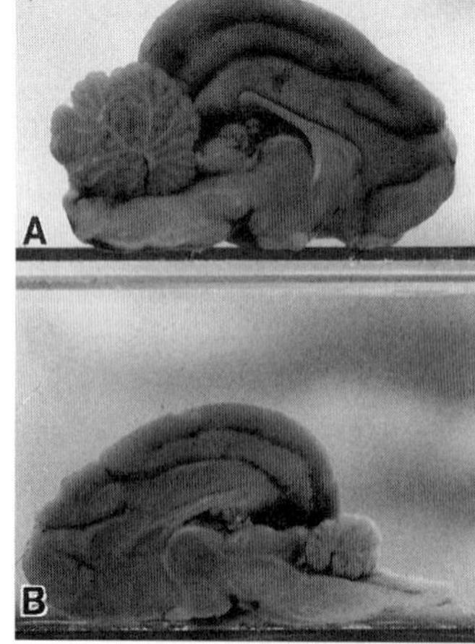

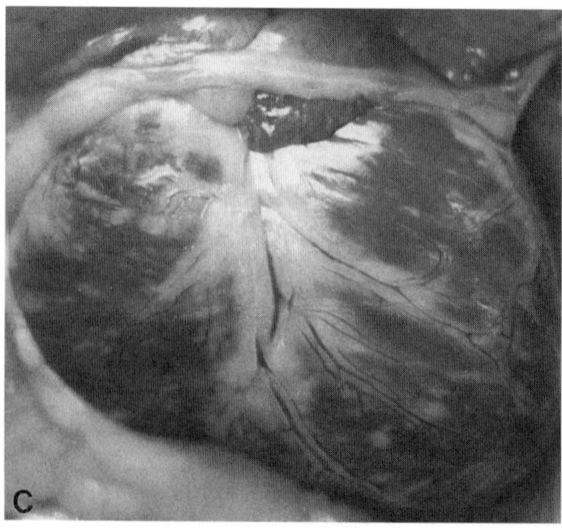

(A) Normal brain of a 3-month-old kitten. (B) Cerebellar hypoplasia caused by feline panleukopenia virus infection in a 3-month-old kitten. (C) Canine parvovirus myocarditis showing scar tissue throughout the myocardium. (Courtesy of C. Lenghaus.)

and isolated. For disinfection, 1% sodium hypochlorite applied to clean surfaces will destroy residual contaminating virus, but it is ineffective in the presence of much organic matter. Organic iodine-, phenolic, and glutaraldehyde-based disinfectants, together with thorough cleaning with detergent-based cleansers, are used in these circumstances.

Canine Parvovirus Disease

Canine parvovirus disease, caused by canine parvovirus 2, was first described in several countries in mid-1978. In one of the most dramatic events in the history of infectious diseases, the virus spread rapidly around the world, causing a virgin-soil pandemic that was marked by high incidence rates and high mortality rates. Retrospective serologic studies have indicated that the apparent immediate ancestor of the virus began infecting dogs in Europe during the early or mid-1970s; this conclusion is based on the finding of antibodies in sera from dogs in Greece, The Netherlands, and Belgium in 1974, 1976, and 1977, respectively. During 1978, antibodies were found in Japan, Australia, New Zealand, and the United States, suggesting that the virus spread around the world in less than 6 months. The stability of the virus, its efficient fecal–oral transmission, and the near-universal susceptibility of the dog population of the world accounted for this pandemic.

All members of the family *Canidae* (dogs, wolves, coyotes) are known to be susceptible to natural infection. In fact, canine parvovirus 2 has been a major problem in gray and red wolf conservation and captive breeding/release programs. In these programs, pups may be recaptured and vaccinated, but when programs are aimed at reintroducing wolves into very remote areas, this becomes unfeasible and represents an unsolved dilemma.

Canine parvovirus 2 is distinct genetically from a previously described parvovirus of dogs, minute virus of canines, which is now called canine parvovirus 1.

Clinical Features

Three distinct age-related canine parvovirus disease syndromes have been recognized in dogs (Table 21.3). The generalized neonatal disease syndrome is rare. The myocarditis syndrome is usually recognized in pups by sudden death, usually without preceding clinical signs. Even though damage to the myocardium may be extensive, some pups may survive with lifelong cardiac problems. This syndrome is seen predominantly in pups at 4 to 8 weeks of age and was common when the virus first emerged in 1978–1979. Today, the widespread use of vaccine and its induction or boosting of maternal antibody has made the generalized neonatal disease syndrome and the myocarditis syndrome less common.

The leukopenia/enteritis syndrome parallels that seen in cats precisely (however, the cerebellar hypoplasia seen in cats has not been recognized in dogs). The incidence of the leukopenia/enteritis syndrome has fallen since the virus first emerged, but is still an important cause of morbidity. This syndrome is seen most commonly in pups at 8 to 12 weeks of age. Vomiting is often the initial sign and can be severe and protracted. There is anorexia, lethargy, and diarrhea leading to rapid dehydration. The feces are often streaked with blood or frankly hemorrhagic and remain fluid until recovery or death. Death is uncommon except in young pups.

Pathogenesis, Pathology, and Immunity

The pathogenesis of canine parvovirus infection in the dog is similar to that of feline parvovirus infection in the cat, but the absence of cerebellar hypoplasia and the occurrence of myocarditis are somewhat surprising, as myocardial cells are not normally considered as rapidly dividing and thereby susceptible to viral infection (see Chapter 10). In the myocarditis syndrome, pulmonary edema is a prominent finding (Figure 21.7). Histologically, there is focal myocardial necrosis with fiber loss and intranuclear basophilic inclusions in cardiac muscle cells. In animals that survive for some time, there are extensive lymphocytic infiltrations and fibrosis in the myocardium.

In the panleukopenia/enteritis syndrome, there is intestinal congestion or blanching in pups that die acutely. When pups live longer the small intestines are thickened and inelastic and the serosal surface has a granular appearance. Histologically, there may be thymic atrophy and rarefaction of lymphoid follicles in the spleen and lymph nodes as well as necrosis of intestinal epithelial cells in the crypts of Lieberkühn with associated villus blunting.

Following natural infection there is a rapid immune response. Neutralizing antibodies can be detected within 3 to 5 days of infection and may rise rapidly to very high titers (Figure 21.8). Immunity after natural infection appears to be lifelong. Some maternal antibody may be transferred transplacentally but most is transferred with colostrum. The titer of natural passive antibody in pups parallels the maternal antibody titer and is therefore quite variable, providing protection for only a few weeks or for as long as 22 weeks (see later). Cytotoxic T cells are also generated after both infection and vaccination.

FIGURE 21.8.

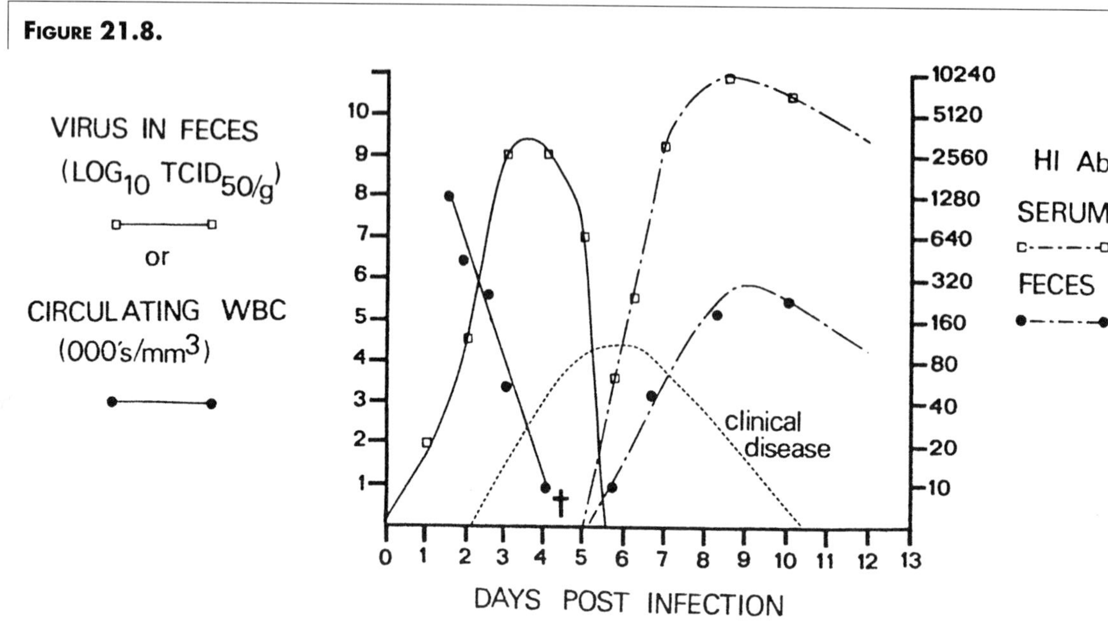

Overview of the pathogenesis of canine parvovirus enteritis/leukopenia syndrome. The time between infection and the onset of clinical signs is variable and may be delayed until 4–7 days postinfection, by which time an antibody response, which rises very rapidly to high titer, is underway and the virus can no longer be detected in feces. Severe disease and leukopenia are more likely to occur in pups 3–6 months of age that completely lack maternal antibody and are maintained under stressful conditions, such as may occur with early weaning, poor diet, and unhygenic conditions (e.g., in large breeding kennels, pet shops, shelters).

Laboratory Diagnosis

The simplest procedure for the laboratory diagnosis of canine parvovirus infection is hemagglutination of pig or rhesus monkey red blood cells (pH 6.5, 4°C) by virus present in fecal extracts. The specificity of this hemagglutination is determined by titrating the fecal specimen in parallel in the presence of normal and immune dog serum. Fecal samples from dogs with acute enteritis may contain up to 20,000 hemagglutinating units of virus, equivalent to about 10^9 virions, per gram. Electron microscopy, virus isolation, enzyme immunoassay, and amplification of viral DNA using the polymerase chain reaction are also used for laboratory confirmation of clinical diagnosis. Serologic diagnosis is also used in some settings, with the IgM-capture enzyme immunoassay used to determine recent infection.

Epidemiology, Prevention, and Control

When canine parvovirus disease was first recognized in 1978 the canine population throughout the world was completely susceptible. Generalized neonatal disease was recognized rarely but myocarditis and leukopenia/enteritis syndromes were common. Myocarditis is now rare, as passively acquired maternal antibody usually protects pups beyond the period when they are most susceptible. The leukopenia/enteritis syndrome is now endemic worldwide.

Problems in parvovirus disease prevention and control are encountered commonly in large, crowded breeding colonies where hygiene is difficult to maintain. Subclinical infection is more common in single dog households where pups are well cared for, again emphasizing the importance of hygiene and general good health in mitigating disease incidence and severity.

Attenuated virus vaccines and inactivated virus vaccines are used universally. Maternal antibody interference during immunization is the most common cause of vaccine failure in weanling pups. Pups receive about 10% of their maternal antibody via transplacental transfer and 90% through colostrum (the half-life of canine IgG is 10 days). It has been determined that an antibody titer of 80 or greater is protective (as measured by the hemagglutination–inhibition assay); thus pups born to bitches with low antibody titers may become susceptible to wild-type virus as early as 4–6 weeks after birth whereas pups born to bitches with high titers may be immune to infection for 12–20 weeks. Of course, pups born to seronegative bitches are susceptible at birth.

The level of maternal antibody that is able to protect pups against infection by the wild-type virus is different than that which interferes with an attenuated vaccine virus. In addition to the difference in their intrinsic properties, the wild virus may be introduced in a much larger dose. In effect, as maternally acquired immunity wanes, there is a 2- to 10-week time period when antibody titers have declined to levels where pups are susceptible to wild virus but are still refractory to immunization (Figure 21.9A). This gap can be determined precisely for each pup by serologic testing, but this is expensive and, in most instances, impractical (see Chapter 13). The usual approach is to administer pups a series of vaccinations at 2- to 3-week intervals, starting at 6 to 8 weeks of age and continuing through 18 to 20 weeks of age. Another approach has been to use very high-titered vaccine, thereby partially overcoming immune interference. Yet another approach has been to use vaccine containing a lower passage "hotter" virus, favoring more virus replication in the recipient and a better chance to overcome interference (Figure 21.9B).

Along with any vaccination strategy, it is also important to isolate pups to minimize their chances of becoming infected during their vulnerable period. It is

FIGURE 21.9.

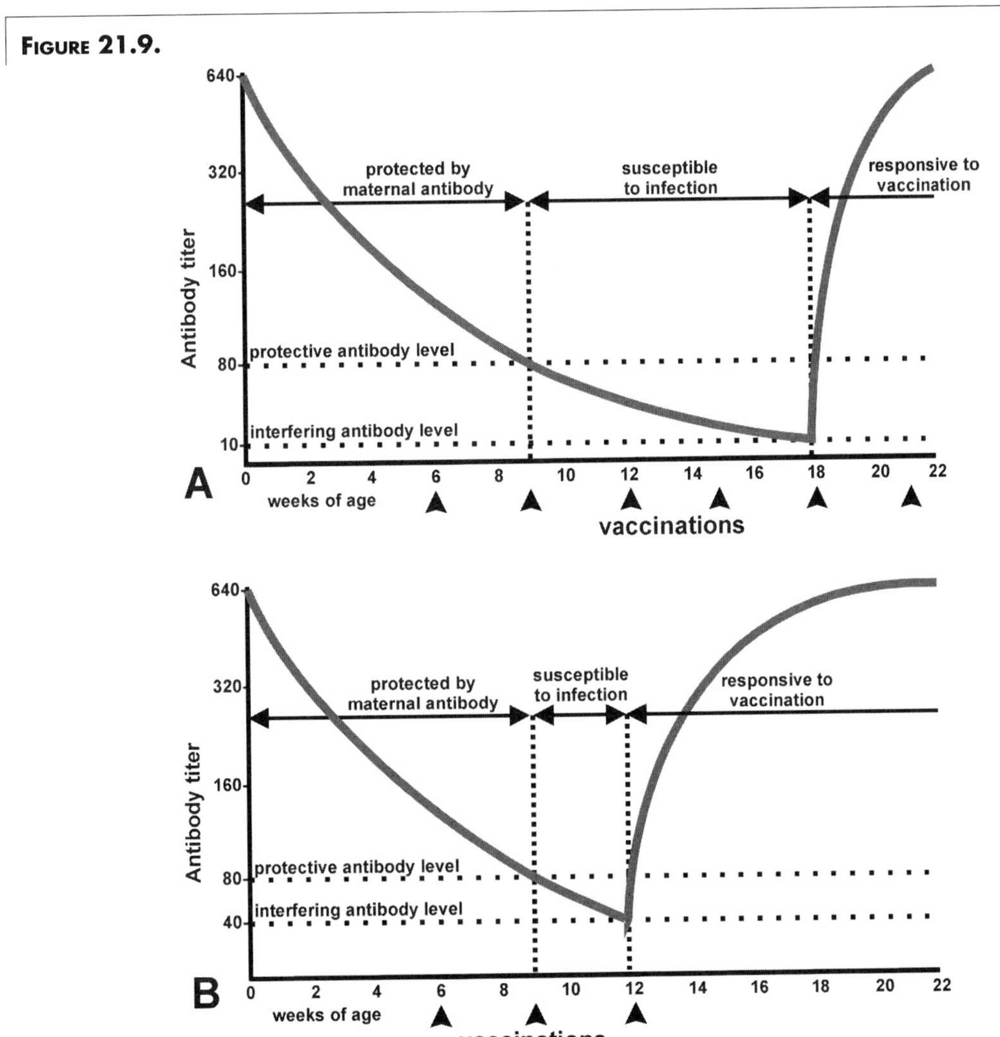

Most attenuated virus vaccines leave pups susceptible to canine parvovirus disease for several weeks between the time when maternal antibodies are no longer protective but still interfere with vaccination. (A) Decline of maternal antibody from a usual level, falling to a level where it is no longer protective (80) at 9 weeks of age and to a level where it no longer interferes with vaccination (10) at 18 weeks. To deal with this, six doses of vaccine, given at the times indicated (arrowheads), are recommended by some vaccine manufacturers. (B) With a high-titered or low-passage vaccine, the maternal antibody reaches a level where it no longer interferes with vaccination (40) at 12 weeks of age. The window of susceptibility is shortened and, as indicated, some vaccine manufacturers recommend only three doses of vaccine.

especially important in kennels to isolate pups from other dogs beginning at 4 to 6 weeks of age and continuing until their vaccination series is complete. In household settings, if true isolation is not possible, pups should at least be kept from areas where dogs congregate, such as parks and recreational sites.

Porcine Parvovirus Disease

Porcine parvovirus disease is the most important infectious cause of reproductive failure in swine throughout the world. When the virus is introduced into a fully susceptible breeding herd it can have devastating effects. Some manifestations of the disease are captured in its acronym, SMEDI (*s*tillbirth, *m*ummification, *e*mbryonic *d*eath, *i*nfertility). Infection has also been associated with respiratory disease and vesicular disease, neonatal systemic disease, and low fertility in boars. A single serotype of porcine parvovirus is recognized.

Clinical Features

The stage of gestation at which infection of gilts or sows occurs determines the particular clinical signs seen. The first sign of infection in a herd is frequently an increase in the number of gilts or sows returning to estrus 3 to 8 weeks after breeding. Some sows may remain "endocrinologically pregnant," not returning to estrus until after the expected time of farrowing. These clinical features are caused by fetal infection and resorption. Infection occurring later in gestation is evidenced at farrowing by smaller than normal litters and mummified fetuses. This is because only a proportion of fetuses are infected and the course of infection in those infected is variable (Figure 21.10). In addition, some piglets at birth may be smaller than normal or so weak that they do not survive. In young pigs, infection has been associated with a vesicular disease of the feet and mouth.

Pathogenesis, Pathology, and Immunity

It has been shown experimentally that it takes about 15 days after maternal infection for the virus to reach the fetus. When infection occurs less than 30 days after conception the fetus dies and is resorbed; when infection occurs between 30 and 70 days after conception the fetus is usually affected severely and is likely to die. Fetuses infected 70 or more days after conception, although frequently developing lesions, are affected less severely and mount an immune response (immunocompetence of swine fetuses starts at 55–70 days). The virus replicates in lymph nodes, tonsils, thymus, spleen, lungs, salivary glands, and other organs. It replicates well in peripheral blood lymphocytes (T, B, and null cells) and stimulates these cells to proliferate, thereby increasing the viral load. Monocytes and macrophages phagocytose virus, but then become infected and are destroyed, again contributing to the viral load and, in this case, to the leukopenia. More than with the other parvoviruses, swine parvovirus causes persistent infection with chronic shedding.

FIGURE 21.10.

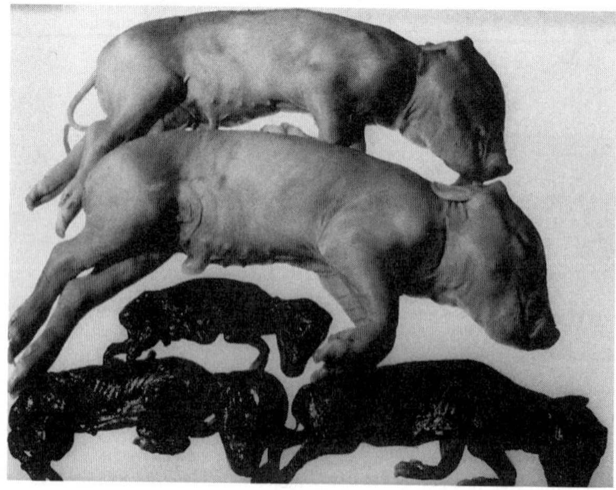

Porcine parvovirus infection. Infected fetuses in various stages of mummification compared with normal fetuses. (Courtesy of R. H. Johnston and H. S. Joo.)

Laboratory Diagnosis

Frozen-section immunofluorescence of fetal tissues using standardized reagents is rapid and reliable and the preferred diagnostic test. Hemagglutination of guinea pig red blood cells by virus contained in extracts of fetal tissues may also be used. The polymerase chain reaction is also used in some settings. Serologic tests are of limited value because the virus is so widespread. Diagnosis is difficult if infection occurs in the first few weeks of gestation; commonly, fetuses are resorbed completely and there may be no suspicion of the presence of the virus and hence no specimens collected for laboratory diagnosis.

Epidemiology, Prevention, and Control

Porcine parvovirus occurs worldwide and is endemic in many herds. Because the virus is so stable, premises may remain infected for many months even where hygiene appears satisfactory. Losses are most extreme if the virus is introduced into a seronegative herd at a time when many sows are pregnant. There is a possibility that some pigs infected *in utero* may survive as long-term immunotolerant carriers, but this is unproven. A large proportion of gilts are infected naturally before they conceive and hence are immune. Passively acquired maternal antibody can persist for up to 6 months or more, which interferes with active immunization following either natural infection or vaccination. Consequently, some gilts may conceive and then, when their residual maternal antibody levels decline to unprotective levels, their pregnancy is at very high risk. Boars play a significant role in the dissemination of virus in that they may shed virus in semen for protracted periods.

Vaccination is practiced widely as the only means of assuring that all gilts are protected. Inactivated and attenuated virus vaccines are used. There is often only a brief window of opportunity to immunize gilts that are bred before 7 months of age. The duration of immunity is uncertain, but there seems to be good immunological memory, and infection in vaccinated pigs rarely leads to fetal disease.

Mink Enteritis

Mink enteritis is caused by a parvovirus that is related very closely to feline panleukopenia virus. In mink, the virus produces a syndrome similar to that caused by feline panleukopenia virus in cats, except that cerebellar hypoplasia has not been recognized. The disease in mink appears to have been due to the introduction of feline panleukopenia virus into commercial mink farms in Ontario, Canada, in about 1946.

Aleutian Disease of Mink

Aleutian disease of mink is characterized by chronic plasmacytosis, hypergammaglobulinemia, splenomegaly, lymphadenopathy, glomerulonephritis, arteritis, focal hepatitis, anemia, and death. Lesions are the result of chronic infection in which there is a sustained production of virus and a failure to eliminate virus–antibody complexes. Despite extremely high levels of virus-specific antibody, the virus is not neutralized and infectious virus can be recovered from circulating immune complexes. Plasmacytosis, antibody-specific hypergammaglobulinemia and immune complex-mediated disease follow. The disease occurs primarily in mink that are homozygous for the recessive gene for a commercially desirable pale ("Aleutian") coat color. This gene is linked to a gene associated with a lysosomal abnormality of the Chediak-Higashi type, whereby following phagocytosis immune complexes are not destroyed. The level of the hypergammaglobulinemia is cyclical, with death occurring during a peak response, between 2 and 5 months after infection. Immunization of mink carrying the Aleutian gene with inactivated virus vaccine increases the severity of the disease. Conversely, immunosuppression diminishes the severity of the disease.

Rodent Parvovirus Diseases

Over 30 distinct parvoviruses, falling into 13 serogroups, have been isolated from laboratory rodents; of these, 3 occur endemically in rodent colonies: rat virus (also called Kilham's rat virus), H-1 virus of rats, and minute virus of mice. Serological surveys have indicated that these viruses are very common in laboratory colonies and that once they are present they are extremely difficult to eliminate. For example, in one survey, 38 of 44 conventional mouse colonies, 3 of 8 specific pathogen-free colonies, and none of 5 germ-free colonies were found to harbor minute virus of mice. There is also a high prevalence of minute virus of mice, rat virus, and H-1 virus in wild mice and rats, respectively. The major importance of these viruses is their confounding effect on research, especially immunology and cancer research. They are infamous for contaminating tumor cell lines and tumor virus stocks.

Rodent parvoviruses most commonly cause subclinical infection; they are, however, also the cause of fetal and neonatal abnormalities. As with the other parvoviruses, they destroy dividing cells—the result may be fetal death, runting, cerebellar hypoplasia and ataxia (as seen in kittens infected with feline panleukopenia virus), periodontal deformities, hemorrhagic encephalopathy (rat virus in rats), hepatitis, and enteritis.

One consequence of rodent parvovirus infections seems to be persistent viral carriage even in the presence of high titers of neutralizing antibody. This is important because some experimental manipulations, especially those that are immunosuppressive, may cause viral reactivation and recrudescent shedding. In turn, infection can be immunosuppressive (e.g., abrogating Tc lymphocyte responses and Th-dependent B cell responses), again affecting experiments in which infected animals are used unknowingly.

Diagnosis is based on serology (hemagglutination–inhibition, indirect immunofluroescence, neutralization, or enzyme immunoassay) and virus isolation in rodent cell cultures. Reference reagents are used to identify particular virus strains.

In laboratory colonies, these viruses are transmitted horizontally by contact and fomites. Young animals are protected by maternal antibody for the first few weeks of life, but then are infected via the oronasal route. As with other parvoviruses, rodent viruses are extremely stable and resistant to desiccation and may be carried between rodent colonies by unsuspected fomites (such as the shoes of laboratory animal veterinarians)—accordingly, the strictness of facility quarantine must be rigorous. When virus is detected, the colony must be depopulated, the premises disinfected meticulously, and new founding stock screened for the presence of virus and/or antibody. Unlike the situation in rebuilding a colony after eliminating some other rodent viruses, colonies that have had parvovirus infections cannot be repopulated by cesarean section and use of foster mothers. Importantly, serological surveillance is required to monitor the presence of rodent parvoviruses—this is required in the United States for mice and rats used in federally funded biomedical research.

Goose Parvovirus Disease

Goose parvovirus causes a lethal disease in goslings 8 to 30 days of age that is characterized by focal or diffuse hepatitis and widespread acute degeneration of striated, smooth, and cardiac muscle. Inclusion bodies are found mainly in the liver, but also in the spleen, myocardium, thymus, thyroid, and intestines. Control is achieved by the vaccination of laying geese with attenuated virus vaccine; maternal antibody persists in goslings for at least 4 weeks, the period of maximum vulnerability.

Duck Parvovirus Disease

A seemingly new disease affecting muscovy ducklings was described in France in 1989. Surprisingly, the virus is related most closely to adeno-associated virus 2. Mortality has been high and clinical and postmortem findings have resembled those found in geese infected with goose parvovirus. Ducks that survive are stunted and feathering is delayed. Effective vaccines, including one derived from VP2 and VP3 antigens expressed in a baculovirus system, are available.

Further Reading

Berns, K. I. (1996). Parvoviridae: The viruses and their replication. *In* "Fields Virology" (B. N. Fields, D. M. Knipe, P. M. Howley, R. M. Chanock, J. L. Melnick, T. P. Monath, B. Roizman, and S. E. Straus, eds.), 3rd ed., pp. 2173–2198. Lippincott-Raven, Philadelphia, PA.

Le Gall-Recule, G., Jestin, V., Chagnaud, P., Blanchard, P., and Jestin, A. (1997). Expression of muscovy duck parvovirus capsid proteins (VP2 and VP3) in a baculovirus expression system and demonstration of immunity induced by the recombinant proteins. *J. Gen. Virol.* 77, 2159–2163.

Mengeling, W. L. (1992). Porcine parvovirus infection. *In* "Diseases of Swine" (A. D. Leman, B. Straw, W. L. Mengeling, S. D'Allaire, and D. J. Taylor, eds.), 7th ed., pp. 299–325. Iowa State University Press, Ames.

Parker, J. S. L., and Parrish, C. R. (1997). Canine parvovirus host range is determined by the specific conformation of an additional region of the capsid. *J. Virol.* **71**, 9214–9222.

Parrish, C. R. (1990). Emergence, natural history, and variation of canine, mink and feline parvoviruses. *Adv. Virus Res.* **38**, 403–450.

Parrish, C. R. (1994). The emergence and evolution of canine parvovirus—an example of recent host range mutation. *Semin. Virol.* **5**, 121–132.

Parrish, C. R. (1995). Pathogenesis of feline panleukopenia virus and canine parvovirus. *Bailliere's Clin. Haematol.* **8**, 57–71.

Tijssen, P., ed. (1990). "Handbook of Parvoviruses," Vol. 1 and 2. CRC Press, Boca Raton, FL.

Truyen, U., Gruenberg, A., Chang, S. F., Obermaier, B., Veijalainen, P., and Parrish, C. R. (1995). Evolution of the feline subgroup parvoviruses and the control of canine host range *in vivo*. *J. Virol.* **69**, 4702–4710.

Tsao, J., Chapman, M. S., Agbandje, M., Keller, W., Smith, K., Wu, M. L., Smith, T. J., Rossman, M. G., Compans, R. W., and Parrish, C. R. (1991). The three-dimensional structure of canine parvovirus and its functional implications. *Science* **251**, 1456–1464.

CHAPTER 22

Circoviridae

The family *Circoviridae* was established recently after several previously unclassified viruses were found to share common physicochemical and genomic properties. The family presently includes psittacine beak and feather disease virus, porcine circovirus, and chicken anemia virus. Curiously, several plant viruses share the same properties and are included in the family. These are the smallest known viruses of vertebrates and of plants.

Properties of Circoviruses

Classification

The member viruses of the family *Circoviridae* have somewhat similar virion and genome properties, but are ecologically, biologically, and antigenically quite distinct—in fact, there are no common antigenic determinants and no sequence homology between the viruses. Presently, the family contains one genus, *Circovirus,* with chicken anemia virus as the type virus and psittacine beak and feather disease virus and two porcine circoviruses as members. However, it is being suggested on the basis of recent sequencing studies that there should be at least two genera—porcine circovirus and psittacine beak and feather disease virus employ an ambisense transcription strategy but chicken anemia virus, which is also larger, does not. Virus-like particles resembling circoviruses have been visualized by electron microscopy in diagnostic specimens from other host species, e.g., in cattle feces. They have not been isolated and their role in animal disease is unknown.

Although the viruses of vertebrates share no common antigenic determinants or genomic sequence homologies, surprisingly, one protein (M_r 35,700) of porcine circovirus is quite similar to a homologue in some plant circoviruses that have multipartite genomes, i.e., viruses that encapsidate each of their genomic segments in separate particles. This observation raises questions as to the origin of the circoviruses.

Virion Properties

Circovirus virions are nonenveloped, spherical in outline, with icosahedral symmetry, 17–22 nm in diameter (psittacine beak and feather disease virus and porcine circovirus are 17 nm in diameter and are the smallest viruses of vertebrates known; chicken anemia virus is 22 nm in diameter) (Figure 22.1). Characteristically, virions often appear in infected cells and free in diagnostic specimens in rather stable linear arrays—"strings of pearls." The genome consists of a single molecule of circular (covalently closed ends) single-stranded ambisense or positive-sense DNA, 1.7–2.3 kb in size (Figure 22.2). The complete sequences of porcine circovirus (1759 nucleotides), psittacine beak and feather disease virus (1993 nucleotides), and chicken anemia virus (2319 nucleotides) have been determined.

Psittacine beak and feather disease virus and porcine circovirus, but not chicken anemia virus, employ an ambisense transcription strategy, i.e., some genes are encoded in the viral sense DNA and others in the complementary strand (Figure 22.2). Chicken anemia virus genes are all encoded in the positive-sense strand. Chicken anemia virus has three open reading frames, each encoding a protein found in virions; one is the major capsid protein (M_r 52,000)

FIGURE 22.1.

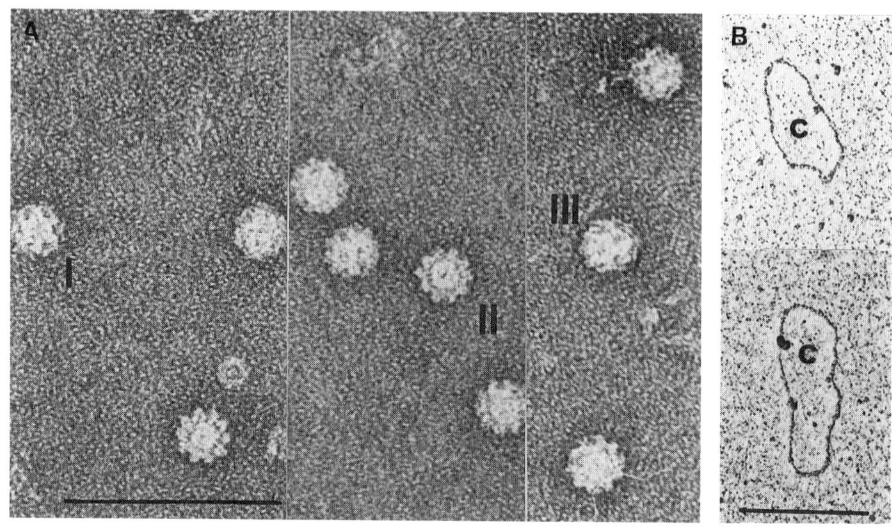

(A) Virions of chicken anemia virus as seen by negative staining. Bar 100 nm. (B) Kleinschmidt preparation showing the circular DNA of chicken anemia virus. Bar 50 nm. (Courtesy of R. Lurz and H. Gelderblom.)

and another (called apotin, M_r 13,000) by itself induces apoptosis of T lymphocytes and is considered an important factor in the pathogenesis of infections in chickens. Psittacine beak and feather disease virus has three open reading frames and porcine circovirus has four; in each case there is one major capsid protein. The viruses are very stable in the environment; they resist heating at 60°C for 30 minutes.

Viral Replication

Viral replication occurs in the nucleus and, similar to parvoviruses, probably depends on cellular proteins produced during the S phase of the cell cycle. The double-stranded DNA replicative intermediates of porcine circovirus and chicken anemia virus are infectious. Replication of the genome is believed to occur via a rolling

FIGURE 22.2.

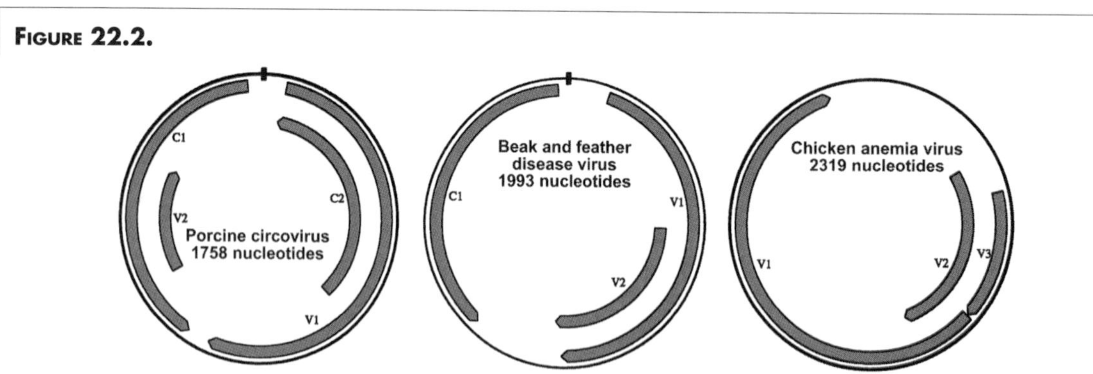

The genome of three circoviruses, psittacine beak and feather disease virus, porcine circovirus, and chicken anemia virus. The outer circles represent the genomes; stem-loop structures, represented by boxes at the top of the circular DNAs, are concerned with the initiation and termination of transcription. Open reading frames on the viral sense DNA strands are labeled as V1, V2, and so on; those on the complementary strands as C1, C2, and so on. The outer partial circles represent map positions of the three major open reading frames coding for VP1, VP2, and VP3; transcription start sites for the three proteins are at nucleotides 386, 486, and 853, respectively, and the positions of the stop codons are also indicated. [From F. D. Niagro, A. N. Forsthoefel, R. P. Lawther, L. Kamalanathan, B. W. Ritchie, K. S. Latrimer, and P. D. Lukert. Beak and feather disease virus and porcine circovirus genomes: Intermediates between the geminiviruses and plant circoviruses. *Arch. Virol.* (1998) **143,** 1723–1744.]

Table 22.1
Properties of Circoviruses

Virions are nonenveloped, spherical in outline, with icosahedral symmetry, 17–22 nm in diameter (psittacine beak and feather disease virus and porcine circovirus are 17 nm in diameter; chicken anemia virus is 22 nm in diameter)
Virions often appear in infected cells and free in diagnostic specimens in rather stable linear arrays—"strings of pearls"
The genome consists of a single molecule of circular (covalently closed ends) single-stranded ambisense or positive-sense DNA, 1.7–2.3 kb in size
Chicken anemia virus codes for a protein that induces apoptosis in T lymphocytes of chickens
Replication takes place in the nucleus of cycling cells, producing large intranuclear inclusion bodies
Virions are very stable, resisting 60°C for 30 minutes and pH 3 to pH 9

circle that originates at a stem-loop structure. In chicken anemia virus, one product of translation is a polyprotein that is cleaved to form mature proteins (Figure 22.2) (Table 22.1).

Psittacine Beak and Feather Disease

It had long been known that many species of Australian parrots undergo permanent loss of feathers and develop beak and claw deformities when in captivity. In 1984, thin section electron microscopy of affected tissues from such birds revealed large numbers of virions that were later found to resemble those of porcine circovirus in size and genome structure.

Clinical Features

Psittacine beak and feather disease is a debilitating disease of cockatoos, parrots, and budgerigars. Although principally a disease of cockatoos, many other psittacine species are susceptible. The natural infection occurs primarily in birds less than 5 years of age, most often in young birds during first feather formation. Typical findings include feather loss, abnormal pin feathers (constricted, clubbed, or stunted), abnormal mature feathers (blood in shaft), and various beak abnormalities (Figure 22.3). Beaks are described as shiny, overgrown, broken, or with palatine necrosis. Birds may have feather lesions, beak lesions, or both.

Pathogenesis, Pathology, and Immunity

The disease can be reproduced experimentally by exposing psittacine birds to homogenates of feather follicles from affected birds. Basophilic intracytoplasmic inclusions are found in follicular epithelium, which by electron microscopy contain masses of virions. The disease is relentlessly progressive; some birds die after the first appearance of malformed feathers or beak whereas others may live for years in a featherless state. Immunosuppression is part of the syndrome, so affected birds are often also infected and damaged by opportunistic pathogens.

Laboratory Diagnosis

Diagnosis is based on gross appearance of the bird and biopsy of affected feather follicles, which by histopathologic examination contain basophilic intracytoplasmic inclusion bodies. Electron microscopy is used for confirmation of the diagnosis.

Epidemiology, Prevention, and Control

The contagious nature of psittacine beak and feather disease and its persistent, progressive course may lead to requests for euthanasia of infected birds. Strict hygiene, screening protocols, and lengthy quarantines are used in cockatoo breeding colonies to prevent introduction of the virus.

Chicken Anemia Virus Disease

Chicken anemia virus disease was first recognized in Japan in 1979; it is now known to occur worldwide and is a problem in all countries with industrial poultry industries. The virus is not known to infect birds other than chickens and only a single serotype has been recognized.

Clinical Features

Chicken anemia virus disease is an acute, immunosuppressive disease of young chickens characterized by anorexia, lethargy, depression, anemia, atrophy or hypoplasia of lymphoid organs, cutaneous, subcutaneous and intramuscular hemorrhages, and increased mortality. Disease occurs in chicks hatched to silently infected breeder hens that have been infected as adults. At 2–3

FIGURE 22.3.

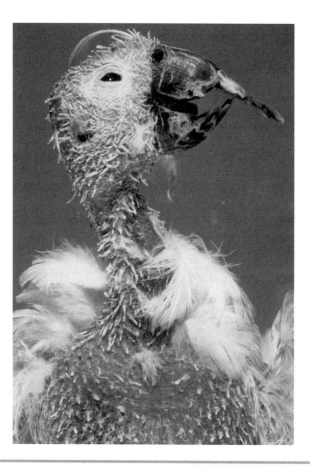

Psittacine beak and feather disease. There is loss of feathers and beak abnormalities due to the destruction of rapidly dividing cells at the base of these structures that are responsible for the continuous replacement and form of the beak and feathers throughout life. (Courtesy of D. Pass.)

weeks of age chicks become anorectic, lethargic, depressed, and pale. They are anemic and develop bone marrow aplasia and atrophy of the thymus, bursa of Fabricius, and spleen. Disease is most severe in chicks that are also infected with other viruses such as avian reoviruses, avian adenoviruses, reticuloendotheliosis virus, Marek's disease virus, or infectious bursal disease virus. There is usually no illness or loss of egg production when adult chickens are infected.

Pathogenesis, Pathology, and Immunity

When 1-day-old susceptible chicks are inoculated with the virus, viremia occurs within 24 hours and virus can be recovered from most organs and rectal contents for up to 35 days. Anemia results from decreased erythropoiesis. Packed cell volumes are low and blood smears often reveal anemia and leukopenia. Blood may be watery and clot slowly. Mortality rates usually are about 10%, but may be higher than 50%. Histologically, there is depletion of lymphoid cells in all lymphoid organs. Secondary bacterial infection is common. Age resistance to disease (not infection) begins at about 1 week of age and is complete by 2 weeks after hatching. However, the protective effects of maternal antibody and age resistance can be overcome where there is coinfection with immunosuppressive viruses. Infection with chicken anemia virus has been shown to suppress the immune system of chickens, a finding that helps explain why dual infections involving the virus and other avian pathogens are often more severe than would otherwise be expected.

Laboratory Diagnosis

A presumptive diagnosis is based on history, clinical signs, and gross and microscopic pathologic findings. Confirmatory diagnosis requires virus isolation, which is usually done in MDCC-MSB1 cells (a Marek's disease tumor-derived lymphoblastoid cell line) or in 1-day-old chicks or chick embryos (which must be virus and antibody negative). Because the virus is noncytopathic in low passage, immunologic methods must be used to determine the presence of virus. Serologic methods include indirect immunofluorescence and virus neutralization. Electron microscopy is also used to detect virions in chick tissues or blood.

Epidemiology, Prevention, and Control

Chicken anemia virus is transmitted horizontally by direct contact and contaminated fomites and vertically through the egg. Breeder flocks may become infected before they begin to lay fertile eggs; in this case the virus is transmitted vertically for as long as the hen is viremic. If hens are seropositive, maternal antibody generally protects chicks from disease but not from infection. Many flocks of otherwise specific pathogen-free chickens carry chicken anemia virus.

A vaccine has been developed and is available in Germany, but not in many other countries. In some areas, young breeder hens are infected deliberately with wild virus by adding crude homogenates of tissues from affected chickens to drinking water—this ensures infection and seroconversion before hens begin to lay eggs—but this procedure is not recommended by most authorities. Because severe disease results from coinfection with immunosuppressive viruses, control of each of such pathogens is important.

Porcine Circovirus Infection

Porcine circovirus 1 was first isolated in Germany in 1974 from a pig kidney cell line (PK15) infected persistently with this virus. Serologic evidence indicates that the virus is widespread in swine populations wherever it has been searched for. Of various animals tested, only domestic swine, minipigs, and wild boars have antibodies. Although early investigation suggested that the virus may be nonpathogenic for pigs, recent isolation of the virus from stillborn piglets implicates the virus as a possible fetal pathogen.

Porcine circovirus 2, an antigenically distinct virus originally isolated in France in 1997, has been isolated from young pigs with wasting disease syndromes in Canada, the United States, Spain, Denmark, and Northern Ireland. By sequence analysis, isolates of this virus from different countries are 96% similar but less than 80% similar to porcine circovirus 1.

Further Reading

Allan, G., Meehan, B., Todd, D., Kennedy, S., McNeilly, F., Ellis, J. Clark, E. G., Harding, J., Espuna, E., Botner, A., and Charreyre, C. (1998). Novel porcine circoviruses from pigs with wasting desease syndromes. *Vet. Rec.* **142,** 467.

Calnek, B. W., and Barnes, H. J., eds. (1998). "Diseases of Poultry," 10th ed. Iowa State University Press, Ames.

McNulty, M. S., McIlroy, S. G., Bruce, D. W., and Todd, D. (1991). Economic effects of subclinical chicken anemia agent infection in broiler chickens. *Avian Dis.* **35,** 263–268.

Meehan, B. M., Greelan, J. L., McNulty, M. S., and Todd, D. (1997). Sequence of porcine circovirus DNA: Affinities with plant circoviruses. *J. Gen. Virol.* **78,** 221–227.

Niagro, F. D., Forsthoefel, A. N., Lawther, R. P., Kamalanathan, L., Ritchie, B. W., Latrimer, K. S., and Lukert, P. D. (1998). Beak and feather disease virus and porcine circovirus genomes: Intermediates between the geminiviruses and plant circoviruses. *Arch. Virol.* **143,** 1723–1744.

Noteborn, M. H. M., de Boer, G. E., van Roozelaar, D. J., Karreman, C., Kranenburg, O., Vos, J. G., Jeurissen, S. H. M., Hoeben, R. C., Zanlema, A., Koch, G., van Ormondt, H., and van der Eb, A. J. (1991). Characterization of chicken anemia agent virus DNA that contains all elements for the infectious replication cycle. *J. Virol.* **65,** 3131–3138.

Ritchie, B., Niagro, F., Lukert, P., Steffens, W., and Latimer, K. (1989). Characterization of a new virus from cockatoos with psittacine beak and feather disease. *Virology* **171,** 83–88.

Tischer, I., Gelderblom, H., Vetterman, W., and Koch, M. (1982). A very small porcine virus with circular single-stranded DNA. *Nature (London)* **295,** 64–66.

Todd, D. (1995). The genome of chicken anemia virus. *Avian Pathol.* **24,** 349–363.

Todd, D., Niagro, F., Ritchie, B., Curran, W., Alan, G., Lukert, P., Latimer, K., and McNulty, M. (1991). Comparison of three animal viruses with circular single-stranded DNA genomes. *Arch. Virol.* **117,** 129–135.

CHAPTER 23

Retroviridae

Diseases caused by retroviruses have long been important in veterinary medicine. The veterinarians Ellerman and Bang in Denmark in 1908 and the medical pathologist Rous in the United States in 1911 demonstrated that avian leukosis and avian sarcoma could be transmitted from one chicken to another by inoculation of cell-free filtrates derived from tumor tissues obtained from diseased birds. The two related viruses—avian leukosis and avian sarcoma viruses—are prototypic of the etiologic agents of similar infectious malignant tumors now recognized in many other animal species, including cattle, cats, mice, and primates. These viruses are now classified as members of the family *Retroviridae,* a large family that includes many viruses of veterinary importance. The name *retro* (reverse, backward) derives from the reverse transcriptase (RNA-dependent DNA polymerase) that is found within the virions of all members of the family. Because the recognition that a number of human diseases, including leukemias and, most notably, acquired immunodeficiency disease (AIDS), are caused by retroviruses, no group of animal viruses has been the subject of such intense study. The enormous tragedy of human AIDS necessitates that such intense study be continued and, as begun by Ellerman and Bang, the comparative aspects of retrovirus diseases in animals and humans in such studies continue to be utilized for the advance of veterinary as well as medical science (see Chapter 1).

Properties of Retroviruses

Classification

The family *Retroviridae* is subdivided into seven genera: the genus *Alpharetrovirus,* comprising the avian type C retroviruses, such as avian leukosis virus; the genus *Betaretrovirus,* comprising the mammalian type B and type D retroviruses, such as mouse mammary tumor virus and Mason–Pfizer monkey virus; the genus *Gammaretrovirus,* comprising the mammalian and reptilian type C retroviruses, such as murine leukemia virus; the genus *Deltaretrovirus,* comprising the bovine leukemia and human T lymphotropic viruses; the genus *Epsilonretrovirus,* comprising the fish retroviruses, such as walleye epidermal sarcoma virus; the genus *Lentivirus,* comprising several important pathogens, including human immunodeficiency viruses 1 and 2, several simian immunodeficiency viruses (African green monkey, sooty mangabey, stump-tailed macaque, pig-tailed macaque, Rhesus, chimpanzee, and mandrill viruses), equine infectious anemia virus, maedi/visna virus, caprine arthritis–encephalitis virus, feline immunodeficiency virus, and bovine immunodeficiency virus; and the genus *Spumavirus,* comprising the foamy viruses (Table 23.1). The spumaviruses are not known to be pathogenic and have been recognized only when they are found in cultured cells.

The first classification of the retroviruses was based on their host species and on virion morphology and morphogenesis. Four types of particle, designated A, B, C, and D, were recognized and the viruses were classified accordingly—elements of this classification are still found in the way the various viruses are described. For example, type C retrovirus morphogenesis involves the formation at the cell membrane of distinctive crescent-shaped nascent nucleocapsids (hence the name *type C retrovirus*). More recently, the characterization of virion RNA has been used in the classification of the viruses: virion RNAs of different oncogenic retroviruses from the same species of animal show extensive homologies, whereas those of different species (e.g., chicken, cow, cat, and mouse) show virtually no sequence identity.

The antigenic relationships between different retroviruses are complicated. Various envelope glycoprotein epitopes are type specific, whereas others are strain specific; antibodies to the envelope glycoproteins neutralize viral infectivity. Core protein epitopes specified by the *gag* gene are common to the retroviruses of particular animal species, i.e., they are group specific. Some epitopes (e.g., those of reverse transcriptases) are shared by viruses associated with several animal species (interspecies antigens), but are distinguishable between avian and mammalian type C retroviruses. The internal proteins of different lentiviruses (*gag* and *pol* gene products) show extensive, but again complex patterns of cross-reactivity.

Table 23.1
Retrovirus of Animals

Genus	Virus
Alpharetrovirus	Avian leukosis viruses, avian carcinoma viruses, avian sarcoma viruses, avian myeloblastosis viruses, Rous sarcoma virus, duck spleen necrosis virus
Betaretrovirus	Mouse mammary tumor virus, ovine pulmonary adenomatosis virus (Jaagsiekte), Mason–Pfizer monkey virus, simian type D virus 1, langur type D virus, squirrel monkey type D virus
Gammaretrovirus	Feline leukemia virus, feline sarcoma viruses, porcine type C virus, many murine leukemia viruses, many murine sarcoma viruses, gibbon ape leukemia virus, woolly monkey sarcoma virus, guinea pig type C virus, viper type C virus (and avian reticuloendotheliosis viruses)
Deltaretrovirus	Bovine leukemia virus, human T lymphotropic viruses 1 and 2, simian T lymphotropic viruses
Epsilonretrovirus	Walleye dermal sarcoma virus, walleye epidermal hyperplasia viruses 1 and 2
Lentivirus	Human immunodeficiency viruses 1 and 2, simian immunodeficiency viruses (African green monkey, sooty mangabey, stump-tailed macaque, pig-tailed macaque, rhesus macaque, chimpanzee, and mandrill viruses), maedi/visna virus, caprine arthritis–encephalitis virus, feline immunodeficiency virus, equine infectious anemia virus, bovine immunodeficiency virus
Spumavirus	Bovine, feline, simian, and human foamy viruses (which are a problem when they contaminate cultured cells but are not known to cause disease)

Virion Properties

Retrovirus virions are enveloped, 80–100 nm in diameter, and have a unique three-layered structure (Figures 23.1, 23.2, and 23.3). Innermost is the genome–nucleoprotein complex, which includes about 30 molecules of reverse transcriptase, and has helical symmetry. This structure is enclosed within an icosahedral capsid, about 60 nm in diameter, which in turn is surrounded by a host cell membrane-derived envelope from which glycoprotein peplomers project. The lentiviruses bear approximately 72 knob-like peplomers, each about 10 nm long with an ovoid distal knob.

The genome is diploid, consisting of an inverted dimer of two molecules of linear positive-sense, single-stranded RNA; each monomer is 7–11 kb in size and has a 3′-polyadenylated tail and a 5′-cap; details of the organization of the genomes of the various viruses vary widely, as shown in Figure 23.4.

The retrovirus genome is unique in several respects:

FIGURE 23.1.

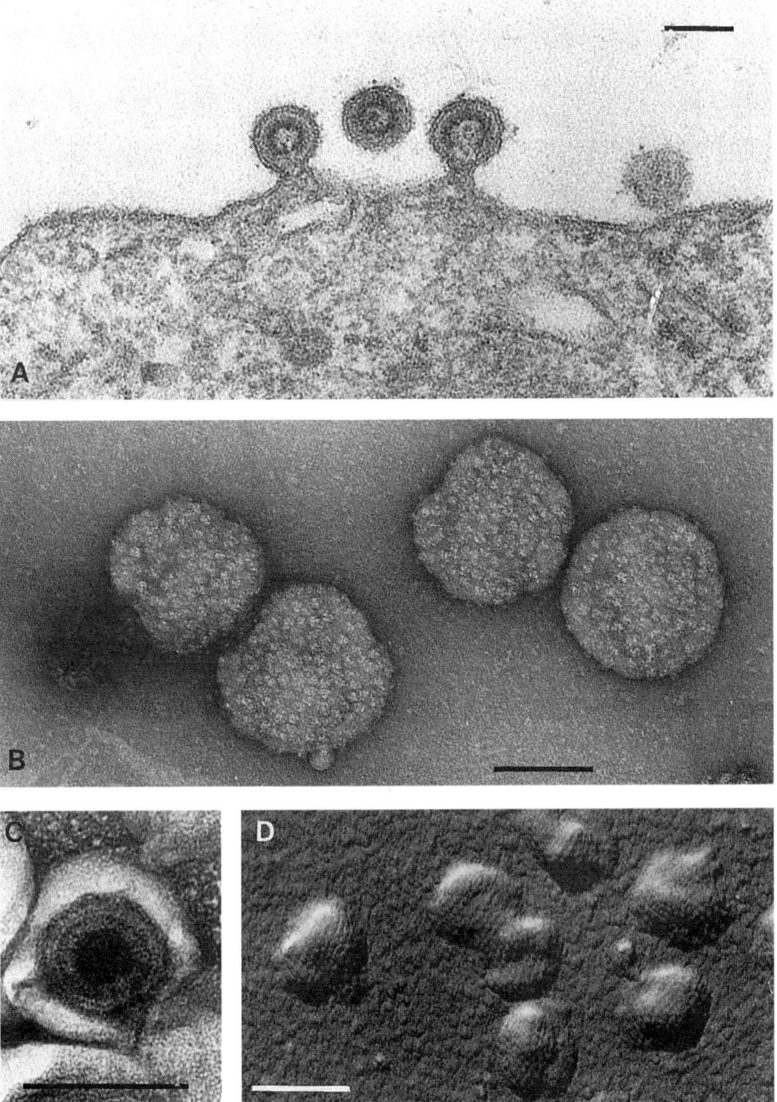

Family *Retroviridae*, genus *Gammaretrovirus* (comprising mammalian and reptilian type C retroviruses): murine leukemia virus. (A) Budding of typical type C retrovirus virions from a mouse embryo cell. (B) Virions stained negatively with uranyl acetate, showing peplomers on their surface. (C) Virion somewhat damaged and penetrated by uranyl acetate so that the concentric arrangement of core, shell, and nucleocapsid becomes visible. (D) Cores isolated by ether treatment of virions, freeze-dried and shadow-cast. The hexagonal arrangement of the subunits of the shell around the nucleocapsid is recognizable. Bars: 100 nm. (Courtesy of H. Frank and W. Schafer.)

FIGURE 23.2.

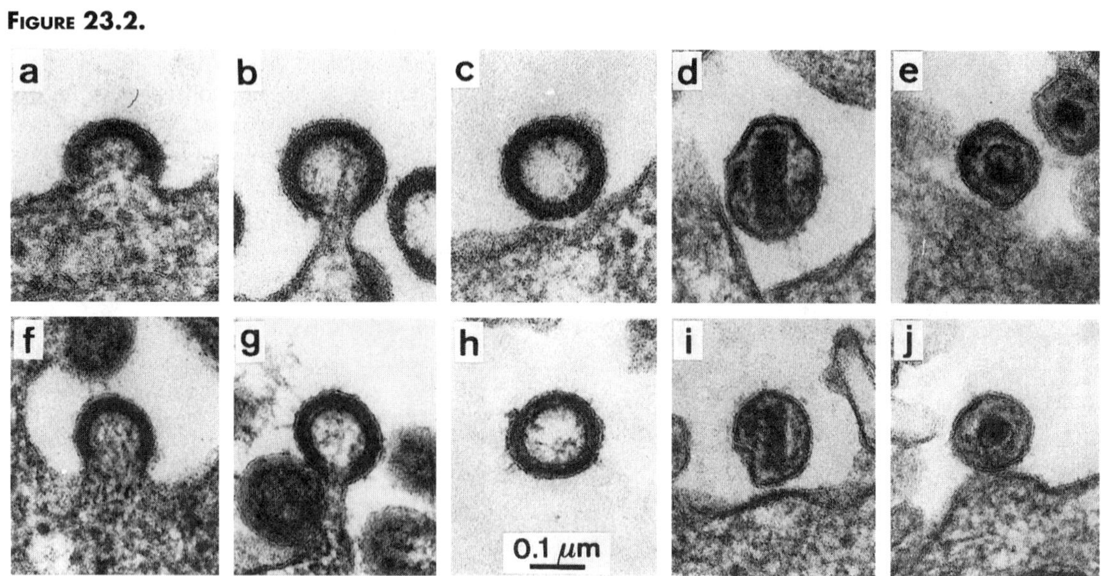

Family *Retroviridae,* genus *Lentivirus:* the structural details of lentiviruses are different from those of other retroviruses. (a to e) Human immunodeficiency virus (HIV) showing the progression of the budding process and the continuing maturation of the core structure of the virus after budding. (f to j) Maedi/visna virus showing the same progression. It was this precise similarity in morphology that first suggested that HIV is a lentivirus. Thin section electron microscopy. (Courtesy of M. A. Gonda.)

FIGURE 23.3.

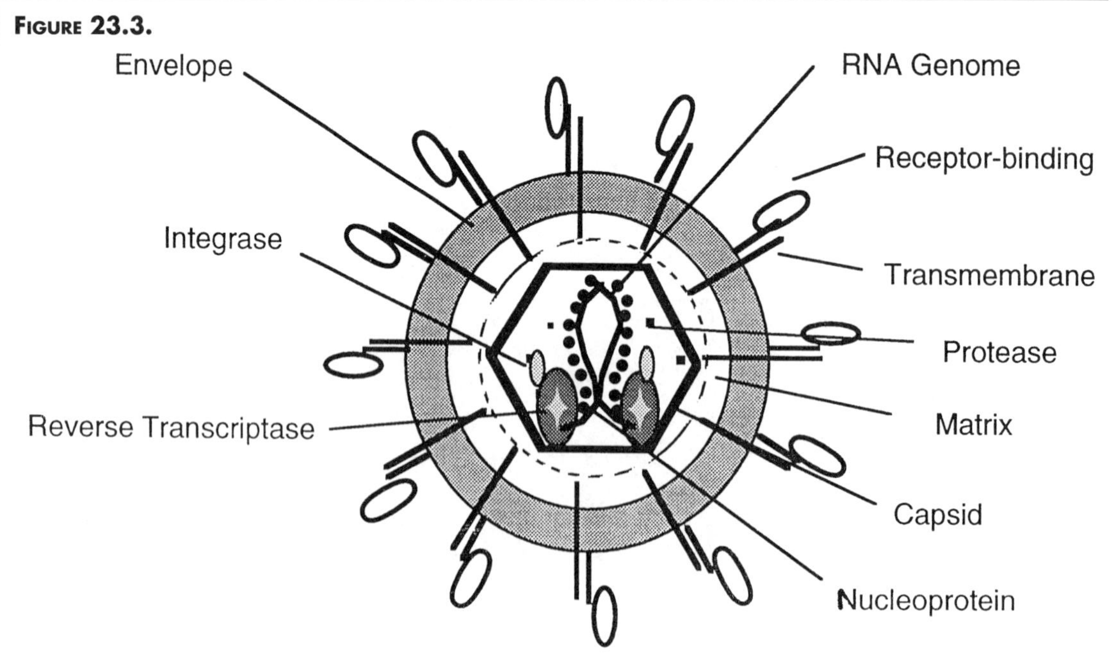

Schematic diagram of a retrovirus virion indicating various structures and proteins. [From J. M. Coffin, Retroviridae: The viruses and their replication. *In* "Fields Virology" (B. N. Fields, D. M. Knipe, P. M. Howley, R. M. Chanock, J. L. Melnick, T. P. Monath, B. Roizman, and S. E. Straus, eds.), 3rd ed., pp. 1767–1848. Lippincott-Raven, Philadelphia, PA, 1996.]

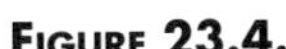

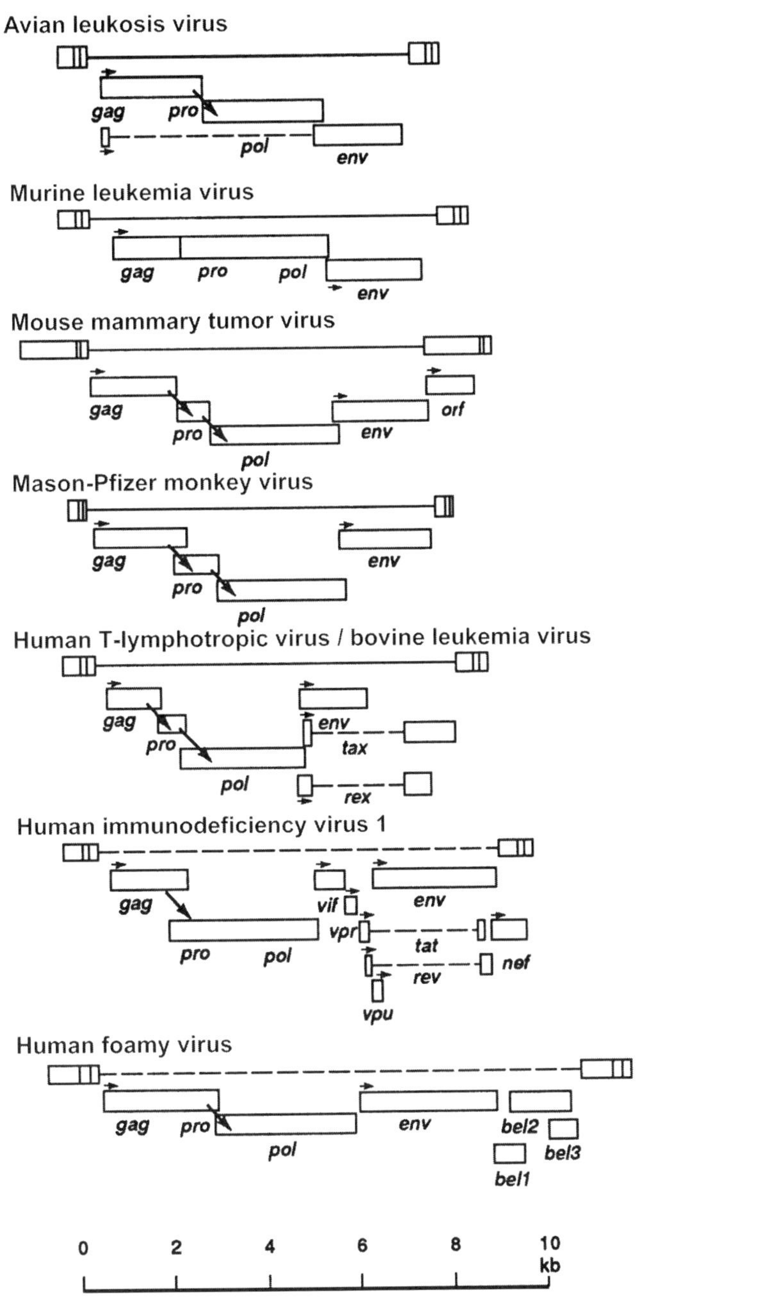

Genomes of representative retroviruses showing coding regions. The top lines depict proviral DNAs with their LTRs shown as terminal boxes. Under them are the coding regions, with each box corresponding to a separate open reading frame. Horizontal arrows indicate sites of initiation of translation, diagonal arrows indicate sites of frame-shifting, and dashed lines indicate split reading frames joined by splicing events [From J. M. Coffin, Structure and classification of retroviruses *in* "The Retroviridae" (J. Levy, ed.), Vol. 1. pp. 19–50. Plenum, New York, 1992]

(1) It is the only diploid genome. (2) It is the only viral RNA that is synthesized and processed by host cell mRNA-processing machinery. (3) It is the only genome associated with a specific transfer RNA whose function is to prime replication. (4) It is the only positive-sense, single-stranded RNA genome that does not serve as mRNA soon after infection. (5) It is the only genome to encode a reverse transcriptase, which in itself is unique. Among its many functions, the reverse transcriptase serves as an RNA-dependent DNA polymerase, a DNA-

Figure 23.5.

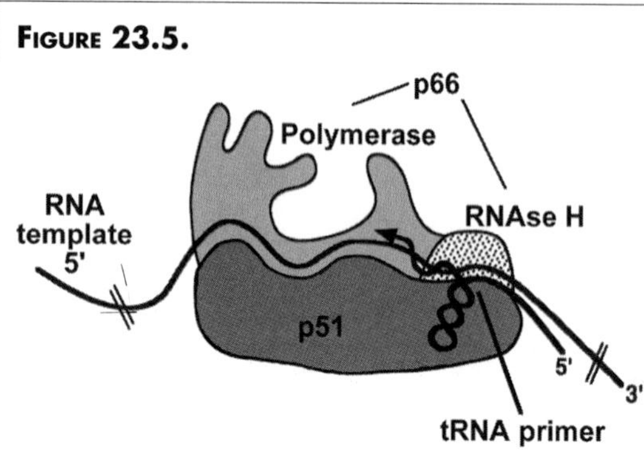

Schematic diagram of a reverse transcriptase molecule showing its multiple functional domains. The virion reverse transcriptase is coded for as a component of the Gag-Pol precursor and is processed by a viral-coded protease to yield a homodimer of p66 molecules; a portion of the C terminus is subsequently cleaved from one subunit to produce a heterodimer, composed of one molecule of p66 and one of p51. Because of its three-dimensional structure the molecule has been compared to a clenched right hand—specific domains are designated as the palm, thumb, and fingers. A short connection joins the reverse transcriptase domain to the RNase H domain. The viral RNA template and the tRNA primer are positioned within the palm. [From J. M. Coffin, Retroviridae: The viruses and their replication. *In* "Fields Virology" (B. N. Fields, D. M. Knipe, P. M. Howley, R. M. Chanock, J. L. Melnick, T. P. Monath, B. Roizman, and S. E. Straus, eds.), 3rd ed., pp. 1767–1848. Lippincott-Raven, Philadelphia, PA, 1996.]

dependent DNA polymerase, an integrase, and an RNase, with each distinctive function being carried out by a different part of the protein molecule (Figure 23.5). The enzymatic activities of the reverse transcriptase also work with various nonviral substrates hence reverse transcriptase is an important tool in many recombinant DNA technologies.

The genome of nondefective retroviruses contains three major genes, each encoding two or more proteins. The *gag* gene (standing for *g*roup-specific *a*nti*g*en) encodes the virion core (capsid) proteins, the *pol* gene encodes the reverse transcriptase (*pol*ymerase), and the *env* gene encodes the virion peplomer proteins (*env*elope). Genome termini have several distinctive components, each of which is functionally important.

The genome of the rapidly transforming retroviruses contains a fourth gene, the viral oncogene (v-*onc*) (see Chapter 11, Table 11.5). The presence of the v-*onc* gene is usually associated with deletions elsewhere in the genome, usually in the *env* gene, so that most v-*onc*-containing viruses are unable to synthesize a complete envelope and are therefore replication defective. They are always found associated with nondefective viruses that are replication competent; the latter act as helpers (see later). Rous sarcoma virus is an exception; its genome contains the viral oncogene v-*src*, but it also contains complete *gag, pol,* and *env* genes and is therefore replication competent.

In addition to encoding *gag, pol,* and *env* genes, which are common to all retroviruses, lentiviruses encode several other genes, referred to as accessory genes (Figure 23.6). These include (1) *tat,* which encodes a potent transactivator that, in association with cellular factors, enhances the efficiency of transcription by cellular RNA polymerase 1000-fold, mainly by preventing premature termination of transcription; (2) *rev,* which encodes a protein that is involved in the splicing of viral RNA transcripts and their export from the nucleus to the cytoplasm, making the full range of mRNAs available for translation; (3) *nef,* which is not required for viral replication in cultured lymphocytes but is essential for

Figure 23.6.

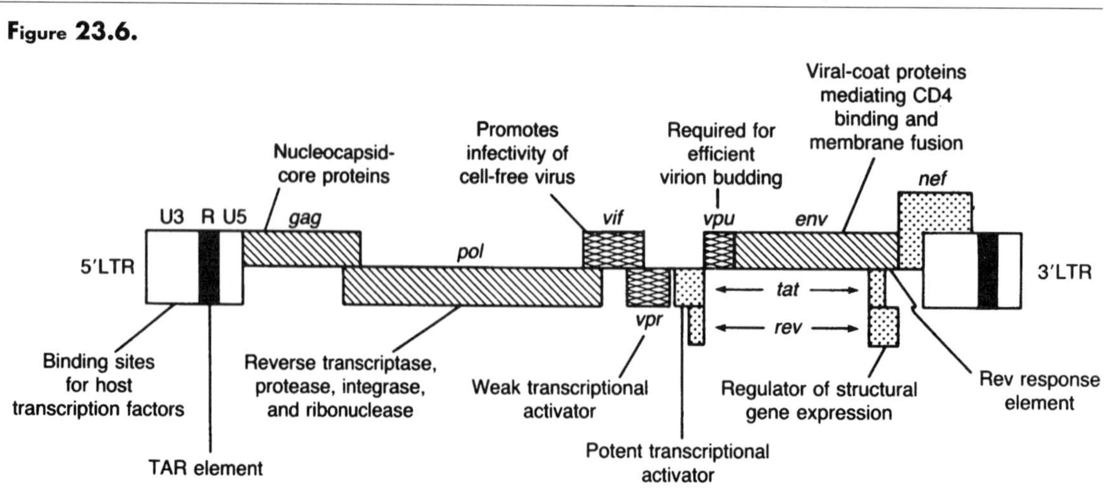

Genomic organization of human immunodeficiency virus 1, with an overview of some of the known functions of each gene product. [From W. C. Greene, The molecular biology of human immunodeficiency virus type 1 infection. *N. Engl. J. Med.* **324,** 308–317 (1991).]

replication in macrophages and also for the development of disease in simian immunodeficiency virus (SIV)-infected rhesus monkeys; the Nef protein also down-regulates expression of CD4 and IL-2 and may also alter the state of activation of target cells *in vivo*; and (4) *vif*, which encodes a protein (viral infectivity factor) that is required for some step in virion morphogenesis that determines infectivity. *vpu, vpr,* and *vpx* are found in primate lentiviruses: Vpu promotes maturation of the viral glycoprotein and release of virions by budding; Vpr is a weak transcriptional activator; and Vpx seems to be required for efficient replication in T lymphocytes and macrophages.

Retroviruses are inactivated by lipid solvents and detergents and by heating at 56°C for 30 minutes, but are more resistant than other viruses to UV- and X-irradiation, probably because of their diploid genomes.

Viral Replication

Retrovirus replication is unique and complex: in overview, replication starts with reverse transcription of virion RNA into double-stranded DNA by the reverse transcriptase. These linear double-stranded DNA intermediates are circularized, integrated into the host chromosomal DNA, and then used for transcription, including the transcription of full-length genomic RNA and various mRNAs. The essential features in the replication cycle of a nondefective retrovirus are shown in Figure 23.7. Aspects of retrovirus replication that relate to the role of the integrated provirus in oncogenesis are discussed in Chapter 11.

Depending on the virus, virions attach to a number of different specific cellular receptors via their envelope glycoproteins. In most instances the virus envelope and the cell membrane fuse, allowing the virion core to enter the cytoplasm; in fewer instances, entry involves receptor-mediated endocytosis. In the cytoplasm, but still within the capsid, a double-stranded DNA copy of the virion RNA is synthesized by the virion-associated reverse transcriptase. In the process, 300 to 1300 bp are added to each end of each genomic RNA molecule—these termini, called *long terminal repeats* (LTRs), have a complex secondary structure formed by base pairing and are central in the replication strategy of all retroviruses (see Chapter 11). The capsid is removed and the double-stranded DNA moves to the nucleus; it circularizes by noncovalent binding of the LTRs, and several such molecules become integrated as provirus at different sites in the cellular DNA. Transcription by cellular RNA polymerase, initiated in the 5′-LTR and ending in the 3′-LTR, generates new virion RNA.

FIGURE 23.7.

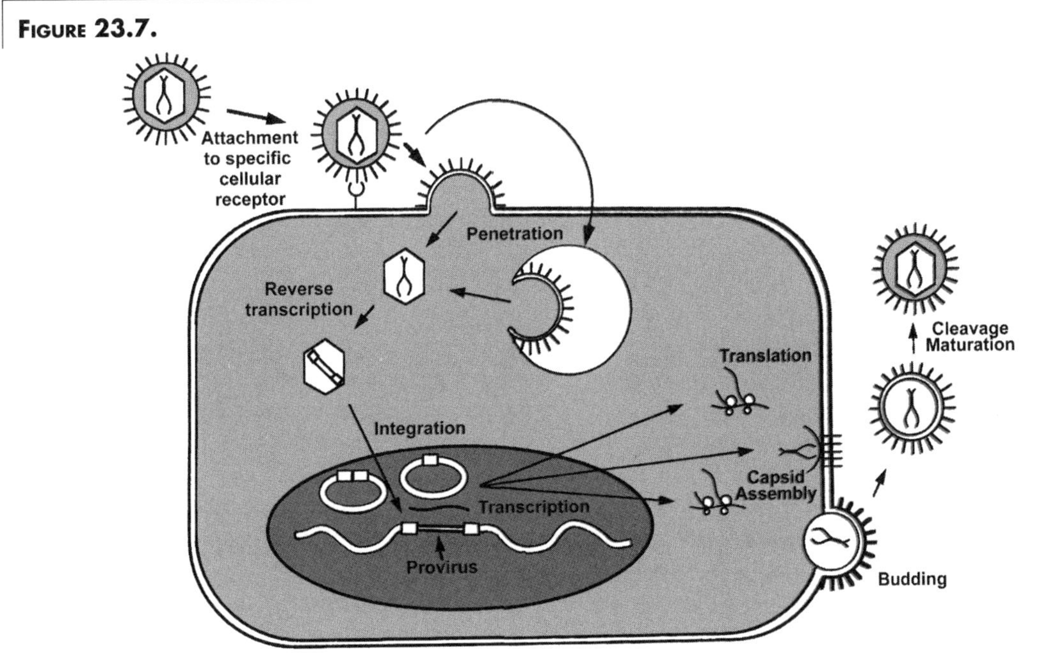

An overview of the replication cycle of retroviruses. Virions enter their host cells either by fusion or by receptor-mediated endocytosis (top) and mature by budding through the plasma membrane (bottom, right). [From J. M. Coffin, *Retroviridae:* The viruses and their replication. *In* "Fields Virology" (B. N. Fields, D. M. Knipe, P. M. Howley, R. M. Chanock, J. L. Melnick, T. P. Monath, B. Roizman, and S. E. Straus, eds.), 3rd ed., pp. 1767–1848. Lippincott-Raven, Philadelphia, PA. 1996.]

Synthesis of viral proteins occurs at the same time as virion RNA synthesis. Two major mRNAs are transcribed: (1) a 35S RNA, which is probably the same as full-length virion RNA, encodes the Gag protein; the same RNA is translated in a different reading frame to produce the Pol protein. (2) a 25S mRNA, spliced from the 35S RNA, is translated to produce a precursor of Env protein; this translation also involves a different reading frame. The *pol* and *env* genes are separate in lentiviruses. The major polyproteins are cleaved posttranslationally by a viral protease to yield mature viral proteins.

The Env protein enters the cisternae of the endoplasmic reticulum during synthesis and moves to the Golgi complex where it is glycosylated. It then moves to the plasma membrane. A fraction of the Gag polyprotein follows the same pathway and is glycosylated and reaches the plasma membrane. Together with viral RNA, Gag and Gag-Pol precursors begin to assemble nucleocapsids on the inner side of the plasma membrane; the polyproteins are cleaved during the process. Budding proceeds with nucleocapsids binding to Env proteins already fixed as peplomers in the plasma membrane. Many retroviruses, including lentiviruses, replicate only in dividing cells. Many retroviruses are not cytopathic and do not dramatically alter the metabolism of the cells that they infect; others, such as the lentiviruses, cause cell death in a number of ways, including syncytium formation (an inherently unstable event) and apoptosis. In some instances, infected cells may continue to divide while budding large numbers of virions.

Replication of retroviruses is accompanied by a high mutation frequency—one in 10^{-4} to 10^{-5} of progeny virions per replication cycle—suggesting frequent errors by reverse transcriptase. The sites of mutation are distributed unevenly; *gag, pol,* and *onc* genes are conserved as are certain parts of *env* genes; other parts of *env,* particularly those regions coding for sites to which antibody binds, are highly variable. There is also a high frequency of recombination between retrovirus genomes in doubly infected cells. Recombination is an early event occurring prior to integration during reverse transcription to form viral DNA. Together, the mutation and recombination frequencies far exceed those of any other animal virus. This genetic instability accounts for the variation in the types of tumors produced by the acutely transforming oncogenic retroviruses. It makes classification of retrovirus species and subtypes difficult, a reality that is compounded by the occurrence of phenotypic mixing of envelope proteins, producing pseudotypes, which have the genome of one virus or subtype and the envelope antigens of another. Pseudotypes have the ability to invade cells via the receptor specificity of their envelope, but their progeny behave according to their genome specificity—this may be one basis for retrovirus species jumping (see Chapter 4).

Exceptional Aspects of Lentivirus Replication

Because human immunodeficiency virus 1 has been studied in such detail, further review of its replication cycle is instructive for understanding the replication of the lentiviruses of animals (Figure 23.8).

1. $CD4^+$ T lymphocytes support human immunodeficiency virus replication only when dividing, yet most T lymphocytes in the body are at rest at any particular time; therefore, many human immunodeficiency virus–host cell interactions result in a long-standing subclinical infection that takes years to progress to clinical disease. T lymphocyte proliferation is stimulated by mitogens, cytokines, antigenic stimulation, and transactivating proteins encoded by certain other viruses; hence, the onset of clinical disease is often precipitated by seemingly unrelated infections or other stimuli. The same phenomena explain the long preclinical course and triggering events seen in many animal lentivirus infections.

2. Human immunodeficiency virus ligands, contained on exposed loops on their gp120 peplomers, designated V1, V2, V3, V4, and V5 (Figure 23.9), bind to CD4, which is the primary viral receptor. CD4 is expressed on cells of the macrophage lineage, including bone marrow precursors and dendritic cells in the skin, lymph nodes, and spleen, and on astroglia in the brain. B lymphocytes, colonic epithelial cells, and some other lymphocytes also carry CD4 receptors and are also targets of initial infection. In many of the lentivirus infections of animals (e.g., maedi/visna virus infection of sheep, caprine arthritis–encephalitis virus infection of goats, equine infectious anemia virus infection of horses) macrophages are not only the essential initial target in the pathogenesis of systemic infection, but are also the central target throughout the entire course of infection. In other lentivirus infections of animals (e.g., feline immunodeficiency virus infection in cats and simian immunodeficiency virus infection of nonhuman primates), the main target cells are $CD4^+$ T lymphocytes. Macrophage-tropic viruses are present early and late in infection and are primarily responsible for animal-to-animal transmission.

3. The recognition of human immunodeficiency virus coreceptors or secondary receptors has provided important advances in our understanding of the pathogenesis of lentivirus infections. Such receptors broaden the tropism of the lentiviruses and, when acting together with the primary receptor, serve to increase the strength

FIGURE 23.8.

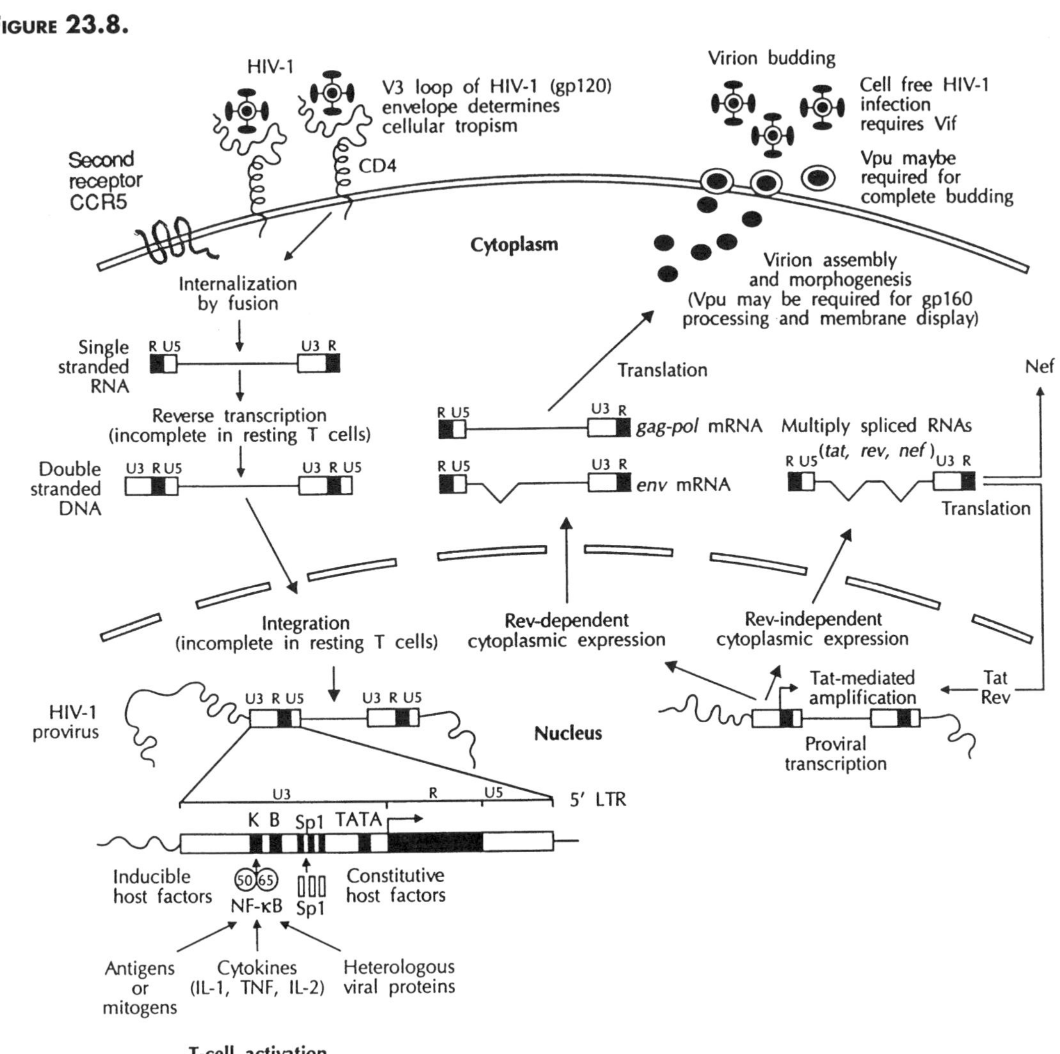

An overview of the replication cycle of human immunodeficiency virus 1 in a CD4⁺ T cell. Infection begins (top, left) with attachment of the virion via gp120 to its major receptor, CD4, followed by the binding of SU to its secondary chemokine receptor, CCR5. The double receptor binding of SU exposes the transmembrane subunit and brings it into direct contact with the cell membrane, allowing it to penetrate the cell membrane and create a channel through which the virus penetrates into the cytoplasm of the cell. Following entry the genome is released from the core and becomes available for reverse transcription to produce a double-stranded DNA with added long terminal repeats (LTRs) composed of sequences duplicated from the 3′ (U3) and 5′ (U5) ends of the viral RNA. Complete reverse transcription and integration of the DNA provirus into a chromosome occur efficiently only in activated, proliferating cells. Transcriptional activity of the HIV provirus is regulated by constitutive host cell transcription factors (Sp1 and TATA-binding factors) and by activation-inducible members of the NF-κB family of host transcription factors, both of which bind to specific sequences in the regulatory region of the LTR in its integrated proviral state (an enlarged version of which is shown in the bottom left of the diagram). The virus-coded regulatory protein, Tat, is one of the early gene products; Tat binds to the TAR region in the LTR and greatly amplifies transcription of all the viral genes (bottom, right). Following synthesis of a full-length RNA transcript, an array of alternatively spliced viral mRNAs is produced. The differential expression of distinct species of viral mRNAs is controlled by a second regulatory protein, Rev. Early in infection, when the level of Rev is low, only the multiply spliced mRNAs for the regulatory proteins Tat, Rev, and Nef are exported to the cytoplasm for translation. Once a sufficient level of Rev accumulates, the unspliced and singly spliced mRNAs that drive the synthesis of new viral genomes and structural proteins are exported to the cytoplasm and translated. These include mRNAs that encode Gag, Env, Pol, and the remaining accessory proteins Vif, Vpr, and Vpu. Encapsidation of the viral genome into the virion core structure is followed by budding from the plasma membrane (top, right). [From M. B. Feinberg and W. C. Greene, Molecular insights into human immunodeficiency virus type 1 pathogenesis. *Curr. Opin. Immunol.* **4,** 466–474 (1992).]

FIGURE 23.9.

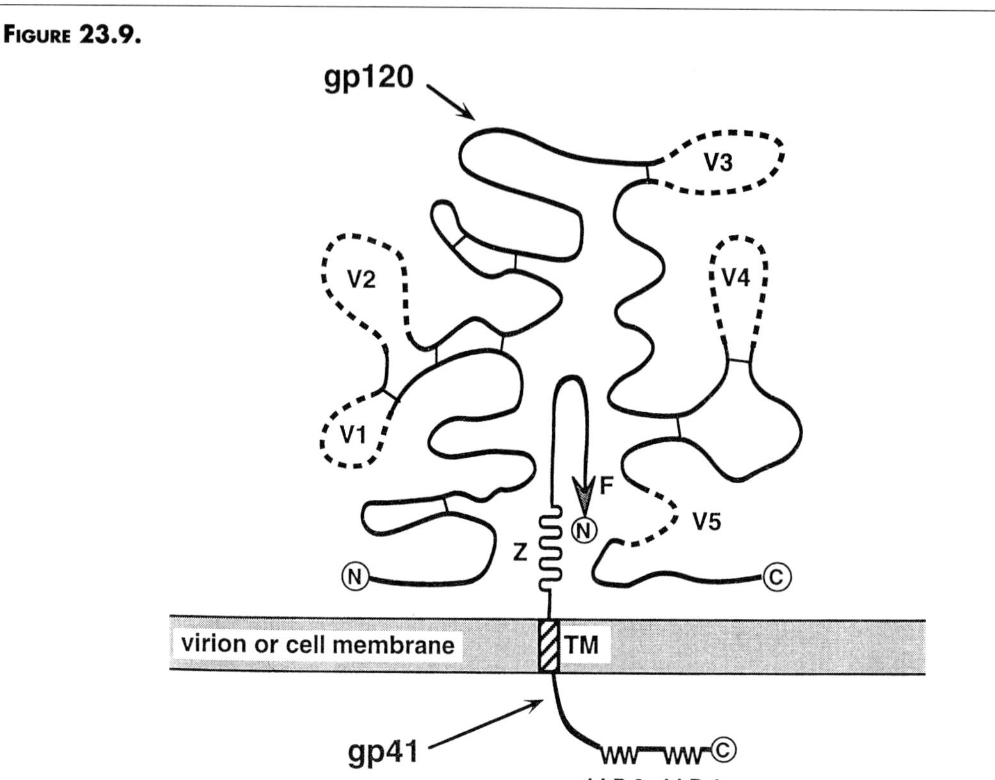

The human immunodeficiency virus 1 peplomer glycoproteins, gp120 and gp41, showing their predicted folding patterns and the major loops on gp120, designated V1, V2, V3, V4, and V5, which contain epitopic sites that bind to CD4, the primary receptor on T lymphocytes. These loops are hypervariable, accounting for much of the serologic heterogeneity between strains of the virus. [From P. A. Luciw, Human immunodeficiency viruses and their replication. *In* "Fields Virology" (B. N. Fields, D. M. Knipe, P. M. Howley, R. M. Chanock, J. L. Melnick, T. P. Monath, B. Roizman, and S. E. Straus, eds.), 3rd ed., pp. 1881–1952. Lippincott-Raven, Philadelphia, PA, 1996.]

of viral binding to target cells. First, it was found that the infection of $CD4^+$ lymphocytes was not sufficient to explain dynamic patterns of HIV infection in humans. Next, two coreceptors, CXCR-4 and CCR-5, were found. Early in infection, mildly virulent viruses use CCR-5 to gain entry into cells and these viruses evolve slowly into more highly virulent variants that prefer the CXCR4 receptor. Then another receptor, CCR8, was discovered—this molecule is abundant on the surface of thymocytes and it has been hypothesized that it is important in infection in babies and children. Subsequently, more than a dozen coreceptors have been described, with two obvious consequences: (1) it seems clear that the pattern of human immunodeficiency virus infection in various target tissues and over time is far more complex than earlier appreciated and (2), it seems clear that the development of therapeutic agents that block viral binding to receptors is a much more unlikely notion than it was when CD4 seemed to be the only receptor human immunodeficiency virus employed.

4. Human immunodeficiency virus transcription and translation are more complex than that of other retroviruses. Both cellular and viral proteins are involved in complex pathways regulating every step in the replication cycle. Transcriptional events are modulated by the binding of certain regulatory proteins (e.g., Tat and Rev), not to the DNA provirus but to their RNA transcripts. There are multiple splicing arrangements that, in the case of human immunodeficiency virus and the primate lentiviruses, yield over 30 distinct RNA species. This extra complexity contributes to the success of human immunodeficiency virus and the animal lentiviruses as pathogens, but the viral genes and proteins that direct this modulation also represent unique targets for antiviral chemotherapy. Inhibitors of viral reverse transcriptase and protease have proven their worth in treating AIDS patients, and inhibitors of some accessory genes and their encoded proteins seem promising in nonhuman primate experiments; however, although reverse transcriptase inhibitors are already in use in veterinary medicine, such therapies are unlikely to be adopted very widely because of their very high cost.

5. Contrary to an earlier view which held that during their long incubation period lentiviruses remained

latent, it is now known that rates of viral replication and cell destruction in lymphoid tissues are extraordinarily high. Throughout most of its incubation period, human immunodeficiency virus RNA can be detected in only a small fraction of peripheral blood leukocytes, typically about 1 in 10,000; however, 10^{10} or more virions may be produced and cleared from the plasma each day. As noted earlier, triggers of lymphoid cell proliferation are of critical importance in determining the level of viral replication and hence the onset and progression of disease. The close confinement of Icelandic sheep that facilitated the spread of respiratory pathogens provided the antigenic stimulus for the replication of maedi/visna virus and the consequent spread of the virus until it became a major problem. Coinfection with feline leukemia virus is a major precipitating factor in the progression of feline immunodeficiency virus infection to clinical immunodeficiency disease. Some lentiviruses, such as bovine immunodeficiency virus and equine infectious anemia virus, may remain silent throughout the life of their host animal, creating a major dilemma for "test-and-slaughter" eradication programs, especially when individual animals may have high monetary value. In all animal lentivirus infections the difference between events pertinent to the health of the individual animal and the health of the population are such that clinicians and disease control specialists may be at odds.

6. Human immunodeficiency virus and other lentiviruses spread efficiently by cell–cell fusion, forming syncytia as they spread; however, most of our knowledge of the cell biology of lentivirus infections comes from cell culture studies involving conventional infection by free virions—there are probably important differences between the two that must be taken into account in future vaccine and antiviral drug research aimed at preventing and treating the important lentivirus infections of animals as well as humans.

7. In common with other retroviruses, the mutation rates of human immunodeficiency virus are very high—point, deletion, and insertional mutations occur frequently. Rates are estimated to be 3×10^{-5} mutations per nucleotide per replication cycle and rates are likely similar in animal lentivirus infections. Given the chronicity of lentivirus infections, these mutation rates become a central feature in the pathogenesis of the diseases caused by these viruses, influencing tropism, transmissibility, and the immunological control of opportunistic infections, as well as the progression of lesions per se. Mutations occur randomly across the whole genome, but only those that confer replicative advantages or escape from host immune reactions become fixed into the prevailing genotype—the largest number of mutations are found in the *env* gene where they give rise to immune-escape variants (Table 23.2).

Table 23.2
Properties of Retroviruses

Virions are enveloped, 80–100 nm in diameter, and have a three-layered structure: an innermost genome–nucleoprotein complex with helical symmetry, surrounded by an icosahedral capsid, in turn surrounded by an envelope with glycoprotein peplomers

The genome is diploid, consisting of a dimer of two molecules of linear positive-sense, single-stranded RNA, each 7–11 kb in size. Genomic RNA has a 3′-polyadenylated tail and a 5′-cap

All retroviruses have *gag, pol,* and *env* genes; some acquire an oncogene and are usually defective in their own replication as a consequence; lentiviruses have a complex array of up to six accessory genes

Viral reverse transcriptase transcribes DNA from virion RNA following the formation of long terminal repeats; circular double-stranded DNA is formed and integrates into cellular chromosomal DNA as a provirus

In productive infections, virions assemble at and bud from plasma membrane

Some retroviruses produce tumors, particularly leukemias and sarcomas; members of the genus *Lentivirus* produce slow demyelinating neurologic disease, arthritis, generalized chronic debilitating disease, or acquired immunodeficiency syndromes

Diseases Caused by Members of the Genus *Alpharetrovirus*

Much of our understanding of the biology of oncogenic retroviruses derives from research on the viruses affecting birds. Retrovirus infections of chickens fall into two distinct groups: (1) the avian leukosis, myeloblastosis, and sarcoma viruses, which belong to the genus *Alpharetrovirus,* and (2) the avian reticuloendotheliosis viruses, which belong to the genus *Gammaretrovirus,* comprising mostly mammalian type C retroviruses (Table 23.1). Each of these groups of viruses, especially the first, is large and complex, and the diseases they cause are of considerable economic importance.

There are three classes of avian viruses involved (see Chapter 11): *endogenous, exogenous replication competent,* and *exogenous replication defective.* Endogenous avian leukosis viruses occur in the genome of every chicken as DNA proviruses. They are rarely expressed, but if induced by various manipulations they are nonpathogenic. Exogenous avian leukosis viruses are replication competent and have a standard complement of *gag, pol,* and *env* genes. For the most part they are nonpathogenic, but in the course of lifetime infection a small percentage of infected birds develop leukemia or lymphoma. Finally, some exogenous viruses acquire an oncogene (v-*onc*) from a cellular *onc* (c-*onc*) gene and then induce malignant tumors rapidly. The great majority of such rapidly transforming viruses lose part of their genome when they acquire their oncogene, so that they become replication defective and dependent on the helper activity of a replication-competent virus. A few viruses, however, like Rous sarcoma virus, have a full complement of viral genes plus a v-*onc* gene—they are rapidly oncogenic while at the same time capable of replication without a helper virus.

Oncogenic retroviruses may be transmitted from one chicken to another horizontally or vertically, and vertical transmission may occur through infectious virus (complete virions) or through provirus integrated into the DNA of the host germplasm (Figure 23.10). All routes of transmission occur, although germ plasm transmission is restricted to nonpathogenic endogenous viruses.

With most of the avian retroviruses, if chickens are infected horizontally when more than 5 or 6 days of age they are unlikely to develop leukemia; instead they develop a transient viremia and produce neutralizing antibody. If virus is transmitted congenitally via the egg or within the first few days of life, the chicken becomes viremic. The viremia persists for life because of the induction of immunological tolerance. Such birds may appear to grow normally but they frequently develop leukemia and associated diseases and are a major source of exogenous virus that is shed continuously and transmitted horizontally. Genetic (germ line) transmission occurs when germ cells, ova and sperm, contain endogenous

FIGURE 23.10.

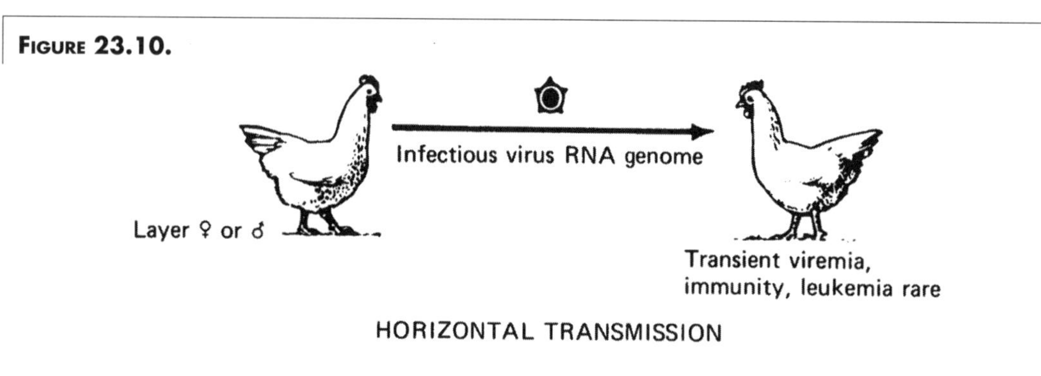

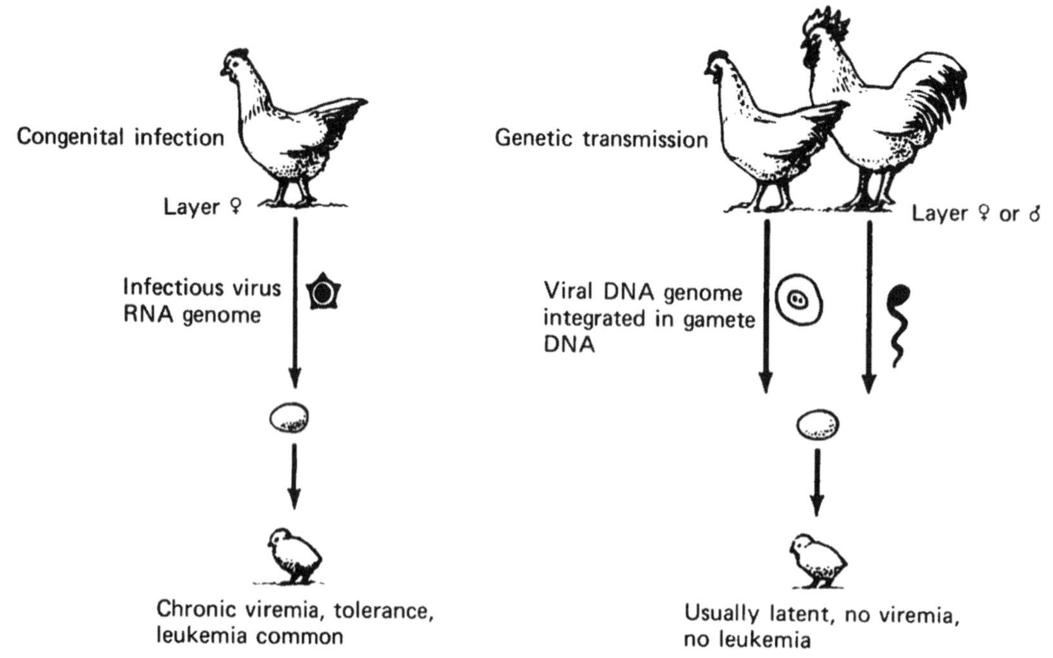

Horizontal and vertical transmission of avian leukosis viruses. (Courtesy of R. A. Weiss.)

virus. Presumably this infection pattern is initiated when the provirus is integrated into the genome of germ line cells following horizontal transmission.

Avian Leukosis and Sarcoma

Clinical Features

Avian leukosis viruses are endemic in virtually all flocks of chickens and most chickens in a flock will have been infected within a few months of hatching. If rapidly transforming viruses are not present, disease occurs sporadically in birds over 14 weeks of age, with an overall incidence of about 3%, but sometimes the incidence of disease may be as high as 20%. The variety of syndromes produced by avian leukosis/sarcoma viruses is shown in Table 23.3.

Diseases Due to Exogenous Nondefective Viruses

Lymphoid Leukosis (syn., Visceral Lymphomatosis)

This is the commonest form of avian leukosis and occurs in chickens 14 to 30 weeks of age. Clinical signs are nonspecific. The comb may be pale, shriveled, and occasionally cyanotic. Inappetence, emaciation, and weakness occur and the abdomen may be enlarged. Tumors may be present for some time before clinical illness is recognized, although the course may be rapid from the onset of disease. Hematological changes are inconsistent; leukemia is uncommon and lymphoblastoid cells are rarely seen in the circulating blood. Tumors are usually present in the liver, spleen, and bursa of Fabricius and may occur in other internal organs. Microscopically the lesions are focal multicentric aggregates of lymphoblasts—these cells express B lymphocyte markers. They may secrete large amounts of IgM, but their capacity to differentiate into IgG-, IgA- or IgE-producing cells is arrested. The primary target cells are poststem cells in the bursa of Fabricius, from where transformed cells invade blood vessels and metastasize. Bursectomy, even up to 5 months of age, abrogates the development of lymphoid leukosis.

Osteopetrosis (syn., Thick Leg)

In this form of the disease the bones are affected by a uniform or irregular diaphyseal or metaphyseal thickening. In advanced cases, osteoma, osteogenic sarcoma, and chondrosarcoma may occur. Lesions are usually most obvious in the long bones of the leg, but may also be present in the pelvis, shoulder girdle, and ribs. Birds with osteopetrosis frequently also have anemia and often have lesions of lymphoid leukosis.

Table 23.3
Syndromes Produced in Chickens by Avian Retroviruses

Virus[a]	Syndrome	Rate of Tumor Development	Viral Oncogene	Cell First Affected	Type of Lesion
Replication-competent (avian leukosis viruses)					
	Lymphoid leukosis	Slow	—	Lymphoblast	Lymphoid cell infiltrations of various organs
	Osteopetrosis	Slow	—	Osteoclast or osteoblast	Thickened long bones
	Renal tumors	Slow	—	Renal cells	Nephroblastoma, carcinoma
Replication-defective (avian erythroblastosis, avian myeloblastosis, avian myelocytomatosis viruses)					
	Erythroblastosis	Rapid	v-*erbB*	Erythroblast	Anemia
	Myeloblastosis	Rapid	v-*myb*	Myeloblast	Anemia, leukemia
	Myelocytomatosis	Rapid	v-*myc*	Myelocyte	Carcinoma, sarcoma
	Hemangioma	Rapid	?	Capillary endothelium	Hemangioma
	Sarcomas	Rapid	v-*fps*, v-*yes*	Various mesenchymal cells	Sarcoma, carcinoma
Replication-competent rapidly transforming (Rous sarcoma virus)					
	Sarcoma	Very rapid	v-*src*	Various mesenchymal cells	Sarcomas

[a]In addition to these exogenous viruses, all chickens carry endogenous retroviral DNA as part of their genome.

Renal Tumors

These are usually found coincidentally at slaughter, but may be associated with emaciation and weakness before death. Two forms occur: nephroblastomas, which originate from embryonic nephrogenic buds in the kidneys, and carcinomas, which originate from tubular epithelium. In this disease, by electron microscopy, numerous typical retrovirus virions are seen budding from transformed renal cells.

Diseases due to Defective Viruses

Erythroblastosis

In this form of disease the incubation period may be as short as 21 days. Two patterns are recognized: a proliferative form characterized by the presence of many erythroblasts in the blood and an anemic form in which the predominant feature is anemia with few circulating erythroblasts. The primary target cells are erythroblasts, which resemble normal erythroblasts in appearance except that retrovirus particles can be demonstrated either within cytoplasmic vacuoles or budding from their plasma membranes. Lesions are mainly attributable to hemostasis because of the accumulation of erythroblasts in the blood vessels, particularly capillaries and sinusoids.

Myeloblastosis

In this form of disease, clinical signs are similar to those of erythroblastosis and develop after an incubation period that may be as short as 10 days. The target cells are myeloblasts in the bone marrow. The features of myeloblastosis and erythroblastosis overlap. In myeloblastosis, leukemia is a major feature; up to 10^9 myeloblasts per milliliter are present in the blood—when a hematocrit is done there may be more buffy coat cells than red cells. Bone marrow displacement may result in secondary anemia.

Myelocytomatosis

In this form of disease, signs similar to those seen in erythroblastosis develop after an incubation period of 3 to 11 weeks. Target cells, which are nongranulated myelocytes (morphologically distinct from myeloblasts), proliferate to occupy much of the bone marrow, and tumor growth may extend through the bone and periosteum. The tumors are distinctive and characteristically occur on the surface of bone, in association with the periosteum, and near cartilage, although any organ or tissue may be affected. Visceral organs may be infiltrated with myelocytes. Histologically, the tumors consist of compact masses of strikingly uniform myelocytes with very little stroma, similar to normal bone marrow myelocytes.

Hemangioma

In this form of disease, after an incubation period of less than 3 weeks, a hemangioma develops, usually as a single tumor in the skin or on the surface of the viscera. The lesion takes the form of a "blood blister," which may rupture, causing death from acute hemorrhage. The visibility of these lesions in the skin encourages cannibalism. The target in this case is endothelial cells.

Connective Tissue Tumors

A variety of malignant tumors, including fibrosarcoma, fibroma, myxosarcoma, myxoma, histiocytic sarcoma, osteoma, osteogenic sarcoma, and chondrosarcoma, are caused by avian retroviruses containing v-*onc* genes, such as defective viruses acting in concert with a helper virus or Rous sarcoma virus.

Pathogenesis, Pathology, and Immunity

In chickens infected with exogenous nondefective viruses, tumors occur only when infection occurs congenitally and there is persistent viremia. Over the course of the life of the chicken proviral DNA is integrated into many different kinds of cells, sometimes, by chance, in a location where the activity of a c-*onc* gene is disturbed in such a way as to initiate tumor production (see Chapter 11). Because lymphoid cells represent 10% of all the cells in the animal and have a very high rate of cell division, particularly in the early weeks of life, the probability that lymphoid cells that have appropriate receptors will become infected and transformed by leukosis viruses is higher than for most other cell types.

A variety of neoplasms are generated by replication-defective leukemia viruses propagated by coinfection with a nondefective helper, which is usually an exogenous avian leukemia virus. These defective viruses, for the most part, arise as a rare event in each individual bird in which they are found; because they are defective in their own replication and are so rapidly fatal, they are seldom, if ever, transmitted horizontally or from generation to generation. They can be divided into three groups—avian erythroblastosis, avian myeloblastosis, and avian myelocytomatosis—on the basis of the nature of the causative virus and the character of the tumors produced. The different pathogenic potential of the various viruses is due to the different v-*onc* genes they carry (Table 23.3).

Laboratory Diagnosis

History, clinical signs, the location of tumors, and gross and histopathologic postmortem findings are usually enough to make a diagnosis of avian leukosis. As far as differential diagnosis is concerned, the most important disease is Marek's disease, a distinction that is important because Marek's disease can be controlled by vaccination. Viral isolation is rarely required in veterinary practice, but is used for research purposes.

When an unusual episode of oncogenic disease occurs in chickens, specialized reference diagnostic procedures are undertaken in specialty laboratories. Rous sarcoma virus and other replication-competent, acutely transforming avian retroviruses are assayed directly by proliferative focus formation assays in chick embryo fibroblast cell cultures. Because they produce infectious virions, these are recovered readily and can then be characterized in detail. Replication-defective rapidly transforming viruses, which carry v-*onc* genes, can also be assayed by focus formation, but virions can only be obtained in cells carrying a replication-competent leukosis virus; the yield always consists of a mixture. Replication-competent leukosis viruses do not transform cells *in vitro;* because they interfere with transformation by viruses that carry a v-*onc* gene, interference assays are used. Assays for the presence of leukosis viruses can also be carried out by serologic methods using enzyme immunoassay or radioimmunoassay.

Epidemiology, Prevention, and Control

Transmission may occur horizontally or vertically (Figure 23.10). Horizontal transmission is relatively inefficient, requiring prolonged, close contact, and was not of major significance in the natural transmission of the disease until intensive chicken production began in the 1940s. This led to the appearance of lymphoid leukosis as an economically important disease, as horizontal transmission via saliva led to conditions that promoted egg-borne vertical transmission. Individual infected hens may transmit virus via ova either continuously or intermittently, although some known infected hens do not transmit virus at all, and transmission is less efficient in hens more than 18 months of age. Congenitally infected chickens may be immunologically tolerant and their blood may contain up to 10^9 ID_{50} per milliliter. They excrete virus in saliva and feces, but are otherwise healthy, although some eventually develop leukosis. These hens transmit virus horizontally throughout their lives and, more importantly, they also transmit virus vertically, the virus infecting cells of the blastocyst from the eight-cell stage onward. During embryogenesis the pancreas is particularly favored as a site of replication, and large amounts of virus accumulate in the albumen. At hatching, large amounts of virus are shed in the meconium, resulting in heavy environmental contamination.

Most 1-day-old chicks have maternal antibody titers between 1 and 10% of those of their dams. Thus the efficiency of passive antibody transfer is low, and the titer declines so that chicks are seronegative by 4 to 7 weeks of age. Then, if they have not been infected congenitally, they become infected by horizontal transmission and develop a transient viremia followed by high levels of antibody; virus is usually eliminated and the antibody persists for life. However, some birds remain persistently infected and act as a source of virus for both horizontal and vertical transmission. Roosters may be involved in the germ line transmission of endogenous (nonpathogenic) retroviruses, but play no part in congenital infection as sperm cells are acytoplasmic.

Hygiene is important in minimizing the level of virus contamination, particularly in the immediate posthatching period when the age, population density, and levels of virus are highly conducive to horizontal transmission. The "all-in-all-out" management system, with thorough cleaning and disinfection of incubators, hatcheries, brooding houses, and equipment, is standard practice. The risk of introducing additional strains of virus is minimized if stock are obtained from a single source.

When intensive methods for broiler and egg production were introduced in the 1940s, there was an unwitting selection of genetically susceptible chicken lines. Today, most commercial flocks consist of genetically resistant lines and, accordingly, there has been a sharp reduction in the incidence of leukosis. Resistance correlates with the viral subgroup and with the absence of receptors for viral envelope glycoproteins; the genes for virus receptors are located on an autosomal chromosome. It is possible to select for genetically resistant birds by challenging chorioallantoic membranes or chick embryo fibroblast cell cultures derived from leukosis-free birds with appropriate pseudotypes of Rous sarcoma virus. Failure to produce foci of cell transformation correlates with resistance, and lines of chickens can be bred that are homozygous for the resistance allele. Viral mutants able to bypass resistance emerge frequently, so that in practice genetic resistance as a basis for control requires an ongoing selection program.

Eradication of horizontally transmitted virus has been accomplished in poultry flocks, especially those used as a source of eggs for vaccine production. This is the case whether the eggs are for human, domestic mammal, or avian virus vaccines. Establishment and maintenance of leukosis-free flocks, which still carry endogenous avian retrovirus genes, is expensive, but is being developed more and more. In addition to eliminating the occurrence of tumors, eradication has a number of other benefits, including reduced mortality from other causes, improved growth rate, and improved production, quality, fertility, and hatchability of eggs. Using either inactivated or attenuated virus vaccines, immunization has met with limited success.

Diseases Caused by Members of the Genus *Betaretrovirus*

Ovine Pulmonary Adenomatosis (Jaagsiekte)

The most studied retrovirus diseases of sheep are those due to lentiviruses (maedi/visna virus, also known as ovine progressive pneumonia virus; see later), but oncogenic retroviruses belonging to the genus *Deltaretrovirus,* comprising bovine leukemia and human T-lymphotropic viruses, also occur. In fact, some ovine retroviruses are related antigenically to bovine leukemia virus. However, little is known about these ovine viruses and there is no evidence that they are transmitted naturally between sheep and cattle.

A more common retroviral disease in sheep, ovine pulmonary adenomatosis (also called ovine pulmonary carcinoma), produces signs similar to those of maedi (ovine progressive pneumonia; see later). The causative virus is a type D retrovirus (or a B/D retrovirus chimera), but little is known of its molecular biology because the virus cannot be cultivated in cell culture. Originally described in South Africa, where it was called Jaagsiekte, the disease occurs worldwide except in Australia where it has never occurred and Iceland where it was eradicated in 1952. It occurs sporadically in the Americas and in some countries in Europe. In Peru it is responsible for about a quarter of the annual mortality in adult sheep. There is also evidence that the virus infects and causes disease in goats in southern Africa.

The incubation period varies from 1 to 3 years—it may be shorter when young lambs are infected. The onset of disease is insidious, with progressive respiratory distress, bouts of spasmodic coughing, and the production of large amounts of surfactant-containing viscous fluid (produced by tumor cells), leading to blockage of small airways and death from anoxia and secondary bacterial pneumonia. In affected sheep, pea-sized nodular lesions are found scattered through the lungs. Histologically, these lesions are adenomas and adenocarcinomas; they represent neoplastic transformation of type II secretory epithelial cells and possibly nonciliated bronchiolar epithelium. There are also metastases to regional lymph nodes. Diagnosis is made by histopathology.

Outbreaks occur when infected sheep are introduced into uninfected flocks; where sheep are confined, about 5 to 8 months elapse between the introduction of an infected sheep and the appearance of new cases, but in range-reared sheep the interval may be years. Infected animals shed virus in saliva and respiratory secretions; infection is presumed to be acquired via the respiratory route.

Eradication in Iceland involved the near depopulation of the entire sheep population of the country; in the absence of a sensitive test to detect preclinical cases, eradication in other countries has proven unfeasible. Nevertheless, the incidence of the disease can be reduced greatly by strict isolation of flocks and removal of sick animals (ewes and their lambs) immediately upon the onset of clinical signs.

Type D Retrovirus Disease of Macaques

The first type D retrovirus described was Mason–Pfizer monkey virus; it was isolated in 1983 from a macaque and is now recognized as the cause of a severe, often fatal, immunosuppressive disease (as well as a severe retroperitoneal fibromatosis). This disease was the first to be called simian-acquired immunodeficiency syndrome (SAIDS), but because simian immunodeficiency viruses (lentiviruses) also cause a similar syndrome, the term has become too vague to be useful.

The type D retroviruses seem to be restricted to various species of the genus *Macaca* (subfamily *Cercopithecinae*) and to squirrel monkeys (*Saimiri sciureus*) and langurs (*Presbytis obscurus*). There are seven recognized viruses, each named for the primate center of origin (e.g., SAIDS-D/CA, from the California Regional Primate Research Center). Sequence data have been used for a more comprehensive naming system [e.g., SAIDS-D/CA has become simian retrovirus 1 (SRV 1)]. Members of the group include exogenous and endogenous viruses. At present, primate type D retrovirus disease is seen mainly in primate research centers in the United States. The viruses are undoubtedly more widespread, although their distribution has not yet been fully investigated.

Transmission of these exogenous viruses requires close contact, with virus being present in saliva and blood and spread occurring via biting, grooming, and fighting. Infection leads to viral replication and damage in several organs, including lymph nodes, salivary gland, spleen, thymus, and brain. When infected as juveniles, rhesus macaques may die within 1 year, although other infection courses are also seen (fulminant infection and death, self-limiting infection and chronic immunodeficiency with wasting, chronic diarrhea, splenomegaly, generalized lymphadenopathy, and anemia).

Effective inactivated virus vaccines have been produced against three of the viruses; their use has been limited, but in any case would be complementary to strict isolation of colonies, serological screening, removal of infected animals, and good sanitation.

Diseases Caused by Members of the Genus *Gammaretrovirus* (Including Avian Reticuloendotheliosis Viruses)

Feline Leukemia and Feline Sarcoma

Feline retroviruses may be endogenous, exogenous replication competent (feline leukemia virus), or exogenous defective (feline sarcoma virus)—they may be nonpathogenic or the cause of leukemia and sarcoma, respectively. Neoplastic and nonneoplastic diseases due to feline leukemia virus occur worldwide and are the most common nonaccidental cause of death in cats. In a survey in California, the incidence of feline leukemia virus neoplasms was found to be 41 per 100,000 cats per year, and it has been estimated that deaths from all feline leukemia virus-related diseases are 250 per 100,000 cats per year. The prevalence of antibody to feline leukemia virus varies from 6% in isolated populations to 50% in urban and colony cats.

The feline leukemia virus was first recovered in 1964; remarkably only a few other isolates have been obtained—it has proved impossible to isolate the virus from the majority of tumors that would be expected to contain it. However, the presence of the viral genome is demonstrable by hybridization and transfection. It has therefore been suggested that viral replication and release are not required to produce disease.

Feline sarcoma virus is known to be defective, carrying the v-*onc* gene v-*fms* and lacking an *env* gene. All strains that have been recovered from fibrosarcomas are pseudotypes with envelopes provided by feline leukemia virus and all feline sarcoma virus stocks contain feline leukemia virus. Besides being important as pathogens of cats, several aspects of feline leukemia virus/feline sarcoma virus have attracted the attention of research workers concerned with human oncology and immunodeficiency diseases. There is no evidence that the feline viruses can infect humans, but in many places, women of child-bearing age, children, and immunocompromised persons have been advised that they should avoid close contact with cats showing signs of disease.

Clinical Features

The feline retroviruses are responsible for a variety of disease syndromes, some neoplastic and others relating to effects on hematopoietic cells and the immune system. Three types of neoplasia are recognized—lymphosarcoma, myeloproliferative disease and fibrosarcoma, along with two types of nonneoplastic disease—anemia and an immunopathologic disease.

Feline Lymphosarcomas

Feline lymphosarcoma is the most common naturally occurring mammalian lymphosarcoma and accounts for some 30% of all feline tumors. About one-third of all cats with lymphosarcoma have no demonstrable feline leukemia virus antigens and, as noted earlier, the virus can rarely be isolated. However, epidemiological evidence supports the view that feline leukemia virus causes the vast majority of cases of feline lymphosarcoma.

Four major forms of lymphosarcoma are recognized based on the location of the primary tumor: (1) *multicentric lymphosarcoma,* in which tumors occur in various lymphoid and nonlymphoid tissues; (2) *thymic lymphosarcoma,* occurring particularly in kittens; (3) *alimentary lymphosarcoma,* usually occurring in older cats in which lymphoid tissues of the gastrointestinal tract and/or mesenteric lymph nodes are affected; and (4) *unclassified lymphosarcomas,* an uncommon finding in which tumors are seen in nonlymphoid tissues such as the skin, eyes, and central nervous system. The lymphosarcomas are predominantly T lymphocyte tumors, except the alimentary tract form, which is a B lymphocyte tumor.

Feline Myeloproliferative Diseases and Anemia

In this group of diseases, transformation of one or a combination of bone marrow cell types is induced by feline leukemia virus. Four types are recognized: (1) *erythromyelosis,* in which the target is an erythroid cell; (2) *granulocytic leukemia,* in which a granulocytic myeloid cell, usually a neutrophil, is targeted; (3) *erythroleukemia,* in which both erythroid and granulocytic myeloid precursors become neoplastic; and (4) *myelofibrosis,* a proliferation of fibroblasts and cancellous bone resulting in medullary osteosclerosis and myelofibrosis. These diseases, which are similar to those produced by the acutely transforming avian retroviruses, are characterized by the presence of large numbers of neoplastic cells in the bone marrow, a nonregenerative anemia and immunosuppression. Transformation of erythropoietic cells may produce erythroblastosis, erythroblastopenia, or pancytopenia, all of which are associated with anemia.

Immunopathologic Disease

This group of diseases includes both immune complex diseases and immunodeficiency diseases. Sometimes persistent high levels of feline leukemia virus antigens are produced, which, when bound in immune complexes, produce glomerulonephritis. In other cases, lymphoid cells are depleted greatly, in part by antibody-dependent cytotoxicity, with feline oncovirus membrane-associated antigens (FOCMA) being the target. This leads to a variety of secondary infections in which the cat fails to thrive, growth is stunted, the hair coat is harsh, there is intercurrent and repeated infection, chronic stomatitis, and gingivitis, nonhealing skin lesions, subcutaneous abscesses, chronic respiratory disease, and a high incidence of feline infectious peritonitis (see Chapter 33). Toxoplasmosis and infection with *Hemobartonella felis* are much more common in feline leukemia virus-infected than in normal cats. Poor reproductive performance, including infertility, fetal deaths, and abortions, is also attributed to feline leukemia virus infection.

Feline Fibrosarcoma

Feline fibrosarcoma accounts for 6 to 12% of all feline tumors, usually seen as solitary tumors in older cats. In young feline leukemia virus-infected kittens, feline sarcoma virus may, on rare occasions, induce a multifocal subcutaneous fibrosarcoma, which is anaplastic, rapidly growing, and frequently metastatic. One strain of feline sarcoma virus induces melanoma as well as fibrosarcoma. There is no evidence that feline sarcoma virus is transmitted horizontally; the tumors and the virus appear to arise *de novo* following feline leukemia virus infection.

Pathogenesis, Pathology, and Immunity

There are three antigenic types of feline leukemia virus—A, B, and C—based on differences in envelope antigens. Cells transformed by either feline leukemia virus or feline sarcoma virus, unlike infected, nontransformed cells, express a novel viral antigen (FOCMA) in their plasma membrane, antibodies to which, like antibodies to envelope antigens, protect cats against disease. Antibodies to the internal proteins and the reverse transcriptase are not protective but may be involved in immune complex disease.

Within 6 weeks of infection with feline leukemia virus, one of two host–virus relationships develops: persistent active infection or a self-limiting infection. Persistent active infection is recognized by the presence of persistent viremia. The serum of persistently infected cats lacks both neutralizing and FOCMA antibodies. Viremia persists for months and is usually terminated by feline leukemia virus-related disease. Persistently infected cats shed virus in secretions and represent the most important source for the dissemination of feline leukemia virus. Immunosuppression is the most common sequel to persistent feline leukemia virus viremia and accounts for most feline leukemia virus-related deaths. Strains of virus from immunosuppressive illness infect $CD4^+$ and $CD8^+$ T lymphocytes, B lymphocytes, and myeloid cells. Viremic cats have suppressed blastogenic responses to T cell mitogens, suppressed antibody responses, prolonged allograft rejection times, hypocomplementemia, thymic atrophy, depletion of paracortical zones of lymph nodes, and an almost total failure of interferon production. Age appears to have some influence on the disease pattern, perhaps because of an association between the virus and dividing cells.

The vast majority of cats exposed to infection with feline leukemia virus develop a self-limiting infection. They remain nonviremic, develop neutralizing and FOCMA-specific antibodies, do not shed virus, and do not develop leukemia. Sometimes there is a transient viremia, which disappears with the development of neutralizing and FOCMA-specific antibodies.

Finally, in some cats persistent viremia is initially accompanied by high FOCMA-specific antibody. This is an unstable condition; such cats either develop neutralizing antibody or the FOCMA-specific antibody declines and the cats develop feline leukemia virus-related disease.

Laboratory Diagnosis

Viral isolation is rarely possible, but a number of diagnostic tests have been developed based on detecting viral proteins in cells in the blood, either by indirect immunofluorescence or enzyme immunoassay. The indirect immunofluorescence test is performed on blood smears on glass slides, which may be mailed to an appropriate laboratory. Enzyme immunoassay is performed on plasma or buffy coat cells and is available commercially in kit form that can be used in the veterinary clinic. Both tests detect a group-specific antigen within the viral core.

Epidemiology, Prevention, and Control

Only the nonpathogenic endogenous type of feline leukemia virus is transmitted vertically, via the germ plasm. Although many cats are exposed to horizontally transmitted, pathogenic feline leukemia virus, relatively few become infected, despite the fact that the saliva of persistently infected and viremic cats may contain 10^6 infectious virions per milliliter. Prolonged, direct exposure is usually required for transmission, which may occur by mutual grooming or possibly via fleas. Circumstantial evidence suggests that biting, such as occurs during fighting, is probably the most important method of transmission, which may also occur iatrogenically via blood transfusion, reused syringes and needles, and surgical instruments.

The prevalence of feline leukemia virus infection and disease parallels the opportunities for exposure. The prevalence of infection in single, confined, household cats is about 1%; infection rates rise progressively if cats also go outside, particularly to shows, live in a multiple cat household, or in breeding colonies. Infection rates may be as high as 33% in colonies in which the virus is endemic.

Using immunofluorescence or enzyme immunoassay procedures for detecting viral antigens, it is possible with a test and removal program to establish feline leukemia virus-free cat colonies. Such programs may be undertaken by large catteries, particularly where the incidence of infection is high and there is clinical evidence of disease due to feline leukemia virus. Laboratory tests aid in identifying preclinical or subclinical infections and in confirming clinical diagnosis.

At least two inactivated whole virus vaccines derived from infected cultured cells are available. Clinical trials have indicated that these vaccines reduce the incidence of disease by about 70%. A subunit vaccine based on a nonglycosylated subunit (p45) of the SU (gp70) envelope protein of a subgroup A virus, expressed in *Escherichia coli* and administered with two adjuvants, is also available. Various antiviral drugs, including azidothymidine, which is used in cancer therapy in humans, have been tried in particularly valuable cats, with limited success.

Murine Leukemias/Sarcomas

Murine leukemia/sarcoma viruses were identified originally in the 1920s and 1930s; several viruses were isolated and passaged in mice, each somewhat different, each given the name of the person identifying it—Gross, Friend, Moloney, Rauscher, and many other murine leukemia/sarcoma viruses. The different viruses induce distinct tumors: Gross and Moloney viruses induce T cell lymphomas, whereas Friend and Rauscher viruses induce erythroleukemia. Some viruses are immunosuppressive—infected animals may develop both B and T cell hyporesponsiveness. This has been referred to as murine acquired immunodeficiency syndrome (MAIDS).

All mice carry endogenous murine leukemia/sarcoma virus sequences in their chromosomes. Most of these are replication defective, although some inbred mouse strains (e.g., AKR) express replication-competent endogenous viruses spontaneously. Murine leukemia/sarcoma viruses induce tumors with latencies ranging from 2 to 18 months, depending on the strain of virus and strain of mouse. Neonatal infection is most efficient for leukemogenesis, whereas infection of adults usually does not lead to disease.

Murine leukemia/sarcoma viruses are widely distributed in laboratory and wild mice. The wild mouse viruses have been important because they have shown new receptor specificities and distinct lesion patterns; the laboratory mouse viruses have been the cause over the years of many compromised experiments, especially long-term experiments and experiments in which mouse strains that express high levels of virus must be used (e.g., AKR, C58, PL, HRS, CWD). The effect on experiments of the immunosuppression caused by some murine leukemia/sarcoma viruses has not been as well appreciated, but is another reason for choosing, where possible, strains of mice that express low levels of virus for experiments. Unlike the situation with other important murine viruses, there is no way to eliminate murine leukemia/sarcoma viruses from a colony; nevertheless, in some circumstances, testing is warranted to assess virus load.

Porcine Lymphosarcoma

A retrovirus has been isolated from porcine lymphosarcomas, which occur at a rate of 0.3 to 5 per 100,000 animals at slaughter and account for 25% of all porcine tumors known. Most porcine cell lines contain this virus, a host-specific type C retrovirus. There is evidence of the presence of the genome of this virus in wild Old World but not in New World species of the family *Suidae,* suggesting that the virus originated as an endogenous virus in Old World wild pigs. Two porcine endogenous retrovirus have been described recently, which will have to be accounted for in the breeding of retrovirus-free pigs for human xenotransplantation purposes.

Avian Reticuloendotheliosis

Reticuloendotheliosis viruses are pathogenic avian retroviruses that are antigenically and genetically unrelated to the avian leukosis/sarcoma retroviruses, but genetically similar to the mammalian and reptilian type C retroviruses. Five viruses have been recognized. The prototype of the group, reticuloendotheliosis virus-T, was isolated from an adult turkey that died of visceral reticuloendotheliosis and nerve lesions. Reticuloendotheliosis virus-T is replication defective and carries a v-*onc* gene, v-*rel*. The other avian reticuloendotheliosis viruses are reticuloendotheliosis-associated virus, duck infectious anemia virus, Trager duck spleen necrosis virus, and chick syncytial virus. These viruses are replication competent.

When inoculated into 1-day-old chicks, reticuloendotheliosis virus-T produces severe hepatosplenomegaly with either marked necrosis or lymphoproliferative lesions. Reticuloendotheliosis virus-T pseudotypes with avian leukosis virus envelopes are produced in chickens that carry the latter viruses. Some major outbreaks of reticuloendotheliosis virus-T disease, involving the deaths of several million chickens, have occurred as a consequence of contamination of turkey herpesvirus Marek's disease vaccine with reticuloendotheliosis virus-T virus. There is some evidence that the virus may be transmitted mechanically by mosquitoes.

Diseases Caused by Members of the Genus *Deltaretrovirus*

Bovine Leukemia

Bovine leukemia (*syn.*, enzootic bovine leukosis) attracted attention early in this century in several European countries, notably Denmark and Germany, where clusters of herds with a high incidence of disease suggested a viral etiology. Herds and areas characterized by a high prevalence are recognized in most countries. Overall prevalence figures for particular countries vary between 4 and 165 per 100,000 cattle per year, reflecting the great difference between low and high prevalence herds.

Sheep and goats can be infected with bovine leukemia virus, with most sheep developing lymphosarcoma. All evidence indicates that the virus does not spread from cattle to sheep (or from sheep to cattle) by normal contact. Neither is there any evidence that the bovine virus is transmissible to humans.

Clinical Features

Most bovine leukemia virus infections are asymptomatic and are recognized only by serological testing. Of infected cattle, about 30% develop persistent lymphocytosis, but this is not associated with any clinical signs. In those few animals that do develop disease, clinical signs are seen at 4 to 8 years of age; there are lymphoid tumors (i.e., lymphosarcomas or malignant lymphomas) in lymph nodes, abomasum, heart, spleen, kidneys, uterus, spinal meninges, and brain, but not any consistent presence of large numbers of malignant cells in the blood as suggested by the name of the disease and the virus.

Pathogenesis, Pathology, and Immunity

Oncogenesis probably depends on the integration of a bovine proviral v-*onc* gene(s) into cellular DNA. The course of infection suggests a multistage process. The major target cells are B lymphocytes. In an animal destined to develop disease, infection is at first inapparent, then may progress to a persistent lymphocytosis, and finally to neoplasia. The latter is marked by enlarged lymph nodes and leukemic infiltrations into a variety of organs and tissues. Some tumors, particularly those from terminal cases, do not contain the virus or viral antigens. However, cocultivation of lymphocytes with susceptible cells, with or without mitogens, results in the production of infectious virus.

Laboratory Diagnosis

Enzyme immunoassay, agar gel diffusion, and syncytium–inhibition assays are used for diagnosis. Test and removal programs have been adopted by several European countries, including Denmark and Germany, and these countries require that imported cattle be serologically negative using standardized tests. In other countries, including the United States and Canada, individual owners have undertaken test and removal programs on a voluntary basis, but national programs are not in place.

Epidemiology, Prevention, and Control

Bovine leukemia virus, like other retroviruses, is not highly transmissible. Virus is transmitted horizontally within herds but does not extend readily to neighboring herds, suggesting that close and prolonged direct exposure is required. Overall national incidence rates seldom exceed a few percent. For particular herds the incidence may be much higher, which should signal the possibility of iatrogenic transmission. The high incidence of infection in Denmark earlier in the 20th century was probably iatrogenic, linked to whole-blood vaccines used for the control of babesiosis and anaplasmosis.

Transmission of bovine leukemia virus occurs primarily by the transfer of lymphocytes between animals via trauma, restraint devices, gloves used for rectal examination, reuse of needles and surgical instruments, and rarely by insects acting as mechanical vectors. The virus can be transmitted to the fetus, but usually less than 10% of calves born to infected dams are infected at birth.

Virus may be eliminated from a herd if all cattle are tested serologically at 2- to 3-month intervals and positive animals removed immediately. The length of time required to obtain a virus-free herd varies, depending on the initial prevalence of infection, but in most herds the elimination can be accomplished in 1 year. If the prevalence of infection is too high to permit removal of all serologically positive animals, segregation of seropositive and seronegative animals may be attempted. Calves from infected dams should be isolated, tested, and only allowed to enter the seronegative cohort if seronegative at 6 months of age. An inactivated vaccine, which has been shown to prevent disease following virus challenge in clinical trials, has been used on an experimental basis.

Diseases Caused by Members of the Genus *Epsilonretrovirus*

Retrovirus Diseases of Fish

Walleye dermal sarcoma virus is a newly described retrovirus that is associated etiologically with a multifocal skin tumor of the walleye (*Stigostedium vitreum*), an important North American sport fish. Tumor prevalence ranges from 27% of adult walleyes in a densely populated lake, Oneida Lake, New York, to 1% in less populated waters. Phylogenetic analysis of isolates from different regions of North America has indicated that there are distinct genotypic clusters matching geographic origins suggesting that the various genotypes have a long association with fish in various lakes. Two other retroviruses have been isolated from walleyes, walleye epidermal hyperplasia viruses 1 and 2, and other retroviruses have been isolated from snakeheads, sea bass, and salmon. The sea bass virus has been associated with an erythrocytic disease and the salmon virus with leukemia. Because the discovery of these viruses occurred only recently, little is known of their overall importance, but already there is a sense that there are many more fish retroviruses awaiting discovery and epidemiologic study.

Diseases Caused by Members of the Genus *Lentivirus*

Since the discovery in 1983 that human acquired immunodeficiency syndrome (AIDS) is caused by human immunodeficiency virus (HIV) and that this virus is a lentivirus, these viruses have become the most intensively studied viruses of all time. There has been remarkable progress in defining their basic properties and the pathogenesis of the diseases they cause. Human acquired immunodeficiency syndrome now serves as a model for the lentivirus diseases of veterinary importance, and the lentivirus diseases of animals are used as models for the study of the human disease. This "cross-fertilization" even involves the surrogate testing of drugs and vaccines in primate and feline models with the aim of developing preventive and therapeutic regimens for animals as well as humans. In this regard all of the animal lentiviruses and the diseases they cause are of interest, each providing particular lessons and particular experimental advantages. The complex interrelationships among these viruses are shown in Figure 23.11.

Maedi/Visna (Ovine Progressive Pneumonia)

In 1933, 20 karakul sheep were imported into Iceland from Germany, and within 2 years two diseases, called *maedi* (dyspnea) and *visna* (wasting) emerged, which in the following years were responsible for the deaths of 105,000 sheep. A further 600,000 sheep were slaughtered in 1965, when the diseases were declared eradicated. These diseases have an incubation period of over 2 years, an insidious onset, and a protracted clinical course, lasting 6 months to several years, unless terminated by intercurrent disease. Sigurdsson, who demonstrated that both Icelandic diseases were transmissible with cell-free filtrates, described the diseases as "slow virus infections," thus introducing into virology a term that has been widely used for other infections as well.

Visna, in which the lesions occur in the central nervous system, has rarely been described in sheep outside Iceland, although a few cases have been reported in The Netherlands. However, maedi occurs in several countries in Europe (where in The Netherlands it is called Zwoegerziekte and in France La Bouhite), in South Africa (where it is called Graaf Reinet), and in the United States (where it is called ovine progressive pneumonia). Maedi does not occur in Australia or New Zealand. It is now clear that maedi and visna are caused by the same or very closely related lentiviruses.

Clinical Features

Maedi (Progressive Pneumonia)

The onset of clinical signs in maedi is insidious and is seldom detected in sheep less than 3 years of age. Incubation periods of up to 8 years have been recorded. There is progressive weight loss, and dyspnea, initially detectable only after exercise, becoming progressively more apparent over time. Affected sheep straggle when the flock is driven. The head may jerk rhythmically with each inspiration, nostrils are flared, there may be a slight nasal discharge and a cough. Severely dyspneic sheep spend much time lying down. The clinical course may last 3 to 8 months; it may be prolonged by careful nursing

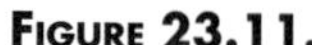

FIGURE 23.11.

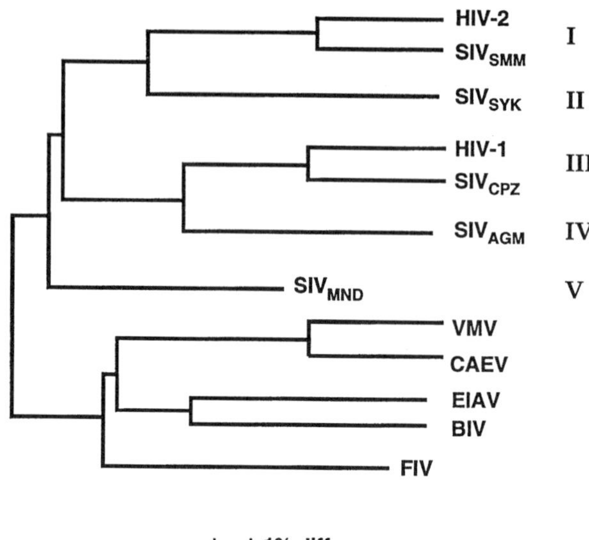

The close phylogenetic relationship among animal lentiviruses. Representative viruses were compared using *pol* gene nucleotide sequences. Five groups of primate lentiviruses are shown (roman numerals), along with the lentiviruses of other animals. HIV 1, human immunodeficiency virus 1; HIV 2, human immunodeficiency virus 2; SIVsmm, simian immunodeficiency virus from sooty mangabey monkey; SIVsyk, simian immunodeficiency virus from Sykes monkey; SIVcpz, simian immunodeficiency virus from chimpanzee; SIVagm, simian immunodeficiency virus from African green monkey; SIVmnd, simian immunodeficiency virus from mandrill; VMV, maedi/visna virus; CAEV, caprine arthritis–encephalitis virus; EIAV, equine infectious anemia virus; BIV, bovine immunodeficiency virus; and FIV, feline immunodeficiency virus. The branching order of the primate lentiviruses is controversial. The scale indicates percentage difference in nucleotide sequences in the *pol* gene. [From P. A. Luciw, Human immunodeficiency viruses and their replication. *In* "Fields Virology" (B. N. Fields, D. M. Knipe, P. M. Howley, R. M. Chanock, J. L. Melnick, T. P. Monath, B. Roizman, and S. E. Straus, eds.), 3rd ed., pp. 1881–1952. Lippincott-Raven, Philadelphia, PA, 1996.]

or shortened by pregnancy, stress such as occasioned by inclement weather or poor nutrition, or intercurrent disease, particularly pneumonia due to *Pasteurella* spp. Pregnant ewes may abort or deliver weak lambs.

Visna

The incubation period of visna varies from a few months to 9 years. The onset of clinical signs is insidious and usually begins with slight weakness of the hind legs. Affected sheep may not be able to keep up with the flock and may stumble and fall for no apparent reason. There is progressive weight loss and trembling of facial muscles and lips. The paresis eventually leads to paraplegia. There is no fever, appetite is maintained, and sheep remain alert. The clinical course may last several years, with periods of remission. The cerebrospinal fluid contains up to 200 mononuclear cells per milliliter (normal: 50 per milliliter).

Pathogenesis, Pathology, and Immunity

Prior to 1933, Icelandic sheep were genetically isolated for 1000 years and it has been suggested, but not proven, that there may be a genetic predisposition to lentivirus disease, especially visna. The virus is probably acquired most commonly by droplet infection via the respiratory tract. A lymphocyte-associated viremia occurs, in which about 1 in every 10^6 peripheral blood leukocytes is infected.

Apart from neurogenic muscle atrophy, no gross lesions are found in visna and histologically lesions are usually confined to the central nervous system, although occasionally minor lesions are seen in the lungs. The characteristic lesion in the central nervous system is a demyelinating leukoencephalomyelitis. The meninges and subependymal spaces are infiltrated with mononuclear cells, mainly lymphocytes, with some plasma cells and macrophages. There is perivascular cuffing, neuronal necrosis, malacia, and demyelination scattered patchily throughout the central nervous system.

Gross findings in maedi are restricted to the lungs and associated lymph nodes. The lungs show extensive consolidation and do not collapse when the thoracic cavity is opened. Bronchial and mediastinal lymph nodes are enlarged greatly. Histologically there is hyperplasia of the fibrous tissue and muscle of the alveolar septa and a mononuclear cell inflammatory infiltration.

Lentiviruses are exceptionally resistant to interferon, and despite a diverse range of immune responses, including the production of neutralizing antibodies and a cell-mediated immune response, neither virus nor infected cells are eliminated. Immune suppression abrogates or delays the progress of degenerative changes, indicating that there is an immunopathologic element in lesions in both the lungs and central nervous system. In infected sheep, antigenic variation in the envelope antigens of the virus occurs over time—this may be an important mechanism for circumventing viral elimination and a key in the pathogenesis of the disease.

Laboratory Diagnosis

The most widely used diagnostic tests for the detection of antibody are enzyme immunoassays in which either or both core and surface antigens are present. Western blots are more sensitive and are used frequently to confirm a diagnosis. Antigen may be detected in peripheral blood leukocytes by enzyme immunoassay and viral DNA may be detected in these cells by *in situ* hybridization, directly or following viral RNA amplification using the reverse-transcriptase polymerase chain reaction. Virus can be isolated by cocultivation of gradient-purified peripheral blood leukocytes with mitogen-stimulated purified sheep peripheral blood leukocytes in the presence of interleukin 2. Reverse transcriptase assays performed at various times on the supernatants from these cultures provide an indication of virus growth and are used to guide virus isolation methods.

Epidemiology, Prevention, and Control

Maedi/visna virus is present in a variety of body fluids, including blood, semen, bronchial secretions, tears, saliva, and milk. Droplet transmission is facilitated by housing and close confinement and was important in Iceland, where sheep are housed for 6 months of the year. Transmission is usually direct, although infection via drinking water or from fecal or urine contamination seems to occur as well. Asymptomatic sheep are rarely a source of virus for infection of other sheep, with the possible exception of ewe to lamb transmission via milk. Evidence for transplacental infection is conflicting but virus may be shed in semen of rams with a high virus load. Biting arthropods and surgical equipment readily transmit virus mechanically from viremic sheep.

Maedi/visna was eradicated from Iceland by a drastic slaughter policy, before the availability of any diagnostic test. Test and removal programs are used in Norway and The Netherlands. Enzyme immunoassays, agar gel diffusion, and a syncytial plaque reduction assay are used for antibody detection in support of these programs.

Caprine Arthritis–Encephalomyelitis

First recognized in the United States in 1974, caprine arthritis–encephalomyelitis is now known to occur worldwide. In the United States, the disease is now the most important disease of goats; infection rates as high as 80% have been reported in some herds and the economic loss from the disease is substantial. The virus is most closely related to North American isolates of maedi/visna virus. Two syndromes are recognized: encephalomyelitis in kids 2 to 4 months of age and more commonly arthritis in goats from about 12 months of age onward. The virus is not known to be transmitted naturally to other animal species. Experimentally, the virus infects sheep and causes arthritis; however, despite the high incidence of infection in goats in Australia and New Zealand, infection of sheep has not been reported in these countries.

Clinical Features

The central nervous system disease is a progressive leukoencephalomyelitis associated with ascending paralysis. Affected goats also show progressive wasting and trembling and the hair coat is dull, but they remain afebrile, alert, and usually maintain good appetite and sight (Figure 23.12). Terminally there is paralysis, deviation of the head and neck, and paddling. The onset of arthritis is usually insidious and progresses slowly over months to years, but in some cases disease may appear suddenly and remain static. The joints are swollen and painful, particularly the carpal joints but also hock, stifle, shoulder, fetlock, and vertebral joints. Cold weather exacerbates the signs. Bursae, particularly the atlantooccipital, and tendon sheaths are thickened and distended with fluid. Thickening of the joint capsules results in restricted movement and flexion contracture.

Pathogenesis, Pathology, and Immunity

At autopsy, central nervous system lesions may be visible as focal malacia in white matter, but are identi-

FIGURE 23.12.

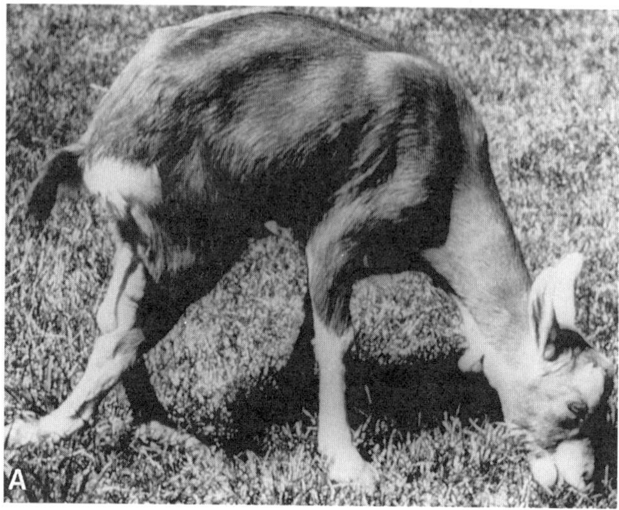

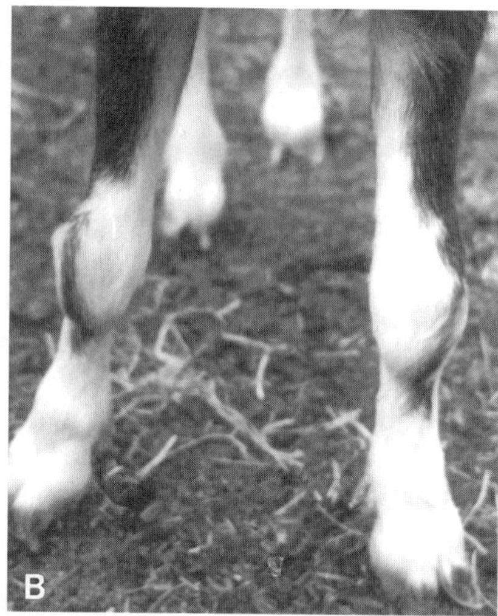

Caprine arthritis–encephalomyelitis. (A) Kid goat with paralyzed hind quarters, but alert and attempting to graze. (B) Enlarged carpal joints in a 5-year-old goat. (Courtesy of J. R. Gorham and T. H. Crawford.)

fied more reliably microscopically as foci of mononuclear cell inflammation and demyelination. The basic joint lesion is a proliferative synovitis; tendon sheaths and bursae are characterized by villus hypertrophy, synovial cell hyperplasia, and infiltration with lymphocytes, plasma cells, and macrophages. Progression is accompanied by degenerative changes including fibrosis, necrosis, mineralization of synovial membranes, and osteoporosis. Mild interstitial pneumonia and hyperplasia of pulmonary lymphoid tissue may be seen at necropsy.

Laboratory Diagnosis

Antibodies can be detected by agar gel diffusion, indirect immunofluorescence, or enzyme immunoassays and form the basis of voluntary control programs based on test and removal.

Epidemiology, Prevention, and Control

Virus is acquired during the neonatal period, via colostrum or milk. The rate of infection of newborn goats can be reduced by more than 90% by removing kids from infected does as they pass from the birth canal, providing them with colostrum that has been heated to 56°C for 1 hour, feeding them pasteurized goat or cow's milk, and raising them in isolation from infected goats. Serological tests such as the agar gel immunodiffusion test can be used to monitor herd status.

Equine Infectious Anemia

Equine infectious anemia is an important disease of horses that occurs worldwide. The disease may vary from an acute syndrome that ends fatally within a month of onset to a chronic relapsing disease. It may also remain silent for the life of the infected horse.

Clinical Features

Following primary infection, most horses develop fever after an incubation period of 7–21 days. The disease is recognized as four interchanging, overlapping syndromes. In acute equine infectious anemia there is a marked fever, weakness, severe anemia, jaundice, blood-stained feces, tachypnea, and petechial hemorrhages of the mucosae. As many as 80% of acute cases are fatal; others pass into the subacute form, in which continuing moderate fever is followed by recovery. Recovery from either the acute or the subacute disease is followed by lifelong persistent infection. Recovered viremic horses may appear and perform well, but some experience recurrent episodes of disease whereas others develop chronic disease that varies from mild signs of illness and failure to thrive to episodic or persistent fever, cachexia, anemia, and ventral edema.

Pathogenesis, Pathology, and Immunity

The disease is due to initial infection of macrophages and then lymphocytes, in which degenerative or proliferative responses may occur. Lifelong, cell-associated viremia develops in all infected horses. It is uncertain whether anemia develops as a consequence of bone marrow suppression, increased clearance of red cells from the circulation, or autoimmune destruction of erythrocytes. Vasculitis, including glomerulonephritis, is mediated by immune complexes. Hemorrhages may be a consequence of thrombocytopenia. During the course of infection and linked to recurrent episodes of disease, significant genomic variations, including deletions, have been mapped to the principal neutralizing domain of the SU (gp90) envelope protein.

Laboratory Diagnosis

Clinical diagnosis is confirmed by the immunodiffusion or "Coggins test," a simple and highly accurate serological test to detect infection. Foals nursing infected dams test positive temporarily, and recently infected horses may test negative.

Epidemiology, Prevention, and Control

Tabanid flies and stable flies (*Stomoxys* spp.), mosquitoes, and possibly *Culicoides* spp. can serve as mechanical vectors for equine infectious anemia virus. Transmission occurs particularly in the summer months in low-lying, humid, swamp areas such as occur in the Mississippi delta region of the United States and in parts of South and Central America, South Africa, and northern Australia. National prevalence figures are geographically uneven and reflect the importance of insect transmission. On farms where infection has been endemic for many years the prevalence may be as high as 70%. Iatrogenic transmission by the use of nonsterile equipment has been responsible for some major outbreaks. Transplacental infection has been recognized; colostrum and milk, saliva, urine, and semen are other unproved but possible modes of transmission.

In endemic areas the rate of transmission may be reduced by insect-proof stabling of horses during those times of the year (summer) and that time of the day (dusk) when insects are most active. Iatrogenic transmission is avoided by careful hygiene.

The development in 1970 of the agar gel diffusion test for detecting antibodies to equine infectious anemia virus was followed in the United States by regulations, promulgated by federal and state agencies and some breed associations, to limit the movement of seropositive horses. In some instances a negative test has been required as a condition of entry to racetracks, sale yards, and shows. Buyers of horses have also increasingly sought negative test certification. The United States Department of Agriculture introduced regulations relating to the licensing and operation of laboratories authorized to conduct the agar gel diffusion test, and horses imported into the United States and some other countries are now required to have a negative test certificate from an authorized laboratory. For horses remaining within a state, testing is not compulsory nor is it compulsory for an owner to destroy a horse giving a positive test. A reportedly efficacious vaccine has been used in China since 1983.

Feline Immunodeficiency Virus Disease

Since its first isolation in California in 1987 and the development of enzyme immunoassays for its diagnosis, feline immunodeficiency virus (FIV) has been identified in many countries. It probably has a worldwide distribution. Most isolates have come from domestic cats; however, related but distinguishable isolates have also been made from lions, puma, Pallas' cat, and bobcat; antibodies have been found in the sera of more than 18 different feline species. The seroprevalence varies from 1% in random surveys to 30% in sick domestic cats. It is now clear that many of the signs of disease in cats formerly associated with aging more recently, with feline leukemia virus infection may be due to FIV infection. As noted earlier, it is likely that the clinical features of feline leukemia virus infection given earlier in this chapter may require further revision as the two infections are better distinguished.

Clinical Features

The clinical disease may be described as having three stages: an acute stage marked by lymphadenopathy and fever, a long subclinical stage, and a terminal stage marked by degenerative disease and opportunistic infections. Common presenting clinical signs include an insidious onset of recurrent fever of undetermined origin, lymphadenopathy, leukopenia, anemia, weight loss, and nonspecific behavioral changes.

In the terminal stage, opportunistic bacterial and fungal infections are especially common in the mouth, periodontal tissue, cheeks, and tongue. About 25% of cats have chronic respiratory disease, and a lesser number have chronic enteritis, urinary tract infection, dermatitis, and neurologic signs. The terminal disease resembles advanced human AIDS. Terminally, about 5% of cats have serious neurologic disease, although histology studies reveal that a higher proportion have central nervous system lesions at necropsy.

Pathogenesis, Pathology, and Immunity

The incubation period of FIV infection may last for several years; progression of the disease that follows parallels the decline in $CD4^+$ T lymphocytes. Infected cats have a higher than expected incidence of feline leukemia virus-negative lymphomas, usually of the B cell type, and myeloproliferative disorders (neoplasias and dysplasias). Of affected cats, about 5% have central nervous system lesions that are associated with behavioral abnormalities, psychomotor disturbances, dementia, and convulsions. Cats remain infected for life; the presence of serum antibodies is correlated directly with the ability to isolate virus from blood cells and saliva.

Laboratory Diagnosis

Virus antigen can be detected by enzyme immunoassay or proviral DNA by the polymerase chain reaction in peripheral blood leukocytes of infected cats. In experimental infections, antibodies can be detected within 2 to 4 weeks of infection using enzyme immunoassay, immunofluorescence, or Western blotting. False-positive enzyme immunoassay results range from 2 to 20%, probably because of the use in cats of vaccines that have been produced in feline cell cultures and the presence in these products of allotypic antigens; vigorous attempts are under way to improve the specificity of enzyme immunoassays.

Epidemiology, Prevention, and Control

Feline immunodeficiency virus is shed mainly in the saliva, and the principal mode of transmission is through bites. Because of this, free-roaming (feral and pet), male, and aged cats are at the greatest risk of infection. Feline immunodeficiency virus infection is uncommon in closed purebred catteries. Neither sexual contact nor maternal grooming appears to be significant modes of transmission, although virus may be shed in semen. However, the virus is transmitted to kittens from acutely infected queens through colostrum and milk.

Drugs directed against the viral reverse transcriptase, such as azidothymidine, have been used with modest success. Appropriate test and removal programs and certification at the point of sale can be applied to control the infection. A wide range of experimental vaccines have been developed, including products made from whole inactivated virus, whole inactivated infected cells, a variety of recombinant DNA-produced antigens [SU protein, peptides to the VR3 region, p24 (capsid) protein], and "naked DNA." Some of these vaccines have enhanced disease and no feline immunodeficiency virus vaccine is in wide clinical use. A fully infectious DNA clone of FIV has been made and will enhance vaccine development and other research. No human public health risks have been identified in association with the infection in cats.

Simian Immunodeficiency Virus Disease

There is a high prevalence of persistent infection of several African nonhuman primate species with lentiviruses that seem to have evolved separately with their host species (Table 23.1). For example, a high proportion of African green (*Cercopithecus aethiops*) monkeys in the wild in Africa (as well as in colonies in other areas) are infected. In most cases these viruses do not cause overt disease in their natural hosts; however, when some of these viruses gain entry into other species of monkeys, there may be severe, even fatal, disease. For example, when virus from African green monkeys (simian immunodeficiency virus SIV_{agm}) infects rhesus macaques (*Macaca mullata*), it causes an AIDS-like disease.

Simian immunodeficiency virus SIV_{mac} has not been identified in rhesus monkeys in the wild in Asia but it is transmitted among animals in colonies where it causes an AIDS-like disease. Months after exposure, the first signs of infection are an inguinal rash and lymphadenopathy. This progresses to a wasting syndrome, chronic enteritis, and the onset of opportunistic infections caused by organisms such as *Toxoplasma gondii, Pneumocystis carinii, Cryptosporidium* spp., *Salmonella* spp. and adenoviruses, papovaviruses, and cytomegaloviruses. There is often an encephalopathy with neural lesions similar to those seen in humans with AIDS dementia.

Following the discovery of a similar virus (SIV_{stm}) in stump-tailed macaques (*Macaca arctoides*) in the California Regional Primate Research Center in the 1970s, infected animals were found to develop lymphomas, progressive multifocal leukoencephalopathy (a fatal disease of the central nervous system caused by any of several papovaviruses), tuberculosis, and other diseases seen typically in human AIDS patients.

Human Infection

Two workers have been reported as having developed antibodies to simian immunodeficiency viruses following exposures in the laboratory and in the course of handling monkeys (one via a needle stick, one from bleeding an infected monkey). Recommendations for workers are now the same as for working with nonhuman primates infected with HIV.

Bovine Immunodeficiency Virus Disease

Bovine immunodeficiency virus was isolated from peripheral blood leukocytes in 1972 and for the next 20 years received little attention. It causes a nonacute disease and can be grown in monolayer cell cultures from a variety of bovine embryonic tissues, producing a cytopathic effect characterized by syncytium formation. The genome is the most complex of the nonprimate lentiviruses in that in addition to *tat, rev,* and *vif,* the genome also contains three other accessory genes designated *vpy, vpw,* and *tmx.* When transmitted to calves by intravenous inoculation there is an immediate leukopenia followed within 15–20 days by lymphocytosis that persists. The virus infects a wide spectrum of cells; proviral DNA has been detected in $CD3^+$, $CD4^+$, and $CD8^+$ cells as well as γ/δ and B lymphocytes, null cells, and monocytes. Virus persists in naturally infected cows for at least 12 months, but neither the prevalence of the infection nor its economic significance has been determined.

Jembrana Disease

In contrast to the somewhat benign nature of bovine immunodeficiency virus infection in European cattle, a related virus has been established as the cause of a peracute disease of Bali cattle (*Bos javanicus*) in Indonesia. The disease, called Jembrana disease for the district, was recognized in 1964. Within 12 months, 26,000 of 300,000 cattle in the area died. The disease remains endemic on Bali and has spread to Sumatra, Java, and Kalimantan. The origin of the virus has not been established. Disease is characterized by high morbidity and high mortality rates. After a very short incubation period of 5 to 12 days there is fever, lethargy, anorexia, and pronounced swelling of lymph nodes and panleukopenia. About 17% of acutely ill cattle die. Postmortem findings include widespread hemorrhages, lymphadenopathy, and splenomegaly. Histologically, many lymphoblastoid cells are found in the lymphoid tissues. The viral genome has been sequenced completely and is similar to, but distinguishable from, other isolates of bovine immunodeficiency virus.

Further Reading

Anonymous. (1991). Colloquium on feline leukemia virus/feline immunodeficiency virus: Tests and vaccination. *J. Am. Vet. Med. Assoc.* **199**, 1271–1485.

Biggs, P. M. (1991). Lymphoproliferative diseases of turkeys. *In* "Diseases of Poultry" (B. W. Calnek, ed.), 10th ed., pp. 485–489. Iowa State University Press, Ames.

Cheevers, W. P., and McGuire, T. C. (1985). Equine infectious anemia virus: Immunopathogenesis and persistence. *Rev. Infect. Dis.* **7**, 83–88.

Cheevers, W. P., and McGuire, T. C. (1988). The lentiviruses: Maedi/visna, caprine arthritis-encephalitis, and equine infectious anemia. *Adv. Virus Res.* **34**, 189–215.

Coffin, J. M. (1996). Retroviridae: The viruses and their replication. *In* "Fields Virology" (B. N. Fields, D. M. Knipe, P. M. Howley, R. M. Chanock, J. L. Melnick, T. P. Monath, B. Roizman, and S. E. Straus, eds.), 3rd ed., pp. 1767–1848. Lippincott-Raven, Philadelphia, PA.

Coffin, J. M., Hughes, A. H., and Varmus, H. E., eds. (1997). "Retroviruses." Cold Spring Harbor Laboratory Press, Cold Spring Harbor, NY.

Fauci, A. S. (1996). Host factors and the pathogenesis of HIV-induced disease. *Nature (London)* **384**, 529–534.

Hoover, E. A., Mullins, J. I., Quackenbush, S. L., and Gasper, P. W. (1987). Experimental transmission and pathogenesis of immunodeficiency syndrome in cats. *Blood* **70**, 1880–1892.

Jarrett, O. (1996). The relevance of feline retroviruses to the development of vaccines against HIV. AIDS *Res. Hum. Retroviruses* **20**, 385–387.

Joag, S. V., Stephens, E. B., and Narayan, O. (1996). Lentiviruses. *In* "Fields Virology" (B. N. Fields, D. M. Knipe, P. M. Howley, R. M. Chanock, J. L. Melnick, T. P. Monath, B. Roizman, and S. E. Straus, eds.), 3rd ed., pp. 1977–1996. Lippincott-Raven, Philadelphia, PA.

Levy, J. A. (1997). "HIV and the Pathogenesis of AIDS," 2nd ed. American Society for Microbiology Press, Washington, DC.

Luciw, P. A. (1996). Human immunodeficiency viruses and their replication. *In* "Fields Virology" (B. N. Fields, D. M. Knipe, P. M. Howley, R. M. Chanock, J. L. Melnick, T. P. Monath, B. Roizman, and S. E. Straus, eds.), 3rd ed., pp. 1881–1952. Lippincott-Raven, Philadelphia, PA.

Neil, J. C., Fulton, R., Rigby, M., and Stewart, M. (1991). Feline leukemia virus: Generation of pathogenic and oncogenic variants. *Curr. Top. Microbiol. Immunol.* **171**, 67–93.

Payne, L. N., and Fadly, A. M. (1991). Leukosis/sarcoma group. *In* "Diseases of Poultry" (B. W. Calnek, ed.), 10th ed., pp. 414–420. Iowa State University Press, Ames.

Pedersen, N. C., Ho, E. W., Brown, M. L., and Yamamoto, J. K. (1987). Isolation of a T-lymphotropic virus from domestic cats with immunodeficiency-like syndrome. *Science* **235**, 790–793.

Sparkes, A. H. (1997). Feline leukaemia virus: A review of immunity and vaccination. *J. Small Anim. Pract.* **38**, 187–194.

van der Marten, M. J., and Miller, J. M. (1990). Bovine leukosis virus. *In* "Virus Infections of Vertebrates" (Z. Dinter, and B. Morein, eds.), vol. 3, pp. 419–425. Elsevier, Amsterdam.

Wilcox, G. R. (1997). Jembrana disease. *Aust. Vet. J.* **75**, 492–493.

Willett, B., Flynn, J. N., and Hosie, M. J. (1997). FIV infection of the domestic cat: An animal model for AIDS. *Immunol. Today* **18**, 182–189.

Witter, R. L. (1997). Reticuloendotheliosis. *In* "Diseases of Poultry" (B. W. Calnek, ed.), 10th ed., pp. 467–470. Iowa State University Press, Ames.

CHAPTER 24

Reoviridae

The family *Reoviridae* is one of the most complex in all of virology, comprising nine genera that variously contain viruses of mammals, birds, reptiles, amphibians, fish, invertebrates, and plants. The root term *reo,* an acronym for "*r*espiratory *e*nteric *o*rphan," was coined because the first members of the family were found in the respiratory and the enteric tracts of animals and humans as "orphans," i.e., not associated with any disease. These viruses are now members of the genus *Orthoreovirus.* The later inclusion in the family of the genera *Orbivirus, Coltivirus, Rotavirus,* and *Aquareovirus* added important animal and human pathogens. The diversity of the hosts infected and the variety of transmission patterns employed by the member viruses raise, but do not answer, the question of where these fascinating viruses might have originated.

The distribution of the member viruses of the genus *Orthoreovirus* is ubiquitous. Although their host range includes cattle, sheep, swine, humans, monkeys, bats, and birds, associated diseases are usually rather insignificant—some diarrhea, some respiratory illness, and some neurologic disease. Only the infection of laboratory rodents, chickens, and turkeys is of clinical significance.

The distribution of the member viruses of the genus *Orbivirus,* as is typical of arthropod-borne viruses, is much more circumscribed than that of other genera; each virus is limited by the distribution of its particular vector. There is much diversity in vectors, however, with some viruses being transmitted by mosquitoes, some by *Culicoides* spp., and some by black flies, sandflies, and ticks. The most important members of this genus, bluetongue viruses and African horse sickness viruses, have been the cause of economically important diseases in South Africa since the early days of European settlement—in recent years bluetongue has been recognized as a *nontariff trade barrier* in North and South America and Australia, and African horse sickness has been recognized as a substantial problem in the Iberian peninsula.

Rotaviruses are also widespread; essentially every species of domestic animal and bird has been found to harbor at least one indigenous rotavirus, in most cases causing diarrhea ("scours") in newborn animals. Considering all animal species and humans together, rotavirus diarrhea, which is often more severe than diarrhea caused by other viruses, is one of the most important diseases in the world. It is the proximal cause of death of millions of children in developing countries and the cause of great economic loss in many livestock industries.

Properties of Reoviruses

Classification

All viruses of animals with segmented double-stranded RNA genomes, except the birnaviruses (see Chapter 25), have been placed in the family *Reoviridae*. Consequently, the family is quite complex (Table 24.1). The genus *Orthoreovirus* comprises 3 viruses of mammals, reoviruses 1, 2, and 3, a few other viruses of mammals that will not be mentioned further, and 11 avian viruses, which are designated by serial numbers.

The genus *Orbivirus* is divided into 14 distinct subgroups, of which 5 include viruses that cause disease in domestic animals. Separate subgroups encompass bluetongue viruses 1 to 25, African horse sickness viruses 1 to 9, epizootic hemorrhagic disease of deer viruses 1 and 2, Ibaraki virus, equine encephalosis viruses 1 and 2, and other viruses affecting various animal species. The subgroups have been defined serologically and genotypically—viruses within each subgroup have a common antigen demonstrable by serologic tests. Low-level serological cross-reactions do occur between individual viruses in different subgroups, but the confusion that this once caused has now been obviated by genotyping (e.g., partial sequencing).

The classification of the member viruses of the genus *Rotavirus* is based on genotypic and serologic analyses. Variance in the group-specific capsid antigen on VP6 is used to define major groups. Rotavirus group A includes important pathogens of humans, cattle, and other animals; group B includes only pathogens of humans; groups C and E include only pathogens of swine; and groups D and F include only pathogens of fowl. Differentiation into serotypes is based on neutralization tests. Because both outer capsid proteins (VP4 and VP7) carry type-specific epitopes recognized by neutralizing antibodies, a binary system of classification of serotypes has been developed, akin to that used for influenza viruses. For example, in group A, 14 serotypes have been defined on the basis of different VP7 antigens and 8 serotypes on the basis of different VP4 antigens. Mono-

Table 24.1
Diseases Caused by Members of the Family *Reoviridae*

Genus	Virus	Principal species affected	Disease
Orthoreovirus			
	Mammalian reoviruses 1–3	Isolated from many species of mammals	Hepatoencephalomyelitis in mice
	Avian reoviruses 1–11	Chickens, turkeys, and geese	Arthritis, nephrosis, enteritis, chronic respiratory disease, myocarditis
Orbivirus			
	Bluetongue viruses 1–25	Sheep, cattle, and deer	Bluetongue
	African horse sickness viruses 1–9	Horses, donkeys, mules, and zebras	African horse sickness
	Equine encephalosis viruses 1–5	Horses	Abortion and encephalitis
	Epizootic hemorrhagic disease of deer viruses 1–7	Deer	Epizootic hemorrhagic disease
	Ibaraki virus	Cattle	Acute febrile disease similar to bluetongue
	Palyam viruses 1–6	Cattle	Abortion, congenital abnormalities
Rotavirus			
	Rotaviruses: many different viruses, often host specific	Virtually all animals	Enteritis
Coltivirus			
	Colorado tick fever virus, Eyach virus	Zoonotic, small mammals, and humans	Colorado tick fever
Aquareovirus			
	Many viruses of fish, shellfish	Fish, shellfish	Not certain

clonal antibodies, polyacrylamide gel electrophoresis of viral RNA segments, and partial sequencing can be used to make even finer distinctions as may be necessary in molecular epidemiology studies.

There are only a few members of the genus *Coltivirus*—in fact for many years Colorado tick fever virus had no relatives. Eyach virus is the European counterpart of the prototype virus, and other distinct coltiviruses have been isolated in California, Indonesia, and China.

The genus *Aquareovirus* contains a large number of viruses isolated from saltwater fish (various species of Atlantic and Pacific salmon, smelt), freshwater fish (bass, catfish), and oysters and other shellfish. The pathogenic and economic significance of many of these viruses remains unknown.

Virion Properties

Reovirus virions are nonenveloped, nearly spherical in outline, and have a diameter of 80 nm. Virions consist of an outer, middle, and inner capsid, each with icosahedral symmetry, the precise morphology varying with the genus (Figure 24.1). The genome consists of linear double-

FIGURE 24.1.

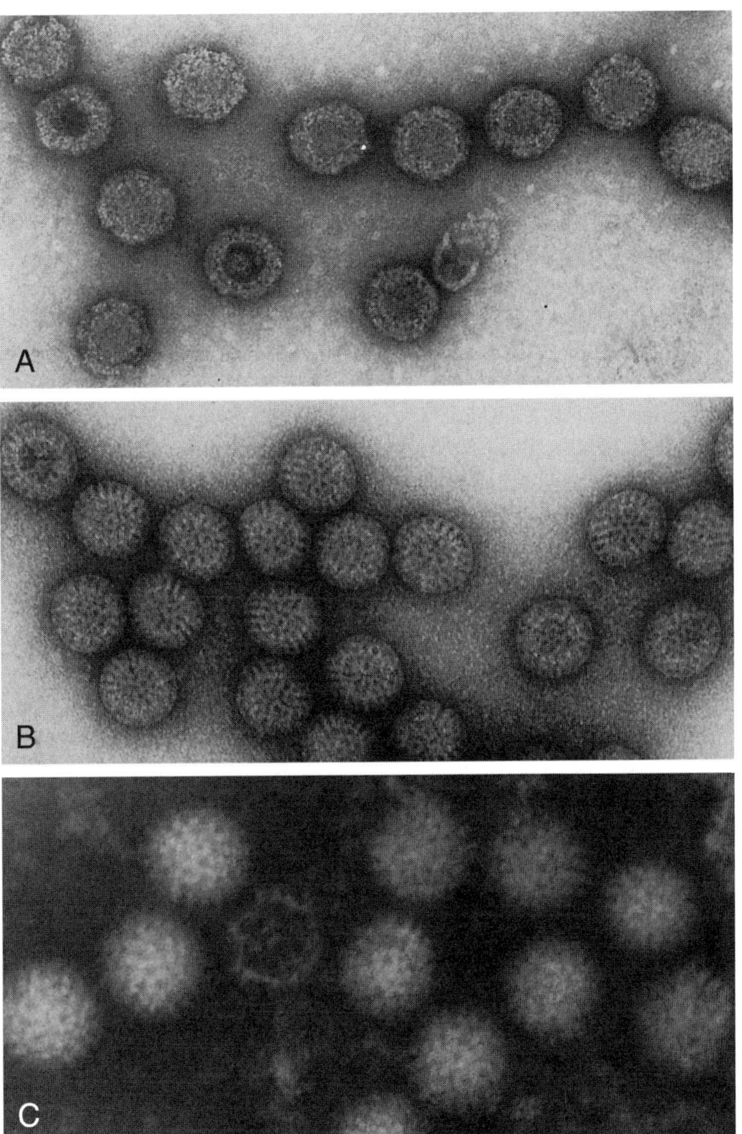

Family *Reoviridae;* representative viruses visualized by negative contrast electron microscopy. (A) Genus *Orthoreovirus,* mammalian reovirus 3. (B) Genus *Rotavirus,* simian rotavirus SA11. (C) Genus *Orbivirus,* bluetongue virus 11. Bars: 100 nm.

stranded RNA divided into 10 (genus *Orthoreovirus* and *Orbivirus*), 11 (genus *Rotavirus* and *Aquareovirus*), or 12 (genus *Coltivirus*) segments. The overall genome size is 23 (genus *Orthoreovirus*), 18 (genus *Orbivirus*), 16–21 (genus *Rotavirus*), 27 (genus *Coltivirus*), or 15 (genus *Aquareovirus*) kbp. The positive strands of each double-stranded segment have 5′-terminal caps (type 1 structure), and the negative strands have phosphorylated 5′-termini. The 3′-termini of both strands lack 3′-poly(A) tails. Each RNA segment is present in equimolar proportion in virions. Further detail requires separate mention of each genus.

Genus *Orthoreovirus:* The outer capsid forms a nearly spherical icosahedron, consisting predominantly of complexes of the proteins $\sigma 3$ and $\mu 1C$ (see Figure 7.3). In addition to intact virions, there are two stable subviral particles. The first of these is missing only its outer capsid (i.e., it is lacking $\sigma 3$ and contains cleaved forms of $\mu 1$ protein); this particle is called the *infectious subviral particle* (ISVP). The second subviral particle is missing both its outer and its middle capsids and is called the *core particle.* The protein by which virions attach to host cells, $\sigma 1$, forms spikes that project through the outer capsid at each of the 12 vertices of the virion. Most importantly, when the outer capsid layer is removed, $\sigma 1$ protein molecules remain attached to the infectious subviral particle and form extended fibers containing the cellular attachment domain at their tips. The core contains the viral RNA polymerase (transcriptase) and consists of three major proteins ($\lambda 1$, $\lambda 2$, $\sigma 2$) and two minor proteins ($\lambda 3$, $\mu 2$). The 10 genome segments of the orthoreoviruses fall into three size classes: large, medium, and small. Each segment encodes a single protein, except for one that is cleaved cotranslationally to form two proteins. Each genome segment can be differentiated by size, using polyacrylamide gel electrophoresis, forming reproducible gel patterns. These patterns are used to type isolates of mammalian and avian viruses.

Genus *Orbivirus:* The outer capsid consists of a diffuse layer formed by two proteins, VP2 and VP5; it is dissociated readily from the middle and inner capsids. The main capsid layer is constructed from VP7 molecules arranged in ring-like structures. Both VP2 and VP5 are attached to VP7, which in turn is associated with a subcore composed of VP3 and the genomic RNA segments. As with the orthoreoviruses, the core contains an RNA polymerase and other proteins involved in transcription. Surface projections are only observed on virions that have been stabilized (e.g., frozen for cryoelectron microscopy). Otherwise, the surface of virions appears rather smooth and unstructured. The 10 genome segments of the orbiviruses are all monocistronic; as with the orthoreoviruses, they form distinct size patterns in polyacrylamide gel electrophoresis that can be used to type isolates.

Genus *Rotavirus:* The outer capsid forms a nearly spherical icosahedron; it consists of the glycoprotein VP7 from which dimers of VP4 extend. The outer capsid and the middle capsid, which is composed of VP6, are dissociated readily from the core, which is composed of three proteins, VP1, VP2, and VP3. The 11 genome segments of the rotaviruses encode 13 proteins, 2 of which are formed by posttranslational cleavage. Again, each genome segment can be differentiated by size, using polyacrylamide gel electrophoresis, and these patterns are used to type isolates (Figure 24.2).

Genus *Coltivirus:* The outer and middle capsids appear nearly smooth, with faint markings showing their icosahedral symmetry. The inner capsid resembles that of the orbiviruses. Virions are nearly always associated with host cell membranes, prominent intracytoplasmic filaments, and granular inclusion bodies.

Genus *Aquareovirus:* Virions resemble those of the orthoreoviruses.

Orthoreoviruses and rotaviruses are resistant to lipid solvents and are stable over a wide pH range, but orbiviruses and coltiviruses have a narrower zone of pH stability (pH 6–8) and lose some but not all infectivity on exposure to lipid solvents. Proteolytic enzymes increase the infectivity of orthoreoviruses and rotaviruses (e.g., chymotrypsin in the small intestine removes the outer capsid, thereby enhancing infectivity). Orbiviruses are remarkably stable in the presence of protein—bluetongue viruses have been reisolated from blood held for 25 years at room temperature.

Viral Replication

Orthoreovirus virions or infectious subviral particles attach to sialylated glycoprotein receptors on cells via the spikes at each of their 12 vertices (Figure 24.3). Variations in the $\sigma 1$ protein making up the spikes determine the cell and tissue tropism of each virus. Virions or infectious subviral particles enter cells by receptor-mediated endocytosis. In the cytoplasm, virions are degraded to core particles, within which virion-associated RNA polymerase (transcriptase) and capping enzymes repetitively transcribe 5′-capped mRNAs, which are extruded into the cytoplasm through channels at core particle vertices. RNA polymerase (transcriptase) utilizes the negative strands of each of the double-stranded RNA segments as templates; only certain genes are transcribed initially, four mRNAs appearing before the other six. The proportion of the various mRNAs found in infected cells varies

FIGURE 24.2.

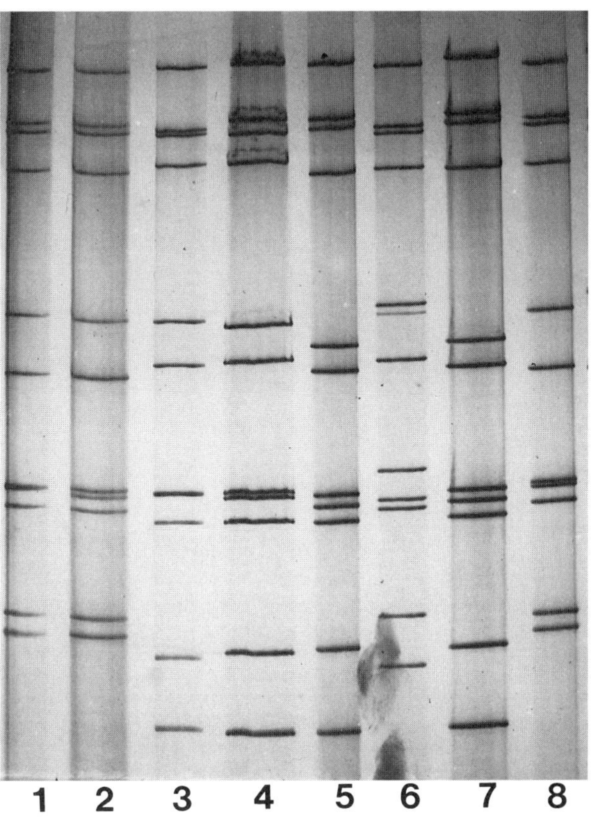

Rotavirus typing by electrophoresis of the RNA from isolates. Seven fecal isolates of rotavirus were analyzed by polyacrylamide gel electrophoresis of their RNA. Tracks 5 and 7 contain two samples of the same type. This kind of analysis is rather simple to do and is used widely to support molecular epidemiology studies, such as those done to trace the origin of virus newly appearing in a herd or flock. (Courtesy of G. Panon and I. H. Holmes.)

and the efficiency of the translation of each also varies (over a 100-fold range). How this regulation is mediated is not known.

After early mRNA synthesis, genomic RNA replication takes place in the cytoplasm within nascent progeny subviral particles. The mechanism of genomic RNA replication is complex and not fully understood. Newly synthesized, double-stranded RNA in turn serves as a template for the transcription of more mRNAs, which this time are uncapped. These mRNAs are translated preferentially to yield a large pool of viral structural proteins that self-assemble to form virions. The mechanism that ensures that one copy of each double-stranded RNA segment is encapsidated into nascent virions is not known.

Shortly after viral entry, host–cell protein synthesis decreases; one proposed mechanism is that the cap-dependent host-cell mRNAs are less efficient in driving protein translation than uncapped viral mRNAs. Structures, termed viroplasms or virus factories, form in localized areas of the cytoplasm—in many cases these intracytoplasmic inclusion bodies can be dramatic in size and number of associated virions (Figure 24.4). Inclusion bodies have a granular and moderately electron-dense appearance in thin section electron microscopy. Progeny virions tend to remain cell associated but are eventually released by cell lysis.

While the replication of orbiviruses and rotaviruses has not been studied in as much detail as that of orthoreoviruses, it is apparent that the processes are quite similar. Rotaviruses require that their outer capsid be removed before attachment—their outer capsid protein, VP4, is cleaved by chymotrypsin in the small intestine, increasing their infectivity greatly. Rotavirus progenitor particles bud into cisternae of the endoplasmic reticulum of infected cells, acquiring a temporary envelope, which then breaks down, allowing VP7 to form the outer capsid (Table 24.2).

FIGURE 24.3.

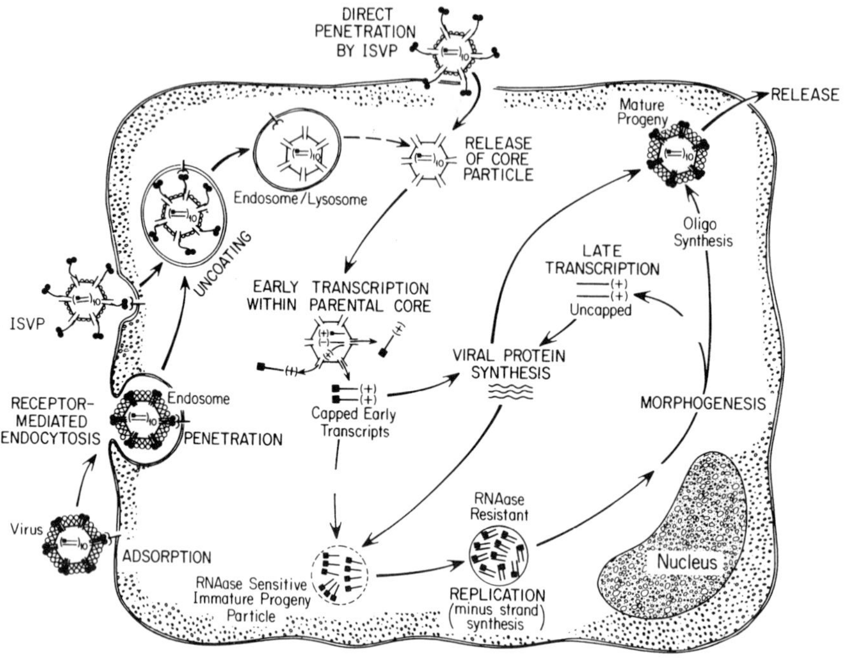

Schematic diagram of the reovirus replication cycle. After entry by receptor-mediated endocytosis of an intact virion or an infectious subviral particle (ISVP) produced outside the cell by intestinal proteases, the viral core particle is released. Within cores mRNAs are transcribed and capped; mRNAs enter the cytoplasm and early proteins are synthesized. After synthesis of new double-stranded RNA segments, late, uncapped mRNAs are produced—these direct the synthesis of the structural proteins. Maturation occurs by self-assembly and virions are released by cell lysis. [From M. L. Nibert, L. A. Schiff, and B. N. Fields, Reoviruses and their replication. *In* Fields Virology. (B. N. Fields, D. M. Knipe, P. M. Howley, R. M. Chanock, J. L. Melnick, T. P. Monath, B. Roizman, and S. E. Straus, eds.), 3rd ed., pp. 1557–1596. Lippincott-Raven, Philadelphia, PA, 1996.]

TABLE 24.2
Properties of Reoviruses

Virions are nonenveloped, spherical in outline, 80 nm in diameter

Virions are composed of three concentric capsid layers, all with icosahedral symmetry; the outer capsid differs in appearance in the various genera

Genome is composed of double-stranded RNA, divided into 10–12 segments, total size 18–27 kbp: genus *Orthoreovirus,* 10 segments, 23 kbp; genus *Orbivirus,* 10 segments, 18 kbp; genus *Rotavirus,* 11 segments, 16–21 kbp; genus *Coltivirus,* 12 segments, 27 kbp; genus *Aquareovirus,* 11 segments, 15 kbp

Cytoplasmic replication

Genetic reassortment occurs between viruses within each genus or serogroup

Diseases Caused by Members of the Genus *Orthoreovirus*

Orthoreovirus Infections of Mammals and Birds

The host range of reoviruses includes a variety of vertebrate species (cattle, sheep, swine, humans, monkeys, bats, chickens, turkeys, and geese). Only infections in laboratory rodents and chickens and turkeys are clinically significant, but respiratory or enteric infections in other species may present diagnostic difficulties.

Clinical Features

Orthoreoviruses, especially reovirus 3, cause a disease syndrome in laboratory mice that is characterized by

FIGURE 24.4.

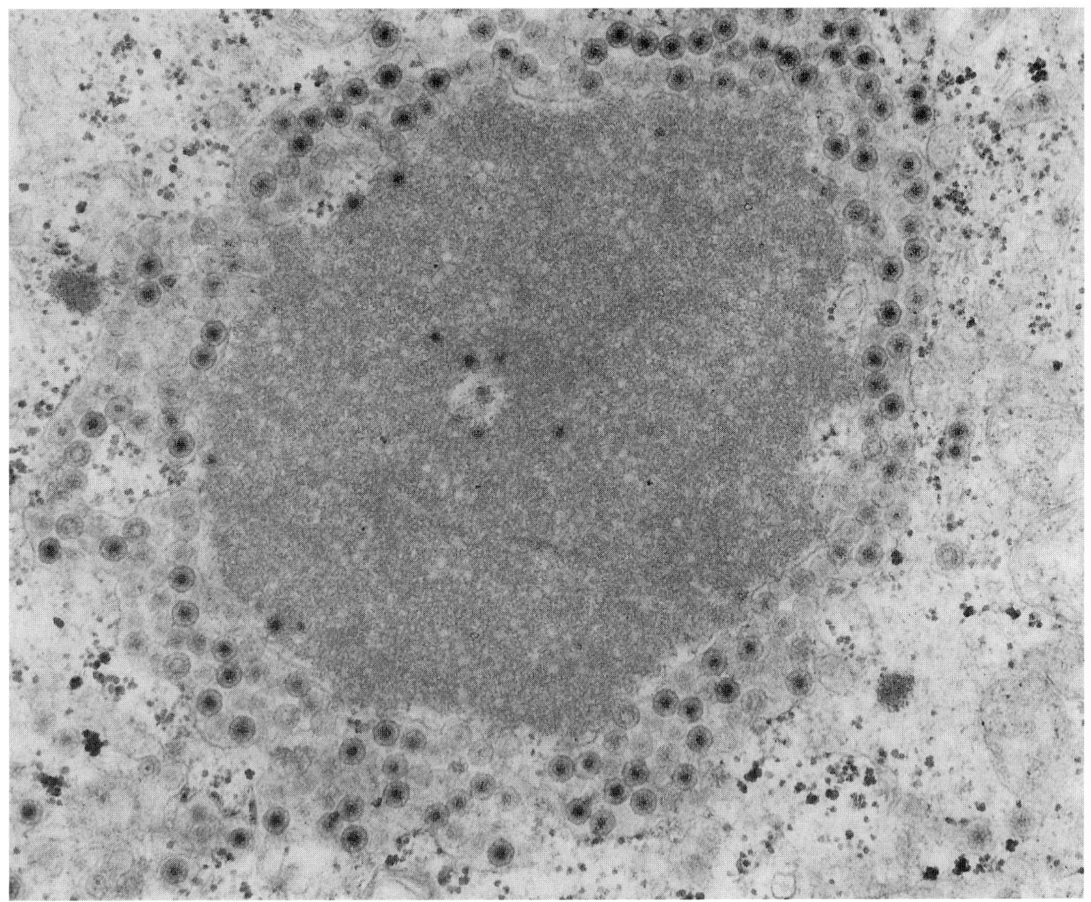

Cytoplasm of a cell infected with simian rotavirus SA11 showing a granular intracytoplasmic inclusion body (viroplasm or virus factory) with a large number of virions self-assembling at its margin. In many cases these inclusions can be dramatic in size and number of associated virions. Virions are largely cell associated and are released by cell lysis. Thin section electron microscopy. Magnification: ×25,000.

jaundice, diarrhea, runting, oily hair and skin, and neurologic signs (e.g., ataxia). There is hepatitis, myocarditis, and pancreatitis. In horses, these viruses cause upper and lower respiratory illness (laryngitis, rhinitis, conjunctivitis, and cough) and in cattle, sheep, swine, and dogs the same and also diarrhea. In monkeys there may also be hepatitis and meningitis.

The outcome of avian orthoreovirus infection in birds ranges from inapparent to fatal. Infection in some chicken, turkeys, and goose flocks may be subclinical, whereas in others there may be chronic respiratory disease, feathering abnormalities, gastroenteritis, malabsorption syndrome, hepatitis, myocarditis, tenosynovitis, arthritis, weight loss, stunted growth, and excess mortality. Tenosynovitis and arthritis usually occur in meat-producing birds over 5 weeks of age. Morbidity is often 100%, and mortality is usually less than 2%. In some turkey flocks infection may be indicated only by enteritis.

Pathogenesis, Pathology, and Immunity

Although the pathogenesis of orthoreovirus infections in mice has been studied extensively as a model system, little is known of the pathogenetic events in the disease seen in naturally infected mouse colonies. Virus is acquired via a fecal–oral transmission cycle and infection is systemic, but lesions are rather nondescript, often appearing as focal necrosis and inflammatory infiltrations into the parenchyma of organs. Avian orthoreovirus infections cause similar lesions in the bursa of Fabricius and other lymphoreticular tissues, the intestine, heart, kidney, liver, pancreas, and tendon sheaths.

Laboratory Diagnosis

Orthoreovirus infections in mice are diagnosed serologically, usually by enzyme immunoassay. Such assays are included in the battery of tests done regularly as part of the surveillance programs used to assure that mice used in research are free of intercurrent infections. Similar assays as well as immunofluorescence are used for avian orthoreoviruses; in addition, virus isolation using avian cell cultures is employed when serology proves inadequate. Isolates produce vacuoles and syncytia and are typed by neutralization assay.

Epidemiology, Prevention, and Control

The practices used in mouse colonies to maintain specific pathogen-free status are adequate to prevent the introduction of orthoreoviruses—the key is good sanitation, regular serologic testing, quarantine and testing before introducing new stock, and rodent control to prevent contact with wild mice. Similar methods are effective in preventing the introduction of avian orthoreoviruses into breeder and layer flocks.

Diseases Caused by Members of the Genus *Orbivirus*

Bluetongue

Until the 1940s bluetongue was recognized only in Africa; then following a major epidemic in 1956–1957 in Portugal and Spain the disease was recognized in the United States, the Middle East, Asia, and later in Australia. Today it is recognized that the viruses are present in most, if not all, countries in the tropics and subtropics. Bluetongue is of most importance in sheep, in which its severity varies, depending on the virus, the breed of sheep, and environmental stresses. Economic losses result from death and loss of conditioning in sheep that survive, but more importantly the disease has emerged as a major non-tariff trade barrier, i.e., suspicion of its presence is used at the convenience of importing countries to limit live sheep, lamb, and mutton imports.

Clinical Features

In sheep, bluetongue is characterized by fever that may last several days before hyperemia, excess salivation, and frothing at the mouth are noticed; a nasal discharge, initially serous but becoming mucopurulent and speckled with blood, is common. The tongue may become cyanosed, hence the name "bluetongue." There is a marked loss of condition and the sheep may die, often through aspiration pneumonia. The coronary bands of the feet may exhibit hyperemia and may be painful. Edema of the head and neck is not uncommon; animals with coronitis are often reluctant to walk and tend to be recumbent (Figures 24.5A–24.5C).

Hyperemia of the skin may occur, leading to "wool break" some weeks later. Muscle degeneration occurs and, in many sheep, convalescence is protracted. Morbidity may be as high as 80% and in Africa the mortality rate may reach 30%, but in the United States the disease is usually not associated with death. Convalescence may be protracted and wool growth may be impaired. Some bluetongue virus strains (possibly of attenuated virus vaccine origin, but transmitted by arthropod vectors) may cause abortion and congenital abnormalities (arthrogryposis, hydranencephaly, ataxia) (Figure 24.5D).

Infection in cattle and goats is usually subclinical, but again, in Africa, some cattle develop clinical signs similar to those seen in sheep. In white-tailed deer (*Odocoileus virginianus*) and pronghorn antelope (*Antilocapra americana*), the North American bluetongue viruses often cause a peracute fatal hemorrhagic disease.

Pathogenesis, Pathology, and Immunity

Bluetongue viruses replicate in hematopoietic cells and endothelial cells of the blood vessels. Adult sheep sometimes remain viremic for 14 to 28 days, and in cattle the viruses can persist for as long as 10 weeks. Rarely, and only when the bull is viremic, bluetongue viruses may be recovered from semen. The notion that this might lead to the transmission of virus to cows and their offspring in the absence of arthropod transmission and the additional notion that such infections might be persistent, even lifelong and tolerogenic (infection in the absence of an immune response), were the bases for severe limits on the movement of sheep and cattle (mostly breeding bulls) from bluetongue endemic countries. However, it has been shown that transmission via semen is a very rare event and that there are no lifelong shedders or tolerogenic infections.

Laboratory Diagnosis

Bluetongue viruses are often difficult to isolate in the laboratory. The success of virus isolation is enhanced if blood is collected from animals showing early clinical

FIGURE 24.5.

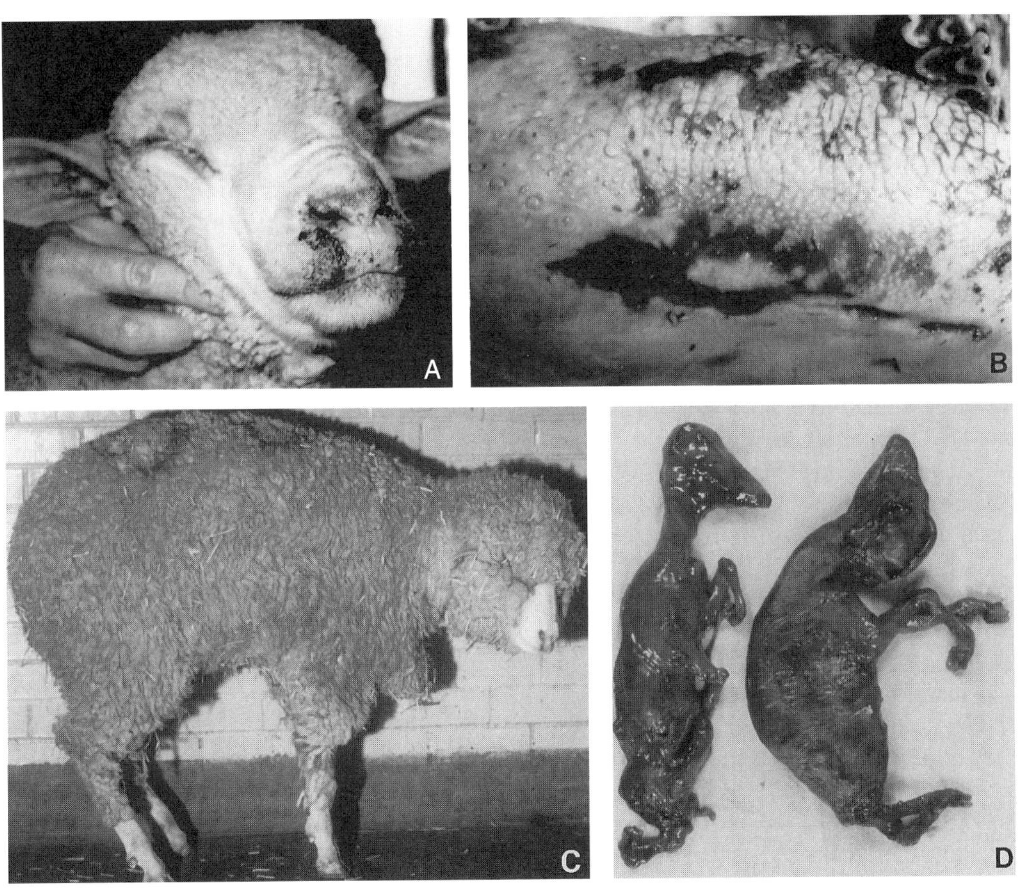

Bluetongue in sheep. (A) The muzzle is swollen and has erosions (B) Erosion of the lateral margins of the tongue, which is swollen greatly and cyanosed. (C) Lameness due to hyperemia of the coronary band of the hoofs. (D) Mummified fetal lambs aborted at 135 days gestation. The ewe was infected about the 60th day of gestation. (A, B, and D, courtesy of B. Erasmus; C, courtesy of the United States Department of Agriculture.)

signs or a pronounced fever and if the buffy coat is used as the specimen of choice. Virus isolation is done in embryonated eggs or in cell cultures (usually by blind passage) but both systems are quite insensitive. Viremia is primarily associated with red blood cells and leukocytes, and the viruses can coexist in infected animals with high concentrations of neutralizing antibody. Therefore, washed blood cells are often used for virus isolation.

Serologic techniques, most notably enzyme immunoassays, based on the detection of a group antigen have been used where required in the certification of animals as "bluetongue free." However, indeterminate serologic reactions have been a major problem—such reactions led to the use of terms such as "positive for bluetongue-like virus" and "suspected positive for bluetongue-related virus." Such results have been especially troublesome when testing has been done for regulatory purposes involving international livestock trade. This is a situation where more sensitive and specific assays, such as those based on antigens produced by recombinant DNA technologies and the polymerase chain reaction (with specific identification of amplified products), should prove useful. However, such methods to date are only available at a few national reference diagnostic centers and their use in the certification of animals for international movement is still uncertain.

Epidemiology, Prevention, and Control

Bluetongue viruses are transmitted by *Culicoides* spp. (no-see-ums, midges; different species serving as vectors in different parts of the world). The epidemiology and natural history of the disease depend on interactions of vector, host, climate, and virus. Disease occurs most commonly in late summer when vectors are most numerous.

Culicoides spp. breed in many habitats, particularly in damp muddy areas and in cow dung, but some species may be found in apparently arid areas and others can breed in highly saline water. Female *Culicoides* take a blood meal every 3–4 days throughout their life, which can be as long as 70 days. If one blood meal contains virus the arthropod becomes infected and after an extrinsic incubation period of 7 to 10 days virus is shed in saliva in every subsequent blood meal. There is no evidence of transovarial viral transmission in arthropods and not all species of *Culicoides* in a given area serve as vectors; nevertheless, because *Culicoides* may reach incredible densities, sheep and cattle are often bitten many times each day. Over time, nearly every animal in a flock or herd becomes infected in such circumstances. When the climate changes, the vectors may no longer be able to survive and the viruses may "die out." Long-range, windborne dispersal of infected *Culicoides* may occur, introducing or reintroducing the viruses to distant areas.

The attenuated virus vaccines available for the control of bluetongue in South Africa have several disadvantages: (1) they have been associated with fetal death and cerebral abnormalities in sheep in the United States and (2) their use may lead to the emergence of genetic reassortants. In addition, *Culicoides* transmission of vaccine viruses can occur, with possible reversion to virulence. Research on various recombinant DNA-based vaccines has progressed to a stage that suggests that a safe vaccine that will protect sheep and cattle from infection can be developed.

Control by vaccination is necessary where virulent bluetongue viruses are endemic; however, it is important to minimize the use of vaccines in nonendemic areas. In view of the widespread distribution of bluetongue viruses in the tropics and subtropics, the control of their movement between countries by testing and certification of livestock and germ plasm may not appear, at first glance, to have been effective. However, this impression is probably erroneous. In retrospect, most of the geographic expansion of bluetongue viruses probably occurred before animals were certified by other than clinical examination. The limited number of different bluetongue viruses in the United States, a country that until recently has had a very restrictive policy regarding the importation of livestock, testifies to the probable success of the policy.

African Horse Sickness

African horse sickness occurs in horses, mules, and donkeys with up to 95% mortality. Apart from Venezuelan equine encephalitis, this is the most important and lethal viral disease of horses. Epidemics of African horse sickness have been recognized in South Africa since 1780. More recently, major epidemics have occurred in the Middle East, the Indian subcontinent, North Africa, Spain, and Portugal. African horse sickness viruses were considered endemic only in sub-Saharan Africa, but since 1987 they have also become endemic in the Iberian peninsula. In this latter area the number of horses dying has been relatively low, due, in part, to the widespread use of vaccines. However, the true epidemic potential of these viruses may be seen in earlier epidemics; for example, in one epidemic in the Middle East and Indian subcontinent, over 300,000 horses, donkeys, and mules were reported to have died. African horse sickness has never been recognized in the Western Hemisphere, eastern Asia, or Australasia.

Nine African horse sickness viruses are recognized in South Africa and additional viruses are suspected to occur elsewhere in Africa. There is no significant serologic or genetic relationship between African horse sickness viruses and other orbiviruses of veterinary importance.

Clinical Features

The severity of clinical disease in horses, donkeys, and mules varies with the strain of virus. Horses are generally the most susceptible, with high morbidity and mortality rates; there is also substantial morbidity in mules but mortality is low, whereas donkeys are the least affected, usually developing only a mild febrile illness. In acute cases, the disease is characterized by severe and progressive respiratory disease leading to death. After an incubation period of 3 to 5 days, horses develop fever for 1 to 2 days, the respiration rate then increases, often to 70 per minute, and affected animals stand with their forelegs apart, head extended, and nostrils dilated. Spasmodic coughing may occur terminally, accompanied by profuse sweating and a discharge of frothy fluid from the nostrils. This pulmonary form is seen most commonly in completely susceptible horses infected with a highly virulent virus.

In contrast, some cases are mild and easily overlooked. Apart from fever, which may last for 5 to 8 days, there are few other clinical signs other than conjunctival injection. This form of disease, often called the cardiac form, is seen most commonly in donkeys and in vaccinated horses infected with a virus not covered by the vaccine. Disease of intermediate severity is seen in some animals. The incubation period is 7 to 14 days, followed by fever, which persists for 3 to 6 days. As the temperature falls, characteristic edema appears involving the supraorbital fossae and eyelids (Figure 24.6). Subsequently

FIGURE 24.6.

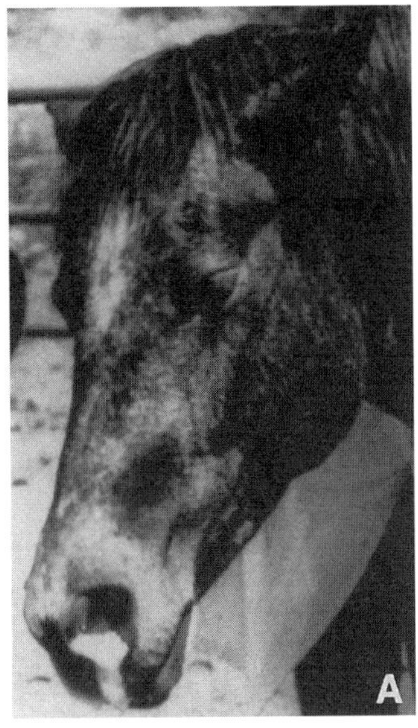

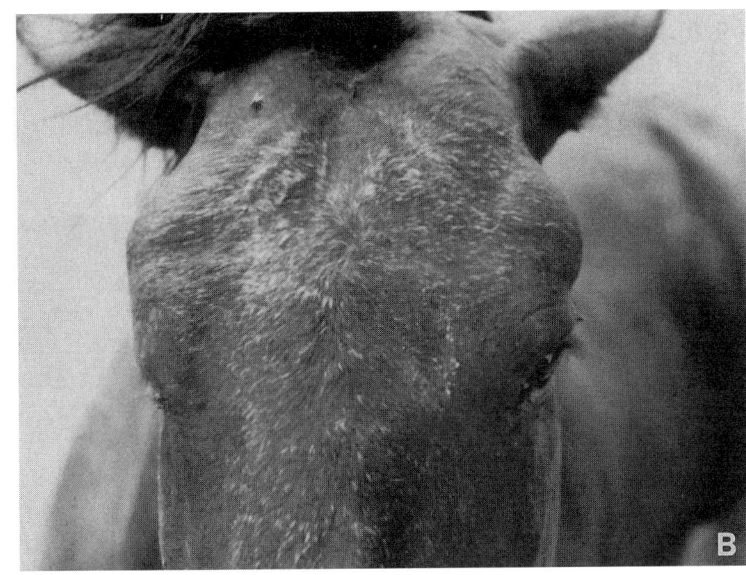

African horse sickness. (A) Respiratory form, with profuse frothy nasal discharge. (B) Characteristic edema of the supraorbital fossae and eyelids. (Courtesy of B. Erasmus.)

the edema extends to affect the lips, tongue, intermandibular space, and the laryngeal region. Subcutaneous edema may also track down the neck toward the chest. Mortality rates for such cases may be as high as 50%; death occurs within 6 to 8 days of onset of fever. Terminally, affected animals have signs of colic.

Pathogenesis, Pathology, and Immunity

After the bite of an infective arthropod, the virus replicates in the local lymph node before producing a transient primary viremia, which leads to infection of other tissues and organs in the reticuloendothelial system and then a secondary viremia. As with bluetongue, the precise mechanisms by which the viruses cause disease are unknown, but the vasculitis of small- and medium-sized blood vessels is clearly central to the development of clinical signs and lesions.

At necropsy, in horses infected with the most virulent viruses there is pulmonary edema, which is especially visible in the intralobular spaces. The lungs are distended and heavy, and frothy fluid may be found in the trachea, bronchi, and bronchioles. This frothy exudate may ooze from the nostrils. There may be pleural effusion. Thoracic lymph nodes may be edematous, and the gastric fundus congested. Petechial hemorrhages are found in the pericardium and there is an increase in pericardial fluid. In horses infected with less virulent viruses and having a longer clinical course, there are yellow, gelatinous infiltrations into subcutaneous tissues, especially along the jugular veins and ligamentum nuchae. The pulmonary form is occasionally seen in dogs.

Laboratory Diagnosis

African horse sickness is considered an exotic disease outside Africa. Clinical diagnosis of the pulmonary and cardiac forms is not difficult; the edema of the supraorbital fossae is characteristic of the disease. Excess pleural and pericardial fluid at postmortem provides a further reason to suspect the disease, especially in endemic areas and in the appropriate season. The viruses are isolated most easily by intracerebral inoculation of 2- to 6-day-old mice with blood or a spleen suspension from the suspect animal, using washed cell fractions to remove any early antibody. Identification of the particular virus (e.g., African horse sickness viruses 1 to 9) is done by neutralization assays in mice or cell culture.

Epidemiology, Prevention, and Control

African horse sickness is usually seasonal, occurring in the late summer on swampy low-lying farms and especially affecting horses that are not stabled at night. This indicates that crepusculid and night-flying insects are the vectors. The viruses can infect mosquitoes, but *Culicoides* spp. are thought to be the principal vectors. The original reservoir host of African horse sickness viruses may be the zebra, in which clinical disease is unusual, but virus persists longer than in horses.

Attenuated virus vaccines have been used in South Africa for many years. The polyvalent vaccine containing all nine viruses is generally unsatisfactory as it fails to protect all horses and can cause neurologic disease. An inactivated vaccine containing some of the viruses is available.

Vigilance in monitoring the worldwide incidence of African horse sickness is important. The explosive epidemics of the disease outside continental Africa in the 1960s and its reintroduction into Spain and Portugal have demonstrated its invasive potential. Recognition that bluetongue viruses have established endemic infection cycles in the Americas, Asia, and Australia serves as a reminder that, contrary to previous experience in the Middle East and Mediterranean areas, African horse sickness viruses could become endemic if introduced into a new area such as the Americas.

Human Disease

Very rarely, African horse sickness can be zoonotic. The first evidence of this came when laboratory workers, exposed to the virus during vaccine manufacture, developed encephalitis, chorioretinitis, and disseminated intravascular coagulation.

Equine Encephalosis

Prior to 1967, African horse sickness viruses were the only orbiviruses known to cause clinical disease in horses. In that year, sporadic cases of peracute deaths, preceded by alternating periods of hyperexcitement and depression, hence the name encephalosis, occurred in horses in various parts of South Africa. At necropsy, general venous congestion, fatty liver degeneration, cerebral edema, and enteritis were observed, and isolations of orbiviruses were made from various organs and blood collected from affected horses.

Serum neutralization tests have shown that there are at least five viruses involved; serologic surveys have indicated a high incidence of infection with each of them. Encephalosis viruses have been recognized only in South Africa; further work is needed to define their origin, geographic distribution, and veterinary importance.

Ibaraki Disease of Cattle and Epizootic Hemorrhagic Disease of Deer

Viruses related closely to bluetongue viruses, Ibaraki virus and epizootic hemorrhagic disease of deer viruses 1 and 2, have been isolated from cattle and deer, respectively, affected with a disease clinically indistinguishable from bluetongue. Epizootic hemorrhagic disease viruses have also been isolated from cattle, which appear to be their reservoir host. Bluetongue and epizootic hemorrhagic disease are regarded as the most important diseases of *Cervidae* in North America.

Ibaraki disease was first recorded as an acute, febrile disease of cattle in Japan in 1959; the virus is now known to be present in many parts of South East Asia.

Epizootic hemorrhagic disease of deer was first shown to have a viral etiology in 1955 in the United States and in 1964 in Alberta, Canada. The viruses have been isolated from cattle and arthropods in the United States and Canada and arthropods in Africa. Similar viruses exist in Australia.

Palyam Virus Disease of Cattle

Abortions in cattle in southern Africa and an epidemic of congenital abnormalities in calves in Japan, characterized by hydranencephaly and cerebellar hypoplasia, have been shown to be caused by Palyam virus. Similar diseases associated with related viruses have been recorded in Australia.

Diseases Caused by Members of the Genus *Rotavirus*

Rotavirus Infections of Mammals and Birds

Rotaviruses have been recovered from diarrheal feces of a multitude of animal species, including bovine, ovine, porcine, equine, canine, feline, lapine, murine, simian, and avian species. Rotaviruses are a major cause of diarrhea in intensively reared farm animals throughout the world. The clinical signs, diagnosis, and epidemiology of disease are similar in all species; the severity of disease ranges from subclinical, through enteritis of varying severity, to death. Disease is usually seen only in young animals, 1 to 8 weeks of age, but only rarely during the first week of life. Rotaviruses isolated from animals, even those indistinguishable from human viruses, rarely infect humans in nature.

Clinical Features

Rotavirus diarrhea in calves, piglets, foals, and lambs is often referred to as "white scours" or "milk scours." The incubation period is 16 to 24 hours. Affected animals are only moderately depressed and often continue to suckle or drink milk. The feces are voluminous, soft to liquid, and often contain large amounts of mucus. Ingestion of a large volume of milk is a contributory factor to the severity of the diarrhea as the reduced production of lactase caused by rotavirus infection exacerbates osmotic dysregulation. Other factors, particularly reduced colostrum intake, but also pathogenic *E. coli*, poor hygiene, chilling, and overcrowding, may contribute to the severity of disease. Young animals may die as a result of dehydration or secondary bacterial infection but most recover within 3 to 4 days.

Pathogenesis, Pathology, and Immunity

The pathogenesis of rotavirus infection was discussed in Chapters 9 and 10—infection leads to the destruction of epithelial cells at the apices of villi in the small intestine. Villi become shortened and covered with cuboidal epithelial cells that migrate from the crypts. These cells secrete reduced levels of disaccharidases such as lactase and are less able to carry out glucose-coupled sodium transport. Undigested lactose in the milk promotes bacterial growth and exerts a further osmotic effect; both mechanisms contribute to the diarrhea.

Laboratory Diagnosis

Rotaviruses were discovered by electron microscopy and this remains a satisfactory approach to rapid diagnosis (see Chapter 12); the virions are plentiful in feces and are so distinctive that they cannot be mistaken for anything else. The main disadvantage is that a high concentration of virions is required (at least 10^5 per gram of feces), but this can be offset somewhat by using immunoelectron microscopy. However, enzyme immunoassay is a more practicable and more sensitive method for the detection of rotaviruses in feces in most laboratories. The specificity of enzyme immunoassays can be manipulated by selecting either type-specific or broadly cross-reactive antibodies as capture and/or indicator antibodies in an antigen-capture assay. Recently, attention has turned to improving the sensitivity of diagnostic tests by identifying the viral genome in RNA extracted directly from feces. For example, polyacrylamide gel electrophoresis can distinguish rotavirus groups A, B, and C by RNA pattern alone. Finally, the polymerase chain reaction can be used to amplify viral RNA extracted from feces; the RNA is purified and then used as a template for reverse transcription and polymerase amplification using primer pairs appropriate for the degree of specificity desired.

Rotaviruses are difficult to isolate in cell culture. One secret of success is that trypsin must be incorporated in (serum-free) medium to cleave the relevant outer capsid protein (VP4) and thus facilitate entry and uncoating of the virus; immunofluorescence is used to identify rotavirus antigen in infected cells. Most bovine, porcine, and avian rotaviruses are not cytopathic initially, but can be passaged serially if grown in epithelial cells of intestinal or kidney origin in media containing trypsin. Neutralization tests using appropriate polyclonal antisera or monoclonal antibodies can be used to determine the serotype of isolates. Serum antibodies can be measured by enzyme immunoassay or neutralization tests.

Epidemiology, Prevention, and Control

Rotaviruses are excreted in the feces of infected animals in high titer (10^{11} viral particles per gram); maximum shedding occurs on the third and fourth days postinfection. Rotaviruses survive in feces for several months so gross contamination of rearing pens can occur, which explains why intensively reared animals are commonly affected. Some rotaviruses are highly resistant to chlorination and can survive for long periods in water, so that waterborne transmission is also a risk.

Although the management of intensive rearing units can be improved to reduce the incidence of disease, there is little likelihood that improved hygiene alone can completely control rotavirus infections. Local immunity in the small intestine is more important than systemic immunity in providing resistance to infection. In domestic mammals, rotavirus antibodies present in colostrum are particularly important in protecting neonatal animals. Although much of the colostral antibody enters the circulation, serum antibody levels are not critical for protection; far more important is the presence of antibody in the gut lumen. Ingestion of large volumes of colostrum for a short period gives protection for only 48 hours after suckling ceases, whereas continuous feeding of smaller amounts of colostrum can provide protection for as long as it is available. Inoculation of the dam with inactivated virus vaccine promotes higher levels of antibody in the colostrum and milk and a longer period of antibody secretion, with a corresponding decrease on the incidence of disease in neonates.

Recovery in affected calves can be helped by feeding them water instead of milk for 30 hours at the onset of diarrhea. Antibiotics to control secondary bacterial diarrhea and oral electrolyte solutions containing glucose to offset dehydration may also be useful.

Diseases Caused by Members of the Genus *Coltivirus*

Colorado Tick Fever

Colorado tick fever is a zoonotic disease that occurs in forest habitats at 1000 to 3000 m elevation in the Rocky Mountain region of North America. The vector is the wood tick, *Dermacentor andersoni;* virus is transmitted transstadially and overwinters in hibernating nymphs and adults. Some rodent species have prolonged viremia (more than 5 months), which may also facilitate virus persistence. Nymphal ticks feed on small mammals such as squirrels and other rodents, which serve as the reservoir for the virus. Adult ticks feed on larger mammals, including humans, during the spring and early summer. Eyach virus fills the same niche in Europe: it is widespread in ticks and antibodies have been reported in patients with meningoencephalitis and polyneuritis as well as a syndrome resembling that caused by Colorado tick fever virus.

The disease in humans is characterized by an incubation period of 3 to 6 days, followed by a sudden onset of illness. There is "saddle-back" fever, headache, retroorbital pain, severe myalgia in the back and legs, and leukopenia; convalescence can be protracted, particularly in adults. More serious forms of the disease, notably meningoencephalitis and hemorrhagic fever, occur in perhaps 5% of cases, mainly in children. Virus can be isolated from red blood cells or detected inside them by immunofluorescence even several weeks after symptoms have disappeared. This is a remarkable situation, as erythrocytes have no ribosomes and cannot support viral replication; however, the virus replicates in erythrocyte precursors in bone marrow, then persists in mature erythrocytes throughout their life span, protected from antibody during a viremia that can be as long as 100 days.

Further Reading

Coetzer, J. A. W., and Erasmus, B. J. (1994). African horsesickness and equine encephalosis. *In* "Infectious Diseases of Livestock with Special Reference to Southern Africa" (J. A. W. Coetzer, G. R. Thompson, and R. C. Tustin, eds.), Vol. 1, pp. 460–479. Oxford University Press, Cape Town.

Desselberger, U. (1997). Viral factors determining rotavirus pathogenicity. *Arch. Virol. Suppl.* **13**, 131–139.

Estes, M. K. (1996). Rotaviruses and their replication. *In* "Fields Virology" (B. N. Fields, D. M. Knipe, P. M. Howley, R. M. Chanock, J. L. Melnick, T. P. Monath, B. Roizman, and S. E. Straus, eds.), 3rd ed., pp. 1625–1665. Lippincott-Raven, Philadelphia, PA.

Gibbs, E. P. J., and Greiner, E. C. (1989). Bluetongue and epizootic hemorrhagic disease. *In* "The Arboviruses: Epidemiology and Ecology" (T. P. Monath, ed.), Vol. 2, pp. 39–60. CRC Press, Boca Raton, FL.

Gibbs, E. P. J., and Greiner, E. C. (1994). The epidemiology of bluetongue. *Comp. Immunol. Microbiol. Infect. Dis.* **17**, 207–220.

Kapikian, A. Z., and Chanock, R. M. (1996). Rotaviruses. *In* "Fields Virology" (B. N. Fields, D. M. Knipe, P. M. Howley, R. M. Chanock, J. L. Melnick, T. P. Monath, B. Roizman, and S. E. Straus, eds.), 3rd ed., pp. 1657–1708. Lippincott-Raven, Philadelphia, PA.

Laegrid, W. W. (1996). African horsesickness. *In* "Virus Infections of Vertebrates" (M. J. Studdert, ed.), Vol. 4, pp. 101–123. Elsevier, Amsterdam.

Laegrid, W. W. (1996). Equine encephalosis. *In* "Virus Infections of Vertebrates" (M. J. Studdert, ed.), Vol. 4, pp. 125–135. Elsevier, Amsterdam.

MacLachlan, N. J. (1994). The pathogenesis and immunology of bluetongue virus infection of ruminants. *Comp. Immunol. Microbiol. Infect. Dis.* **17**, 197–206.

Monath, T. P., and Guirakhoo, F. (1996). Orbiviruses and coltiviruses. *In* "Fields Virology" (B. N. Fields, D. M. Knipe, P. M. Howley, R. M. Chanock, J. L. Melnick, T. P. Monath, B. Roizman, and S. E. Straus, eds.), 3rd ed., pp. 1735–1766. Lippincott-Raven, Philadelphia, PA.

Nibert, M. L., Schiff, L. A., and Fields, B. N. (1996). Reoviruses and their replication. *In* "Fields Virology" (B. N. Fields, D. M. Knipe, P. M. Howley, R. M. Chanock, J. L. Melnick, T. P. Monath, B. Roizman, and S. E. Straus, eds.), 3rd ed., pp. 1557–1596. Lippincott-Raven, Philadelphia, PA.

Ramig, R. F. (1997). Genetics of the rotaviruses. *Annu. Rev. Microbiol.* **51**, 225–255.

Roy, P. (1996). Orbiviruses and their replication. *In* "Fields Virology" (B. N. Fields, D. M. Knipe, P. M. Howley, R. M. Chanock, J. L. Melnick, T. P. Monath, B. Roizman, and S. E. Straus, eds.), 3rd ed., pp. 1709–1734. Lippincott-Raven, Philadelphia, PA.

Saif, L. J., and Thiel, K. W. (1989). "Viral Diarrheas of Man and Animals." CRC Press, Boca Raton, FL.

Tyler, K. L., and Fields, B. N. (1996). Reoviruses. *In* "Fields Virology" (B. N. Fields, D. M. Knipe, P. M. Howley, R. M. Chanock, J. L. Melnick, T. P. Monath, B. Roizman, and S. E. Straus, eds.), 3rd ed., pp. 1597–1624. Lippincott-Raven, Philadelphia, PA.

Verwoerd, D. W., and Erasmus, B. J. (1994). Bluetongue. *In* "Infectious Diseases of Livestock with Special Reference to Southern Africa" (J. A. W. Coetzer, G. R. Thompson, and R. C. Tustin, eds.), Vol. 1, pp. 443–459. Oxford University Press, Cape Town.

Walton, T. E., and Osburn, B. I., eds. (1992). "Bluetongue, African Horse Sickness and Related Orbiviruses." CRC Press, Boca Raton, FL.

CHAPTER 25

Birnaviridae

The family *Birnaviridae* was established to bring together viruses with two segments of double-stranded RNA. There are two important member viruses: infectious bursal disease virus of chickens and infectious pancreatic necrosis virus of fish.

Infectious bursal disease was first recognized in 1962 in an outbreak in Gumboro, Delaware; further outbreaks were subsequently referred to as "Gumboro disease." The most prominent lesion was found in the bursa of Fabricius, hence the present name of the disease. Initial attempts to identify the causative virus involved electron microscopy—large numbers of virions were observed in the bursa of infected birds, but for some years they were classified improperly as picornavirus, adenovirus, or reoviruses. In retrospect, given the morphological differences among these viruses, it is hard to imagine how this happened.

Infectious pancreatic necrosis was first described in Canada in 1940; today the disease is recognized as the cause of considerable economic loss in salmonid aquaculture in many regions of the world.

Birnavirus-like virions have been observed in fecal samples of humans, rats, guinea pigs, and swine. Differences from true birnaviruses have been noted in size, length of genome segments, and so on; the designation "picobirnaviruses" has therefore been proposed. The role of these agents as the cause of diarrhea is still uncertain.

Properties of Birnaviruses

Classification

The family *Birnaviridae* comprises three genera: *Avibirnavirus*, *Aquabirnavirus*, and *Entomobirnavirus*. Infectious bursal disease virus is the sole member of the genus *Avibirnavirus*. Members of the genus *Aquabirnavirus* include infectious pancreatic necrosis virus of salmonid fish and related viruses of oysters and crabs. Members of the genus *Entomobirnavirus* infect only insects. The classification of the "picobirnaviruses," i.e., viruses that resemble birnaviruses but are smaller (35-nm diameter compared with 60 nm for the birnaviruses), has not been resolved.

Virion Properties

Birnavirus virions are nonenveloped, hexagonal in outline, 60 nm in diameter, with a single shell having icosahedral symmetry (Figure 25.1). The genome consists of two molecules of linear double-stranded RNA, designated A and B (Figure 25.2), 6 kbp in overall size. Segment A is 3.2 kbp in size and contains two open reading frames, the largest of which encodes a polyprotein that is processed to form two structural proteins, VP2 and VP3, and a putative viral protease, VP4. VP2 contains the major antigenic site responsible for eliciting neutralizing antibodies and VP3 contains group-specific antigenic determinants and a minor neutralizing site. Segment B is 2.8 kbp in size and encodes VP1, which is the RNA polymerase. VP1 exists as a genome-linked protein (VPg) circularizing segments A and B by tightly binding to their ends. Termini of the genome segments resemble those of other segmented RNA viruses such as reoviruses and influenza viruses where both 5′ and 3′ ends are homologous between the segments. At both ends of both segments there are direct terminal and inverted repeats that are predicted to form stem and loop secondary structures and likely contain important signals for replication,

Figure 25.1.

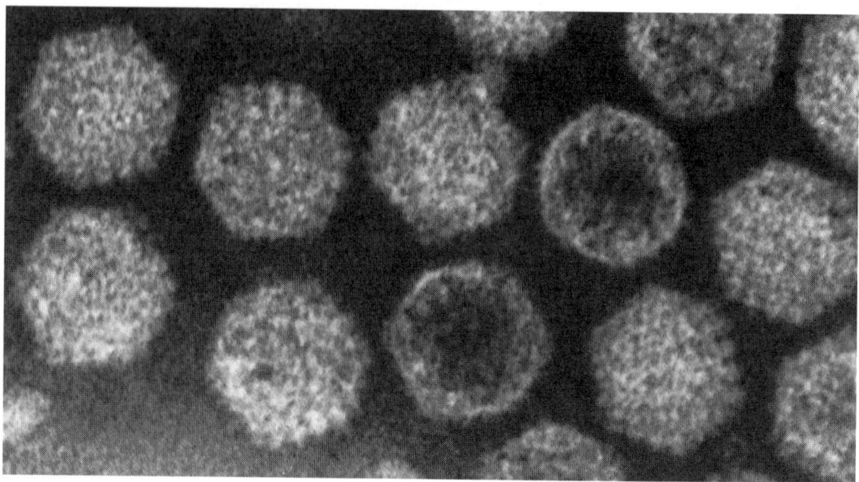

Family *Birnaviridae*, genus *Birnavirus*. Virions of infectious bursal disease virus. Negative stain electron microscopy. Bar: 100 nm.

transcription, and encapsidation—it is possible that virulence variations are due to mutations in these regions.

Virions are relatively heat stable, and their infectivity is resistant to exposure at pH3 and to ether and chloroform.

Viral Replication

Infectious bursal disease virus replicates in both chicken and mammalian cells; however, highly pathogenic strains are often difficult to cultivate. Infectious pancreatic necrosis virus replicates in fish cell lines incubated below 24°C. Both viruses grow to high titer and produce cytopathic effects 1 to 2 days after inoculation. Birnaviruses replicate in the cytoplasm without greatly depressing cellular RNA or protein synthesis. The viral mRNA is transcribed by a virion-associated RNA-dependent RNA polymerase (transcriptase). RNA replication is thought to be initiated independently at the ends of the segments and to proceed by strand displacement, with the inverted terminal repeats at the ends of each segment playing a role in replication (Table 25.1).

Infectious Bursal Disease of Chickens

Infectious bursal disease occurs worldwide and few commercial flocks are free of the virus. It is of considerable economic importance and is of scientific interest because

Figure 25.2.

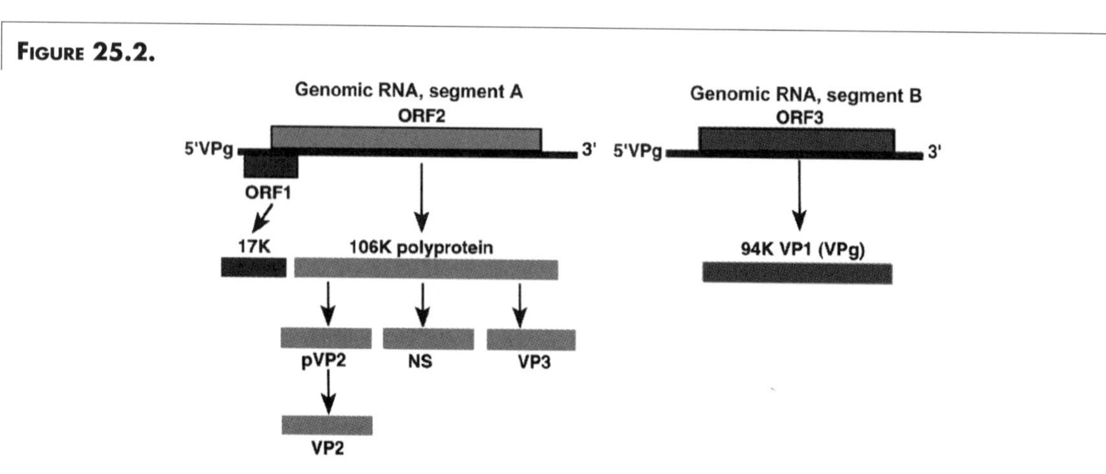

Genome of infectious pancreatic necrosis virus: its organization and transcription strategy.

TABLE 25.1
Properties of Birnaviruses

Virions are nonenveloped, hexagonal in outline, 60 nm in diameter, with a single shell having icosahedral symmetry
The genome consists of two molecules of linear double-stranded RNA, designated A and B, 6 kbp in overall size (A, 3.2 kbp; B, 2.8 kbp)
Four structural proteins, one nonstructural protein [RNA polymerase (transcriptase)]
Cytoplasmic replication
Survives at 60°C for 60 minutes; stable at pH 3 to pH 9
Member viruses occur in chickens (infectious bursal disease virus), fish (infectious pancreatic necrosis virus), molluscs, and insects

of the nature of the virus and its affinity for replicating in dividing pre-B lymphocytes in the bursa of Fabricius, leading to acquired B lymphocyte deficiency in affected birds.

Two serotypes of the virus show minimal cross-protection; only serotype 1 is pathogenic. Beginning in 1990 in the United States, western Europe, and parts of southeast Asia, variant strains of serotype 1 virus emerged that are more virulent than older strains. These have been officially designated in Europe as *very virulent strains* and have caused mortality rates of over 50%. These viruses have been isolated from flocks vaccinated with classical strain vaccines.

Clinical Features

When infectious bursal disease virus is newly introduced into a flock, morbidity approaches 100% and mortality may be up to 90%. Disease is most severe in chicks 3 to 6 weeks of age, when the target organ, the bursa of Fabricius, reaches its maximal stage of development. Accordingly, chicks 1 to 14 days of age are less sensitive; in addition they are usually protected by maternal antibodies. Birds older than 6 weeks rarely develop signs of disease, although they produce antibodies to the virus. After an incubation period of 2 to 3 days, chicks show distress, depression, ruffled feathers, anorexia, diarrhea, trembling, and dehydration; usually 20 to 30% die. The clinical disease lasts for 3 to 4 days, after which surviving birds recover rapidly.

Pathogenesis, Pathology, and Immunity

The most striking feature of the pathogenesis and pathology of infectious bursal disease is the selective replication of virus in the bursa of Fabricius, which early in infection becomes enlarged up to five times its normal size and becomes edematous, hyperemic, and cream colored, with prominent longitudinal striations (Figures 25.3A and 25.3B). Lymphoid follicles of the bursa become totally necrotic as a consequence of both necrosis and apoptosis, and in surviving birds they are devoid of lymphoid cells. Very virulent virus strains also produce depletion of cells in the thymus, spleen, and bone marrow. Hemorrhages occur beneath the serosa and there are necrotic foci throughout the bursal parenchyma. At the time of death the bursa may be atrophied and gray and the kidneys are usually enlarged, with accumulation of urates due to dehydration and possibly with immune complexes in the glomeruli.

Following oral infection, the virus replicates in gut-associated macrophages and lymphoid cells from which it enters the portal circulation, leading to primary viremia. Within 11 hours of infection, viral antigen is detectable in the bursal lymphoid cells, but not in lymphoid cells of other tissues. Large amounts of virus released from the bursa produce a secondary viremia, resulting in localization in other tissues.

The central role of the bursa in these events is made clear by the fact that bursectomized birds survive otherwise lethal infection without any clinical manifestations at all. The stage of differentiation of B lymphocytes that occurs in the bursa is crucial in supporting maximum viral replication—stem cells and peripheral B cells do not support replication of the virus. Interestingly, when lymphoid cells from the bursa are maintained in culture, only a fraction can be infected, but when the bursa is examined directly (by frozen section immunofluorescence or electron microscopy), nearly every cell is found to be infected productively (Figure 25.3C). This phenomenon has been interpreted as indicating that the microenvironment of the bursa is important in maintaining just the right level of differentiation of B lymphocytes to support viral replication. It is this exquisite viral tropism for only lymphocytes at a certain stage of differentiation that accounts for the age-dependent clinical disease in chicks.

The predilection of the virus for bursal lymphocytes leads to an important immunopathological manifestation in birds that recover from the infection. What has been called "viral bursectomy" results in a diminished antibody response and increased susceptibility to a wide range of opportunistic infectious agents, including *Salmonella* spp. and *Escherichia coli.* In addition, the immunosuppression leads to diminished antibody production after vaccinations so that outbreaks of other viral diseases may occur. These effects are most obvious in the weeks immediately following recovery from infection with the virus. There is a correlation between the variety and severity of opportunistic infections and the

FIGURE 25.3.

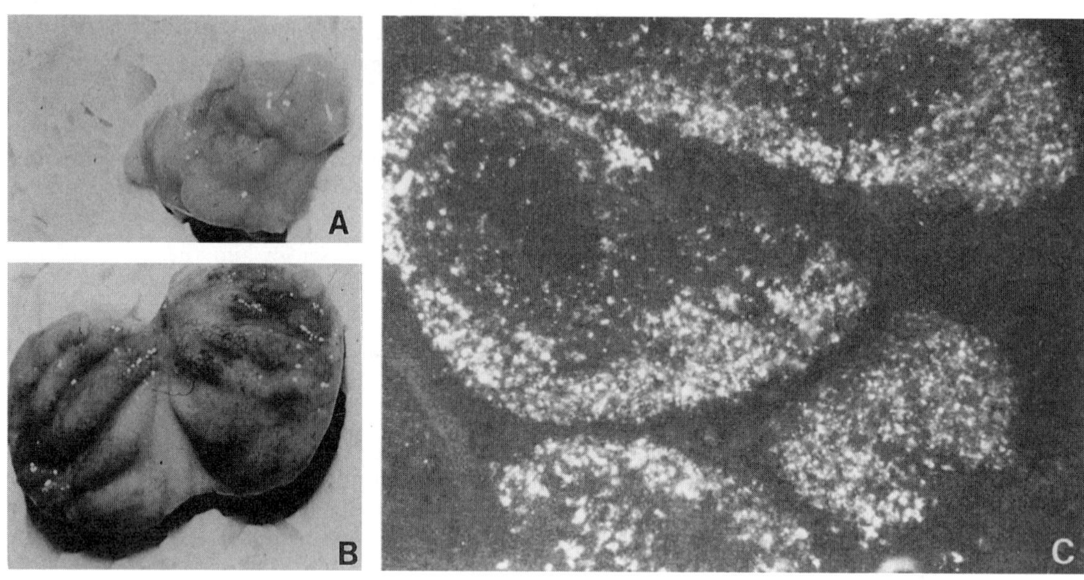

Infectious bursal disease. (A) Normal bursa of Fabricius. (B) Enlarged, hemorrhagic bursa of Fabricius of a diseased chick. (C) Specific immunofluorescence in the follicles of the bursa of Fabricius in a chick infected with infectious bursal disease virus at 24 hours postinfection. (C, courtesy of H. Becht.)

age of bird at the time of the viral infection: younger birds are affected more severely. Paradoxically, recovered birds develop high levels of antibody to the virus itself because their mature peripheral B lymphocytes are still functional.

Laboratory Diagnosis

Immunofluorescence of impression smears of bursal tissue, gel diffusion tests with infected bursal tissue as the antigen, electron microscopy of bursal specimens, and viral isolation in embryonated eggs are all useful in confirming the clinical diagnosis. The presence of virus or viral antigen can be detected in bursal tissue by immunofluorescence for 3 to 4 days after infection, for 5 to 6 days by immunodiffusion, and for up to 14 days by viral isolation. Neutralization tests and enzyme immunoassays are reliable methods for serodiagnosis.

Epidemiology, Prevention, and Control

Infectious bursal disease virus is excreted in the feces for 2 to 14 days; it is highly contagious and transmission occurs directly through contact and oral uptake. The disease is most severe when the virus is introduced into an uninfected flock. If the disease then becomes endemic, its course is much milder and its spread is slower.

The virus is extremely stable and persists for over 4 months in pens and for some 7 weeks in feed. Usual cleaning and disinfection measures often do not lead to elimination of the virus from contaminated premises, hence indirect transmission via contaminated feed, water, dust, litter, and clothing or mechanical spread through insects may reintroduce the virus. Vertical transmission probably occurs via the egg.

No fully satisfactory regimen of vaccination is yet available. Breeding stock is vaccinated by adding vaccine virus to drinking water in the hope that passively transferred maternal antibody will prevent infection of the newly hatched chicks at the time of their maximum susceptibility. An increasingly common practice is to follow oral live-virus vaccination of breeding stock, after they have reached the age of about 18 weeks, with an injection of inactivated vaccine in oil adjuvant just before they begin laying. Vaccination is repeated a year later. This results in a well-maintained high level of neutralizing antibody throughout the laying life of the birds. Maternal antibody provides effective protection for chicks for between 4 and 7 weeks after hatching. In situations where chicks have low or inconsistent levels of maternal antibodies, vaccination is carried out with an attenuated virus vaccine, starting at 1 to 2 weeks of age.

The gene for VP2 has been expressed in yeast, in a baculovirus system, and in a recombinant fowlpox virus; these experimental products induce high titers of neutralizing antibody but they have not yet displaced conventional vaccines. A major challenge is to continue to modify vaccines so that they are effective against antigenic variants as they emerge.

Infectious Pancreatic Necrosis of Fish

Infectious pancreatic necrosis is a highly contagious and lethal disease of salmonid fish (e.g., brook trout, rainbow trout) reared in hatcheries. Considerable economic loss can occur mainly in fish less than 6 months of age. The virus has also been isolated from Atlantic salmon, but its pathogenic significance for this fish remains uncertain. Other subclinically infected fish species such as pike, carp, and barbels are considered as carriers and a potential source of contagion. First recognized in North America in 1941, the disease now occurs in many countries, probably because of the worldwide shipment of eggs and live fish. There are three serotypes of infectious pancreatic necrosis virus, all pathogenic.

Clinical Features

Disease is usually observed in trout fingerlings shortly after they commence to feed. With increasing age, the infection becomes subclinical. Affected fish are dark in color, with a swollen abdomen, exophthalmus, ventral cutaneous hemorrhages, and are described as frantically whirling on their long axis and then lying quietly on the bottom. Mortality varies between 10 and 90%.

Pathogenesis, Pathology, and Immunity

Affected fish have a pale liver and spleen and visceral organs are often covered with multiple petechiae. A clear or milky mucus is seen in the stomach and anterior intestine. Histologically, there are necrotic foci in acinar and islet tissue of the pancreas.

Laboratory Diagnosis

Clinical diagnosis is confirmed by virus isolation in standard fish cell cultures; high-virus titers are usually present in kidney tissue so this organ is preferred as inoculum. Virus can be titrated in fish cells by plaque assay. Immunofluorescence (frozen sections or tissue smears) is also used diagnostically, with large amounts of viral antigen being present in internal organs, especially kidneys.

Epidemiology, Prevention, and Control

Surviving fish become lifelong carriers of the virus, which they shed in feces, eggs, sperm, and genital fluids. The virus is highly stable under various environment conditions; for example, it can survive for months in fresh water or sea water. Control is based on hygiene, water disinfection with iodophores, and, if an outbreak occurs, complete destocking.

Vaccine development has been hampered by the circumstance that during their most susceptible period, young fish are not protected by maternal antibodies or by effective active immunocompetence (young fish become immunocompetent to some extent by 30 days of age). Further, the lack of cross-protection between serotypes makes the requirements for an effective vaccine even more demanding.

Because international commerce in live fish and eggs is an important mode of spread of infection, the *Code Zoosanitaire International* has established guidelines for export that specify freedom from clinical disease or pathologic changes in the farm of origin for at least 12 months, and negative results from attempts to isolate infectious pancreatic necrosis virus from pond water, eggs, sperm, and fish.

Further Reading

Bernard, J., and Brémont, M. (1995). Molecular biology of fish viruses: A review. *Vet. Res.* **26,** 341–351.

Dobos, P., Hill, B. J., Hallet, R., Kells, D. T. C., Becht, H., and Teninges, D. (1979). Biophysical and biochemical characterization of five animal viruses with bisegmented, double-stranded RNA genomes. *J. Virol.* **32,** 593–605.

Lasher, H. N., and Davis, V. S. (1997). History of infectious bursal disease in the U.S.A.—the first two decades. *Avian Dis.* **41,** 11–19.

Lukert, P. D., and Saif, Y. M. (1997). Infectious bursal disease. *In* "Diseases of Poultry" (B. W. Calnek, ed.), 10th ed., pp. 721–728. Iowa State University Press, Ames.

Nagarajan, M. M., and Kibenge, F. S. B. (1997). Infectious bursal disease virus: A review of the molecular basis for variations in antigenicity and virulence. *Can. J. Vet. Res.* **61,** 81–88.

Sharma, J. M., Karaca, K., and Pertile, T. (1994). Virus-induced immunosuppression in chickens. *Poult. Sci.* **73,** 1082–1086.

Wolf, K. (1988). "Fish Viruses and Fish Viral Diseases." Cornell University Press, Ithaca, NY.

CHAPTER 26

Paramyxoviridae

Several of the most devastating viral disease of animals and humans are caused by members of the family *Paramyxoviridae*. Rinderpest, canine distemper, Newcastle disease, measles, and mumps have arguably caused more morbidity and mortality than any other group of related diseases in recorded history. However, these diseases are only part of the threat represented by the member viruses of this family: bovine parainfluenza virus 3 disease and bovine respiratory syncytial disease are major contributors to the bovine pneumonia complex known as shipping fever and murine parainfluenza virus 1 (Sendai virus) disease is a major problem in mouse colonies. Moreover, important new, emerging diseases of animals, such as equine morbillivirus disease and phocine, dolphin, and porpoise distemper, have raised the question of whether additional new diseases will be found.

The family *Paramyxoviridae,* together with the families *Rhabdoviridae, Filoviridae,* and *Bornaviridae,* form the order *Mononegavirales.* This order was established to bring together viruses with distant, ancient phylogenetic relationships that are reflected in some conserved genomic domains, similar strategies of gene expression and replication, and similar gene order. All the viruses are enveloped, covered with peplomers, and

Table 26.1
Distinguishing Characteristics of Four Families of the Order *Mononegavirales*

Characteristic	Family *Paramyxoviridae*	Family *Rhabdoviridae*[a]	Family *Filoviridae*	Family *Bornaviridae*
Genome size (kb)	15–16	11–15	19	9
Morphology	Pleomorphic virions	Bullet-shaped virions	Filamentous virions	90-nm-diameter spherical virions
Site of replication	Cytoplasm	Cytoplasm	Cytoplasm	Nucleus
Mode of transcription	Polar with nonoverlapping signals (except pneumoviruses) and stepwise attenuation	Polar with nonoverlapping signals and stepwise attenuation	Polar with nonoverlapping signals and stepwise attenuation	Complex with mRNA splicing and overlapping start/stop signals
Host range	Vertebrates	Vertebrates	Humans, unknown	Horses, sheep, cats, ostriches, (humans?)
Pathogenic potential	Mainly respiratory disease	Mild febrile to fatal neurological disease	Hemorrhagic fever	Immune-mediated neurological disease

[a]Vertebrate virus members.

all have genomes consisting of a single molecule of negative-sense, single-stranded RNA. The features that differentiate the individual families of the order are summarized in Table 26.1. These include genome size, nucleocapsid structure, site of genome replication and transcription, manner and extent of mRNA processing, virion morphology, tissue specificity, host range, and pathogenic potential.

Properties of Paramyxoviruses

Classification

The family *Paramyxoviridae* is subdivided into the subfamilies *Paramyxovirinae* and *Pneumovirinae*, the former containing the genera *Respirovirus*, *Rubulavirus*, and *Morbillivirus*, the latter containing the genera *Pneumovirus* and *Metapneumovirus* (Table 26.2) (see Figure 26.1 for an example of how some important members of the family are related). In addition to the viruses covered in more detail in this chapter, there are several members of the family that have not been characterized fully: for example, fer-de-lance virus of reptiles, Mapuera virus of chiropteran bats, Nariva virus of rodents, and several viruses of penguins that are distinct from avian paramyxoviruses 1–9.

Virion Properties

Paramyxovirus virions are pleomorphic in shape (spherical as well as filamentous forms occur), 150–300 nm in diameter (Figure 26.2). Virions are enveloped, covered with large peplomers (8–20 nm in length), and contain a "herringbone-shaped" helically symmetrical nucleocapsid, 600–800 nm in length and 18 (*Paramyxovirus*, *Rubulavirus*, *Morbillivirus*) or 13 (*Pneumovirus*) nm in diameter. The genome consists of a single linear molecule of negative-sense, single-stranded RNA, 15–16 kb in size. There are 6 to 10 genes separated by conserved noncoding sequences that contain termination, polyadenylation, and initiation signals. The gene order is generally conserved within the family, although member viruses of the genera *Paramyxovirus* and *Morbillivirus* contain 6, *Rubulavirus* contain 7, and *Pneumovirus* contain 10 genes. Whereas the 10 pneumovirus genes encode 10 proteins, the 6 or 7 genes of the other genera encode 10 to 12 proteins (Figure 26.3). Most of the gene products are structural proteins found in virions.

The peplomers are composed of two glycoproteins: a hemagglutinin–neuraminidase protein (HN) (the equivalent protein of pneumoviruses, G, lacks neuraminidase activity) and a fusion protein (F) (Table 26.3). Both proteins play key roles in the pathogenesis of all paramyxovirus infections. Cell attachment is mediated via the hemagglutinin–neuraminidase protein. This glycoprotein elicits neutralizing antibodies that inhibit adsorption of virus to cellular receptors.

The fusion protein is present on newly formed virions in an inactive precursor form that is activated by proteolytic cleavage by a cellular protease. After cleavage, the newly generated amino-terminal sequence of the protein has a hydrophobic domain and it is postulated that this is involved directly in fusion. Cleavage of

Table 26.2
Paramyxoviruses and the Diseases They Cause

Subfamily/Genus and Virus	Animal Species Affected	Disease
Paramyxovirinae/Respirovirus		
Bovine parainfluenza virus 3	Cattle, sheep, other mammals	Respiratory disease in cattle and sheep
Murine parainfluenza virus 1 (Sendai virus)	Mice, rats, rabbits	Severe respiratory disease in laboratory rats and mice
Human parainfluenza viruses 1 and 3	Humans	Respiratory disease
Paramyxovirinae/Rubulavirus		
Newcastle disease virus (avian paramyxovirus 1)	Domestic and wild fowl	Severe generalized disease with central nervous system signs
Avian paramyxoviruses 2–9	Fowl	Respiratory disease
Canine parainfluenza virus 2 (SV5)	Dogs	Respiratory disease
Porcine rubulavirus (La-Piedad-Michoacan-Mexico virus)	Swine	Encephalitis, reproductive failure, corneal opacities
Mumps virus	Humans	Parotitis
Human parainfluenza viruses 2, 4a, and 4b	Humans	Respiratory disease
Paramyxovirinae/Morbillivirus		
Rinderpest virus	Cattle, wild ruminants	Severe generalized disease
Peste des petits ruminants virus	Sheep, goats	Severe generalized disease such as rinderpest
Canine distemper virus	Dogs and members of families *Procyonidae, Mustelidae, Felidae*	Severe generalized disease with central nervous system signs
Phocine distemper virus	Seals and sea lions	Severe generalized disease with respiratory system signs
Dolphin distemper virus	Dolphins	Severe generalized disease with respiratory system signs
Porpoise distemper virus	Porpoises	Severe generalized disease with respiratory system signs
Bovine morbillivirus (MV-K1)	Cattle	Poorly characterized—significance unknown
Measles virus	Humans	Measles, severe systemic disease with respiratory and central nervous system signs
Possible genus, equine morbillivirus		
Equine morbillivirus	Horses and humans	Acute respiratory distress syndrome in horses and humans
Pneumovirinae/Pneumovirus		
Bovine respiratory syncytial virus	Cattle, sheep	Respiratory syncytial disease
Pneumonia virus of mice	Mice	Respiratory syncytial disease
Human respiratory syncytial virus	Humans	Respiratory syncytial disease
Pneumovirinae/Metapneumovirus		
Turkey rhinotracheitis virus	Turkeys, chickens	Severe respiratory disease in turkeys, swollen head syndrome of chickens

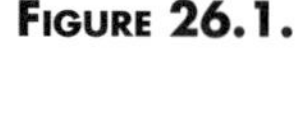

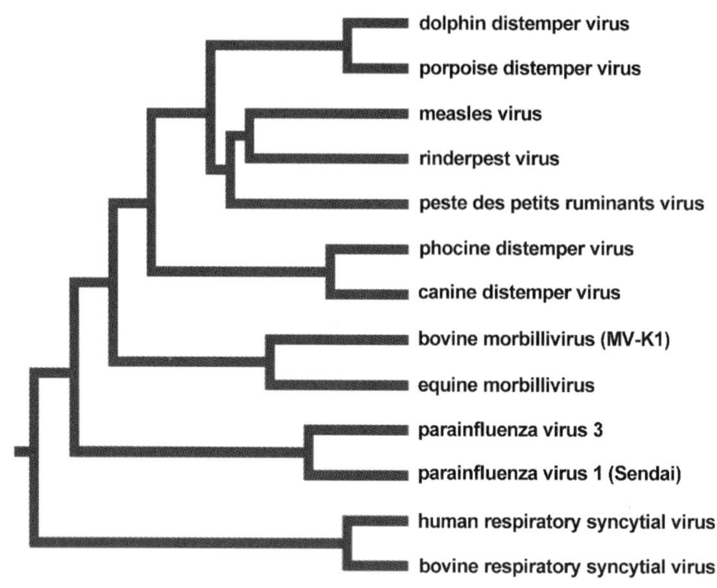

Phylogenetic relationships among member viruses of the family *Paramyxoviridae* based on the nucleotide sequences of their matrix protein and hemagglutinin genes. Member viruses of the subfamily *Pneumovirinae* are most distant from the others. Members of the genus *Respirovirus* and *Rubulavirus* each form rather homogeneous clusters, as do the members of the genus *Morbillivirus*. Of all the morbilliviruses, the Australian equine morbillivirus and bovine morbillivirus are most distant. Not to scale—the relationships between the subfamilies are more distant than indicated. (Adapted from the work of D. E. Griffin, W. J. Bellini, A Gould, B. Eaton, P. Young, and P. K. Murray.)

the fusion protein is essential for viral infectivity; when a host cell does not contain appropriate proteases the virus formed is not infectious. Further, viral virulence has been correlated with the presence or absence of specific amino acid protease recognition motifs. Because the fusion protein is essential for viral infectivity and for direct cell-to-cell spread via fusion, it plays a key role in the pathogenesis of paramyxovirus infections, including persistent infections. To be maximally effective, paramyxovirus vaccines must elicit antibodies against the fusion protein as well as against the hemagglutinin–neuraminidase protein.

FIGURE 26.2.

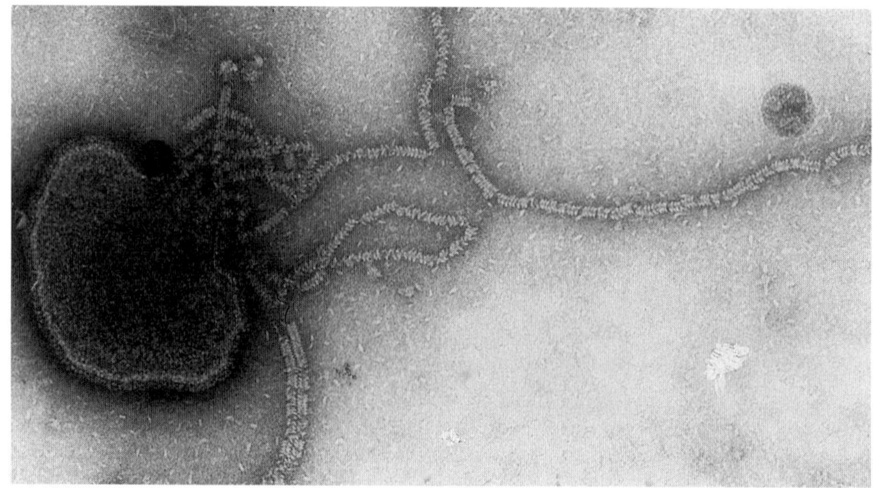

Family *Paramyxoviridae*, subfamily *Paramyxovirinae*, genus *Respirovirus*, parainfluenza virus 3. A single partially disrupted virion, with peplomers visible at its edge and its herringbone-shaped nucleocapsid spilling out. Negative stain electron microscopy. Magnification: ×50,000.

FIGURE 26.3.

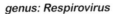

genus: Respirovirus

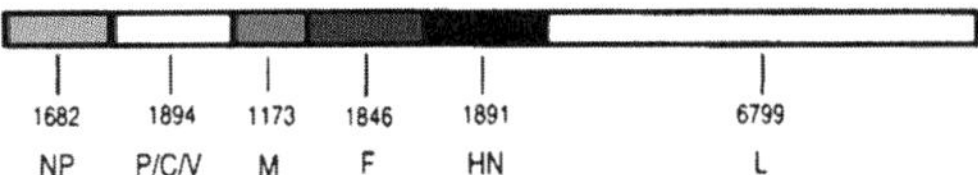

genus: Rubulavirus

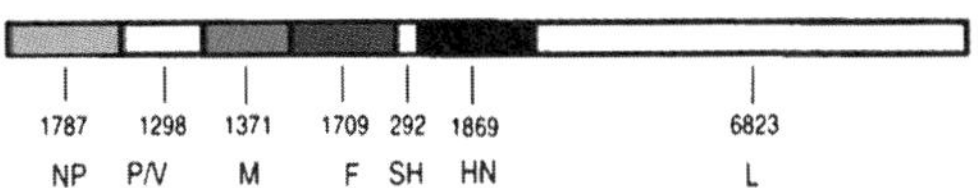

genus: Morbillivirus

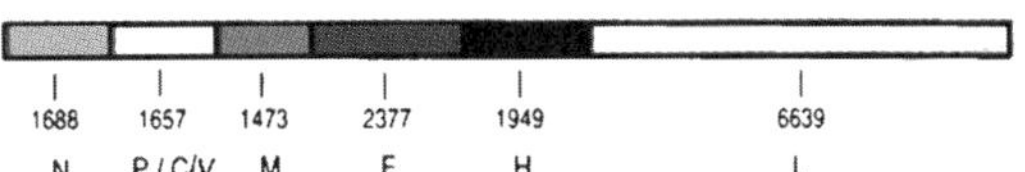

genus: Pneumovirus

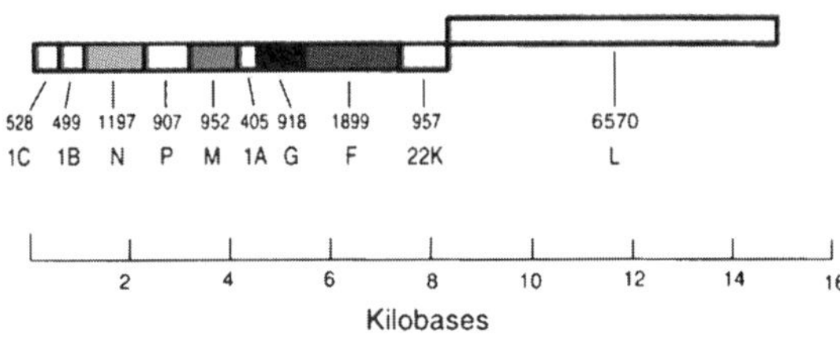

Genetic maps of some typical members of the family *Paramyxoviridae*. Homologous genes are indicated by the style of shading; the number beneath each gene indicates the number of nucleotides comprising the gene. [Adapted from R. L. Lamb and D. Kolakofsky, Paramyxoviridae: The viruses and their replication. *In* "Fields Virology" (B. N. Fields, D. M. Knipe, P. M. Howley, R. M., Chanock, J. L. Melnick, T. P. Monath, B. Roizman, and S. E. Straus, eds.), 3rd ed., pp. 1177–1204. Lippincott-Raven, Philadelphia, PA, 1996.]

TABLE 26.3
Functions and Terminology of Virion Proteins in the Family *Paramyxoviridae*

FUNCTION	GENUS *RESPIROVIRUS* AND *RUBULAVIRUS*	GENUS *MORBILLIVIRUS*	GENUS *PNEUMOVIRUS*
Attachment protein: hemagglutinin, induction of productive immunity	HN	H	G[a]
Neuraminidase: virion release, destruction of mucin inhibitors	HN	None	None
Fusion protein: cell fusion, virus penetration, cell–cell spread, contribution to induction of protective immunity	F	F	F
Nucleoprotein: protection of genome RNA	NP	N	N
Transcriptase: RNA genome transcription	L and P	L and P	L and P
Matrix protein: virion stability	M	M	M
Other	(SH)	—	SH, 22 K

[a]No hemagglutinating activity.

Viruses have narrow host ranges and have only been identified in vertebrates, primarily in mammals and birds. They are labile to the effects of heat or desiccation and are destroyed easily by common disinfectants and lipid solvents.

Viral Replication

Several different cell types are used to grow different paramyxoviruses. Cell cultures derived from homologueous species are usually used for morbilliviruses and pneumoviruses, but these viruses are not cultivated readily and adaptation by passage is usually necessary. Viral replication in cell cultures is usually lytic, but carrier cultures arise readily in many virus–host cell systems. Syncytium formation in cell cultures and *in vivo* is a characteristic feature of infection, as is the formation of acidophilic inclusions in the cytoplasm. Even though their replication is entirely cytoplasmic, morbilliviruses also produce acidophilic intranuclear inclusions. Hemadsorption is demonstrated readily with parainfluenza viruses and some morbilliviruses, but not with pneumoviruses.

Paramyxoviruses replicate within the cytoplasm, indeed some have been shown to replicate in enucleated cells. Virions attach via their hemagglutinin–neuraminidase protein to cellular sialoglycoprotein or glycolipid receptors. The fusion protein then mediates fusion of the viral envelope with the plasma membrane, at physiologic pH. The liberated nucleocapsid remains intact, with all three of its associated proteins (N, P, and L) being required for transcription by the virion-associated, RNA-dependent RNA polymerase (transcriptase). The genome is transcribed progressively into some 6 or 10 discrete unprocessed mRNAs by sequential interrupted synthesis from a single promoter. Full genome-length positive-sense RNA is also synthesized and serves as a template for the replication of negative-sense genomic RNA. Control of these processes is mainly at the level of transcription.

Whereas most genes encode a single protein, the P gene of the member viruses of the subfamily *Paramyxovirinae* encodes two to five distinct P/V/C proteins (see Figure 26.3 and Table 26.3). Remarkably, different strategies for maximizing the coding potential of this gene complex have evolved in the different genera of the subfamily. For example, the gene complex of the member viruses of the genera *Morbillivirus* and *Paramyxovirus* encodes four proteins, the production of which entails two distinct transcription mechanisms: (1) internal initiation of translation and (2) insertion of nontemplated G residues into mRNA to shift the reading frame to that of an otherwise inaccessible open reading frame. Whereas the P protein itself is translated from a faithful mRNA copy of the complete gene, the smaller C protein is read in a different reading frame following initiation of translation from an internal initiation codon. Quite separately, the transcription of the V gene involves the insertion of an extra G nucleotide into its mRNA by polymerase site-specific stuttering ("editing")—this results in the production of a protein that displays N-terminal homology with the P protein but downstream has a distinct amino sequence. Because the reading frame used to transcribe the V gene is also distinct, all three reading frames are utilized in the transcription of the P/C/V gene complex. In the case of parainfluenza virus 3, a fourth protein, D, is translated by insertion of two nontemplated G residues. In the genus *Rubulavirus* there are additional variations in the transcription of the P/V/C gene complex and the products formed, and in the genus *Pneumovirus* each of the 10 genes encodes a single protein with little sense of genomic coding economy.

During infection, as the concentration of N protein builds up in the cell, these molecules are believed to associate either with the viral RNA polymerase (transcriptase) or with nascent positive-sense RNA intermediates, thereby preventing the polyadenylation, termination, and reinitiation events that characterize the *transcription mode* of the infection cycle. This enables a switch to a *replication mode* in which more full-length positive-sense intermediates are synthesized. These, in turn, serve as a template for RNA replication. Newly synthesized negative-sense RNA associates with N protein and transcriptase to form nucleocapsids. Virion maturation involves (1) the incorporation of viral glycoproteins into patches on the host cell plasma membrane, (2) the association of matrix protein (M) and other nonglycosylated proteins with this altered host cell membrane, (3) the alignment of nucleocapsid beneath the M protein, and (4) the formation and release via budding of mature virions (Table 26.4).

Diseases Caused by Members of Subfamily *Paramyxovirinae*, Genus *Respirovirus*

Bovine Parainfluenza Virus 3 Disease

Whether bovine parainfluenza virus 3 causes disease in cattle and sheep independently of its role of predisposing to secondary bacterial infections of the respiratory tract has been debated for many years. However, it is its role in shipping fever that has prompted most attention and

Table 26.4
Properties of Members of the Family *Paramyxoviridae*

Two subfamilies: *Paramyxovirinae* containing the genera *Respirovirus, Rubulavirus,* and *Morbillivirus,* and *Pneumovirinae* containing the genera *Pneumovirus* and *Metapneumovirus*

Virions are enveloped, pleomorphic (spherical as well as filamentous forms occur), and 150–300 nm in diameter. They are covered with large peplomers (8–20 nm in length)

Virions contain a "herringbone-shaped" helically symmetrical nucleocapsid, 600–800 nm in length, and 18 (genera *Respirovirus, Rubulavirus, Morbillivirus*) or 13 (genera *Pneumovirus* and *Metapneumovirus*) nm in diameter

Virion envelope contains two viral glycoproteins and one or two nonglycosylated proteins

Genome consists of a single linear molecule of negative-sense, single-stranded RNA, 15–16 kb in size, with seven to eight open reading frames encoding 10 to 12 proteins, including NP (or N), P, M, F, L, and HN (or H or G), which are common to all genera

Cytoplasmic replication, budding from the plasma membrane

Syncytium formation, intracytoplasmic and intranuclear inclusion bodies (genus *Morbillivirus*)

controversy. Shipping fever occurs as a consequence of transportation and other stressful situations; the term refers to an ill-defined respiratory syndrome caused by a variety of agents acting in concert or in sequence. The syndrome is an economically important problem, particularly in feedlots and large-scale breeding facilities in regions where climate provides additional stress. The virus can infect many other species, including dogs, horses, monkeys, and humans; it is found worldwide.

Clinical Features

In calves and lambs, infection is marked by fever, lacrimation, serous nasal discharge, depression, dyspnea, and coughing. Many animals may exhibit minimal clinical signs, but some may develop interstitial pneumonia, in which inflammatory consolidation is usually present only in the anterior lobes of the lungs.

The uncomplicated respiratory infection caused by parainfluenza 3 runs a clinical course of 3 to 4 days with complete recovery the rule. However, in stressful circumstances, many cattle and sheep develop interstitial pneumonia, i.e., shipping fever. In this case the infection alone or in concert with other viral infections (adenovirus, infectious bovine rhinotracheitis virus, bovine respiratory syncytial virus infections) predisposes to secondary bacterial infection, especially *Pasteurella hemolytica* infection. This syndrome is marked by purulent nasal discharge, cough, rapid respiration, anorexia, fever, and general malaise. Poor hygiene, crowding, transport, harsh climatic conditions, and other causes of stress exacerbate this syndrome (see Chapter 10).

Pathogenesis, Pathology, and Immunity

Under farm conditions, clinical signs of infection are usually distorted by intercurrent infections with several different agents. Upon intranasal or intratracheal inoculation of parainfluenza virus 3 alone, calves show only mild fever and serous nasal discharge, whereas cattle infected with a mixture of virus and bacteria and variously stressed develop pneumonia that is often intractable in regard to economically feasible management. In shipping fever, the lesions are those of lobular pneumonia; there is massive inflammatory infiltration, necrosis, and caseation and marked lobar hepatization (lungs resembling liver). Syncytium formation and intracytoplasmic inclusion bodies are encountered in bronchiolar and alveolar epithelial cells.

Convalescent animals develop a strong immune response, evidenced by the presence of hemagglutination inhibition, neuraminidase inhibition, and neutralizing antibodies. These antibodies are all directed against the hemagglutinin–neuraminidase protein. The role of the cellular immune system has not been determined. Immunity is short lived, and animals become susceptible to reinfection after several months.

Laboratory Diagnosis

Because of the variety of agents that can cause shipping fever and the common occurrence of the virus without disease, diagnosis is difficult. Virus can be recovered from the nasal discharges for 7 to 9 days after infection by cultivation in bovine cell cultures or it may be identified in nasal discharges or respiratory tissues by immunofluorescence or enzyme immunoassay, but interpretation of results requires an assessment of the overall clinical condition in the individual animal and the herd.

Epidemiology, Prevention, and Control

The most important transmission routes are by aerosol and fomites contaminated with nasal discharges. The virus has been recovered also from intestinal contents, milk, and aborted fetuses but the importance of these sources of contagion is unknown.

Several attenuated virus vaccines for intranasal and parenteral use are available that are able to induce protective mucosal IgA antibodies. Typically, combined vaccines are formulated, containing infectious bovine rhinotracheitis virus, bovine adenovirus, and bovine viral diarrhea virus antigens. However, it is widely acknowledged that better vaccines are needed—vaccines that provide longer-lasting immunity. Even more important is the need for good vaccines against *Pasteurella hemolytica*. In the absence of the latter, antibiotics are used to treat the pneumonia, but with limited success. Many cattle surviving the acute and subacute manifestations of shipping fever become unthrifty and are eliminated from production units.

Canine Parainfluenza Virus 2 Disease

Canine parainfluenza virus 2 is closely related to if not identical to simian virus 5 (SV5); the virus causes inapparent infections or mild respiratory disease in dogs and may be the cause of central nervous system disease as well. The prevalence of antibodies indicates its worldwide distribution in dog populations. Infections play a role in the kennel cough syndrome, and more serious, chronic respiratory disease may develop when additional microbial or viral agents, poor hygiene, or stress complicate infections. Infection is characterized by the sudden onset of serous nasal secretion, cough, and fever, lasting 3–14 days. In severe cases (mostly in malnourished or young dogs) there is also conjunctivitis, tonsillitis, anorexia, and lethargy. Because a number of other infections can induce similar clinical signs, definitive diagnosis depends on virus isolation from nasal or throat swabs. Vaccines are available; they are usually used in various combination formulations containing antigens of other canine viral and microbial pathogens. The virus also infects humans, monkeys, probably cattle, sheep, swine, and cats, and an antigenically related virus has been isolated from chickens.

Murine Parainfluenza Virus 1 (Sendai Virus) Disease

Parainfluenza virus 1, also known as Sendai virus, produces natural infections in mice, rats, guinea pigs, hamsters, rabbits, monkeys, and humans. Whereas in most species infection remains subclinical, severe respiratory disease with high mortality can occur in breeding colonies of laboratory mice and rats used for biomedical research. In this setting it is a substantial problem, particularly difficult to control or eliminate because of cross-infection between different rodent species.

Clinical Features

In epidemics, affected mice are characterized by a roughened hair coat, crusting of the eyes, neonatal mortality, retarded growth, weight loss, and prolonged gestation. In endemic situations, where there is some background immunity, most animals are infected subclinically shortly after weaning. Nude mice develop a chronic wasting disease characterized by decreased activity, weight loss, sniffling, and wrinkled skin; there is no evidence of chronic or persistent infection in immunocompetent mice, but in nude mice virus has been demonstrated for up to 27 days postinfection.

Pathogenesis, Pathology, and Immunity

After natural infection, the virus replicates for 6 to 7 days primarily in respiratory epithelium. In mice, the epidemic form is generally acute, morbidity is high, and mortality varies between 0 and 100%, depending on the mouse strain. Following recovery, virus is no longer detectable and antibodies persist throughout life. In the absence of clinical signs, there are no gross lesions, with the exception of adhesions between the serosa of lung and pleura (as a result of secondary bacterial infection). In ill animals, areas of congestion and consolidation are seen throughout the lungs, which are replaced by grayish fibrotic tissue upon recovery. Histologically, there are lesions in the upper and lower respiratory tract (acute rhinitis with focal ulcerative lesions, epithelial necrosis in the trachea). Intracytoplasmic eosinophilic inclusion bodies surrounded by a clear halo are present in epithelial cells of the trachea.

Laboratory Diagnosis

Of the serological tests available to diagnose Sendai virus infections in laboratory rodent colonies, enzyme immunoassays are most often used. Antibodies are detected as early as 7 days postinfection but their presence may not be indicative of an ongoing outbreak in a colony unless regular, serial testing is done and the colony is otherwise negative. Histologic demonstration of lesions and electron microscopic demonstration of virions in lung homogenates are used to confirm diagnoses. The use of sentinel animals is useful: mice put in contact with bedding material develop antibody if the virus is present.

The virus can be isolated in numerous cell culture systems (monkey kidney, Vero, and BHK-21 cells) and embryonated eggs; the presence of virus is demonstrated by hemadsorption of guinea pig erythrocytes to infected cell monolayers and/or by hemagglutination of type O human red blood cells by the supernatant fluids from such cultures. Immunofluorescence staining of tracheal smears collected from suspect animals between 48 hours and 12 days after infection is also a convenient method of detecting the presence of virus in a colony.

Epidemiology, Prevention, and Control

Sendai virus disease has a worldwide distribution in laboratory mice and rats. In colonies, the infection is perpetuated by the introduction of susceptible animals, which become infected from animals in the colony that are infected either acutely or inapparently. The same infection pattern can occur in rat colonies. When epidemic or endemic infection has been diagnosed, elimination of affected animals, disinfection of the premises, and screening of incoming animals are needed for control. Infected colonies must be reestablished, either by cesarean section and foster mothers or by embryo transfer. Importantly, serological surveillance is required to monitor the success of such efforts—this is required in the United States for mice used in federally funded biomedical research.

Diseases Caused by Members of Subfamily *Paramyxovirinae*, Genus *Rubulavirus*

Newcastle Disease

Newcastle disease has been one of the most important diseases of poultry worldwide ever since the advent of high-density, confinement husbandry systems. The disease was first observed in Java in 1926 and in the same year it spread to England, where it was first recognized in Newcastle, hence the name. The disease is one of the most contagious of all viral diseases, spreading rapidly among susceptible birds, in some cases seemingly in mysterious fashion. As threatening as most strains of the virus are, the threat of exotic velogenic (viscerotropic) strains represents another order of magnitude of risk. Newcastle disease virus and perhaps related viruses also cause disease in wild species including cockatoos, cockatiels, parakeets, and finches, which are transported around the world legally and illegally.

Clinical Features

In chickens, respiratory, circulatory, gastrointestinal, and nervous signs are seen; the particular set of clinical manifestations depends on the age and immune status of the host and on the virulence and tropism of the infecting strain. A combination of inspiratory dyspnea (gasping), cyanosis of comb and wattles, and clonic muscular spasm is indicative. The average incubation period is 5 days. There is a loss of appetite, listlessness, abnormal thirst, huddling, weakness, and somnolence. Intestinal symptoms may include crop dilatation, presence of foamy mucus and fibrinous exudate in the pharynx, a similar discharge from the beak, and yellow-green diarrhea. Nervous system involvement is indicated by paralysis of wings and/or legs, torticollis, ataxia or circular movements, bobbing-and-weaving movements of the head, and clonic spasms. In layers there is a sudden decrease in egg production together with depigmentation and/or loss of shell and reduction in the albumen quality of eggs.

The disease in turkeys is similar; there are signs of respiratory and nervous system involvement. Airsacculitis rather than tracheitis is the most common lesion. In ducks and geese most infections are inapparent.

Pathogenesis, Pathology, and Immunity

Initially the virus replicates in the mucosal epithelium of the upper respiratory and intestinal tracts; shortly after infection, virus spreads via the blood to the spleen and bone marrow, producing a secondary viremia. This leads to infection of other target organs: lung, intestine, and central nervous system. Respiratory distress and dyspnea result from congestion of the lungs and damage to the respiratory center in the brain. Gross pathologic findings include ecchymotic hemorrhages in the larynx, trachea, esophagus, and throughout the intestine. The most prominent histologic lesions are necrotic foci in the intestinal mucosa and the lymphatic tissue and hyperemic changes in most organs, including the brain.

Strains of Newcastle disease virus differ widely in virulence, depending on the cleavability and activation of their hemagglutinin–neuraminidase and fusion glycoproteins. Avirulent strains produce inactive precursor proteins; in virulent strains these precursors are cleaved and activated readily. Cleavage activation must occur in the same tissues in which initial viral replication occurs if the infection is to be progressive—the presence of cellular proteases as well as the strain-based cleavability of the viral glycoprotein precursors defines the tissue tropism of various viral strains and their capacity to spread rapidly.

The terms velogenic (viscerotropic), mesogenic, and lentogenic are applied to Newcastle disease virus strains of high, intermediate, and low virulence. Whereas velogenic strains kill virtually 100% of infected fowl, naturally avirulent strains have even been used as vaccines. Virulent velogenic strains cause predominantly hemorrhagic lesions, in particular at the esophagus/proventriculus and proventriculus/gizzard junctions and in the posterior half of the duodenum, the jejunum, and ileum. These lesions are virtually pathognomonic for velogenic strains. In severe cases, hemorrhages are also present in subcutaneous tissues, muscles, larynx, tracheal/esophageal tissues, serous membranes, trachea, lungs, airsacs, pericardium, and myocardium. In adult hens, hemorrhages are present in ovarian follicles. Lesions can develop into diphtheroid inflammatory foci and later into necrotic foci. In the central nervous system, lesions are those of encephalomyelitis—neuronal necrosis, perivascular cuffing, and interstitial inflammatory infiltration.

Antibody production is rapid. Hemagglutination-inhibiting antibody can be detected within 4 to 6 days of infection and persists for at least 2 years. The level of hemagglutinating-inhibiting antibody is a measure of immunity. Maternal antibodies protect chicks for 3 to 4 weeks after hatching. IgG is confined to the circulation and does not prevent respiratory infection, but it does block viremia; locally produced IgA antibodies play an important role in protection in both the respiratory tract and the intestine.

Laboratory Diagnosis

Because clinical signs are relatively nonspecific and because the disease is such a threat, diagnosis must be confirmed by virus isolation and serology. The virus may be isolated from spleen, brain, or lungs by allantoic inoculation of 10-day-old embryonated eggs, with the virus being differentiated from other viruses by hemadsorption– and hemagglutination–inhibition tests. Diagnosis can be attempted about 1 week after onset of the symptoms and repeated 1 week later in case of inconclusive results. Virus can be isolated from the gut when circulating antibodies are already present. Immunofluorescence on tracheal sections or smears is rapid although less sensitive. Demonstration of antibody is diagnostic only in unvaccinated flocks; hemagglutination inhibition is the test of choice. The hemagglutination–inhibition test is also used for surveillance of chronic Newcastle disease in countries where this form of the disease is endemic.

Determination of virulence is essential for field isolates. In addition to the "neuropathic index" and the mean death time of chicken embryos, plaque formation in chicken cells in the presence or absence of trypsin is used as an index for virulence determination.

Epidemiology, Prevention, and Control

In addition to chickens, turkeys, pheasants, guinea fowl, ducks, geese, and pigeons, a wide range of captive and free-ranging semidomestic and free-living birds, including migratory waterfowl, are susceptible but the role of the latter in long-distance transmission is not clear.

In birds that survive, virus is shed in all secretions and excretions for at least 4 weeks. Transmission occurs by direct contact between birds by the airborne route via aerosols and dust particles and via contaminated feed and water. Mechanical spread between flocks is favored by the relative stability of the virus and its wide host range. With lentogenic strains, transovarial transmission is important, and virus-infected chicks may hatch from virus-containing eggs.

Trade in infected avian species and products plays a key role in the spread of Newcastle disease from infected to noninfected areas. Caged or aviary birds imported from endemic regions constitute a risk for the introduction of exotic velogenic strains of the virus into areas where there are commercial poultry industries. Some psittacine species may become persistently infected with velogenic virus and excrete it intermittently for more than 1 year without showing clinical signs. Virus may also be disseminated by frozen chickens, uncooked kitchen refuse, foodstuffs, bedding, manure, and transport containers.

Because Newcastle disease is a notifiable disease in most developed countries, legislative measures constitute the basis for control. Where the disease is endemic, control can be achieved by good hygiene combined with immunization, both live-virus vaccines containing naturally occurring lentogenic virus strains and inactivated virus (injectable oil emulsions) being commonly used. These vaccines are effective and safe, even in chicks, and may be administered via drinking water or by aerosol, eye or nostril droplets, or beak dipping. Laying hens are revaccinated every 4 months. Protection against disease can be expected about a week after vaccination. Vaccinated birds excrete the vaccine virus for up to 15 days after vaccination, hence in some countries birds cannot be moved from vaccinated flocks until 21 days after vaccination. Furthermore, infected birds can shed wild-type virus for up to 40 days even after being vaccinated and may thus represent an important virus reservoir. Inactivated vaccine, administered subcutaneously, is usually used for pigeons.

Human Disease

Newcastle disease virus can produce a transitory conjunctivitis in humans; the condition has been seen primarily in laboratory workers and vaccination teams exposed to large quantities of virus and, before vaccination was widely practiced, in workers eviscerating poultry in processing plants. The disease has not been reported in individuals who rear poultry or consume poultry products.

Other Avian Rubulavirus Diseases

Serologically distinct rubulaviruses have been isolated from birds; their significance is usually not made clear by the circumstances. One was isolated in the 1960s, in Yucaipa, California, where it caused outbreaks of serious systemic disease in turkeys. Another was isolated from turkeys in Canada in 1967 and the United States in 1968, again causing systemic disease. In the following decades, many isolations of serologically distinct viruses were reported worldwide, most as a consequence of testing associated with the quarantine of imported birds that was implemented after the 1970–1974 Newcastle disease pandemic.

Porcine Rubulavirus Disease (La-Piedad-Michoacan-Mexico)

A rubulavirus has been isolated from numerous outbreaks of a disease in young pigs in Mexico that is characterized by encephalomyelitis, reproductive failure, and corneal opacity, which may be the only clinical sign in older pigs, hence the common name for the disease, "blue eye." There is no serologic cross-reactivity with any other paramyxovirus, but analysis of the genome suggests that it is related most closely to mumps virus.

In 1997 an apparently new paramyxovirus was isolated from mummified and stillborn deformed piglets in Australia. Abnormalities included arthrogryposis and craniofacial deformities, including undershot jaw. Sera from two humans on the property who had experienced undiagnosed febrile illnesses coincidentally with the recognition of the disease in the pigs were positive for antibody to the new virus.

Diseases Caused by Members of Subfamily *Paramyxovirinae*, Genus *Morbillivirus*

Rinderpest

Rinderpest is one of the oldest recorded plagues of livestock. It is of Asiatic origin, first described in the 4th century. In the 18th and 19th centuries it was the cause of devastating epidemics that swept across Europe and in the early part of the 20th century across sub-Saharan Africa. The 1920 outbreak in Europe led to the founding of the *Office International des Épizooties,* in Paris, the organization that today brings together animal infectious disease authorities globally, especially to facilitate international trade. Today, it is still the cause of great economic loss in Africa, the Middle East, and parts of Asia.

The causative agent was first shown to be filterable virus in 1902. On the basis of phylogenetic analysis, it has been suggested that rinderpest virus is the archetype morbillivirus, having given rise to canine distemper and human measles viruses some 5000 to 10,000 years ago.

Clinical Features

In its typical manifestation, rinderpest is an acute febrile disease with morbidity in susceptible populations approaching 100% and mortality 90–100%. Indigenous cattle breeds in Africa have a lower mortality, up to 50%. After an incubation period of 3–5 days, a rapid rise in temperature is seen, called the prodromal phase. This is followed by the mucosal phase in which nasal and ocular mucopurulent secretions caused by severe mouth lesions (erosions) are observed. Depression and anorexia characterize this stage. This is followed by a phase of severe bloody diarrhea and prostration, during which animals may die from dehydration and shock.

Convalescence may take many weeks during which pregnant animals may abort. Strains prevalent in eastern

Africa are generally mild and there may be no clinical signs, only seroconversion.

Pathogenesis, Pathology, and Immunity

After nasal entry, virus replicates in tonsils and mandibular and pharyngeal lymph nodes. Viremia develops within 2 to 3 days, after which virus can be demonstrated in lymph nodes, spleen, bone marrow, and mucosa of the upper respiratory tract, lung, and the digestive tract. Thereafter, virus replicates in the nasal mucosa, causing necrosis, erosions, and fibrinous exudation. Leukopenia is profound as a result of viral replication and destruction of lymphoid organs, especially the mesenteric lymph nodes and gut-associated lymphoid tissue. The immunodeficiency that develops often results in the activation of latent or intercurrent viral infections and opportunistic bacterial infections.

Virulent virus strains also infect the epithelial layers of the upper respiratory, urogenital, and alimentary tracts. Less virulent strains induce less extensive mucosal lesions, which may account for their reduced ability to transmit by contact. In the cecum, colon, and rectum, "zebra" stripes are commonly found; these are caused by distended capillaries packed with erythrocytes. Intracytoplasmic and intranuclear eosinophilic inclusion bodies are found commonly in infected epithelial cells.

Dehydration in acute infections due to profuse diarrhea causes changes in hematological findings and blood chemistry. As a consequence, total serum proteins and serum chloride levels drop. There is an apparent increase in the packed cell volume of 40 to 65%. At death the blood is dark, thick, and slow to coagulate.

Cattle that survive rinderpest have lifelong immunity. Neutralizing antibodies appear 6 to 7 days after the onset of clinical signs, and maximum titers are reached during the third and fourth weeks postinfection.

Laboratory Diagnosis

In countries where rinderpest is endemic, clinical diagnosis is usually considered sufficient. In countries free of the disease but subject to occasional importations, it can be confused with other diseases affecting the mucosa, such as bovine viral diarrhea and malignant catarrhal fever. In the early stages, differentiation from infectious bovine rhinotracheitis and foot-and-mouth disease is difficult. The virus infects a wide range of cells, but isolation for laboratory diagnosis is carried out routinely in primary bovine kidney cell cultures. A marmoset lymphoblastoid cell line (B95a) and a *Theileria parva*-transformed bovine lymphocyte cell line are also used. The best specimens for virus isolation are tissues from mucosal lesions or lymph nodes; cocultivation of washed buffy coat cells from suspect animals with bovine kidney cells may be used to avoid the effects of the presence of early antibody. Cytopathology is evident in 3 to 12 days. Neutralization and enzyme immunoassays are used to confirm the identity of isolates and for serologic diagnosis.

Epidemiology, Prevention, and Control

The host range includes domestic cattle, water buffalo, sheep, and goats. Domestic pigs can develop clinical signs and are regarded as an important virus reservoir in Asia. Among wild animals, wildebeest, deer, antelope, and hippopotamuses are susceptible.

In endemic areas the disease spreads from animal to animal by contact, with infection occurring through aerosol droplets. Virus is shed in secretions from the nose, throat, and conjunctiva as well as in feces, urine, and milk. Infected cattle excrete virus during the incubation period, before clinical signs occur, and in Africa and Asia such animals are an important source for the introduction of rinderpest into disease-free areas. The disease is also introduced into new areas by importation of live, subclinically infected sheep, goats, and possibly other ruminants. Subclinically infected swine may act as a source of infection for cattle; only Asian breeds of swine and warthogs show clinical signs, although all species of pigs are susceptible. Because the virus is thermolabile, indirect spread via fresh meat and meat products, food, and transport vehicles is unusual.

Outbreaks have often followed wars and civil disturbance where movements of troops and refugees with live food animals disseminates the virus. A recent outbreak in Sri Lanka followed 40 years of freedom from the disease; the likely source was live goats introduced from India by soldiers. Rinderpest also reappeared in Turkey in the 1990s, possibly a consequence of the Gulf War.

In rinderpest-free countries, veterinary public health measures are designed to prevent introduction of the virus. Importation of uncooked meat and meat products from infected countries is forbidden, and zoo animals must be quarantined before being transported to such countries. In countries with endemic rinderpest and where the disease has a high probability of being introduced, attenuated virus vaccines are used.

Early rinderpest vaccine strains were produced by virus passage in rabbits (lapinized vaccine), embryonated eggs (avianized vaccine), or goats (caprinized vaccine). The latter vaccine, attenuated inadequately may have been responsible for the circulation of rinderpest in small ruminants in India.

In the 1960s an attenuated virus vaccine produced in cell culture (Plowright vaccine) was developed and used throughout Africa in a program that almost succeeded in eliminating the disease from the continent. However, political instability, lack of funds, and the persistence of relatively avirulent strains resulted in a resurgence of disease in the 1980s. This vaccine is efficacious because it induces lifelong immunity and it is inexpensive to produce. In fact, it is still one of the best vaccines available for any animal disease, but it is thermolabile and requires a well-maintained "cold chain," a difficult practical problem in many areas where rinderpest occurs. To remedy this, a vaccinia virus recombinant carrying the genes for the rinderpest virus hemagglutinin–neuraminidase and fusion proteins is currently in field trials in Africa; it is very thermostable.

Peste des Petits Ruminants

Peste des petits ruminants is a highly contagious, systemic disease of goats and sheep very similar to rinderpest and caused by a closely related morbillivirus. Unlike rinderpest, however, many infections are subclinical. It occurs mainly in West Africa, although outbreaks have also been described elsewhere. After an incubation period of 5 or 6 days, clinical signs develop, including fever, anorexia, a necrotic stomatitis with gingivitis, and diarrhea. Bronchopneumonia is a frequent complication. The course of the disease may be peracute, acute, or chronic; however, the virus does not persist. Peste des petits ruminants has economic consequences, in that mortality in goats can reach 95% and in sheep only slightly less. Transmission of the virus is similar to that of rinderpest. Wild animals are not believed to play a role in the spread of virus. Primary lamb kidney cells are used for virus isolation. Rinderpest vaccine has been used to control spread of the disease, but an homologueous vaccine is now being field tested in West Africa.

Canine Distemper

Canine distemper is the most important viral disease of dogs, producing high morbidity and mortality in unvaccinated populations worldwide. It is a highly contagious acute or subacute, febrile disease, which has been known since 1760. Edward Jenner first described the course and clinical features of the disease in 1809; its viral etiology was demonstrated in 1906 by Carré. It is now comparatively rare in many industrialized countries, being well controlled by vaccination. However, in recent years it has emerged as a significant pathogen of the large species in the family *Felidae*. In the 1990s, thousands of African lions have died, contracting the virus via contact with free-roaming canids (hyenas, feral dogs).

Clinical Features

The disease occurs in several forms. In the rare peracute form of the disease there is sudden onset of fever and sudden death. In the most common acute form of the disease, after an incubation period of 3 to 6 days, infected dogs develop a biphasic rise of temperature up to 41°C, with the second peak corresponding to the onset of severe leukopenia and other clinical signs. Anorexia, catarrh, conjunctivitis, and depression are common during this stage. Some dogs show primarily respiratory signs, others gastrointestinal signs. The pulmonary disease is characterized by catarrhal inflammation of the larynx and bronchi, tonsillitis, and a cough. Later, bronchitis or catarrhal bronchopneumonia develop, sometimes with pleuritis. The gastrointestinal disease is characterized by severe vomiting and watery diarrhea. After the onset of the disease, central nervous system signs may occur: behavioral changes, forced movements, local myoclony, tonic–clonic spasms, epileptic-like attacks, ataxia, and paresis. The duration of disease varies, depending on complications caused by secondary bacterial infections.

The subacute neurological form of the disease may follow any of the acute manifestations of infection or may appear after subclinical infection: there is frank encephalitis with convulsions and seizures and most surviving dogs have permanent central nervous system sequelae such as nervous "ticks" or involuntary leg movements.

Finally, there are two late forms of the disease seen in old dogs, one called *old dog encephalitis* in which there is slowly progressive loss of neurologic functions, the other called *hard-pad disease,* in which hyperkeratosis of foot pads and the nose occurs. These late manifestations of canine distemper may occur in dogs with no history of earlier acute or subacute disease. Neurological signs include (1) localized twitching of a muscle or group of muscles (chorea, flexor spasm, hyperkinesia), such as in the leg or facial muscles; (2) paresis or paralysis, often beginning in the hind limbs and evident as ataxia, followed by ascending paresis and paralysis; and (3) convulsions characterized by salivation and chewing movements (petit mal). The seizures may become more frequent and severe, and the dog may then fall on its side and paddle its legs, with involuntary urination and defecation (grand mal). Both of these late diseases may occur together and both may end in death. The mortality rate of all forms of the disease, taken together, ranges between 30 and 80%.

Pathogenesis, Pathology, and Immunity

The first pathogenetic event is the local replication of the virus for 2 to 4 days in cells of the upper respiratory tract or in conjunctival epithelium. After further multiplication in regional lymph nodes, the virus enters the bloodstream, carried within lymphocytes, to produce a primary viremia (synchronous with the first bout of fever) that spreads the virus to the reticuloendothelial system. The effects of viral replication at these sites are manifested by hyperplasia and by the presence of multinucleated giant cells in lymphoid organs. Virions formed in these sites are carried by lymphocytes and monocytes to produce a secondary viremia, coincident with the second peak of fever.

In acute distemper a serous inflammation of respiratory mucosal membranes associated with interstitial pneumonia occurs. Intestinal and neurologic (nonsuppurative encephalitis) signs also characterize the pathology of this disease.

For protection and survival, cell-mediated immunity is important in morbillivirus infections in general. In human measles, persons with agammaglobulinemia can overcome the infection but those with inherited or acquired deficiencies in their cell-mediated immune system are at extreme risk. However, animals with any detectable neutralizing antibody are immune and immunity following morbillivirus infections is lifelong.

Laboratory Diagnosis

Clinical diagnosis of canine distemper has been made difficult by its rarity where vaccination is widely practiced. Laboratory diagnosis is necessary to exclude infectious canine hepatitis, canine parvovirus disease, leptospirosis, toxoplasmosis, and rabies. Virus isolation is done by cocultivation of lymphocytes from suspect animals with mitogen-stimulated canine or ferret lymphocytes. After passage the virus can then be adapted to grow in MDCK, Vero, or primary dog lung cells. Typical cytopathic effects such as the formation of stellate cells and syncytia can be observed 3 to 12 days after infection. Several blind passages may be necessary before cytopathic changes are observed. Immunohistologic methods are useful for demonstrating the presence of viral antigen in impression smears of the conjunctiva or in peripheral blood lymphocytes (antemortem) or in lung, stomach, intestinal, and bladder tissue (postmortem).

Epidemiology, Prevention, and Control

The host range of canine distemper virus embraces all species of the families *Canidae* (dog, dingo, fox, coyote, jackal, wolf), *Procyonidae* (raccoon, coati mundi, panda), *Mustelidae* (weasel, ferret, mink, skunk, badger, marten, otter), the large members of the family *Felidae* (lions, leopards, cheetahs, tigers), and the collared peccary (*Tayassu tajacu*). The highly publicized outbreak of distemper in lions in the Serengeti National Park in Tanzania and cases in the Chinese leopard and other large cats in zoos have underlined the capacity of the virus to invade new hosts.

The virus is shed in all secretions and excretions from the fifth day after infection, which is before the onset of clinical signs, and continues, sometimes for weeks. Transmission is mainly via direct contact, droplet and aerosol. Young dogs are more susceptible than older dogs, with the highest susceptibility being between 4 and 6 months of age, after puppies have lost their maternal antibody.

There are differences between urban and isolated dogs with respect to the epidemiologic pattern of canine distemper. In the absence of vaccination, infections are frequent in urban dogs, in kennels, and in other situations where close contact between dogs occurs. This leads to a high level of herd immunity. For example, serologic studies have show that 80% of puppies born to vaccinated urban bitches have antibodies to distemper virus at 8 weeks of age; this rate decreases to 10% by 4 or 5 months of age. This percentage then increases slowly, reaching 85% at the age of 2 years. In rural areas the number of dogs is too small to support a continuing chain of infection, so that highly susceptible dog populations develop, a situation that leads to catastrophic epidemics affecting dogs of all ages.

Control is based on adequate diagnosis, quarantine, sanitation, and vaccination. The virus is extremely fragile, and disinfection of premises is achieved easily with any standard disinfectant. Successful immunization of pups with canine distemper attenuated virus vaccines depends on the absence of interfering maternal antibody. The age at which pups can be immunized can be predicted from a nomograph if the serum antibody titer of the mother is known; this service is available in some diagnostic laboratories. Variations in colostrum uptake among pups in a litter limit the value of this procedure. Alternatively, pups can be vaccinated with modified live-virus vaccine at 6 weeks of age and then at 2- to 4-week intervals until 16 weeks of age. For treatment, hyperimmune serum or immune globulin can be used prophylactically immediately after exposure. Antibiotic therapy generally has a beneficial effect by lessening the effect of secondary opportunistic bacterial infections.

Equine Morbillivirus Disease

In 1994 an outbreak of severe respiratory disease occurred in thoroughbred horses stabled in Brisbane, Queensland, Australia; within 2 weeks, 14 horses had died. Two persons at the stable developed a severe influenza-like disease and one died after 6 days in intensive care. A new virus was isolated from both the horses and the trainer, and the syndrome could be reproduced experimentally in horses using this isolate. Another human case was reported a year later: at about the time of the outbreak in Brisbane, 2 horses died on a farm in Mackay, 1000 km north of Brisbane. The owners, a veterinarian and her husband, performed necropsies on the 2 horses; soon afterward the husband became ill with a mild meningoencephalitis and then seemed to recover. However, 12 months later he developed severe encephalitis and died. Serum stored from the time of his first illness contained a low titer and serum from the time of his fatal illness contained very high titers of antibody to the equine virus. The diagnosis was confirmed by immunofluorescence and polymerase chain reaction assays on postmortem tissues from the human and stored tissues from the 2 horses.

Antibody was detected in all recovered horses and humans, but not in other persons, horses, or a variety of terrestrial animals tested in the course of an extensive serological survey. Remarkably, in 1996, neutralizing antibody was found in four species of fruit bats (flying foxes, suborder *Megachiroptera*) collected along the whole of the eastern coast of Queensland, from Cairns to Brisbane. Later, virus was isolated from a bat. Studies are underway to unravel the context of these findings. The virus is the first morbilli-like virus found to infect and cause disease in horses. Although related most closely to the morbilliviruses, this virus is different enough to possibly warrant placement in a new genus within the family *Paramyxoviridae*.

Clinical Features

Affected horses were anorectic, depressed, febrile, had increased respiratory and heart rates, and some had paroxysms of coughing. Ataxia, head pressing, a frothy nasal discharge, and collapse occurred as the disease progressed. The clinical course was short, with 10 of the 20 naturally infected horses dying within 36 hours of onset of clinical signs; 7 of these deaths occurred within 12 hours of onset. The incubation period in experimentally infected horses was from 6 to 10 days.

Pathogenesis, Pathology, and Immunity

The most important lesions involved the lungs; they were congested, firm, and fluid filled with dilated lymphatics, and some had fibrin tags on the pleura. Naturally occurring cases had a thick, foamy hemorrhagic exudate in the airways; the pericardial sac contained serous fluid. There was histological evidence of interstitial pneumonia with proteinaceous alveolar edema associated with hemorrhage, dilated lymphatics, alveolar thrombosis and necrosis, and necrosis of the walls of small blood vessels. Syncytial giant cells were detected in the endothelium of lung capillaries and arterioles; within these, cytoplasmic inclusion bodies consistent with the ultrastructure of massed viral nucleocapsids were observed by electron microscopy. Sera from horses surviving the disease had high neutralizing antibody titers. Cats and guinea pigs but not rabbits and mice were found to be susceptible to experimental infection, with cats developing a fatal pneumonia identical to that seen in the equine disease.

Laboratory Diagnosis

Virus isolation is done by inoculating Vero monolayer or primary equine fetal kidney cell cultures with filtered lung homogenates from fresh cases. A syncytial cytopathology develops in about 3 days, and the virus can be identified by serological and molecular biologic methods. Serological testing involves virus neutralization and fluorescent antibody blocking tests, and an enzyme immunoassay is available for routine screening and surveillance.

Epidemiology, Prevention, and Control

Transmission requires direct contact, e.g., with saliva or nasal secretions. The first outbreak was controlled by euthanasia and deep burial of all infected horses, quarantine and control of the movement of horses within a defined zone, and serological surveillance to determine the extent of infection. Surveillance indicated that the disease had not spread beyond the original 20 infected horses. The reservoir source of the virus in fruit bats (flying foxes) raises many questions in regard to possible future prevention and control strategies.

Human Disease

Equine morbillivirus is clearly a dangerous zoonotic pathogen. Care must be taken when its presence is suspected and adequate biocontainment facilities, equipment, and practices must be used in the laboratory.

Phocine, Dolphin, and Porpoise Distemper

In 1987 and 1988, serious disease outbreaks were observed among the seal populations of Lake Baikal and along the sea shores of the Baltic and North Sea (western Europe), respectively. The European epidemic became conspicuous by the appearance of large numbers of aborted harbor seal (*Phoca vitulina*) pups, as well as the stranding of many adolescent and adult animals. Clinical signs resembling those of distemper in dogs, such as serous nasal discharge, conjunctivitis, gastrointestinal disturbances, cutaneous lesions, and central nervous signs, gave the first clues as to the nature of the etiological agent. The animals died within 2 weeks of disease onset from respiratory distress or central nervous system disease. Virologic investigations that followed upon these episodes uncovered a diverse global morbillivirus disease problem involving many marine mammal species. Several closely related morbilliviruses have been shown to be involved in disease episodes in pinnipeds and cetaceans.

Phocine distemper virus has been associated not only with massive epidemics in harbor seals in Europe, but also in harbor porpoises (*Phocoena phocoena*) along the Irish coast and in striped dolphins (*Stenella coeruleoalba*) in the Mediterranean Sea. Phocine distemper virus has been shown by molecular biologic methods to be a new member of the genus *Morbillivirus*. The virus infecting Lake Baikal seals (*Phoca sibirica*) has been shown to be very similar, if not identical, to canine distemper virus (Figure 26.1).

Dolphin distemper virus has been associated with a massive epidemic in bottlenose dolphins along the Atlantic coast from New Jersey to Florida. More than half of the inshore population of this species may have died in the early 1990s. Deaths have occurred along the coast of Alabama, Mississippi, and Texas as well. Porpoise distemper virus is related very closely to the dolphin virus, so in many cases a distinction is not made, except in recording the species involved. In any case, disease has been seen in several species of dolphins in several ocean regions. In a recent study, serological evidence of morbillivirus infection was found in 11 of 15 cetacean species in the western Atlantic. Neutralizing antibody titers were higher against the dolphin and porpoise viruses than the seal (phocine) virus. A high prevalence of antibody was found in two species of pilot whale (*Globicephala melas* and *G. macrorhynchus*); of interest is the notion that pilot whales might serve as long-distance vectors between America and Europe, carrying viruses to otherwise isolated populations of marine mammals.

Pathological changes in these diseases are similar to those observed in distemper virus-infected canids. The most prominent finding is an acute hemorrhagic pneumonia with interstitial edema and emphysema. As also observed in influenza virus infections, many seals show swollen necks due to the escaping of air from the damaged lung parenchyma. Demyelinating encephalitis with necrotic degeneration of neurons in the cerebral cortex and perivascular infiltration of lymphocytes and macrophages is also common. Cytoplasmic inclusion bodies are found in apparently normal neurons, astrocytes, microglia cells, and above all in the urinary bladder. In demyelinated areas, astrocyte proliferation and syncytia are seen. In the spleen, bronchial lymph nodes and Peyer's patches, lymphocyte depletion, and necrosis are prominent.

Diagnosis has been made using immunofluorescence on sections of the respiratory tract and other infected organs of suspect animals. Morbillivirus RNA has been demonstrated in spleen and liver samples from affected animals by hybridization techniques using molecular probes.

Diseases Caused by Members of Subfamily *Pneumovirinae*, Genus *Pneumovirus*

Bovine Respiratory Syncytial Disease

Bovine respiratory syncytial virus was first detected in Japan, Belgium, and Switzerland in 1967, and was isolated a little later in England and the United States. It is now known to occur worldwide in all bovine species as well as in sheep, goats, and other animals. The virus is related closely to human respiratory syncytial virus. In many settings the bovine virus causes inapparent infection, but especially in recently weaned calves and young cattle it is the cause of pneumonia, interstitial pulmonary edema, and emphysema. There is also evidence that, like bovine parainfluenza virus 3, the virus is a major initiating factor in the development of shipping fever.

Clinical Features

Respiratory syncytial disease is particularly important in recently weaned calves and young cattle, especially when they are maintained in closely confined conditions. Infection is characterized by a sudden onset of fever, hyperpnea, abdominal breathing, lethargy, rhinitis, nasal discharge, and cough. Bronchiolitis and multifocal and interstitial pneumonia may be associated with interstitial edema and emphysema, and cases progressing to severe bronchopneumonia may end in death. Secondary bacterial pneumonia, especially that caused by *Pasteurella hemolytica,* is common. The highest mortality often occurs in calves on a high plane of nutrition, leading to the speculation that certain feedstuffs such as corn silage may predispose cattle to the effect of infection. In general, in outbreak situations morbidity is high but mortality is low.

Pathogenesis, Pathology, and Immunity

In calves infected experimentally, the virus causes complete loss of the ciliated epithelium 8 to 10 days after infection so that pulmonary clearance is compromised, with consequent secondary infections. At necropsy, pleural and interstitial emphysema may be seen in all lobes of the lungs; if secondary bacterial infection is present there may be areas of consolidation. A characteristic finding is the presence of syncytial cells in the lungs, which are usually larger than those seen in parainfluenza virus 3 infection.

After a primary natural infection, protection is short lived and reinfections are common. In vaccination studies, increased lung pathology was observed after application of formalin-inactivated preparations, an observation following similar findings in humans. An Arthus-type reaction, antibody-mediated enhancement of macrophage infection, complement activation, and hypersensitivity reactions have all been postulated to play a role in the pathogenesis of the respiratory disease. Disease may be a consequence of a predominant Th2 response of helper cells with the preferential release of inflammatory cytokines.

Laboratory Diagnosis

Diagnosis is made difficult by the common presence of the virus in many calves—interpretation of clinical and laboratory data must be done prudently. Because interpretation of virus isolation data is so difficult and because viral infectivity is very labile, virus isolation is not attempted very often. The virus may be isolated in a variety of bovine cell cultures, best in those derived from the respiratory tract. The cytopathic effect is similar to that of parainfluenza virus 3; syncytia and intracytoplasmic inclusions are prominent. Immunofluorescence on nasal swab material has rarely been successful, whereas cells obtained by lung lavage and at necropsy are more useful. The classical retrospective method to diagnose the infection has been serology on paired serum samples, but again, interpretation of findings is difficult.

Epidemiology, Prevention, and Control

Most commonly, the infection occurs during the winter months when cattle and sheep are housed in confined conditions. However, there have been substantial outbreaks in cow–calf operations in summer as well. The virus spreads rapidly, probably through aerosols or droplets of respiratory tract excretions. Reinfection of the respiratory tract is not uncommon in calves with antibody. Preexisting antibody, whether derived passively from maternal transfer or actively by prior infection or vaccination, does not prevent viral replication and excretion, although clinical signs may be lessened or inapparent if the antibody titer is high. The virus persists in herds, most probably through continuous subclinical reinfections or in carriers; stress of transport and so on may trigger acute disease in such circumstances.

Several inactivated and attenuated virus vaccines have been developed, but information on their efficacy in calves with maternal antibodies and about the duration of the immunity they evoke is lacking. Experimentally, a novel recombinant vaccine employing a bovine herpesvirus as the vector for the G protein of bovine respiratory syncytial virus has been found to induce mucosal immunity and to protect cattle. A DNA vaccine has also shown promise in the experimental setting.

Pneumonia Virus of Mice Disease

Pneumonia virus of mice is widespread in mouse colonies; it also infects rats, cotton rats, hamsters, gerbils, and guinea pigs. However, for many years it was not clear what effect infection has on the health of these species other than when it is introduced experimentally into the respiratory tract. More recently, studies have shown that the virus is capable of causing significant lesions in the lungs of infected mice, thereby interfering with a wide range of scientific investigations. Control is based on depopulation, disinfection of the premises, and screening of incoming animals. Serological surveillance is required in the United States for mice used in federally funded biomedical research.

Diseases Caused by Members of Subfamily *Pneumovirinae*, Genus *Metapneumovirus*

Turkey Rhinotracheitis

First described in South Africa in 1978, turkey rhinotracheitis or coryza has now been recognized in many countries. In young turkeys the disease is characterized by catarrh, rales, sneezing, frothy nasal discharge, foamy conjunctivitis, swelling of the infraorbital sinuses, and submandibular edema. These signs are exacerbated by secondary infections. In laying birds, a drop in egg production is associated with slight respiratory distress. Morbidity is often 100%; mortality ranges from 0.4 to 90% and is highest in young poults. A milder form of the disease occurring in chickens is termed "swollen head syndrome." This disease is characterized by swelling of the infraorbital sinuses, torticollis, disorientation, and general depression, sometimes also with respiratory distress.

Histologically, the disease is distinguished by destruction of the tracheal epithelium beginning about 48 hours after infection, followed by mucosal thickening, congestion, and infiltration with lymphocytes, plasma cells, and neutrophils. Cytoplasmic eosinophilic inclusions are seen in epithelial cells of the airways and nasal cavities.

Diagnosis of both the turkey and the chicken disease is based most commonly on enzyme immunoassay. Virus isolation is difficult, but can be achieved by serial passage in 6- to 7-day-old turkey or chicken embryos or in chicken embryo tracheal organ cultures. Antibodies can be measured by enzyme immunoassay. Attenuated virus vaccines are available commercially.

Further Reading

Barrett, T. (1998). Rinderpest and distemper viruses. *In* "Encyclopedia of Virology" (R. G. Webster and A. Granoff, eds.), 2nd ed. (CD-ROM). Academic Press, London.

Collins, P. L., Chanock, R. M., and McIntosh, K. (1996). Parainfluenza viruses. *In* "Fields Virology" (B. N. Fields, D. M. Knipe, P. M. Howley, R. M. Chanock, J. L. Melnick, T. P. Monath, B. Roizman, and S. E. Straus, eds.), 3rd ed., pp. 1205–1242. Lippincott-Raven, Philadelphia, PA.

Collins, P. L., McIntosh, K., and Chanock, R. M. (1996). Respiratory syncytial virus. *In* "Fields Virology" (B. N. Fields, D. M. Knipe, P. M. Howley, R. M., Chanock, J. L. Melnick, T. P. Monath, B. Roizman, and S. E. Straus, eds.), 3rd ed., pp. 1313–1352. Lippincott-Raven, Philadelphia, PA.

Descoteaux, J.-P. (1994). Myxovirus parainfluenza type 1 (Sendai). *In* "Virus Infections of Vertebrates" (A. D. M. E. Osterhaus, ed.), Vol. 5, pp. 285–291. Elsevier, Amsterdam.

Kimman, T. G., and Westenbrink, F. (1990). Immunity to human and bovine respiratory syncytial viruses, brief review. *Arch. Virol.* **112,** 1–25.

Kouwenhoven, B. (1993). Newcastle disease. *In* "Virus Infections of Vertebrates" (J. B. McFerran and M. S. McNulty, eds.), Vol. 4, pp. 341–361. Elsevier, Amsterdam.

Lamb, R. A., and Kolakofsky, D. (1996). Paramyxoviridae: The viruses and their replication. *In* "Fields Virology" (B. N. Fields, D. M. Knipe, P. M. Howley, R. M. Chanock, J. L. Melnick, T. P. Monath, B. Roizman, and S. E. Straus, eds.), 3rd ed., pp. 1177–1204. Lippincott-Raven, Philadelphia, PA.

Murray, K., Rogers, R., Selvey, L., Selleck, P., Hyatt, A., Gould, A., Gleeson, L., Hooper, P., and Westbury, H. (1995). A novel morbillivirus pneumonia of horses and its transmission to humans. *Emerg. Infect. Dis.* **1,** 31–33.

Rossiter, P. B. (1994). Rinderpest. *In* "Infectious Diseases of Livestock with Special Reference to Southern Africa" (J. A. W. Coetzer, G. R. Thompson, and R. C. Tustin, eds.), Vol. 2, pp. 733–757. Oxford University Press, Cape Town.

Rossiter, P. B., and Taylor, W. P. (1994). Peste des petits ruminants. *In* "Infectious Diseases of Livestock with Special Reference to Southern Africa" (J. A. W. Coetzer, G. R. Thompson, and R. C. Tustin, eds.), Vol. 2, pp. 758–765. Oxford University Press, Cape Town.

Shibuta, H. (1998). Animal parainfluenzaviruses. *In* "Encyclopedia of Virology" (R. G. Webster and A. Granoff, eds.), 2nd ed. (CD-ROM). Academic Press, London.

Westbury, H. A., and Murray, P. K. (1996). Equine morbillivirus pneumonia (acute equine respiratory syndrome). *In* "Virus Infections of Vertebrates" (M. J. Studdert, ed.), Vol. 6, pp. 225–233. Elsevier, Amsterdam.

Wright, P. F. (1997). Viral respiratory diseases. *In* "Viral Pathogenesis" (N. Nathanson, R. Ahmed, F. Gonzalez-Scarano, D. E. Griffin, K. V. Holmes, F. A. Murphy, and H. L. Robinson, eds.), pp. 703–712. Lippincott-Raven, Philadelphia, PA.

CHAPTER 27

Rhabdoviridae

The family *Rhabdoviridae* encompasses more than 175 viruses of vertebrates, invertebrates (mostly arthropods), and plants. Virions have a distinctive bullet-shaped morphology. The family comprises several important animal pathogens, including rabies virus, vesicular stomatitis viruses, bovine ephemeral fever virus, and several rhabdoviruses of fish.

Rabies is the cause of one of the oldest and most feared diseases of humans and animals—it was recognized in Egypt before 2300 B.C. and in ancient Greece, where it was well described by Aristotle. Perhaps the most lethal of all infectious diseases, rabies also has the distinction of having stimulated one of the great early discoveries in biomedical science. In 1885, before the nature of viruses was comprehended, Louis Pasteur developed, tested, and applied a rabies vaccine, thereby opening the modern era of infectious disease prevention by vaccination.

Vesicular stomatitis of horses, cattle, and swine was first distinguished from foot-and-mouth disease early in the 19th century—it was recognized as the cause of periodic epidemics throughout the Western hemisphere. The disease was a significant problem in artillery and cavalry horses during the American Civil War. The first large epidemic to be described in detail occurred in 1916; the disease spread rapidly from Colorado to the east coast of the United States, affecting large numbers of horses and mules and, to a lesser extent, cattle. Large epidemics have continued to occur in the United States on an approximately 5- to 10-year cycle.

Bovine ephemeral fever was first recognized in Africa in 1867 and is now known to be widespread across Africa, most of southeast Asia, Japan, and Australia. Several rhabdoviruses are the cause of serious losses in the aquaculture industries of North America, Europe, and Asia.

Properties of Rhabdoviruses

Classification

Based on virion properties and serologic relationships, four genera containing animal viruses have been recognized in the family *Rhabdoviridae,* the genera *Lyssavirus, Vesiculovirus, Ephemerovirus,* and *Novirhabdovirus.* There are also several important viruses, mostly of fish, that have not yet been placed in genera (Table 27.1). Rhabdovirus species are distinguished genetically (by partial sequencing) and serologically, most importantly by neutralization tests.

The genus *Lyssavirus* comprises rabies virus and closely related viruses, including Mokola virus, Lagos bat virus, and Duvenhage virus from Africa, European bat viruses 1 and 2, and Australian bat lyssavirus. Each of these viruses is considered capable of causing rabies-

Table 27.1
Rhabdoviruses That Affect Animals

Virus	Geographic Distribution
Genus *Lyssavirus*	
Rabies virus	All continents except Antarctica
Mokola virus	Central Africa
Lagos bat virus	Central and southern Africa
Duvenhage virus	South Africa
European bat lyssaviruses 1 and 2	Europe
Australian bat lyssavirus	Australia
Genus *Vesiculovirus*	
Vesicular stomatitis–Indiana virus	North, Central, and South America
Vesicular stomatitis–New Jersey virus	North, Central, and South America
Vesicular stomatitis–Alagoas virus	Argentina, Brazil
Cocal virus	Trinidad, Brazil
Piry virus	Brazil
Chandipura virus	India, Nigeria
Isfahan virus	Iran
Pike fry rhabdovirus	Europe
Spring viremia of carp virus	Widespread
Genus *Ephemerovirus*	
Bovine ephemeral fever virus	Asia, Africa, Australia
Genus *Novirhabdovirus*	
Infectious hematopoietic necrosis virus	North America, Europe, Asia
Ungrouped fish rhabdoviruses	
Viral hemorrhagic septicemia virus of salmon (Egtved virus)	Europe, North America

like disease in animals and humans. Rabies virus and the rabies-like viruses, including European bat viruses 1 and 2, Lagos bat virus, Duvenhage virus, and Australian bat lyssavirus use bats as reservoir hosts; several other members of the family *Rhabdoviridae* have been isolated from bats. The genus *Vesiculovirus* contains about 35 serologically distinct viruses, most importantly vesicular stomatitis–Indiana virus and vesicular stomatitis–New Jersey virus, as well as six other viruses that are known to cause vesicular disease in horses, cattle, swine, and humans. Several fish and eel rhabdoviruses are also members of this genus, including pike fry rhabdovirus (also called grass carp rhabdovirus) and spring viremia of carp virus. The genus *Ephemerovirus* contains bovine ephemeral fever virus and many other serologically distinct viruses, including several that can cause bovine ephemeral fever-like disease in cattle. The genus *Novirhabdovirus* contains infectious hematopoietic necrosis virus of fish. Among the ungrouped rhabdoviruses is the important fish pathogen, viral hemorrhagic septicemia virus (Egtved virus) of salmon.

Virion Properties

Rhabdovirus virions are 70 nm in diameter and 170 nm long (although some are longer and some shorter) and consist of an envelope with large peplomers within which is a helically coiled cylindrical nucleocapsid. The precise cylindrical form of the nucleocapsid is what gives the viruses their distinctive bullet or conical shape (Figure 27.1). The genome is a single molecule of linear, negative-sense, single-stranded RNA, 11 to 15 kb in size. For example, 11,932 nucleotides make up the genome of rabies virus. The genome encodes five genes in the order 3′-N-NS-M-G-L-5′; some viruses have additional genes

FIGURE 27.1.

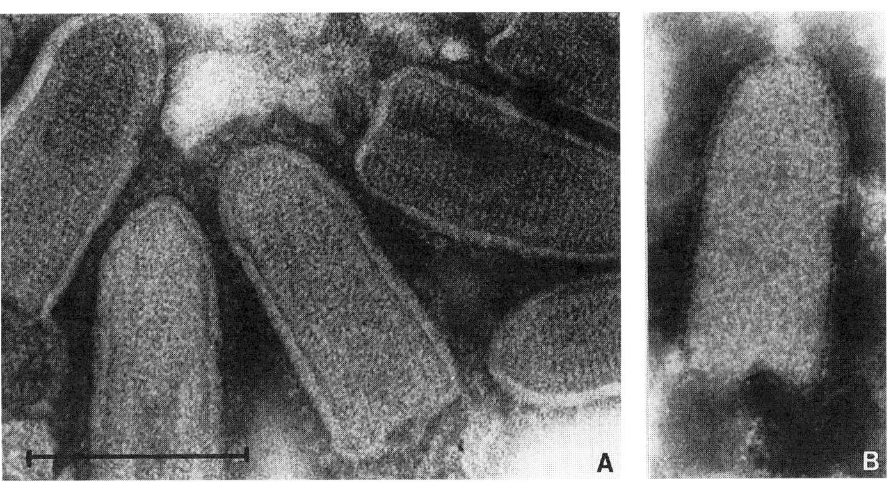

Family *Rhaddoviridae*, genus *Vesiculovirus* and *Lyssavirus*. (A) Vesicular stomatitis Indiana virus showing characteristic bullet-shaped virions. (B) Rabies virus. Negative stain electron microscopy. Bar: 100 nm.

or pseudogenes interposed (Figure 27.2). The viruses generally have five proteins (the following values are for rabies virus): L (2142 amino acids), the RNA-dependent RNA polymerase that functions in transcription and RNA replication; G (505 amino acids), the glycoprotein that forms trimers that make up the peplomers (spikes); N (450 amino acids), the nucleoprotein, the major component of the viral nucleocapsid; NS (297 amino acids)

FIGURE 27.2.

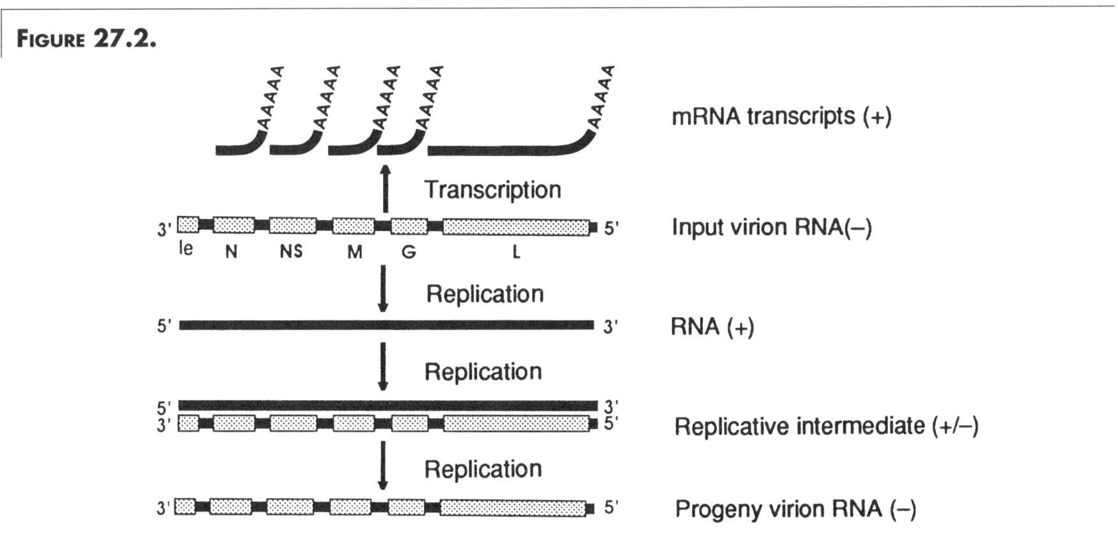

Genome structure of vesicular stomatitis virus and its mode of replication. Wide bars indicate genes and their relative sizes. Replication first involves mRNA transcription from the genomic RNA; later, using the protein products of this transcription, there is production of full-length, positive-stranded template, which in turn is used for the synthesis of genomic RNA. Using virion RNA as template, the viral transcriptase transcribes five subgenomic mRNA species (top). The N protein-RNA nucleocapsid plus the NS and L proteins comprise the transcription complex. There is only a single promoter site, located at the 3′ end of the viral genome; the polymerase (transcriptase) attaches to the genomic RNA template at this site and, as it moves along the viral RNA, it encounters stop/start signals at the boundaries of each of the viral genes—only a proportion of polymerase molecules move past each junction and continue the transcription process. This is called *stop–start* or *stuttering transcription*—it also accounts for the addition of poly(A) tails on the 3′ ends of each mRNA. Le, leader; N, nucleoprotein; NS, component of the viral polymerase; M, matrix protein; G, peplomer glycoprotein; L, RNA-dependent RNA polymerase (transcriptase).

(also called P or M1), a component of the viral polymerase; and M (202 amino acids) (or M2 for rabies virus), a protein that facilitates virion budding by binding to the nucleocapsid and to the cytoplasmic domain of the glycoprotein. Three proteins (N, NS, and L), in association with viral RNA, constitute the nucleocapsid. The glycoprotein contains neutralizing epitopes, which are targets of vaccine-induced immunity; it and the nucleoprotein have epitopes involved in cell-mediated immunity. Virions also contain lipids, their composition reflecting the composition of host cell membranes, and carbohydrates as side chains on the glycoprotein. Rhabdovirus infectivity is rather stable in the environment, especially when the pH is alkaline—vesicular stomatitis viruses can contaminate water troughs for many days—but the viruses are thermolabile and sensitive to the UV irradiation of sunlight. In clinical practice, rabies and vesicular stomatitis viruses are inactivated easily by detergent-based disinfectants.

Viral Replication

Viral entry into its host cell occurs via fusion of the viral envelope with the cell membrane; all replication steps occur in the cytoplasm. Replication first involves mRNA transcription from the genomic RNA via the virion polymerase; later, using the protein products of this transcription, there is production of full-length, positive-stranded templates, which in turn are used for the synthesis of genomic RNA. Using virion RNA as a template, the viral transcriptase transcribes five subgenomic mRNA species (Figure 27.2). There is only a single promoter site, located at the 3′ end of the viral genome; the polymerase attaches to the genomic RNA template at this site and as it moves along the viral RNA, it encounters stop/start signals at the boundaries of each of the viral genes. Only a proportion of polymerase molecules move past each junction and continue the transcription process. This mechanism, called attenuated transcription (or stop-start transcription, or stuttering transcription) results in more mRNA being made from genes that are located at the 3′ end of the genome and a gradient of less and less mRNA from downstream genes: N>P>M>G>L. This allows large amounts of the structural proteins such as the N (nucleocapsid) protein to be produced relative to the amount of the L (RNA polymerase) protein.

Attachment of nucleoprotein molecules to newly formed genomic RNA molecules leads to the self-assembly of helically wound nucleocapsids. Through the action of M protein, nucleocapsids are in turn bound to cell membranes at sites where viral peplomers are inserted. Virions are formed by the budding of nucleocapsids through cell membranes. Rabies virus budding takes place mostly on intracytoplasmic membranes of infected neurons, but almost exclusively on plasma membranes of salivary gland epithelial cells. Vesicular stomatitis viruses bud from basal plasma membranes. Vesicular stomatitis viruses usually cause rapid cytopathology—perhaps the most rapid of any viruses, but the replication of rabies and bovine ephemeral fever viruses is slower and usually noncytopathic because these viruses do not shut down host cell protein and nucleic acid synthesis. Rabies virus produces prominent cytoplasmic inclusion bodies (Negri bodies) in infected cells.

Laboratory-adapted ("fixed") rabies virus and vesicular stomatitis viruses replicate well in many kinds of cell cultures: Vero (African green monkey kidney) cells and BHK-21 (baby hamster kidney) cells, which are the most common substrate for animal rabies vaccines. Rabies and vesicular stomatitis viruses, as well as adapted bovine ephemeral fever virus, replicate to high titer in suckling mouse and suckling hamster brain.

During rhabdovirus replication, defective interfering (DI) virus particles are commonly formed. These are complex deletion mutants, having greatly truncated genomic RNA, which interfere with normal viral replication processes (see Chapter 4) (Table 27.2).

Rabies

Rabies virus can infect all warm-blooded animals, and in nearly all instances the infection ends in death. The disease occurs throughout the world, with certain

Table 27.2
Properties of Rhabdoviruses

Virions are enveloped, bullet shaped, 70 nm in diameter and 170 nm long (although some are longer, some shorter), and consist of an envelope with large peplomers within which is a helically coiled cylindrical nucleocapsid
The genome is a single molecule of linear, negative-sense, single-stranded RNA, 11 to 15 kb in size
Cytoplasmic replication
Viral RNA-dependent RNA polymerase (transcriptase) transcribes five subgenomic mRNAs, which are translated into five proteins: L, the RNA-dependent RNA polymerase (transcriptase); G, the glycoprotein that forms the peplomers; N, the nucleoprotein, the major component of the viral nucleocapsid; NS, a component of the viral polymerase; and M, the protein that facilitates virion budding
Maturation is by budding through the plasma membrane
Some viruses, such as vesicular stomatitis viruses, cause rapid cytopathology, whereas others, such as street rabies virus strains, are noncytopathogenic

exceptions: (1) there is no rabies in Japan, the United Kingdom, New Zealand, Antarctica, and many smaller islands such as Hawaii and most of the islands of the Caribbean basin; (2) there had been no rabies in Australia until recently when a lyssavirus, called Australian bat lyssavirus, was discovered; and (3) there is no rabies in Switzerland and large areas of France and southern Germany as a result of recent wildlife vaccination programs. The number of human deaths caused each year by rabies is estimated to be 40,000–50,000 worldwide. An estimated 10 million people receive postexposure treatments each year after being exposed to rabies-suspect animals. Dog rabies is still most important in many parts of the world and the cause of most human rabies cases. Cattle rabies is important in Central and South America. In many countries, wildlife rabies has become of increasing importance as a threat to domestic animals and humans.

Clinical Features

The clinical features of rabies are similar in most species, but there is great variation between individuals. Following the bite of a rabid animal the incubation period is usually between 14 and 90 days, but may be considerably longer. Human cases have been observed in which the last opportunity for exposure occurred from 2 to 7 years before the onset of clinical disease. In each of these human cases the virus was shown to be a dog genotype from a developing country. Such data are not generally available for domestic animals, but an incubation period of 2 years has been reported in a cat.

There is a prodromal phase prior to overt clinical disease that often is overlooked in animals or is recalled only in retrospect as a change in temperament. Two clinical forms of the disease are recognized: furious and dumb or paralytic. In the furious form, the animal becomes restless, nervous, aggressive, and often dangerous as it loses all fear of humans and bites at anything that gains its attention. The animal often cannot swallow water, giving rise to the old name for the disease, "hydrophobia." There is often excessive salivation, exaggerated responses to light and sound, and hyperesthesia (animals commonly bite and scratch themselves). As the encephalitis progresses, fury gives way to paralysis, and the animal presents the same clinical picture as seen in the dumb form of the disease. Terminally, there are often convulsive seizures, coma, and respiratory arrest, with death occurring 2 to 14 days after the onset of clinical signs. A higher proportion of dogs, cats, and horses exhibit fury than is the case for cattle or other ruminants or laboratory animal species.

Pathogenesis, Pathology, and Immunity

The proportion of animals that develop rabies after exposure depends on the location and severity of the bite and the species of animals involved (foxes can carry up to 10^6 infectious units of virus per milliliter of saliva). The bite of a rabid animal usually delivers virus deep into striated muscles and connective tissue, but infection can also occur, albeit with less certainty, after superficial abrasion of the skin. From its entry site, virus must gain entry into peripheral nerves; recent evidence indicates that this may happen directly, but in many instances virus is amplified by first replicating in muscle cells. It invades the peripheral nervous system through sensory or motor nerve endings. The virus binds specifically to the receptor for the neurotransmitter acetylcholine at neuromuscular junctions, facilitating its entry into nerve endings. The virus also employs other receptors (gangliosides, phospholipids). Neuronal infection and centripetal passive movement of the viral genome within axons deliver virus to the central nervous system, usually via the spinal cord. An ascending wave of neuronal infection and neuronal dysfunction then occurs. Virus reaches the limbic system of the brain, where it replicates extensively, and causes the release of cortical control of behavior—this leads to the fury seen clinically. Spread within the central nervous system continues, and when replication occurs in the neocortex, the clinical picture changes to the dumb or paralytic form of the disease. Depression, coma, and death from respiratory arrest follow.

In animal species that serve as reservoir hosts of rabies virus, late in infection viral genome moves centrifugally from the central nervous system through peripheral nerves to a variety of organs: the adrenal cortex, pancreas, and, most importantly, the salivary glands. In the nervous system most virus is formed by budding on intracytoplasmic membranes; however, in the salivary glands, virions bud on plasma membranes at the apical (lumenal) surface of mucous cells and are released in high concentrations into the saliva. Thus, at the time when viral replication within the central nervous system causes the infected animal to become furious and bite indiscriminately, the saliva is highly infectious.

On histopathologic examination there is only modest evidence of a level of neuronal damage that would correspond to the lethality of the infection. Electron microscopy, immunofluorescence, or immunohistochemistry prove that many neurons are infected, but there is no frank cytopathology and little inflammatory cell infiltration—this has always been considered a great paradox—minimal target damage but lethal neurologic dysfunction.

Although rabies proteins are highly immunogenic, neither humoral nor cell-mediated responses can be detected during the stage of movement of virus from the site of the bite to the central nervous system, probably because very little antigen is delivered to the immune system—most is sequestered in muscle cells or within nerve axons. However, this early stage of infection is accessible to antibody, hence the efficacy in exposed humans of the classical Pasteurian postexposure vaccination, especially when combined with the administration of hyperimmune globulin. Immunologic intervention is effective for some time during the long incubation period because of the delay between the initial viral replication in muscle cells and the entry of virus into the protected environment of the nervous system.

Laboratory Diagnosis

In most countries, laboratory diagnosis of rabies is done only in approved laboratories by qualified, experienced personnel. The most common request is to determine whether an animal known to have bitten a human is rabid. If rabies is suspected, the suspect animal must be killed and brain tissue collected for testing. Postmortem diagnosis involves direct immunofluorescence to demonstrate rabies antigen in touch impressions of brain tissue (medulla, cerebellum, and hippocampus). In some laboratories, under some circumstances, postmortem diagnosis can also be performed using the reverse transcription–polymerase chain reaction (RT-PCR) to test for the presence of viral RNA in the brain of the suspect animal; this is done with primers that amplify both genomic RNA and viral mRNA sequences. The method is 100- to 1000-fold more sensitive than standard methods and is a great benefit when specimens are unsuitable for other testing (e.g., when the suspect animal has been buried for some time). Using immunofluorescence or RT-PCR assays, antemortem diagnosis is only done in suspected human rabies cases. For this, skin biopsy, corneal impression, or saliva specimens are used. Only positive results are of diagnostic value, as the choice of specimens for these procedures is never optimum and sites of infection may be missed.

Epidemiology, Prevention, and Control

In usual circumstances the only risk of rabies virus transmission is by the bite or scratch of a rabid animal, although in bat caves, where the amount of virus may be very high and the extremely high humidity may stabilize the virus, transmission may occur via aerosol.

The control of rabies in different regions of the world poses very different problems, depending on which reservoir hosts are present and the level of infection in such hosts.

Rabies-Free Countries

Rigidly enforced quarantine of dogs and cats for various periods before entry has been used effectively to exclude rabies from Japan, the United Kingdom, Australia, New Zealand, Hawaii, and several other islands. Rabies had never become endemic in wildlife in the United Kingdom and was eradicated from dogs in that country in 1902 and again in 1922 after its reestablishment in the dog population in 1918. Since then, there had been no rabies in the United Kingdom until recently when a single bat was found infected with European bat virus 1—this isolated incident has not changed the rabies-free status of that country. In contrast, rabies had not been recognized in Australia until recently when a lyssavirus, called Australian bat lyssavirus, was discovered. The virus has been found to be endemic in several areas and there have been two human deaths. In this case, the maintenance of strict quarantine for imported dogs and cats is still key to preventing the virus from becoming endemic in terrestrial wild and domestic animals.

Developing Countries

In most countries of Asia, Latin America, and Africa, endemic dog rabies is a serious problem, marked by significant domestic animal and human mortality. In these countries, very large numbers of doses of human vaccines are used and there is a continuing need for comprehensive, professionally organized and publicly supported rabies control agencies. That such agencies are not in place in many developing countries is a reflection of their high cost; nevertheless, progress is being made. For example, a substantial decrease in rabies incidence has been reported in recent years in China, Thailand, and Sri Lanka following the implementation of programs for the vaccination of dogs and improved post-exposure prophylaxis of humans. Similarly, the number of rabies cases in Latin America is declining significantly; the Pan American Health Organization has implemented a vaccination program to eliminate urban dog rabies from the hemisphere by the year 2000.

Developed Countries

In most developed countries, even those with modest disease burden, publicly supported rabies control agencies operate in the following areas: (1) stray dog and cat removal and control of the movement of pets (quarantine is used in epidemic circumstances, but rarely); (2) immunization of dogs and cats so as to break the chain of virus transmission; (3) laboratory diagnosis to confirm clinical observations and obtain accurate incidence data;

(4) surveillance to measure the effectiveness of all control measures; and (5) public education programs to assure cooperation.

European Countries

Historically, in developed countries, rabies control in wildlife was based on animal population reduction by trapping and poisoning, but in recent years the immunization of wild animal reservoir host species, especially foxes, by the aerial distribution of baits containing attenuated virus vaccine has become the method of choice. Since 1990, fox rabies, the only endemic rabies in much of Europe, has been eliminated from Switzerland and large areas of France and southern Germany and is being dealt with rapidly in Belgium and other western European countries (Figure 27.3). Extending this approach to eastern European countries poses a much more difficult problem.

North American Countries

In North America, there are six rabies virus genotypes in terrestrial animals (and many more in various species of bats): (1) a skunk genotype in north-central states of the United States and south-central Canada; (2) a second skunk genotype in south-central states and California; (3) an arctic fox and red fox genotype in Alaska and Canada; (4) a gray fox genotype in Arizona and western Texas; (5) a dog/coyote genotype in southern Texas and northern Mexico; and (6) a raccoon genotype in eastern states extending to the Canadian border. These genotypes reflect the evolutionary consequence of host preference: "raccoons-bite-raccoons-bite-raccoons," and after an unknown number of passages the virus becomes a distinct genotype, still able to kill other species but transmitted most efficiently within its own reservoir host population (Figure 27.4).

In recent years, there has been a significant increase in the numbers of animal rabies cases reported in the

Figure 27.3.

A

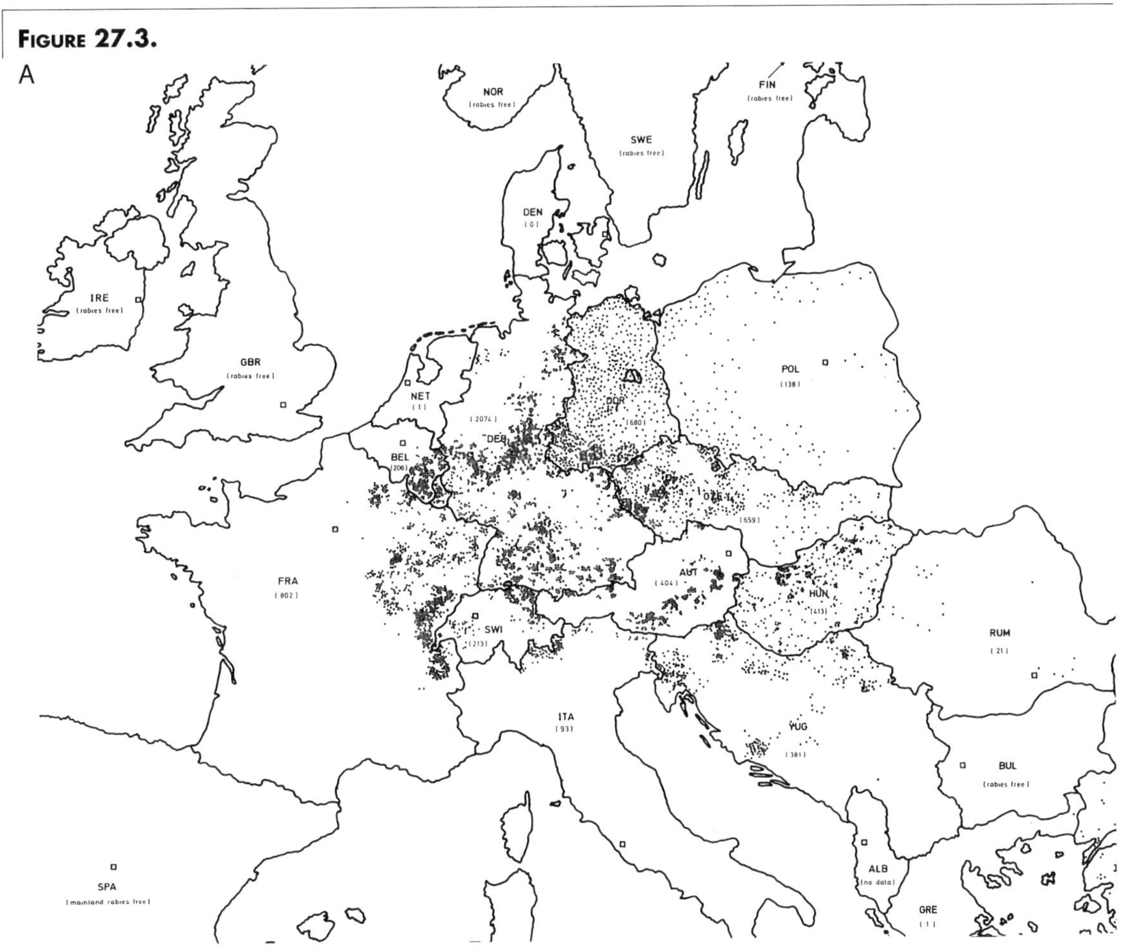

Occurrence of fox rabies in Europe during the (A) last quarter of 1983 (6606 cases reported to WHO).

Figure 27.3. (continued)

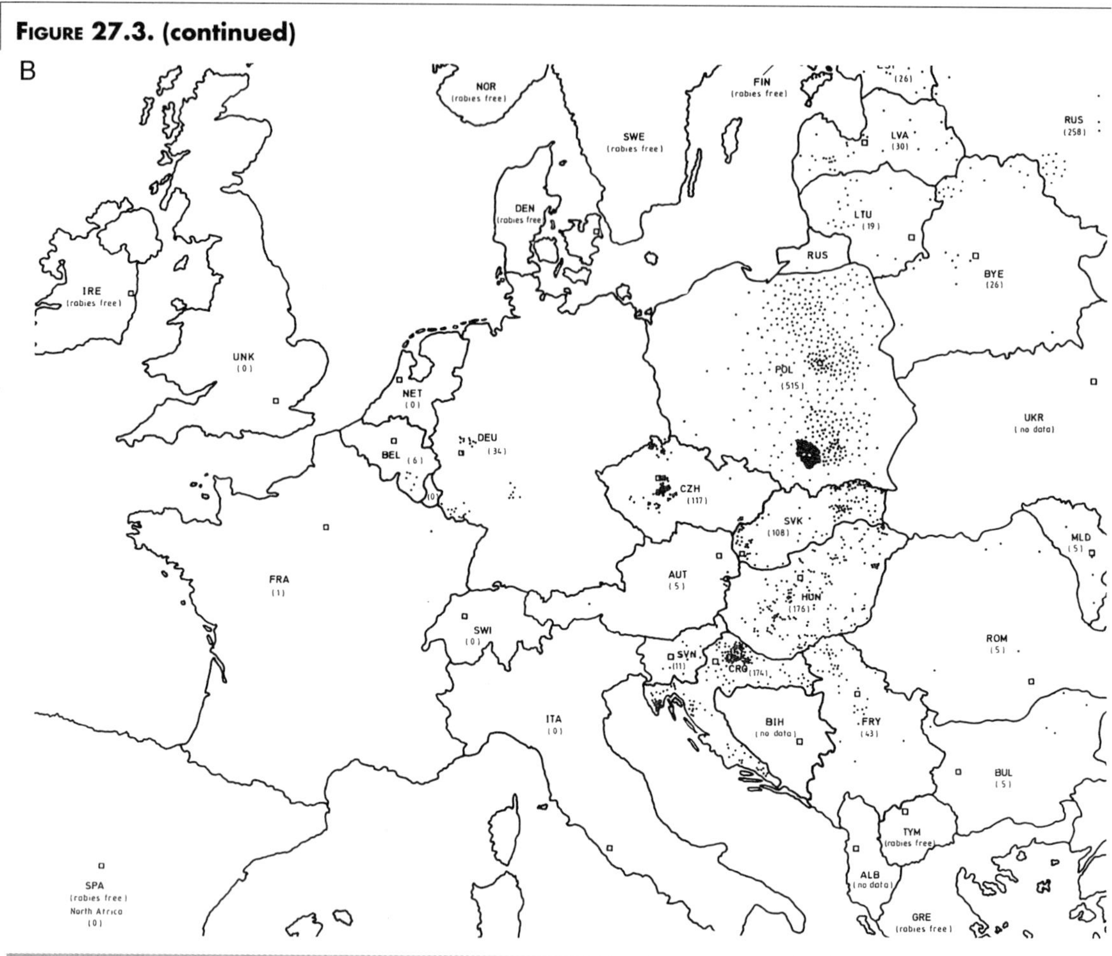

(B) Fox rabies during the first quarter of 1997 (1583 cases reported). During this interval, endemic rabies was eliminated from Switzerland, France, and most of Germany by compaigns to vaccinate foxes. A few imported cases continue to occur in these countries from foci in eastern Europe. (Courtesy of W. W. Müller, World Health Organization Collaborating Centre for Rabies Surveillance and Research, Tübingen, Federal Republic of Germany.)

United States (Figure 27.5), mostly because of the epidemic of raccoon rabies, but also because of increases in coyote rabies in southern Texas and arctic fox rabies in Alaska. Rabies in arctic foxes is an endemic, refractory problem extending across most areas of the northern polar regions of the world; it periodically extends into regions of Canada and the United States inhabited by the red fox, resulting in wavefront epidemics. Skunk rabies in central North America, from Texas to Saskatchewan, is the principal cause of rabies in cattle. The epidemic of raccoon rabies in eastern United States has been traced to the translocation of raccoons from an old rabies endemic area in Florida to West Virginia in 1977. Its continuing spread, by 1997 as far as the Canadian border and across the Appalachian mountains into Ohio, is the cause of massive prevention and control efforts (Figure 27.6).

Fox rabies had been a problem in eastern United States and Canada, but since the mid-1990s, especially in Ontario, aerial distribution of vaccine-containing baits has largely eliminated the problem. The great merit of this approach over animal population reduction is that the econiche remains occupied, in this case by an immune population, and is not subject to the sort of reproductive "population boom" that the fox is capable of when faced with an empty niche. The same approach has also been very successful in intercepting the northern movement toward large population centers of the coyote rabies epidemic in southern Texas. Attenuated virus rabies vaccine is quite immunogenic in foxes and coyotes when administered *per os* in baits, but not so in raccoons or skunks. Further, the habits of the latter two species requires use of much higher baiting densities, thereby greatly increasing the cost of control programs. Never-

Figure 27.4.

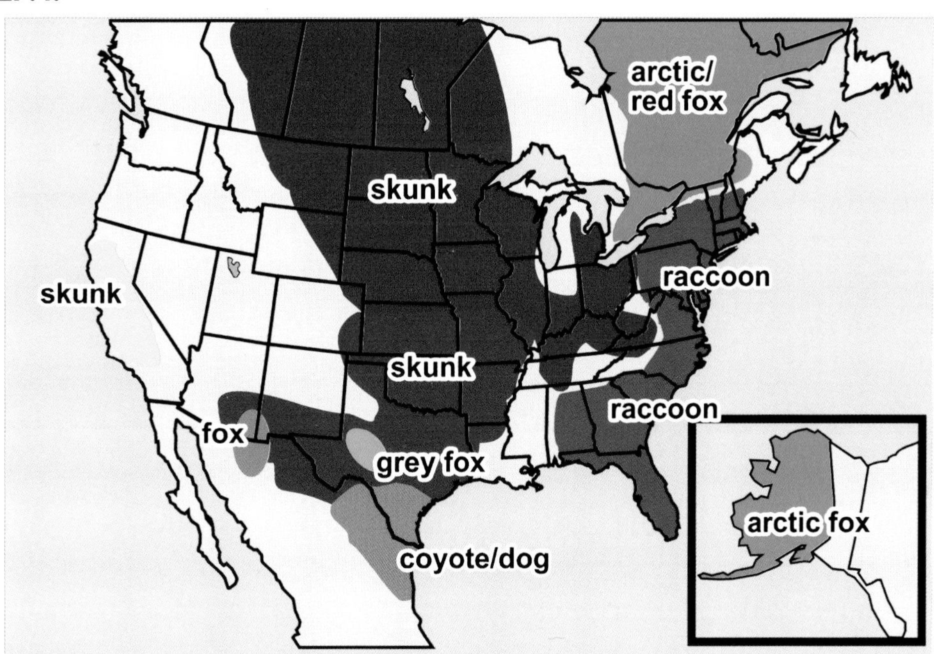

Distribution of genotypic/antigenic variants of rabies in the United States and Canada. There are two different skunk genotypes; the one in California is the same as that in south-central United States. The newest foci involve a coyote/dog genotype in Texas and northern Mexico and a raccoon genotype in eastern United States. (Courtesy of J. S. Smith and C. Rupprecht.)

FIGURE 27.5.

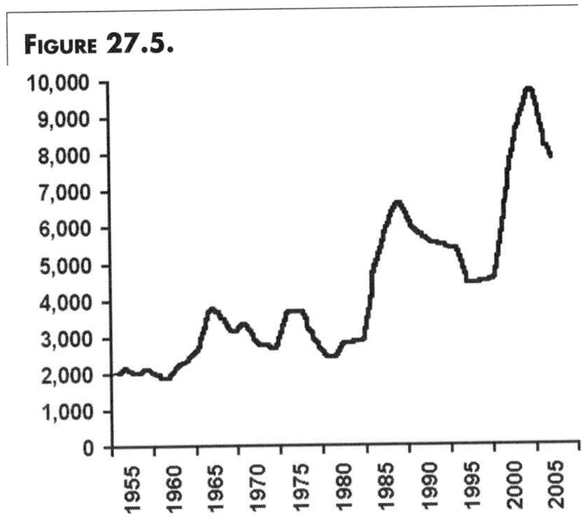

Actual and projected increasing incidence of rabies in animals in the United States, cumulatively due to epidemics in raccoons in the east, coyotes in Texas and endemic increases in cases in skunks in the Midwest, and arctic and red foxes in Alaska. (Data from the Centers for Disease Control and Prevention.)

FIGURE 27.6.

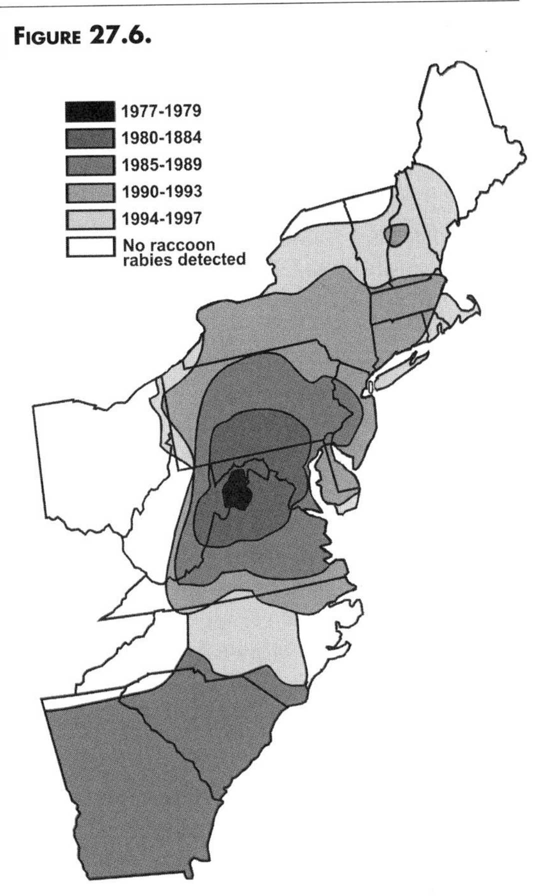

The raccoon rabies epidemic in the United States from its beginning in 1977, caused by translocation of animals from Florida to West Virginia, to its extension to the Canadian border and into Ohio in 1997. (Data from the Centers for Disease Control and Prevention.)

theless, raccoon vaccination programs are now in progress in New York, New Jersey, Massachusetts, and Florida, employing novel vaccinia or canarypox-rabies glycoprotein recombinant virus vaccines that have been proven in the laboratory to be effective.

Special Case of Bat Rabies

In the United States and Canada, bat rabies represents a unique problem: (1) a total of 700–800 cases are reported annually in all species of bats; (2) more than 40 species of insectivorous bats are involved; and (3) distribution is wide, indeed, being documented in all 48 contiguous states of the United States and most provinces of Canada. Bat rabies occurs in areas where there is no other rabies transmission. Moreover, bats have been the source of most human rabies cases in recent years, and in many of these cases there has been no history of a bite. Of 38 human rabies deaths in the United States between 1976 and 1995, an animal bite was reported in only 13—of the other 27 more than half were attributed (by viral genomc sequence analysis) to various bat genotypes. Further, an inordinate number of the most recent cases have been attributed to a genotype carried by the silver-haired bat (*Lasionycteris noctivagans*), a species that is uncommon and submitted infrequently for rabies diagnosis. It has been suggested that this viral genotype might have enhanced invasiveness, causing infection even after the most trivial, unrecognized bite (bat incisors may leave a wound as invisible as a 30-gauge needle puncture).

In the past 20 years, more than 500 cases of bat rabies have been reported in Europe, mostly in Denmark, Germany, The Netherlands, and Russia, mostly involving serotine bats (especially *Eptesicus serotinus*) and causing at least three human deaths. A single isolate of European bat virus 1 has been reported from the United Kingdom in 1996, while 1800 other bats tested were negative.

In several countries of Latin America, vampire bat rabies is a problem for livestock industries (and humans). There are three species of vampire bats, the most important being *Desmodus rotundus*. Here, control efforts have depended on the use of bovine vaccines and on the use of anticoagulants such as diphenadione and warfarin. These anticoagulants are either fed to cattle as slow-release boluses (cattle are very insensitive to their anticoagulant effect) or mixed with grease and spread on the backs of cattle. When vampire bats feed on the blood of treated cattle or preen themselves and each other to remove the grease they suffer fatal hemorrhages in their wing capillaries.

In 1996, a new virus was discovered in a black flying fox (fruit bat, *Pteropus alecto*) in Queensland, Australia. The virus, called Australian bat lyssavirus, now appears to extend along the entire east coast of Australia and has been found in three of the four species of flying foxes (gray-headed flying fox, *Pteropus poliocephalus;* little red flying fox, *Pteropus scapulatus*). The virus has also been found in an insectivorous bat, the yellow-bellied sheath-tailed bat (*Saccolaimus flaviventrus*). The virus is a lyssavirus, closely related to rabies virus, exhibiting only an 8% sequence difference in its N gene. There have been two human infections which were fatal, both in people who had been exposed to a number of bats.

Vaccines and Their Use

Animal rabies vaccines (either inactivated virus vaccines or attenuated virus vaccines) are efficacious and safe. Many different formulations are available. A compendium, updating the indications and contraindications for the use of each of these vaccine, is published annually in the United States by the National Association of State Public Health Veterinarians (see Further Reading).

Human Disease

Public health veterinarians are called on regularly to provide advice on rabies postexposure prophylaxis, preexposure vaccination, and other matters pertaining to the risk of rabies in humans. Further, practicing veterinarians represent a major risk group for rabies infection in many areas of the world. Therefore, this section is more extensive than might otherwise be expected in a book on veterinary and zoonotic virology.

The first step in dealing with a possible human rabies exposure is thorough cleansing of the wound—immediate vigorous washing and flushing with soap and water is crucial. The next step is an appraisal of the nature of the exposure (Table 27.3). In a rabies endemic area, if the individual has simply touched the suspect animal treatment is not recommended. If the individual has been scratched or bitten or if there are skin abrasions present, treatment is started. Where possible exposure involves a dog or cat, treatment may be stopped if the animal remains healthy throughout a 10-day observation period or if the animal is euthanized and found to be negative by appropriate laboratory testing. Where possible exposure involves any other domestic or wild animal, the animal is euthanized immediately and its brain examined using appropriate laboratory techniques. In the United States, because of recent experiences, more conservative recommendations have been made when exposure involves bats—bat exposures are treated as if the bat is rabid (until proved negative by laboratory tests) and extra consideration is given to the possibility that exposure may have occurred even when a bite wound is not evident. In areas where there is little or no rabies, the decision to treat or not is adjusted accordingly, but again extra consideration is given to bat exposures, given the fact that bat rabies may occur in the absence of rabies in terrestrial species and the fact that rabies surveillance in bats is not commonly done. Exposure to rodents, rabbits, and hares seldom, if ever, requires specific antirabies treatment.

Postexposure prophylaxis consists of hyperimmune globulin and a course of vaccine. In the United States, human rabies immune globulin (HRIG) is used at 20 IU/kg of body weight, half infiltrated around the wound, half injected intramuscularly. In the United States there are two licensed human rabies vaccines: human diploid cell-culture vaccine (HDCV) and rhesus kidney cell-culture adjuvanted vaccine (RVA)—these vaccines are used in many other developed countries as well. The vaccination regimen consists of five 1.0-ml doses given intramuscularly in the deltoid area, one each on days 0, 3, 7, 14, and 28. If the exposed person has been vaccinated previously, no human rabies immune globulin is used and only two doses of vaccine are given, one each on days 0 and 3. Slightly different regimens are recommended in different countries. Remarkably, these regimens have reduced the mortality from this frightening disease virtually to zero. A comprehensive guide on human postexposure treatment is provided by the World Health Organization (see Further Reading).

Preexposure vaccination of veterinarians and other individuals occupationally or otherwise at risk (e.g., laboratory personnel working with rabies virus, animal control and wildlife workers in rabies-endemic areas, and certain international travelers) has become a standard of practice in developed countries. Because of several variables in the level and nature of risk and the likelihood of immediate availability of postexposure prophylaxis, an algorithm is used to guide recommendations for primary vaccination and boosters (Table 27.4). The vaccination regimen consists of three 1.0-ml doses given intramuscularly in the deltoid area, one each on days 0, 7, and 28. Because of the high cost of human vaccines, there is an alternate regimen consisting of four 0.1-ml doses given intradermally, one each on days 0, 7, 21, and 28. Boosters (or serologic confirmation of adequate antibody level) are given depending on the individual's continuing risk category.

Biohazard: Laboratory and clinically associated rabies infections are extremely rare. Nevertheless, infected animals, their tissues, and their excretions contain

TABLE 27.3
Rabies: Guide for Human Postexposure Prophylaxis

ANIMAL SPECIES	EVALUTION AND DISPOSITION OF ANIMAL	RECOMMENDATIONS FOR TREATMENT OF EXPOSED PERSON[a]
Dog, cat	Healthy and available for 10 days of observation	None, unless animal develops signs of rabies[b]
	Rabid or suspected rabid	Immediate rabies immune globulin[c] and vaccine[d]
	Unknown (escaped)	Consult public health official. If treatment is indicated, give rabies immune globulin and vaccine
Bat	Regard as rabid and consider that exposure may have occurred even if a bite wound is not evident, unless proved negative by laboratory tests[e]	Rabies immune globulin[c] and vaccine[d]
Skunk, fox, coyote, raccoon, bobcat, woodchuck, other carnivores	Regard as rabid unless proved negative by laboratory tests[e] or from geographic area known to be rabies free	Rabies immune globulin[c] and vaccine[d]
Livestock, rodents, rabbits, hares	Consider individually. Public health officials should be consulted about the need for rabies prophylaxis. Bites of squirrels, hamsters, guinea pigs, gerbils, chipmunks, rats, mice, other rodents, rabbits, and hares almost never call for antirabies prophylaxis	

[a]These recommendations derive from those used in the United States; there are some differences in other countries. In applying these recommendations, take into account the animal species involved, the circumstances of the bite or other exposure, the vaccination status of the animal, and presence of rabies in the region. Public health officials should be consulted if questions arise about the need for rabies prophylaxis. All bites and wounds should immediately be thoroughly cleansed with soap and water. If antirabies treatment is indicated, both rabies immune globulin and vaccine should be given as soon as possible, regardless of the interval from exposure.
[b]If during the 10-day observation period a dog or cat exhibits clinical signs of rabies, it should be killed and tested immediately, and treatment of the exposed individual with human rabies immune globulin (HRIG) and vaccine should be started.
[c]If rabies immune globulin is not available, use antirabies serum, equine. Do not use more than the recommended dosage. Anticipate a possible need to treat for serum sickness.
[d]Five 1.0-ml intramuscular doses to be given on days 0, 3, 7, 14, and 28. WHO recommends an optimal sixth dose at 90 days. Local reactions to vaccines are common and do not contraindicate continuing treatment. Discontinue vaccine if fluorescent antibody tests of the animal are negative.
[e]The animal should be killed and tested as soon as possible; holding for observation is not recommended.

virus and should be handled only with gloves. Decontamination of pens, stalls, and cages should be done with standard disinfectants and suspect carcasses should be incinerated or buried after diagnostic specimens have been obtained.

Vesicular Stomatitis

Originally, vesicular stomatitis was considered of interest only because of its role in the differential diagnosis of foot-and-mouth disease in cattle and the debilitating lameness it can cause in horses. More recently, however, the disease has been recognized as the cause of economically important losses in conditioning and milk production in cattle, especially as more dairying is undertaken in warmer climates.

Clinical Features

The clinical features of vesicular stomatitis infection vary greatly among animals in a herd. Lesions develop quickly after an incubation period of 1 to 5 days. Excess salivation and fever often are the first signs of infection in cattle and horses, and lameness is often the first sign in swine. Vesicular lesions on the tongue, the oral mucosa, teats, and coronary bands of cattle may progress to total epithelial denudation with secondary bacterial infection. Lesions may cause profuse salivation and anorexia, lameness, and rejection of the suckling calf. In horses, tongue lesions are most pronounced, often progressing to complete sloughing of the epithelium. In swine, vesicular lesions are most common on the snout and coronary bands. Lesions usually heal within 7 to 10 days and there are no sequelae.

Table 27.4
Rabies: Guide for Human Preexposure Prophylaxis

Risk category	Nature of risk	Typical populations at risk	Preexposure vaccination
Continuous	Virus present continuously, often in high concentrations. Aerosol, mucous membrane, bite, or nonbite exposure. Specific exposures may go unrecognized	Rabies research laboratory workers;[a] rabies biologics production workers	Primary course. Serologic testing every 6 months; booster vaccination when antibody level falls below acceptable level[b]
Frequent	Exposure usually episodic, with source recognized, but exposure may also be unrecognized. Aerosol, mucous membrane, bite, or nonbite exposure	Veterinarians and staff, animal-control and wildlife workers, rabies diagnostic laboratory workers, spelunkers in rabies endemic areas. Certain travelers visiting areas of endemic rabies	Primary course. Serologic testing or booster vaccination every 2 years
Infrequent (but greater than the population at large)	Exposure nearly always episodic with source recognized. Mucous membrane, bite, or nonbite exposure	Veterinarians and staff, animal-control and wildlife workers in areas of low rabies endemicity. Veterinary students	Primary course. No serologic testing or booster vaccination
Rare (population at large)	Exposure always episodic. Mucous membrane, bite, or nonbite exposure	Developed countries, populations at large, including persons in rabies epidemic areas	No vaccination necessary

[a]In laboratories, judgment of relative risk and extra monitoring of vaccination status is a responsibility of the laboratory supervisor.
[b]Standards for minimum acceptable antibody level vary with the test used—in the United States, complete virus neutralization at a 1 : 5 serum dilution by the official rabies immunofluorescent focus-inhibition test (RIFFIT) assay is considered adequate—a booster dose of vaccine should be administered if the titer falls below this level.

Pathogenesis, Pathology, and Immunity

The virus probably enters the body through breaks in the mucosa and skin, due to the minor abrasions caused, for example, by rough forage or by the bites of arthropods. There does not seem to be a systemic, viremic phase of infection except in swine and small laboratory animals. Local vesiculation and epithelial denudation follow epithelial cell destruction and interstitial edema, which separates the epithelium from underlying tissues. Spread of such lesions occurs by extension, such that it is common for the entire epithelium of the tongue or teat to be sloughed. High titers of infectious virus are present, usually for a short time, in vesicular fluids and in tissues at the margins of lesions. From this source, virus may be transmitted by fomites, such as contaminated food, milking machines, and restraint devices. The virus may also be transmitted mechanically by arthropods. Despite the extent of epithelial damage, healing is usually rapid and complete. Cattle with high levels of neutralizing antibodies are often susceptible to reinfection, suggesting that such antibodies have a limited protective effect. This may be explained by the majority of viral replication being localized in the epithelium. There is little heterologous immunity (e.g., between vesicular stomatitis–New Jersey and vesicular stomatitis–Indiana viruses).

Laboratory Diagnosis

Virus can be recovered from vesicular fluids and tissue scrapings by standard virus isolation techniques in cell culture (or in embryonated eggs or in suckling mice by intracerebral inoculation). Virus isolates are usually identified by conventional serologic methods. Because diagnosis involves differentiation from foot-and-mouth disease, these procedures should be carried out in an authorized reference laboratory.

Epidemiology, Prevention, and Control

Epidemics of vesicular stomatitis occur in the United States, Canada, Mexico, regions of the Caribbean, Central America, Panama, Venezuela, Colombia, Ecuador, Peru, Brazil, and Argentina. Epidemics occur annually or at intervals of 2 or 3 years in tropical and subtropical countries and at intervals of 5 to 10 years in temperate zones. Vesicular stomatitis–New Jersey virus is the most common and has the widest distribution, with isolations as far north as Canada and as far south as Peru. Vesicular stomatitis–Indiana virus has a similar wide geographical distribution but is encountered less frequently.

Genomic analysis of large numbers of vesicular stomatitis–New Jersey and vesicular stomatitis–Indiana isolates has indicated that temperate zone epidemics are caused by a single viral genotype, suggesting spread from a common origin. For example, vesicular stomatitis–Indiana isolates from the United States and Mexico always derive from a recent common ancestor. Epidemic isolates from different geographic areas, such as the temperate zones of North and South America, have been shown to be distinct, indicating spatial genetic isolation. Isolates from different endemic foci in the tropics are also distinct, but they reflect a more complex genetic diversity, including multiple phylogenetic lineages. For example, multiple genotypes of vesicular stomatitis–Indiana virus coexist in Costa Rica, Panama, and adjacent countries of South America. Within even small endemic foci these variants may be maintained over an extended period of time. Endemic foci of vesicular stomatitis–Indiana and–New Jersey occur in southeastern Mexico, Venezuela, Colombia, Panama, and Costa Rica, mostly in wet lowland areas. In the United States, a band of endemic vesicular stomatitis–New Jersey formerly existed across the coastal plains of South Carolina, Georgia, and Florida; currently, only one focus remains, on Ossabaw Island, Georgia.

Even though the geographic range of the vesicular stomatitis viruses is large, disease problems are restricted to favorable habitats: for example, in the upper Mississippi valley in the United States, disease appears regularly in aspen park lands, the narrow zone separating hardwood forest from open prairies. In the western mountainous regions of the United States, disease seems to move up and down valleys, not along roads, rarely reaching higher pastures. Seasonally, outbreaks begin in the late spring, peak in the late summer, and cease with the first frosts of late fall/early winter. The disease may appear almost simultaneously over large areas or in multiple spreading foci, suggesting that the virus might be arthropod-borne. In more tropical regions, outbreaks appear frequently at the cessation of rainy seasons.

Vesicular stomatitis viruses can be stable in the environment for days, e.g., on milking machine parts where transmission results in teat and udder lesions, in water troughs, in soil, and on vegetation where transmission results in mouth lesions.

Several lines of evidence suggest that vesicular stomatitis viruses are arthropod-borne in nature. In tropical and subtropical areas, there is evidence for transmission by sandflies (*Lutzomyia* spp.), with transovarial transmission in sandflies contributing to the perpetuation of the viruses in endemic foci—transovarial transmission is considered evidence of a long-standing evolutionary relationship. Sandflies have also been incriminated in maintaining the endemic focus of vesicular stomatitis–New Jersey on Ossabaw Island, Georgia. Isolates have also been made from *Simulidae* (black flies), *Culicoides* (midges), *Culex nigripalpus* (mosquitoes), *Hippilates* spp. (eye gnats), *Musca domestica* (houseflies), and *Gigantolaelap* spp. (mites). There has also been seroconversion of caged sentinel animals placed in endemic areas. In a large epidemic of vesicular stomatitis–New Jersey that occurred in the western United States in 1982, many virus isolates were made from flies, mostly from the common house fly, *M. domestica,* but it is not clear how flies might fulfill known patterns of virus transmission between herds and between individual animals. The manner by which vesicular stomatitis viruses are transmitted over long distances also remains controversial despite years of study. Arthropod involvement is also suggested here.

Outbreaks of disease may be explosive, so avoidance of pastures known as sites of transmission may help avoid infection, but in general little is usually done even in the face of an epidemic. In temperate zones, epidemics occur at such infrequent intervals that the index of suspicion falls to a low level during interepidemic periods. Both inactivated and attenuated virus vaccines are available, but neither is used much.

Human Disease

Vesicular stomatitis viruses are zoonotic, being transmissible to human (typically, farmers and veterinarians) from vesicular fluids and tissues of infected animals, but there are no practical measures for preventing occupational exposure. The disease in human resembles influenza, presenting with an acute onset of fever, chills, and muscle pain. It resolves without complications within 7 to 10 days. Human cases are not uncommon during epidemics in cattle and horses, but because of lack of awareness, few cases are reported. Human cases can be diagnosed retrospectively by serologic methods.

Bovine Ephemeral Fever

Bovine ephemeral fever, also called 3-day sickness, is a widespread disease of cattle, spanning tropical and subtropical zones of Africa, Australia, and Asia. From these endemic sites the disease extends intermittently into temperate zones in major or minor epidemics. The disease has never been reported in North or South America or in Europe.

Clinical Features

Clinical signs in cattle are characteristic but all are not seen in an individual animal. Onset is sudden; the disease is marked by a biphasic or polyphasic fever with an immediate drop in milk production. Other clinical signs are associated with the second and later febrile phases: these include depression, stiffness, and lameness, and less often nasal and ocular discharges, cessation of rumination, and constipation. Infrequently there is diarrhea and temporary or permanent paresis. Usually, recovery is dramatic and complete in 3 days (range 2 to 5 days). Morbidity rates often approach 100%, and the mortality rate in an outbreak is usually 1 to 2%, but can reach 10 to 20% in mature, well-conditioned beef cattle and high-producing dairy cattle. Subclinical cases do occur, but their relative rate is unknown because antibody testing is confounded by intercurrent infections in the same areas by related but nonpathogenic rhabdoviruses.

Pathogenesis, Pathology, and Immunity

The pathogenesis of the disease is complex; it seems clear that pathophysiologic and immunologic effects on host inflammatory response, mediated by the release of lymphokines, are involved in the expression of disease. There is no evidence that the virus causes widespread tissue destruction. In all cases there is an early neutrophilia with an abnormal level of immature neutrophils in the circulation ("left shift"). There is a rise in plasma fibrinogen and a significant drop in plasma calcium. Therapeutically, there is a dramatic response to nonsteroid anti-inflammatory drugs and often to calcium infusion. Infection results in solid immunity; because outbreaks tend to involve most animals in a herd, repeat clinical episodes usually involve young animals born since previous outbreaks.

Laboratory Diagnosis

Laboratory diagnosis is difficult; the "gold standard" is virus isolation by blind passage in mosquito (*Aedes albopictus*) cells or suckling mouse brain. Detection of a rise in antibody is the most practical diagnostic technique available; this is done by enzyme immunoassay or neutralization assays, which are virus specific, or by immunofluorescence or agar gel precipitin tests, which are cross-reactive with related rhabdoviruses.

Epidemiology, Prevention, and Control

Bovine ephemeral fever virus is transmitted by two types of arthropod vectors, *Culicoides* and culicine and anopheline mosquitoes: endemic and epidemic spread is limited to the distribution of vectors. There is epidemiologic evidence that more arthropod vector species remain to be identified. Prevention by vector control is impractical in the areas of the world where this disease is prevalent. In Japan, South Africa, and Australia, inactivated and attenuated virus vaccines have been used. Problems with conventional vaccines stem from lack of potency—inactivated vaccines require more antigenic mass than it has been possible to achieve economically, and attenuated virus vaccines suffer from a loss in immunogenicity linked with the attenuation process. A recombinant DNA-derived G protein vaccine has also been developed.

Rhabdovirus Diseases of Fish

At least nine distinct rhabdoviruses cause economically important diseases in fish (Table 27.5). These viruses are antigenically distinguishable by neutralization tests. The viruses may be propagated in a variety of piscine cell lines and also in mammalian, avian, and reptilian cells, with the optimal growth temperatures and the temperature range for growth differing from one virus to another.

Viral Hemorrhagic Septicemia

Viral hemorrhagic septicemia, a systemic infection of various salmonid and a few nonsalmonid fishes, is caused by viral hemorrhagic septicemia virus. The infection occurs in fish of any age and may result in significant cumulative mortality. Fish that survive may become carriers. Viral hemorrhagic septicemia has been reported under various names, of which Egtved disease is the best known.

Clinical Features

There are acute, chronic, and latent forms of infection. Acutely infected fish are lethargic, dark in color, exophthalmic, anemic, and there is a high mortality rate. Hemorrhages are evident in the eyes, skin, and gills and at

TABLE 27.5
Rhabdoviruses of Fish

VIRUS	SPECIES AFFECTED	GEOGRAPHIC DISTRIBUTION	GROWTH TEMPERATURE[a] (°C)	
			RANGE	OPTIMUM
Viral hemorrhagic septicemia virus (Egtved virus)	Salmonids, pike, sea bass, turbot, Pacific and Atlantic cod	Europe, west coast of United States	6–20	10–15
Infectious hematopoietic necrosis viruses	Salmonids	Western North America, France, Italy, Japan, China, Taiwan	4–20	13–18
Hirame rhabdovirus	Japanese flounder	Japan	5–20	15–20
Spring viremia of carp virus	Cyprinids	Europe	4–32	Variable[b]
Pike fry rhabdovirus	Northern pike, guppies, cyprinids, pike	Europe, including Russia	10–31	21–28
Eel rhabdovirus	American, European eels, rainbow trout fry[c]	Japan and Europe	15–20	15
Perch rhabdovirus	Perch	Europe	10–20	15
Rio Grande cichlid rhabdovirus	Rio Grande cichlid	United States	23–30	?
Ulcerative syndrome and snakehead rhabdovirus	Snakehead	Southeast Asia	18–35	24–30

[a]Measured in cultured piscine cells.
[b]Depends on cell line.
[c]Experimental infections only.

the bases of the fins. Internally, hemorrhages are evident and the liver appears mottled and hyperemic. Chronically infected fish have a markedly distended abdomen due to edema of the liver, kidneys, and spleen, but there is little hemorrhage.

Pathogenesis, Pathology, and Immunity

The virus is transmissible readily to fish of all ages, and survivors of infection can become lifelong carriers that shed virus in urine and semen and on the surface of eggs. In aquaculture settings, virus transmission occurs by cohabitation or by fomites. The virus has been isolated from wild fish in waters receiving hatchery effluent. Epidemic losses occur at temperatures below 12°C (mortality is greatest at 3 to 5°C); mortality and the proportion of fish that become virus carriers decrease at higher temperatures. Deaths rarely occur at temperatures above 15°C.

Laboratory Diagnosis

Diagnosis is based on virus isolation in any of several regularly used piscine cell lines. The virus may also be grown in mammalian cells such as BHK 21 (baby hamster kidney) and WI 38 (human diploid fibroblasts) maintained at low temperature. Fluorescent antibody, immunodiffusion, and enzyme immunoassays are available. There are at least three virus serotypes distinguishable by neutralization assay.

Epidemiology, Prevention, and Control

Viral hemorrhagic septicemia is endemic in most countries of continental eastern and western Europe, and the virus has been isolated in the Puget Sound area of Washington in the United States. In Europe, epidemics occur primarily in rainbow trout, *Oncorhynchus mykiss*, and brown trout, *Salmo trutta*. In the United States, infection is most common in chinook salmon, *O. tshawytscha*, coho salmon, *O. kisutch*, and steelhead (which is actually a sea-run rainbow trout). Isolation of fish in hatcheries and aquaculture facilities is the most effective method for preventing infection—hatchery disinfection, followed by restocking with specific pathogen-free fish and eggs, has been successful in breaking the transmission chain. There are several experimental vaccines under study, including attenuated virus vaccines.

Infectious Hematopoietic Necrosis

This disease of salmonids is caused by a group of serologically related viruses, each infecting particular species of salmon or trout. The disease causes frequent losses in hatcheries along the Pacific coast of North America from Alaska to northern California, in France and Italy, and in Japan and Taiwan. Epidemics usually involve juvenile fish at water temperatures below 15°C; mortality may reach 50 to 90%. Survivors become lifelong carriers and shed large amounts of virus in urine and feces and in ovarian and seminal fluids at spawning. Fish infected acutely are dark in color, lethargic, and show anemia, exophthalmia, distention of the abdomen, and hemorrhages at the base of fins. Diagnosis is made by virus isolation and serology. Control measures center on isolation of premises and are similar to those for viral hemorrhagic septicemia. Elevation of water temperature to at least 18°C is very effective in controlling the disease, but is usually not feasible economically. Inactivated and attenuated virus vaccines have been developed, but the most promising control measure for the future is selective breeding for resistance.

Spring Viremia of Carp

This disease occurs in European countries when the water temperature rises in spring. Diseased fish excrete large amounts of virus and the virus can be spread by a bloodsucking ectoparasite, *Argils* spp. Infected fish become lethargic, have abdominal swelling indicative of visceral organ edema, and hemorrhages. Control is possible by isolation of premises. A vaccine has been developed, but must be injected.

Other Rhabdovirus Diseases of Fish

Pike fry rhabdovirus causes a disease similar to spring viremia of carp virus in hatchery-reared pike fry in The Netherlands, where it is controlled primarily by isolation and by iodophor treatment of eggs to remove surface virus contamination. Rhabdoviruses with similar serologic properties to the pike fry rhabdovirus have been found in several species of cyprinids, including the grass carp. Five rhabdoviruses have been isolated from eels that are serologically distinct from other known fish rhabdoviruses. None of the eel viruses has been demonstrated to cause disease in the freshwater stages of eel but certain isolates are pathogenic for rainbow trout fry. In Japan, hirame (a flounder-like flatfish) and ayu (a trout-like species) have suffered severe hemorrhagic disease with pathologic characteristics resembling viral hemorrhagic septicemia and infectious hematopoietic necrosis in salmonids. The disease is caused by hirame rhabdovirus, which is isolated readily in piscine cell culture. Perch and Rio Grande cichlid rhabdoviruses have been isolated from fish cell lines and induce clinical diseases similar to those occurring naturally. The perch rhabdovirus appears to be serologically distinct from any other known fish rhabdovirus. Rhabdoviruses belonging to the genus *Vesiculovirus* and others as yet ungrouped have been isolated from snakeheads, an important food fish in Thailand. However, it has yet to be demonstrated whether they have a role in the chronic ulcerative syndrome often suffered by this species.

Further Reading

Baer, G. M., ed. (1991). "The Natural History of Rabies," 2nd Ed., 2 vol. CRC Press, Boca Raton, FL.

Banerjee, A. K., and Barik, S. (1992). Gene expression of vesicular stomatitis virus genome. *Virology* **188**, 417–428.

Bernard, J., and Bréamont, M. (1995). Molecular biology of fish viruses: A review. *Vet. Res.* **26**, 341–351.

Calisher, C. H., Karabatsos, N., Zeller, H., Digoutte, J.-P., Tesh, R. B., Shope, R. E., Travasoos da Rosa, A. P. A., and St. George, T. D. (1989). Antigenic relationships among rhabdoviruses from vertebrates and hematophagous arthropods. *Intervirology* **30**, 241–257.

Dietzschold, B., Rupprecht, C. E., Fang Fu, Z., and Koprowski, H. (1996). Rhabdoviruses. *In* "Fields Virology" (B. N. Fields, D. M. Knipe, P. M. Howley, R. M. Chanock, J. L. Melnick, T. P. Monath, B. Roizman, and S. E. Straus, eds.), 3rd ed., pp. 1137–1159. Lippincott-Raven, Philadelphia, PA.

Jackson, A. C. (1997). Rabies. *In* "Viral Pathogenesis" (N. Nathanson, R. Ahmed, F. Gonzalez-Scarano, D. E. Griffin, K. V. Holmes, F. A. Murphy, and H. L. Robinson, eds.), pp. 575–592. Lippincott-Raven, Philadelphia, PA.

Leong, J.-A., and Munn, C. B. (1991). Potential uses of recombinant DNA in the development of fish vaccines. *Bull. Eur. Assoc. Fish Pathol.* **11**, 30–35.

National Association of State Public Health Veterinarians. (1997) (published annually). Compendium of animal rabies control. *Morbid. Mortal. Wkly. Rep. Recommend. Rep.* **46**, RR-4.

Rupprecht, C. E., and Smith, J. S. (1994). Raccoon rabies: The re-emergence of an epizootic in a densely populated area. *Semin. Virol.* **5**, 155–164.

Rupprecht, C. E., Smith, J. S., Fekadu, M., and Childs, J. E. (1995). The ascension of wildlife rabies: A cause for public health concern or intervention? *Emerg. Infect. Dis.* **1**, 107–114.

Smith, J. S. (1989). Rabies virus epitopic variation: Use in ecologic studies. *Adv. Virus Res.* **36,** 215–254.

St. George, T. D. (1988). Bovine ephemeral fever. *In* "The Arboviruses: Epidemiology and Ecology" (T. P. Monath, ed.), Vol. 2, pp. 71–83. CRC Press, Boca Raton, FL.

Tsiang, H. (1993). Pathophysiology of rabies virus infection of the nervous system. *Adv. Virus Res.* **42,** 375–412.

Wagner, R. R., and Rose, J. K. (1996). Rhabdoviridae: The viruses and their replication. *In* "Fields Virology" (B. N. Fields, D. M. Knipe, P. M. Howley, R. M. Chanock, J. L. Melnick, T. P. Monath, B. Roizman, and S. E. Straus, eds.), 3rd ed., pp. 1121–1135. Lippincott-Raven, Philadelphia, PA.

Wandeler, A., Nadin-Davis, S. A., Tinline, R. R., and Rupprecht, C. E. (1994). Rabies epizootiology: An ecological and evolutionary perspective. *In* "Lyssaviruses" (C. E. Rupprecht, B. Dietzschold, and H. Koprowski, eds.), pp. 297–324. Springer-Verlag, New York.

World Health Organization. (1997). "WHO Recommendations on Rabies Post-Exposure Treatment and the Correct Technique of Intradermal Immunization Against Rabies." World Health Organization, Geneva.

Chapter 28

Filoviridae

In 1967, 31 cases of hemorrhagic fever, with 7 deaths, occurred among laboratory workers in Germany and Yugoslavia who were processing kidneys from African green monkeys (*Cercopithecus aethiops*) that had been imported from Uganda. A new virus was isolated from patients and monkeys; it was named Marburg virus, now the prototype member of the family *Filoviridae*. Nine years later two further extraordinary epidemics of hemorrhagic fever occurred, one in villages in the rain forest of Zaire (now the Democratic Republic of Congo) and the other in southern Sudan, 700 km away. Altogether there were more than 550 cases and 430 deaths. A virus morphologically identical to but antigenically distinct from Marburg virus was isolated; it was named Ebola virus. Later, the viruses from Zaire and Sudan were found to be genetically distinct and are now designated Ebola virus, subtypes Zaire and Sudan. Since 1976, there have been more than 18 episodes of Ebola hemorrhagic fever, caused by three genetically distinct viruses (subtypes Zaire, Sudan, and Côte d'Ivoire), representing an ever-increasing geographic range within Africa. In 1989 and 1990, monkeys imported from the Philippines into an import quarantine facility in Reston, Virginia, were found to have been infected with a another new virus, now called Ebola virus, subtype Reston. Infected monkeys at the facility became ill and many died. Four animal caretakers were infected but there was no clinically apparent disease. This virus reappeared in imported monkeys in Italy in 1992 and Texas in 1996.

The member viruses of the family *Filoviridae* intrigue us for several reasons: (1) the viruses, although similar in genomic organization and mode of replication to other members of the order *Mononegavirales* (the viruses comprising the families *Paramyxoviridae, Rhabdoviridae, Filoviridae,* and *Bornaviridae*) are morphologically the most bizarre of all viruses; (2) the viruses have caused large outbreaks and therefore are recognized as having substantial epidemic potential; (3) the viruses cause a most devastating clinical disease in humans, with extremely rapid and florid tissue damage and with a very high mortality rate; and (4) most intriguing of all, the viruses, although clearly zoonotic, occupy a still unknown ecologic niche(s) involving a still unknown reservoir host(s). In fact, the family *Filoviridae* is the only virus family containing pathogens of domestic animals or humans for which the ecologic niche(s) and reservoir host(s) remain unknown.

Properties of Filoviruses

Classification

All nonsegmented negative-sense RNA viruses share several characteristics: (1) a similar genome organization and roughly the same gene order, (2) a virion-associated RNA polymerase (transcriptase), (3) a helical nucleocapsid, (4) transcription of mRNAs by sequential interrupted synthesis from a single promoter, and (5) virion maturation via budding of preassembled nucleocapsids from plasma membrane at sites containing patches of viral glycoprotein peplomers. These characteristics and conserved ancient domains found in genomic nucleotide sequences support the notion of a common ancestry as reflected in the establishment of the order *Mononegavirales.* Conserved domains in nucleoprotein and polymerase genes suggest that the family *Filoviridae* is related most closely to the genus *Pneumovirus* in the family *Paramyxoviridae* rather than to the family *Rhabdoviridae* as might be expected from their similar helically wound nucleocapsid structures.

The family *Filoviridae* contains two genera, both unnamed, one comprising the Marburg-like viruses, the other the Ebola-like viruses, the latter with four subtypes,

Ebola virus subtypes Zaire, Sudan, Côte d'Ivoire, and Reston. The degree of genetic stability of the filoviruses overall and the absence of genetic variability among Ebola virus isolates obtained within an outbreak match the character of other member viruses of the order *Mononegavirales* (see Chapter 26, Table 26.1). Ebola virus isolates made recently during human disease outbreaks in Gabon are very similar to isolates from the Democratic Republic of Congo.

Virion Properties

Filovirus virions are pleomorphic, appearing as long filamentous, sometimes branched forms, or as "U"-shaped, "6"-shaped, or circular forms. Virions have a uniform diameter of 80 nm and vary greatly in length (particles may be up to 14,000 nm long, but have unit nucleocapsid lengths of about 800 nm for Marburg and 1000 nm for Ebola virus). Virions are composed of a lipid envelope covered with peplomers, surrounding a helically wound nucleocapsid (50 nm in diameter) (Figure 28.1). The genome is composed of a single molecule of negative-sense, single-stranded RNA, 19.1 kb in size, the largest of all negative-sense RNA viruses. The gene order is 3′-untranslated region—NP (the nucleoprotein)–VP35 (part of nucleocapsid)—VP40 (membrane-associated matrix protein)—GP (the glycoprotein)–VP30 (part of nucleocapsid)—VP24 (membrane-associated protein)—L (the RNA polymerase or transcriptase)—5′-untranslated region. Genes are separated either by intergenic sequences or by overlaps, i.e., short (17–20 bases) regions where the transcription start signal of the downstream gene overlaps the transcription stop signal of the upstream gene. Ebola virus has three overlaps that alternate with intergenic sequences, whereas Marburg virus has a single overlap (Figure 28.2).

FIGURE 28.1.

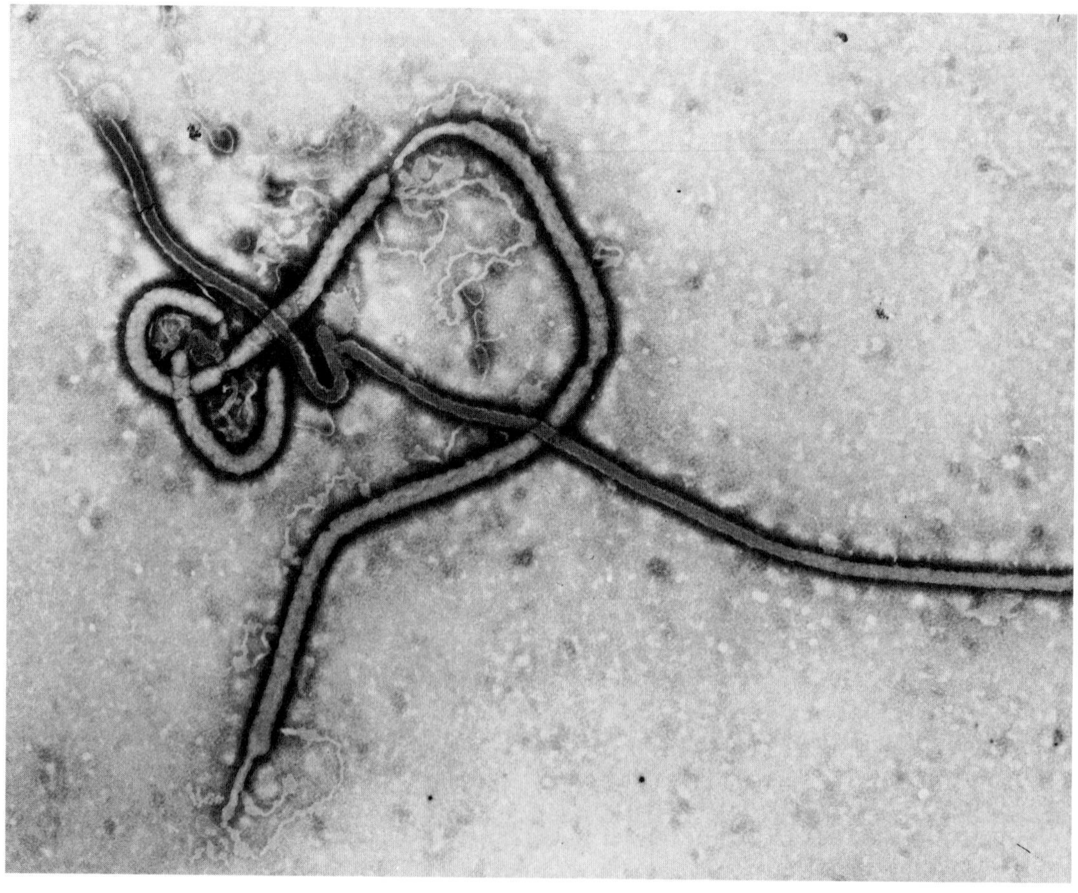

Family *Filoviridae*, genus, unnamed, comprising the Ebola-like viruses, Ebola virus (subtype Zaire). Virions in a diagnostic specimen (human tissue passaged once in Vero cells for 2 days); negative stain electron microscopy. Magnification: ×62,000.

FIGURE 28.2.

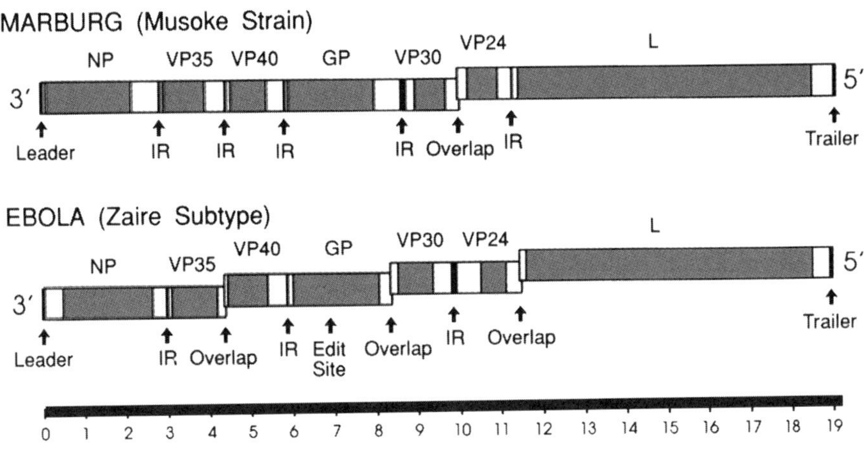

Genome organization of Ebola and Marburg viruses. Genes for the structural proteins associated with the virion RNA are identified as (1) nucleoprotein (NP), (2) VP30, (3) VP35, and (4) polymerase (L) protein. Genes for the membrane-associated proteins are identified as (5) matrix (VP40), (6) VP24, and (7) glycoprotein (GP). Shaded areas denote the coding regions and white areas denote noncoding sequences. Genes begin with a conserved transcriptional start site and end with a transcriptional stop (polyadenylation) signal; adjoining genes are either separated from one another by an intergenic region (IR) or overlap one another. The primary gene product of the GP gene of Ebola virus is SGP, a nonstructural secreted glycoprotein. At the extreme 3′ and 5′ ends of the genomes are complementary leader and trailer sequences. Scale: kb. (Courtesy of A. Sanchez.)

The Marburg virus glycoprotein is encoded in a single open reading frame, whereas the Ebola virus glycoprotein in encoded in two reading frames. Expression of Ebola virus glycoprotein involves site-specific RNA transcriptional editing and translational frame-shifting that joins the two open reading frames.

Filovirus virions contain seven proteins. The Ebola virion glycoprotein (M_r 120,000–170,000) forms the surface peplomers, whereas a second glycoprotein (M_r 60,000), made in large amounts, is secreted extracellularly. The nature of the participation of this soluble glycoprotein in the pathogenesis of Ebola virus disease is unknown, but it may serve as some sort of immune decoy, minimizing the immune response to the virus, and/or it may be immunosuppressive, affecting the host response to infection. Virions also contain lipids, their composition reflecting the composition of host cell membranes, and large amounts of carbohydrates as side chains on the glycoproteins. Viral infectivity is quite stable at room temperature, but sensitive to UV- and γ-irradiation, detergents, and common disinfectants.

Viral Replication

Filoviruses replicate well in cell cultures, such as Vero (African green monkey kidney) cells; infection is characterized by rapid cytopathology and large intracytoplasmic inclusion bodies (composed of masses of viral nucleocapsids). Virions enter cells by endocytosis and replication occurs in the cytoplasm.

Transcription is initiated at a single promoter site, located at the 3′ end of the viral genome. Transcription yields monocistronic mRNAs, i.e., separate mRNAs for each protein. This is accomplished by conserved transcriptional stop and start signals that are located at the boundaries of each viral gene. As the viral polymerase moves along the genomic RNA, these signals cause it to pause and sometimes to fall off the template and terminate transcription (called stuttering or stop/start transcription). The result is that more mRNA is made from genes that are located close to the promoter and less from downstream genes. This regulates the expression of genes, producing large amounts of structural proteins such as the nucleoprotein and smaller amounts of proteins such as the RNA polymerase. Replication of the genome is mediated by the synthesis of full-length complementary-sense RNA, which then serves as the template for the synthesis of virion-sense RNA. This requires that the stop/start signals needed for transcription be overridden by the viral polymerase—the immediate envelopment of newly formed viral-sense RNA by nucleoprotein seems to mediate this. Maturation of virions occurs via budding of preassembled nucleocapsids from the plasma membrane at sites already containing patches of viral glycoprotein peplomers (Table 28.1).

Table 28.1
Properties of Filoviruses

Virions are pleomorphic, appearing as long filamentous forms and other shapes; virions have a uniform diameter of 80 nm and vary greatly in length (unit nucleocapsid lengths of about 800 nm for Marburg and 1000 nm for Ebola virus)
Virions are composed of a lipid envelope covered with peplomers surrounding a helically wound nucleocapsid
The genome is composed of a single molecule of negative-sense, single-stranded RNA, 19.1 kb in size, the largest of all negative-sense RNA viruses
Infection is extremely cytopathic in cultured cells and in target organs of host
Cytoplasmic replication, large intracytoplasmic inclusion bodies, budding from the plasma membrane

Marburg and Ebola Hemorrhagic Fevers

There has been an increasing incidence of Ebola hemorrhagic fever in West Africa since the mid-1990s, evident as large and small outbreaks, involving an ever-increasing geographic range. Because the reservoir host(s) is not known, ecological, environmental, and human behavioral changes that might have increased the opportunities for emergence are still matters of speculation, matters needing more study.

Clinical Features

Because the reservoir host(s) of the filoviruses remains unknown, nothing can be said about the clinical features of infections in nature. Nevertheless, many experimental animals have been studied, including guinea pigs and hamsters and several species of monkeys, in most instances with infection ending in death. In rhesus (*Macaca mulatta*), cynomolgus (*Macaca fascicularis*), African green monkeys (*Cercopithecus aethiops*) and baboons (*Papio* spp.) inoculated with Marburg virus or the Zaire subtype of Ebola virus, the incubation period is 4 to 6 days, followed by an abrupt onset of clinical disease marked by petechiae, ecchymoses, hemorrhagic pharyngitis, hematemesis, melena, and prostration. Infection nearly always ends in death. There is considerable similarity in the way filoviruses attack these nonhuman primates and humans. The Sudan and Reston subtypes of Ebola virus are least pathogenic for primates and guinea pigs, killing only a fraction of animals inoculated with unpassaged virus—serial passage increases the virulence of these viruses for these hosts.

Pathogenesis, Pathology, and Immunity

In experimentally infected rhesus, cynomolgus, and African green monkeys, filoviruses replicate to high titer in the reticuloendothelial system (especially Kupffer cells and macrophages in lymph nodes and spleen), endothelium, liver, and lungs; there is severe necrosis of these target organs, which is most evident in liver, and there is interstitial hemorrhage, which is most evident in the gastrointestinal tract (Figure 28.3). Virus shedding from infected primates occurs from all body surfaces and orifices, including the skin and mucous membranes, and especially from hemorrhagic diatheses. Of all the hemorrhagic fever agents, filoviruses cause the most severe hemorrhagic manifestations and the most pronounced liver necrosis (the latter perhaps matched only by Rift Valley fever virus infection in target species). There is an early and profound leukopenia, followed by a dramatic neutrophilia with a shift to the left, and very little inflammatory infiltration in sites of parenchymal necrosis in the liver. There is no evidence for latency or persistence in any filovirus infection in any experimental animal.

The filoviruses outmaneuver specific host defense mechanisms of experimental animals by (1) their speed—animals often die before it might be expected that an effective primary specific inflammatory/immune response would be elicited, and (2) their tropism(s)—early reticuloendothelial and lymphoid tropisms likely minimize the response that might be elicited otherwise. Abnormalities in coagulation parameters include the appearance of fibrin split products in the blood and prolonged prothrombin and partial thromboplastin times; disseminated intravascular coagulation is a common terminal event.

Laboratory Diagnosis

Diagnosis of filovirus infections has been based on virus isolation from blood or tissues in cell culture, such as Vero (African green monkey kidney) cells or MA-104 (fetal rhesus monkey kidney) cells, with detection of the presence of virus by immunofluorescence or electron microscopy. Diagnosis is also based on the direct detection of viral antigen in tissues by immunofluorescence

FIGURE 28.3.

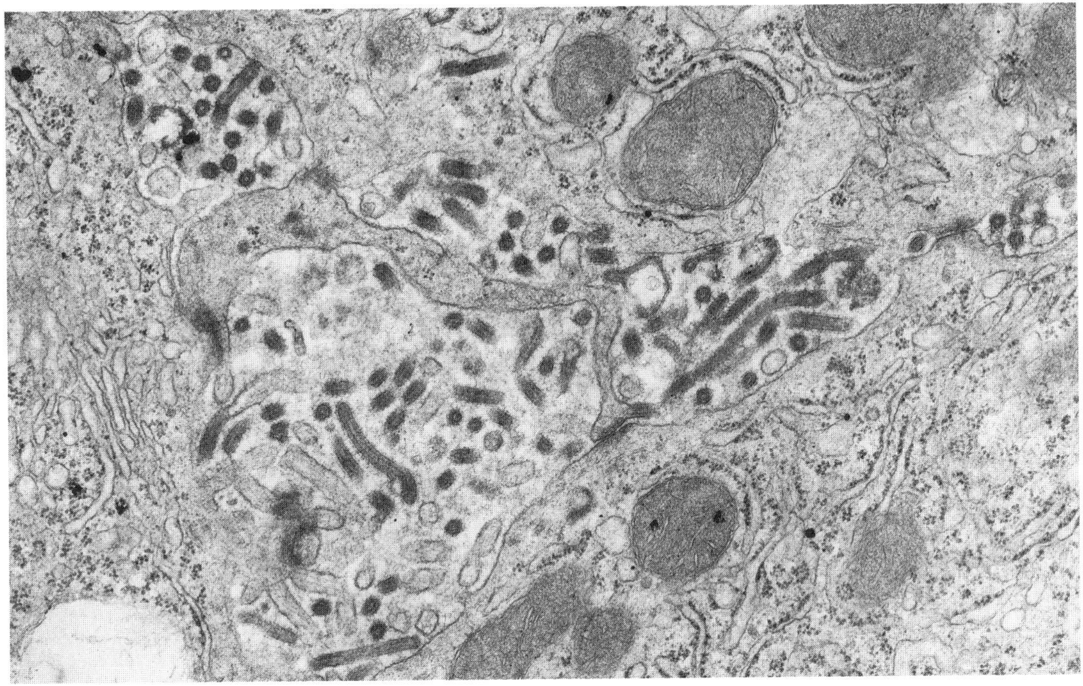

Liver from a *Cercopithecus aethiops* (African green) monkey inoculated with Marburg virus and sacrificed at day 7 postinfection when clinically ill. This image depicts an area where hepatocytes are still intact; at this site, virions fill the intercellular space as a result of budding from plasma membranes. Thin section electron microscopy. Magnification: ×39,000.

or antigen-capture enzyme immunoassay. A reverse transcriptase–polymerase chain reaction assay has proven useful as well. Serological diagnostics have been fraught with problems—indirect immunofluorescence suffers from many false positives, especially when used for serosurveys of filovirus infection rates in captive monkeys. An IgM capture enzyme immunoassay has proven much more reliable than other serological methods and has become the standard for human and primate serological diagnosis.

Epidemiology, Prevention, and Control

The fact that the Ebola virus subtypes that have caused human disease episodes have been different from each other makes it clear that a common source transmission chain extending across sub-Saharan Africa is not the case—rather, virus subtypes lodged at or near each site of human disease episodes have been responsible (Figure 28.4). Human index cases have often occurred in or near the end of the tropical rainy season and all have been associated with the tropical forest or the marginal zone between tropical forest and savanna. This puts the search for the reservoir host(s) of the viruses in the most biologically diverse of all econiches. Further, it must be recognized that within the ecosystems under consideration, there is great micro-niche isolation and ecologic insularity, i.e., there are many sites within larger geographical areas in which the filoviruses may coexist invisibly with their reservoir host(s). Candidate reservoir hosts include all mammals (particularly monkeys and rodents), birds, reptiles, amphibians, and arthropods. Particular attention is being given to bats; following experimental virus inoculation, several species of bats have been found to support the growth of Ebola virus very well, sustaining virus in their tissues and blood for as long as 3 weeks.

In all Ebola hemorrhagic fever outbreaks, secondary spread between humans appears to have been due principally to contact with body fluids from an acute case. In the major African epidemics in 1976, spread was largely within hospitals due to the reuse of blood-contaminated syringes and/or needles and, more recently, due to close contact without gloves, mask, or protective clothing. Recent episodes, including those in Zaire in 1995 and Gabon in 1996, were controlled with relatively simple sanitary measures: strict barrier nursing practices, patient isolation, and rigorous decontamination of all materials and equipment used in patient care.

Filovirus disease prevention and control strategies have not been widely adopted in Africa—in fact, there are still arguments about approaches, resources, and

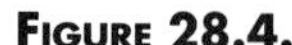

FIGURE 28.4.

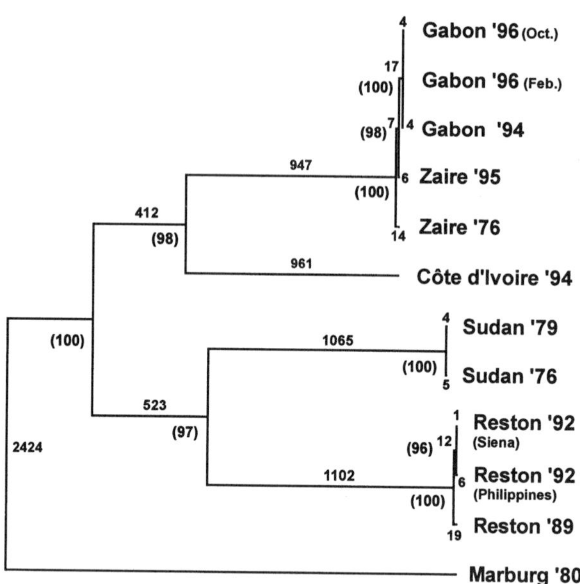

Phylogenetic tree showing the relationship between Ebola virus subtypes and Marburg virus. The various isolates of each subtype, in some cases made over long intervals and from distant geographic locals, are remarkably similar and yet different enough to indicate that each subtype exists separately in its locale. The entire coding region for the glycoprotein gene of the viruses shown was used in maximum parsimony analysis, and a single most parsimonious tree was obtained. Numbers in parentheses indicate bootstrap confidence values for branch points and were generated from 500 replicates. Branch length values are also shown. (Courtesy of A. Sanchez.)

training. In contrast, the episodes in the United States and Italy from 1989 onward, involving the Reston subtype of Ebola virus, have refocused attention on the risk of importation of filoviruses into countries outside endemic zones in West and Central Africa and the Philippines. Despite export prohibitions established by source countries for conservation purposes, large numbers of wild-caught monkeys are still imported into many countries, primarily for vaccine production and medical research. Today, most importing countries operate import quarantine facilities and adhere to international primate transport and import standards. These standards include testing for the presence of filoviruses and protocols to prevent infection in primate facility workers. Similarly, guidelines are in place to minimize risk in caring for filovirus hemorrhagic fever patients in hospitals in non-endemic areas.

Human Disease

Marburg and Ebola virus subtypes Zaire, Sudan, and Côte d'Ivoire cause severe hemorrhagic fever in humans—it has been said that "the evolution of disease often seems inexorable and invariable." Following an incubation period of usually 4 to 10 days (extreme range 2 to 21 days for infection by the Zaire subtype of Ebola virus), there is an abrupt onset of illness with initial nonspecific signs and symptoms, including fever, severe frontal headache, malaise, and myalgia. There is a profound leukopenia, bradycardia, and conjunctivitis and there may be a macropapular rash. Deterioration over the following 2 to 3 days is marked by pharyngitis, nausea and vomiting, prostration, and bleeding, which is manifested as petechiae, ecchymoses, uncontrolled bleeding from venepuncture sites, and melena. Abortion is a common consequence of infection, and infants born to mothers dying of infection invariably die. Death usually occurs 6 to 9 days after the onset of clinical disease (range 1 to 21 days). The mortality rate has been very high: 25% with Marburg virus, 60% with the Sudan subtype of Ebola virus, and 88–90% with the Zaire subtype of Ebola virus. Convalescence is slow and marked by prostration, by weight loss, and often by amnesia for the period of acute illness.

Marburg and Ebola viruses cause similar pathological changes in humans. The most striking lesions are found in liver, spleen, and kidney. These lesions are characterized by focal hepatic necrosis with little inflammatory response and by follicular necrosis in lymph nodes and spleen. Treatment of patients is nonspecific and supportive: therapeutic approaches such as convalescent human plasma, interferon α, and antiviral drugs such as Ribavirin have proven ineffective. Recently, hyperimmune equine globulin has been developed in Russia and use of whole blood from convalescent patients has been tried in Zaire, but these therapeutic modalities are still under investigation.

Biohazard: Marburg and Ebola viruses are *restricted pathogens* and their importation or possession is regulated by most national governments. The viruses are restricted to certain national laboratories for all research and diagnostic procedures; the viruses are also Biosafety Level 4 pathogens; they must be handled in the laboratory under maximum containment conditions to prevent human exposure.

Further Reading

Centers for Disease Control and Prevention. (1995). Update: Management of patients with suspected viral hemorrhagic fever—United States. *Morbid. Mortal W. Rep.* **44,** 475–479.

Johnson, K. M., Webb, P. A., Lange, J. V., and Murphy, F. A. (1977). Isolation and characterization of a new virus, Ebola virus, causing acute hemorrhagic fever in Zaire. *Lancet* **1,** 569–571.

Murphy, F. A., and Nathanson, N. (1997). An atlas of viral disease pathogenesis. *In* "Viral Pathogenesis" (N. Nathanson, R. Ahmed, F. Gonzalez-Scarano, D. E. Griffin, K. V. Holmes, F. A. Murphy, and H. L. Robinson, eds.), pp. 433–463. Lippincott-Raven, Philadelphia, PA.

Murphy, F. A., and Peters, C. J. (1998). Ebola virus: Where does it come from and where is it going? *In* "Emerging Infections" (R. Krause and A. Fauci, eds.), pp. 375–410. Academic Press, New York.

Nathanson, N., and Murphy, F. A. (1997). Evolution of viral diseases. *In* "Viral Pathogenesis" (N. Nathanson, R. Ahmed, F. Gonzalez-Scarano, D. E. Griffin, K. V. Holmes, F. A. Murphy, and H. L. Robinson, eds.), pp. 353–370. Lippincott-Raven, Philadelphia, PA.

Pattyn, S. R., ed. (1978). "Ebola Virus Hemorrhagic Fever." Elsevier/North-Holland, Amsterdam.

Peters, C. J. (1997). Pathogenesis of viral hemorrhagic fevers. *In* "Viral Pathogenesis" (N. Nathanson, R. Ahmed, F. Gonzalez-Scarano, D. E. Griffin, K. V. Holmes, F. A. Murphy, and H. L. Robinson, eds.), pp. 779–800. Lippincott-Raven, Philadelphia, PA.

Peters, C. J., Sanchez, A., Feldmann, H., Rollin, P. E., Nichol, S., and Ksiazek, T. G. (1994). Filoviruses as emerging pathogens. *Semin. Virol.* **5,** 147–154.

Peters, C. J., Sanchez, A., Rollin, P. E., Ksiazek, T. G., and Murphy, F. A. (1996). Filoviridae: Marburg and Ebola viruses. *In* "Fields Virology" (B. N. Fields, D. M. Knipe, P. M. Howley, R. M. Chanock, J. L. Melnick, T. P. Monath, B. Roizman, and S. E. Straus, eds.), 3rd ed., pp. 1161–1176. Lippincott-Raven, Philadelphia, PA.

Swanepoel, R., Leman, P. A., Burt, F. J., Zachariades, N. A., Braack, L. E., Ksiazek, T. G., Rollin, P. E., Zaki, S. R., and Peters, C. J. (1996). Experimental inoculation of plants and animals with Ebola virus. *Emerg. Infect. Dis.* **2,** 321–325.

Zaki, S., and Kilmarx, P. (1997). Ebola virus hemorrhagic fever. *In* "Pathology of Emerging Infections" (C. R. Horsburgh and A. M. Nelson, eds.) pp. 299–312. American Society for Microbiology Press, Washington, DC.

CHAPTER 29

Bornaviridae

Borna disease is named for the town of Borna in Saxony, Germany, where at least since 1895 devastating epidemics of a naturally occurring, infectious, usually fatal, neurological disease of horses and occasionally sheep have occurred. The viral etiology of the disease was established as early as 1925. With improved understanding of the virus and increased surveillance there is evidence that the virus may have a very wide, perhaps worldwide, distribution and there are suggestions that infection of humans with Borna disease virus may be linked to specific neuropsychiatric illnesses.

Properties of Borna Disease Virus

Classification

The virus is the sole member of the genus *Bornavirus*, family *Bornaviridae*, order *Mononegavirales*. A disease of horses of unproved etiology, termed Near East encephalitis and possibly transmitted by ticks, is similar in many ways to Borna disease.

Virion Properties

Borna disease virus virions are spherical, enveloped, about 90 nm in diameter and contain a core that is about 50–60 nm in diameter (Figure 29.1). The genome is a single molecule of negative-sense, single-stranded RNA, 8.9 kb in size (Figure 29.2). The genome contains five open reading frames that code for six proteins through polymerase readthrough and posttranscriptional RNA splicing. Virion proteins are of the following sizes: M_r 190,000, 57,000, 40,000, 23,000, 18,000, and 16,000. The M_r 190,000 protein is the RNA-dependent RNA polymerase and the M_r 18,000 protein is a glycoprotein. The virus is sensitive to heat, acid, lipid solvents, and usual disinfectants (Table 29.1).

Viral Replication

Borna disease virus differs from other members of the order *Mononegavirales* in that transcription and replication occur in the host cell nucleus. The virus is also unusual in its transcriptional strategy. The genome is transcribed into six primary transcripts, two of which are modified posttranslationally by splicing to yield two additional mRNA species. Three transcription initiation and four transcription termination signals have been identified in the genome and these differ from other negative-stranded viruses in the configuration of their initiation and termination signals, their intergenic regions, and overlaps at gene boundaries.

Primary embryonic brain cell cultures including neural cells, astrocytes, and oligodendrocytes prepared from various animal species can be infected. In cell cultures the virus spreads mainly by cell-to-cell contact; infectivity remains highly cell associated. The virus can be adapted to canine kidney and Vero (African Green monkey kidney) cells; infection becomes persistent in these cells. Virus replication can be detected by immunofluorescence as brightly fluorescent granules of various sizes in the nucleus of infected cells.

Figure 29.1.

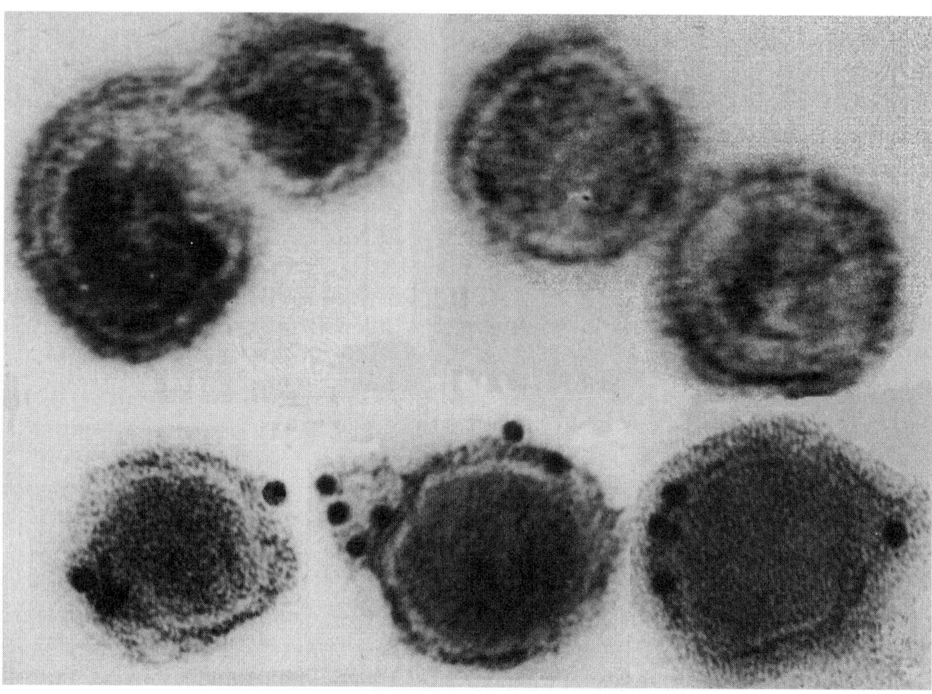

Family *Bornaviridae*, genus *Bornavirus*, Borna disease virus virions. Negative stain, immunogold label; because virions are so nondescript, specific antibody conjugated to gold microspheres was used to identify them. (Courtesy of H. Ludwig.)

Borna Disease

Clinical Features

The incubation period is usually about 4 weeks but varies from a few days up to 12 months or even longer. Initial clinical signs in the horse are variable and may include general fatigue, attacks of colic, coughing, icterus, and mild fever. This prodrome is followed by alternating phases of excitability and somnolence, ataxia, hyperesthesia, and difficulty in coordination. There is often an abnormal positioning of the fore and hind legs—legs may be spread apart or remain crossed for long periods while the horse stands motionless with its head down (Figure 29.3). Many horses refuse to eat or may suddenly stop chewing and swallowing and there may be constipation or diarrhea. Early neurological signs are mainly attributable to dysfunctions in the limbic system, whereas during later stages of the disease dysfunctions of motor systems causing paralysis and pareses predominate. Ophthalmologic disorders including nystagmus, pupillary reflex dysfunction, and blindness may occur in advanced stages. The course of the disease is 3 to 20 days and usually ends in death; surviving horses usually have permanent sensory and or motor deficits.

Figure 29.2.

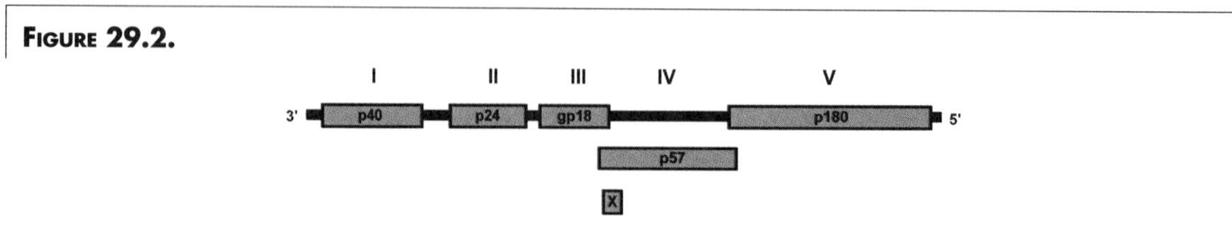

Genome of Borna disease virus. There are five open reading frames in the negative-sense, single-stranded RNA genome; reading frame IV overlaps with II and V. (Courtesy of S. Briese and I. Lipkin.)

TABLE 29.1
Properties of Borna Disease Virus

Virions are 90 nm in diameter, enveloped with an inner core, 50–60 nm in diameter
The genome is a single molecule of negative-sense, single-stranded RNA, 8.9 kb in size
The genome has six main open reading frames coding for six proteins, including a glycoprotein and an RNA-dependent RNA polymerase
Viral replication takes place in the nucleus
Infection in cell culture characteristically produces intranuclear inclusion bodies

Pathogenesis, Pathology and Immunity

Natural infection has been shown to occur in horses, sheep, cattle, and rabbits. Recently, ostriches have been identified as possible hosts as well. Experimentally, the host range is wide, from chickens to primates. The most thoroughly investigated experimental model infection is in the rat. The intranasal route seems to be most likely in natural infection, with virus passing intraaxonally to the olfactory bulbs of the brain from olfactory nerve endings in the nares. In the brain the virus infects neurons, astrocytes, and oligodendrocytes.

FIGURE 29.3.

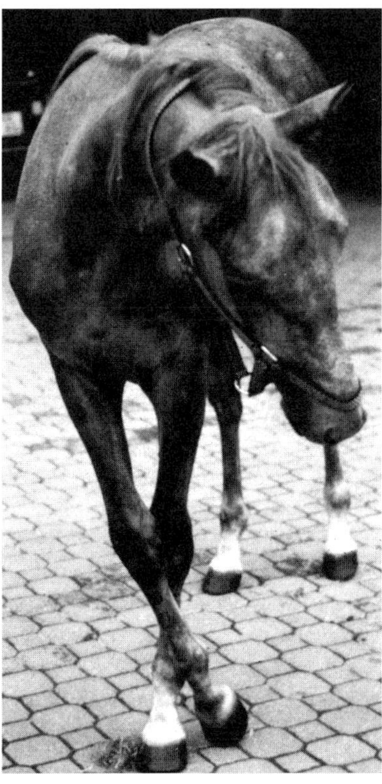

An advanced case of Borna disease, characterized by an abnormal positioning of the fore and hind legs–legs may be spread apart or remain crossed for long periods while the horse stands motionless with its head down. [Courtesy of S. Herzog.]

There is a severe encephalomyelitis but no neuronal necrosis; histologically, there is perivascular cuffing consisting mainly of lymphocytes and plasma cells. Intranuclear eosinophilic inclusions, called Joest-Degen bodies, are characteristic, even pathognomonic of Borna disease, although they cannot be demonstrated in all cases. Lesions are prominent in the gray matter of the olfactory bulb, basal cortex, caudate nucleus, and hippocampus. The necrotic process results in a dilatation of the lateral ventricles, resulting in marked hydrocephalus accompanied by severe cortical atrophy, most probably due to a progressive loss of neurons.

Infection does not elicit a protective immune response, but rather a cell-mediated immunopathological reaction. Experimentally, whereas infection of adult immunocompetent animals regularly results in disease, infection of neonatal or immunocompromised animals leads neither to encephalitis nor disease, despite the persistence of the virus. Antibodies do not participate in this pathogenetic process: antibodies lack neutralizing capacity and adoptive transfer of immunoglobulins from infected animals to immunocompromised recipients does not induce pathological changes or disease.

Laboratory Diagnosis

Even "typical" clinical manifestations do not justify more than the suspicion of Borna disease. Rabies, tetanus, equine herpesviruses, and other diseases have to be considered in the differential diagnosis. Diagnosis is usually confirmed by the demonstration of antibodies in the serum or preferably in the cerebrospinal fluid. This is done routinely by indirect immunofluorescence, where persistently infected Madin–Darby canine kidney cells are used as substrate. Antibody titers are relatively low, ranging from 1:10 to 1:64.

Other methods are also used in reference laboratories. Virus isolation in sensitive cultured cells can be used to confirm infection. The presence of virus is usually detected by direct immunofluorescence. Enzyme immunoassay methods are sensitive and reliable if purified antigen is used and monoclonal antibodies are used for antigen capture. The reverse transcriptase–polymerase chain reaction, using standard Borna disease virus primers, has become a valuable tool for diagnosis—viral RNA may be detected in conjunctival or nasal secretions or saliva. Postmortem diagnosis relies on immunohistochemistry to demonstrate viral antigen in the brain.

Epidemiology, Prevention, and Control

For many years Borna disease was considered sporadically endemic only in certain areas of central Europe. However, recent seroepidemiological investigations have indicated that infection in horses is much more widespread. Antibodies have been found in about 12% of horses in Germany, Switzerland, and The Netherlands and antibodies have also been found in horses in the United States. Most of the animals surveyed were without clinical signs, but most exhibited disease within 1 year. Because the opportunity for contact between horses has been expanded tremendously in recent years by international racing and other activities, the virus may just now be spreading after many years of relative confinement in traditionally endemic areas. Equine vaccination has been attempted but its value has been questionable and, given the immunopathologic nature of the disease, it may even be dangerous.

No data are available on reservoirs that might transmit the virus to horses on a regional or international basis. Whether the only important source of virus is inapparently infected horses or whether other species may contribute, such as sheep, is unknown. Because persistent-tolerant infections can be established in rats and these animals shed virus continuously, it seems clear that the question of an inapparently infected reservoir host must be pursued. In any case, an essential step in the control of the disease is the identification and quarantine of carrier animals.

Human Disease

When the tree shrew (a primate, *Tupaia glis*) was infected experimentally with Borna disease virus, the only change noted was aberrant social behavior and reduced reactions toward environmental stimuli. This finding motivated the search for evidence of infection in human patients with behavioral or neuropsychiatric disorders. Antibodies were found in the serum and cerebrospinal fluid of up to 7% of patients with specific behavioral and cognitive dysfunctions in Germany, the United States, and Japan, with the highest incidence in regions where Borna disease was known to be endemic in horses. Antibody prevalence has been found to be highest in patients with recurrent bipolar disorder (depression) and schizophrenia. Although it is still premature to call Borna disease a zoonosis, appropriate care is indicated when handling infected animals.

Further Reading

Becht, H., and Richt, J. A. (1996). Borna disease. *In* "Virus Infections of Vertebrates" (M. J. Studdert, ed.), Vol. 6, pp. 235–244. Elsevier, Amsterdam.

Briese, T., de la Torre, J. C., Lewis, A. J., Park, Y. S., Kim, S., Ludwig, H., and Lipkin, W. I. (1994). Genomic organization of Borna disease virus. *Proc. Natl. Acad. Sci. U.S.A.* **91**, 4362–4367.

Briese, T., Lipkin, W. I., and de la Torre, J. C. (1995). Molecular biology of Borna disease virus. *Curr. Top. Microbiol. Immunol.* **190**, 1–16.

Daubney, R., and Mahlau, E. A. (1967). Viral encephalomyelitis of equines and domestic ruminants in the Near East. *Res. Vet. Sci.* **8**, 375–397.

Lipkin, W. I., and Koprowski, H., eds. (1995). Borna disease. *Curr. Top. Microbiol. Immunol.* **190**, 1–134.

Ludwig, H., Bode, L., and Gosztonyi, G. (1988). Borna disease: A persistent virus infection of the central nervous system. *Prog. Med. Virol.* **35**, 107–151.

Rott, R., Herzog, S., Bechter, K., and Frese, K. (1991). Borna disease, a possible hazard for man? *Arch. Virol.* **118**, 143–149.

CHAPTER 30

Orthomyxoviridae

Influenza viruses are important pathogens of animals, but only rarely are they zoonotic, i.e., they are not transmitted directly from animals each time there is a human infection. Instead, they are the ultimate species jumpers, forever evolving host range variants in animals that become epidemic and even pandemic when they invade humans. For this reason, veterinary and human concerns over influenza are tightly linked.

The reservoir of influenza A viruses is in aquatic birds, especially ducks, shorebirds, and gulls; the viruses replicate in intestinal epithelium and are excreted in high concentrations in feces, resulting in an efficient fecal–oral transmission pattern. Migrating aquatic birds carry viruses between the continents and thereby play a key role in the continuing process of virus evolution. There are periodic exchanges of viral genes or whole viruses between these reservoirs and other species: domestic fowl, especially ducks, and mammals such as swine, horses, mink, seals, whales, and humans. Domestic swine are important intermediate hosts (in the United States, turkeys may also serve as intermediate hosts) and China is the epicenter for viral movement from reservoir hosts through intermediate hosts and into horses, swine, and humans. There are human epidemics nearly every year and pandemics whenever a major antigenic variant virus emerges. The "Spanish flu" pandemic that swept the world in 1918, just as World War I ended, killed 25–40 million people—more than the war itself.

Phylogenetic analyses have indicated that influenza viruses have evolved into five host-specific lineages: an old equine lineage, which has not been seen in over 15 years, a separate recent equine lineage, a lineage in gulls, another in swine, and another in humans. The lineages in swine and humans are closely related, derived from a common avian ancestor. In fact, the viruses currently circulating in swine in Europe and horses in China derived all of their eight genomic segments from avian viruses. The dates when some lineages diverged from their ancestors can also be estimated: the ancestor of the human virus that caused the 1918 pandemic diverged from a classic swine virus between 1905 and 1914. Avian viruses, unlike mammalian viruses, show low evolutionary rates; in fact, viruses in aquatic birds appear to be in evolutionary stasis. Nucleotide changes have continued to occur at a similar rate in avian and mammalian influenza viruses, but these changes no longer result in amino acid changes in avian viruses. This suggests that avian viruses are approaching or have reached a state of adaptation where further changes provide no selective advantage. This also means that the source of genes for future epidemics in domestic fowl, horses, and humans already exist in the aquatic bird reservoir.

Given our new understanding of the natural history of influenza viruses as species jumpers, prevention efforts might become more focused: for example, live-bird markets that bring together a wide variety of avian species (chickens, ducks, turkeys, pheasants, guinea fowl, and chukars) and provide opportunity for genetic mixing might be monitored to reduce the emergence of reassortant viruses. Changes in agricultural practices to separate swine and turkeys from aquatic birds and other species might break the evolutionary progression of new variants. Of course, such measures are not likely to be feasible on a global scale—instead, new variant influenza viruses will continue to emerge.

Properties of Orthomyxoviruses

Classification

The family *Orthomyxoviridae* comprises the genera *Influenzavirus A, Influenzavirus B, Influenzavirus C,* and *Thogotovirus*. Influenza A viruses are pathogens of horses, swine, mink, seals, whales, fowl, and humans. Influenza B viruses are pathogens of humans only, and although influenza C viruses infect humans and swine, they rarely causes serious disease. The thogotoviruses are a little-known group of tick-borne arboviruses infecting livestock and humans in Africa, Europe, and Asia. The name of the family is derived from the Greek *myxa,* meaning mucus, and *orthos,* meaning correct or right. The name originated to distinguish these viruses from the *para*myxoviruses. *Influenza* is the Italian form of Latin, from *influentia,* "influence," so used because epidemics were thought to be due to astrological or other occult influences.

The classification of the influenza viruses is influenced greatly by the practical need for assessment of the risk represented by the emergence of new variant viruses and the question of whether herd immunity against previously circulating strains will dampen spread and whether existing vaccines will need to be reformulated. The emergence of variant viruses not only depends on *genetic drift,* i.e., point mutations (nucleotide substitutions, insertions, deletions), but also on *genetic shift,* i.e., genomic segment reassortment. Drift and shift of two genes, the viral hemagglutinin and the neuraminidase are most important—in the classification system, influenza A viruses are categorized into 15 hemagglutinin and 9 neuraminidase types. Viruses are further categorized by their host (swine, horses, birds, etc.), geographic origin, strain number, and year of isolation. Thus, the full identification of an influenza virus looks like a secret code but is precise and informative:

Influenza virus A/equine/Prague/1/56 (H7N7), the prototypic equine influenza virus 1

Influenza virus A/equine/Miami/1/63 (H3N8), the prototypic equine influenza virus 2

Influenza virus A/swine/Iowa/15/30 (H1N1), the prototypic strain of swine influenza virus

Influenza virus A/Hong Kong/1/68 (H3N2), the virus that caused the human pandemic of 1968 (when the host of origin is not specified it indicates human origin)

Although any gene constellation and any combination of H and N genes can arise by genetic reassortment, only a limited range of combinations are recognized as important as pathogens: (1) H7N7 and H3N8 viruses (previously designated equine influenza viruses 1 and 2) cause respiratory disease in horses; (2) H1N1 and H3N2 viruses are isolated often from swine; (3) H7N7 and H4N5 viruses cause respiratory and systemic disease in seals; (4) H10N4 viruses cause respiratory disease in mink; (5) H1N1, H2N2, H3N2, recently H5N1, and possibly H3N8 viruses cause respiratory disease in humans; and (6) nearly all combinations occur in birds, particularly H5N2 and H7N1 (the major causes of avian influenza, also called fowl plague, in chickens).

Virion Properties

Orthomyxovirus virions are pleomorphic, often spherical but predominantly filamentous in fresh isolates, 80–120 nm in their smallest dimension (Figure 30.1). Virions consist of an envelope with large peplomers surrounding eight (genera *Influenzavirus A* and *Influenzavirus B*), seven (genus *Influenzavirus* C), or six (genus *Thogotovirus*) helically symmetrical nucleocapsid segments of different sizes. There are two kinds of glycoprotein peplomers: (1) homotrimers of the hemagglutinin protein and (2) homotetramers of the neuraminidase protein (Figure 30.2). Influenza C viruses have only one type of glycoprotein peplomer, consisting of multifunctional hemagglutinin-esterase molecules (HE). Genomic segments have a loop at one end and consist of a molecule of viral RNA enclosed within a capsid composed of helically arranged nucleoprotein (NP). Associated with the RNA are three proteins that make up the viral RNA polymerase (PB1, PB2, and PA). Virion envelopes are lined by the matrix protein (M1) and are spanned by a small number of ion channels composed of tetramers of a second matrix protein, M2. The genome in eight, seven, or six segments consists of linear negative-sense, single-stranded RNA, 10–13.6 kb in overall size. The genome segments have terminal repeats at both ends, with those on the 3′ ends being identical on all segments.

Influenza viruses are sensitive to heat (56°C, 30 minutes), acid (pH 3), and lipid solvents and are thus very labile under ordinary environmental conditions.

Viral Replication

In permissive cells, the viral hemagglutinin is activated by cleavage into two parts—HA1 and HA2—which remain linked by disulfide bonds. Virions attach to cells via the binding of their activated hemagglutinin to sialic acid receptors on the plasma membrane (different orthomyxoviruses use sialic acid molecules with different carbohydrate side chains as their receptors). Entry is via receptor-mediated endocytosis; transcription complexes (nucleocapsids with associated RNA polymerase) are re-

FIGURE 30.1.

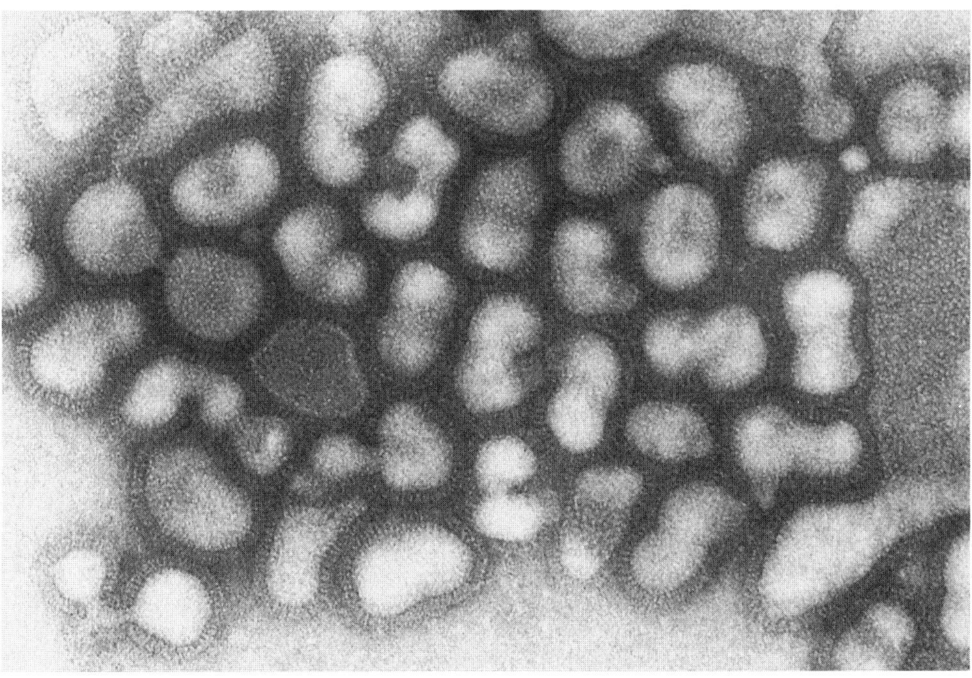

Family *Orthomyxoviridae,* genus *Influenzavirus A,* influenza virus A/Hong Kong/1/68 (H3N2). Virions showing distinct peplomers, which are actually of two kinds: hemagglutinin and neuraminidase. Negative stain electron microscopy. Magnification: ×70,000.

FIGURE 30.2.

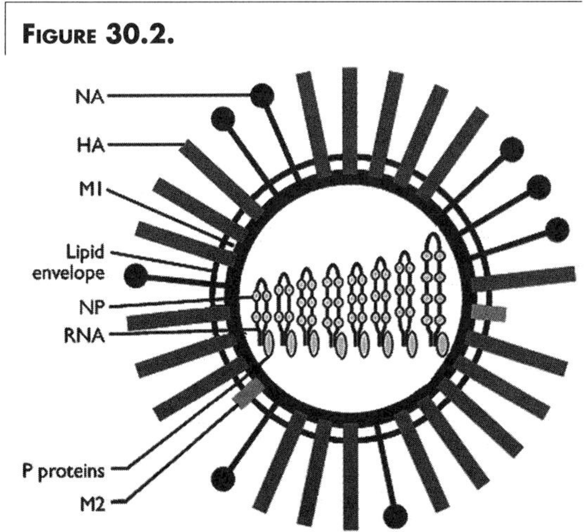

Schematic representation of an influenza A virion showing the envelope in which three different types of transmembrane proteins are anchored: the hemagglutinin (HA) and the neuraminidase (NA) form the characteristic peplomers and the M2 protein, which is short and not visible by electron microscopy. Inside the envelope there is a layer of M1 protein that surrounds eight ribonucleoprotein (RNP) structures, each of which consists of one RNA segment covered with nucleoprotein (NP) and associated with the three polymerase (P) proteins. The RNA segments exist in a circular conformation stabilized by base pairing between their 3′ and 5′ ends. [Adapted from P. Palese and A. Garciá-Sastre. Influenza viruses. *In* "Encyclopedia of Virology" (R. G. Webster and A. Granoff, eds.), 2nd ed. (CD-ROM. Academic Press, London, 1998].

leased into the cytoplasm after fusion between the viral envelope and the endosomal membrane (Figure 30.3). This fusion is triggered by the low pH in the endosome, which causes another conformational activation of the hemagglutinin. Transcriptional complexes are transported into the nucleus where transcription and RNA replication take place.

As with all other viruses with negative-sense RNA genomes, the genome of orthomyxoviruses serves two functions; (1) a template for the synthesis of mRNAs and (2) a template for the synthesis of positive-sense replicative intermediate RNA, which serves as template for progeny genomic RNA synthesis. Primary transcription involves a unusual phenomenon known as *cap-snatching:* the viral endonuclease (PB2) cleaves the 5′-methylguanosine cap plus about 10–13 nucleotides from heterogeneous cellular RNAs, and these caps are then used by the virus as primers for transcription by the viral RNA polymerase (transcriptase; PB1). Of the primary RNA transcripts produced from the eight gene segments of influenza A and B viruses, six are monocistronic and are translated directly. The other two undergo splicing, each yielding two mRNAs, which are translated in different reading frames, each producing two proteins. Influenza B virus uses a different strategy, involving alternative translation start sites and reading frames. Viral mRNAs are 3′-polyadenylated and lack the 5′-terminal

Figure 30.3.

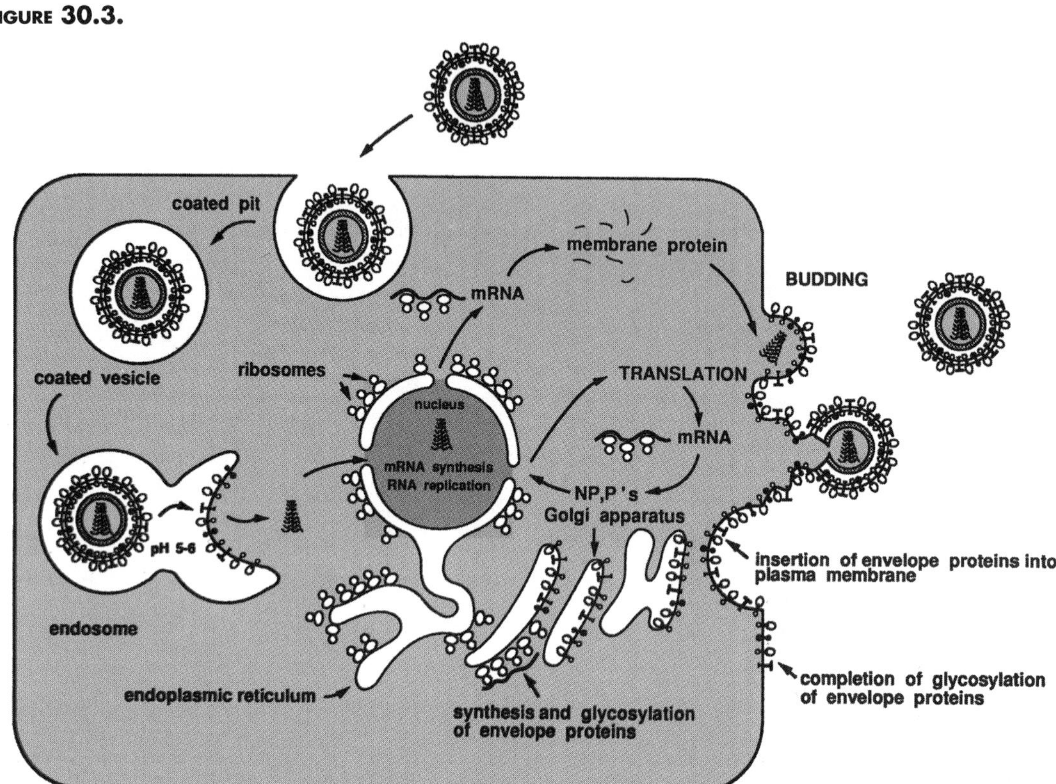

Replication of influenza virus. (1) *Adsorption:* the virus interacts with sialic acid-containing cell receptors via its hemagglutinin and enters via endocytosis. (2) *Fusion and uncoating:* the hemagglutinin undergoes a conformational change mediated by the acid environment of the endosome, which leads to the fusion of viral and cellular membranes. The ribonucleoprotein complexes are then transported into the nucleus. (3) *Transcription and replication:* the viral RNA is transcribed and replicated in the nucleus by the viral RNA polymerase. Two different species of RNA are synthesized from the viral RNA template: (a) full-length, positive-sense replicative intermediate RNAs, which are used by the polymerase to produce virion RNA and (b) mRNAs. (4) *Translation:* the mRNAs are translated in the cytoplasm to form viral proteins. The membrane proteins (the hemagglutinin, neuraminidase, and M2) are transported to the plasma membrane. The viral proteins possessing nuclear signals (PB1, PB2, PA, NP, M1, NS1, and NS2) are transported into the nucleus. (5) *Packaging and budding:* the newly synthesized membrane protein facilitates the transport of nucleocapsids from the nucleus into the cytoplasm, where they interact with viral membrane proteins already inserted into patches in the plasma membrane. Virions bud from the host cell membrane. [From R. A. Lamb, and R. M. Krug. Orthomyxoviridae: The viruses and their replication. *In* "Fields Virology (B. N. Fields, D. M. Knipe, P. M. Howley, R. M. Chanock, J. L. Melnick, T. P. Monath, B. Roizman, and S. E. Straus, eds.), 3rd ed., pp. 1353–1395. Lippincott-Raven, Philadelphia, PA, 1996.]

16 nucleotides of the corresponding genomic RNA segment.

Viral protein synthesis occurs in the cytoplasm using cellular translation machinery. Interestingly, the orthomyxoviruses have evolved several mechanisms to increase their coding capacity: splicing of mRNAs, coupled stop–start translation of tandem genes, and frame shifting. The proteins associated with the virion RNA are transported to the nucleus during the first hours postinfection, then migrate to the cytoplasm.

Replication of genomic RNA segments requires the synthesis of full-length, positive-sense RNA intermediates, which unlike the corresponding mRNA transcripts, must lack 5′-caps and 3′-poly(A) tracts. Newly synthesized nucleoprotein binds to these RNAs, facilitating their use as templates for the synthesis of genomic RNAs. Late in infection, the matrix protein M1 enters the nucleus and binds to nascent genomic RNAs, thereby down-regulating transcription and permitting export from the nucleus and assembly into virions.

Virions are formed by budding, incorporating M protein and nucleocapsids that have aligned below patches on the plasma membrane in which hemagglutinin and neuraminidase have been inserted. It is not known by what mechanism one copy of each RNA segment is incorporated into each virion. One possibility is that the segments are linked loosely by RNA/protein recognition signals. Alternatively, the segments may be packaged almost at random, with most virions encapsidating extra segments to ensure viability. As virions bud, the neuraminidase peplomers facilitate the "pinching off" and release of virions by destroying receptors on

Table 30.1
Properties of Influenza Virus

Four genera: *Influenzavirus A, Influenzavirus B, Influenzavirus C,* and *Thogotovirus*
Virions are pleomorphic, spherical, or filamentous, 80–120 nm in diameter, and consist of an envelope with large peplomers surrounding eight (genera *Influenzavirus A* and *Influenzavirus B*), seven (genus *Influenzavirus C*), or six (genus *Thogotovirus*) helically symmetrical nucleocapsid segments of different sizes
The genome consists of linear negative-sense, single-stranded RNA, divided into eight or seven or six segments, 10–13.6 kb in overall size
There are two kinds of peplomers: rod shaped, consisting of homotrimers of the hemagglutinin glycoprotein, and mushroom shaped, consisting of homotetramers of the neuraminidase protein
Transcription and RNA replication occur in the nucleus; capped 5′-termini of cellular RNAs are cannibalized as primers for mRNA transcription; budding takes place on the plasma membrane
Defective interfering particles and genetic reassortment occur frequently

the plasma membrane that would otherwise recapture virions and hold them at the cell surface. Transmission is by aerosol, droplets, and fomites and is water borne among ducks. Thogoto and Dhori viruses are transmitted by ticks and replicate in both ticks and mammals (Table 30.1).

Equine Influenza

The differentiation of equine influenza from other equine respiratory diseases was established in 1956 when influenza virus A/equine/Prague/1/56 (H7N7) (equine influenza virus 1) was isolated in an epidemic in central Europe and subsequently in the United States; a second virus, A/equine/Miami/1/63 (H3N8) (equine influenza virus 2), was first isolated in 1963. Since then, the disease has been reported in horses and also in donkeys and mules in all parts of the world except Australia, New Zealand, and Iceland. H3N8 virus has been identified in all recent outbreaks; the last outbreak caused by subtype H7N7 virus was in 1979, but antibody has been detected in unvaccinated horses since then, suggesting that the virus still circulates. H3N8 virus has undergone only modest genetic drift since it was first isolated, yet it continues to cause disease and to affect the performance of racehorses.

Clinical Features

In susceptible horses, influenza spreads rapidly and causes disease of high morbidity 24 to 48 hours after infection; the rapid spread is a valuable diagnostic indicator. The clinical signs are due to infection of the respiratory tract: there is reddening of the nasal mucosa, conjunctivitis, and serous, later mucopurulent nasal discharge. The serous nasal discharge develops at the same time as a characteristic harsh, dry paroxysmal cough that may persist for up to 3 weeks. Infected horses develop fever (39.5 to 41°C) lasting for 4 to 5 days and become inappetent and depressed. Mortality is rare, but prolonged fever in pregnant mares may result in abortion. Clinical diagnosis of acute cases is straightforward, but diagnosis in partially immune horses is more difficult, as the disease must be differentiated from other respiratory infections, including those caused by equine herpesviruses 1 and 4, equine adenoviruses, and rhinoviruses. Secondary bacterial infections may occur, characterized by purulent nasal exudates and bronchopneumonia. In the absence of such complications the disease is self-limiting, with complete recovery occurring within 2 to 3 weeks after infection.

Pathogenesis, Pathology, and Immunity

Equine influenza viruses replicate in epithelial cells of the upper and lower respiratory tract. Infection causes inflammation, which leads to serous nasal discharge. The most important changes occur in the lower respiratory tract and include laryngitis, tracheitis, bronchitis, bronchiolitis, and interstitial pneumonia accompanied by congestion and alveolar edema. Myocarditis has been reported rarely. Secondary infections may result in conjunctivitis, pharyngitis, bronchopneumonia, chronic pulmonary disease, guttural pouch infections, purpura, and strangles.

Factors contributing to innate resistance include (1) the mucus blanket that protects the underlying epithelium and the continuous beating of cilia that clears virus from the respiratory tract; (2) soluble lectins, lung surfactants, and sialoglycoproteins present in mucus and transudates that bind virions; and (3) alveolar macrophages.

If the horse has been infected previously, antihemagglutinin antibodies may intercept and neutralize invading virions—secretory IgA is generally believed to be the most relevant antibody, in the upper respiratory tract at least, but serum IgG may provide protection in the lung especially after infection and the inflammatory response have progressed. In laboratory animal models, it has been shown that activated macrophages and natural killer cells, plus two important cytokines, interferon-γ and interleukin-2, as well as immunologically-specific CD4 and CD8 T lymphocytes, are crucial in clearing virus from the lower respiratory tract. Class I-restricted CD8 cytotoxic T cells are most effective in ensuring cross-protection when long-lived memory T cells are reactivated by a new infection caused by a different strain of virus. Class II-restricted $CD4^+$ T cells are important in secreting cytokines that attract and activate macrophages, NK cells, and other T cells.

Laboratory Diagnosis

The best material for viral isolation from horses is nasal mucus taken early in the course of the infection or lung material obtained at necropsy. The viruses replicate well in 10-day-old embryonated eggs, using either the amniotic or the allantoic route of inoculation, and incubating at 35°–37°C for 3 to 4 days. The same may be done in cell culture systems, including chick embryo fibroblasts and the canine kidney cell line, MDCK. Viral replication is detected by the demonstration of hemagglutinating activity in the harvested amniotic or allantoic fluid or cell culture fluid and isolates are identified by hemagglutination–inhibition, using a panel of subtype-specific reference antisera. Retrospective serologic diagnosis can be done using hemagglutination–inhibition and paired serum samples; sera must be suitably treated to eliminate nonspecific inhibitors.

Epidemiology, Prevention, and Control

Equine influenza viruses are highly contagious and are spread rapidly in stables or studs by infectious exudate that is aerosolized by frequent coughing. Virus is excreted during the incubation period and horses remain infectious for at least 5 days after clinical disease begins. Close contact between horses seems to be necessary for rapid transmission; however, contaminated clothing of stable personnel, equipment, and transport vehicles may also contribute to virus distribution. Equine populations that are moved frequently, such as racehorses, breeding stock, show jumpers, and horses sent to sales, are at special risk. The rapid international spread of equine influenza is caused by the year-round transport of horses for racing and breeding purposes between Europe, North America, Japan, Hong Kong, and elsewhere. Although clinical manifestations normally begin in the cold season, epidemics occur mostly during the main racing season, i.e., between April and October in the northern hemisphere.

Apart from one outbreak in China that was derived from an avian source, equids are the only known reservoir of equine influenza viruses; however, that outbreak provides insight into the pathogenic potential of these viruses. In 1989 a severe outbreak of influenza A occurred in horses in northeastern China, with morbidity of 80% and mortality of 20%. In a second outbreak a year later, the morbidity was about 50% and there was no mortality, probably because of the immune status of horses in the region. Of particular interest was the discovery that although the causative virus had the same antigenic composition as viruses circulating among horses in other parts of the world, its genes were of recent avian origin. Serological studies indicated that the virus was not present in China before 1989; thus, it represents the transfer of an avian influenza virus to mammals without reassortment. Of course, predicting the epidemic potential of viruses like this is impossible—only ongoing surveillance can indicate spread.

Control involves isolation and vaccination. Stables and courses where equine influenza outbreaks occur are put under quarantine for at least 4 weeks. After all horses have recovered, cleaning and disinfection of boxes and stables, equipment, and transport vehicles is necessary.

Vaccination is done with inactivated vaccine containing A/equine (H7N7) and A/equine (H3N8) viruses, the latter preferably also including strains to match the prevalent field virus. Oil and polymer-adjuvanted preparations and Quil-A-based immune-stimulating complexes (ISCOMs) have resulted in more durable responses as compared with previous whole virus and subunit vaccines. Vaccine is given in multiple doses according to risk; for example, some racehorses are revaccinated every 3 to 9 months. The 1989 epidemic in Europe highlighted an additional problem: while vaccination reduced the severity of disease, it failed to limit transmission—after many years of genetic stability, antigenic drift had occurred, compromising vaccine efficacy. An effective vaccination policy requires the regular updating of vaccine; however, some vaccine manufacturers have continued to use only prototype strains.

Swine Influenza

Swine influenza was first observed in the north central United States at the time of the catastrophic 1918 pandemic of human influenza, and for a long time was reported only from this area where annual outbreaks occurred each winter. Today, it is one of the most prevalent respiratory diseases in swine in North America. In Europe, the disease was observed in the 1950s in Czechoslovakia, the United Kingdom, and West Germany; then the virus apparently disappeared. It reappeared again in 1976 in northern Italy and spread to Belgium and southern France in 1979; since then it has occurred in Europe rather regularly.

Two distinct variants of swine influenza virus, both H1N1, are presently circulating in the world: (1) the variant found in Europe (except Italy) since 1979 and (2) the variant found in the United States (and Italy) that is similar to classical strains. Swine may also be infected with H3N2 strains, either from humans or birds, but such infections are inapparent. Reassortants have been detected in parts of Japan where both H1N1 and H3N2 strains occur among swine, but so far these have not spread among humans or caused serious disease in swine.

Clinical Features

After an incubation period of 24 to 72 hours, the onset of disease is abrupt, often appearing in many animals in a herd at the same time. There is fever (>42°C), apathy, inappetence, huddling and a reluctance to move, and signs of respiratory distress: paroxysmal coughing, sneezing, rhinitis with nasal discharge, labored breathing, and bronchial rales at auscultation. After 3 to 6 days, swine usually recover quickly, eating normally by 7 days after appearance of the first clinical signs. If sick swine are kept warm and free of stress the course of disease is benign with very few complications and a case-fatality rate of less than 1%, but some animals develop severe bronchopneumonia, which may result in death. Even when they recover, the economic consequences of swine influenza are considerable in that sick swine either lose weight or their weight gains are reduced.

Pathogenesis, Pathology, and Immunity

The infection follows the usual pattern for respiratory infections: viral entry is via aerosol and there is a rapid progression of infection in the epithelium of the nasal, tracheal, and bronchial airways. Infection may progress to involve all airways in just a few hours. Sharply demarcated lung lesions are encountered, mostly in apical and cardiac lobes, with hyperemia, consolidation, and the presence of exudates in airways. Histologically, epithelial surfaces may be totally denuded and the debris of this necrosis may plug small bronchioles. This may progress to alveolar atelectasis, interstitial pneumonia, and emphysema.

Laboratory Diagnosis

Traditionally, the chick embryo was the standard host for cultivation of influenza viruses and is still used in addition to cell culture (MDCK cells) by some reference laboratories. Cytopathology is usually not conspicuous, but growth of virus may be recognized after 3 to 7 days by hemadsorption and the isolate identified immunologically (immunofluorescence or enzyme immunoassay using enzyme-labeled monoclonal antibodies specific for influenza types and subtypes).

Epidemiology, Prevention, and Control

The coincidence of the first swine influenza outbreaks with the 1918 human influenza pandemic has led to suspicion that the causative viruses might be related. Recent phylogenetic studies based on sequence analysis of polymerase chain reaction products from formalin-fixed, paraffin-embedded archival lung tissue from human patients who died during the 1918 pandemic have confirmed that the human virus was related most closely to swine influenza virus. Apart from classical H1N1-like viruses, H3N2 strains also cocirculate in swine populations.

Outbreaks are observed mostly in late fall and winter, after the introduction of new swine into susceptible herds. Frequently the disease appears simultaneously on several farms within an area; outbreaks are explosive, with all swine in a herd becoming sick at the same time. The problem of the interepidemic survival of swine influenza virus has been a matter of intensive investigation for many years, but is still unsolved. Recent investigations suggest that the virus circulates in swine throughout the year and that some swine become carriers, manifesting disease only when the weather becomes colder. Vaccines have been developed, but have not been widely applied. Swine influenza virus also infects turkeys: there can be respiratory disease or a decline in egg production and an increase in the number of abnormal eggs.

Human Disease

Infection of humans with swine influenza virus is relatively common, especially among abattoir workers, and may cause respiratory disease, but cases in other settings are rare and person-to-person spread is limited. However, the fear of another pandemic like that of 1918 has always made human cases the subject of public concern. For example, the isolation of swine influenza virus from military recruits at Fort Dix in the United States in 1976 led to a massive human immunization campaign in the United States.

Avian Influenza

The devastating form of influenza in chickens known as "fowl plague" was recognized as a distinct disease entity as early as 1878. The isolation of an avian influenza virus in 1901 preceded the discovery of mammalian and human influenza viruses, but it was not until 1955 that it was recognized that avian and mammalian influenza viruses are closely related. From the 1970s onward, avian influenza came into ecological focus when surveillance indicated the ubiquitous presence of viruses in waterfowl and the risk these birds pose to commercial chicken industries. A very large epidemic centered in the broiler industry of Pennsylvania in 1983, which cost $61 million to control, brought substance to this risk. A repeat of this kind of epidemic in the commercial broiler industry of Mexico in the 1990s showed that the risk continues.

Clinical Features

The disease caused in chickens and turkeys by highly pathogenic avian influenza viruses has historically been called "fowl plague." Today, the term should be avoided except where it is part of the name of well-characterized strains [e.g., A/fowl plague virus/Dutch/27 (H7N7)]. Highly virulent strains cause sudden death without prodromal symptoms. If birds survive for more than 48 hours (which is more likely in older birds), there is a cessation of egg laying, respiratory distress, lacrimation, sinusitis, diarrhea, edema of the head, face and neck, and cyanosis of unfeathered skin, particularly the comb and wattles. Less virulent viruses may also cause considerable losses, particularly in turkeys, because of anorexia, decreased egg production, respiratory disease, and sinusitis. Clinical signs in chickens and turkeys may be exacerbated greatly by concurrent infections (e.g., Newcastle disease and various bacterial and mycoplasma infections), the use of live-virus vaccines, or environmental stress (e.g., poor ventilation and overcrowding).

Pathogenesis, Pathology, and Immunity

The pathogenic mechanisms responsible for the extraordinary virulence of some avian influenza virus strains and the avirulence of others were unraveled through the outstanding work of Rudolf Rott, Christof Scholtissek, and colleagues at the Faculty of Veterinary Medicine of the Justus Liebig University, Giessen, Germany. They found that although the viral hemagglutinin is of paramount importance in determining virulence, a combination or constellation of genes contributes, including the nucleoprotein and polymerase genes.

Virions with uncleaved hemagglutinin are noninfectious. Hemagglutinin cleavability is dependent on its primary structure at the site where cleavage occurs and the presence of the right proteases in target tissues that can carry out that cleavage. In epithelial cells lining the respiratory and intestinal tracts, the hemagglutinin of all incoming avian influenza viruses is cleaved by host proteases, thereby activating its fusion activity and allowing its entry; however, in other tissues, only the hemagglutinin of virulent viruses is cleaved, leading to systemic disease and death. This phenomenon accounts not only for viral strain differences but also for the susceptibility or resistance of different avian species. For example, A/chicken/Scotland/59 (H5N1) virus is more virulent for chickens whereas A/turkey/Ontario/7732/66 (H5N9) virus is more virulent for turkeys. In nature, ducks are refractory to even the most virulent viruses.

The pathogenesis of avian influenza is quite different from that in mammals in that viral replication occurs in the intestinal tract as well as the respiratory tract. In infections with the most virulent strains there is viremia and multifocal lymphoid and visceral necrosis, leading to pancreatitis, myocarditis, myositis, and encephalitis. Chickens and turkeys succumbing after several days of illness exhibit petechial hemorrhages and serous exudates in respiratory, digestive, and cardiac tissues. Turkeys may also have air sacculitis and pulmonary congestion. In all avian species, neutralizing antibodies are detectable within 3 to 7 days after the onset of disease, reaching a peak during the second week and persisting for up to 18 months.

Laboratory Diagnosis

Clinical diagnosis is usually not possible except in an epidemic because of the variability of clinical signs. Virus isolation is essential not only to establish the cause of an outbreak but to assess objectively the virulence of the causative virus. Virus is best isolated from cloacal swabs; specimens are inoculated into the allantoic cavity of 8- to 10-day-old embryonated eggs and the presence of virus is indicated by hemagglutinating activity using allantoic fluid and chicken red blood cells. Isolates are roughly identified using hemagglutination–inhibition, enzyme immunoassay, or single radial diffusion and broadly reactive antisera. Finally, isolates may be typed and subtyped using hemagglutination– and neuraminidase–inhibition assays; due to antigenic drift, a broad range of antisera is used in reference laboratories. To assess the virulence of isolates, intracerebral and intravenous pathogenicity indices are determined using 1 day-old chicks and 6-week-old chickens, respectively. The cleavability of the hemagglutinin of isolates is assessed by the production of plaques in cell cultures that are permissive for virulent viruses but not permissive for avirulent viruses.

Epidemiology, Prevention, and Control

Avian influenza virus is shed in high concentrations in the feces and survives for long periods, especially in water at low temperature. The virus is introduced into susceptible flocks periodically by interspecies transmission, i.e., between chickens and turkeys and from wild birds, especially wild ducks. Influenza in turkeys is seen principally in countries where they are raised in facilities where wild birds have access.

It is unclear how all of the subtypes of avian influenza A viruses are maintained in wild birds from year to year; it is hypothesized that the viruses are maintained by circulation at low levels in large wild bird populations even during migration and overwintering. Studies of wild ducks in Canada have shown that up to 20% of juvenile birds are already infected silently as they congregate prior to their southern migration. Avian influenza viruses have also been isolated in many countries from imported caged birds. The epidemiologic importance of live bird markets should not be underestimated: a H5N2 virus similar to that responsible for the epidemic in chickens in Pennsylvania in 1983 reappeared later in caged bird markets in New York City.

Avian influenza control activities operate at international, national, and local levels:

1. At the international level, countries must be willing to report disease outbreaks. The "fowl plague" form of avian influenza appears in list A of the International Animal Health Code of the Office International des Épizooties; the disease is thereby notifiable and restrictions apply to the movement of birds or avian products. In addition, the code defines freedom from fowl plague. Of course the success of international oversight depends on the willingness of countries to report outbreaks.

2. At the national level, many countries have regulations aimed at preventing the introduction and spread of virus; these regulations are often primarily concerned with Newcastle disease. Policies usually involve trade embargoes to guard against importation of infected birds or avian products from countries not declared "virus free." In the United States, Australia, and most European countries, virulent avian influenza virus is handled as an exotic pathogen: once diagnosed, quarantine and removal programs are implemented. To minimize secondary spread, strict hygienic measures are required, which include cleaning and disinfection, an interval between slaughter and repopulation, and controlled movement of humans and animals.

3. At the local farm-based level, efforts are aimed at preventing virus introduction into chicken and turkey flocks from wild birds. Today, commercial chicken facilities are always made wild bird proof but turkeys are often still raised in the open.

Vaccination has not been used to control outbreaks in most developed countries because of traditional conservatism and problems pertaining to international trade. In fact, the real potential of vaccination has not really been tested: criticisms leveled at vaccines in the past, such as failure to prevent shedding and transmission, failure to match the antigenic profile of current viral variants, high cost, and failure to be able to adequately measure vaccine potency and efficacy, still prevail. Potency, efficacy, safety, and practicality have not been assessed for any product based on modern vaccine design strategy. Nonetheless, in the epidemic that swept the commercial broiler industry of Mexico in the early 1990s, conventional vaccines were used and after potency assays were standardized they proved very valuable.

Human Disease

It is now clear that avian influenza viruses are zoonotic. After a massive epidemic in chickens in China in 1997, a child who had contact with pet chickens died in Hong Kong with influenza-like clinical signs. An H5N1 virus subtype, previously known to occur only in birds, was isolated at autopsy. Within a short time additional cases were reported and by the time the episode ended in early 1998 there were 18 confirmed cases, many of which involved severe disease and 6 of which were fatal.

Epidemiological investigations indicated that there was widespread transmission in the area among chickens, ducks, and geese. Investigations also showed that there was some human-to-human transmission, but most human infections occurred through contact with infected chickens. Surveillance in the area was increased, all 1.2 million chickens in Hong Kong were slaughtered, premises were disinfected, and strategies were developed for production of a human vaccine.

The hemagglutinin of the virus was found to contain multiple basic amino acids adjacent to its cleavage site and an insert at the same site, a feature characteristic of highly pathogenic avian influenza A viruses; experimentally, the virus was found to be highly pathogenic for chickens. The fact that the virus remained lethal to chickens even after it had passed through a human raised the possibility that a few infected people traveling beyond Hong Kong could spread this virus to chickens in other countries—intense surveillance of poultry flocks at possible risk was initiated quickly.

Further Reading

Alexander, D. J. (1993). Orthomyxovirus infection. *In* "Virus Infections of Vertebrates" (J. B. McFerran and M. S. McNulty, eds.), Vol. 4, pp. 287–316. Elsevier, Amsterdam.

Bachmann, P. A. (1989). Swine influenza virus. *In* "Virus Infections of Vertebrates" (M. B. Pensaert, ed.), Vol. 2, pp. 193–207. Elsevier, Amsterdam.

Easterday, B. C., Hinshaw, V. S., and Halvorson, D. A. (1997). Influenza. *In* "Diseases of Poultry" (B. W. Calnek, ed.), 10th ed., pp. 583–589. Iowa State University Press, Ames.

Klenk, H.-D., and Rott, R. (1988). The molecular biology of influenza virus pathogenicity. *Adv. Virus Res.* **34**, 247–282.

Lamb, R. A., and Krug, R. M. (1996). Orthomyxoviridae: The viruses and their replication. *In* "Fields Virology" (B. N. Fields, D. M. Knipe, P. M. Howley, R. M. Chanock, J. L. Melnick, T. P. Monath, B. Roizman, and S. E. Straus, eds.), 3rd ed., pp. 1353–1395. Lippincott-Raven, Philadelphia, PA.

Mumford, J. A., and Hannant, D. (1996). Equine influenza. *In* "Virus Infections of Vertebrates" (M. J. Studdert, ed.), Vol. 6, pp. 285–293. Elsevier, Amsterdam.

Mumford, J. A., Jessett, D., Dunleavy, U., Wood, J., Hannant, D., Sundquist, B. and Cook, R. F. (1994). Antigenicity and immunogenicity of experimental equine influenza ISCOM vaccines. *Vaccine* **12**, 857–863.

Murphy, B. R., and Webster, R. G. (1996). Orthomyxoviruses. *In* "Fields Virology" (B. N. Fields, D. M. Knipe, P. M. Howley, R. M. Chanock, J. L. Melnick, T. P. Monath, B. Roizman, and S. E. Straus, eds.), 3rd ed., pp. 1397–1446. Lippincott-Raven, Philadelphia, PA.

Webster, R. G., and Kawaoka, Y. (1994). Influenza—an emerging and re-emerging disease. *Semin. Virol.* **5**, 103–111.

CHAPTER 31

Bunyaviridae

The family *Bunyaviridae* is the largest virus family, with more than 350 member viruses. The common features of the viruses pertain both to the nature of the virions and to their biological properties. Nearly all of the viruses are arboviruses, maintained in arthropod–vertebrate–arthropod cycles, which have great specificity in regard to both arthropod vectors and vertebrate reservoir hosts. This specificity is the basis for the usually narrow geographic and ecologic niches occupied by each virus. The important exception is the hantaviruses, which are transmitted in vertebrate–vertebrate cycles without arthropod vectors; still, the hantaviruses also exhibit great specificity in vertebrate reservoir hosts and therefore also have narrow geographic and ecologic niches.

Particular bunyaviruses are transmitted by specific mosquitoes, ticks, culicoides, or flies and particular hantaviruses by specific rodents. The viruses cause transient infection in their vertebrate hosts, whether this be a mammal or bird, and lifelong persistent infection in their arthropod vectors—again, hantaviruses are exceptional in that infection in their rodent reservoir hosts is persistent and often lifelong. Most bunyaviruses never infect domestic animals or humans, but those that do cause important diseases, varying from encephalitis to hepatitis, nephritis, acute respiratory distress syndrome, and undifferentiated multiorgan syndromes. Three important zoonotic bunyaviruses, Rift Valley fever virus, Crimean-Congo hemorrhagic fever virus, and Nairobi sheep disease virus, command particular attention from national and international disease control agencies. These viruses are restricted to certain national laboratories for all research and diagnostic procedures; they are Biosafety Level 4 pathogens and must be handled in the laboratory only under maximum containment conditions to prevent human exposure.

Properties of Bunyaviruses

Classification

The very large number and diversity of the bunyaviruses offer a taxonomic challenge. Genomic features are used to define genera, particularly the organization of each RNA genome segment and the sequences of conserved nucleotides at the termini of each segment. Classical serological methods are used to define serogroups within each genus. In general, antigenic determinants on the nucleocapsid protein are rather conserved and so serve to define broad groupings among the viruses, whereas shared epitopes on the envelope glycoproteins, which are the targets in neutralization and hemagglutination–inhibition assays, define narrow groupings. Unique epitopes on envelope glycoproteins, also determined by neutralization assays, define individual viruses. With few exceptions, viruses within a given genus are related antigenically to each other but not to viruses in other genera.

Genetic reassortment occurs when cultured cells or mosquitoes are coinfected with closely related bunyaviruses and this has probably played some part in the evolution of the family in nature. Within its particular ecologic niche, each bunyavirus evolves by genetic drift and Darwinian selective forces; for example, isolates of La Crosse virus from different regions in the United States differ considerably due to cumulative point mutations and nucleotide deletions and duplications, such mutations are stabilized by niche isolation. The evolution of La Crosse virus has also involved genome segment reassortment—reassortant viruses have been isolated from mosquitoes in the field.

The more than 350 distinct bunyaviruses are grouped into more than 30 serogroups, which in turn fall into four genera of interest (a fifth genus, *Tospovirus*, contains plant viruses). Additionally, more than 80 viruses have not yet been assigned to a genus or serogroup (Table 31.1).

Genus *Bunyavirus* contains 18 serogroups and at least 160 viruses, most of which are mosquito borne, but some of which are transmitted by sandflies or *Culicoides* spp. The genus includes more than 30 pathogens of domestic animals and humans, including Akabane, Cache Valley, La Crosse, Bunyamwera, and Oropouche viruses.

Genus *Hantavirus* contains 22 viruses, many of which have been discovered just in the past few years. All are transmitted by persistently infected reservoir rodent hosts via urine, feces, and saliva; the same transmission pattern has occurred among rats in laboratory colonies. In humans, several of these viruses cause hemorrhagic fever with renal syndrome whereas others cause acute respiratory distress syndrome (hantavirus pulmonary syndrome).

Genus *Phlebovirus* contains two serogroups (and many serologic subgroups) and at least 50 viruses, all of which are transmitted by sandflies or mosquitoes. The genus contains important pathogens, including Rift Valley fever virus and the sandfly fever viruses.

Genus *Nairovirus* contains seven serogroups and at least 33 viruses, nearly all of which are tick borne, including the pathogens Nairobi sheep disease, Crimean-Congo hemorrhagic fever, and Dugbe viruses.

Virion Properties

Bunyavirus virions are spherical, approximately 80–120 nm in diameter, and are composed of an envelope with glycoprotein peplomers inside of which there are three circular, helical nucleocapsid segments (Figure 31.1). Nucleocapsid circles are formed by panhandles, i.e., non-

TABLE 31.1
Family *Bunyaviridae*: Pathogens of Animals and Humans

GENUS	VIRUS	GEOGRAPHIC DISTRIBUTION	ARTHROPOD VECTOR	TARGET HOST SPECIES OR AMPLIFIER HOST	DISEASE IN ANIMALS	DISEASE IN HUMANS
Phlebovirus	Rift Valley fever virus	Africa	Mosquitoes	Sheep, cattle, buffalo, humans	Systemic disease, hepatitis, abortion	Flu-like illness, hepatitis, hemorrhagic fever, retinitis
Nairovirus	Nairobi sheep disease virus	Eastern Africa	Mosquitoes	Sheep, goats, humans	Hemorrhagic enteritis	Hepatitis, hemorrhagic fever
	Crimean-Congo hemorrhagic fever virus	Africa, Asia	Ticks	Sheep, cattle, goats, humans	Nil-zoonosis	Hemorrhagic fever, hepatitis
Bunyavirus	Akabane virus	Australia, Japan, Israel, Africa	Mosquitoes	Cattle, sheep	Arthrogryposis, hydranencephaly	None
	Cache Valley virus	United States	Mosquitoes	Cattle, sheep	Arthrogryposis hydranencephaly rarely	Very rarely congenital infection
	La Crosse and other California encephalitis group viruses	North America	Mosquitoes	Mammals, humans	Nil-zoonosis	Encephalitis
Hantavirus (see Table 31.3)						

FIGURE 31.1.

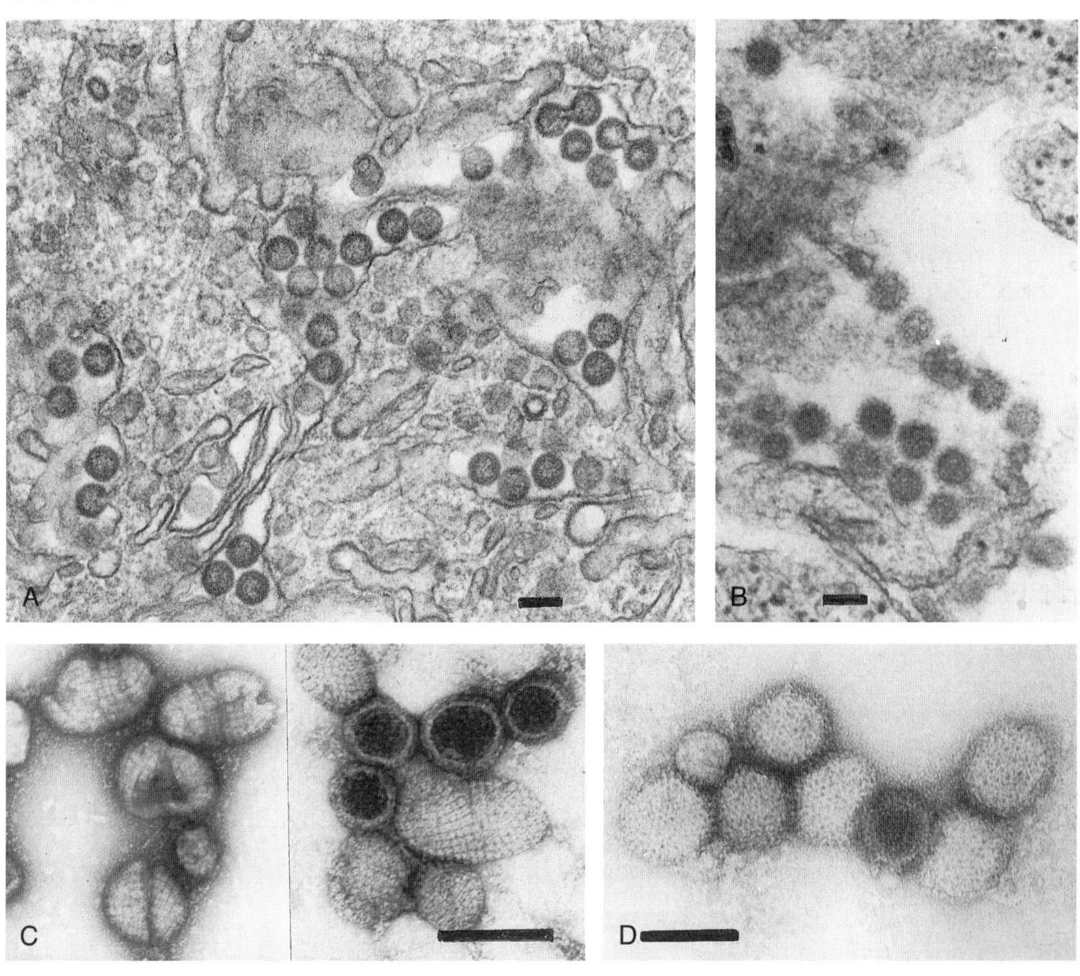

Family *Bunyaviridae*. (A) Hepatocyte of a rat infected with Rift Valley fever virus showing virions budding in Golgi vesicles. (B) Thin section of mouse brain infected with California encephalitis virus showing extracellular virions. (C) Negatively stained Hantaan virus virions showing the pattern of peplomer placement in squares that is characteristic of all hantaviruses. (D) Negatively stained Rift Valley fever virus virions showing the delicate peplomer fringe, Bars: 100 nm. (A, courtesy of T. W. Geisbert; C and D, courtesy of E. L. Palmer and J. M. Dalrymple.)

covalent bonds between palindromic sequences on the 3′ and 5′ ends of each RNA genome segment. The terminal sequences are identical for all three RNA segments for all members of each genus, but they differ among the genera.

The genome consists of three segments of negative-sense (or ambisense), single-stranded RNA, designated large (L), medium (M), and small (S). The RNA segments differ in size among the genera: the L RNA segment ranges in size from 6.3 to 12 kb, the M RNA segment from 3.5 to 6 kb, and the S RNA segment from 1 to 2.2 kb. Complete (or M and S segment) nucleotide sequences have been determined for many viruses, including representative viruses of each genus.

The L RNA encodes a single large protein, the RNA-dependent RNA polymerase (transcriptase). The M RNA encodes a polyprotein that is processed to form two glycoproteins (G1 and G2) and a nonstructural protein (NSm). The S RNA encodes the nucleocapsid (N) protein and a nonstructural (NSs) protein—its translation strategy differs among the genera. In the genera *Bunyavirus* and *Phlebovirus* the S RNA encodes two overlapping reading frames for the N and NSs proteins, but in the genera *Nairovirus* and *Hantavirus* the S RNA encodes only one open reading frame; the N and NSs proteins are formed by cotranslational processing (Figure 31.2).

An exception to the usual coding strategy of negative-sense RNA viruses occurs in the S RNA of the mem-

Figure 31.2.

Bunyavirus, Hantavirus, Phlebovirus, Nairovirus: L Genome Segment

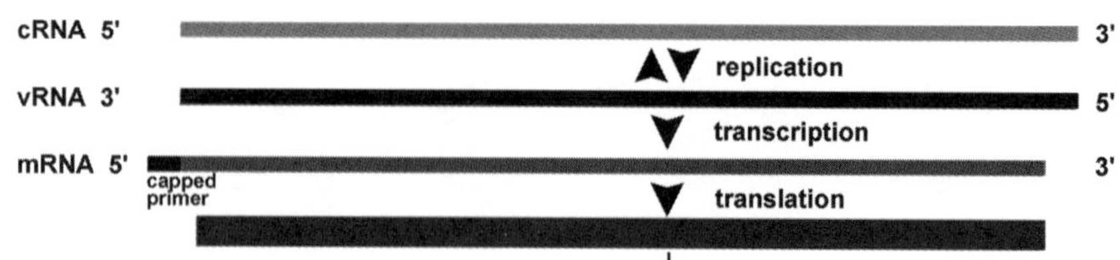

Bunyavirus, Hantavirus, Phlebovirus, Nairovirus: M Genome Segment

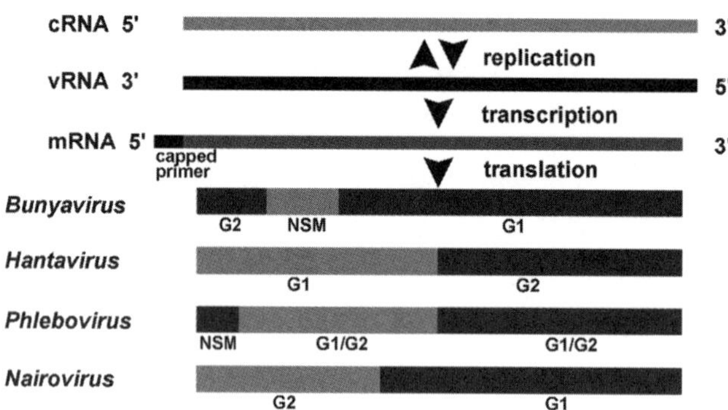

Bunyavirus, Hantavirus, Nairovirus: S Genome Segment

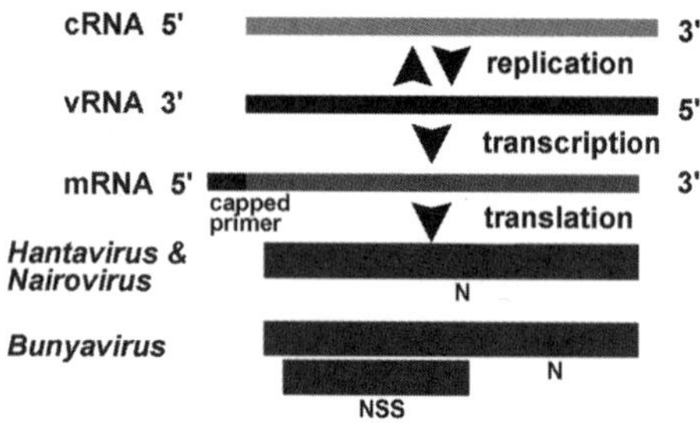

Phlebovirus: S Genome Segment

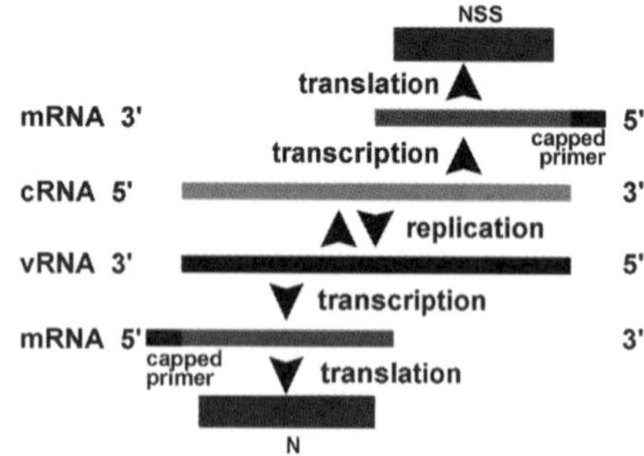

Coding, transcription, translation, and replication strategies employed in the various genera of the family *Bunyaviridae*. Most of the steps are typical of other negative-sense RNA viruses, but a unique sequence of events is necessary to obtain viral proteins from the ambisense S segment of the phlebovirus genome (see text): (1) first, the open reading frame at the 3′ end of the phlebovirus genomic S segment is transcribed (from its 3′ end) by the viral RNA-dependent RNA polymerase (transcriptase) to produce a subgenomic mRNA of complementary sense that is capped at its 5′-terminus by a primer obtained from cellular mRNAs (viral cap snatching); (2) this mRNA is translated into the nucleoprotein (N); (3) genomic replication produces full-length, complementary-sense RNA (cRNA); (4) the open reading frame in the complementary-sense RNA then serves as a template for transcription, from its 3′ end, of mRNA that is translated to produce the nonstructural protein (NSs). [Adapted from C. S. Schmaljohn, Bunyaviridae: the viruses and their replication. *In* "Fields Virology" (B. N. Fields, D. M. Knipe, P. M. Howley, R. M. Chanock, J. L. Melnick, T. P. Monath, B. Roizman, and S. E. Straus, eds.), 3rd ed., pp. 1447–1471. Lippincott-Raven, Philadelphia, PA, 1996.]

ber viruses of the genus *Phlebovirus*. The S RNA encodes the N and NSs proteins, each translated from a separate subgenomic mRNA. The N protein is encoded in the 3′ half of the S RNA, as usual its mRNA is transcribed using genomic RNA as template; however, the NSs protein, occupying the 5′ half of the same S RNA, is encoded in the complementary-sense RNA species and is translated only after the synthesis of full-length RNA intermediates—the S RNA is therefore said to exhibit an *ambisense* coding strategy.

The four major virion proteins differ in size among the genera: the L protein [the RNA-dependent RNA polymerase (transcriptase)] has an M_r of 150,000 to 200,000, the N protein (nucleoprotein) has an M_r of 25,000 to 50,000 and G1 and G2, the two glycoproteins have M_r values of 40,000 to 120,000. Virions also contain lipids, with their composition reflecting the composition of host cell membranes and carbohydrates as side chains on the glycoproteins.

The viruses are quite sensitive to heat and acid conditions and are inactivated readily by detergents, lipid solvents, and common disinfectants.

Viral Replication

Bunyaviruses replicate well in many kinds of cells: Vero E6 (African green monkey) cells, BHK-21 (baby hamster kidney) cells, and mosquito (*Aedes albopictus*) cells. Hantaviruses do not replicate in mosquito cells. The viruses are cytolytic for mammalian cells (except for hantaviruses and some nairoviruses), but are noncytolytic for invertebrate cells. Most of the viruses also replicate to high titer in suckling mouse brain.

Viral entry into its host cell is by receptor-mediated endocytosis; all subsequent steps take place in the cytoplasm. Because the genome of the single-stranded, negative-sense RNA viruses cannot be translated directly, the first step after penetration of the host cell and uncoating is the activation of the virion RNA polymerase (transcriptase) and its transcription of viral mRNAs from each of the three virion RNAs (the exception, as noted earlier, is that in the genus *Phlebovirus* the 5′ half of the S RNA is not transcribed directly; instead, the mRNA for the NSs protein is transcribed following synthesis of full-length complementary RNA). The RNA polymerase also has endonuclease activity, cleaving 5′-methylated caps from host mRNAs and adding these to viral mRNAs to prime transcription (this is called cap snatching). After primary viral mRNA transcription and translation, replication of the virion RNA occurs and a second round of transcription begins, amplifying in particular structural proteins for virion synthesis.

Virions mature by budding through intracytoplasmic vesicles associated with the Golgi complex and are released by the transport of vesicles through the cytoplasm and release by exocytosis from the basolateral plasma membrane (Table 31.2).

Rift Valley Fever

Rift Valley fever virus, a member of the genus *Phlebovirus*, is one of the most important veterinary pathogens in the world—it has great potential to cause lethal epidemic disease in sheep and cattle far beyond its usual habitat in sub-Saharan Africa and great potential to cause severe human disease in such epidemics.

Table 31.2
Properties of Bunyaviruses

Four genera infect vertebrates: *Bunyavirus*, *Phlebovirus*, and *Nairovirus*, all arthropod-borne; *Hantavirus*, nonarthropod-borne
Virions are spherical, enveloped, 80–100 nm in diamter
Virions have glycoprotein peplomers but no matrix protein in their envelope
Three nucleocapsid segments with helical symmetry
Segmented negative-sense, single-stranded RNA genome; three segments: L, 6.3 to 12 kb; M, 3.5 to 6 kb; and S, 1 to 2.2 kb in size
The S segment of the genomic RNA of the member viruses of the genus *Phlebovirus* has an *ambisense* coding strategy
Capped 5′-termini of cellular RNAs cannibalized as primers for mRNA transcription
Cytoplasmic replication; budding into Golgi vesicles
Generally cytocidal for vertebrate cells but noncytocidal persistent infection in invertebrate cells
Genetic reassortment occurs between closely related viruses

Clinical Features

Infected sheep develop fever, inappetence, mucopurulent nasal discharge, and bloody diarrhea. Under field conditions, 90–100% of pregnant ewes abort ("abortion storm") and there is a mortality rate of 90% in lambs and 20–60% in adult sheep. The clinical disease and outcome are similar in goats. In cattle the disease is somewhat less severe, with mortality rates in calves and cows of 10–30%, but again, 90–100% of pregnant cows abort.

Pathogenesis, Pathology, and Immunity

Rift Valley fever virus is one of the most prolific viruses known—in its target tissues it replicates very quickly and to very high titer. After entry by mosquito bite or through the oropharynx, there is an incubation period of 30 to 72 hours, during which virus invades the parenchyma of the liver and reticuloendothelial organs, leading to widespread severe cytopathology. At necropsy of terminally affected sheep, it is not uncommon to find nearly total hepatocellular destruction. The spleen is enlarged and there are gastrointestinal and subserosal hemorrhages. Encephalitis, evidenced by neuronal necrosis and perivascular inflammatory infiltration, is a late event, seen in a small proportion of animals surviving the hepatic infection. In sheep, hepatic necrosis and hemorrhagic complications are the primary cause of death. In survivors, recovery is rapid and immunity is long-lasting. Experimentally, the virus infects a wide variety of laboratory and domestic animals and is often lethal. In experimentally infected animals the two most frequent syndromes are hepatitis and encephalitis.

Laboratory Diagnosis

Because of its broad geographic distribution and its explosive potential for invading new areas where livestock husbandry is extensive, the laboratory confirmation of the presence of Rift Valley fever virus is treated as a diagnostic emergency. Diagnosis depends on virus isolation in mice or in cell culture. The virus replicates in a variety of cell cultures such as Vero E6 (African green monkey) and BHK-21 (baby hamster kidney) cells—the virus is rapidly cytopathic and causes plaques. Immunologic methods are used to prove the identity of isolates. Serologic diagnosis is done by IgM capture enzyme immunoassay on single acute sera or by usual enzyme immunoassays, neutralization, or hemagglutination–inhibition assays on paired sera from surviving animals. Veterinarians and field and laboratory workers need to exercise caution to not become infected during postmortem examination of animals or processing diagnostic materials in the laboratory. There is an inactivated vaccine available for laboratory and field workers at high risk of infection.

Epidemiology, Prevention, and Control

Epidemics in sheep, goats, and cattle have been recognized in southern and eastern African countries from the time when intensive livestock husbandry was introduced at the beginning of the 20th century. Between 1950 and 1976 there were at least 16 major epidemics in livestock at various places in sub-Saharan Africa. An exceptionally devastating epidemic occurred in Egypt in 1977 and 1978, resembling the biblical description of one of the plagues of ancient Egypt. There were many hundreds of thousands of cases in sheep and cattle and more than 200,000 human cases with 600 deaths. The extent and severity of this epidemic may have been due to the high population densities of fully susceptible animals and humans. In 1988–1989, further virus activity was detected in eastern Africa and in western Africa, with hundreds of human deaths in Senegal and Mauritania. In 1993, epidemic Rift Valley fever returned to Egypt—molecular epidemiologic studies suggest that the virus was reintroduced from an unknown habitat in the Sudan.

In late 1997 and 1998 a major epidemic spread from Somalia through Kenya into Tanzania, causing the death of many thousands of sheep, goats, and camels. By March of 1998 there had been more than 90,000 human cases and more than 500 deaths. This epidemic, considered the largest ever seen in eastern Africa, was blamed on exceptional rainfall as a result of an El Nino weather pattern.

In eastern, western, and southern Africa, Rift Valley fever virus survives in a minimally evident endemic cycle for years; then, when there is a period of exceptionally heavy rainfall, the virus explodes in epidemics of great magnitude. Although such epidemics had been studied for many years, it was not until the late 1980s that the mechanism of this phenomenon was discovered. It was found that the virus is transmitted transovarially among floodwater *Aedes* spp. mosquitoes; the virus survives for very long periods in mosquito eggs laid at the edges of usually dry depressions, called "dambos," which are common throughout grassy plateau regions. When the rains come and these dambos flood, the eggs hatch and infected mosquitoes emerge and infect nearby wild and domestic animals. This discovery involved one of the first successful applications of satellite remote sensing and geographic information system technology.

In an epidemic, virus is amplified in wild and domestic animal populations by many species of *Culex* spp. and other *Aedes* spp. mosquitoes. These mosquitoes become very numerous after heavy rains or when improper irrigation techniques are used; they feed indiscriminately on viremic sheep and cattle (and humans). A very high level of viremia is maintained for 3 to 5 days in infected sheep and cattle, allowing many mosquitoes to become infected. This amplification, together with mechanical transmission by biting flies, results in infection and disease in a very high proportion of animals (and humans) at risk. In its epidemic cycles, Rift Valley fever virus is also spread mechanically by fomites and by blood and tissues of infected animals. Infected sheep have a very high level of viremia and transmission at the time of abortion via contaminated placentae and fetal and maternal blood is a particular problem. Abattoir workers and veterinarians (especially those performing necropsies) are often infected directly.

The capacity of Rift Valley fever virus to be transmitted without the involvement of an arthropod vector raises concerns over the possibility for its importation into nonendemic areas via contaminated materials, animal products, viremic humans, or nonlivestock animal species. Although the virus has never appeared outside Africa, it poses a great threat to the Tigris-Euphrates basin, other areas of the Middle East, and everywhere else where livestock are raised. As was the case in Egypt in 1977–1978 and more recently, many mosquito species capable of efficient virus transmission are present in most of the livestock-producing areas of the world; for example, experimental mosquito transmission studies have shown that more than 30 common mosquitoes in the United States could serve as efficient vectors.

Control is based primarily on livestock vaccination, but vector control (via mosquito larvicide and insecticide use) and environmental management play roles too: agricultural development projects in Africa must take into account the danger of creating new larval habitats (water impoundments, artificial dambos).

Vaccination

Attenuated virus Rift Valley fever vaccines for use in sheep, produced in mouse brain and in embryonated eggs, are effective and inexpensive, but they cause abortions in pregnant ewes. Inactivated virus vaccines produced in cell cultures avoid the problem of abortion, but are expensive. Both types of vaccines have been produced in Africa in large quantities, but to be effective vaccines must be delivered in a systematic way to entire animal populations, preferably on a regular schedule before the start of the mosquito season or at least at the first indications of viral activity (as determined by sentinel surveillance). However, after an epidemic has been detected, viral movement is so rapid that it is difficult to administer enough vaccine fast enough. Even when vaccine is delivered quickly, there is often not enough time for protective immunity to develop. Thus, disease control is expensive, rather ineffective, and very demanding in terms of fiscal and human resources—these realities have led to resistance to vaccination among farmers and ranchers in most areas of southern Africa. Because of the great risk of introduction of the virus outside Africa, veterinary vaccine should be stockpiled, but this has not been done in any developed country.

Vector Control

Mosquito larvicide and insecticide use is virtually impossible in most areas of Africa—the involvement in epidemics of a wide range of vector species with different habits and econiche preferences, the usual wide geographic distribution of epidemics, and the need to intervene throughout long vector breeding seasons contribute to this reality. However, vector control would be a major element in control programs were the virus to be introduced outside Africa.

Human Disease

Rift Valley fever virus is zoonotic and causes an important human disease that occurs coincidentally with outbreaks in sheep, cattle, and camels. The human disease begins after a very short incubation period (2 to 6 days) with fever, severe headache, chills, "back-breaking" myalgia, diarrhea, vomiting, and hemorrhages. Usually the clinical disease lasts 4 to 6 days, followed by a prolonged convalescence and complete recovery. A small percentage of infected humans develop more severe disease, with liver necrosis, hemorrhagic pneumonia, meningoencephalitis, and retinitis with vision loss. The case-fatality rate is about 1–2%, but in patients with hemorrhagic disease, it may reach 10%. Prevention of disease in humans at particular risk, such as veterinarians and livestock and abattoir workers, can be achieved with vaccine. An improved inactivated virus vaccine has been produced by the U.S. Army, but it has not been commercialized and supplies are limited.

Biohazard: Rift Valley fever virus is a restricted animal pathogen and its importation or possession is prohibited by law or regulation by most national governments. The virus is restricted to certain national laboratories for all research and diagnostic procedures; the virus is a Biosafety Level 4 pathogen; it must be handled in the laboratory under maximum containment conditions to prevent human exposure.

Akabane Disease (Arthrogryposis-Hydranencephaly)

Seasonally, in some years, in Australia, Japan, and Israel, there are epidemics in cattle of fetal or newborn arthrogryposis and hydranencephaly, abortions, and fetal death caused by Akabane virus, a mosquito- and *Culicoides*-borne member of the Simbu serogroup in the genus *Bunyavirus*. The virus can cause the same disease in sheep and goats. Evidence shows that the virus is also present in other countries of the southwest Pacific region and in Turkey, Kenya, and South Africa. A less common related virus, Aino virus, is known to cause similar disease in the same areas. In the United States, outbreaks of arthrogryposis-hydranencephaly in sheep have been associated with another related virus, Cache Valley virus.

Clinical Features

Bovine fetuses infected early in pregnancy (second trimester) are often born with rigid fixation of the limbs, usually in flexion due to a loss of spinal motor neurons—this is called arthrogryposis. They also exhibit neurogenic torticollis, kyphosis, and scoliosis. Fetuses infected earlier (late first trimester) often die shortly after birth, and those that survive exhibit sensory, motor, and optical nerve damage.

Pathogenesis, Pathology, and Immunity

Following the bite of an infected mosquito, the virus infects the pregnant cow without producing clinical signs and reaches the fetus from the maternal circulation. The primary fetal infection is an encephalomyelitis and polymyositis. Severely affected fetuses usually die and are aborted; survivors often develop large cavitations of the cerebrum, hydranencephaly, and neurogenic arthrogryposis (Figure 31.3).

Laboratory Diagnosis

Diagnosis may be suggested by clinical, pathologic, and epidemiologic observations, but most often by gross pathologic examination. Diagnosis is confirmed by the detection of a specific neutralizing antibody in serum taken from aborted fetuses or from newborn calves before suckling. Alternatively, diagnosis may be made by detecting a titer rise between paired maternal sera. Virus is difficult to isolate after calves are born, but can be recovered from the placenta or fetal brain or muscle of calves taken by cesarean section or after slaughter of the dam. Virus isolation is done in cell cultures or by intracerebral inoculation of suckling mice.

Epidemiology, Prevention, and Control

In Japan, Akabane virus is transmitted by *Aedes* spp. and *Culex* spp. mosquitoes, and in Australia by the midge,

FIGURE 31.3.

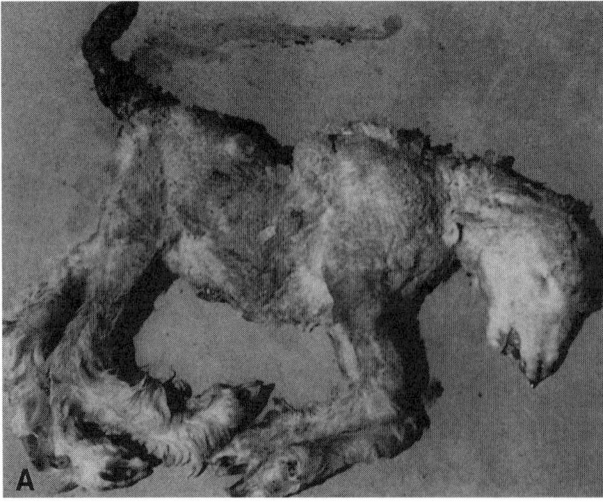

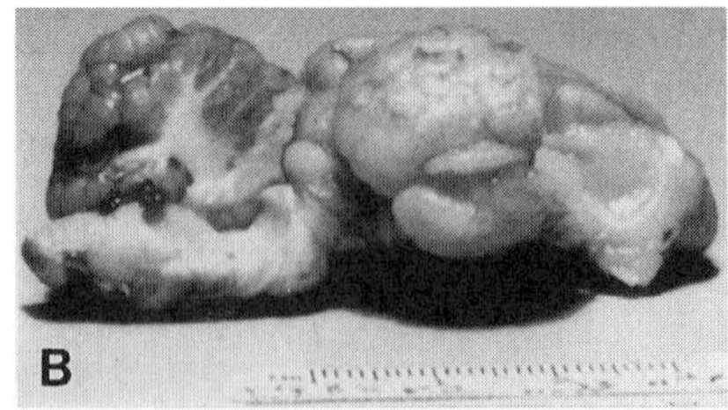

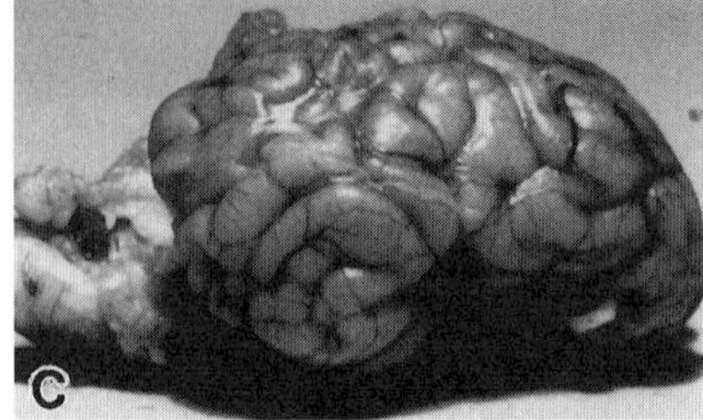

Akabane virus infection. (A) Arthrogryposis in a lamb born during an outbreak of Akabane infection in Australia. (B) Microencephaly involving mainly the cerebral hemispheres. (C) Normal brain for comparison with B (part of the cerebellum has been removed). (C, Courtesy of I. M. Parsonson.)

Culicoides brevitarsis. An inactivated virus vaccine produced in cell culture has proved safe and efficacious and is used widely in Japan and Australia.

Nairobi Sheep Disease

Nairobi sheep disease virus, a member of the genus *Nairovirus,* is possibly the most pathogenic virus known for sheep and goats. It is endemic in eastern Africa and related viruses occur in Nigeria (Dugbe virus in cattle) and India (Ganjam virus in sheep and goats). The virus is transmitted by all stages of the brown ear tick, *Rhipicephalus appendiculatus,* in which there is transovarial and transstadial infection and very long-term carriage in adult ticks (up to 2 years). The vertebrate reservoir host of the virus remains unknown; the virus has not been found in wild ruminants or other animals in endemic areas.

In Kenya, sheep and goats acquire the infection when they are transported from northern districts to the Nairobi area. After a short incubation period there is high fever, hemorrhagic enteritis, and prostration. Affected animals may die within a few days and pregnant ewes abort. Mortality in sheep is 30–90%. Subclinical infections also occur and recovered animals are immune. Diagnosis is made clinically and by gross pathologic examination and may be confirmed by virus isolation in cell culture and identification of isolates immunologically. Control depends primarily on dipping to control the vector tick, which is also the vector of the economically important protozoan disease, East Coast fever. Vaccines are effective in preventing the disease in sheep. Although the virus is zoonotic, human infections are rare.

Biohazard: Nairobi sheep disease virus is a restricted animal pathogen; its importation or possession is prohibited by law or regulation by most national governments. The virus is restricted to certain national laboratories for all research and diagnostic procedures; the virus is a Biosafety Level 4 pathogen; it must be handled in the laboratory under maximum containment conditions to prevent human exposure (see Chapter 12).

Crimean-Congo Hemorrhagic Fever

Crimean-Congo hemorrhagic fever virus, a member of the genus *Nairovirus,* is the cause of an important zoonotic disease that had been recognized for many years in central Asia and eastern Europe. However, this recognition was just the tip of the iceberg—today, the disease is known to extend from China through central Asia to India, Pakistan, Afghanistan, Iran, Iraq, other countries of the Middle East, eastern Europe, and most of Saharan and sub-Saharan Africa. In recent years, there have been repeated outbreaks in the countries of the Persian Gulf, especially in connection with traditional sheep slaughtering and butchering practices.

Clinical Features

There is no evidence that there is any clinical disease in animals other than humans, but the infection in domestic animals is the basis for the overall importance of this disease.

Pathogenesis, Pathology, and Immunity

The virus is maintained by a cycle involving transovarial and transstadial transmission in *Hyalomma* spp. and many related ticks. Larval and nymphal ticks become infected when feeding on small mammals and ground-dwelling birds and adult ticks when feeding on wild and domestic ruminants (sheep, goats, and cattle). Infection in wild and domestic ruminants is very productive, resulting in viremia levels high enough that ticks become infected when feeding.

Laboratory Diagnosis

Diagnosis is made by the detection of antigen in tissues (usually by immunofluorescence) or IgM antibody (by antigen-capture enzyme immunoassay). A recently developed reverse transcriptase–polymerase chain reaction assay is also valuable. Virus isolation has proven difficult: the virus is very labile, shipping of diagnostic specimens from usual sites of disease is often less than satisfactory, and all laboratory work must be done under maximum containment conditions (see Chapter 12).

Epidemiology, Prevention, and Control

Crimean-Congo hemorrhagic fever is an emerging problem, with more and more cases being reported each year from many parts of the world and more and more antibody being found in animal populations. For example, in serosurveys, more than 8% of cattle in several regions of Africa have been shown to be seropositive. There is no vaccine, and prevention based on vector control is difficult because of the large areas of wooded and brushy tick habitat involved. One important prevention approach would be the enforcement in endemic areas of Asia, the Middle East, and Africa of occupational safety standards on farms and in livestock markets, abattoirs, and other workplaces where there is routine contact with sheep, goats, and cattle.

Human Disease

The disease in humans is a severe hemorrhagic fever. The incubation period is 3 to 7 days; onset is abrupt with fever, severe headache, myalgia, back and abdominal pain, nausea and vomiting, and marked prostration. It is the most dramatic of all human hemorrhagic fevers in the amount of hemorrhaging and the extent of subcutaneous, mucosal, gastroenteric, and genitourinary ecchymoses. There is a necrotizing hepatitis and damage to the heart and central nervous system; the case-fatality rate is commonly 15–40%. The disease affects primarily farmers, veterinarians, slaughter-house workers and butchers and others coming in contact with livestock, and woodcutters and others coming in contact with infected ticks. The virus is also transmitted by direct contact with subclinically infected viremic animals, e.g., during sheep docking, shearing, anthelminthic drenching, and veterinary procedures. The virus is also transmitted from human to human, especially in hospitals. Not uncommonly, nosocomial outbreaks are traced to surgical intervention when a patient presents with extensive gastric hemorrhaging—a lack of precautions leaves the surgical team at great risk.

Biohazard: Crimean-Congo hemorrhagic fever virus is a restricted animal pathogen; its importation or possession is prohibited by law or regulation by most national governments. The virus is restricted to certain national laboratories for all research and diagnostic procedures; the virus is a Biosafety Level 4 pathogen; it must be handled in the laboratory under maximum containment conditions to prevent human exposure (see Chapter 12).

Hemorrhagic Fever with Renal Syndrome

The 22 member viruses of the genus *Hantavirus* comprise the only viruses in the family *Bunyaviridae* that are not arthropod-borne—they are transmitted among rodents by long-term shedding in saliva, urine, and feces. Several of the viruses are zoonotic, the cause of severe human disease. Four Old World hantaviruses cause multisystem disease centered on the kidneys (hemorrhagic fever with renal syndrome) and several New World hantaviruses cause multisystem disease centered on the lungs (hantavirus pulmonary syndrome, also known as acute respiratory distress syndrome). The pathogenicity of some of the newly discovered viruses has not yet been determined. Some viruses also infect other mammalian species, such as horses, but this is uncommon and does not contribute to the life cycle of the viruses or to human disease risk (Table 31.3).

One distinction of the hantaviruses has been the level of difficulty surrounding their discovery. For example, during the Korean war of 1950–52, thousands of United Nations troops developed a disease marked by fever, headache, hemorrhagic manifestations, and acute renal failure with shock; the mortality rate following infection was 5–10%. Despite intense research, the etiologic agent of this disease remained a mystery for 28 years when the prototype hantavirus, Hantaan virus, was isolated from the striped field mouse *Apodemus agrarius.* Hantaviruses discovered since then have also been so difficult to isolate in cell culture or experimental animals that reverse transcriptase–polymerase chain reaction assays have become a key tool for obtaining diagnostic sequences from clinical materials (including acute-phase blood) and rodent tissues. More than 200,000 cases of hemorrhagic fever with renal syndrome are reported each year throughout the world, with more than half in China. Russia and Korea report hundreds to thousands of cases; fewer are reported from Japan, Finland, Sweden, Bulgaria, Greece, Hungary, France, and the Balkan countries.

Clinical Features

There is no evidence that there is any clinical disease in animals other than humans; however, the infection in reservoir host animals is the key to dealing with human diseases.

Pathogenesis, Pathology, and Immunity

The pathogenesis of hantavirus infection of reservoir rodent hosts is not well understood. The hallmark of infection is persistent, usually lifelong, inapparent infection and shedding in saliva, urine, and feces. Human disease involves contact with contaminated rodent excreta, usually in winter when human–rodent contact is maximum. In a landmark pathogenesis study, H. W. Lee inoculated the reservoir rodent, *Apodemus agrarius,* with Hantaan virus and followed the course of infection by virus titration of organs, serology, and immunofluorescence. Viremia was found to be brief and disappeared as neutralizing antibodies appeared. However, virus persisted in several organs, including lungs and kidneys. Virus titers in urine and throat swabs were about 100 to

TABLE 31.3
Family *Bunyaviridae*, Genus *Hantavirus*

VIRUS	PRINCIPAL RESERVOIR	DISTRIBUTION	DISEASE
Hantaan	*Apodemus agrarius* (striped field mouse)	China, Russia, Korea	HFRS[a]
Dobrava	*Apodemus flavicollis* (yellow-neck mouse)	Balkans	HFRS
Seoul	*Rattus norvegicus* (Norway rat)	Worldwide	HFRS
Puumala	*Clethrionomys glareolus* (bank vole)	Scandinavia, Europe, Russia	HFRS (NE)[b]
Sin Nombre	*Peromyscus maniculatus* (deer mouse)	United States, Canada	HPS[a]
New York	*Peromyscus leucopus* (white-footed mouse)	United States	HPS
Bayou	*Oryzomys palustris* (rice rat)	United States	HPS
Black Creek Canal	*Sigmodon hispidus* (cotton rat)	United States	HPS
Andes	*Oligoryzomys longicaudatus* (long-tailed pygmy rice rat)	Argentina	HPS
To be named	*Calomys laucha* (vesper mouse)	Paraguay	HPS
Bloodland Lake	*Microtus ochrogaster* (prairie vole)	United States	Unknown[d]
El Moro Canyon	*Reithrodontomys megalotis* (Western harvest mouse)	United States	Unknown
Isla Vista	*Microtus californicus* (California vole)	United States	Unknown
Khabarovsk	*Microtus fortis* (reed vole)	Russia	Unknown
Muleshoe	*Sigmodon hispidus* (cotton rat)	United States	Unknown
Rio Mamore	*Oryzomys microtis* (small-eared pygmy rice rat)	Bolivia	Unknown
Rio Segundo	*Reithrodontomys mexicanus* (Mexican harvest mouse)	Costa Rica	Unknown
Thailand	*Bandicota indica* (bandicoot rat)	Thailand	Unknown
Thottapalayam	*Suncus murinus* (musk shrew)	India	Unknown
Topografov	*Lemmus sibiricus* (Siberian lemming)	Siberia	Unknown
Tula	*Microtus arvalis* (European common vole)	Europe	Unknown
Prospect Hill	*Microtus pennsylvanicus* (meadow vole)	United States, Canada	None

[a]Hemorrhagic fever with renal syndrome in humans.
[b]Nephropathia epidemica, mild form of HFRS in humans.
[c]Hantavirus pulmonary syndrome in humans.
[d]No disease documented.

1000 times higher during the first weeks after inoculation than subsequently and animals were much more infectious for cage mates or nearby mice during this period.

Laboratory Diagnosis

Diagnosis is made by the detection of antigen in tissues (usually by immunofluorescence) or serologically by IgG and IgM capture enzyme immunoassays. The IgM capture enzyme immunoassay is the primary diagnostic tool in reference diagnostics centers, but recently developed reverse transcriptase–polymerase chain reaction assays are being added and are likely to become widely available in the future. Virus isolation has proven very difficult: the viruses must be blind-passaged in cell culture (most commonly Vero E6 cells) and detected by immunologic or molecular means. Shipping of diagnostic specimens from sites of disease is often less than satisfactory and all laboratory work on Hantaan, Dobrava, Sin Nombre, and other highly pathogenic viruses must be done under maximum containment conditions (see Chapter 12).

Epidemiology, Prevention, and Control

A matrix of four characters is needed to define the global context of the disease hemorrhagic fever with renal syndrome (Table 31.1): (1) the viruses, per se; (2) their reservoir rodent hosts; (3) the locale of human cases; and (4) the severity of human cases. Four viruses are involved: Hantaan, Dobrava, Seoul, and Puumala viruses. Hantaan and Dobrava viruses cause severe disease with mortality rates of 5–15%; Seoul virus causes less severe disease and Puumala virus causes the least severe form of the disease (mortality rate less than 1%), which is known in Scandinavia as nephropathia epidemica. There are three disease locale patterns: rural, urban, and laboratory acquired. Rural disease is caused by Hantaan virus, which is widespread in China, Asian Russia, and Korea, and Dobrava virus in the Balkans and Greece. Rural disease is also caused by Puumula virus in northern Europe, especially in Scandinavia and Russia. Urban disease is caused by Seoul virus; it occurs in Japan, Korea, China, and South and North America. Each virus has a specific reservoir rodent host: Hantaan virus, the striped field mouse, *Apodemus agrarius;* Dobrava virus, the yellow-neck mouse, *Apodemus flavicollis;* Seoul virus, the Norway rat, *Rattus norvegicus;* and Puumala virus, the bank vole, *Clethrionomys glareolus.* The relationship between each virus and its host defines the geographical limits of disease and confirms ancient virus–host relationships. For example, the relationship between Seoul virus and the Norway rat explains its worldwide distribution and presence in seaports. A major scientific challenge is to understand the Darwinian forces that drive the long-standing maintenance of these relationships.

From the veterinary point of view, the most important disease pattern is that involving laboratory rats (and wild rodents brought into laboratories) and transmission to animal caretakers and research personnel. There have been episodes of human disease in Belgium, Korea, the United Kingdom, and Japan, totaling more than 100 cases and one death. Prevention of introduction of virus into laboratory rat colonies requires quarantined entry of new stock (or entry only of known virus-free stock), prevention of access by wild rodents, and regular serologic testing. Cesarean derivation and barrier rearing of valuable rat strains can eliminate the virus from infected colonies. Prevention of viral spread should also involve the testing of all rat-origin cell lines before their release from cell culture collections or other laboratories.

Control of the wide-ranging rodent reservoirs of Hantaan, Seoul, and Puumala viruses is not possible in most settings where disease occurs, but in some situations their entry into dwellings can be minimized. Vaccine development has been hampered by the lack of animal models of disease. Nevertheless, a vaccinia virus vector, containing the two glycoprotein genes of Hantaan virus, has been developed and is currently in phase II clinical trials. Korean and Chinese investigators have developed inactivated whole virus vaccines that are also currently in human trials.

Human Disease

The clinical course of severe hemorrhagic fever with renal syndrome in humans involves five overlapping stages: febrile, hypotensive, oliguric, diuretic, and convalescent stages, not all of which are seen in every case. The onset of the disease is sudden with intense headache, backache, fever, and chills. Hemorrhage, if it occurs, is manifested during the febrile stage as a flushing of the face and injection of the conjunctiva and mucous membranes. A petechial rash may also appear. Sudden and extreme hypotension, albuminuria, and nausea and vomiting around day four are characteristic of severe disease. One-third of deaths occur during this stage because of vascular leakage and acute shock. Deaths also occur during the subsequent (oliguric) stage because of hypervolemia. Patients who survive and progress to the diuretic stage show improved renal function but may still die of shock or pulmonary complications. The convalescent stage can last weeks to months before recovery is complete. The disease is believed to be mediated immunopathologically as antibodies are present usually from the first day that the patient presents for medical care.

Supportive therapy, with particular constraint in the use of fluids and, in some cases, the use of hemodialysis, has resulted in a decline of the mortality rate from 15 to 5% or less. The antiviral drug Ribavirin has resulted in a further fall in mortality.

Hantavirus Pulmonary Syndrome

In 1993 a new zoonotic hantavirus disease was recognized in the southwestern region of the United States. The disease was manifest not as hemorrhagic fever with renal syndrome, but rather as an acute respiratory distress syndrome. Through December 1997, a total of 172 cases had been reported in 28 states of the United States with a mortality rate of 45%. About 75% of patients were residents of rural areas. At least six viruses have been associated etiologically with the pulmonary syndrome, with more than 400 cases reported from Canada, Argentina, Bolivia, Brazil, Canada, Chile, Paraguay, Peru, and Uruguay as well as the United States. Other New World hantaviruses have been discovered recently; their pathogenicity has not yet been determined.

Clinical Features

There is no evidence that there is any clinical disease in animals other than humans; however, the infection in reservoir host animals is the key to dealing with the human disease.

Pathogenesis, Pathology, and Immunity

Little is known about the pathogenesis of New World hantavirus infections in reservoir rodent hosts. Similarly, little is know about the pathology of infection; the viruses seem to be minimally deleterious to the survival or reproduction of their reservoir rodent hosts, but virus is shed in saliva, urine, and feces of these animals for at least many weeks and likely the lifetime of the animal. Transmission from rodent to rodent is believed to occur after weaning by contact, perhaps aggressive contact, biting, and scratching. Transmission (and human infection) likely also occurs by the inhalation of aerosols or dust containing infected dried rodent saliva or excreta.

Laboratory Diagnosis

During 1993, before the virus causing the human disease outbreak in southwestern United States had been isolated, serologic tests (using surrogate antigens from related hantaviruses) and molecular biologic tests were developed and used to prove that the etiologic agent was a previously unknown virus. Viral RNA was amplified from human autopsy tissues and peripheral blood mononuclear cells using the reverse transcriptase–polymerase chain reaction, followed by partial sequencing of amplified products. Where specimens were unsuitable for the reverse transcriptase–polymerase chain reaction, immunohistochemical staining was used to detect viral antigens in fixed lung tissues. Later, polymerase chain reaction-amplified products were extended, i.e., overlapping amplified products were sequenced and aligned until the entire genome of the new viruses had been determined. Sequences encoding the G1 glycoprotein of Sin Nombre virus were then used in expression systems to produce homologous antigens and in turn to produce reference antisera for further diagnostic studies and services. The same methods were applied to specimens from large numbers of rodents collected in the areas where patients lived. This proved that at least eight species of rodents were involved, the primary reservoir host in the southwest being *Peromyscus maniculatus,* the deer mouse (10 to 30 and even up to 50% of these animals were found to harbor Sin Nombre virus in areas where there was human disease). Comparing sequences obtained from specimens from different areas indicated that several different variant viruses, all previously unknown, were active in the United States (Table 31.1). These diagnostic methods have now been standardized and made available in regional laboratories serving populations at risk.

Epidemiology, Prevention, and Control

Sin Nombre virus and other New World hantaviruses have been present for eons in the large area of western United States inhabited by *P. maniculatus* and other reservoir rodent species; they were recognized in 1993 only because of the number and clustering of human cases. A great increase in rodent numbers following two especially wet winters and a consequent increase in piñon seeds and other rodent food contributed to the number of human cases. The temporal distribution of human disease reflects a spring–summer seasonality (although cases have occurred throughout the year), again matching rodent reservoir host behavior. Just as with Old World hantaviruses, each New World virus has a specific reservoir rodent host: Sin Nombre virus, the deer mouse, *P. maniculatus;* New York virus, the white-footed mouse, *P. leucopus;* Black Creek Canal virus, the cotton rat, *Sigmodon hispidus;* Bayou virus, the rice rat, *Oryzomys palustris;* Andes virus, the long-tailed pygmy rice rat, *Oligoryzomys longicaudatus;* and an unnamed virus from Paraguay, the vesper mouse, *Calomys laucha.*

Extensive public education programs have been developed to advise people about reducing the risk of infection, mostly by reducing rodent habitats and food supplies in and near homes and taking precautions when cleaning rodent-contaminated areas. The latter involves rodent proofing food and pet food containers, trapping and poisoning rodents in and around dwellings, eliminating rodent habitats near dwellings, use of respirators, and wetting down areas with detergent, disinfectant, or hypochlorite solution before cleaning areas that may contain rodent excreta. Recommendations have also been developed for specific equipment and practices to reduce risks when working with wild-caught rodents, especially when this involves obtaining tissue or blood specimens: these include use of live-capture traps, protective clothing and gloves, suitable disinfectants, and safe transport packaging.

Human Disease

Hantavirus pulmonary syndrome typically starts with fever, myalgia, headache, nausea, vomiting, nonproductive cough, and shortness of breath. As disease progresses, there is radiological evidence of bilateral interstitial pulmonary edema and pleural effusions. There is thrombocytopenia, a left shift in the myeloid series, and large immunoblasts in the circulation. The course of the disease progresses rapidly, with death often following in hours to days. Recovery can be as rapid as the development of life-threatening clinical signs. Functional impairment of vascular endothelium and shock are central to the pathogenesis of the disease. Histopathologic lesions include interstitial pneumonitis with congestion, edema, and mononuclear cell infiltration. Current therapy includes aggressive management of cardiovascular abnormalities and the pulmonary edema. Investigation of an epidemic in Argentina in 1995 provided strong evidence for person-to-person transmission; strict barrier nursing techniques are now recommended for management of suspected cases.

California (La Crosse Virus) Encephalitis

The California serogroup in the genus *Bunyavirus* includes 14 viruses, each of which is transmitted by mosquitoes, has a narrow range of vertebrate hosts, and a limited geographic distribution. There is no evidence that there is any clinical disease associated with these viruses in animals other than humans; however, the infection in reservoir host animals and mosquito hosts is the key to dealing with human diseases. The most important zoonotic pathogen in the California serogroup is La Crosse virus, which is maintained by transovarial transmission in *Aedes triseriatus,* a tree-hole breeding woodland mosquito, and is amplified by a mosquito–vertebrate–mosquito cycle involving silent infection of woodland rodents, such as squirrels and chipmunks. The virus occurs throughout the eastern and midwestern United States, whereas a closely related virus, snowshoe hare virus, occupies a similar niche in Canada. Most cases occur during the summer months in children and young adults who are exposed to vector mosquitoes in wooded areas. Humans are dead-end hosts, and there is no human-to-human transmission. The encephalitis caused by La Crosse virus is relatively benign; about 10% of children develop seizures during the acute disease, a few develop persistent paresis and learning disabilities, and the mortality rate is about 0.3%.

California encephalitis caused by La Crosse virus is a classical example of a disease that was not recognized until the development of laboratory methods permitting a specific etiologic diagnosis. The virus was first isolated in 1964 from a fatal case of encephalitis in a 4-year-old child. Using this isolate as a source of antigen, retrospective serological surveys showed that the virus was an important cause of disease previously listed under the heading "viral meningitis of undetermined etiology." It is now estimated that annually there are well over 100,000 human infections and at least 100 cases of encephalitis in the United States—this disease had been occurring regularly for many decades, long before the time when the virus came to light.

Further Reading

Gonzalez-Scarano, F., and Nathanson, N. (1996). Bunyaviridae. *In* "Fields Virology" (B. N. Fields, D. M. Knipe, P. M. Howley, R. M. Chanock, J. L. Melnick, T. P. Monath, B. Roizman, and S. E. Straus, eds.), 3rd ed., pp. 1473–1504. Lippincott-Raven, Philadelphia, PA.

Johnson, K. M. (1997). Hantaviruses. *In* "Viral Infections of Humans: Epidemiology and Control" (A. S. Evans and A. Kaslow, eds.), 4th ed., pp. 341–355. Plenum, New York.

Karabatsos, N., ed. (1985). "International Catalogue of Arboviruses Including Certain Other Viruses of Vertebrates," 3rd Ed. American Society of Tropical Medicine and Hygiene, San Antonio, TX.

Kolakofsky, D., ed. (1991). Bunyaviridae. *Curr. Top. Microbiol. Immunol.* **169**, 1–256.

Lee, H. W., and van der Groen, G. (1989). Hemorrhagic fever with renal syndrome. *Prog. Med. Virol.* **36**, 62–102.

Meegan, J. M. (1979). The Rift Valley fever epizootic in Egypt 1977–78. I. Description of the epizootic and virological studies. *Trans. R. Soc. Trop. Med. Hyg.* **73**, 618–623.
Monath, T. P., ed. (1988). "The Arboviruses: Epidemiology and Ecology," 5 vol. CRC Press, Boca Raton, FL.
Parsonson, I. M., and Patterson, J. L. (1985). Bunyavirus pathogenesis. *Adv. Virus Res.* **30**, 279–316.
Schmaljohn, C. S. (1996). Bunyaviridae: The viruses and their replication. *In* "Fields Virology" (B. N. Fields, D. M. Knipe, P. M. Howley, R. M. Chanock, J. L. Melnick, T. P. Monath, B. Roizman, and S. E. Straus, eds.), 3rd ed., pp. 1447–1471. Lippincott-Raven, Philadelphia, PA.
Schmaljohn, C. S., and Hjelle, B. (1997). Hantaviruses: A global disease problem. *Emerg. Infect. Dis.* **3**, 95–104.

CHAPTER 32

Arenaviridae

The fundamental determinant in the ecology of the member viruses of the family *Arenaviridae* and their importance as zoonotic pathogens is their ancient coevolutionary relationships with their reservoir rodent hosts. The risk of transmission of each virus to humans relates to the nature of the infection of its rodent host (usually persistent asymptomatic infection with lifelong viral shedding), as well as to rodent population dynamics and behavior and human occupational and other risk factors that lead to exposure to virus-laden rodent excreta. The consequences of human exposure include some of the most lethal hemorrhagic fevers known: Lassa, Argentine, Bolivian, Venezuelan, and Brazilian hemorrhagic fevers. The viruses that cause these diseases are Biosafety Level 4 pathogens; they must be handled in the laboratory under maximum containment conditions to prevent human exposure (see Chapter 12).

The prototype arenavirus, lymphocytic choriomeningitis virus, has over many years played two disparate roles in comparative virology: wild-type strains are zoonotic pathogens and the subject of public health surveillance in some countries, whereas laboratory strains have provided much of the conceptual basis for our understanding of viral immunology and pathogenesis, including: (1) immunological tolerance, (2) virus-induced immunopathology, (3) immune complex disease, (4) virus-specific cytotoxic T lymphocytes as mediators of viral clearance and immunopathology, (5) major histocompatibility complex (MHC) restriction in T lymphocyte recognition, (6) natural killer cell activation and proliferation, and (7) infection-induced pathophysiologic impairment of specialized cell functions. Conceptual advances continue to flow from research with the lymphocytic choriomeningitis virus model, including vaccine development based on antiviral T lymphocyte epitopes and cytokine and lymphokine modulation of viral infections.

Properties of Arenaviruses

Classification

The family *Arenaviridae* contains a single genus, *Arenavirus,* which is divided into two evolutionary subgroups based on genetic and serologic characteristics. The first subgroup includes lymphocytic choriomeningitis virus, which is allied with the common house mouse, *Mus musculus,* in North and South America, Europe, and perhaps elsewhere, and the Old World arenaviruses, which are associated with *Mastomys* spp. and *Paromys* spp. in Africa. This subgroup contains Lassa virus, which produces severe disease in humans and a few other viruses that infect humans but are not known to cause disease. The second subgroup includes the New World arenaviruses (also called the Tacaribe complex), which are associated with particular cricetids (many different rodents, muskrats, and gerbils) in North, Central, and South America. This subgroup contains the important human pathogens Junin, Machupo, Guanarito, and Sabiá viruses and several other viruses that are not known to be pathogenic for humans (Table 32.1).

Virion Properties

Arenavirus virions are pleomorphic in shape, ranging in diameter from 50 to 300 nm, although most virions have

Table 32.1
Natural History and Zoonotic Disease Potential of Arenaviruses

Virus	Natural host	Geographic distribution	Human disease
Lymphocytic choriomeningitis virus	*Mus musculus*	Western hemisphere, Europe, perhaps worldwide	Grippe-like disease, meningitis, meningoencephalitis
Old World arenaviruses			
Lassa virus	*Mastomys natalensis*	West Africa	Hemorrhagic fever (Lassa fever)
Mopeia virus	*Mastomys natalensis*	Southern Africa	Infection, no disease
Mobala virus	*Praomys jacksoni*	Central African Republic	Infection, no disease
Ippy virus	*Arvicanthus* spp.	Central African Republic	Infection, no disease
New World arenaviruses			
Junin virus	*Calomys musculinus, C. laucha, Akodon azarae*	Argentina	Hemorrhagic fever (Argentine hemorrhagic fever)
Machupo virus	*Calomys callosus*	Bolivia	Hemorrhagic fever (Bolivian hemorrhagic fever)
Guanarito virus	*Zygodontomys brevicauda, Oryzomys* spp.	Venezuela	Hemorrhagic fever (Venezuelan hemorrhagic fever)
Sabiá virus virus	?	Brazil	Hemorrhagic fever (Brazilian hemorrhagic fever)
Tacaribe virus	*Artibeus literatus* and *A. jamaicensis* (bats)	Trinidad	None, except for one laboratory-acquired case of systemic disease
Pirital virus	*Sigmodon alstoni*	Venezuela	Unknown
El-Arroyo virus	?	United States	Unknown
Oliveros virus	*Bolomys obscurus*	Argentina	Unknown
Amapari virus	*Oryzomys goeldi, Neacomys guinae*	Brazil	None
Flexal virus	*Oryzomys* spp.	Brazil	None
Latino virus	*Calomys callosus*	Bolivia	None
Parana virus	*Oryzomys buccinatus*	Paraguay	None
Pichinde virus	*Oryzomys albigularis*	Colombia	None
Tamiami virus	*Sigmodon hispidus*	Florida, United States	None

a diameter of 110–130 nm (Figure 32.1). Virions are composed of an envelope covered with club-shaped glycoprotein peplomers 8–10 nm in length, within which are two circular helical nucleocapsid segments, each looking like a string of beads. The nucleocapsids are circular as a consequence of forming panhandles, i.e., noncovalent bonds between conserved complementary nucleotide sequences at the 3′ and 5′ ends of each RNA genome segment. The family derives its name from the presence within virions of cellular ribosomes, which by thin section electron microscopy resemble grains of sand (*arena*, sand). The genome consists of two segments of single-stranded RNA, designated large (L) and small (S), 7.2 and 3.4 kb in size, respectively. Virions may contain multiple copies of the two genome segments, often with more copies of the S RNA segment.

Most of the genome is of negative sense, but the 5′ half of the S segment and the 5′ end of the L segment are of positive sense; the term *ambisense* is used to describe this unusual genome arrangement, which is also found in some members of the family *Bunyaviridae* (see Chapter 31 and Figure 32.2). Specifically, the nucleoprotein is encoded in the 3′ half of the complementary-sense S RNA, whereas the viral glycoprotein precursor

FIGURE 32.1.

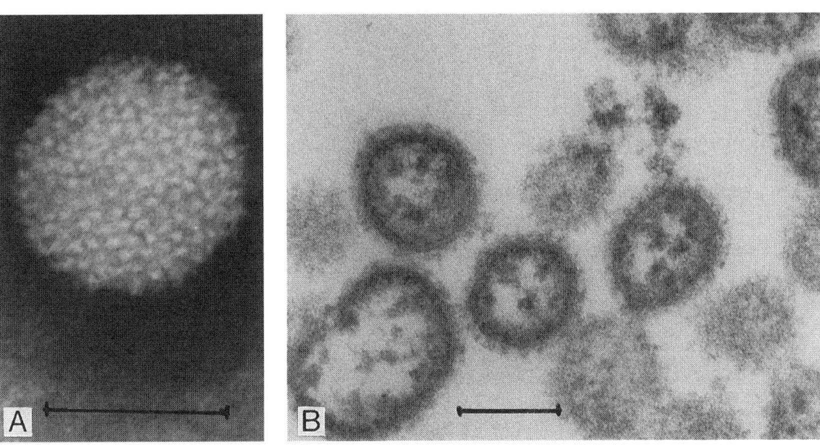

Family *Arenaviridae*, genus *Arenavirus*. (A) Tacaribe virus, negative stain electron microscopy. (B) Lassa virus—the presence of nonfunctioning host cell ribosomes within virions is a characteristic of all arenaviruses; thin section electron microscopy. Bars: 100 nm.

is encoded in the 5′ half of the viral-sense S RNA. The L protein is encoded in the 3′ end of the complementary-sense L RNA and a zinc-binding protein is encoded in the 5′ end of the viral-sense L RNA. RNAs contain hairpin configurations between the genes that function to terminate transcription from viral and viral-complementary RNAs. The mRNAs are capped—5′-methylated caps are cleaved from host mRNAs by the viral RNA-dependent RNA polymerase (transcriptase), which also has endonuclease activity, and are added to viral mRNAs to prime transcription (called cap snatching).

The viruses are quite sensitive to heat and acid conditions and are inactivated readily by detergents, lipid solvents, and common disinfectants.

Viral Replication

Arenaviruses replicate to high titer in many kinds of cells: Vero E6 (African green monkey) cells and BHK-21 (baby hamster kidney) cells. They replicate in the cytoplasm. Because the genome of the single-stranded, negative-sense RNA viruses cannot be translated directly, the first step after attachment to yet unknown cellular receptors and penetration of the host cell and uncoating, is the activation of the virion RNA polymerase (transcriptase). Because of the ambisense coding strategy, only nucleoprotein and polymerase mRNAs are transcribed directly from genomic RNAs prior to translation. Newly synthesized polymerase and nucleocapsid proteins facilitate the synthesis of full-length, complementary-sense RNA, which then serves as template for the transcription of glycoprotein and zinc-binding protein mRNAs and the synthesis of more full-length, negative-sense RNA. Budding of virions occurs from the plasma membrane (Figure 32.3). Arenaviruses have limited lytic capacity, usually producing a carrier state in which defective-interfering particles are produced. After an initial period of active viral transcription, translation, genome replication, and production of progeny virions, viral gene expression is down-regulated and cells enter a state of persistent infection wherein virion production continues for an indefinite period but at a greatly reduced rate (Table 32.2).

TABLE 32.2
Properties of Arenaviruses

One genus, *Arenavirus*, with two subgroups, one for Old World and one for New World (Tacaribe complex) viruses

Virions are pleomorphic, enveloped, 50–300 (generally 110–130) nm in size

Virion contains nonfunctional host cell ribosomes

Virions contain two circular helical nucleocapsids with associated RNA-dependent RNA polymerase (transcriptase)

Genome consists of two segments, large (L, 7.2 kb) and small (S, 3.4 kb), of single-stranded RNA, both ambisense

Viral proteins: nucleoprotein, RNA-dependent RNA polymerase, two glycoproteins, zinc-binding protein, plus minor proteins

Replication occurs in the cytoplasm, generally noncytocidal, persistent infections

Maturation occurs by budding from the plasma membrane

Genetic reassortment occurs between closely related viruses

FIGURE 32.2.

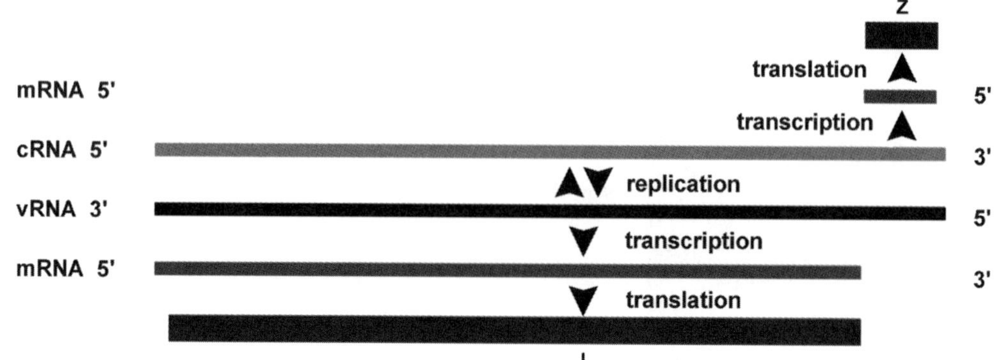

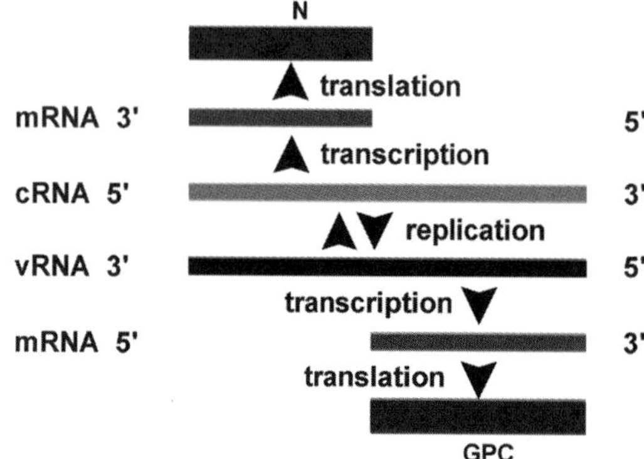

The transcription, translation, and replication of arenavirus S and L RNA segments. Both segments employ an ambisense transcription strategy. Four protein are synthesized: Z, a zinc-binding protein; L, the RNA-dependent RNA polymerase (transcriptase); N, the nucleoprotein; and GPC, the precursor of the two envelope glycoproteins. The sequence and amount of synthesis of each protein are controlled by this strategy: (1) proteins encoded in complementary RNAs (cRNA) are produced immediately (Z, which functions early in the replication cycle, and N, which binds to nascent RNAs); (2) the cRNAs direct the synthesis of more viral RNAs (vRNA); and (3) proteins encoded in the viral sense RNAs (L and GPC) are synthesized later. GPC is cleaved posttranslationally, forming the mature peplomer glycoproteins, GP1 and GP2. [Adapted from P. J. Southern, Arenaviridae: The viruses and their replication. *In* "Fields Virology" (B. N. Fields, D. M. Knipe, P. M. Howley, R. M. Chanock, J. L. Melnick, T. P. Monath, B. Roizman, and S. E. Straus, eds.), 3rd ed., pp. 1505–1520. Lippincott-Raven, Philadelphia, PA, 1996.]

Lymphocytic Choriomeningitis Virus Infection

Lymphocytic choriomeningitis virus presents two zoonotic disease problems. First, the virus causes human disease when infected wild mice invade dwellings and farm buildings where dried virus-laden excreta may be transmitted by aerosols or fomites. Second, the virus causes major problems when it becomes established in mouse and hamster colonies, where it then poses a zoonotic threat and confounds research results dependent on virus-free animals or cell cultures derived from these animals. For example, infected mouse tumors have been implicated in infections of laboratory workers. Mice and hamsters are the only species in which long-term, asymptomatic infection is known to exist, but guinea pigs, rabbits, rats, dogs, swine, and primates may also become infected in laboratory settings.

Clinical Features

Clinical signs of lymphocytic choriomeningitis in mice depend on age, route of infection, and immunological status at the time of infection (Figure 32.4). Most laboratory mouse strains infected *in utero* or during the first

FIGURE 32.3.

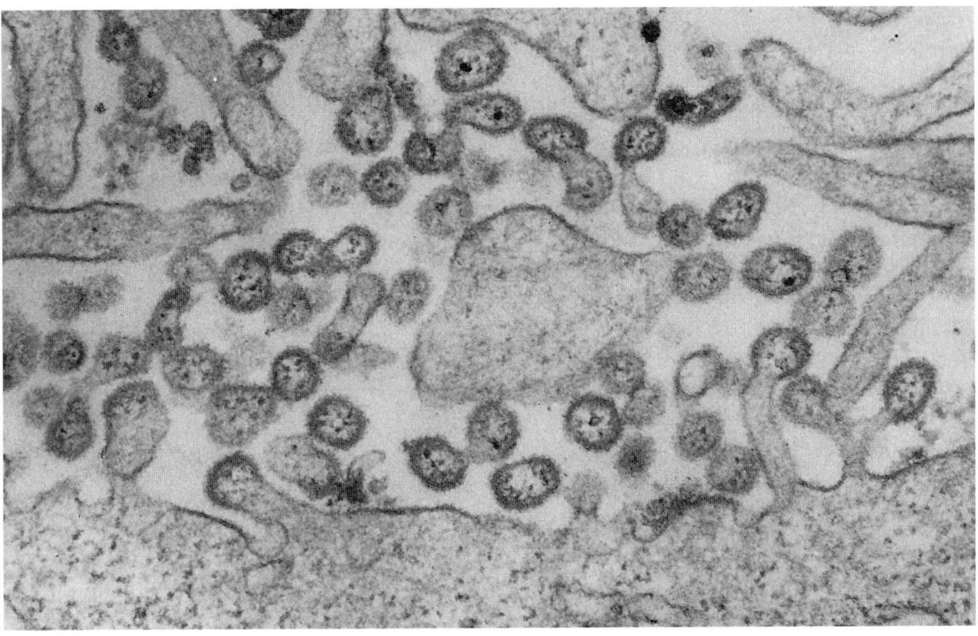

Prolific budding of Lassa virus from the plasma membrane of an infected Vero cell. Magnification: ×70,000.

48 hours after birth develop a persistent tolerant infection. This infection may be asymptomatic, or over the course of several weeks to a year may become evident by weight loss, runting, blepharitis, and impaired reproductive performance. Terminal immune complex glomerulonephritis is a common result of the breakdown of tolerance. Animals infected peripherally after the first few days of life may overcome the infection or may show decreased growth, rough hair coat, hunched posture, blepharitis, weakness, photophobia, tremors, and convulsions over a period of weeks. The visceral organs of these animals, including the liver, kidneys, lungs, pancreas, and major blood vessels, become infiltrated by large numbers of lymphocytes. Animals inoculated intra-

FIGURE 32.4.

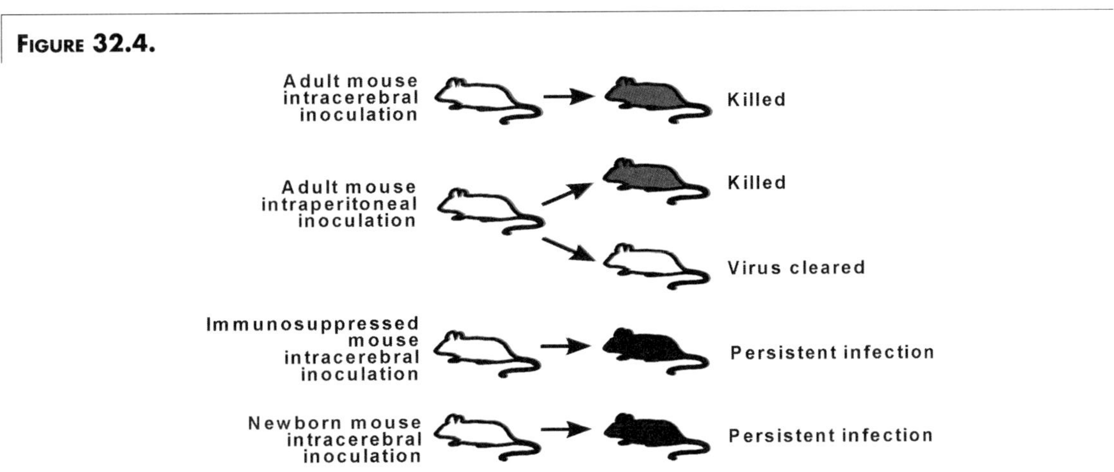

Various outcomes of lymphocytic choriomeningitis virus infection in mice, depending on age, route of infection, and immunological status at the time of infection.

cerebrally (such as when the virus contaminates materials being used in research) usually develop an acutely fatal choriomeningoencephalitis, marked by florid accumulations of lymphocytes at all brain surfaces (meninges, choroid plexus, ependyma, and ventricles). Clinical disease is rare in hamsters, again depending on age at time of infection. As in mice, infection of young hamsters may lead to growth retardation, unthriftiness, weakness, conjunctivitis, dehydration, occasional tremors, and prostration. Lesions include vasculitis, glomerulonephritis, choriomeningoencephalitis, and lymphocytic infiltrations in visceral organs.

Pathogenesis, Pathology, and Immunity

Because the lymphocytic choriomeningitis virus has been such an important model, a great deal is known about the pathogenesis, pathology, and immunology of the infection in mice. Burnet and Fenner first postulated the concept of immunological tolerance after studying the infection in mice: they concluded that exposure to viral antigens before the maturation of the immune system results in mice becoming tolerant and thus unable to clear the infection. Subsequent work showed that persistently infected mice do make antiviral antibodies; most of these antibodies are complexed with virus and complement and contribute to the progressive degenerative disease in mice, including glomerulonephritis, arteritis, and chronic inflammatory lesions.

Persistently infected mice were eventually shown to have *split-tolerance* to the virus; although they mount an antibody response, they do not generate specific cytotoxic T lymphocytes that are needed to clear the infection. In contrast, in acutely infected mice, both the clearance of virus and the lethal choriomeningoencephalitis are due to an overly exuberant cytotoxic T lymphocyte response. The accumulation of T lymphocytes results in neuronal dysfunction and osmotic disturbances, often ending with fatal convulsions. In fact, antiviral cytotoxic T lymphocytes were first demonstrated in the lymphocytic choriomeningitis virus model; Doherty and Zinkernagel earned the Nobel Prize in medicine for work using this model to demonstrate the concept of major histocompatibility complex (MHC) restriction in antigen recognition by T lymphocytes.

One additional pathogenetic characteristic of lymphocytic choriomeningitis virus is its ability to cause the loss of specialized cellular functions, i.e., functions required not for cell survival but for homeostasis of the whole animal. For example, persistent infection in mice results in reduced neurotransmitter activity and reduced levels of growth and thyroid hormones. Reduced growth hormone synthesis is associated with runting in young mice.

Laboratory Diagnosis

For many years, the serological diagnosis of lymphocytic choriomeningitis was done by indirect immunofluorescence, using inactivated cell culture "spot slides" as antigen substrate. Such tests were also set up to measure IgM antibody so as to indicate recent infection. In recent years, in national reference laboratories, IgM capture enzyme immunoassays have become the standard to detect recent infection and IgG capture enzyme immunoassays to detect the presence of the virus in mouse and hamster colonies. Virus is cultivated easily in a wide variety of mammalian cells, particularly Vero E6 (African green monkey kidney) cells and BHK-21 (baby hamster kidney) cells. Primary isolates often do not produce a cytopathic effect so cultures are assayed for antigen by immunofluorescence or enzyme immunoassay. With proper sampling, virus isolation may also be used to confirm the presence of virus in animal colonies.

Epidemiology, Prevention, and Control

Lymphocytic choriomeningitis virus is maintained in nature by persistent infection of mice with long-term, even lifelong virus shedding in urine, saliva, and feces. Vertical transmission occurs by transovarial, transuterine, and various postpartum routes, including milk, saliva, and urine. Human infections derive from contaminated food and dust, the handling of dead mice, and mouse bites. The distribution of human cases is focal and seasonal, probably because mice move into houses and barns in winter. Wild mice may also introduce the virus into laboratory and commercial mouse, rat, hamster, guinea pig, and primate colonies. In the United States, the virus has been a particular problem in hamster colonies and immunocompromised (nude, SCID, etc.) mouse colonies, resulting in contaminated diagnostic reagents, failed research protocols, and clinical disease in laboratory and animal care personnel. Infection can be eradicated by cesarean derivation of mouse and hamster breeding stock and by the modification of facilities to prevent the entry of wild mice. Animals, cell cultures, and tumors and tumor cell lines derived from them must be subjected to regular testing so as to recognize any reintroduction of the virus. The increasing popularity of hamsters as pets has also resulted in many human disease episodes, some involving hundreds of cases. Again, similar attention to breeding stock, facilities, and testing is necessary to prevent this zoonotic problem.

Lymphocytic choriomeningitis virus poses a particular threat to the golden lion tamarin (*Leontopithecus rosalia*), an endangered primate currently found only in a small area of Brazil. There are only about 600 of these animals left in the wild and, because of habitat destruction, the number keeps declining. A global captive-breeding, habituation, and reintroduction program had been developed, involving zoos in several countries, but for several years episodic mortality due to a disease called marmoset (callitrichid) hepatitis threatened its success. It was found that this mortality was due to the exquisite susceptibility of these tamarins (and other tamarins and marmosets) to virus that was introduced into primate facilities by wild mice. Rodent-proofing facilities has succeeded in stopping this mortality; recently 140 captive-bred tamarins have been released into the reserve in Brazil where the habitat will be maintained in perpetuity.

Human Disease

Of the many latent viruses present in mice, only lymphocytic choriomeningitis virus infects humans naturally. Human infection may be asymptomatic or may present as one of three syndromes: (1) most commonly as an influenza-like illness with fever, headache, myalgia, and malaise; (2) less often as an aseptic meningitis; and (3) rarely as a severe encephalomyelitis. Most rare, intrauterine infection has resulted in fetal and neonatal death, as well as hydrocephalus and chorioretinitis in infants. Because it is uncommon, nothing is done to prevent or control human exposure, except in laboratory animal facilities.

Biohazard: Lymphocytic choriomeningitis virus isolates from nature (wild-type isolates), including those from laboratory rodent colonies, require adequate containment facilities, usually at Biosafety Level 3. Classical laboratory-adapted strains, such as the Armstrong strain, which is used in immunology and pathogenesis research, usually require Biosafety Level 2 containment.

Lassa Fever

In 1969, a nurse from a missionary hospital in Lassa, Nigeria, died, a nurse who attended her also died, and another nurse who had assisted at her autopsy became desperately ill but recovered after evacuation to the United States. A new virus was isolated from her blood by virologists at Yale University, one of whom died and another of whom became severely ill but survived following transfusion with immune plasma from the surviving nurse. In succeeding years, Lassa fever, caused by Lassa virus, was found to be a rather common zoonotic disease in West Africa. The only known reservoir of the virus is the multimammate mouse, *Mastomys natalensis,* one of the most commonly occurring rodents in Africa.

Clinical Features

There is no evidence that there is any clinical disease in animals other than humans, but the infection in the reservoir rodent host, *M. natalensis,* is the basis for the overall importance of this disease.

Pathogenesis, Pathology, and Immunity

Lassa virus infection in *M. natalensis* is similar in character to lymphocytic choriomeningitis virus infection in mice—it is persistent and leads to chronic viral shedding in urine, saliva, and feces. In experimentally infected rhesus monkeys there is anorexia, progressive wasting, vascular collapse, and shock, with death occurring at 10–15 days postinfection. The pathophysiologic basis for the disease is not well understood, although there is some hepatocellular necrosis, platelet dysfunction, and endothelial damage. Antibodies are found in recovered humans and experimental animals, but they usually do not neutralize the virus in standard assays—it is presumed that cell-mediated immunity is key in recovery and protection against reinfection.

Laboratory Diagnosis

Diagnosis is now based on the demonstration of IgM antibodies using an IgM capture enzyme immunoassay. Virus antigen may also be detected in liver tissue in fatal cases by immunofluorescence or enzyme immunoassay and virus may be isolated from blood or lymphoreticular tissues using Vero E6 cells and immunological detection of viral growth.

Epidemiology, Prevention, and Control

Risk factors for human infection include contact with rodents (practices such as catching, cooking, and eating rodents), the presence of rodents in dwellings, direct contact with patients, and reuse of unsterilized needles and syringes. Serologic surveys have shown that millions of people in west Africa have antibody; there are over 100,000 new human infections per year, and at least 1000 to 3000 deaths. Ecologic changes account for much of the increasing occurrence of the disease; for example, in Sierra Leone, diamond mining has led to the building of primitive villages in which *M. natalensis* populations flourish. In several areas of West Africa, demonstration projects have shown the value of rodent elimination in villages; however, these programs have been difficult to sustain. Similarly, demonstration projects have shown the efficacy of Ribavirin in the treatment of patients, but unfortunately the drug is not usually available for use in endemic areas. Finally, a vaccinia virus-vectored vaccine carrying the genes for the glycoproteins and nucleoprotein of Lassa virus has been shown to be protective in experimental animals; unfortunately, there are no plans for its commercialization and use in west Africa.

Human Disease

Lassa fever is variable in its presentation, making it difficult to diagnose, whether in endemic areas or in returning travelers. It usually starts with fever, headache, and malaise and progresses to sore throat, back, chest and joint pain, and vomiting. In severe cases, there is conjunctivitis, pneumonitis, carditis, hepatitis, encephalopathy, nerve deafness, and some hemorrhages; death occurs in about 20% of hospitalized cases, usually following cardiovascular collapse. Mortality is very high in pregnancy and fetal loss is almost invariable.

Biohazard: Lassa virus is a restricted pathogen and its importation or possession is regulated by most national governments. The virus is restricted to certain national laboratories for all research and diagnostic procedures; the virus is a Biosafety Level 4 pathogen; it must be handled in the laboratory under maximum containment conditions to prevent human exposure (see Chapter 12).

Argentine, Bolivian, Venezuelan, and Brazilian Hemorrhagic Fevers

Each of the four South American arenavirus hemorrhagic fevers occupies a separate geographical range, each is associated with a different reservoir host, and each represents an expanding zoonotic disease threat. The four viruses have similar natural histories: they cause persistent, lifelong infections in their reservoir rodent hosts, with long-term shedding of large amounts of virus in urine, saliva, and feces. The natural history of each human diseases is determined by the pathogenicity of the virus, its geographic distribution, the habitat and habits of the rodent reservoir host, and the nature of the human–rodent contact. Human disease is usually rural and often occupational, reflecting the relative risk of exposure to virus-contaminated dust and fomites. During the past few years several other newly recognized rodent-borne arenaviruses have been identified in South America, including some that have been associated with human disease. Changes in ecology and farming practices throughout the region have increased concerns over the potential public health threat posed by these viruses (see Table 32.1).

Clinical Features

Unlike lymphocytic choriomeningitis and Lassa viruses, Junin and Machupo viruses are pathogenic in their reservoir rodent hosts. Junin causes up to 50% mortality among infected suckling *Calomys musculinus* and *C. laucha* and stunted growth in others. Machupo virus induces hemolytic anemia, splenomegaly, and fetal death in its rodent host, *Calomys callosus.* Nothing is known about the nature of the infection in reservoir hosts caused by Guanarito or Sabiá viruses.

Pathogenesis, Pathology, and Immunity

As with other arenavirus pathogens, the pattern of infection in reservoir hosts caused by the South American viruses differs with age, host genetic determinants, route of exposure and viral entry, and the dose and genetic character of the virus. Transmission from rodent to rodent is horizontal, not vertical, and occurs through contaminated saliva, urine, and feces. Junin and Machupo viruses not only cause disease in their reservoir hosts, they also induce sterility in neonatally infected females, thereby minimizing their role in producing offspring that are chronic viral shedders. Complex cyclic fluctuations in infection rates and population densities are thought to be a consequence of this. Again, nothing is known about the pathogenesis of Guanarito or Sabiá virus infections in their reservoir hosts.

Laboratory Diagnosis

Diagnosis of Junin and Machupo virus infections is now based on the demonstration of IgM antibodies using an IgM capture enzyme immunoassay. Virus antigen may also be detected in liver tissue in fatal human cases, and virus isolation may be done using Vero E6 cells and immunological detection of viral growth. Methods for the diagnosis of Guanarito or Sabiá virus infections are the same, but reagents are still under development.

Epidemiology, Prevention, and Control

Argentine Hemorrhagic Fever

Argentine hemorrhagic fever, caused by Junin virus, was first recognized in the 1950s in a grain-farming region of Argentina. Most commonly affected are farm workers, which is explained by the behavior of the rodent hosts, *Calomys musculinus* and *C. laucha*. These rodents are not peridomestic, but rather occupy grain fields, exposing humans through contact with virus-infected dust and grain products. Virus is acquired through cuts and abrasions or through airborne dust generated primarily when rodents are caught up in harvesting machinery. Since the 1950s the disease has spread from an area of 16,000 km^2 to 120,000 km^2 containing a population of over 1 million persons. There is a 3- to 5-year cyclic trend in the incidence of human cases, which exactly parallels cyclic changes in the density of *Calomys* spp.

Strategies for the prevention and control of Argentine hemorrhagic fever through rodent control are unrealistic; human exposure during grain harvesting will increase as more and more rodents thrive in grain fields. However, much progress has been made using vaccine; an attenuated virus vaccine is now in use throughout the endemic area in Argentina and has been a great success. Administered intravenously in high dosage, Ribavirin is used as a secondary complement to this vaccine.

Bolivian Hemorrhagic Fever

Machupo virus emerged in Bolivia in 1952 when a revolution forced people to attempt subsistence agriculture at the borders of tropical grassland and forest; by 1962 more than 1000 cases of Bolivian hemorrhagic fever had been identified, with a 22% case-fatality rate. *Calomys callosus*, a forest rodent and the reservoir host of Machupo virus, adapts well to human contact—invasion of villages resulted in clusters of cases in particular houses in which substantial numbers of infected rodents were subsequently trapped. Control of *C. callosus* in dwellings in the endemic area by trapping resulted in the disappearance of the disease for many years, but in the 1990s cases reappeared, again starting on farms and then moving into villages. In one instance there was secondary spread to six of eight family members, all of whom died. As in the past, disease prevention could be facilitated by rodent trapping; however, such programs are difficult to sustain except for short periods in villages with exceptional transmission rates.

Venezuelan Hemorrhagic Fever

Venezuelan hemorrhagic fever was first recognized in rural areas of Venezuela in 1989; it appeared to result from clearing of forest and subsequent preparation of land for farming. In 1990–1991, a total of 104 cases was seen, with 26 deaths, but fewer cases have been seen since then. An arenavirus, Guanarito virus, was isolated from cases and traced to a reservoir rodent host, *Zygodontomys brevicauda*. In the same area another new arenavirus, Pirital virus, was isolated from the rodent *Sigmodon alstoni;* its association with human disease is under investigation. Given the similarities between the natural history of Guanarito and Machupo viruses, disease prevention in Venezuela might be facilitated by rodent trapping, but this has not been done to date.

Brazilian Hemorrhagic Fever

Sabiá virus was isolated from a fatal case of hemorrhagic fever in Sao Paulo, Brazil, in 1990; subsequently there have been two additional cases, one a naturally acquired fatal infection in an agricultural engineer and the second a nonfatal infection in a virologist who was working with the virus. The latter suffered a severe illness characterized by 15 days of fever, headache, chills, myalgia, sore throat, conjunctivitis, nausea, vomiting, diarrhea, bleeding gums, and leukopenia. Given the lack of knowledge of the natural history and epidemiology of Sabiá virus, nothing can be said in regard to disease prevention and control.

Human Disease

The South American hemorrhagic fevers are typical hemorrhagic fevers; prominent features are hemorrhage, thrombocytopenia, leukopenia, hemoconcentration, and proteinuria; some cases are associated with pulmonary edema, with some cases culminating in death from hypotension and hypovolemic shock. Lesions are confined largely to the circulatory system. Isolation and barrier nursing are required to prevent nosocomial spread of the viruses to other patients and nursing staff.

Biohazard: Lassa, Junin, Machupo, Guanarito, and Sabiá viruses are restricted pathogens and their importation or possession is regulated by most national governments. The viruses are restricted to certain national laboratories for all research and diagnostic procedures; the viruses are Biosafety Level 4 pathogens; they must be handled in the laboratory under maximum containment conditions to prevent human exposure.

Further Reading

Borrow, P., and Oldstone, M. B. A. (1997). Lymphocytic choriomeningitis. *In* "Viral Pathogenesis" (N. Nathanson, R. Ahmed, F. Gonzalez-Scarano, D. E. Griffin, K. V. Holmes, F. A. Murphy, and H. L. Robinson, eds.), pp. 593–628. Lippincott-Raven, Philadelphia, PA.

Buchmeier, M. J., and Zajac, A. J. (1998). Lymphocytic choriomeningitis virus. *In* "Persistent Virus Infections" (R. Ahmed and I. Chen, eds.) pp. 575–605. Wiley, Chichester, Sussex.

Childs, J. E., and Peters, C. J. (1993). Ecology and epidemiology of arenaviruses and their hosts. *In* "The Arenaviridae" (M. S. Salvato, ed.) pp. 331–373. Plenum, New York.

Peters, C. J. (1997). Pathogenesis of viral hemorrhagic fevers. *In* "Viral Pathogenesis" (N. Nathanson, R. Ahmed, F. Gonzalez-Scarano, D. E. Griffin, K. V. Holmes, F. A. Murphy, and H. L. Robinson, eds.), pp. 779–800. Lippincott-Raven, Philadelphia, PA.

Peters, C. J., Buchmeier, M., Rollin, P. E., and Ksiazek, T. G. (1996). Arenaviruses. *In* "Fields Virology," (B. N. Fields, D. M. Knipe, P. M. Howley, R. M. Chanock, J. L. Melnick, T. P. Monath, B. Roizman, and S. E. Straus, eds.), 3rd ed., pp. 1521–1552. Lippincott-Raven, Philadelphia, PA.

Salvato, M. S., ed. (1993). "The Arenaviridae." Plenum, New York.

Southern, P. J. (1996). Arenaviridae: The viruses and their replication. *In* "Fields Virology" (B. N. Fields, D. M. Knipe, P. M. Howley, R. M. Chanock, J. L. Melnick, T. P. Monath, B. Roizman, and S. E. Straus, eds.), 3rd ed., pp. 1505–1520. Lippincott-Raven, Philadelphia, PA.

Chapter 33

Coronaviridae

The family *Coronaviridae* comprises two genera: one, the genus *Coronavirus,* contains over a dozen major pathogens of mammals and birds causing respiratory disease (e.g., avian infectious bronchitis virus), enteritis (transmissible gastroenteritis virus of swine), polyserositis (feline infectious peritonitis virus), myocarditis (rabbit coronavirus), sialodacryadenitis (sialodacryadenitis virus of rats), hepatitis (mouse hepatitis virus), encephalomyelitis (mouse hepatitis virus), nephritis (avian infectious bronchitis virus), immunopathologic disease (feline infectious peritonitis), and various other disorders. In humans, coronaviruses are part of the spectrum of viruses that cause the common cold. The second genus, *Torovirus,* contains two viruses of animals: Berne virus, which was first isolated from a horse with diarrhea, and Breda virus, which was first isolated from neonatal calves with severe diarrhea. Torovirus-like particles have also been observed by electron microscopy in feces of swine, cats, and humans.

Properties of Coronaviruses

Classification

Despite differences in virion structure and genome size, coronaviruses, toroviruses, and arteriviruses exhibit similarities in genome organization and replication strategy. In infected cells, all these viruses employ a nested set transcription strategy, i.e., the expression of their genes is mediated via a set of several 3′-coterminal subgenomic mRNAs. This unique strategy has been recognized by the establishment of the order *Nidovirales* (from the Latin *nidus,* nest), encompassing two families: the family *Coronaviridae* with two genera, *Coronavirus* and *Torovirus,* and the family *Arteriviridae,* with one genus, *Arterivirus.* Although conspicuous only in one of the open reading frames encoding the viral RNA-dependent RNA polymerase (transcriptase), the 1b gene, sequence similarities confirm that the member viruses of the order likely evolved from a common ancestor. Extensive genome rearrangements through heterologous RNA recombination have resulted in the variations seen, i.e., viruses with similar replication and transcription strategies but disparate structural features.

The genus *Coronavirus* can be subdivided into three groups on the basis of genetic and serologic properties (Table 33.1). Group I includes transmissible gastroenteritis virus of swine, porcine respiratory coronavirus, canine coronavirus, feline infectious peritonitis virus, feline enteric coronavirus, and human coronavirus 229E. Group II includes mouse hepatitis virus, bovine coronavirus, sialodacryadenitis virus of rats, rabbit coronavirus, turkey bluecomb coronavirus, and human

TABLE 33.1
Antigenic Groups and Diseases Caused by Coronaviruses[a]

ANTIGENIC GROUP	VIRUS	DISEASE
Group I (mammalian viruses)	Transmissible gastroenteritis virus of swine	Gastroenteritis
	Porcine epidemic diarrhea virus	Gastroenteritis
	Feline infectious peritonitis virus	Peritonitis, pneumonia, meningoencephalitis, panophthalmitis, wasting syndrome
	Feline enteric coronavirus	Diarrhea in kittens
	Canine coronavirus	Enteritis
	Human coronavirus 229 E	Common cold
Group II (mammalian and avian)	Mouse hepatitis virus (many types)	Hepatitis, enteritis, encephalomyelitis
	Sialodacryadenitis virus (rats)	Sialodacryadenitis
	Bovine coronavirus	Gastroenteritis (winter dysentery)
	Porcine hemagglutinating encephalomyelitis virus	Vomiting, wasting, and encephalomyelitis
	Human coronavirus OC43	Common cold
	Bluecomb virus of turkeys	Enteritis
Group III (avian)	Infectious bronchitis virus (at least eight serotypes)	Tracheobronchitis, nephritis
Ungrouped	Rabbit coronavirus	Enteritis

[a]Coronaviruses have been associated with infections of the respiratory and enteric tracts and with central nervous system disease in monkeys, rats, and other species.

coronavirus OC43. Group III includes avian infectious bronchitis virus.

Virion Properties

Member viruses of the family *Coronaviridae* are enveloped, 80–220 nm in size, and roughly spherical in shape (coronaviruses) or 120–140 nm in size and disc, kidney, or rod shaped (toroviruses). Coronavirus virions have large (20 nm long) club-shaped peplomers enclosing what appears to be an icosahedral internal core structure within which is a helical nucleocapsid (Figure 33.1). Some coronaviruses also have a second fringe of shorter (5 nm long) peplomers. Toroviruses also have large club-shaped peplomers but they are more pleomorphic and have a tightly coiled tubular nucleocapsid bent into a doughnut-shape (Figure 33.2A). By thin section electron microscopy, because of various planes of section, torovirus nucleocapsids appear as kidney-, disc-, or rod-shaped forms (Figure 33.2B).

The genome consists of a single molecule of linear positive-sense, single-stranded RNA, 27–32 kb in size, the latter being the largest RNA virus genomes known. The genomic RNA is 5′-capped and 3′-polyadenylated and is infectious.

The major virion proteins of the member viruses of the genus *Coronavirus* include a nucleocapsid protein (N, M_r 50,000) and several envelope/peplomer proteins: (1) the major peplomer glycoprotein (S, M_r 180,000 to 200,000); (2) a triple-spanning transmembrane protein (M, M_r 25,000 to 30,000); and (3) a minor transmembrane protein (E, M_r 9,000), which together with M is essential for virion assembly. The secondary, smaller peplomers, seen in group II coronaviruses, consist of a dimer of a class I membrane protein (M_r 65,000), a hemagglutinin-esterase (HE) that shares 30% sequence identity with the N-terminal subunit of the hemagglutinin-esterase fusion protein (HEF) of influenza C virus.

Torovirus virions also have a nucleocapsid protein (N, M_r 19,000), a major peplomer glycoprotein (S, M_r 180,000), and a triple-spanning transmembrane protein (M, M_r 26,000). Although there is no sequence similarity between these proteins and their coronavirus counterparts, they are similar in structure and function and seem to be related phylogenetically. Toroviruses lack a

Figure 33.1.

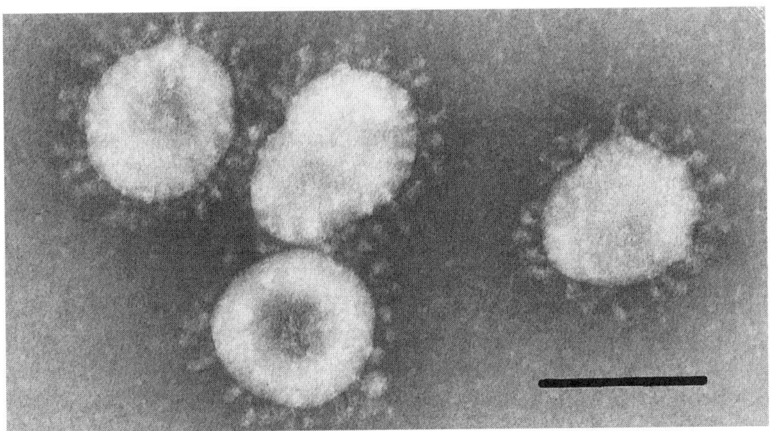

Family *Coronaviridae*, genus *Coronavirus*. Negatively stained virions. Bar: 100 nm.

homologue of the coronavirus E protein—this may relate to the structural differences between the viruses. Bovine toroviruses contain a third transmembrane protein, a hemagglutinin-esterase (M_r 65,000). Sequence comparisons indicate that the HE gene in coronaviruses, toroviruses and orthomyxoviruses has been acquired by independent, non-homologous recombination events (probably from the host cell).

Viral Replication

The strategy of expression of the coronavirus genome is complex (Figure 33.3). First, the viral RNA serves as mRNA for synthesis of the RNA-dependent RNA polymerase. The two large open reading frames (totaling 20 kb in size) encoding the units of the polymerase are translated, the larger via ribosomal frame shifting, as a single polyprotein that is then cleaved. These proteins then assemble to form the active RNA polymerase.

This enzyme is then employed to transcribe full-length complementary (negative-sense) RNA, from which in turn is transcribed not only full-length genomic RNA, but also a 3′-coterminal nested set of subgenomic mRNAs. The nested set comprises five to seven (differing in the various viruses) overlapping mRNAs that extend for different lengths from common 3′ ends and share a common 5′-leader sequence. They are generated by a leader-primed mechanism of discontinuous transcrip-

Figure 33.2.

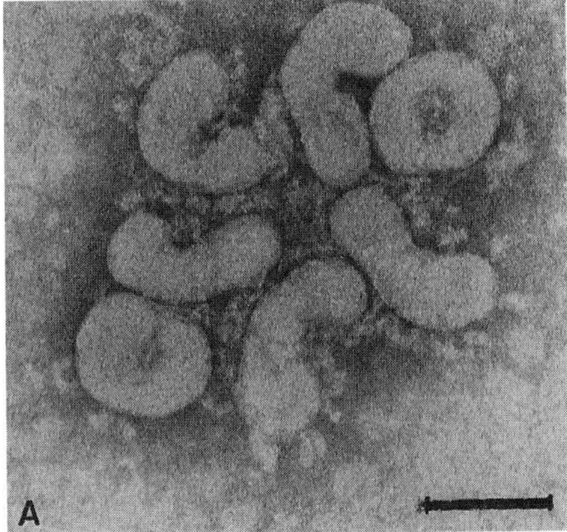

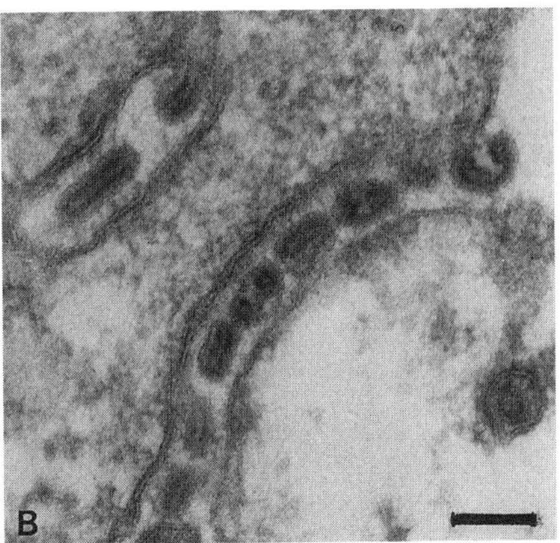

Family *Coronaviridae*, genus *Torovirus*. (A) Negatively stained virions. (B) Thin-sectioned virions in an infected cell. Bar: 100 nm.

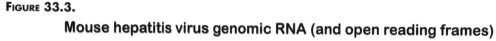

Figure 33.3.

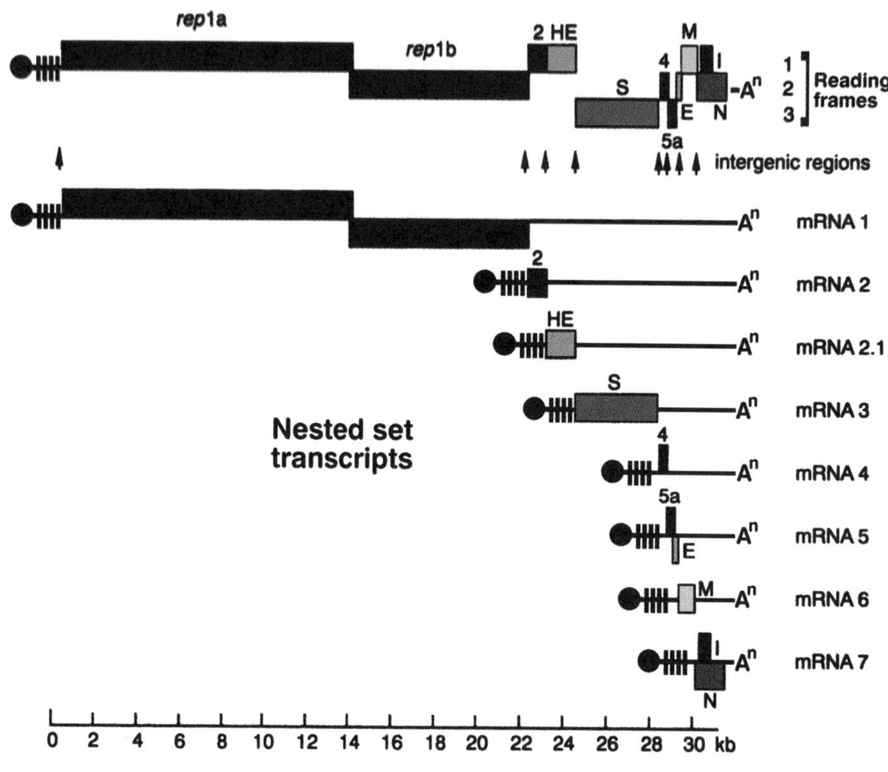

The genome and transcription strategy of mouse hepatitis virus, a typical member of the genus *Coronavirus* (the organization of the genome of toroviruses is slightly different). Genomic and mRNAs are capped (black circles), have leader sequences (vertical lines representing about 70 nucleotides encoded by the 3′ end of the negative strand template), and are polyadenylated (A^n). After release of the positive-sense genomic RNA in the cytoplasm, the viral RNA-dependent RNA polymerase is synthesized; it directs the transcription of a full-length complementary (negative-sense) RNA, from which (1) new genomic RNA, (2) an overlapping set of subgenomic mRNAs, and (3) leader RNA are synthesized. The mRNA transcripts form a nested set with common 3′ ends and common leader sequences on their 5′ ends. Only the unique sequences at the 5′ end of the mRNAs are translated, producing the various proteins: rep1a and rep1b, the two units of the RNA-dependent RNA polymerase; HE, the hemagglutinin-esterase glycoprotein; S, the major peplomer glycoprotein; M, a transmembrane glycoprotein; N, the nucleoprotein; and several nonstructural proteins. [Adapted from S. G. Siddell and E. J. Snijder. Coronaviruses, toroviruses and arteriviruses. *In* "Topley and Wilson's Microbiology and Microbial Infections" (B. W. J. Mahy and L. H. Collier, eds.), Vol. 1, pp. 463–484. Edward Arnold, London, 1998.]

tion: the polymerase first transcribes the noncoding leader sequence from the 3′ end of the complementary (negative-sense) RNA. Then, the capped leader RNA dissociates from the template and reassociates with a complementary sequence at the start of any one of the genes to continue copying the template right through to its 5′ end. Only the unique sequence that is not shared with the next smallest mRNA in the nested set is translated; this strategy yields the various viral proteins in regulated amounts. Intergenic sequences serve as promoters and attenuators of transcription.

Torovirus transcription and replication seems to be similar to that of coronaviruses, except that there are no common 5′-leader sequences on the mRNAs. A puzzling finding is that subgenomic negative-sense RNAs complementary to the nested set of mRNAs are also present in coronavirus- infected cells. The fact that these subgenomic RNAs contain 5′- and 3′-terminal sequences that are identical to those of genomic RNA implies that they may function as replicons.

The synthesis, processing, oligomerization, and transport of the several envelope glycoproteins of coronaviruses display some unusual features. For example, the envelope protein M, which in some coronaviruses contains O-linked rather than N-linked glycans, is directed exclusively to cisternae of the endoplasmic reticulum. As a result of this, virions bud only there and not from the plasma membrane. Virions are then transported in vesicles to the plasma membrane and are released by exocytosis (Figure 33.4). Following their release, many of the mature enveloped virions remain adherent to the outside of the cell. The whole of the replication cycle is

FIGURE 33.4.

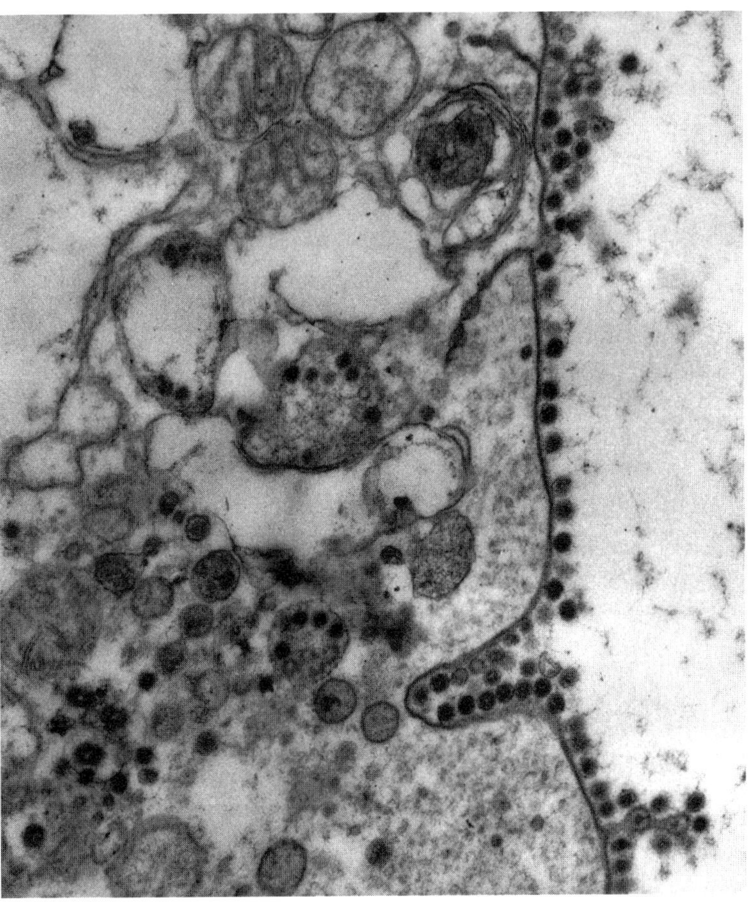

Mouse hepatitis virus infection in the duodenum of a 1-week-old mouse. Virions are transported to the plasma membrane from their site of formation in the endoplasmic reticulum in vesicles and are released by exocytosis. Following their release, many virions remain adherent to the outside of the cell. Thin section electron microscopy. Magnification: ×30,000.

confined to the cytoplasm, indeed it can occur in enucleated cells.

Genetic recombination occurs at high frequency between the genomes of different but related coronaviruses. This may be an important mechanism for the generation of the genetic diversity seen with these viruses in nature (Table 33.2).

Transmissible Gastroenteritis of Swine

There are four distinct coronavirus disease patterns in swine, referred to as (1) vomiting and wasting disease, (2) porcine epidemic diarrhea, (3) transmissible gastroenteritis, and (4) respiratory disease. The respiratory variant of transmissible gastroenteritis virus was discovered in 1986 when seroconversion was seen in swine herds in countries (e.g., Denmark) known to be free of porcine coronaviruses; the virus causing this disease pattern has been shown to be a deletion mutant that has completely lost its enterotropism and has acquired a respiratory tropism and transmission pattern. When this mutant appeared it served as a reminder of the pathogenic potential of continuing coronavirus evolution.

Clinical Features

Clinical signs are most severe in very young piglets. Most, if not all, neonates succumb, whereas few deaths occur in animals more than 3 weeks of age. Piglets present with vomiting followed by profuse yellowish diarrhea, weight loss, and dehydration. Time until death is 2 to

Table 33.2
Properties of Coronaviruses and Toroviruses

Virions are pleomorphic or spherical (genus *Coronavirus*) or disc, kidney, or rod shaped (genus *Torovirus*); 80–220 (genus *Coronavirus*) or 120–140 (genus *Torovirus*) nm in diameter. Virions are enveloped with large club-shaped peplomers

Virions have an icosahedral internal core structure within which is a helical nucleocapsid (genus *Coronavirus*) or a tightly coiled tubular nucleocapsid bent into a doughnut-shape (genus *Torovirus*)

The genome consists of a single molecule of linear positive-sense, single-stranded RNA, 27–32 kb in size; the genome is 5′-capped, 3′-polyadenylated, and infectious

Coronavirus virions contain three or four structural proteins: a major peplomer glycoprotein (S), transmembrane glycoproteins (M and E), a nucleoprotein (N), and, in some viruses, a hemagglutinin-esterase (HE). Torovirus virions contain analogous proteins, but there is no E protein

Viruses replicate in the cytoplasm; the genome is transcribed, forming a full-length complementary RNA from which is transcribed a 3′-coterminal nested set of mRNAs, only the unique sequences of which are translated

Virions are formed by budding into the endoplasmic reticulum and are released by exocytosis

7 days after the onset of clinical signs in piglets less than 1 week of age. In older animals, the duration of diarrhea is shorter and vomiting is seen only rarely. Exceptions to these disease patterns pose important clinical diagnostic problems: in some outbreaks there is high mortality in adult swine, in others sows may show anorexia, fever, vomiting, diarrhea, and agalactia, and in yet others infection may be inapparent.

Pathogenesis, Pathology, and Immunity

The virus enters the body by ingestion, and after an incubation period of 18 to 72 hours it causes clinical signs that vary according to the age of the animal infected. There are several reasons for the susceptibility of very young piglets: (1) their gastric secretions are not yet as acid as those of older animals and the virus is rather acid labile and (2) their diet of milk buffers gastric acid, thereby protecting the virus. Virus is therefore free to reach and infect villous enterocytes of the small intestine. These cells are destroyed by the infection, resulting in shortening and blunting of villi. Villous enterocytes are the source of lactase and other disaccharidases needed in the digestion of milk—absence of enzymes results in an increased osmolarity of the intestinal contents, resulting in water transport from tissues into the intestinal lumen. The consequence is diarrhea. Crypt epithelial cells remain uninfected so recovery of the integrity and function of villi is rather rapid.

Gross pathology (except for the dehydration) is restricted to the gastrointestinal tract and consists of a distended stomach and small intestine, often containing yellowish undigested milk. The destruction of villi, which can be best seen when the gut is submerged in isotonic buffer, results in a thinning of the intestinal wall.

Maternal IgA antibodies, passed to piglets in colostrum and milk, provide protection against infection; systemic IgG antibody does not protect. IgA antibodies are also more resistant to proteolytic degradation in the intestine and adhere more firmly to the gut epithelium. The gut–mammary link of lymphocyte trafficking results in local IgA production in the mammary gland. Immunity cannot be stimulated by parenteral immunization, only by mucosal immunization.

Laboratory Diagnosis

Mucosal impression smears or cryostat sections of intestinal tissue prepared from piglets in early stages of the disease may be examined by immunofluorescence or immunoperoxidase staining—these methods provide rapid results. Virus isolation is carried out in porcine thyroid or testicle cells; there is cytopathology and isolates are identified by serology, usually using an enzyme immunoassay. Using paired serum samples and either serum neutralization or enzyme immunoassay, serology allows retrospective diagnosis and is also valuable in epidemiological investigations.

Epidemiology, Prevention, and Control

Between epidemics, transmissible gastroenteritis virus probably persists in some swine, as a reservoir in another host species seems unlikely. When the virus is introduced into a nonimmune herd there is epidemic spread among animals of all ages with 100% mortality in newborn piglets and variable, usually less severe disease in older animals. When no susceptible swine are left and no new animals are reintroduced, the epidemic terminates, usually within a few weeks.

Another epidemiologic pattern occurs in intense production facilities where the farrowing system makes susceptible piglets available continuously. Endemic infection and background immunity usually lead to low mortality that is most pronounced shortly after weaning when maternally acquired IgA-based immunity has waned.

Protection of swine by attenuated virus vaccines has not been very effective: the best protection has been obtained when virulent virus has been administered to pregnant sows, thereby boosting lactogenic immunity in piglets. Control also involves good sanitation and management practices: for example after an outbreak in a 650 sow farrowing unit in Ireland, which supplied piglets to a 12,000 head fattening unit, endemic disease was eliminated by depopulation of all pens where clinical cases had occurred and all pens housing seropositive sows. Control was maintained by extensive serological monitoring.

Porcine Hemagglutinating Encephalomyelitis Virus Disease

Porcine hemagglutinating encephalitis virus causes vomiting and wasting disease. This disease was first reported in Canadian swine in 1958, but it is now recognized in the United States and Europe as well.

Many of the clinical and pathologic features of this disease are indistinguishable from those of porcine polioencephalomyelitis, which is caused by a picornavirus. The disease, seen principally in piglets under 2 weeks of age, is characterized by anorexia, hyperesthesia, muscle tremors, paddling of the legs, vomiting, and depression, often leading to emaciation and death. In contrast to transmissible gastroenteritis, diarrhea is not common. Mortality in young piglets is high; older animals often survive but remain permanently stunted. Serologic surveys indicate that the virus is present in many herds in many countries; in many settings the disease is not diagnosed and goes unrecognized while causing substantial morbidity and economic loss.

The virus multiplies first in the nasal mucosa, tonsils, lung, and small intestine and then spreads to the central nervous system via peripheral nerves. Viremia is not important in the pathogenesis of this disease. In the central nervous system, virus is first detected in the sensory nuclei of the trigeminal and vagus nerves, with subsequent spread to the brain stem, cerebrum, and cerebellum. The infection of other organs does not contribute significantly to the pathogenesis of the disease. One characteristic clinical sign, vomiting, is due to virus replication in the *ganglion distale vagi*; the other, wasting, is due to neurologic disturbance of the vomition center. Severe, unremitting vomiting leads to malnutrition.

A clinical diagnosis of porcine hemagglutinating virus encephalomyelitis may be confirmed by the isolation of virus in primary porcine cell culture; growth of the virus is detected by hemagglutination. Because no vaccines are available, good husbandry is essential for the prevention and control of the disease.

Porcine Epidemic Diarrhea

Porcine epidemic diarrhea, described in several countries of western Europe, is clinically similar to transmissible gastroenteritis, but spreads more slowly. The virus that causes this disease is unrelated to the other porcine coronaviruses. The main clinical sign in piglets is watery diarrhea, sometimes preceded by vomiting. In adult swine the infection may remain asymptomatic or may be limited to depression, anorexia, and vomiting. The mortality rate in piglets is usually about 50% but may be as high as 90%. Older pigs recover after about 1 week of illness. A diagnosis may be confirmed by the isolation of virus in primary porcine cell culture or by the demonstration of antibodies in convalescent swine. Vaccines are not available.

Bovine Coronavirus Enteritis (and Winter Dysentery)

Coronaviruses are second to rotaviruses as the major cause of diarrhea in young calves. Coronaviruses were first reported as a cause of diarrhea in calves in the United States in 1973, and since then they have been recognized worldwide. Initially, diagnosis was based on the detection of virus by electron microscopy, but subsequently the addition of trypsin to bovine cell culture medium was shown to facilitate the isolation of virus. Today, for many virus strains, a variety of bovine cells and human HRT-18 cells are used for primary isolation. Viral growth may be recognized by hemadsorption.

The pathogenesis of bovine coronavirus enteritis is similar to that of rotavirus diarrhea. Disease is seen most commonly in calves at about 1 week of age, the time when antibody in the dam's milk starts to wane and exposure is maximal. The diarrhea usually lasts for 4 or 5 days. The destruction of the absorptive cells of the intestinal epithelium of the small intestine and, to a lesser extent, the large intestine leads to the rapid loss of water and electrolytes. Glucose and lactose metabolism are affected; hypoglycemia, lactic acidosis, and hypervolemia can lead to acute shock, cardiac failure, and death. Bovine coronaviruses may cause diarrhea in humans.

Available vaccines are not effective because they do not appear to contain sufficient antigenic mass and they cannot be given early enough to evoke protection at the time of maximum risk. One alternative to vaccinating calves is to immunize the dam, thereby promoting elevated antibody levels in the colostrum. Another alternative is to feed calves colostrum and milk from hyperimmunized cows used as donors.

Winter dysentery is a sporadic acute disease of adult cattle that occurs in many countries throughout the world. It is believed to be caused by one or more coronaviruses, but this is still debated. The syndrome is characterized by explosive, often bloody diarrhea accompanied by decreased milk production, depression, and anorexia.

Feline Infectious Peritonitis

Feline infectious peritonitis is arguably the most enigmatic coronavirus disease of all. Its pathogenesis involves immunopathologic mechanisms such as antibody-dependent enhancement of infection and immune complex-induced lesions (see Chapter 10). Feline enteric coronavirus has been proven to play a crucial role in the pathogenesis of this disease. The sporadic occurrence of the disease is the result of *in vivo* mutations of the enteric virus, resulting in an acquired macrophage tropism. Two serotypes of feline enteric coronavirus have been identified, both being able to cause feline infectious peritonitis via this mechanism. Type 2 is a recombinant with genetic information acquired from canine coronavirus, which is the cause of a generally benign diarrheal disease in pups.

Clinical Features

Feline infectious peritonitis is a progressive, debilitating lethal disease of domestic and wild members of the family *Felidae*. The initial clinical signs are not very distinguishing. Affected cats present with anorexia, chronic fever, and malaise. Occasionally, ocular and neurological manifestations are seen. In classical "wet" or effusive feline infectious peritonitis, these signs are accompanied by a gradual abdominal distention due to the accumulation of a viscous yellow ascitic fluid. The quantity of fluid can vary from a few milliliters to well over a liter. There is also a "dry" or noneffusive form of disease with little or no exudate. The wet and dry forms are different manifestations of the same infection.

Pathogenesis, Pathology, and Immunity

The key pathogenic event in feline infectious peritonitis is the infection of monocytes and macrophages. Experimentally, the virulence of strains of feline enteric coronavirus has been correlated with their ability to infect cultured peritoneal macrophages, avirulent isolates infecting fewer macrophages and producing lower virus titers than virulent isolates. Avirulent isolates are also less able to sustain viral replication and spread between macrophages. This is a quantitative phenomenon, seen as a gradient from rather benign isolates to exceptionally virulent isolates.

The ubiquitous avirulent feline enteric coronavirus is not confined to the digestive tract; rather, it spreads beyond the intestinal epithelium and regional lymph nodes. Therefore, the mutations that transform this virus into pathogenic feline infectious peritonitis virus can occur in several organs and tissues, each the basis for some variation in the clinical manifestations of the disease.

Gross lesions in feline infectious peritonitis appear as multiple grayish-white nodules (<1 to 10 mm in diameter) in the serosa of the liver, lungs, spleen, omentum, intestines, and kidneys. Microscopically, the primary lesion is an acute, immune-mediated, perivascular necrosis, which progresses to a chronic pyogranulomatous lesion (foci of macrophages, neutrophils, and lymphocytes). Lesions may appear in various tissues, but omentum, peritoneal serosa, liver, kidney, pleura, lung parenchyma, pericardium, meninges, brain, and uvea are common sites.

Although the vascular and perivascular lesions in feline infectious peritonitis are clearly immune mediated, there is uncertainty about the actual pathogenetic mechanisms involved. Some vascular injury may be attributed to the immune-mediated lysis of infected white blood cells; such events have been detected in the lumen, intima, and wall of veins and in perivascular tissues. Furthermore, inflammatory mediators such as cytokines, leukotrienes, and prostaglandins that are released by infected macrophages may play a role in the development of perivascular inflammatory lesions. These host-response molecules may induce changes in vascular permeability and provide chemotactic stimuli for neutrophils and monocytes. In response to the inflammation, the attracted cells may release additional mediators and cytotoxic substances. Invading monocytes may also serve as new virus targets, thereby amplifying the infection further. The end result is enhanced local virus production and increased tissue damage.

Deposition of immune complexes and subsequent complement activation exacerbate the inflammatory response that extends across involved blood vessel walls. The resulting vascular damage permits leakage of fluid into perivascular spaces and leads to the accumulation of thoracic and abdominal transudates/exudates. Morphologic features of the vascular lesions (necrosis, neutrophil infiltration around small veins and venules) indicate an Arthus-type reaction. The lesions contain focal deposits of virus–IgG–C3 complexes. There is complement depletion and circulating immune complexes in cats with terminal feline infectious peritonitis.

Although feline infectious peritonitis virus does not infect T cells, depletion and programmed cell death (apoptosis) have been observed in lymphoid organs of infected cats. Apoptosis is mediated by the immune complexes present in the serum and ascitic fluid of diseased cats. T cell destruction and consequent immunosuppression lead to the opportunistic infections that characterize the late stages of this disease.

Humoral immunity is not protective: cats that are seropositive to feline enteric coronavirus, when challenged experimentally with virulent feline infectious peritonitis virus, develop an accelerated, fulminant disease, leading to an "early death syndrome." Clinical signs and lesions develop earlier, and the mean survival time is reduced as compared to seronegative cats. Direct evidence for the involvement of antibodies in this phenomenon was obtained in experiments in which purified IgG from cats infected with feline enteric coronavirus was transfused into uninfected cats, which where then challenged with virulent virus. These cats developed an accelerated, fulminant disease identical to that seen naturally.

Diagnosis

Serology, usually done using indirect immunofluorescence or enzyme immunoassay, generally shows moderate to high antibody titers in infected cats. However, some cats with the disease remain seronegative or have only a very low antibody titer, and some healthy cats with no clinical signs of disease have high titers. Therefore, interpretation of serology data is not possible for an individual cat. Biopsy of affected organs not only confirms the diagnosis, but also reveals the extent and stage of the disease.

Epidemiology, Prevention, and Control

The scenario leading to fatal feline infectious peritonitis may be described as follows: a kitten, suckled by its seropositive queen, is protected by colostral antibody during the first few weeks of life. As maternal antibody wanes, mucosal protection ebbs and, during an episode of maternal feline enteric coronavirus shedding, the kitten becomes infected. A bout of diarrhea may be the only sign that this has happened. The kitten now develops an active immune response, but in most cases not a sterilizing response. Virus and antibodies continue to coexist in the kitten's tissues, modulated by an efficient cell-mediated immune response that keeps infected macrophages and monocytes in check. In a small, socially stable cat community, this animal may remain healthy. However, problems occur when the kitten is stressed or when there is another cause of immunosuppression. Infections with feline leukemia virus or feline immunodeficiency virus are the most common immunosuppressive events. However, crowding, displacement to a new location, and social/territorial factors (e.g., changes in group hierarchy, dominance) are becoming recognized as important stressors as well. Failing immune surveillance allows viral mutants to flourish—more macrophage-tropic mutants emerge. Among these mutants and some that grow to high titers and out-compete less pathogenic viruses. This is the point when immunopathogenetic events begin.

Feline infectious peritonitis is not controlled easily; control requires the elimination of the virus from the local environment, whether this be the household or the cattery. This requires a high level of hygiene, strict quarantine, and immunoprophylactic measures. Because kittens acquire the infection from their queens, early weaning programs have also been used in attempts to interrupt virus transmission.

The only commercially available feline infectious peritonitis vaccine contains a temperature-sensitive mutant virus. The vaccine is applied to the nasal mucosa where conditions favor a low level of viral replication without antibody formation. Under these conditions, a cellular immune response is favored, and some protection is achieved. Vaccination of infected, seropositive adult cats (and these are most cats) is not effective.

Canine Coronavirus Diarrhea

Canine coronavirus usually produces a mild gastroenteritis. Although originally described before the first occurrence of canine parvovirus enteritis in 1978, the disease now commonly occurs in association with canine parvovirus infection, which causes a more severe and sometimes fatal diarrhea. The virus commonly infects pups and is probably worldwide in distribution. Epidemics of coronavirus enteritis have also been recorded in wild dogs. The disease is similar to that caused by enteric coronaviruses in other species, such as calves. Although canine coronavirus does not infect swine, transmissible gastroenteritis virus can infect dogs.

Because there are many causes of diarrhea in dogs, clinical suspicion of canine coronavirus infection should be confirmed by laboratory-based procedures. The virus may be visualized by electron microscopy or may be isolated in primary canine cell culture. Detection of antibody in the sera of pups is of limited value because it may be of maternal origin and unrelated to the cause of the diarrhea. An inactivated vaccine is available for the control of canine coronavirus diarrhea, but its protective value is doubtful.

Mouse Hepatitis (Lethal Intestinal Virus Disease of Infant Mice)

The various diseases caused by mouse hepatitis virus represent the most important infectious disease problems encountered in mouse colonies throughout the world. Mouse hepatitis virus is extremely contagious, in some settings causing explosive epidemics and high mortality and in others causing endemic infection that may go unrecognized. There are many different virus strains, each with characteristic tissue tropisms, resulting in varying clinical manifestations. The nature and severity of disease are also influenced greatly by the strain of mouse. Mouse hepatitis virus infection alters a wide variety of immunological and other physiological parameters—it can be a major confounding factor in research undertaken using mice from infected colonies.

Clinical Features

Although mouse hepatitis virus strains have been characterized very well, both antigenically and genetically, the various patterns of disease caused by each strain are complex, not easily predicted, subject to overlap, and dependent on the age and strain of the mouse. Infection with different virus strains can cause enteritis, hepatitis, demyelinating encephalomyelitis, and nephritis. Disease may be precipitated by any immunosuppressive drug or procedure or by concomitant infection with K virus (a papovavirus) or *Eperythrozoon coccoides*.

Most important in mouse colonies are virus strains that are enteropathogenic: infection of suckling mice with these strains produces a syndrome known previously as *lethal intestinal virus (disease) of infant mice*. When these strains first gain entry into a mouse colony there is widespread diarrhea, which may spread throughout the colony in a few days, with nearly 100% mortality. Older mice lose weight, cease breeding, often exhibit jaundice, and many die. Other clinically important strains of mouse hepatitis virus are the cause of respiratory and central nervous system diseases in mouse colonies. The latter may be seen as paralysis, caused by demyelination.

Pathogenesis, Pathology, and Immunity

Gross lesions in infected suckling mice dying of enteritis are characteristic: their intestines are distended flaccidly with bright yellow fluid and, as a result of stasis, there is an accumulation of bile pigments, epithelial destruction, and osmotic diarrhea (Figure 33.5). The pathophysiologic effects of viral diarrhea are a consequence of rapid infection and destruction of epithelial cells and their replacement by immature, transitional cells that cannot carry out normal absorptive, resorptive, and enzyme secretory functions. Glucose-coupled sodium transport is impaired, disaccharidase (lactase, sucrase) activities are diminished, and, in some cases, adenylate cyclase and cyclic AMP levels are increased (the latter causing a hypersecretion of water and chlorides). The osmotic disequilibrium is most severe in infant mice because of the normal presence of high concentrations of milk lactose in the intestinal lumen. Osmotic equilibrium returns when the regenerating intestinal epithelium matures sufficiently to produce lactase and to absorb the hexoses produced by the enzyme's action.

Histological lesions are characteristic: intestinal villi are blunted and club shaped and there is massive syncytium formation (seen as large clumps of nuclei of epithelial cells) (Figure 33.6). This status gives way to cytonecrosis and massive desquamation of epithelium. Infection is nearly universally lethal. Even in infections caused by enteropathogenic strains of virus, there is also evidence of acute hepatitis (focal hepatocellular necrosis and inflammatory infiltration).

Laboratory Diagnosis

A presumptive diagnosis may be made on the detection of characteristic gross lesions and confirmed by histopathology, immunohistochemistry, and serology using an enzyme immunoassay. Most strains of the virus can be grown in any of several mouse cell lines. Characteristically, infection is evidenced by the formation of large syncytia. Laboratory-based diagnostics are a key element in surveillance systems for many mouse viruses, including mouse hepatitis virus; such diagnostic systems are required in all research protocols funded in the United States by the National Institutes of Health.

Epidemiology, Prevention, and Control

Epidemic mouse hepatitis virus disease in a mouse colony typically follows the introduction of new mice, say a shipment of inbred mice from a new source. Epidemics are devastating, resulting in the rapid death of a high

FIGURE 33.5.

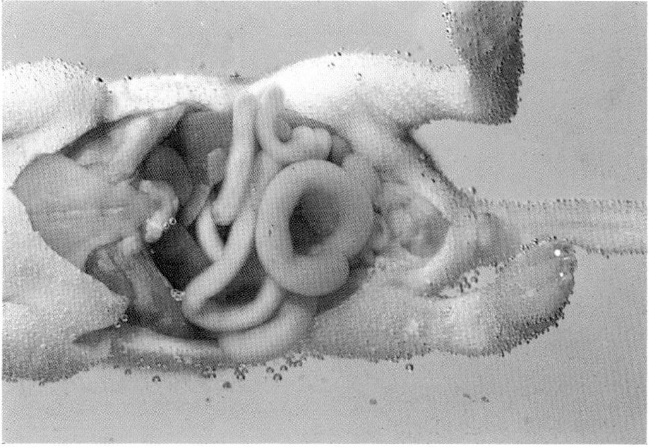

Enteropathogenic mouse hepatitis virus infection in a 10-day-old mouse. The intestines are distended flaccidly and filled with yellowish fluid.

FIGURE 33.6.

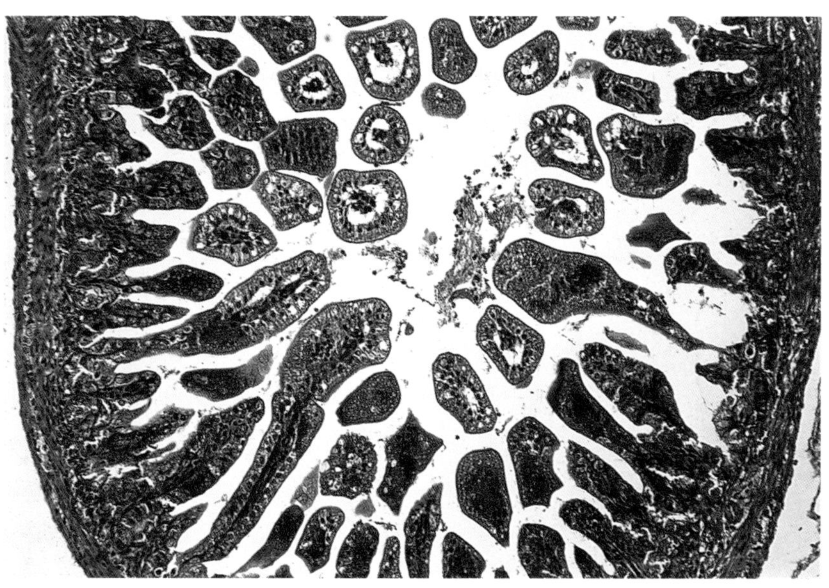

Cross section of the jejunum of a 10-day-old mouse infected with enteropathogenic mouse hepatitis virus. Villi are blunted and club shaped and there is massive syncytium formation (seen as large clumps of nuclei of epithelial cells). This status gives way to cytonecrosis and massive desquamation of epithelium. Infection is nearly universally lethal.

proportion of animals at risk. Following this epidemic phase, surviving mice may maintain the virus and continually infect new, susceptible mice, either those introduced from outside or bred in the colony. If new susceptible mice are introduced into this setting as weanlings, they may sustain subclinical infection, contributing to the endemic persistence of the transmission chain and serving as the source of virus when removed to other rooms or to other colonies.

Control is achieved by breaking the transmission cycle, but this is very difficult. Often, after unsuccessful efforts based on cessation of breeding, quarantine, and care in introducing new mice, the decision is made to depopulate, thoroughly decontaminate the facility, and repopulate from clean sources. When valuable inbred strains of mice are involved, less drastic methods are often tried, usually unsuccessfully. When a colony is returned to a virus-free status, the prevention of any reintroduction of virus is a matter of the strictest quarantine systems, rigorous testing of mice before introducing them into the colony (this requires totally separate holding quarters), prevention of the entry of wild mice, and control of personnel access. In some cases, mice from infected colonies are used for experimental purposes; this decision, of course, must depend on the nature of the studies to be done and the risk of spread of the virus.

Sialodacryadenitis of Rats

Sialodacryoadenitis is a common disease of laboratory rats marked by severe, self-limiting inflammation and necrosis of the salivary and nasolacrimal glands. It is especially severe in young rats. The etiologic agent, sialodacryoadenitis virus, is highly contagious; when the virus invades a rat colony there is a high incidence of morbidity, but little mortality. During epidemics there may be a high incidence of anesthetic deaths. Clinical signs of infection include excessive lacrimation, exophthalmus, squinting, excessive blinking, and swollen face and neck. Lesions in the lacrimal duct may result in corneal drying with severe secondary ocular lesions. The disease is self-limiting, and most lesions resolve within 2 weeks. Transmission is by direct contact, by fomites (such as inadequately sterilized cages and water bottles), and by aerosol. Control is the same as for mouse hepatitis virus in mouse colonies.

Avian Infectious Bronchitis

Infectious bronchitis was the term coined in 1931 to describe the principal clinical–pathological feature of a transmissible respiratory disease of poultry in the United States. It has now been found in almost every country of the world and is one of the most important viral diseases of chickens. The virus is the prototype of the family *Coronaviridae;* it occurs in many antigenic variants as a consequence of mutations in its large genome.

Clinical Features

The clinical presentation of infectious bronchitis depends on the age of the bird at the time of infection, the route of exposure, the bird's immune status, and the strain of virus. Outbreaks may be explosive, with the virus spreading rapidly to involve the entire flock within a few days. In chicks 1 to 4 weeks of age, virulent virus strains produce gasping, coughing, rales, nasal exudate, and respiratory distress (Figure 33.7).

Chicks demonstrate plaintive, high-pitched cheeps, become lethargic, lose appetite, and may die suddenly. Mortality in young chicks is usually 25–30%, but in some outbreaks can be as high as 75%. Less virulent strains cause few respiratory signs; whether clinical signs are seen or not, infection usually results in retarded growth (stunting).

When uncomplicated by opportunistic bacterial superinfection, respiratory signs last for 5 to 7 days and disappear from the flock in 10 to 14 days. Cessation of growth for several days can still occur at this age, however. High mortality can occur in broilers due to secondary infection with *Escherichia coli* or pathogenic mycoplasmas. There appears to be no effect on the reproductive system of birds near sexual maturity, provided egg production has not started. Birds in egg production show respiratory rales and coughing with prominent involvement of the reproductive tract and a decline or cessation of egg production. When laying is resumed, many eggs show abnormalities: no shells, thin shells, shells with deposits, distortions, dimples, depressions, or ridging; eggs that should be colored are often pale or white. There is loss of albumen quality, sometimes the thick white disappearing almost completely. An additional clinical feature (caused especially by strains of low virulence) is "pasting," i.e., the accumulation of a white, sticky exudate around the vent that can plug the cloaca; after a few days, the plug may slough, leaving a bare patch.

Pathogenesis, Pathology, and Immunity

The virus replicates to high titer first in the respiratory tract (ciliated epithelial cells); this is followed by viremia (within 1 to 2 days of infection), which distributes the

Figure 33.7.

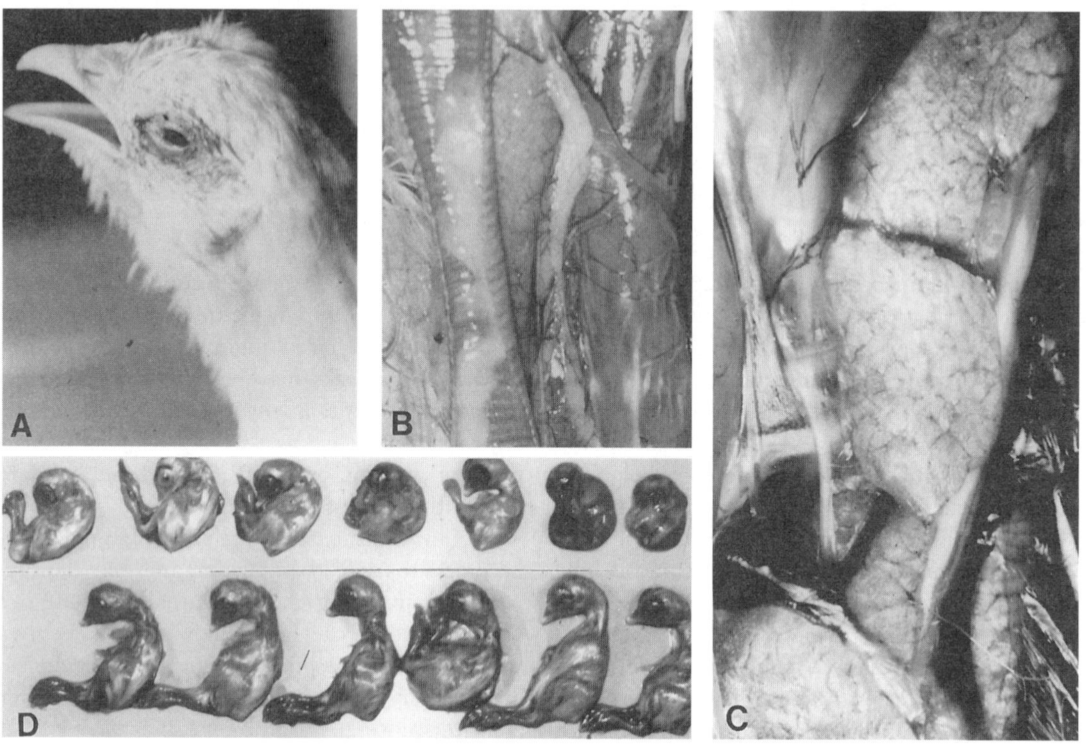

Avian infectious bronchitis. (A) One synonym for the disease is "gasping disease." (B) Thick mucopurulent exudate in the trachea. (C) Nephrosis. The kidney is pale and enlarged to about five times normal size. (D) Embryos from embryonated hen's eggs inoculated via the allantoic cavity with serial dilutions of virus when 9 days old and examined 11 days later. Amounts of virus diminish in pairs from right to left in the top row and from left to right in the bottom row. (Courtesy of R. J. H. Wells.)

virus to many organs. Eventually the virus causes major damage to the reproductive system and the kidneys. The intestinal tract is another site of primary infection. Infections originating in the upper respiratory tract may result in less severe disease than when primary infection occurs in the lower respiratory tract.

Infectivity declines rapidly and isolation of virus beyond 10 days postinfection is uncommon (except from chicks). Rarely, virus may persist for up to 50 days after primary infection. Virus can be isolated from many organs, including the kidneys and bursa of Fabricius (which may be the reason for the immunosuppressive effects noted). Some strains produce permanent anatomical damage to the immature oviduct.

The most frequent gross pathological finding is mucosal thickening with serous or catarrhal exudate in the nasal passages, trachea, bronchi, and air sacs. In very young chicks, the main bronchi may be blocked with caseous yellow casts, which may be the main cause of death. Pneumonia, conjunctivitis, and swollen sinuses are sometimes seen. In laying birds, ova can be congested and sometimes ruptured, with free yolk in the abdominal cavity. Desquamation of respiratory epithelium, edema, epithelial hyperplasia, mononuclear cell infiltration of the submucosa, and regeneration are seen in a various combinations. Repair processes begin after 6 to 10 days, and a return to normal is achieved in 14 to 21 days. Virus strains affecting the kidney occur mostly in Australia, but some degree of nephrotropism (interstitial nephritis) is found worldwide.

Infection induces IgM, IgG, and IgA antibodies. In immune laying hens, the ovum begins to acquire IgG antibody (some of it virus specific) from the blood about 5 days before the egg is layed. As it becomes surrounded with albumen during passage down the oviduct, the ovum acquires both IgM and IgA antibodies, which find their way into the amniotic fluid about halfway through development. During the last third of embryonation, IgG enters the circulation from the yolk; antibody can inhibit virus replication at this time. The chick hatches with a circulating IgG level similar to that of the hen. IgG antibody is metabolized with a half-life of approximately 3 days and may persist for 3 to 4 weeks. The virus may survive until passive immunity declines to a level where it can replicate again, at which time the chicken mounts an active immune response.

Laboratory Diagnosis

Direct immunofluorescence staining of tracheal tissue smears is useful in the diagnosis of early cases before secondary bacterial infection has occurred. For virus isolation, embryonated eggs are inoculated via the intra-allantoic route. Changes suggestive of the presence of a coronavirus include congestion of the main blood vessels in the chorioallantoic membrane and embryo stunting. Identification of virus in the chorioallantoic membrane is usually done by immunofluorescence, gel diffusion, or electron microscopy. In some laboratories the polymerase chain reaction (with appropriate identification of amplified products) or DNA probes are being used. Isolates are usually typed and subtyped by serologic methods.

Epidemiology, Prevention, and Control

Infectious bronchitis virus spreads between birds by aerosol and by ingestion of food contaminated with feces. In the environment the virus can survive on fomites for several days and possibly for weeks, especially at low environmental temperatures. Outbreaks of infectious bronchitis have declined in recent years due to the wide use of vaccines; however, the disease may occur even in vaccinated flocks following the introduction of infected replacement chicks. To minimize this risk, most poultry producers obtain 1-day-old chicks from certified virus-free sources and rear them in isolation.

Attenuated virus vaccines are widely used to protect chicks. These vaccines are derived either from avirulent field isolates or by passage in embryonated eggs. They are administered in drinking water, by coarse spray, or by deposition on the conjunctiva. The vaccine is usually given between 7 and 10 days of age and again at 4 weeks. Vaccination earlier than 7 days may be unsuccessful because of passively acquired maternal antibody. Vaccination breaks are common because of the variable presence of new antigenic variants. Such variants will continue to emerge and spread, posing continuing problems for poultry producers.

Control of infectious bronchitis is difficult because of the presence of persistently infected chickens in many flocks. Eggs have been found to contain virus for approximately 50 days after infection. The domestic chicken is the most important but not the only host for infectious bronchitis virus; infections and disease have been described in pheasants in England, racing pigeons in Australia, and guinea fowl in South America.

Turkey Bluecomb Disease

Bluecomb disease was first recognized in turkeys in the United States in 1951 and has now been recorded in other countries. The disease affects turkeys of all ages but is most severe in 1- to 6-week-old poults. The onset is characterized by loss of appetite, constant chirping, diarrhea, weight loss, and depression. The skin of the head and neck may become cyanotic. Younger poults may die. Lesions in the digestive tract are very similar to those seen in coronavirus infections in mammals. Some turkeys may shed virus in their feces for several months.

Only one serotype of bluecomb virus is recognized; the virus can be isolated in embryonated eggs of turkeys and chickens or in turkey embryo intestinal organ culture. An inactivated virus vaccine is available, but is generally considered to be rather ineffective.

Torovirus Diseases

Thus far, only two toroviruses have been recognized: the equine and bovine toroviruses, better known as Berne virus and Breda virus, respectively. The existence of a torovirus of swine (porcine torovirus), genetically closely related to the equine and bovine viruses, has been demonstrated by molecular techniques.

Clinical Features

Little is known of the disease potential of Berne virus in horses—only a single case has been described, this in a horse with diarrhea that died. Upon postmortem examination, pseudomembranous enteritis and miliary granulomas and necrosis in the liver were seen. Breda virus causes diarrhea in calves and has been recognized as a serious problem in some herds. In swine, torovirus infection has been associated with diarrhea at the time of weaning.

Pathogenesis, Pathology, and Immunity

Breda virus, the bovine torovirus, is pathogenic for newborn gnotobiotic and nonimmune conventional calves; these animals develop watery diarrhea lasting for 4 to 5 days with virus shedding occurring for another 3 to 4 days. In calves with a normal intestinal flora, diarrhea is more severe than in gnotobiotic calves. Histological examination of the intestines has shown villous atrophy and epithelial desquamation from the midjejunum through to the lower small intestine and areas of necrosis in the large intestine. Epithelial cells of crypts and villi are infected. Infection of the former may affect the duration of diarrhea, as regeneration of epithelium starts in the crypts. The germinal centers of the Peyer's patches become depleted of lymphocytes and occasionally develop hemorrhages. Dome epithelial cells, including M cells, exhibit the same cytopathic changes that occur in villi.

Laboratory Diagnosis

Using immunofluorescence, Breda virus antigen can be detected in epithelial cells of the small intestine. Fluorescence is cytoplasmic and is generally most intense in areas of the intestines with the least tissue damage. The midjejunum is the first site to be infected, with viral infection progressing down the small intestine and eventually reaching the large intestine. Given this course of the infection, tissue specimens must be obtained at several levels and as early after the onset of diarrhea as possible. Serum neutralization and enzyme immunoassays are available, using as antigen the equine torovirus, Berne virus.

Epidemiology, Prevention, and Control

Torovirus infections are common. In cattle, 90–95% of randomly sampled cattle have antibodies. Antibody-positive cattle have been identified in every country where tests have been done. Most adult horses in Switzerland possess neutralizing antibodies to Breda virus, which is also true for goats, sheep, pigs, rabbits, and some species of wild mice. Epidemiological surveys have indicated that torovirus infections are involved in two disease entities in cattle: diarrhea in calves up to 2 months of age and winter dysentery of adult cattle in The Netherlands and Costa Rica. In view of their variable role as pathogens, vaccines have not been developed against toroviruses.

Further Reading

Bohl, E. H., and Pensaert, M. B. (1989). Transmissible gastroenteritis virus. *In* "Virus Infections of Vertebrates" (M. B. Pensaert, ed.), Vol. 2, pp. 139–165. Elsevier, Amsterdam.

de Vries, A. A. F., Horzinek, M. C., Rottier, P. J. M., and de Groot, R. J. (1997). The genome organization of the Nidovirales: Similarities and differences between arteri-, toro-, and coronaviruses. *Semin. Virol.* **8**, 33–47.

Homberger, F. R. (1997). Enterotropic mouse hepatitis virus. *Lab. Anim.* **31**, 97–115.

Horzinek, M. C. (1993). Toroviruses—members of the coronavirus superfamily? *Arch. Virol. Suppl.* **7**, 75–80.

Koopmans, M., and Horzinek, M. C. (1994). Toroviruses of animals and humans: A review. *Adv. Virus Res.* **43**, 233–273.

Lai, M. M. C., and Cavanagh, D. (1997). The molecular biology of coronaviruses. *Adv. Virus Res.* **48**, 1–100.

McMartin, D. A., and Faragher, J. T. (1993). Infectious bronchitis. *In* "Virus Infections of Vertebrates" (J. B. McFerran and M. S. McNulty, eds.), Vol. 4, pp. 249–275. Elsevier, Amsterdam.

Pedersen, N. C. (1995). An overview of feline enteric coronavirus and infectious peritonitis virus infections. *Feline Pract.* **23**, 7–20.

Pedersen, N. C., Addie, D., and Wolf, A. (1995). Recommendations from working groups of the international feline enteric coronavirus and feline infectious peritonitis workshop. *Feline Pract.* **23**, 108–111.

Sirinarumitr, T., Paul, P. S., Halbur, P. G., and Kluge, J. P. (1997). An overview of immunological and genetic methods for detecting swine coronaviruses, transmissible gastroenteritis virus, and porcine respiratory coronavirus in tissues. *Adv. Exp. Med. Biol.* **412**, 37–46.

Vennema, H., Poland, E., Floyd Hawkins, K., and Pedersen, N. C. (1995). A comparison of the genomes of feline enteric coronaviruses and feline infectious peritonitis viruses and what they tell us about the relationships between feline coronaviruses and their evolution. *Feline Pract.* **23**, 40–44.

Chapter 34

Arteriviridae

The name of the recently established family *Arteriviridae* is derived from the disease caused by its type species, equine arteritis virus. Apart from horses, arteriviruses infect swine, causing "mystery swine disease," which was first detected in North America in 1987 and in Europe in 1990 and has since then become a major threat to swine industries in many counties. This disease had also been called swine infertility and respiratory syndrome, and porcine epidemic abortion and respiratory syndrome, before being officially named porcine respiratory and reproductive syndrome—it is clear that consensus in naming this disease and its causative virus was only reached with difficulty. Other arteriviruses infect mice (lactate dehydrogenase-elevating virus) and monkeys (simian hemorrhagic fever virus). All arteriviruses have the capacity to establish asymptomatic persistent infections in their natural hosts and to cause severe disease in certain circumstances.

Properties of Arteriviruses

Classification

Member viruses of the family *Arteriviridae* have a genome organization and replication strategy similar to that of member viruses of the family *Coronaviridae*. However, there are major differences: arterivirus virions and genomes are only about half the size of those of coronaviruses. Arterivirus nucleocapsids are isometric, whereas those of coronaviruses are helical, and arterivirus peplomers are inconspicuous whereas those of coronaviruses are the largest of any virus. The major feature in common between the two families is their nested-set transcription strategy—this common feature was the basis for the establishment of the order *Nidovirales* (see Chapter 33) to bring together the families *Coronaviridae* and *Arteriviridae*. The family *Arteriviridae* comprises a single genus, *Arterivirus*, which contains all member viruses (Table 34.1).

Virion Properties

Arterivirus virions are 50–70 nm in diameter and consist of an isometric (probably icosahedral) nucleocapsid, 35 nm in diameter, surrounded by a closely adherent envelope with honeycomb-like surface structures (Figure 34.1). The genome consists of a single molecule of linear positive-sense, single-stranded RNA, 13 to 15 kb in size. Virion RNA has a 5′-type 1 terminal cap and a 3′-terminal poly(A) tract and is infectious. The RNA polymerase gene takes up about 75% of the 5′ end of the genome; genes that encode the viral structural proteins are located in the 3′ end of the genome (Figure 34.2). Virions are composed of a nucleocapsid protein, N (M_r 12,000), a nonglycosylated triple-membrane spanning integral membrane protein, M (M_r 16,000), and at least two N-glycosylated peplomer proteins (G_S, M_r 25,000 and G_L, M_r 42,000).

Viral Replication

Arteriviruses replicate in the perinuclear cytoplasm of their host cells, usually macrophages. Equine arteritis virus replicates to high titer in equine cells. The lactate dehydrogenase-elevating virus replicates to very high ti-

Table 34.1
Arteriviruses of Animals

Virus	Host	Disease
Equine arteritis virus	Horse	Systemic disease, arteritis, abortion, fetal death, pneumonia in foals
Porcine respiratory and reproductive syndrome virus	Swine	Porcine reproductive and respiratory syndrome, a systemic disease characterized by abortion, stillbirth, mummufied fetuses, and respiratory disease in newborn (Europe)
VR2332 virus	Swine	Similar to porcine reproductive and respiratory syndrome (United States)
Lactate dehydrogenase-elevating virus	Mice	Usually none, but the presence of the virus may confound research using infected mice
Simian hemorrhagic fever virus	Macaques	Systemic disease, death

Figure 34.1.

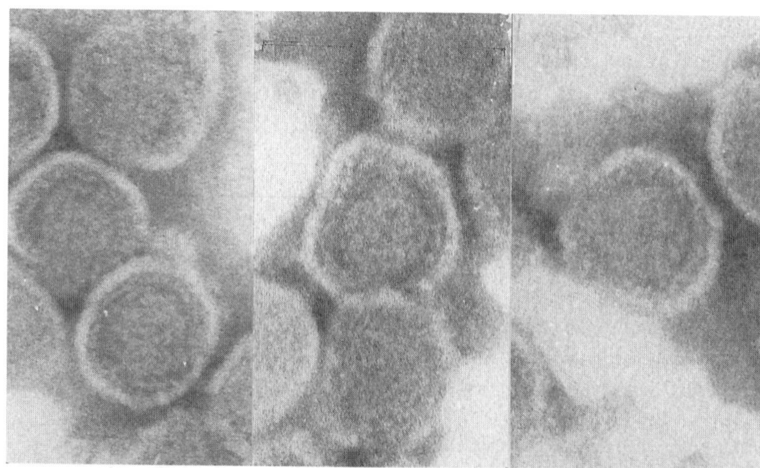

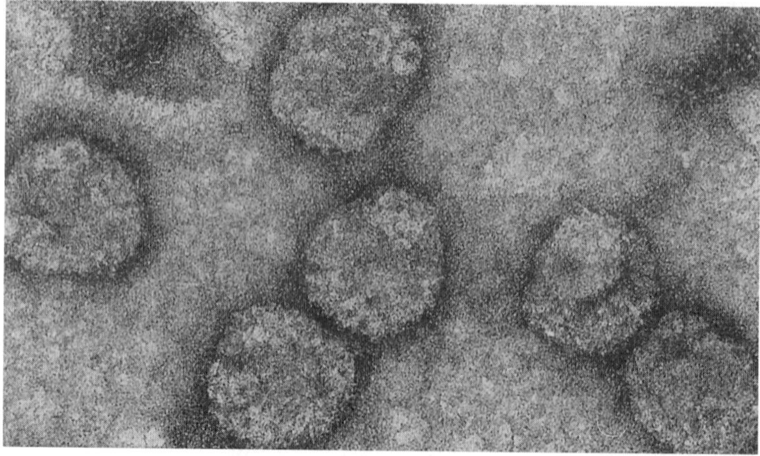

Family *Arteriviridae,* genus *Arterivirus.* (Top) Lactate dehydrogenase-elevating virus showing the nucleocapsid in virions penetrated by the stain. (Bottom) Equine arteritis virus showing ring-shaped structures on the surface of virions. Negative stain electron microscopy. Magnification: ×190,000.

FIGURE 34.2.

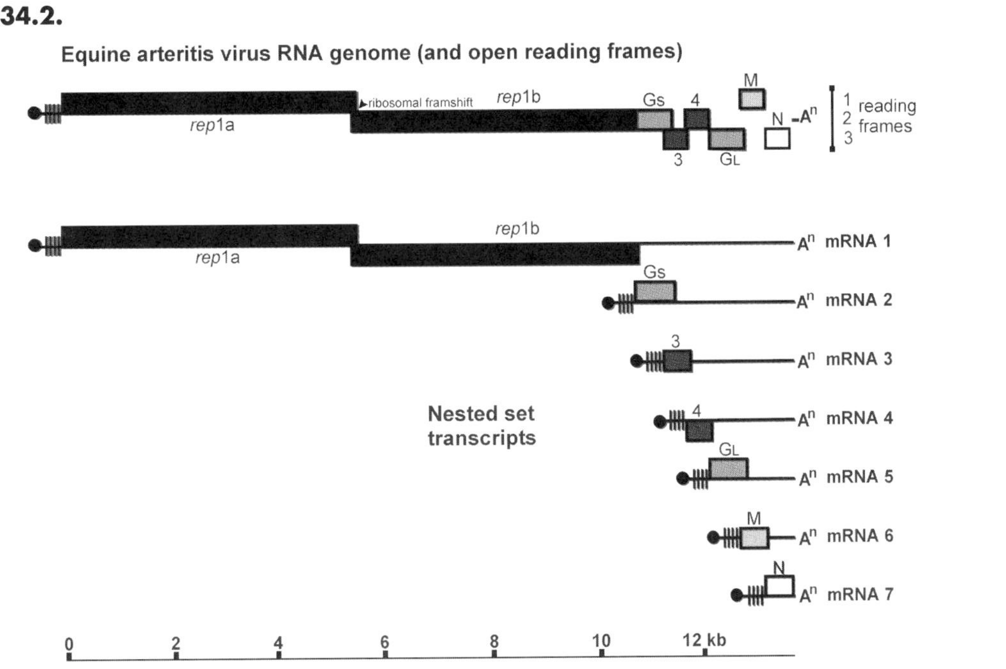

The genome and transcription strategy of the prototype of the family *Arteriviridae*, equine arteritis virus. The genomic and mRNAs are capped (black circles), have leader sequences (vertical lines), and are polyadenylated (A^n). After release of the positive-sense genomic RNA in the cytoplasm, the viral RNA-dependent RNA polymerase is synthesized; it directs the transcription of a full-length complementary (negative-sense) RNA, from which are synthesized (1) new genomic RNA, (2) an overlapping set of subgenomic mRNAs, and (3) leader RNA. The mRNA transcripts form a nested set with common 3′ ends and common leader sequences on their 5′ ends. Only the unique sequences at the 5′ end of the mRNAs are translated, producing the various proteins: rep1a and rep1b, the two units of the RNA-dependent RNA polymerase (synthesized as one large precursor via frameshifting); G_S and G_L, the two N-glycosylated surface proteins; M, a transmembrane glycoprotein; N, the nucleoprotein; and several nonstructural proteins. [Adapted from S. G. Siddell and E. J. Snijder. Coronaviruses, toroviruses and arteriviruses. *In* "Topley and Wilson's Microbiology and Microbial Infections" (B. W. J. Mahy and L. H. Collier, eds.), Vol. 1, pp. 463–484. Edward Arnold, London, 1998.]

ter in mice, reaching a titer of $10^{11}ID_{50}$/ml in plasma within the first few days of infection.

Full-length genomic RNA is synthesized via a full-length, negative-sense replicative intermediate. Transcription involves the synthesis of a nested set of seven or eight 3′-coterminal mRNAs, each reflecting a single open reading frame (Figure 34.2). These subgenomic RNAs are composed of a common leader sequence shared by all mRNAs linked to the unique sequence for each individual mRNA. Thus each protein is not encoded contiguously on the viral genome—the leader sequence of each mRNA is identical and derived from the extreme 5′ end of the genome. Conserved sequence motifs define the junctions where the leader sequence joins the unique part of each subgenomic mRNA. It is not known whether the unique part of each mRNA is derived from a subgenomic negative-strand template or is transcribed individually from a genome-sized negative-stranded template. Some adjacent genes encoded in each subgenomic mRNA are in different reading frames; ribosomal frameshifting is employed to assure that only the 5′-terminal encoded protein is translated from each of the subgenomic mRNAs.

The genome of the prototypic virus, equine arteritis virus, contains eight open reading frames. The 5′-three-fourths of the viral genome is occupied by two large open reading frames, which together encode the viral replicase. The products of both open reading frames are multidomain polyproteins, which are cleaved by viral and host proteases to form the subunits of the mature replicase. Open reading frames 2, 5, and 6, expressed from the subgenomic mRNAs, encode the large and small glycoproteins and the transmembrane protein, respectively. Open reading frame 7 encodes the phosphorylated nucleocapsid protein. Virions bud through membranes of the endoplasmic reticulum into intracellular vesicles; from there they move to the surface of the cell in vesicles and are released by exocytosis (Table 34.2).

Equine Viral Arteritis

Historical documents suggest that the disease now called equine viral arteritis had been recognized in the 19th century. In 1953 the causative virus was isolated from lung tissue of aborted fetuses during an epidemic of

TABLE 34.2
Properties of Arteriviruses

Virions are spherical, 50–70 nm in diameter, with an isometric (probably icosahedral) nucleocapsid and a closely adherent smooth-surfaced envelope

The genome consists of a single molecule of linear positive-sense, single-stranded RNA, 13 to 15 kb in size. Virion RNA has a 5′ cap and its 3′ end is polyadenylated; the genomic RNA is infectious

Replication takes place in the cytoplasm; the genome is transcribed to form full-length negative-sense RNA, from which is transcribed a 3′-coterminal nested set of mRNAs; only the unique sequences at the 5′ end of each mRNA are translated

Virions are formed by budding into the endoplasmic reticulum, from where they are released by exocytosis

abortion and respiratory disease on a breeding farm near Bucyrus, Ohio. The disease is usually observed only on breeding farms; however, serologic studies indicate that infection is usually subclinical and is widespread in equine populations worldwide.

Clinical Features

Most natural infections with equine arteritis virus are asymptomatic. For mares bred to persistently infected stallions the ratio of clinical to inapparent infections may vary widely between epidemics. After an incubation period of 3 to 14 days the onset of frank disease is marked by fever (greater than 41°C), leukopenia, depression, excessive lacrimation, anorexia, conjunctivitis, rhinitis and nasal discharge, urticaria of the head, neck, and trunk, and edema, which is most pronounced over the eyes, the abdomen, including the prepuce, scrotum, and mammary glands, and the hind limbs (often resulting in a stiff gait).

Although naturally infected horses usually recover after cessation of viremia, death as a result of a rapidly progressive bronchointerstitial pneumonia and intestinal necrosis has been reported occasionally in both foals and yearlings. From 40 to 80% of infected pregnant mares may abort ("abortion storms"). Abortion generally occurs 10 to 30 days after infection and is linked closely with the late febrile or early convalescent phase of disease, but can occur even if no clinical signs are noticed.

Fertility problems after infection have not been observed in mares, but stallions may undergo a period of temporary infertility. The reduction of sperm quality and quantity is probably due to scrotal hyperthermia associated with pyrexia; long-term effects on semen quality have not been observed in naturally infected carrier stallions.

Pathogenesis, Pathology, and Immunity

Initial virus replication takes place in alveolar macrophages, and by the second day the bronchial lymph nodes are infected. From there the virus is disseminated throughout the body via the bloodstream, probably both as extracellular virions and infected macrophages. By the third day viremia reaches a high titer, and the virus can be found in practically all body fluids and tissues, with the probable exception of the brain. The primary targets of infection are macrophages and the endothelium and mesothelium of vessels throughout the body; secondary infection targets include the adrenal glands, thyroid gland, kidneys, liver, and seminiferous tubules.

The most conspicuous gross lesions are edema, congestion, and hemorrhage in many tissues. The terminal stage of disease is characterized by infarctions of the intestine, lung, and spleen and by fluid accumulations in the peritoneal and pleural cavities. Infarctions follow on segmental necrosis of small arteries throughout the body. The ultimate consequence of this vascular damage may be the development of fatal hypovolemic–hypotensive shock.

Aborted fetuses are usually expelled together with the fetal membranes and without premonitory clinical signs. Aborted fetuses exhibit mild edema in many tissues, excess fluid in peritoneal and pleural cavities, and petechial hemorrhages in peritoneal and pleural mucosal surfaces.

Most acutely infected stallions shed virus continuously in semen, and a long-term carrier state has been identified. The persistent infection has no obvious negative effect on fertility. The ejaculates of chronic carriers contain virus for years, perhaps even for life. An intermediate carrier state lasting for 3 to 8 months has been found in both adult horses and prepubertal colts. Virus concentration is highest in the accessory sex glands and in the vas deferens. Virus output appears to be testosterone dependent; chronic virus shedding has not been observed in geldings, and persistently infected stallions that are castrated stop secreting virus.

Antibodies may be detected by virus neutralization or enzyme immunoassay within a week after infection, coinciding with virus elimination from the circulation. Vaccination experiments have confirmed the close relationship between neutralizing antibodies and protection. Neutralizing antibodies persist for years, and protection is long-lasting, if not lifelong. Colostrum from immune mares moderates or prevents arteritis in young foals.

Laboratory Diagnosis

Virus isolation was first accomplished in primary equine kidney cell cultures but rabbit kidney cells are used routinely now; not all virus strains cause cytopathology in these cells so the presence of virus must be assayed indirectly (e.g., by immunofluorescence). Virus can be isolated from many body fluids and tissues but only for a few weeks after infection. To detect virus in semen the sperm-rich fraction of full ejaculates is cultured. Because the reverse transcriptase–polymerase chain reaction is as sensitive as virus isolation and has the advantages of being rapid, specific, and applicable to a wide variety of specimens, it is becoming the method of choice for the detection of the virus. For measuring antibodies, most laboratories use virus neutralization tests in microtiter plates; the sensitivity of this method can be increased by the addition of complement and for some virus strains its presence is required.

Epidemiology, Prevention, and Control

Despite its worldwide distribution, equine arteritis virus causes disease outbreaks only occasionally, the most conspicuous of which are "abortion storms." Epidemics occur where horses are congregated from multiple sources, such as at sales and shows and on breeding farms. Transmission occurs through respiratory, sexual, and transplacental routes. Sources for aerosol transmission are aborted fetuses, fetal membranes and amniotic fluids of mares, and genital fluids of infected stallions. Infection may lead to a carrier state, with stallions transmitting the virus chronically via semen.

Immunization of horses with an attenuated virus vaccine or an inactivated virus vaccine prepared from cell cultures produces long-lasting immunity and no untoward effects. In view of the very rare occurrence of clinical outbreaks of disease, the need to immunize is still disputed; nevertheless, because of the impact of the disease on reproductive outcome, immunization of valuable breeding animals is commonly undertaken. To prevent the establishment of persistent infections in stallions that will be used for breeding, vaccination of colts may be done at 6 to 8 months of age (i.e., after maternal antibody has waned but before puberty). To prevent abortions, mares may be vaccinated before or after becoming pregnant.

During outbreaks the spread of virus is best controlled by (1) movement restrictions, (2) isolation of infected horses followed by a quarantine period after recovery, (3) good hygiene, including assignment of separate personnel to work with infected and uninfected animals, and (4) laboratory-supported surveillance.

Porcine Respiratory and Reproductive Syndrome

When porcine respiratory and reproductive syndrome first emerged in the United States and Canada in 1987 and in Europe in the early 1990s it spread quickly—in Europe, reports came from Germany, The Netherlands, England, and Spain in quick succession. The search for a viral etiology resulted in several early false starts until an arterivirus was identified. Today porcine respiratory and reproductive syndrome is recognized as an economically important disease of domesticated and wild pigs in many countries.

The question remains where the virus originated. Genetic analyses of the viruses now linked together in the order *Nidovirales* have shown that coronaviruses and toroviruses (family *Coronaviridae*) are only distantly related phylogenetically to the arteriviruses. Among the arteriviruses, porcine respiratory and reproductive syndrome virus and lactate dehydrogenase-elevating virus of mice are more closely related to each other than either is to equine arteritis virus. From such data it has been suggested, with no further substantiation, that the swine virus may represent the consequence of a species-jumping event of a rodent virus. In any case, the swine virus occurs as two genotypes, European (Lelystad virus) and North American genotypes (VR2332 virus), clearly reflecting another phylogenetic split that perhaps is indicative of recent transmission patterns.

Clinical Features

The disease is characterized by anorexia, fever, a blue discoloration of the ears, snout, and vulva, agalactia, and abortion late in gestation (around day 110). Premature births, stillbirths, and mummified fetuses are observed and, if born alive, piglets are weak, half of them dying during the first week postpartum, often with respiratory distress. Many of these clinical manifestations of infection can also be seen in older swine.

Pathogenesis, Pathology, and Immunity

In infected pigs, viremia may persist for many weeks in the presence of antibody. Antibody-dependent enhancement of infection has been demonstrated, and subneutralizing concentrations of IgG antibody may contribute to the pathogenesis of the disease in other ways as well. Transplacental infection of piglets leads to gross lesions in the umbilical cord, usually segmental hemorrhagic lesions. Histologically, a necrotizing umbilical arteritis with periarterial hemorrhage is seen. In sows, endometritis and myometritis have been observed.

Laboratory Diagnosis

In aborted fetuses the virus is inactivated rapidly so moribund live piglets should be used for virus isolation attempts. The virus is quite fastidious, having been shown to replicate in only a few cell types. The virus grows well in swine lung macrophages and in an African green monkey kidney cell line (MA-104) and its descendant clones. As in equine arteritis virus diagnosis, the sensitivity of neutralization tests can be increased by the addition of guinea pig complement.

Epidemiology, Prevention, and Control

The virus spreads quickly in naive swine populations, with up to 95% of swine in a herd becoming seropositive within 2–3 months after an introduction. The virus has reached high levels of endemicity in many swine-producing countries. At low ambient temperatures the virus survives particularly well in the environment, so epidemic spread is especially efficient in winter months. Contact transmission, airborne, and sexual transmission via semen have been documented. The virus is maintained in persistently infected healthy swine—it has been isolated from the oropharynx more than 5 months after infection.

Lactate Dehydrogenase-Elevating Virus Infection of Mice

The discovery of lactate dehydrogenase-elevating virus was a chance event that occurred during experiments on tumors in mice. The virus generally causes persistent infections that reveal themselves only by elevated levels of certain plasma enzymes, including lactate dehydrogenase. Not only does this characteristic allow virus detection, it has also been used as the end point indicator for virus infectivity titrations. The importance of this infection is that it may confound experiments when mice are unknowingly infected intercurrently by lactate dehydrogenase-elevating virus. For example, the infection can transiently alter the immune response of mice to all kinds of antigens and thereby distort the results of immunological experiments.

Clinical Features

Infected mice usually exhibit no clinical evidence of infection and live a normal life span; however, the virus can induce a poliomyelitis in C58 and AKR mice if these strains are immunosuppressed during the initial stage of the infection.

Pathogenesis, Pathology, and Immunity

Lactate dehydrogenase-elevating virus replicates in all strains of inbred laboratory mice. Even though the virus replicates only in early developmental stage cells of the monocyte/macrophage lineage, it reaches about the highest titers known in animal virology (10^{11} infectious units/ml of plasma) in the first few days postinfection. Viremia persists for the lifetime of the infected mouse; after a week or so of infection the virus circulates as infectious immune complexes.

One isolate (designated LDV-CZ) differs from other strains in its ability to infect the ventral motor neurons of the two most susceptible mouse strains, C58 and AKR. This neurovirulent variant emerged as a "passenger" when transplantable leukemia cells were passaged serially in C58 mice.

Laboratory Diagnosis

It is important for investigators working with laboratory mice or primary murine cell cultures to know whether this virus is present as a contaminant. Lactate dehydrogenase plasma levels increase in all mice infected with this virus, with maximum level being reached about 4 days postinfection. Therefore, virus-free mice are inoculated with material from suspect mice and 4 days later hemolysis-free plasma samples are assayed for the enzyme. Usually an 8- to 10-fold increase over the normal concentration of the enzyme is observed in infected mice.

Epidemiology, Prevention, and Control

The infection was widespread in laboratory mouse colonies but is now rather rare. Natural infections are limited to wild *Mus musculus;* other rodents and lagomorphs are refractory. Transmission probably occurs via contact and biting (saliva contains high titers of virus). Given these facts, prevention of infection in mouse colonies can be accomplished by (1) preventing entry of wild mice, (2) use of barrier-specific, pathogen-free breeding and housing systems, and (3) laboratory test-based surveillance. The virus can be eliminated from valuable mouse tumor cell lines either by passage in another rodent species or by maintenance of the cells in culture. Cells must be passaged several times in order to eliminate any macrophages or macrophage precursors, the only cells that support the replication of the virus.

Simian Hemorrhagic Fever

Simian hemorrhagic fever virus was first isolated in 1964 during devastating epidemics in macaques imported from India into Russia and the United States. Nearly all infected animals died. Similar epidemics have occurred frequently since then; for example, in the United States in 1989 there were epidemics at three primate colonies resulting in the death of more than 600 cynomolgus macaques (*Macaca fascicularis*).

The onset of disease in macaques is rapid, with early fever, facial edema, anorexia, dehydration, skin petechiae, diarrhea, and hemorrhages. Death occurs between 5 and 25 days and mortality approaches 100%. Within a colony, infection spreads rapidly, probably via contact and aerosol. Lesions include hemorrhages in the dermis, nasal mucosa, lungs, intestines, and other visceral organs. Shock is suspected as the underlying cause of death. All species of macaques (genus *Macaca*) are highly susceptible and macaques are the only animals that develop severe or fatal disease. Epidemics in macaque colonies originate from accidental introduction of the virus from other primate species that are infected persistently without showing clinical signs. In captivity, Patas monkeys (*Erythrocebus patas*) have often been implicated as the source of virus, but African green monkeys (*Cercopithecus aethiops*) and baboons (*Papio anubis* and *P. cyanocephalus*) may also carry the virus persistently.

Transmission in primate colonies is facilitated by poor management and improper veterinary practices, such as reusing syringes and needles and tattooing equipment and inadequate cage sterilization. It is not known how the virus is transmitted among nonmacaques or whether the virus exists in nature in macaques—obviously, natural transmission of the virus from persistently infected African monkeys, such as Patas monkeys, to macaques, which come from Asia, is not a factor in the natural history of the virus. Control is based on species separation in colonies and on proper containment facilities and practices.

Further Reading

Brinton, M. A. (1994). Lactate dehydrogenase-elevating virus. *In* "Virus Infections of Vertebrates" (A. D. M. E. Osterhaus, ed.), Vol. 5, pp. 269–279. Elsevier, Amsterdam.

den Boon, J. A., Snijder, E. J., Chirnside, E. D., de Vries, A. A. F., Horzinek, M. C., and Spaan, W. J. M. (1991). Equine arteritis virus is not a togavirus but belongs to the coronavirus-like superfamily. *J. Virol.* **65**, 2910–2920.

de Vries, A. A. F., Rottier, P. J. M., Glaser, A. L., and Horzinek, M. C. (1997). Equine viral arteritis. *In* "Virus Infections of Vertebrates" (M. J. Studdert, ed.), Vol. 6, pp. 171–200. Elsevier, Amsterdam.

MacLachlan, N. J., Balasuriya, U. B., Rossitto, P. V., Hullinger, P. A., Patton, J. F., and Wilson, W. D. (1996). Fatal experimental equine arteritis virus infection of a pregnant mare: Immunohistochemical staining of viral antigens. *J. Vet. Diagn. Invest.* **8**, 367–374.

Meulenberg, J. J., Hulst, M. M., de Meijer, E. J., Moonen, P. L. J. M., den Besten, A., de Kluyver, E. P., Wensvoort, G., and Moormann, R. J. M. (1994). Lelystad virus belongs to a new virus family, comprising lactate dehydrogenase-elevating virus, equine arteritis virus and simian hemorrhagic fever virus. *Arch. Virol., Suppl.* **9**, 441–448.

Meulenberg, J. J., Petersen den Besten, A., de Kluyver, E., van Nieuwstadt, A., Wensvoort, G., and Moormann, R. J. (1997). Molecular characterization of Lelystad virus. *Vet. Microbiol.* **55**, 197–202.

Plagemann, P. G. W., and Moennig, V. (1992). Lactate dehydrogenase-elevating virus, equine arteritis virus, and simian hemorrhagic fever virus, a new group of positive strand RNA viruses. *Adv. Virus Res.* **41**, 99–192.

Thiel, H.-J., Meyers, G., Stark, R., Tautz, N., Ruümenapf, T., Unger, G., and Conzelmann, K. K. (1993). Molecular characterization of positive-strand RNA viruses: Pestiviruses and the porcine reproductive and respiratory syndrome virus (PRRSV). *Arch. Virol., Suppl.* **7**, 41–52.

Timoney, P. J., Klingeborn, B., and Lucas, M. H. (1996). A perspective on equine viral arteritis (infectious arteritis of horses). *Rev. Sci. Tech.* **15**, 1203–1208 (in English).

CHAPTER 35

Picornaviridae

Over 230 viruses in six genera are classified in the family *Picornaviridae,* making it one of the largest virus families; each genus contains viruses causing disease in domestic animals.

Picornaviruses have played an important role in the history of virology and in the history of veterinary medicine. In 1897, Loeffler and Frosch showed that foot-and-mouth disease was caused by an agent that passed through filters that held back bacteria; this was the first demonstration that a disease of animals was caused by a filterable virus. A century later the same virus was among the first animal viruses to have its structure resolved at the atomic level by X-ray crystallography.

In the second half of the 19th century and the first half of the 20th century, repeated rapidly spreading epidemics of foot-and-mouth disease resulted in great losses as increasingly intensive livestock production systems were developed in many countries. Producers demanded of their governments control programs to prevent reintroductions as well as to deal with ongoing epidemics. For example, in 1884, the United States Congress created the Bureau of Animal Industry (BAI) within the Department of Agriculture; its mission was to deal with foot-and-mouth disease and two other diseases, contagious bovine pleuropneumonia and hog cholera. From its beginning, this agency pioneered in the development of veterinarians with special skills in disease control. In 1914, the largest epidemic of foot-and-mouth disease ever recorded in the United States occurred; the epidemic spread rapidly after gaining entry into the Chicago stockyards—more than 3500 herds in 22 states were involved. This episode served to accelerate epidemiologic and disease control programs and the training of more staff veterinarians; eventually, this evolved into the complex field- and laboratory-based systems needed to assure the freedom of domestic livestock industries from foreign animal diseases. Similar developments occurred in other countries with rising intensive livestock industries, in each case advancing the scope of the veterinary medical profession from its roots in equine medicine and surgery.

Properties of Picornaviruses

Classification

The family *Picornaviridae* is divided into six genera: *Aphthovirus, Enterovirus, Cardiovirus, Rhinovirus, Hepatovirus,* and *Parechovirus.* Important member viruses of each genus are listed in Table 35.1 and the phylogenetic relationships between representative members of each genus are shown in Figure 35.1.

An important difference between viruses of the six genera is their stability at low pH; such differences had been used as a factor in the classification of new picornaviruses at one time. The aphthoviruses are unstable below pH 7, the rhinoviruses lose infectivity below pH 5, and the enteroviruses, hepatoviruses, cardioviruses, and

Figure 35.1.

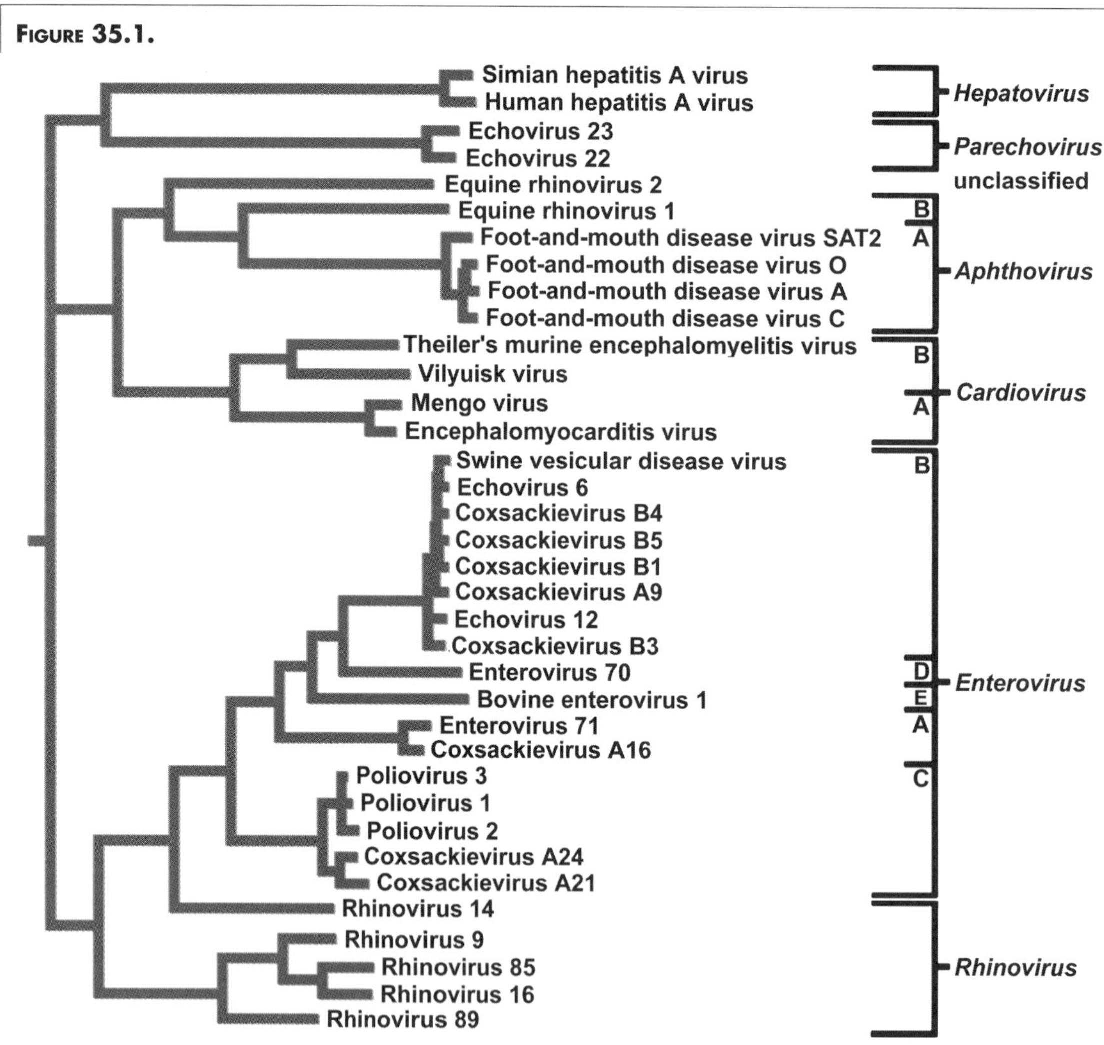

Phylogenetic tree showing the complex interrelationships among the picornaviruses and how this is reflected in the taxonomic structure of the family. Some of the genera are rather narrowly based, but the genera comprising the aphthoviruses (foot-and-mouth disease viruses and equine rhinovirus 1) and especially the enteroviruses reflect the broad genetic diversity of member viruses. In many cases, viruses of veterinary medical importance are interspersed with human pathogens—this is especially the case with swine vesicular disease virus, which is related very closely to important coxsackie B viruses that are human pathogens. Some picornaviruses remain unclassified within the present six-genus taxonomic structure—most notable in this regard is equine rhinovirus 2. This tree is based on amino acid sequence similarities in the 2C, 3C, and 3D regions of the genomes of the picornaviruses shown. Sequences were aligned by reiterative global methods using the Blosum62 scoring tables to maximize the fit between isolates. The 100 most parsimoneous trees, calculated by heuristic methods within the PAUP program package, were averaged, and the result (midpoint rooting) is presented graphically. Branch length is roughly proportional to the distance between any pair of sequences. Genera and taxonomic clusters within genera (designated by letters A–E) are those designated by the Picornavirus Study Group of the International Committee on Taxonomy of Viruses. (Compiled and analyzed by A. Palmenberg and N. Knowles, using data from many sources.)

Table 35.1
Picornviruses of Animals and Humans

Genus	Virus	Principal species affected	Disease
Aphthovirus			
	Foot-and-mouth disease viruses A, O, C, SAT 1, SAT 2, SAT 3, Asia	Cattle, sheep, goats, swine, ruminant wildlife species	Foot-and-mouth disease in ruminants and swine
	Equine rhinovirus 1	Horses	Systemic disease, with respiratory signs
Enterovirus			
	Swine vesicular disease virus	Swine	Swine vesicular disease
	Porcine enterovirus 1	Swine	Polioencephalomyelitis
	Porcine enteroviruses 2–11	Swine	Diarrhea, pericarditis, asymptomatic infection
	Bovine enteroviruses 1–7	Cattle	Usually asymptomatic infection
	Simian enteroviruses 1–18	Monkeys	Usually asymptomatic infection
	Avian enteroviruses	Chickens	Avian encephalomyelitis
		Ducks	Hepatitis
		Turkeys	Hepatitis
	Polioviruses 1, 2, and 3	Humans	Poliomyelitis
	Coxsackieviruses A1–22 and A24 and B1–6	Humans	Aseptic meningitis, poliomyelitis, myocarditis, pleurodynia, hand-foot-and-mouth disease, and other syndromes
	Human echoviruses 1–7, 9, 11–27, and 29–33	Humans	Aseptic meningitis and other syndromes
	Human enteroviruses 68–71	Humans	Poliomyelitis, epidemic keratoconjunctivitis, and other syndromes
Cardiovirus			
	Encephalomyocarditis virus	Swine, elephants, other mammals in contact with rodents	Rarely, encephalomyocarditis in swine and elephants
	Theiler's murine encephalomyelitis virus	Mice	Murine poliomyelitis
Rhinovirus			
	Bovine rhinoviruses 1–3	Cattle	Mild rhinitis
	Human rhinoviruses 1–100+, 1A, 1B	Humans	Common cold
Hepatovirus			
	Simian hepatitis A virus	Monkeys	Hepatitis
	Human hepatitis A virus	Humans	Hepatitis
Parechovirus			
	Human echoviruses 22 and 23	Humans	Aseptic meningitis
Unclassified viruses			
	Equine rhinovirus 2	Horses	Rhinitis

parechoviruses are stable at pH 3. A number of other major differences are recognized. The 5′-untranslated region (5′-UTR) of cardioviruses and aphthoviruses contains a long poly(c) tract that is absent in enteroviruses, parechoviruses, hepatoviruses, and rhinoviruses. Cardioviruses and aphthoviruses are further distinguished by the presence of a leader protein encoded upstream of the capsid proteins.

Aphthoviruses are unique in having three similar, but not identical, VPg-encoding sequences. Equine rhinovirus 1 has been moved into the genus *Aphthovirus;* it shares many genomic characteristics with the aphthoviruses, but its genome encodes only a single copy of the VPg gene.

Virion Properties

Picornavirus virions are nonenveloped, 27 nm in diameter, and have icosahedral symmetry. Virions appear smooth and round in outline in electron micrographs; they appear the same in images reconstructed from X-ray crystallographic analyses (Figures 35.2 and 35.3). The genome consists of a single molecule of linear positive-sense, single-stranded RNA, 7.2–8.4 kb in size. The genomic RNA is polyadenylated at its 3′ end and has a protein, VPg, linked covalently to its 5′ end. Genomic RNA is infectious.

The atomic structure of representative viruses of all genera has been solved; virions are constructed from 60 copies each of four capsid proteins, VP1, VP2, and VP3 (M_r approximately 30,000 for each), and VP4 (M_r 7–8000) and a single copy of the genome linked protein, VPg (M_r variable; aphthoviruses encode three VPgs). Additionally, minor proteins of unknown function have been reported to occur in the virions of many picornaviruses. VP1, VP2, and VP3 are structurally rather similar to one another, each being composed of a wedge-shaped, eight-stranded β barrel and differing primarily in the size and conformation of the loops that occur between the strands and also in the extensions of their amino and carboxyl termini. Amino acid substitutions correlating with antigenic variation occur in the surface-oriented loop regions. The VP1 proteins are located around the fivefold axes of icosahedral symmetry, and VP2 and VP3 alternate around the two- and threefold axes; the amino-terminal extensions of these three proteins form an intricate network on the inner surface of the protein shell. The small, myristylated protein, VP4, is located entirely at the inner surface of the capsid, probably in contact with the RNA.

FIGURE 35.2.

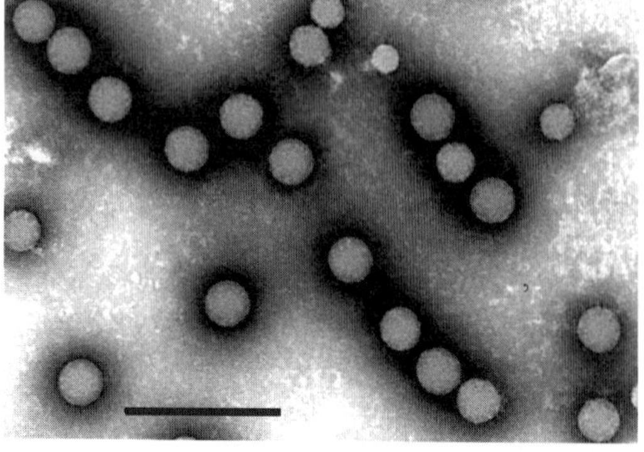

Picornaviridae. Negatively stained foot-and-mouth disease virus virions. Bar: 100 nm. (Courtesy of S. H. Wool.)

In poliovirus and rhinovirus virions the packing together of VP1, VP2, and VP3 results in the formation of a "canyon" around the fivefold axes of the virion (Figure 1.11). The amino acids within the canyon, particularly those on the canyon floor, are conserved but the amino acids on the rim of the canyon are variable. The conserved amino acids on the floor of the canyon are believed to form the points of attachment of the viruses to cell surface receptors and it was proposed that this location might shield attachment sites from immune surveillance because antibody molecules cannot fit into the canyon. Beneath the floor of the canyon in rhinoviruses is a hydrophobic pocket accessible from the surface via a small opening; this pocket has been considered a potential target for chemotherapeutic drugs.

The role of the canyon has been challenged, however. Crystallographic studies suggest that the canyon does not protect the receptor-binding site from antibody binding; indeed it has been shown that the Fab fragment of IgG can penetrate deep into the canyon. In these studies it was concluded that it is unlikely that the viral structure evolves merely to evade immune recognition. Rhinoviruses may resemble foot-and-mouth disease viruses in this respect, with the shape and position of their cellular receptor-binding sites being crucial for binding to cellular receptors but not involved in concealing these sites from immune surveillance. Foot-and-mouth disease viruses have a comparatively smooth surface with no canyon structure; attachment sites for host cell receptors are located at the tips of protuberances on the virion surface. These sites are strongly antigenic, but it seems that nearby structures serve to camouflage them—these sites also have serotype and subtype antigenic specificities that differ among the various foot-and-mouth disease viruses.

The stability of picornaviruses to environmental conditions is important in the epidemiology of the diseases they cause and in the selection of methods of disin-

FIGURE 35.3.

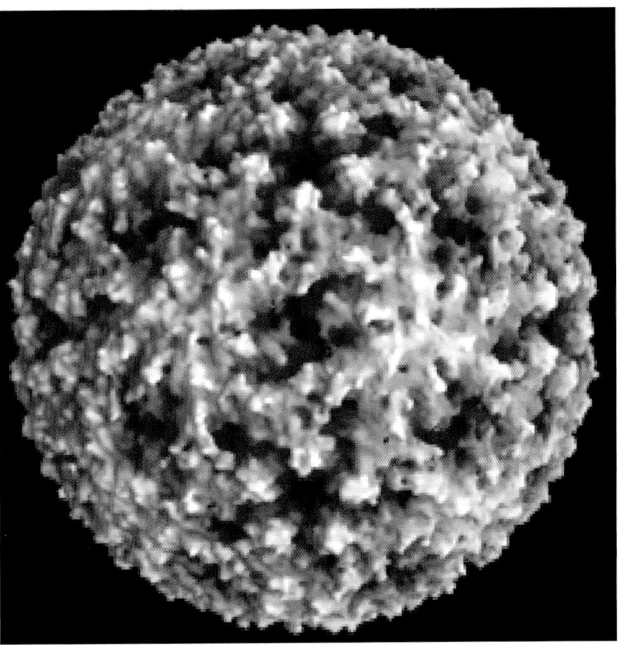

X-ray crystallographic solution of the structure of foot-and-mouth disease virus. [From J. D. Logan, R. Abu-Ghazaleh, W. Blakemore, S. Curry, T. Jackson, A. King, S. Lea, R. Lewis, J. Newman, N. Parry, D. Rowlands, D. Stuart, and E. Fry, *Nature* (*London*) **362,** 566 (1993). Radial depth cue rendering by J.-Y. Sgro.]

fection. For example, if protected by mucus or feces and shielded from strong sunlight, picornaviruses are relatively heat stable at usual ambient temperatures. Enteroviruses may survive for several days and often weeks in feces. Aerosols of rhinoviruses and aphthoviruses are less stable, but under conditions of high humidity they may remain viable for several hours. Because of differences in their pH stability, only certain disinfectants are suitable for use against each virus: for example, sodium carbonate (washing soda) is effective against foot-and-mouth disease viruses but is not effective against the swine vesicular disease virus.

Viral Replication

Polioviruses, which in nature only infect humans and nonhuman primates, have been the principal models for studying the replication of RNA viruses. The poliovirus model serves for understanding the replication of all picornaviruses. The replication of foot-and-mouth disease viruses, which have also been studied in considerable detail, parallels that of poliovirus and provides additional lessons.

The cellular receptors for many picornaviruses are known and are surprisingly diverse. The receptors for polioviruses, coxsackie B viruses, echoviruses, and some human rhinoviruses are members of the immunoglobulin superfamily. Many other cell surface molecules serve as receptors of other picornaviruses, including heparan sulfate, low-density lipoproteins, extracellular matrix-binding proteins, and integrins. Some picornaviruses, including some foot-and-mouth disease viruses, employ two receptors: initial binding involving heparan sulfate followed by high-affinity binding via integrins. Foot-and-mouth disease viruses can also enter cells via Fc receptors if virions are complexed with nonneutralizing IgG molecules. This pathway, termed the antibody-dependent enhancement of infection pathway, is of unknown significance, but may be important in the long-term carrier state that may occur in certain ruminants.

Following adsorption, penetration, and intracellular uncoating, VPg is removed from the virion RNA by cellular enzymes. Picornaviruses have evolved a cap-independent mechanism of translation; normal cellular cap-dependent translation is shut off and viral cap-independent translation takes over. Initiation of translation does not proceed by the well-established Kozak scanning model. Instead, ribosomal binding to viral RNA occurs in a region of the 5′-untranslated region of the genome known as the internal ribosome entry segment (IRES). This segment of the viral genomic RNA is folded into cloverleaf-like structures that bind specifically to host cell proteins, which play key roles in initiating the synthesis of viral protein and RNA. This segment has been recognized as a determinant of the phenotype and neurovirulence of some viruses. All picornavirus genomes have 3′-poly(A) tails that are encoded by the virus rather than added by host cell polyadenylation enzymes. The function of these poly(A) tails is not know, but their length seems to correlate with infectivity, i.e., viruses with shorter tails may be less infectious than viruses with longer tails.

The RNA genome of picornaviruses comprises a single open reading frame that is translated into a single polyprotein. The polyprotein is cleaved posttranslationally by virus-encoded proteinases to produce 11 or 12 proteins (Figure 35.4). The 5′-terminal region of the genome encodes the structural proteins VP4, VP2, VP3, and VP1, in that order. The middle region encodes nonstructural viral proteins including one viral protease. The 3′ end of the genome encodes other nonstructural proteins, including a second protease and the RNA-dependent RNA polymerase.

Viral RNA synthesis takes place in a *replication complex,* which comprises RNA templates and the virus-coded RNA polymerase and several other viral and cellular proteins, tightly associated with newly assembled smooth cytoplasmic membrane structures. Synthesis of the complementary strand is initiated at the 3′-terminus of the virion RNA and uses the protein VPg as a primer. The completed complementary strand in turn serves as a template for the synthesis of virion RNA. Most of the replicative intermediates found within the replication complex consist of a full-length complementary (negative-sense) RNA from which several nascent plus-sense strands are transcribed simultaneously by viral RNA polymerase.

Because of the absence of a 5′ cap on picornavirus mRNAs, these viruses have been able to evolve an unusual mechanism for shutting down the translation of cellular mRNAs; one of the picornavirus proteases inactivates the cellular cap-binding complex that is needed for the binding of cellular mRNAs to ribosomes. Thus, picornavirus replication is not only cytocidal but also very efficient, producing new virions after an eclipse period of less than 3 hours at yields of up to 10^6 virions per cell (Figure 35.5; Table 35.2).

Diseases Caused by Members of the Genus *Aphthovirus*

Foot-and-Mouth Disease

Foot-and-mouth disease is still a major global animal health problem, but its geographic distribution has been

Figure 35.4.

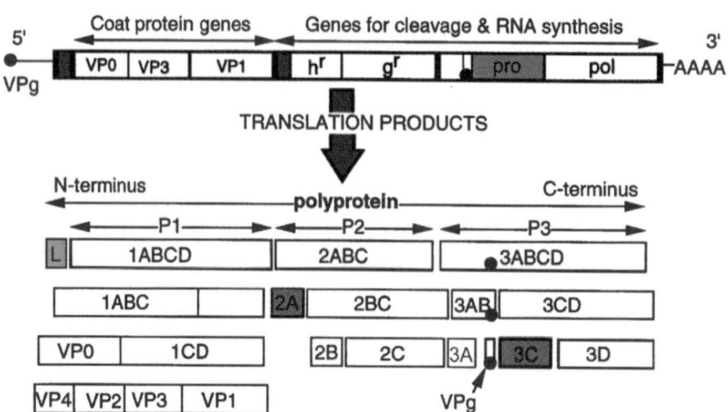

Organization and expression of the genome of poliovirus 1, a typical picornavirus. (Top) Organization of the genome. VPg, at the 5′-terminus, is essential for RNA replication, but the RNA is infectious if it is removed because it can be synthesized from region 3B (black dot). The 3′-terminus is polyadenylated and there are short nontranslated sequences at each end (thin lines). (Bottom) Upon entry into the cell, the virion RNA acting as messenger is translated into a polyprotein. The polyprotein is cleaved rapidly into proteins P1, P2, and P3 by three virus-coded proteinases: the M or maturation proteinase, the early 2A proteinase (inactive in aphthoviruses, which have a unique early proteinase, L, not found in other picornaviruses), and the 3C proteinase. Further cleavages occur as shown in the diagram. VPO is cleaved into VP4 and VP2 by a third protease during capsid formation, so that VP1, VP2, VP3, and VP4 comprise the mature capsid. The organization of the genome and cleavage patterns are slightly different in different genera of picornaviruses. [From R. R. Rueckert, Picornaviridae: the viruses and their replication. *In* "Fields Virology" (B. N. Fields, D. M. Knipe, P. M. Howley, R. M. Chanock, J. L. Melnick, T. P. Monath, B. Roizman, and S. E. Straus, eds.), 3rd ed., pp. 609–654. Lippincott-Raven, Philadelphia, PA, 1996.]

Figure 35.5.

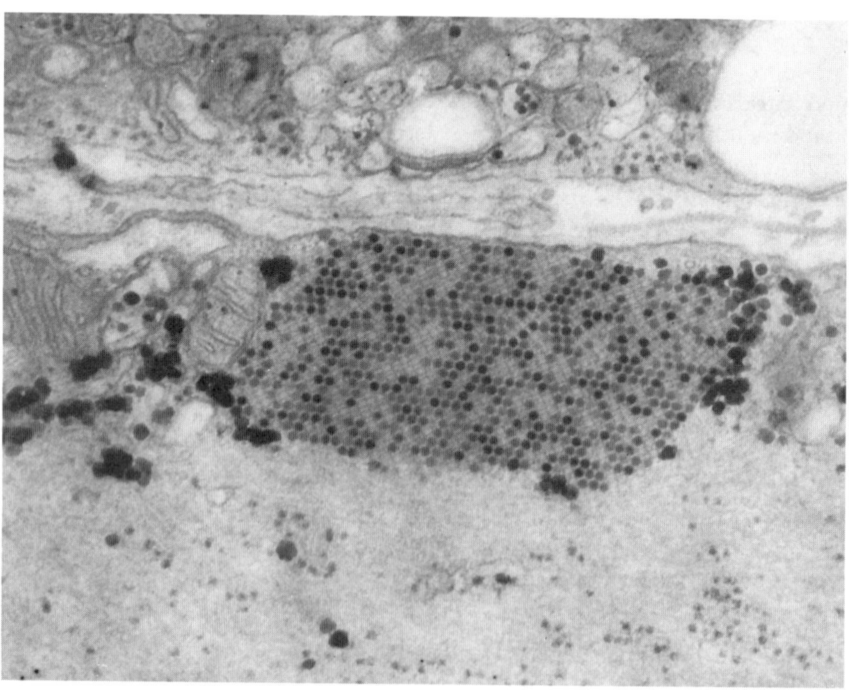

Coxsackie virus B4 in the cytoplasm of a striated muscle cell of a mouse showing a typical large paracrystalline array of virions and associated destruction of contractile fibers. Thin section electron microscopy. Magnification: ×67,000.

Table 35.2
Properties of Picornaviruses

Virions appear smooth and round in outline, are nonenveloped, 27 nm in diameter, and have icosahedral symmetry
The genome consists of a single molecule of linear positive-sense, single-stranded RNA, 7.2–8.4 kb in size
Genomic RNA is polyadenylated at its 3′ end and has a protein, VPg, linked covalently to its 5′ end; genomic RNA is infectious
Virion RNA acts as mRNA and is translated into a polyprotein, which is then cleaved to yield some 11 individual proteins
Cytoplasmic replication

shrinking in recent years as control and elimination programs have been established in more and more countries. Seven serotypes of foot-and-mouth disease virus have been identified by cross-protection and serologic tests; they are designated O, A, C, SAT 1, SAT 2, SAT 3, and Asia 1. At one time or another, these viruses occurred in most parts of the world, often causing extensive epidemics in domestic cattle and swine (Table 35.3). Sheep and many species of wildlife are also susceptible. Mortality is low but morbidity is high; convalescence and virus shedding from affected animals may be protracted and it is these features that make foot-and-mouth disease so important, especially when the virus is introduced into countries previously free of disease (see Chapter 15).

Table 35.3
Geographic Distribution of Foot-and-Mouth Disease[a]

Region	Virus
South America	O, A, C
Europe	O, A, C
Africa	O, A, C, SAT 1, SAT 2, SAT 3
Asia	O, A, C, Asia 1
North and Central America	Virus free
Caribbean	Virus free
Oceania	Virus free

[a]Foot-and-mouth disease-free countries where vaccination is not practiced: Australia, Austria, Belgium, Bulgaria, Canada, Chile, Costa Rica, Croatia, Cuba, Cyprus, Czech Republic, Denmark, Estonia, Finland, France, Germany, Greece, Haiti, Honduras, Hungary, Iceland, Indonesia, Ireland, Italy, Japan, Korea, Lithuania, Luxembourg, Madagascar, Malta, Mexico, Netherlands, New Caledonia, New Zealand, Norway, Panama, Poland, Portugal, Romania, Singapore, Slovakia, Spain, Sweden, Switzerland, United Kingdom, United States, Uruguay, and Vanuatu. Countries having foot-and-mouth disease-free zones where vaccination is not practiced: Colombia, Namibia, and South Africa. Countries having foot-and-mouth disease-free zones where vaccination is practiced: Argentina and Paraguay. Data from the Office International des Épizooties.

During the 19th century, foot-and-mouth disease was widely reported in Europe, Asia, Africa, and South and North America and occurred on one occasion in Australia. From 1880 onward, the control of rinderpest and the improved husbandry in the livestock industries in Europe focused attention on foot-and-mouth disease. Its sequelae were found to be more important than the acute illness. In dairy herds, the febrile disease resulted in the loss of milk production for the rest of the lactation period and mastitis often resulted in a permanent loss of more than 25% of milk production; the growth of beef cattle was retarded. Today, many countries have either eliminated foot-and-mouth disease by compulsory slaughter of infected animals or have reduced its incidence greatly by extensive vaccination programs.

Historically, each virus type has been further subtyped on the basis of quantitative differences in cross-protection and serologic tests. Antigenic variation within a type occurs as a continuous process of antigenic drift without clear-cut demarcations between subtypes. This antigenic heterogeneity has important economic implications for vaccine development and selection, as immunity acquired through infection or use of current vaccines is strictly type specific and, to a lesser degree, subtype specific. Difficulty in defining the threshold at which a new isolate should be given subtype status has always been a problem and current attitudes reflect a pragmatic approach. New strains are now compared with the established vaccine strains of commercial producers, thereby avoiding the complexity of classifying new isolates within an ever increasing catalogue of subtypes, many of which have little relevance to current problems in the field.

Clinical Features

Aphthoviruses infect a wide variety of cloven-hoofed domestic and wild animal species. Although the horse is refractory to infection, cattle, water buffalo, sheep, goats, llamas, camels, and swine are susceptible and develop clinical signs, and more than 70 species of wild mammals belonging to more than 20 families are susceptible. In general, clinical signs are most severe in cattle and swine, but outbreaks have been reported in swine while cattle in close contact with them did not develop clinical disease, such as occurred in Taiwan in 1997 (see Chapter 15). Sheep and goats usually experience subclinical infections. Wild animals show a spectrum of responses ranging from inapparent infection to severe disease and even death.

Cattle

After an incubation period of 2 to 8 days, there is fever, loss of appetite, depression, and a marked drop in milk production. Within 24 hours, drooling of saliva commences and vesicles develop on the tongue and gums (Figure 35.6A). The animal may open and close its mouth with a characteristic smacking sound. Vesicles may also be found in the interdigital skin and coronary band of the feet (Figure 35.6B) and on the teats. The vesicles soon rupture, producing large, denuded ulcerative lesions (Figure 35.6C). Those on the tongue often heal within a few days, but those on the feet and within the nasal cavities often become infected secondarily with bacteria, resulting in prolonged lameness and a mucopurulent nasal discharge. In calves up to 6 months of age, foot-and-mouth disease virus can cause death through myocarditis. The mortality in adult cattle is very low, but although the virus does not cross the placenta, cattle may abort, presumably as a consequence of fever. Also, affected animals become nonproductive or poorly productive for long periods. They may eat little for a week after the onset of clinical signs and are often very lame, and mastitis and abortion further lower milk production. In endemic areas, where cattle may have partial immunity, the disease may be mild or subclinical.

Swine

In swine, lameness is often the first sign. Foot lesions can be severe and may be sufficiently painful to prevent the pig from standing. Denuded areas between the claws usually become infected with bacteria; this causes suppuration and, in some cases, loss of the claw and prolonged lameness. Vesicles within the mouth are usually less prominent than in cattle, although large vesicles, which quickly rupture, often develop on the snout.

Other Animals

The clinical disease in sheep, goats, and wild ruminants is usually milder than in cattle and is characterized by foot lesions accompanied by lameness.

Pathogenesis, Pathology, and Immunity

The main route of infection in ruminants is through the inhalation of droplets, but ingestion of infected food, inoculation with contaminated vaccines, insemination with contaminated semen, and contact with contaminated clothing, veterinary instruments, and so on can all produce infection. In animals infected via the respiratory tract, initial viral replication occurs in the pharynx, followed by viremic spread to other tissues and organs before the onset of clinical disease. Viral excretion commences about 24 hours prior to the onset of clinical disease and continues for several days. Aerosols pro-

Figure 35.6.

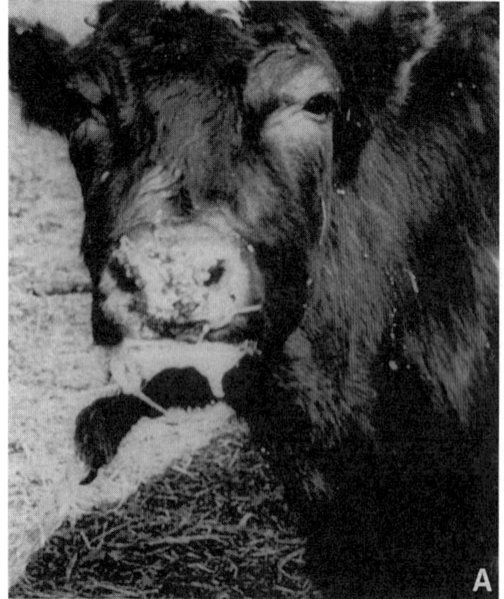

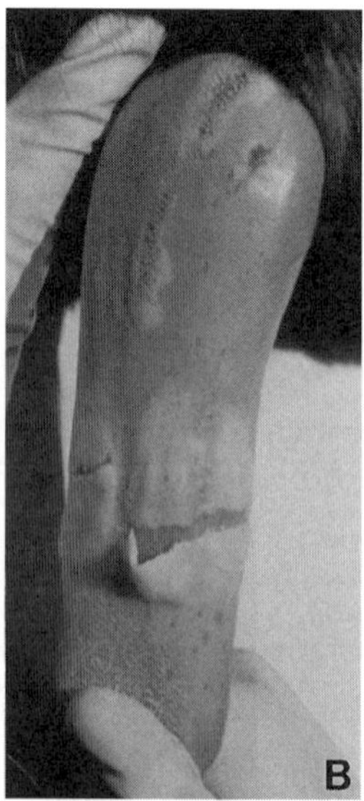

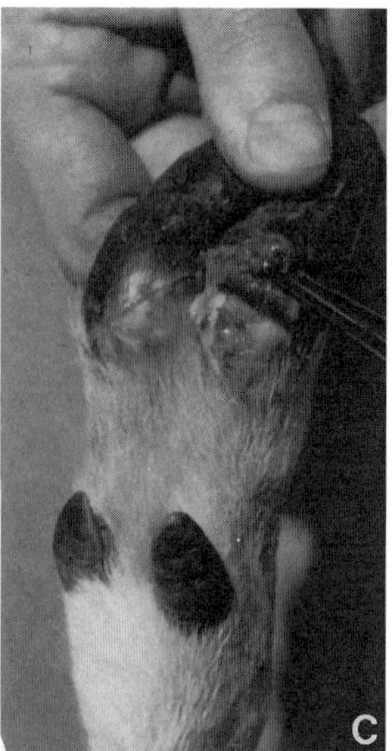

Foot-and-mouth disease. (A) Profuse salivation by a diseased cow. (B) Ruptured vesicles on the tongue of a steer. (C) Vesicular lesions on the foot of a deer.

duced by infected animals contain large amounts of virus, particularly those produced by swine. Large amounts of virus are also excreted in the milk. The excretion of virus in high titer in droplets and in milk has epidemiologic significance and is important for the control of disease (see later).

Foot-and-mouth disease virus may persist in the pharynx of some animals for a prolonged period after recovery. In cattle, virus may be detectable for periods up to 2 years after exposure to infection, in sheep for about 6 months. Viral persistence does not occur in swine. This carrier state has also been observed in wild animals, particularly the African Cape buffalo (*Syncerus caffer*), which is commonly found to be infected with more than one of the SAT virus types even in areas where foot-and-mouth disease does not occur in cattle.

The mechanisms by which the virus produces a persistent infection in ruminants are unknown. The virus is present in the pharynx in an infectious form, for if pharyngeal fluids are inoculated into susceptible animals they develop foot-and-mouth disease. Attempts to demonstrate that carrier cattle can transmit disease by placing them in contact with susceptible animals have given equivocal results, but transmission of virus from persistently infected African Cape buffalo to cattle has been observed.

Recovery from clinical foot-and-mouth disease is correlated with the development of antibody. The early IgM antibodies neutralize the homologous type of virus and may also be effective against heterologous types. In contrast, the IgG produced during convalescence is type specific and, to varying degrees, subtype specific. Little information is available on the role of cell-mediated immunity in recovery from foot-and-mouth disease, but as in other picornavirus infections, it has been assumed to be of minor importance.

Cattle that have recovered from foot-and-mouth disease are usually immune to infection with the same virus type for a year or more, but immunity is not considered lifelong. Recovered animals, however, can be infected immediately with one of the other types of foot-and-mouth disease virus and develop clinical disease.

Table 35.4
Differential Diagnosis of Vesicular Diseases Based on Naturally Occurring Disease in Different Domestic Animal Species[a]

Disease	Cattle	Sheep	Swine	Horse
Foot-and-mouth disease	S	S	S	R
Swine vesicular disease	R	R	S	R
Vesicular stomatitis	S	S	S	S
Vesicular exanthema of swine[b]	R	R	S	R

[a]S, susceptible by natural exposure; R, resistant by natural exposure.
[b]Now extinct in swine, but virus occurs in marine mammals.

Laboratory Diagnosis

Rapid diagnosis of foot-and-mouth disease is of paramount importance, especially in countries that are usually free of infection, so that quarantine and eradication programs can be implemented as quickly as possible. Because three other viruses can produce clinically indistinguishable lesions in domestic animals, confirmation by laboratory diagnosis is essential, although the history of the disease and the involvement of different species can be valuable pointers to the diagnosis (Table 35.4). Foot-and-mouth disease is a notifiable disease in most countries, thus whenever a vesicular disease of domestic animals is seen, it must be reported immediately to the appropriate government authority.

Specimens for diagnosis are collected by government officials from animals with clinical signs; the exact procedure differs in different countries. Usually, samples include vesicular fluid, epithelial tissue from the edge of ruptured vesicles, blood in anticoagulant, serum, and esophageal/pharyngeal fluids collected with a cup-probang. These samples are diluted immediately with an equal volume of cell culture medium containing 10% fetal calf serum. From dead animals, additional tissue samples may be collected from lymph nodes, thyroid, and heart. Samples should be frozen (preferably at −70°C, i.e., the temperature of dry ice) and sent immediately to the laboratory in the frozen state. In places where maintenance of the "cold chain" is difficult, duplicate samples should be collected and transported in glycerol buffer at pH 7.6.

A range of diagnostic tests is available for the differentiation of the vesicular diseases, but an enzyme immunoassay is available commercially and standardized, whereby if vesicular fluid or tissues contain adequate amounts of antigen, a diagnosis is available within a few hours. This test can also be used to identify which of the seven types of foot-and-mouth disease virus is the cause of the disease. Sensitive enzyme immunoassays are also available for specific antibody determinations.

Cell cultures and, on occasion, cattle and swine are used to isolate virus when the concentration of virus in the vesicular epithelium or fluid is low. Cell cultures are generally used to isolate the virus from other tissues, blood, and esophageal or pharyngeal fluids. The isolated virus is identified by the enzyme immunoassay or the neutralization test.

Epidemiology, Prevention, and Control

The recognition of foot-and-mouth disease as the most important viral disease constraining efficient animal production in many parts of the world has resulted in intensive study of its epidemiology.

Countries Free of Endemic Disease

In countries where foot-and-mouth disease either has not existed previously or has been eliminated, a virgin soil epidemic can develop rapidly from introduction of virus on one farm. Within a short period, often measured in days rather than weeks, the outbreak can extend to so many farms that veterinary authorities have difficulty in controlling its spread (see Chapter 15). Reasons for the rapidity of spread in such fully susceptible populations are the highly infectious nature of the virus, the production of high titer virus in respiratory secretions and the large volumes of droplets and aerosols of virus shed by infected animals, the stability of virus in such droplets, the rapid replication cycle with very high virus yields, and the short incubation period.

Foot-and-mouth disease is spread rapidly within a locality by movement of infected animals to market and by mechanical transmission on items such as clothing, shoes, vehicles, and veterinary instruments. The excretion of virus for up to 24 hours prior to the onset of clinical signs means that virus dissemination may have occurred from a farm before any suspicion of disease is raised. Foot-and-mouth disease is commonly shortened to FMD. This abbreviation can also be considered as a mnemonic; namely "fast moving disease" to reflect its rapidity of spread and the consequent need for immediate regulatory action.

It was not until a dramatic epidemic of 1967–1968 in England, in which approximately 634,000 animals were slaughtered before the disease was successfully eradicated, that the importance of long-distance airborne transmission was realized. Long-distance spread is dependent on wind direction and speed and is favored by low temperature, high humidity, and overcast skies. Long-distance spread is therefore more likely to occur in temperate rather than tropical climates. So detailed is the knowledge of the characteristics of aerosols of foot-and-mouth disease virus that computer modeling was used in 1981 to predict the likelihood of spread of disease from France across the English Channel to England (Figure 35.7).

In contrast to humans, who are generally free to move from country to country without extensive health checks, the international movement of domestic food animals and their products is carefully controlled (see Chapter 15). Nowadays, most introductions of foot-and-mouth disease virus to nonendemic countries can be traced either to meat on the bone being fed to swine or rarely to long-distance spread of virus by aerosols.

The use of polymerase chain reaction and partial sequencing of VP1 to compare an isolate causing disease in one country with a possible source of infection in another country can provide strong evidence to link the two events. Using oligonucleotide RNA fingerprinting and sequencing, scientists investigating the 1981 outbreak in England showed that the outbreaks in England and France were caused by a virus that was identical to a strain used in the preparation of inactivated virus vaccine in France.

Countries with Endemic Disease

The introduction of a virus type not present previously in a country may cause a virgin-soil epidemic because livestock will not have acquired immunity either through natural infection or through vaccination. For example, in 1961, the spread of SAT 1 from Africa through the countries of the Near East—where different types of foot-and-mouth disease virus are endemic—was more dramatic than any recorded spread of this type in Africa.

In some countries, particularly those in temperate zones with European breeds of cattle, the severity of disease is modified by vaccination. In subtropical and tropical countries, with predominantly local breeds of cattle, the endemic strains produce only mild disease in indigenous cattle, but cause severe disease in introduced European breeds. There is a greater variety of antigenic types in Africa and Asia than in Europe and South America and, in Africa particularly, there is a large wildlife population that can become involved in the epidemiology. The African Cape buffalo (*Syncerus caffer*) is the natural host for SAT 1, 2, and 3 types of foot-and-mouth disease virus. Transmission of virus occurs between buffalo but clinical disease has not been recorded; the African buffalo does not seem to transmit disease readily to domestic cattle.

Foot-and-mouth disease, more than any other disease, has influenced the development of international regulations designed to minimize the risk of introducing animal diseases into a country. Some countries have successfully avoided the introduction of foot-and-mouth disease by prohibiting the importation of all animals and animal products from countries where disease exists. The United States adopted such a policy from 1929 to 1980; only recently in the light of improved diagnostic

FIGURE 35.7.

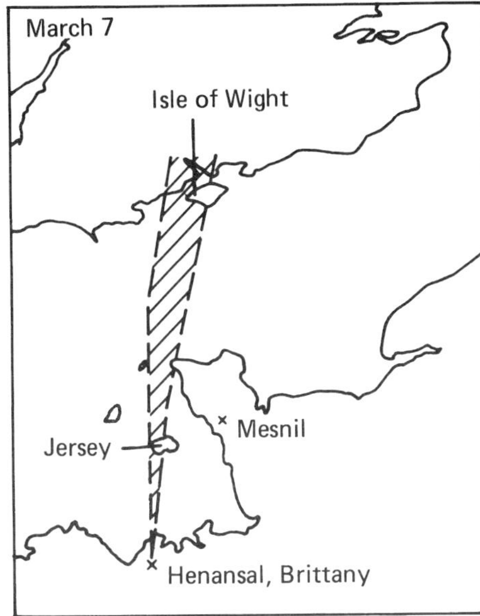

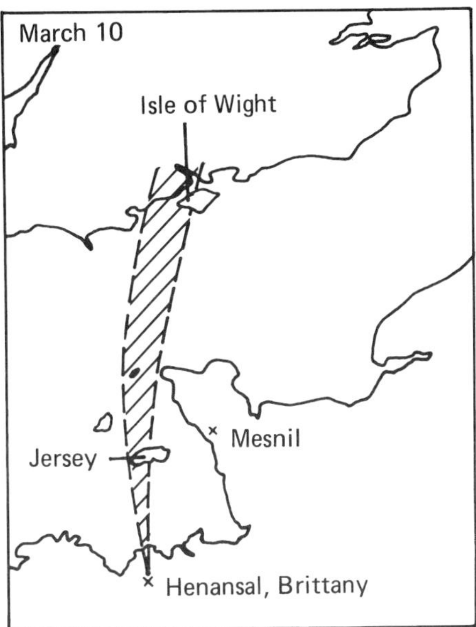

Airborne spread of foot-and-mouth disease. Between March 4 and 26, 1981, French veterinary authorities reported 13 outbreaks of foot-and-mouth disease, virus type O, in Brittany. On March 6, a team of meteorologists and virologists in the United Kingdom began analyses to determine whether weather conditions might be favorable for the airborne spread of the virus from France to England. From this analysis it was considered that the risk for the Channel Islands was high, but that it was low in southern England, as the furthest distance reported previously for airborne spread of the virus was approximately 100 km (from Denmark to Sweden in 1966). Single outbreaks were detected in both the areas predicted, on the island of Jersey and on the Isle of Wight. Analysis of wind direction based on data obtained in Jersey revealed that there were two periods, each 24 hours long, on March 7 and 10 that were ideal for the transmission of virus from Brittany to Jersey and the Isle of Wight. The distance between Henansal, Brittany, and the Isle of Wight is approximately 250 km. (Courtesy of A. I. Donaldson.)

procedures, has it relaxed this embargo to allow small numbers of cattle to be imported, through quarantine, for breeding purposes.

For many countries such as Australia, Canada, United Kingdom, and the United States that have a recent history of freedom from foot-and-mouth disease, cost–benefit analyses justify a "stamping out" policy whenever disease occurs or is suspected. This is based on slaughter of affected animals and exposed animals and rigid enforcement of quarantine and restrictions on movement. Vaccination is not used. To support such policies, legislation is in place, with the most important provision being that foot-and-mouth disease is a notifiable disease. Any suspicion of disease must be brought to the attention of national or state veterinary authorities.

In many countries of the world an eradication policy cannot be pursued because of costs and vaccine is used to reduce the prevalence of disease. Inactivated vaccines, produced by growing virus in suspension cultures of a baby hamster kidney cell line, inactivated with *N*-acetylethyleneimine and used with aluminum hydroxide or double oil emulsion as adjuvants, are now the only vaccines in general use. By systematic use of inactivated vaccines, many countries in Europe have now sufficiently controlled foot-and-mouth disease to discontinue vaccination and adopt an eradication policy whenever clinical disease occurs (see Chapter 15). However, it is difficult to produce a vaccine of consistent potency, and much research continues with peptide and various recombinant DNA-based strategies, including vectored, virus-like particle, and DNA vaccines.

Although less immunogenic than intact inactivated virions, preparations of purified VP1 elicit neutralizing antibody, a discovery that has provided a major impetus for the development of recombinant DNA and synthetic peptide vaccines for foot-and-mouth disease (see Chapter 14).

Human Disease

Foot-and-mouth disease is a zoonosis, although given its incidence in animals in several parts of the world and associated opportunities for human exposure to large amounts of virus, very few human cases are reported. The disease in humans is rather benign: many infections are subclinical, whereas others resemble infection in animals. Clinical signs include fever, anorexia, and vesiculation on the skin and/or mucous membranes. There may be primary vesicular lesions at the site of viral exposure (e.g., abrasion of skin) and secondary vesicular lesions in the mouth and on the hands and feet. Most cases reported over the years have been in persons in close contact with infected animals and in laboratory workers. Laboratory diagnosis is required to confirm human cases. Prevention of human infection is based on control of the disease in animals and use of Biosafety Level 2 practices and equipment in laboratory facilities.

Equine Rhinovirus 1 Infection

It has long been known that equine rhinovirus 1 has physicochemical properties (e.g., acid lability) unlike those of human rhinoviruses, but similar to foot-and-mouth disease viruses. Sequencing of the genome of equine rhinovirus 1 has revealed many other molecular characteristics shared only with the foot-and-mouth disease viruses and a few characteristics that are unique. After assessing these data, in 1998 the International Committee on Taxonomy of Viruses placed equine rhinovirus 1 in the genus *Aphthovirus* and divided the genus into two "clusters," one for the equine virus and the other for the foot-and-mouth disease viruses. The pathogenicity of equine rhinoviruses 1 resembles that of foot-and-mouth disease viruses in cattle in that infection by some strains produces quite severe systemic and respiratory signs. In such infections, there is viremia and the virus can be isolated from feces.

Diseases Caused by Members of the Genus *Enterovirus*

Enteroviruses are ubiquitous and probably occur in all vertebrate species. However, only in swine and poultry do they cause diseases of economic significance. A number of enteroviruses have been recovered from swine, but only two cause diseases of any importance: one causing swine vesicular disease, the major importance of which is its clinical resemblance to foot-and-mouth disease, and the other causing porcine polioencephalomyelitis (Teschen/Talfan disease).

Swine Vesicular Disease

Swine vesicular disease was first recognized in Italy in 1966 and since 1972 has been reported sporadically in many other European and Asian countries.

Clinical Features

Disease is often detected by the sudden appearance of lameness in several swine in a herd. Affected swine have a transient fever, and vesicles appear at the junction between the heel and the coronary band and spread to encircle the digit. In severe cases, the swine are very lame and recovery is protracted. In about 10% of cases, lesions are found on the snout, lips, and tongue. Occasionally, some infected swine develop signs of encephalomyelitis, such as ataxia, circling, and convulsions. Subclinical infections also occur.

Pathogenesis, Pathology, and Immunity

Initial infection with swine vesicular disease virus probably occurs through damaged skin, particularly abrasions around the feet. Infection can also occur if swine eat infected garbage, but the titer of virus required to establish infection is higher. Following infection, there is viremia and large quantities of virus are excreted in the feces, but persistent infection does not occur. Swine that have recovered from disease develop antibody that protects them from reinfection.

Laboratory Diagnosis

Because swine vesicular disease cannot be differentiated clinically from the other vesicular diseases of swine, including foot-and-mouth disease, laboratory diagnosis is essential. A variety of rapid laboratory tests are available to distinguish the vesicular diseases. If sufficient vesicular fluid or epithelium is available, an enzyme immunoassay can be used to detect antigen and establish a diagnosis within 4 to 24 hours; the polymerase chain reaction can also be used for the rapid detection and differentiation of all vesicular diseases. The virus grows well in cultures of swine kidney cells, producing a cytopathic effect, sometimes as early as 6 hours after inoculation. The virus can also be isolated by the intracerebral inoculation of newborn mice, which develop paralysis and die.

Epidemiology, Prevention, and Control

There is no evidence that swine vesicular disease virus exists in any country without clinical disease being reported. Because of its resistance to low pH and ambient temperatures, it is transmitted easily between countries in infected meat. Various pork products that are prepared without heat treatment, such as salami, can harbor virus for several months. Fresh pork infected with swine vesicular disease virus can be an additional hazard within a country and delay eradication of disease, as infected carcasses may be placed unknowingly in cold storage for months or years; when released, such infected meat can give rise to new outbreaks.

At neutral pH and 4°C, the virus has been reported to survive for over 160 days without loss of titer. The conditions found on many swine farms are therefore conducive to gross and persistent contamination of the environment. Because the virus is so stable, it is extremely difficult to decontaminate infected premises, particularly where swine have been housed on soil. The virus has been isolated from the surface and gut of earthworms collected from soil above burial pits containing carcasses of swine slaughtered because of swine vesicular disease.

Swine vesicular disease is not an economically important disease, but it must be controlled so that diagnostic confusion with foot-and-mouth disease can be avoided. For this reason, swine vesicular disease is a notifiable disease and most countries have elected to eliminate the virus by a slaughter program, but this may be difficult.

Human Disease

Swine vesicular disease virus occasionally causes an "influenza-like" illness in humans and is closely related serologically and by RNA hybridization tests to human coxsackievirus B5.

Porcine Polioencephalomyelitis (Caused by Porcine Enterovirus 1)

Porcine polioencephalomyelitis was first recognized in the town of Teschen in 1930 in what is now the Czech Republic. The disease was described as a particularly virulent, highly fatal, nonsuppurative encephalomyelitis in which lesions were present throughout the central nervous system. This severe form of the disease is still recognized, although less severe forms, referred to originally as Talfan disease in the United Kingdom and as endemic posterior paresis in Denmark, are more common and occur worldwide.

Clinical Features

After an incubation period of 4 to 28 days, the initial signs include fever, anorexia, and depression, followed by tremors and incoordination usually beginning with the hind limbs. Initially the limbs may be stiff, then paralysis occurs, leading to prostration followed by convulsions, coma, and death. There may be enhanced responses to touch and sound, paralysis of facial muscles, and loss of voice. In severe outbreaks the mortality may reach 75%. In milder forms of disease the clinical signs are limited to ataxia associated with hind limb paresis from which swine often recover completely in a few days.

Pathogenesis, Pathology, and Immunity

The pathogenicity of strains of porcine enterovirus 1 varies and the severity of the disease is also influenced by age, being most severe in young swine. The virus replicates initially in the alimentary tract and associated lymphoid tissues, followed by viremia and invasion of the central nervous system. Histologically the lesions resemble those of other viral encephalomyelitides, with perivascular cuffing, neuronal degeneration, and gliosis. The extent of the lesions parallels the severity of clinical disease and, in extreme cases, involves the entire spinal cord, brain, and meninges.

Laboratory Diagnosis

Polioencephalomyelitis due to porcine enterovirus 1 must be differentiated from other viral encephalomyelitides, including African swine fever, pseudorabies, hemagglutinating encephalomyelitis, rabies, and hog cholera. The virus is isolated readily in porcine cell cultures, with neutralization assays being used for typing. Immunofluorescent staining of the infected cell culture is preferred for rapid, definitive diagnosis.

Epidemiology, Prevention, and Control

Infection is acquired by ingestion. Inactivated and attenuated virus vaccines, comparable to the Salk and Sabin vaccines for human poliomyelitis, are available commercially. Universal vaccination is not practiced as control in intensive swine units is often achieved satisfactorily by quarantine and hygiene.

Other Porcine Enterovirus Diseases (Caused by Porcine Enteroviruses 2 to 11)

These viruses are isolated frequently from the feces of normal swine, from swine with diarrhea or pericarditis, and from aborted and stillborn fetuses. Several isolates of porcine enteroviruses 2–11 have been shown to cause encephalomyelitis following experimental infection of swine.

Avian Encephalomyelitis

Avian encephalomyelitis was first described in the New England states of the United States in 1932 and is now recognized worldwide. Its natural history parallels closely that of poliomyelitis of humans and polioencephalomyelitis of swine. Avian encephalomyelitis is an important disease of chickens 1 to 21 days of age, but the virus is not pathogenic in older chickens. When the virus is newly introduced into a flock the mortality rate may exceed 50%. There is only a single antigenic type, but strains vary in virulence. Avian encephalomyelitis virus produces relatively mild encephalomyelitis in quail, turkeys, and pheasants; other avian species are susceptible following experimental infection.

Clinical Features

After an incubation period of 1 to 7 days, disease occurs, which is characterized by dullness, progressive ataxia, tremors particularly of the head and neck, weight loss, blindness, paralysis, and, in severe cases, prostration, coma, and death. Birds allowed to recover have deficits of the central nervous system and are usually destroyed.

Pathogenesis, Pathology, and Immunity

No obvious macroscopic lesions are seen at postmortem. Histologic lesions typical of viral encephalitis, but not diagnostic of avian encephalomyelitis, are found throughout the central nervous system, with perivascular cuffing, neuronal degeneration, and gliosis.

Laboratory Diagnosis

Clinical signs and histopathology are suggestive and immunofluorescence is widely used for definitive diagnosis. The virus may be isolated either in cell culture or by inoculating 5- to 7-day-old embryonated hen eggs obtained from antibody-free hens by the yolk sac route; chicks are allowed to hatch and are observed for 7 days for signs of encephalomyelitis. The disease needs to be differentiated from Newcastle disease as well as from a range of nonviral causes of central nervous system disease in chickens.

Epidemiology, Prevention, and Control

High morbidity and mortality occur when avian encephalomyelitis virus is first introduced into a flock. The major mode of transmission is by a fecal–oral route, although transmission via the egg may occur in association with the brief viremic phase of the disease in laying hens. Once established in a flock, losses continue at a greatly reduced incidence because maternal antibody provides protection for chicks during the critical first 21 days after hatching.

The choice for control is either depopulation or vaccination. Attenuated virus vaccines administered in the drinking water are available. The vaccines are administered after chickens reach 10 weeks of age and are designed to provide protection for chicks during the first 21 days after hatching by ensuring that adequate levels of specific antibody are transferred from hens to progeny chicks. They are not administered to chicks because they are not sufficiently attenuated, nor is there sufficient time to provide protection for chicks hatched into a heavily contaminated environment. Inactivated vaccines are also available and are preferred when immunized birds are housed in close proximity to nonimmunized chickens. Vaccines are also used to control avian encephalomyelitis in quail and turkey.

Duck Hepatitis

Duck hepatitis was first recognized in 1945 among ducks reared on Long Island, New York. There is only one serotype, and the natural history of the virus is similar to that of avian encephalomyelitis virus. Goslings, turkey poults, and chicks of guinea fowl and quail, but not chickens, are susceptible to experimental infection.

Clinical Features

Disease occurs in ducks less than 21 days of age, after an incubation period of 1 to 5 days. The course of the disease in a clutch of ducks is often dramatically swift, occurring over a 3-day period with a mortality rate approaching 100%. Affected ducks tend to stand still with partially closed eyes, fall to one side, paddle spasmodically, and die. There may be some diarrhea.

Pathogenesis, Pathology, and Immunity

At postmortem, the liver is enlarged, edematous, and mottled with hemorrhages. Histologically there is extensive hepatic necrosis, inflammatory cell infiltration and proliferation of the bile duct epithelium, and encephalitis with neuronal necrosis, gliosis, and perivascular cuffing.

Laboratory Diagnosis

The history, clinical signs, and characteristic postmortem findings are suggestive; immunofluorescence provides rapid, definitive diagnosis. The virus may be isolated in cell culture or by allantoic inoculation of 10-day-old embryonated hen eggs. When subsequently candled, infected eggs, often show characteristic greenish discoloration of the embryonic fluids and most are dead within 4 days after inoculation. Duck hepatitis needs to be differentiated from duck plague (a herpesvirus infection), influenza, and Newcastle disease.

Epidemiology, Prevention, and Control

Recovered ducks are immune. Hyperimmune serum has been used successfully to reduce losses during outbreaks. Attenuated virus vaccines are available commercially and are used following the same principles as already outlined for avian encephalomyelitis vaccines.

Turkey Hepatitis

Turkey hepatitis was first recognized in 1959 in Canada and the United States. The virus is related antigenically to duck hepatitis virus and the natural history of the disease resembles that of duck hepatitis.

Diseases Caused by Members of the Genus *Cardiovirus*

Encephalomyocarditis Virus Infection

The natural hosts of encephalomyocarditis virus are rodents, including the water rat, *Hydromys chrysogaster*. The virus is transmitted from rodents to humans, monkeys, horses, cattle, and swine. Severe epidemics of myocarditis, with fatalities, have occasionally been reported in swine and other species, such as elephants—notably in Florida, Australia, and South Africa—usually in association with severe mouse or, less commonly, rat infestations. In recent years there have been significant losses of elephants in the Kruger National Park in South Africa attributed to encephalomyocarditis virus infection.

Theiler's Murine Encephalomyelitis Virus Infection

Theiler's murine encephalomyelitis virus, actually a complex (quasispecies) of related viruses, is a common enteric pathogen of mice and rats that can spread to the central nervous system where it causes several neurological syndromes. The most common manifestation is poliomyelitis, but depending on the age and strain of mouse, there is also a chronic inflammatory demyelinating syndrome. This virus is an important problem in mouse colonies where its presence can interfere with research protocols. It is diagnosed along with other important mouse viruses in the usual viral diagnostic panel that is required in the United States for all mice used in federally funded research. Diagnosis involves serology (hemagglutination–inhibition, neutralization, enzyme immunoassay), which may be supported by confirmatory virus isolation in murine cell culture. Control involves a high level of sanitation, diagnostic surveillance, and prevention of entry into colonies of feral rodents.

Diseases Caused by Members of the Genus *Rhinovirus*

Among domestic animals, rhinoviruses are recognized only in cattle. In cattle, only three serotypes have been identified, compared with over 150 serotypes of human rhinovirus. Bovine rhinoviruses are unrelated antigenically to the human rhinoviruses. They are highly host specific and have been isolated from cattle with mild respiratory disease similar to the common cold in humans, but they may predispose to more severe forms of respiratory disease such as shipping fever.

Diseases Caused by Unclassified Picornaviruses

Equine Rhinovirus 2 Infection

Four picornaviruses have been identified in horses. Equine rhinovirus 1 has been classified as a member of the genus *Aphthovirus;* two other viruses seem to be acid-stable enteroviruses of unknown significance as pathogens. The genome of equine rhinovirus 2 has been sequenced and found to be somewhat similar to the cardioviruses, but more or less unique and possibly warranting the construction of another genus. Equine rhinovirus 2 causes respiratory disease in horses; its importance as a pathogen has not been assessed adequately.

Further Reading

Brown, F. (1992). New approaches to vaccination against foot-and-mouth disease. *Vaccine* **10**, 1022–1026.

Calnek, B. W., Luginbuhl, R. E., and Helmboldt, C. F. (1997). Avian encephalomyelitis. *In* "Diseases of Poultry" (B. W. Calnek, ed.), 10th ed., pp. 571–574. Iowa State University Press, Ames.

Carillo, C., Wigdorovitz, A., Oliveros, J. C., Zamarano, P. I., Sadir, A. M., Gomez, N., Salinas, J., Escribano, J. M., and Borca, M. V. (1998). Protective immune response to foot-and-mouth disease virus with VP1 expressed in transgenic plants. *J. Virol.* **72**, 1688–1690.

Derbyshire, J. B. (1992). Porcine enteroviruses. *In* "Diseases of Swine," (A. D. Leman, B. Straw, W. L. Mengeling, S. D'Allaire, and D. J. Taylor, eds.), 7th ed., pp. 263–267. Iowa State University Press, Ames.

Doel, T. R. (1996). Natural and vaccine induced immunity to foot-and-mouth disease: The prospects for improved vaccines. *Sci. Tech. Rev. Off. Int. Épizoot.* **15**, 883–911.

European Commission for the Control of Foot-and-Mouth Disease. Available at: http://www.fao.org/waicent/faoinfo/agricult/aga/agah/eufmd/default.htm

Hunter, P. (1998). Vaccination as a means of control of foot-and-mouth disease in sub-Saharan Africa. *Vaccine* **16**, 261–264.

Hypia, T., Hovi, T., Knowles, N. J., and Stanway, G. (1997). Classification of enteroviruses based on molecular and biological properties. *J. Gen. Virol.* **78**, 1–11.

Institute of Animal Health. Picornaviridae web site. Available at: http://www.iah.bbsrc.ac.uk/virus/picornaviridae/index.htm

Joo, H. S. (1992). Encephalomyocarditis. *In* "Diseases of Swine" (A. D. Leman, B. Straw, W. L. Mengeling, S. D'Allaire, and D. J. Taylor, eds.), 7th ed., pp. 257–260. Iowa State University Press, Ames.

Li, F., Browning, G. F., Studdert, M. J., and Crabb, B. S. (1996). Equine rhinovirus 1 is more closely related to foot-and-mouth disease virus than to other picornaviruses. *Proc. Nat. Acad. Sci. U. S. A.* **93**, 990–995.

McNulty, M. S., and McFerran, J. B. (1996). Diseases associated with Picornaviridae. *In* "Poultry Diseases" (F. T. W. Jordan and M. Pattison, eds.), 4th ed., pp. 187–195. Baillière Tindall, London.

Rueckert, R. R. (1996). Picornaviridae: The viruses and their replication. *In* "Fields Virology" (B. N. Fields, D. M. Knipe, P. M. Howley, R. M. Chanock, J. L. Melnick, T. P. Monath, B. Roizman, and S. E. Straus, eds.), 3rd ed., pp. 609–654. Lippincott-Raven, Philadelphia, PA.

Thomson, G. R. (1994). Foot-and-mouth disease. *In* "Infectious Diseases of Livestock with Special Reference to Southern Africa" (J. A. W. Coetzer, G. R. Thompson, and R. C. Tustin, eds.), Vol. 2, pp. 823–852. Oxford University Press, Cape Town.

Woodcock, P. R., and Fabricant, J. (1997). Duck virus hepatitis. *In* "Diseases of Poultry" (B. W. Calnek, ed.), 10th ed., pp. 661–664. Iowa State University Press, Ames.

Wutz, G., Auer, H., Nowotny, N., Grosse, B., Skern, T., and Kuechler, E. (1996). Equine rhinovirus serotypes 1 and 2: Relationship to each other and to aphthoviruses and cardioviruses. *J. Gen. Virol.* **77**, 1719–1730.

CHAPTER 36

Caliciviridae

The family *Caliciviridae* includes several viruses of veterinary importance: vesicular exanthema of swine viruses and the closely related San Miguel sea lion viruses, feline calicivirus, rabbit hemorrhagic disease virus, European brown hare syndrome virus, and caliciviruses of several other species. Caliciviruses are associated with systemic diseases and gastroenteritis, but one from dogs has been associated with a vesicular genital disease. Probable caliciviruses have also been recovered from monkeys, cattle, mink, dogs, chickens, reptiles, amphibians, and insects.

Vesicular exanthema of swine was first recognized in southern California in 1932 and caused concern because the disease it caused was similar to foot-and-mouth disease; the virus, still the prototype of the family, was eradicated in 1956. Feline calicivirus is one of the two major causes of viral upper respiratory tract disease in cats and has been reported to cause glossitis in dogs. Rabbit hemorrhagic disease first emerged in China in 1984 as an apparently new, usually fatal disease in domestic rabbits; this virus has been introduced into Australia and New Zealand as a biocontrol agent.

Properties of Caliciviruses

Classification

The family *Caliciviridae* comprises four genera, two of which contain viruses of veterinary importance. The genus *Vesivirus* contains the marine animal caliciviruses and the vesicular disease viruses: vesicular exanthema of swine viruses 1–13, San Miguel sea lion viruses 1–17, feline calicivirus, cetacean calicivirus (Tur-1), primate calicivirus (Pan-1), skunk calicivirus, and reptile calicivirus (Cro-1). The genus *Lagovirus* contains rabbit hemorrhagic disease virus and European brown hare syndrome virus. One of the unnamed genera contains important viruses of humans and swine: (SRSV group 1) Norwalk virus, Southampton virus, Snow Mountain virus, Hawaii virus, Taunton virus, and (SRSV group 2) Toronto virus, Lordsdale virus, and several swine caliciviruses. The other unnamed genus contains the classical human enteric caliciviruses such as Sapporo virus and Manchester virus. Many animal caliciviruses are as yet unclassified: bovine enteric caliciviruses, canine calicivirus, mink calicivirus, porcine enteric calicivirus, walrus calicivirus, lion calicivirus, chicken calicivirus, and other caliciviruses of birds. Human hepatitis E virus and a similar virus that causes enteric infection in swine had been included in the family but were removed recently and placed in a floating genus, which is as yet unnamed.

Virion Properties

Calicivirus virions are nonenveloped, 40 nm in diameter, and have icosahedral symmetry. Virions are composed of 180 identical protein molecules (M_r 60,000) arranged in dimers forming 90 arch-like structural units, which in turn form 32 cup-shaped surface depressions that give the viruses their unique appearance (Figure 36.1, top; Figure 36.2). Some calicivirus isolates lack this characteristic surface structure and have a fuzzy appearance—enteric caliciviruses having such an appearance have been referred to as "small round structured viruses" (Figure 36.1, bottom).

FIGURE 36.1.

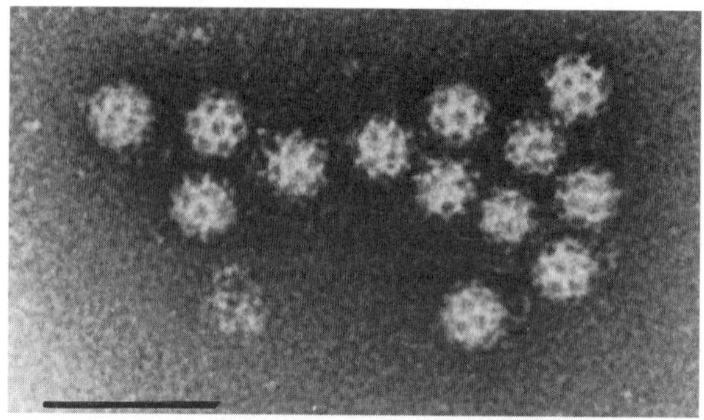

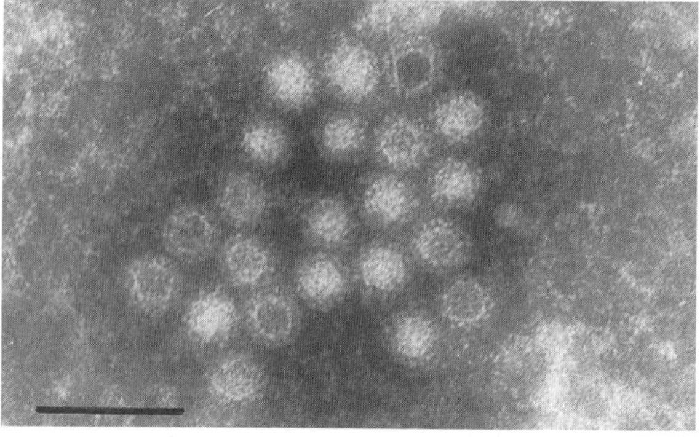

Family *Caliciviridae*. (Top) Vesicular exanthema of swine virus showing the cup-shaped depressions that are characteristic of many of the caliciviruses. (Bottom) An enteric calicivirus showing the lack of surface detail that is characteristic of most of these viruses as seen in diagnostic fecal specimens. Negative stain electron microscopy. Bars: 100 nm. (Top, courtesy of S. S. Breese.)

FIGURE 36.2.

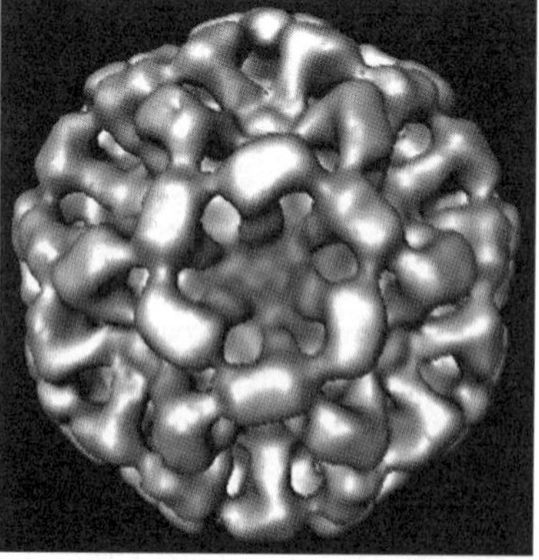

Calicivirus capsid structure, resolved using cryoelectron microscopy and computer analysis of images. The characteristic cup-shaped depressions are seen to reflect the placement of the protein subunits on the surface of the capsid. (Courtesy of J.-Y. Sgro.)

The genome consists of a single molecule of linear positive-sense, single-stranded RNA, 7.4–7.7 kb in size. The 5′ end of the genome is capped by a covalently bound protein (VPg) and the 3′ end is polyadenylated. The viruses are relatively resistant to heat and detergent-based disinfectants, but they are not very resistant to acidic conditions (>99% inactivated at pH 3).

Viral Replication

Caliciviruses replicate in the cytoplasm. Vesicular exanthema of swine virus and feline calicivirus grow well and are rapidly cytopathic in cultured cells derived from tissues of their respective hosts; vesicular exanthema of swine virus also grows well in Vero (African green monkey kidney) cells. Of the growing list of probable caliciviruses, those from gastroenteritis in swine and from vesicular genital disease in dogs have been grown in cell culture whereas most others have proven uncultivable.

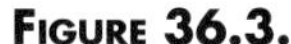

FIGURE 36.3.

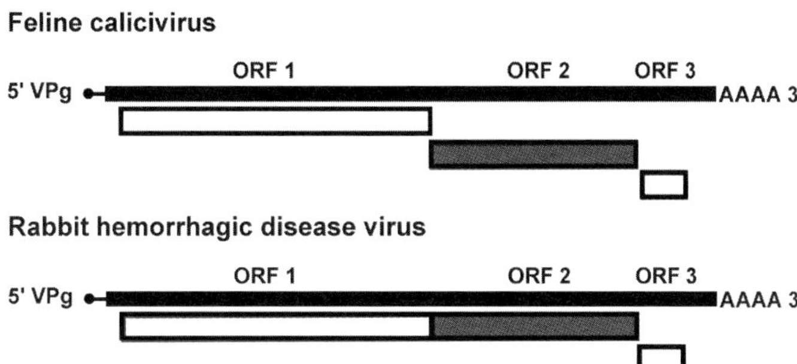

Genome organization of feline calicivirus and rabbit hemorrhagic disease virus. The genomes of all caliciviruses have a 5′ covalently linked protein, VPg, and their 3′ ends are polyadenylated. Open reading frames (ORFs) 1, 2, and 3 are shown. ORF 1 encodes a polyprotein that is cleaved to form the helicase, protease, and the RNA-dependent RNA polymerase. ORF 2 encodes the single capsid protein. ORF 3 encodes a protein of unknown function. ORF 1 and 2 are in different reading frames in feline calicivirus and in the same frame in rabbit hemorrhagic disease virus.

The various caliciviruses use two different transcriptional schemes, as exemplified by feline calicivirus and rabbit hemorrhagic disease virus (Figure 36.3). In rabbit hemorrhagic disease virus the nonstructural proteins and the structural protein are encoded in a single open reading frame, producing a single polyprotein that is cleaved posttranslationally. In feline calicivirus the nonstructural proteins and the structural protein are encoded in two separate open reading frames. The transcription of feline calicivirus (and probably also vesicular exanthema of swine virus) results in two mRNA species: one corresponds to the entire genome and the second is a subgenomic species 2.4 kb in size. The latter is bicistronic, encoding reading frames 2 and 3. Similar RNA species (7.5 and 2.2 kb) are recognized for rabbit hemorrhagic disease virus and it has been shown that both species are probably packaged into either the same or separate virions.

Open reading frame 2 has a minus-1 frame shift relative to open reading frame 1. Open reading frame 3 encodes a basic protein of 116 amino acids of unidentified function that is translated from the 2.4-kb mRNA with a minus-1 frame shift relative to open reading frame 2; it is not necessary for capsid assembly but may itself be a capsid protein. The M_r 10,000 to 15,000 VPg protein is bound to the 5′-terminus of both RNA species. The nonstructural proteins, a 2C helicase, a 3C trypsin-like serine protease, and a 3D polymerase, are similar to those found in picornaviruses. The individual nonstructural proteins are released from the polyprotein by specific viral protease activity in a cascade similar to that of picornaviruses. Genomic RNA is replicated via a negative-sense RNA intermediate. Virions accumulate in the cytoplasm, either scattered or as paracrystalline arrays or as characteristic linear arrays associated with the cytoskeleton; they are released by cell lysis (Table 36.1).

TABLE 36.1
Properties of Caliciviruses

Properties of Caliciviruses
Virions are nonenveloped, 35–40 nm in diameter, with icosahedral symmetry
Some virions have a characteristic appearance, with 32 cup-shaped depressions on their surface
Virions are assembled from one capsid protein (M_r 60,000)
Genome is composed of a single molecule of linear positive-sense, single-stranded RNA, 7.4–7.7 kb in size
Genomic RNA is polyadenylated at its 3′ end and has a protein linked covalently to its 5′ end; genomic RNA is infectious
Cytoplasmic replication. Genomic RNA and several subgenomic mRNAs are produced during replication; mature proteins are produced both by processing of a polyprotein and by translation of subgenomic mRNAs

Vesicular Exanthema of Swine

Vesicular exanthema of swine is now an extinct disease, although the virus is still present in marine mammals.

Its importance derived from the fact that it was indistinguishable clinically from the three other vesicular diseases of swine: foot-and-mouth disease, swine vesicular disease, and vesicular stomatitis. First recognized in swine in southern California in 1932, by 1956 the disease was eradicated from the United States and has not recurred there or been recognized anywhere else.

Clinical Features

Vesicular exanthema of swine was an acute, febrile disease of swine characterized by the formation of vesicles on the snout, tongue, teats, within the oral cavity, and on the feet (between the claws and on the coronary band). In addition, the virus also caused encephalitis, myocarditis, fever, diarrhea, and failure to thrive. Pregnant sows often aborted. Morbidity was often high but mortality low and in uncomplicated cases recovery occurred after 1 to 2 weeks. However, high mortality was associated with infection by some strains of the virus.

Pathogenesis, Pathology, and Immunity

The virus was transmitted by contact and by contaminated fomites, especially feed products derived from contaminated swine meat and offal. The incubation period was as short as 18 to 48 hours, followed by fever, lameness, rapid weight loss, and other signs of systemic infection; recovery was rapid and without sequelae. Pathologic changes seem to have been limited to the involved epithelia, where there was vesiculation, necrosis, sloughing, and rapid healing.

Immunity was solid following infection, but because of the large number of non-cross-protective viral variants, heterologous reinfection was possible.

Laboratory Diagnosis

In most countries, suspected cases of vesicular exanthema must be reported to regulatory authorities. Presumptive diagnosis is based on fever and the presence of typical vesicles, which rupture in 24 to 48 hours and form erosions. Diagnosis if confirmed by virus isolation in swine cell cultures, various serologic tests, and electron microscopy. Vesicular exanthema of swine virus showed a remarkable degree of antigenic heterogeneity; at least 13 distinct antigenic types were identified. Even when recovered concurrently from different swine within a single herd, individual isolates were rarely antigenically identical.

Epidemiology, Prevention, and Control

Initially, in the United States, because of the risk of missing an introduction of foot-and-mouth disease, a slaughter policy was implemented. Although there was a clear link between garbage feeding and outbreaks of the disease, ordinances requiring that all garbage fed to swine should be cooked were not enforced rigorously. However, in 1952 the disease was diagnosed outside California for the first time, initially in Nebraska, and by September 1953 the disease had occurred in 42 states. These experiences led to the rigorous enforcement of infected herd quarantine, garbage cooking laws, and a slaughter program that resulted in a rapid decline in the incidence of disease, such that by 1956 it had disappeared.

San Miguel Sea Lion Virus Disease

Although sometimes listed as separate viruses and for epidemiological reasons usefully considered as such, it is now clear that these viruses are the same as vesicular exanthema of swine viruses and were indeed the source of the disease in swine. Virus was first isolated in 1972 from material obtained from California sea lions inhabiting San Miguel Island, which showed several signs of disease, including abortion and vesicular lesions of the flippers. Although serologically distinguishable from the 13 known vesicular exanthema of swine virus serotypes, these viruses produced lesions when inoculated into swine. In California, dead carcasses of seals and sea lions washed up on mainland beaches were frequently fed to swine, thus providing the opportunity for infection. Retrospective evidence suggested that the multiple antigenic types of vesicular exanthema of swine viruses were generated in the natural hosts of the viruses, sea lions, rather than in swine. Seventeen antigenic types of San Miguel sea lion virus have been isolated since 1972 and these have come from a variety of sea mammals, including northern fur seal, northern elephant seal, Pacific walrus, Atlantic bottle nosed dolphins, and northern sea lion as well as from opal eye fish and sea lion liver fluke. In some of these marine mammals the viruses have been isolated from vesicular lesions.

Feline Calicivirus Disease

Clinical Features

Feline calicivirus is one of the two major causes of respiratory disease in cats and produces an acute or subacute disease characterized by conjunctivitis, rhinitis, tracheitis, pneumonia and vesiculation, and ulceration of the oral epithelium (Figures 36.4 and 36.5). Other common signs are fever, anorexia, lethargy, stiff gait, and sometimes nasal and ocular discharge. Morbidity is high, mortality may reach 30% in very young kittens, and recovery is followed by a prolonged carrier state.

Pathogenesis, Pathology, and Immunity

Natural transmission occurs via aerosol and fomites; the virus is often carried to susceptible cats by human handlers. The incubation period is 2 to 6 days. Lesions are usually confined to the respiratory tract, oral cavity, and eyes; congestion is followed by edema and, in some cases, by epithelial ulceration, especially in the mouth. In severe disease, there may be pulmonary edema and interstitial pneumonia.

Virus is shed in large amounts from infected cats; convalescent cats may continue to shed virus for many months. Stress may precipitate recrudescent disease and further shedding. Different strains of feline calicivirus vary greatly in virulence; some strains are associated mainly with subclinical infection or upper respiratory disease; highly virulent strains regularly produce pneumonia, especially in young kittens.

Laboratory Diagnosis

Presumptive diagnosis is based on clinical presentation; definitive diagnosis is based on isolation of the virus in feline cell culture and its identification by immunofluorescence or enzyme immunoassay. Clinically, feline calicivirus infection cannot be differentiated from feline rhinotracheitis caused by feline herpesvirus 1 (see Chapter 18); these two viruses can be differentiated readily by electron microscopy or lipid solvent sensitivity as well as by immunologic methods.

Epidemiology, Prevention, and Control

Feline calicivirus occurs worldwide and although all *Felidae* are probably susceptible, natural infection has been reported only in domestic cats and cheetahs. Economic losses caused by the death of valuable kittens and the costs of providing supportive treatment for sick cats are substantial. Feline calicivirus can be recovered from about 50% of cats presenting with clinical signs of acute upper respiratory disease, but by the age of 1 year virtually all cats have antibodies to it, and clinical disease is rare in cats over this age. A high percentage of recovered cats remain persistently infected and shed virus from the oropharynx for several years, possibly for life. When antisera raised in rabbits were used for neutralization assays, feline caliciviruses seemed to show a high degree of antigenic heterogeneity. However, when specific pathogen-free cat sera were used and a reasonably large collection of viruses analyzed, a pattern of extensive cross-reactions was found, a finding which paved the way for the development of monotypic vaccines. The molecular basis for these observations is being explored. For control, attenuated virus and inactivated virus feline calicivirus vaccines are widely used, usually in combination with feline herpesvirus 1 vaccine.

Figure 36.4.

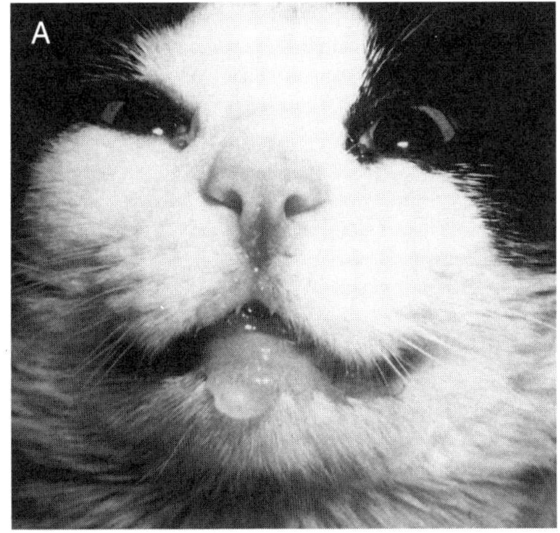

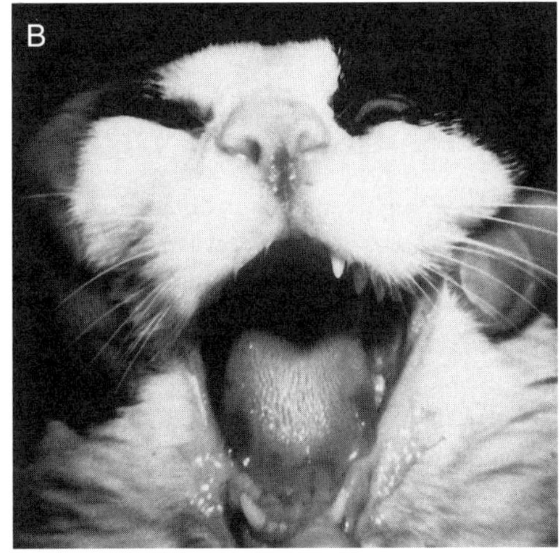

Feline calicivirus infection in a cat showing lesions (A) on the muzzle, and (B) on the tongue. (Courtesy of V. P. Studdert.)

Figure 36.5.

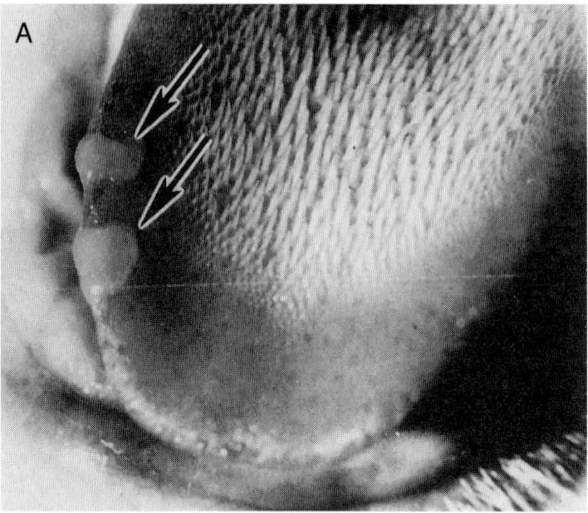

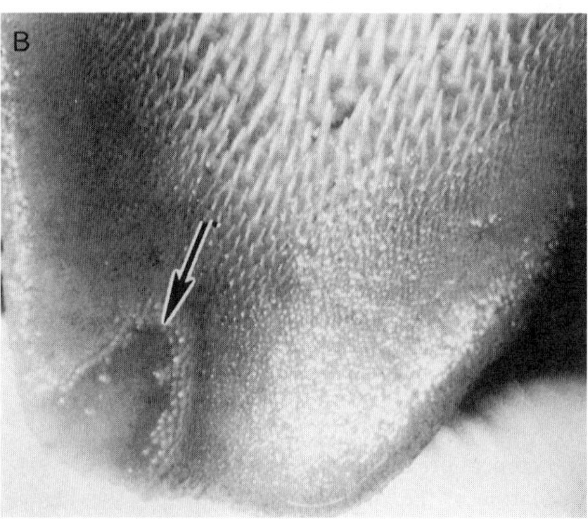

Feline calicivirus infection in a cat showing (A) unruptured and (B) ruptured vesicles on the tongue. (Courtesy of E. A. Hoover and D. E. Kahn.)

Rabbit Hemorrhagic Disease

In 1984 a new, highly infectious disease of the European rabbit, *Oryctolagus cuniculus,* was identified in China. It was characterized by hemorrhagic lesions particularly affecting the lungs and liver and has been called rabbit hemorrhagic disease. It killed some 470,000 rabbits in the first 6 months and by 1985 had spread throughout China. By 1988 it had spread throughout eastern and western Europe and had reached North Africa. In December 1988, cases occurred in Mexico City. Both wild and domestic O. *cuniculus* were affected, but all other species of mammals except the European hare appear to be resistant to infection. The disease was unknown in Europe before 1984; however, a very similar disease called European brown hare syndrome had been recognized in the early 1980s affecting *Lepus europaeus* and subsequently some other *Lepus* spp. Rabbit hemorrhagic disease is caused by a calicivirus that is different from the virus that causes European brown hare syndrome.

Clinical Features

Rabbit hemorrhagic disease affects rabbits over 2 months of age; curiously, rabbits less than 2 months of age do not develop clinical disease following infection. The disease is often peracute, characterized by sudden death following a 6- to 24-hour period of depression

FIGURE 36.6.

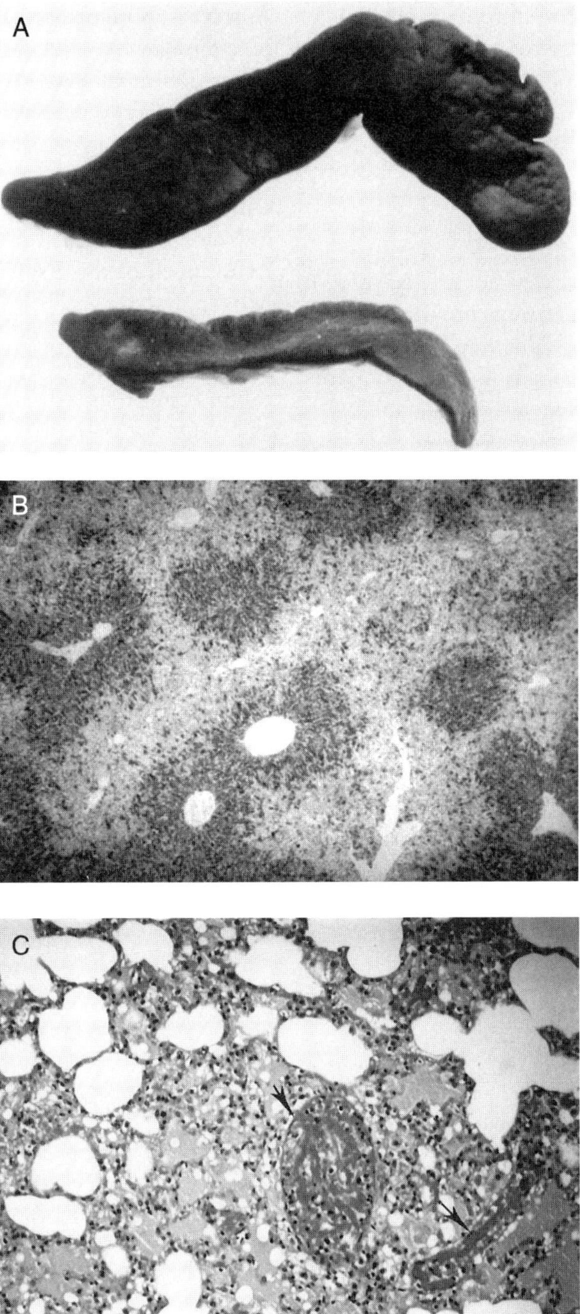

Rabbit hemorrhagic disease. (A) Spleen of an infected rabbit (top), several times larger than normal (bottom), and extremely dark and friable. (B) Massive liver necrosis—midzonal areas are nearly devoid of intact cells. (C) Lung with thrombosis (arrows indicate occlusive thrombi in pulmonary vessels), the result of disseminated intravascular coagulation, triggered by the massive liver necrosis. (Courtesy of C. Lenghaus.)

and fever. In acute and subacute forms of the disease, rabbits have a serosanguinous nasal discharge and develop a variety of nervous signs. Morbidity rates of 100% and mortality rates of 90% are observed in rabbits older than 2 months.

Pathogenesis, Pathology, and Immunity

At postmortem there is congestion and hemorrhage in the lungs, which produces accentuated lobular markings; grossly there is marked splenomegaly and massive necrosis of the liver (Figure 36.6). Large blood clots may be present in major blood vessels on gross examination and evident throughout all tissues on histological examination. The pathogenesis of the disease is linked to disseminated intravascular coagulation, presumably triggered by the massive liver necrosis.

Laboratory Diagnosis

Rabbit hemorrhagic disease virus has not yet been grown in cell culture, but high concentrations of virus occur in tissues of infected rabbits and this source has been used to obtain viral antigens for diagnostic tests. The virus hemagglutinates human erythrocytes; enzyme immunoassay and immunofluorescence are also used for diagnosis.

Epidemiology, Prevention, and Control

Infection is via the fecal–oral route. Preventing entry of virus into commercial rabbit husbandry units, either via fomites or via infected wild rabbits, creates a major challenge in control. Vaccines for the control of the disease are prepared as an inactivated homogenate of infected rabbit tissue mixed with adjuvant. Virus-like particles produced by recombinant DNA technology in baculovirus expression systems are effective as a vaccine following parenteral or oral administration but are not yet available commercially.

Biocontrol of Rabbits in Australia and New Zealand

Rabbit hemorrhagic disease virus was brought into a high security laboratory in Australia in 1991. Australian native animal species susceptibility studies were conducted prior to determining whether the virus would be a safe and effective biocontrol agent. In Australia, rabbits are in plague numbers, perhaps as many as 100 million, and are estimated to cause $600 million in annual losses; some losses, including native species and habitat destruction, may be permanent. The virus was transferred from the high security laboratory to Wardang Island for further pen trials and during these trials it escaped to the mainland, possibly by insect vector transmission (mosquitoes, bush flies) or carrion-eating birds (crows, eagles). Subsequently, it spread to many areas prior to any official release as a biocontrol agent.

In New Zealand the virus was introduced illegally and spread probably by farmers, irate following a decision of the government not to allow legal importation of the virus until more was known about the virus, particularly in relation to its potential host range. In Australia, in many areas, rabbit numbers have declined precipitously (>60%) and there is evidence for the restoration of original habitats and species in unfarmed areas. It is too early to assess the long-term effectiveness and benefits following the introduction of the virus into Australia and New Zealand, but it is likely that it, together with other established methods of control, including myxomatosis (in Australia), will bring long-term benefit. As in much of the rest of the world it is now essential to have effective vaccination programs in place to protect farmed, pet, and laboratory rabbits.

The emergence of a possibly nonvirulent form of rabbit hemorrhagic disease virus in Europe, presumably as a mutation rather than a phenotypic change due to enzymatic digestion of outer peptide residues of the virion surface, may be one of many factors that in the long term will diminish the effectiveness of rabbit hemorrhagic disease virus as a biological control agent.

Other Calicivirus Diseases

Bovine enteric calicivirus and porcine enteric calicivirus infections result in diarrhea and anorexia in young animals. Chicken calicivirus produces stunting and high mortality in chicks. Primate calicivirus produces vesicles and persistent infections. Norwalk virus and other human caliciviruses cause diarrhea, vomiting, fever, nausea, colic, and malaise.

Further Reading

Berke, T., Golding, B., Jiang, X., Cubitt, D. W., Wolfaardt, M. Smith, A. W., and Matson, D. O. (1997). Phylogenetic analysis of the caliciviruses. *J. Med. Virol.* **52**, 419–424.

Clarke, I. N., and Lambden, P. R. (1997). The molecular biology of caliciviruses. *J. Gen. Virol.* **78**, 291–301.

Crandell, R. A. (1988). Isolation and characterization of a calicivirus from dogs with vesicular genital disease. *Arch. Virol.* **98**, 65–71.

Geissler, K., Schneider, K., Platzer, G., Truyen, B., Kaaden, O. R., and Truyen, U. (1997). Genetic and antigenic heterogeneity among feline calicivirus isolates from distinct disease manifestations. *Virus Res.* **48**, 193–206.

Kapikian, A. Z., Estes, M. K., and Chanock, R. M. (1996). Caliciviridae: Norwalk group of viruses. *In* "Fields Virology" (B. N. Fields, D. M. Knipe, P. M. Howley, R. M. Chanock, J. L. Melnick, T. P. Monath, B. Roizman, and S. E. Straus, eds.), 3rd ed., pp. 783–810. Lippincott-Raven, Philadelphia. PA.

Meyers, G., Wirblich, C., and Thiel, H.-J. (1991). Rabbit

hemorrhagic disease virus—molecular cloning and nucleotide sequencing of a calicivirus genome. *Virology* **184**, 664–676.
Morise, J.-P. (1991). Viral hemorrhagic disease of rabbits and European brown hare syndrome. *Rev. Sci. Technol. Off. Int. Épizoot.* **10**, 263–270.
Nowotny, N., BascuÒana, C. R., Ballagi-Pordny, A., and Gamier-Widen, D. M. (1997). Phylogenetic analysis of rabbit hemorrhage disease and European brown hare syndrome viruses by comparison of sequences from the capsid protein gene. *Arch. Virol.* **142**, 657–673.

Chapter 37

Astroviridae

Astroviruses were first described in 1975 when they were observed by electron microscopy in the feces of children with diarrhea. Using the same electron microscopic methods, astroviruses were soon discovered in a range of domestic animals, including cattle, sheep, deer, pigs, dogs, cats, mice, turkeys, and ducks. Astroviruses appear to be virtually ubiquitous in young animals and a fairly common contributor to the overall burden of gastroenteritis, but in contrast to some other viruses, they rarely if ever cause severe disease or death, with ducks an apparent exception.

Properties of Astroviruses

Classification

The family *Astroviridae* comprises one genus, *Astrovirus*, with distinct species-specific viruses identified in humans (seven serotypes), cattle (three serotypes), sheep (one serotype), swine (one serotype), dogs, cats, deer, mice, turkeys, and ducks (one serotype). Astroviruses are so named because the surfaces of some particles have a distinctive five- or six-pointed star-like appearance (*astron*, star). Astroviruses share some properties with caliciviruses and picornaviruses but are distinguished in their virion size, structure, the coding content of their genomes, and replication strategy.

Virion Properties

Astrovirus virions are nonenveloped, 28–30 nm in diameter, and have icosahedral symmetry. As few as 10% of particles in negatively stained preparations have a five- or six-pointed star across their surface (Figure 37.1); the remaining particles appear smooth. The genome consists of a single molecule of linear positive-sense, single-stranded RNA, 6.8 kb in size. The RNA 5′-terminus is linked covalently to a protein, VPg, and the 3′-terminus is polyadenylated. The number of proteins in virions is not clear—there are two major capsid proteins (M_r 90,000 and 27,000 to 30,000) and several minor or nonstructural proteins. Virions are resistant to pH 3 and to 60°C for 5 minutes.

Viral Replication

Bovine, porcine, and human astroviruses have been grown in cell cultures, usually in primary embryonic kidney cells of the homologous host. In each case, trypsin (10 μg/ml) is required to activate virion cell-binding ligands. Virus replication takes place in the cytoplasm, and mature virions accumulate in the cytoplasm in crystalline arrays. Virions are released by cell lysis.

The genomes of astroviruses are unique among the positive-sense, single-stranded RNA viruses of animals in their use of ribosomal frameshifting to express the RNA polymerase and their possession of a serine protease. They are similar only to the luteoviruses, which are plant viruses. There is some evidence for nuclear localization of viral protein and RNA during the replication of bovine astrovirus and possibly other astroviruses—if confirmed, this would represent another major difference between these viruses and picornaviruses and caliciviruses.

The astrovirus genome contains three sequential open reading frames; the two closest to the 5′ end are linked by a ribosomal frameshifting motif and contain sequence motifs indicative of nonstructural virus proteins, the serine protease and an RNA-dependent RNA polymerase. A nuclear addressing sequence is also located here. The 3′-reading frame encodes the virion

FIGURE 37.1.

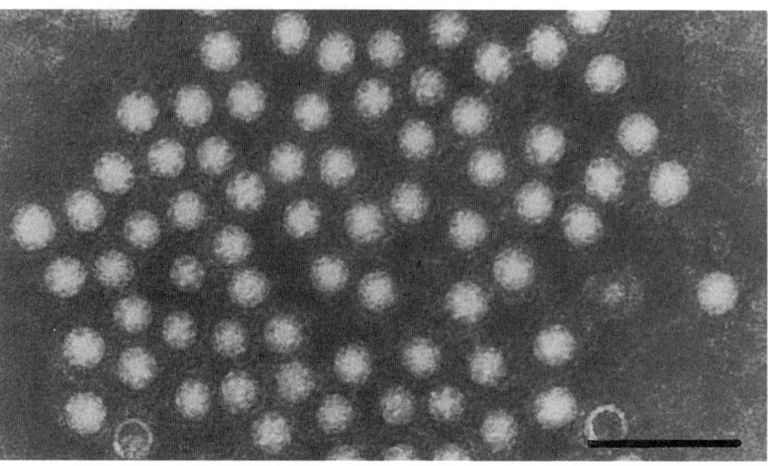

Family *Astroviridae*, genus *Astrovirus*. Typical virions with distinctive five- or six-pointed stars on their surfaces, as found in the feces of many different species of animals with diarrhea. Negative stain electron microscopy. Bar: 100 nm.

structural proteins as a polyprotein precursor (Figure 37.2). Other coding sequences found in picornaviruses and caliciviruses, including an RNA helicase, a methyltransferase, a papain-like protease, and a VPg cap protein, have not been identified in astrovirus genomes.

During infection, two species of RNA are produced, the larger corresponding to full-length genomic RNA, the smaller to a 2.4-kb subgenomic RNA, which encodes the major capsid protein and is produced in large amounts. There in no evidence that the subgenomic RNA species is incorporated into virions, as is the case with some caliciviruses. The three open reading frames overlap and there are frame shifts allowing the production of additional proteins. Translation yields at least two polyproteins, one incorporating the nonstructural proteins and the second incorporating the structural proteins. Both are cleaved posttranslationally (Table 37.1).

Astrovirus Gastroenteritis

Clinical Features

The predominant feature of astrovirus infection in animals is a self-limiting gastroenteritis. Many infections are probably subclinical. Astroviruses appear to be host restricted, so in settings where there are more than one animal species in close contact, infection is manifest as diarrhea in only one species. The incubation period is usually 1 to 4 days, followed by watery diarrhea lasting 1 to 4 days or more. There is often vomiting (in species

FIGURE 37.2.

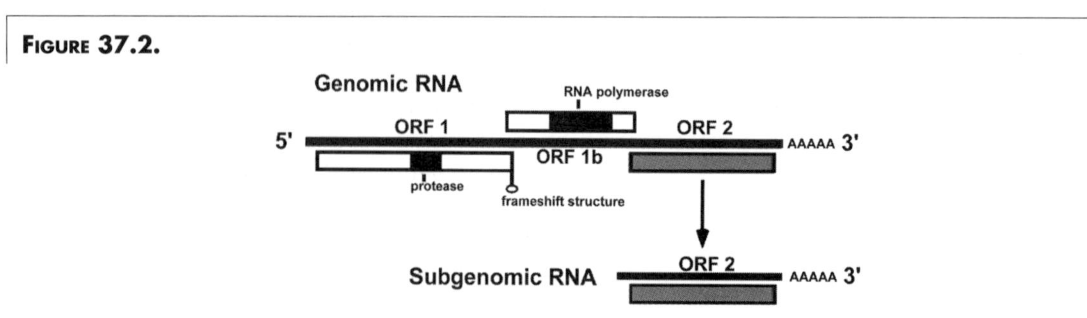

Astrovirus genome organization. Genomic and subgenomic RNAs are depicted. Open reading frames (ORFs) 1, 1b, and 2 are shown. ORF 1 encodes the viral serine protease, a nuclear localization signal, and other nonstructural proteins. ORF 1b encodes the viral RNA-dependent RNA polymerase. ORF 2 encodes the capsid proteins. [Adapted from S. M. Matsui and H. B. Greenberg, Astroviridae: Astroviruses. *In* "Fields Virology" (B. N. Fields, D. M. Knipe, P. M. Howley, R. M. Chanock, J. L. Melnick, T. P. Monath, B. Roizman, and S. E. Straus, eds.), 3rd ed., pp. 811–824. Lippincott-Raven, Philadelphia, PA, 1996.]

TABLE 37.1
Properties of Astroviruses

Virions are nonenveloped, with icosahedral symmetry, 28–30 nm diameter
Some, but not all, virions have a characteristic appearance with five- or six-pointed stars on their surface
Genome is composed of a single molecule of linear positive-sense, single-stranded RNA, 6.8 kb in size. Genomic RNA is polyadenylated at 3′-terminus and is infectious
A subgenomic mRNA is produced during replication; virion structural proteins are produced by translation of subgenomic mRNA and processing and cleavage of precursor polyprotein(s)
Single genus, *Astrovirus;* seven human, three bovine, one ovine, one porcine, and one duck viruses; viruses from different host species are unrelated antigenically

where this occurs). A rapidly fatal hepatitis in ducklings less than 6 weeks of age has been reported in the United Kingdom—mortality rates of up to 50% have been reported.

Pathogenesis, Pathology, and Immunity

Seen principally in young animals, astrovirus gastroenteritis resembles a mild form of rotavirus enteritis. In experimentally infected lambs, the astrovirus destroys mature enterocytes on the apical two-thirds of villi, leading to villus atrophy and crypt hypertrophy. In experimentally infected calves, astrovirus infection is localized to specialized M cells and absorptive enterocytes overlying the dome villi of Peyer's patches. In human volunteer studies involving virus challenge and duodenal biopsies, virions have been detected in epithelial cells in the lower part of villi. In ducks dying of hepatitis there is widespread hepatocellular necrosis; by thin section electron microscopy, large numbers of virions are seen in hepatocytes. Immunity probably lasts for years; anamnestic responses develop following subsequent exposure to a heterologous virus. Most older animals are immune. The viruses of different species are antigenically unrelated to each other.

Laboratory Diagnosis

Although more astrovirus virions are found in feces (up to 10^{10} particles per gram) than is the case in calicivirus infections (usually $<10^6$ particles per gram), electron microscopy is still not optimally sensitive or convenient. Detectable numbers of virions drop off by about 5 days postinfection and frequently several different viruses (including bacteriophage) are present in the same sample. Immunoelectron microscopy is feasible, but requires considerable experience to discriminate among parvoviruses, picornaviruses (enteroviruses), caliciviruses, and the smooth forms of astroviruses. An enzyme immunoassay using polyclonal antibody for antigen capture is feasible, but must be established for each host species of interest. Reverse transcriptase polymerase reactions using primer sets to the more conserved virion polymerase gene are available: this assay is becoming the method of choice in major reference laboratories. Bovine, feline, porcine, and human astroviruses have been isolated in primary embryonic kidney cells, but only the human and porcine viruses have been adapted to growth in established cell lines. Trypsin is required in the growth medium for serial propagation. Duck astrovirus grows in embryonated chicken eggs following blind passage in the amniotic sac. Infected embryos appeared stunted and have greenish, necrotic livers in which virions have been identified. The occurrence of duck astrovirus hepatitis needs to be differentiated from duck hepatitis caused by a picornavirus.

Epidemiology, Prevention, and Control

Astroviruses are distributed worldwide and are probably endemic in many animal husbandry settings. They are transmitted by the fecal–oral route, but also probably via contaminated feed and water. The generally moderate nature of enteric infections is presumably the reason vaccines have not been developed.

Further Reading

Aroonprasert, D., Fagerland, J. A., Kelso, N. E., Zheng, S., and Woode, G. N. (1989). Cultivation and partial characterization of bovine astrovirus. *Vet. Microbiol.* **19,** 113–125.

Belliot, G., Laveran, H., and Monroe, S. S. (1997). Detection and genetic differentiation of astroviruses: Phylogenetic grouping varies by coding region. *Arch. Virol.* **142,** 1323–1334.

Gough, R. E., Collins, M. S., Borland, E., and Keymer, I. F. (1984). Astrovirus-like particles associated with hepatitis in ducklings. *Vet. Rec.* **114,** 279.

Greenberg, H. B., and Matsui, S. M. (1992). Astroviruses and caliciviruses: Emerging enteric pathogens. *Infect. Agents Dis.* **1,** 71–91.

Jiang, B., Monroe S. S., Koonin, E. V., Stine, S. E., and Glass, R. I. (1993). RNA sequence of astrovirus: Distinctive genomic organization and a putative retrovirus-like ribosomal frameshifting signal that directs the viral replicase synthesis. *Proc. Natl. Acad. Sci. U.S.A.* **90,** 10539–10543.

Matsui, S. M., and Greenberg, H. B. (1996). Astroviridae: Astroviruses. *In* "Fields Virology" (B. N. Fields, D. M. Knipe, P. M. Howley, R. M. Chanock, J. L. Melnick, T. P. Monath, B. Roizman, and S. E. Straus, eds.), 3rd ed., pp. 811–824. Lippincott-Raven, Philadelphia, PA.

Monroe, S. S., Jiang, B., Stine, S. E., Koopmans, M., and Glass, R. I. (1993). Subgenomic RNA sequence of human astrovirus supports classification of Astroviridae as a new family of RNA viruses. *J. Virol.* **67,** 3611–3614.

Willcocks, M. M., Carter, M. J., and Madeley, C. R. (1992). Astroviruses. *Rev. Med. Virol.* **2,** 97–106.

CHAPTER 38

Togaviridae

Epidemic equine encephalitis was first recorded in 1831 when an outbreak in Massachusetts resulted in the death of 75 horses. Since then, encephalitis in horses caused by eastern equine encephalitis virus has been described all along the Atlantic seaboard of North America. A similar disease caused by western equine encephalitis virus has been described widely across western North America. This virus was first isolated from the brain of a horse in the San Joaquin Valley of California in 1931 by K. F. Meyer and colleagues, who early on appreciated the role of mosquitoes in the viral transmission cycle and the risk to humans as well—in 1938 both viruses were isolated from human cases of encephalitis occurring in the same regions as equine cases. In 1936 an epidemic of equine encephalitis occurred in Venezuela; the virus isolated was not neutralized by antibodies to the two known viruses and was named Venezuelan equine encephalitis virus. In succeeding years many other arboviruses were characterized; those similar to eastern, western, and Venezuelan equine encephalitis viruses were brought together in the family *Togaviridae*, genus *Alphavirus*.

The togaviruses exist in geographically limited habitats in which specific mosquitoes and vertebrate hosts play roles in virus survival, geographic extension, overwintering, and amplification (see Chapter 14). Vertebrate reservoir hosts include wild birds and mammals; domestic animals and humans are usually not involved in primary transmission cycles in nature, although they may play roles in geographic extension and amplification events that lead to epidemics. For example, in Venezuelan equine encephalitis epidemics, a mosquito–horse–mosquito transmission cycle is responsible for explosive spread.

Properties of Togaviruses

Classification

Based on virion properties and serologic relationships, two genera have been recognized in the family *Togaviridae,* the genera *Alphavirus* and *Rubivirus,* the later containing only one virus, rubella virus, which infects only humans. There are 30 member viruses of the genus *Alphavirus;* 6 of which cause disease in horses and, to a lesser extent, in other domestic animals (Table 38.1)—these 6 viruses and another 7 cause disease in humans. Individual alphaviruses are distinguished serologically, most importantly by neutralization tests and, more recently genetically, by sequencing.

Virion Properties

Togavirus virions are spherical, uniform in appearance, enveloped, and 70 nm in diameter. Virions consist of an envelope with fine peplomers surrounding an isometric nucleocapsid that is 40 nm in diameter (Figure 38.1). Enveloped virions and nucleocapsids have icosahedral (T = 4) symmetry. The peplomers are arranged as 80 trimers, each a heterodimer composed of two glycoproteins, E1 and E2.

The genome is a single molecule of linear, positive-sense, single-stranded RNA, 9.7–11.8 kb in size. The RNA has a 5′-methylated nucleotide cap and its 3′ end is polyadenylated. The 5′ two-thirds of the genome encodes nonstructural proteins; the 3′ one-third is not translated from genomic RNA itself but is expressed as a subgenomic mRNA molecule, which is transcribed from a full-length, negative-sense intermediate. The 26S

Table 38.1
Togaviruses That Cause Disease in Domestic Animals and Zoonotic Disease in Humans[a,b]

Virus	Arthropod vector	Domestic animal host	Disease	Geographic distribution
Eastern equine encephalitis virus	Mosquitoes	Horses (humans)	Encephalitis	Americas
Western equine encephalitis virus	Mosquitoes	Horses (humans)	Encephalitis	Americas
Highlands J virus	Mosquitoes	Horses	Encephalitis	Americas
Venezuelan equine encephalitis	Mosquitoes	Horses (humans)	Febrile disease, encephalitis	Americas
Getah virus	Mosquitoes	Horses	Febrile disease	Southeast Asia
Semliki Forest virus	Mosquitoes	Horses	Febrile disease	Africa

[a]All viruses listed are members of the genus *Alphavirus;* the only member of the second genus, *Rubivirus,* is rubella virus, which infects only humans.
[b]The alphaviruses Sindbis virus (and variants Ockelbo and Babanki viruses), chikungunya virus, o'nyong-nyong virus, Igbo Ora virus, Ross River virus, Mayaro virus, and Barmah Forest virus also cause zoonotic human disease, rarely causing encephalitis, but often causing fever, malaise, arthralgia, and arthritis.

subgenomic mRNA encodes five structural proteins, including a nucleocapsid protein (C, M_r 30–33,000) and two envelope glycoproteins (E1 and E2, M_r 45–58,000). Some alphaviruses have a third envelope protein, E3 (M_r 10,000). Virions contain lipids that are derived from host cell membranes and carbohydrates as side chains on the glycoproteins. The viruses are not very stable in the environment and are inactivated easily by common disinfectants.

Viral Replication

Alphaviruses replicate to very high titers and cause severe cytopathic changes in many kinds of cells: Vero (African green monkey kidney), BHK-21 (baby hamster kidney), and primary chick and duck embryo cells. They also grow, but do not cause cytopathic changes in mosquito cells, such as C6/36, derived from *Aedes albopictus.* In mammalian and avian cells, infection causes a complete

Figure 38.1.

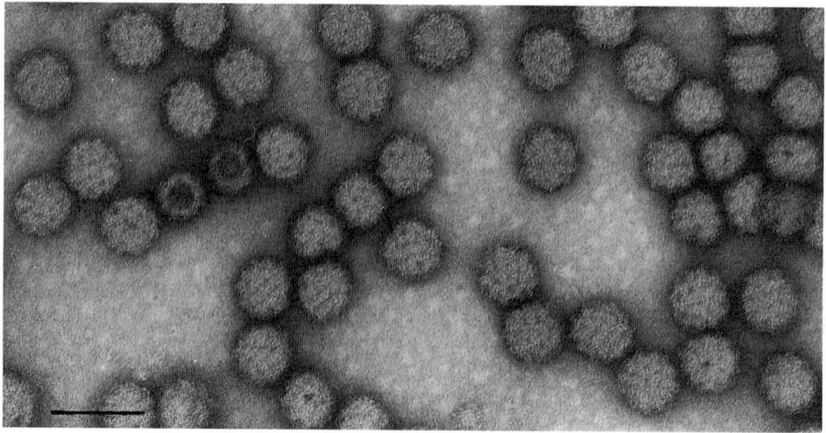

Family *Togaviridae*, genus *Alphavirus*, eastern equine encephalitis virus. Negative stain electron microscopy. Bar: 100 nm.

FIGURE 38.2.

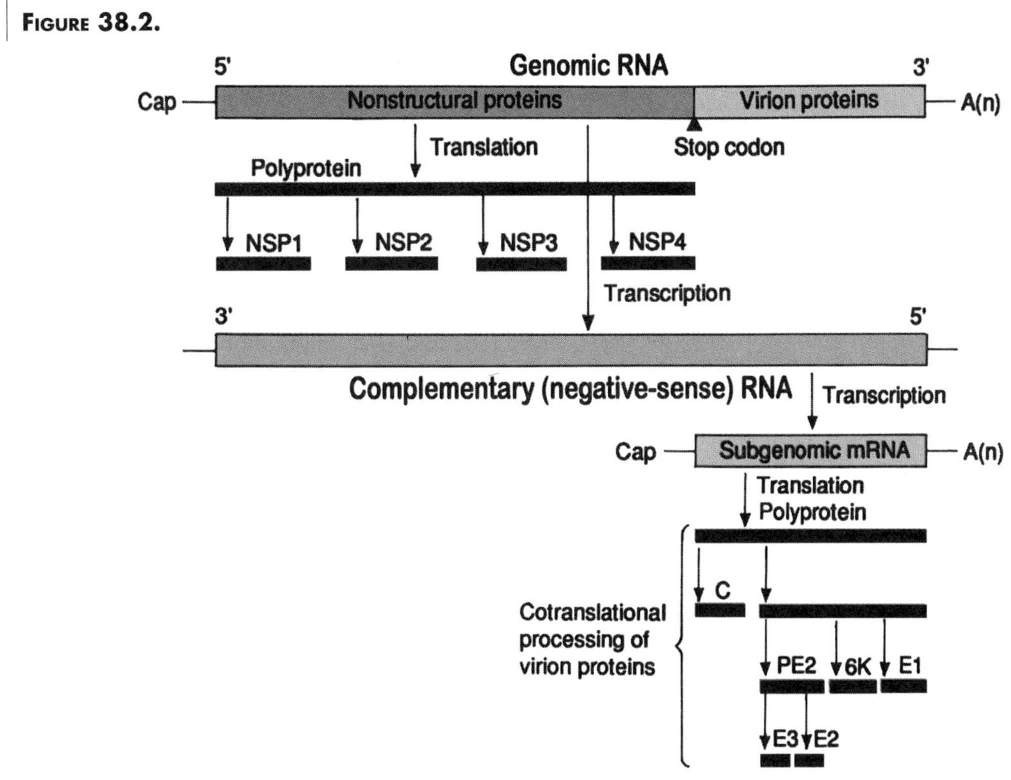

Diagram of the genome of an alphavirus and its transcription and translation strategies. The positive-sense virion RNA is capped and polyadenylated and there are short nontranslated sequences at each terminus (single lines). The 5′ two-thirds of the genome encodes the nonstructural proteins and the 3′-one-third the structural proteins. The portion coding for the nonstructural proteins is translated into a polyprotein, which is cleaved into four nonstructural proteins. Two of these form the RNA polymerase, which transcribes a full-length, negative-sense complementary RNA from the genomic RNA template. Two positive-sense RNA species are transcribed from this complementary RNA: (1) virion RNA (not shown) and (2) a 26S subgenomic mRNA. The latter is identical to the 3′ one-third of the virion RNA; it is translated into a polyprotein that is then cleaved to form the viral structural proteins E1, E2, E3, 6K, and C.

shutdown of host cell protein and nucleic acid synthesis. In mosquito cells there is no shutdown and cell division is unaffected by infection.

Viral attachment to the host cell first involves interaction between the viral E1 glycoprotein with phospholipid receptors on the cell surface; entry involves binding of viral E2 glycoprotein to cellular proteins. This is followed by receptor-mediated endocytosis. Entry of viral nucleocapsids into the cell cytoplasm occurs by fusion of the viral envelope with the endosomal membrane.

Upon entry into the cytoplasm, the virion RNA characteristically directs two rounds of translation (Figure 38.2). First the 5′ end of the genomic RNA, serving as mRNA, is translated to produce a polyprotein that is then cleaved to form four nonstructural proteins, two of which form the viral RNA-dependent RNA polymerase. This enzyme directs the transcription of full-length, negative-sense (complementary) RNA, which is the template for further positive-sense RNA synthesis. Two positive-sense RNA species are synthesized; full-length genomic RNA for amplification of the infection in the cell and for inclusion in progeny virions and 26S subgenomic mRNA. Translation from the subgenomic RNA template results in the production of large amounts of a polyprotein that is cleaved to form the individual structural proteins. Nucleocapsids are assembled in the cytoplasm, upon endoplasmic reticulum membranes, and move to the plasma membrane where they align under patches containing viral glycoprotein peplomers. Finally, virions are formed by budding of nucleocapsids through the peplomer-studded plasma membrane patches (Table 38.2).

Equine Encephalitides

Several alphaviruses cause encephalitis in horses and humans; some also cause nonneurotropic systemic disease in horses, pheasants, and humans (see Table 38.1).

Table 38.2
Properties of Togaviruses

Two genera: *Alphavirus,* arthropod-borne viruses, and *Rubivirus,* rubella virus (human pathogen only)

Virions are spherical, uniform in appearance, enveloped, 70 nm in diameter, and consist of an envelope with fine peplomers surrounding an icosahedral nucleocapsid, 40 nm in diameter

The genome is a single molecule of linear, positive-sense, single-stranded RNA, 9.7–11.8 kb in size; the 5′ end of the genomic RNA is capped whereas the 3′ end is polyadenylated

Genomic RNA is infectious

The 5′ two-thirds of the genome encode nonstructural proteins; the 3′ one-third encodes the structural proteins, which are transcribed from a 26S subgenomic mRNA

Virions contain two (or three) envelope glycoproteins, E1 (M_r 45–53,000), E2 (M_r 53–59,000), and E3 (M_r 1000), which form the peplomers, and one nucleocapsid protein, C (M_r 29–36,000)

Replication occurs in the cytoplasmic, and maturation occurs via budding from the plasma membrane

Clinical Features

Infection of horses with eastern, western, or Venezuelan equine encephalitis viruses produces a range of clinical manifestations—infection may be subclinical or may present with only fever, anorexia, and depression. Progressive systemic disease leading to death with only minor neurologic manifestations is most common in Venezuelan equine encephalitis.

Neurologic disease, which is most severe in eastern equine encephalitis, presents after a 5-day incubation period with fever and signs of drowsiness and incoordination. The disease progresses rapidly to profound depression (typically with wide stance, hanging head, drooping ears, flaccid lips, irregular gait, wandering) and clear signs of encephalitis (impaired vision, photophobia, inability to swallow and other reflex impairment, circling, yawning, grinding of teeth). Constant head pressing against a corner of the stall or fence is a typical presentation. In terminal stages of disease, there is an inability to rise, paralysis, and occasionally convulsions. In horses, the case-fatality rate of eastern equine encephalitis virus infection is 50–90%, western equine encephalitis virus infection is about 20–40%, and Venezuelan equine encephalitis virus (epidemic types) infection is about 50–80%. Mildly affected animals may recover slowly in a few weeks but may have neurological sequelae (dullness, dementia); such horses have been referred to as "dummies." Highlands J virus can cause fatal encephalitis in horses, but this is unusual.

Pathogenesis, Pathology, and Immunity

Following viral entry via the bite of a mosquito vector, viral replication occurs in cells near the entry site and/or in regional lymph nodes. The resulting primary viremia allows virus to invade specific extraneural tissues where further viral replication provides the high titer secondary viremia, which is key to the infection of further mosquitoes and key to the invasion of the central nervous system. The viruses replicate primarily in muscle, connective tissue, and the reticuloendothelial system (especially dendritic reticulum and lymphoid cells). In the central nervous system, infection involves neurons, but also the choroid plexus, ependyma, and meninges. Venezuelan equine encephalitis virus also infects the upper respiratory tract, pancreas, and liver.

Encephalitis due to alphaviruses is due to the hematogenous spread of virus and subsequent entry of the central nervous system by one of several possible routes: (1) passive diffusion of virus through the endothelium of capillaries in the central nervous system; (2) viral replication in vascular endothelial cells and release of progeny into the parenchyma of the central nervous system; (3) viral invasion of the cerebrospinal fluid with infection of the choroid plexus and ependyma; or (4) carriage of virus in lymphocytes and monocytes, which may migrate into the parenchyma of the central nervous system. An alternative possibility, supported by experimental data, is that virus may replicate extensively in the olfactory epithelium in the nares, leading to invasion of the brain parenchyma via axonal spread to the olfactory bulbs. Once in the parenchyma of the brain there are no anatomic or physiologic impediments to viral spread throughout the central nervous system. Typical pathologic features include widespread neuronal necrosis with neuronophagia, intense perivascular and interstitial mononuclear inflammatory infiltration, and interstitial edema. The pathology of Venezuelan equine encephalitis in horses includes cellular depletion of bone marrow, spleen, and lymph nodes, pancreatic necrosis, and, in cases where the animal survives long enough, encephalitis. The immunity that follows clinical or subclinical infection with an alphavirus probably lasts for life. Partial protection may also be conferred against antigenically related viruses.

Laboratory Diagnosis

Diagnosis of the equine encephalitides usually involves serology only—viremia is transient and is usually terminated by the time blood specimens would be drawn for virus isolation. IgM capture enzyme immunoassay is employed routinely to detect IgM antibodies in a single serum sample; the presence of IgG antibodies is much less predictive of recent infection, especially given the background of antibody elicited by equine vaccination. IgM antibodies are almost always detectable before the second week of illness. Where necessary, confirmation of positive results is done by neutralization in cell culture, using paired sera.

The suckling mouse is a particularly sensitive host for virus isolation from clinical specimens (blood, brain) and is still used in some laboratories in the tropics. However, for practical reasons, in most instances cell cultures are used: Vero (African green monkey kidney) or BHK-21 (baby hamster kidney) cells and C6/36 (*Aedes albopictus* mosquito) cells are most popular. Isolates are identified by enzyme immunoassay. Where more than one alphavirus may be circulating in an area, isolate identification is confirmed by neutralization using reference monoclonal antibodies. This is extremely important in one particular circumstance: because Venezuelan equine encephalitis virus occurs as epidemic and endemic types, the identification of isolates to this level of specificity has great epidemiological importance. The types may be differentiated by special hemagglutination–inhibition assays, by neutralization assays, and now most often by partial sequencing. Types IAB and IC are equine virulent and produce high-titered viremia and severe clinical disease in horses, donkeys, and mules. In contrast, type ID, and II-IV viruses are equine avirulent. Type IE had been considered equine avirulent, but in 1993 and 1996 this type was isolated from horses with encephalitis in Mexico.

Epidemiology, Prevention, and Control

Eastern Equine Encephalitis

Eastern equine encephalitis virus is endemic in North America along the Atlantic and Gulf coasts. The virus is also endemic in the Caribbean, Central America, and along the northeastern coast of South America. Less commonly, equine disease occurs inland east of the Mississippi River. In northern regions, cases occur in late summer and up until the time of the first frost, whereas cases can occur throughout the year in southern regions. In the United States the virus is maintained in freshwater marshes by *Culiseta melanura.* This mosquito, which feeds almost exclusively on birds, is also responsible for amplification of the virus during the spring and summer (Figure 38.3). In areas near coastal salt marshes, *Aedes*

FIGURE 38.3.

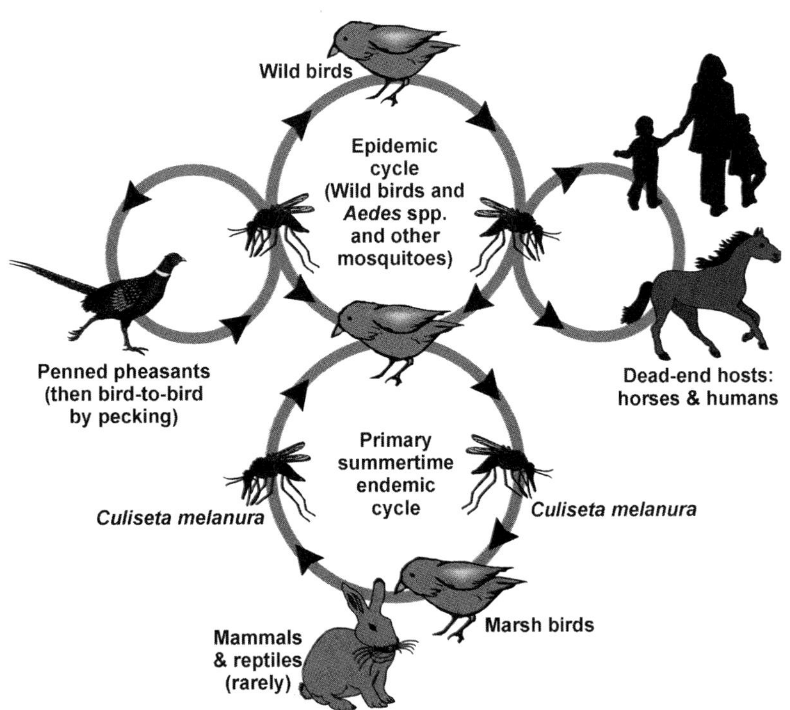

Transmission cycle of eastern equine encephalitis virus in North America. In wild birds, infection is asymptomatic, but in horses, pheasants, and humans, infection is usually devastating, causing in many cases death or neurological sequelae in survivors. The primary summertime endemic cycle takes place mostly in freshwater marshes; the epidemic cycle is often centered in areas near such marshes. Although horses and humans are considered "dead end" hosts from an epidemiological perspective, some horses produce viremia levels high enough to transmit virus to mosquitoes that feed on them. The mode of overwintering of this virus is unknown.

FIGURE 38.4.

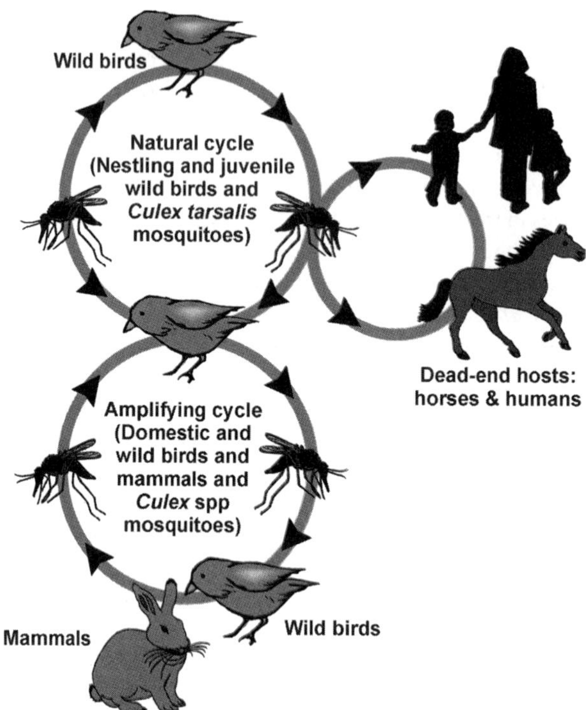

Transmission cycle of western equine encephalitis virus in North America. The cycle in *Culex tarsalis* and nestling and juvenile birds may be amplified by infection of domestic birds and wild and domestic mammals. Because western equine encephalitis virus can replicate in mosquitoes at cooler temperatures than other arboviruses, epidemic disease in horses and humans may occur early in the summer and may extend north into Canada later in the summer and early fall.

sollicitans and *A. vexans* are responsible for transferring the virus from its endemic habitat to nearby horses; these mosquitoes feed indiscriminately on horses as well as birds and occasionally infect humans as well. In some other settings in eastern North America, the mosquito(es) responsible for outbreaks remains a mystery. *Coquillitidea perturbans* has been implicated in some settings by virus isolation and determination of a feeding preference for horses and birds; however, this mosquito does not exist in all sites where equine disease occurs. The mystery is deepened by several lines of evidence opposing an old notion that virus is reintroduced from the tropics each year by migrating birds. Similarly, there is evidence against transovarial transmission and overwintering of virus in mosquitoes. Other notions, such as persistent infection of reptiles, amphibians, or birds, also seem flawed.

Highlands J virus is endemic on the east coast of the United States in the same areas as eastern equine encephalitis virus.

Eastern Equine Encephalitis Infection in Pheasants, Chickens, Emu, and Whooping Cranes

In eastern North America, many outbreaks of eastern equine encephalitis virus infection have occurred in commercial pheasant flocks, resulting in a mortality rate of 50–70%. Introduced into the southern regions of the United States from Australia for commercial husbandry, emu have also succumbed to infection. The virus is introduced into flocks by mosquitoes and is spread when healthy birds peck on sick, viremic birds. Mortality has also been observed in other domestic fowl, such as young broilers and Pekin ducks. Young broilers exhibit somnolence, abdominal distention, and retarded growth; the mortality rate is about 80%. Lesions include multifocal necrosis in the heart and liver, lymphoid depletion, and necrosis in the thymus, spleen, and bursa of Fabricius. Prevention has been attempted by the use of environmental insecticides and vaccine (equine vaccine) in valuable birds, but because of the sporadic occurrence of the disease, usually nothing is done to prevent loss in pheasants or chickens. However, the occurrence of eastern equine encephalitis virus infection in whooping cranes, an endangered species, has led to the systematic vaccination of all chicks at breeding grounds in Texas and Florida—the value of these birds is such that human, not equine, vaccine has been used.

Western Equine Encephalitis

Western equine encephalitis virus is distributed widely throughout the Americas, but especially in the western plains and valleys of the United States and Canada, where it is maintained year round in an endemic cycle involving domestic and passerine birds and *Culex tarsalis,* a mosquito particularly adapted to irrigated agricultural areas (Figure 38.4). Isolations have been made from *Culex stigmatosoma, Aedes melanimon,* and *A. dorsalis,* also competent vectors. *Culex tarsalis* mosquitoes may reach great population densities when climatic conditions or irrigation practices are suitable. For example, in the 1930s, equine epidemics of an enormous scale occurred in western United States: between 1937 and 1939 more than 500,000 cases were reported along with thousands of associated human infections.

Venezuelan Equine Encephalitis

The endemic types of Venezuelan equine encephalitis virus, which are equine avirulent, are perennially active in subtropical and tropical areas of the Americas: type II (Everglades virus) in Florida, and types ID in Central America, and types IF, III, IV, V, and VI in South America. Endemic types occur in silent, stable transmission cycles primarily involving *Culex* (*Melanoconion*) spp. mosquitoes and small mammals in tropical swamps in Central America and northern South America.

Types IAB and IC are equine virulent, producing high-titered viremia in horses, donkeys, and mules—these viruses have been isolated only during epidemics. The epidemic types have been found primarily in Venezuela, Colombia, Peru, and Ecuador, causing major problems at approximately 10-year intervals. In all equid species, these viruses cause severe disease, with survivors often having serious neurological sequelae. During epidemics, horses are an important amplifying host and because nearly every horse in an area becomes infected and there is always substantial associated human disease, the overall consequences may be devastating.

Although the interepidemic maintenance of the epidemic types of the virus had been a long-standing mystery, recent evidence suggests that they emerge each time *de novo* from the mutation of endemic types—the genetic difference between endemic and epidemic viruses is very small indeed. Separately, there is evidence that the use of formalinized vaccines containing residual infectious virus may have been responsible in the past for initiating some type IAB epidemics.

Immunization of horses with inactivated cell culture vaccines for eastern, western, and Venezuelan equine encephalitides is the basis of control programs. Inactivated bivalent or trivalent vaccines are given annually in the spring in two doses 7 to 10 days apart. In areas where mosquitoes are active year round, foals are vaccinated when 3, 4, and 6 months of age and annually thereafter. In Venezuelan equine encephalitis epidemics, an attenuated virus vaccine (TC-83) is also available. In many areas, mosquito control programs are also in place; in short-term emergency situations, such as during an epidemic or when sentinel surveillance indicates the likelihood of an epidemic, vaccination programs are supplemented by aerial spraying with ultra-low volume insecticides, such as malathion or synthetic pyrethrins. Prohibition of the movement of horses is also used in the face of outbreaks.

In an unprecedented event in the history of veterinary medicine, an epidemic of Venezuelan equine encephalitis, which had started in northern South America in 1962–1964 and reemerged in 1969, moved north across Central America and Mexico in 1970 and reached Texas in 1971. There were hundreds of thousands of deaths of horses, mules, and donkeys and a threat of spread further north into the equine industries of the southern United States. There were also many thousands of human infections and many deaths, mostly in children. The epidemic was brought to a halt by an integrated international disease control program that included (1) a surveillance system to target control activities; (2) widespread use of the then experimental attenuated virus vaccine (TC-83); (3) widespread use of ultra-low volume aerial spraying of insecticides; and (4) quarantine and prohibition of the movement of horses. With the end of the 1971 vector season, the virus disappeared. The control program was extremely expensive and demanding of human resources; however, much was learned that has been assimilated into veterinary disease control programs everywhere.

The initial stages of a repeat of these events occurred in 1995: a major epidemic occurred in Venezuela and Colombia, involving an unknown but very large number of horses, mules, and donkeys and an estimated 75,000 to 100,000 humans. This epidemic was remarkably similar in geographic localization and dynamics of spread to an earlier epidemic—one that occurred in the same regions of Venezuela and Colombia in 1962–1964. Viruses isolated during 1995 were antigenically and genetically nearly identical to those obtained during 1962–1964. The lack of genetic change between the 1962–1964 and the 1995 outbreaks is consistent with the slow rate of evolution of endemic alphaviruses. These "molecular epidemiology" findings are consistent with the concept that epidemic type viruses emerge and reemerge via the mutation of endemic types circulating constantly in northern South America and Central America.

Human Disease

Equine encephalitis viruses are zoonotic and cause significant human disease. Eastern equine encephalitis virus infection in humans is characterized by fever, drowsiness, and nucal rigidity. The disease may progress to confusion, paralysis, convulsions, and coma. The overall fatality rate among clinical cases is about 50–75% and many survivors are left with permanent neurologic sequelae, such as mental retardation, epilepsy, paralysis, deafness, and blindness. Western equine encephalitis virus is usually less severe: a high proportion of infections are silent and the case-fatality rate is about 3–10%. Venezuelan equine encephalitis virus (epidemic types) causes a systemic febrile illness in humans and about 1% of those affected develop clinical encephalitis. There is also abortion and fetal death when pregnant women are infected. In the absence of adequate medical care in less developed areas, case-fatality rates as high as 20–30% have been reported in young children with encephalitis.

Zoonotic diseases caused by other alphaviruses are important in various regions of the world, mostly in the tropics and subtropics. Fever, rash, and arthritis form a triad of clinical features in infections caused by chikungunya, o'nyong-nyong, Ross River, Mayaro, Igbo Ora, and Sindbis viruses (and Sindbis virus strains Ockelbo from Scandinavia and Babanki from Africa). Indeed, chikungunya and o'nyong nyong are African terms describing the agony of affected joints.

Biohazard: Laboratory and clinically associated infections are rare, but care should be taken to avoid contact or droplet exposure when working with sick horses or performing equine necropsies when there is suspicion of these infections. Decontamination of pens, stalls, and cages should be done with standard disinfectants and suspect carcasses should be incinerated or buried after diagnostic specimens have been obtained (see Chapter 12).

Further Reading

Johnston, R. E., and Peters, C. J. (1996). Alphaviruses. *In* "Fields Virology" (B. N. Fields, D. M. Knipe, P. M. Howley, R. M. Chanock, J. L. Melnick, T. P. Monath, B. Roizman, and S. E. Straus, eds.), 3rd ed., pp. 843–898. Lippincott-Raven, Philadelphia, PA.

Karabatsos, N., ed. (1985). "International Catalogue of Arboviruses Including Certain Other Viruses of Vertebrates," 3rd Ed. American Society of Tropical Medicine and Hygiene, San Antonio, Texas (and updates published occasionally in the *American Journal of Tropical Medicine and Hygiene*).

Koblet, H. (1990). The "merry-go-round": Alphaviruses between vertebrate and invertebrate cells. *Adv. Virus Res.* **38**, 343–403.

Monath, T. P., ed. (1988). "The Arboviruses: Epidemiology and Ecology," 5 vol. CRC Press, Boca Raton, FL.

Schlesinger, S., and Schlesinger, M. J. (1996). Togaviridae: The viruses and their replication. *In* "Fields Virology" (B. N. Fields, D. M. Knipe, P. M. Howley, R. M. Chanock, J. L. Melnick, T. P. Monath, B. Roizman, and S. E. Straus, eds.), 3rd ed., pp. 825–841. Lippincott-Raven, Philadelphia, PA.

Scott, T. W., and Weaver, S. C. (1989). Eastern equine encephalitis virus: Epidemiology and evolution of mosquito transmission. *Adv. Virus Res.* **37**, 277–328.

Strauss, E. G., Strauss, J. H., and Levine, A. J. (1996). Virus evolution. *In* "Fields Virology" (B. N. Fields, D. M. Knipe, P. M. Howley, R. M. Chanock, J. L. Melnick, T. P. Monath, B. Roizman, and S. E. Straus, eds.), 3rd ed., pp. 153–172. Lippincott-Raven, Philadelphia, PA.

Weaver, S. C. (1997). Vector biology in viral pathogenesis. *In* "Viral Pathogenesis" (N. Nathanson, R. Ahmed, F. Gonzalez-Scarano, D. E. Griffin, K. V. Holmes, F. A. Murphy, and H. L. Robinson, eds.), pp. 329–352. Lippincott-Raven, Philadelphia, PA.

CHAPTER 39

Flaviviridae

The family *Flaviviridae* comprises three genera, the members of which although similar in genomic and physicochemical properties are biologically quite different. The genus *Flavivirus* contains more than 69 viruses; of these about 10 are of veterinary importance, including louping ill, Wesselsbron, and Japanese encephalitis viruses. About 30 of the members of this genus are arthropod-borne zoonotic human pathogens, the causative agents of diseases varying from fevers with rash to life-threatening hemorrhagic fevers, encephalitides, and hepatitides. Members such as yellow fever virus, the four dengue viruses, St. Louis encephalitis virus, Japanese encephalitis virus, Murray Valley encephalitis virus, and several tick-borne encephalitis viruses rank among the most important human viral pathogens in the world. The genus *Pestivirus* contains three viruses, each an important veterinary pathogen: bovine viral diarrhea virus, border disease virus of sheep, and hog cholera virus. The genus *Hepacivirus* contains only the human pathogens hepatitis C and hepatitis G viruses.

Yellow fever virus, the prototype of the genus *Flavivirus*, was the first human virus discovered. In the course of investigating epidemic yellow fever in Havana in 1900, Walter Reed, James Carroll, and colleagues showed that the etiologic agent was a "filterable virus" and that it was transmitted by the mosquito *Aedes aegypti*. Reed acknowledged the role of earlier discoveries by veterinary scientists in this achievement: Loeffler, Frosch, and Koch for their discovery of the first virus of animals, foot-and-mouth disease virus, and Salmon, Smith, Kilborne, and Curtice for their discovery that arthropods can transmit infectious disease among animals (the agent, *Babesia bigemina*, the etiologic agent of Texas fever of cattle; the vector, the tick *Boophilus annulatus*). Yellow fever was one of the great scourges of humankind during the 18th and 19th centuries, with epidemics repeatedly affecting coastal cities in the Americas, Europe, and West Africa. Following the discovery of the virus and its vector, mosquito eradication programs quickly eliminated the disease from cities in the western hemisphere. Hemispheric eradication was envisioned, but in 1932 the zoonotic jungle cycle was discovered, involving monkeys and jungle-canopy mosquitoes, providing uncontrollable potential for initiating urban epidemics.

Members of the genus *Pestivirus* occur worldwide as economically important pathogens. Hog cholera (known in Europe as swine fever or classical swine fever or European swine fever) was first recognized in Ohio in 1833; it has been conjectured that the virus might have emerged at that time by species jumping, i.e., by a host-range mutation of another pestivirus. Early in the 20th century, as intensive swine production expanded, hog cholera became the most important swine disease in all developed countries—subsequently, eradication programs were implemented that have been so successful that today it is breaks and reintroductions rather than endemic disease that attract attention. Bovine viral diarrhea was first described in New York in 1946 as an apparently new cattle disease; then in the 1950s another clinical entity, mucosal disease, was described as somewhat similar yet different in its severity and herd incidence pattern. Viruses isolated from both diseases proved to be virtually identical (see later).

Hepatitis C virus was discovered in 1989 by a *tour de force* of modern molecular biology; even though the virus has never been visualized by electron microscopy or grown in cell culture, its complete genomic nucleotide sequence has been determined, its taxonomic placement in the family *Flaviviridae* decided, and its diagnosis made routine using recombinant DNA-produced reagents. This success now serves as a model for the detection, characterization, and diagnosis of other uncultivable viruses of any animal species.

Properties of Flaviviruses

Classification

The genus *Flavivirus,* with more than 69 members, includes the veterinary pathogens Japanese encephalitis virus, Wesselsbron virus, and louping ill virus. The genus also includes many important human pathogens (Table 39.1). Members of the genus are grouped by genomic similarities (determined by genomic sequencing and partial sequencing) and shared neutralization epitopes into eight complexes, such as the mosquito-borne encephalitis complex and the tick-borne virus complex; there are also several ungrouped viruses, including the prototype, yellow fever virus. Most members of the genus are maintained in nature in arthropod–vertebrate–arthropod cycles, but a few are transmitted directly among bats or rodents.

The genus *Pestivirus* comprises three important veterinary pathogens: bovine viral diarrhea virus, Border disease virus, and hog cholera virus. Genomic sequence analysis indicates that these three viruses are related very closely. Experimentally, the viruses have an overlapping host spectrum: hog cholera virus can be transmitted to cattle and bovine viral diarrhea virus can infect swine, sheep, and goats as well as a wide range of other ungulates. However, in nature the viruses are quite species specific.

A new variant of bovine viral diarrhea virus has been identified as the cause of severe thrombocytopenia and a hemorrhagic syndrome in adult cattle—its overall significance is being assessed. Among Border disease virus isolates from sheep, it has been shown that there are two very similar viruses: true Border disease virus and a bovine viral diarrhea-like virus.

Virion Properties

Flavivirus and pestivirus virions are spherical, 50 nm in diameter, and consist of a tightly adherent lipid envelope covered with indistinct peplomers surrounding a spherical nucleocapsid with probable icosahedral symmetry (Figure 39.1). The genome consists of a single molecule of linear positive-sense, single-stranded RNA, 10.6–10.9 (flaviviruses), 12.5 (pestiviruses), or 9.5 (hepaciviruses) kb in size. Genomic RNA is infectious. The complete nucleotide sequence of several of the viruses has been determined. The 5′ end of the genome is capped and, except for a few of the tick-borne flaviviruses, the 3′ end is not polyadenylated—instead there is a 3′-hairpin loop (Figure 39.2).

The viral genome contains a single long open reading frame encoding about 10 proteins, which are formed by co- and posttranslational processing and cleavage. Virions contain three (genus *Flavivirus*) or four (genus *Pestivirus*) proteins which are encoded in the 5′ end of the genome; the nonstructural proteins are encoded in the 3′ end. Proteins include: C, the nucleocapsid protein; prM, a glycosylated precursor that is cleaved during virus maturation to yield M, the transmembrane protein; and E (E1 and E2 in the genus *Pestivirus*), the major peplomer glycoprotein(s). There are seven or eight nonstructural proteins, including NS5, the RNA-dependent RNA polymerase, and NS3, which functions as a helicase and protease and as part of the RNA polymerase complex. NS3 is responsible for most of the cleavages of the polyprotein, while host cell proteases are responsible for the rest.

The viruses are not very stable in the environment and are inactivated easily by heat and by common disinfectants. However, the stability of hog cholera virus in meat products and offal for weeks or even months has contributed importantly to its spread and reintroduction into virus-free areas.

TABLE 39.1
Flaviviruses That Cause Disease in Domestic Animals and Zoonotic Disease in Humans[a]

VIRUS	HOST OF CONCERN (RESERVOIR HOST)	ARTHROPOD HOST (MODE OF TRANSMISSION)	DISEASE IN DOMESTIC ANIMALS (OR HUMANS)	GEOGRAPHIC DISTRIBUTION
Genus *Flavivirus*				
Japanese encephalitis virus	Swine, humans (birds)	Mosquitoes: *Culex tritaeniorhynchus*	Abortion, neonatal disease (encephalitis)	Asia
Murray Valley encephalitis virus	Humans (birds)	Mosquitoes: *Culex annulirostris*	(Encephalitis)	Australia, New Guinea
St. Louis encephalitis virus	Humans (birds)	Mosquitoes: *Culex tarsalis, C. Pipiens*	(Encephalitis)	United States, Canada, Central and South America
Wesselsbron virus	Sheep	Mosquitoes	Generalized infection, abortion	Africa
Dengue 1, 2, 3, 4 viruses	Humans (humans and monkeys)	Mosquitoes: *Aedes aegypti,* other *Aedes* spp.	(Fever and rash, arthralgia myalgia, hemorrhagic fever)	Tropics worldwide
West Nile virus	Humans (birds)	Mosquitoes: *Culex* spp. (rarely ticks)	(Fever with rash, rarely arthralgia or encephalitis)	Mediterranean, France, Portugal, Cyprus, Russia, CIS, Asia, Africa
Yellow fever virus	Humans (humans and monkeys)	Mosquitoes: *Aedes aegypti, Aedes* spp.	(Hepatitis, hemorrhagic fever)	Tropical Africa and Americas
Russian spring–summer encephalitis virus	Humans (rodents, birds)	Ticks: *Ixodes* spp.	(Encephalitis)	Eastern Russia, CIS
Central European encephalitis virus	Humans (Rodents, birds)	Ticks: *Ixodes* spp. and via ingestion of raw milk	(Encephalitis)	Europe: Scandinavia to Greece
Omsk hemorrhagic fever virus	Humans (muskrats)	Ticks: *Dermacentor* spp.	(Hemorrhagic fever, gastrointestinal disease)	Central Russia, CIS
Kyasanur Forest disease virus	Humans (monkeys, rodents)	Ticks: *Haemaphysalis* spp.	(Hemorrhagic fever, encephalitis)	India (Mysore)
Powassan virus	Small mammals	Ticks: *Ixodes* spp.	Encephalitis	Canada, United States, Russia
Louping ill virus	Sheep	Ticks: *Ixodes ricinus*	Encephalitis	Europe
Genus *Pestivirus*				
Bovine viral diarrhea virus	Cattle Calves	Contact Congenital	Mostly inapparent Congenital disease: generalized persistent infection, mucosal disease	Worldwide
Border disease virus	Sheep Lambs	Contact Congenital	Mostly inapparent Congenital disease—hairy shaker disease	Worldwide
Hog cholera virus	Swine	Contact	Systemic disease Congenital disease	Worldwide, but eradicated in some countries

[a]The genus *Hepacivirus* contains hepatitis C virus, an important cause of human hepatitis.

Figure 39.1.

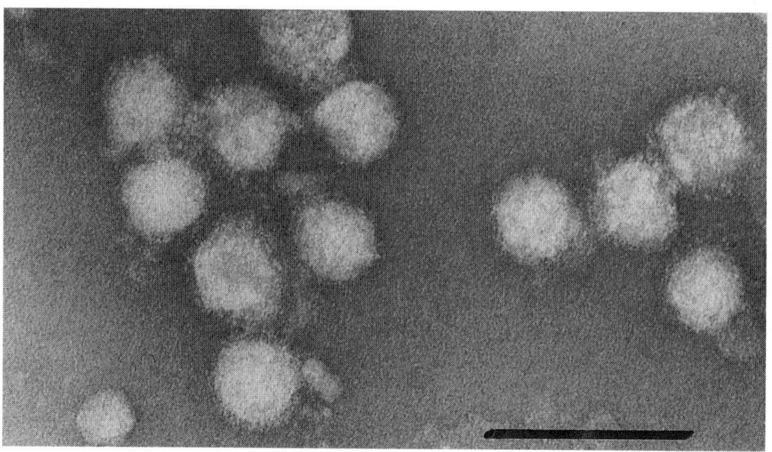

Family *Flaviviridae*, genus *Flavivirus*, central European tick-borne encephalitis virus. Negative stain electron microscopy. Bar: 100 nm.

Viral Replication

Members of the genus *Flavivirus* replicate well and cause cytopathic changes in many kinds of cells: Vero (African green monkey kidney) cells, BHK-21 (baby hamster kidney) cells, and primary chick and duck embryo fibroblasts. Some of the viruses also replicate well in Fc receptor-bearing macrophages and macrophage cell lines where yield is enhanced by the presence of antiviral antibody (called antibody-dependent enhancement). The viruses also replicate in but do not cause cytopathic changes in mosquito cells, such as C6/36 cells, derived from *Aedes albopictus* and AP-61 cells, derived from *A. pseudoscutellaris*. The mosquito-borne viruses are also grown in certain species of very large mosquitoes, such as *Toxorhynchites* spp. The viruses infect and kill newborn mice; in fact, most of the flaviviruses were first isolated in newborn mice.

Members of the genus *Pestivirus* replicate well in primary and continuous cell cultures derived from the principal host species: bovine viral diarrhea virus in bovine embryonic fibroblast or kidney cells and hog cholera virus in porcine lymphoid or kidney cells. Pestiviruses isolated from naturally infected animals are often noncytopathic in cell culture but yield cytopathic variants during passage; however, cytopathic strains of bovine viral diarrhea virus may be isolated directly from cattle with mucosal disease.

Virus attachment is mediated by ligands on the E glycoprotein(s); cellular receptors have not been identi-

Figure 39.2.

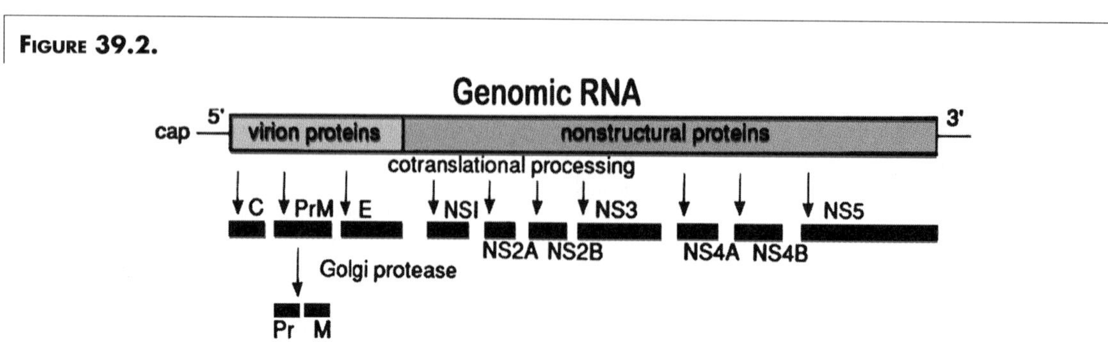

Structure and translation of the flavivirus genome. Virion proteins are encoded in the 5′ end of the genome, the nonstructural proteins in the 3′ end. The RNA is capped at the 5′ end but the 3′ end is not polyadenylated. There are short nontranslated sequences at each terminus (single lines). The genome is the only mRNA found in infected cells and is translated into a single polyprotein that is cleaved cotranslationally by viral and cellular proteases to form the structural proteins C, M, and E and seven nonstructural proteins.

Table 39.2
Properties of Flaviviruses

Genera: *Flavivirus,* mostly arthropod-borne viruses; *Pestivirus,* nonarthropod-borne, includes several veterinary pathogens; *Hepacivirus,* human hepatitis C virus

Virions are spherical, 50 nm in diameter, and consist of a tightly adherent lipid envelope covered with indistinct peplomers surrounding a spherical nucleocapsid with probable icosahedral symmetry

Genome is a single molecule of linear positive-sense, single-stranded RNA, 10.6–10.9 (flaviviruses), 12.5 (pestiviruses), or 9.5 (*hepaciviruses*) kb in size; 5′ end capped, but 3′ end usually is not polyadenylated

Genomic RNA is infectious

Cytoplasmic replication; a single polyprotein is translated from genomic RNA; it is cleaved cotranslationally to yield nonstructural proteins and three or four structural proteins

Maturation occurs on intracytoplasmic membranes without evidence of budding

fied except in the case of antibody-dependent enhancement where Fc receptors mediate viral attachment. The viruses enter cells via receptor-mediated endocytosis and replication takes place in the cytoplasm. The viruses only partially shut off protein and RNA synthesis of mammalian host cells and do not shut off host cell functions in arthropod cells at all. Infection commonly is accompanied by a characteristic proliferation of perinuclear membranes.

Replication involves the synthesis of complementary negative-sense RNA, which in turn serves as a template for positive-sense (genome-sense) RNA synthesis. Positive-sense synthesis is favored, suggesting complex regulatory mechanisms involving host cell constituents. The only viral mRNA is the genome—translation yields a single polyprotein that is cleaved and processed to form virion structural and nonstructural proteins (Figure 39.2). Virion assembly occurs on membranes of the endoplasmic reticulum (and in mosquito cells also on plasma membrane), but preformed capsids and budding are not seen. Instead, fully formed virions appear within the cisternae of the endoplasmic reticulum and are released via exocytosis or cell lysis (Table 39.2).

Diseases Caused by Members of the Genus *Flavivirus*

Japanese Encephalitis

Japanese encephalitis virus is a member of a complex containing three other viruses: St. Louis encephalitis virus, Murray Valley encephalitis virus, and West Nile virus. Each represents an important human disease problem in a different part of the world, but only Japanese encephalitis causes significant disease in domestic animals. A number of animals such as swine, horses, dogs, chickens, ducks, and reptiles are infected in nature. Horses may develop fatal encephalitis, whereas infection in swine is generally inapparent, except for stillbirths and abortions when pregnant sows are infected and aspermia when boars are infected.

Japanese encephalitis virus is the most important mosquito-borne human pathogen in China (where there are 20,000–50,000 cases per year), Korea, Thailand, Indonesia, and other countries of southeast Asia and in the past 20 years it has extended its range westward into India, Nepal, Myanmar, and Sri Lanka and eastward into the Pacific islands of Saipan and the northern Marianas. The human disease is devastating; although there are many silent infections, the case fatality rate is 10–40% and 40–70% of survivors have permanent neurologic sequelae. The mosquito *Culex tritaeniorhynchus,* which breeds in fresh water and irrigated rice fields and feeds on birds, swine, and humans, is the most common vector. Swine are the most abundant species of domestic animal in many parts of Asia; they have a short life span and continuously provide generations of susceptible hosts. The mosquito–swine–mosquito transmission cycle serves as an efficient mode of virus amplification. In tropical areas, outbreaks occur at the end of the wet season and sporadic cases throughout the year. In temperate zones, outbreaks tend to occur in late summer and early autumn.

Japanese encephalitis was a very important disease in Japan; control has involved several integrated approaches, including the draining of rice paddies at the time when *C. tritaeniorhynchus* normally breeds, removal of the principal amplifier host, swine, from areas of human habitation, and widespread vaccination of swine, horses, and children with inactivated virus vaccine produced in mouse brain. Inactivated virus and attenuated virus vaccines produced in cell culture are being used effectively in humans and swine in China. Such low-cost vaccines may be suitable for use in the large areas of southeast Asia where the expensive Japanese vaccines are unaffordable.

Murray Valley (Australian) Encephalitis

Murray Valley encephalitis, another member of the mosquito-borne encephalitis complex, is endemic in Papua New Guinea and northern Australia where cases of encephalitis occur sporadically. The encephalitis in humans is similar to that caused by Japanese encephalitis virus; the case-fatality rate is similar and neurologic sequelae are common in those who recover. Epidemics involving humans occur in the Murray River Valley of southeastern Australia only in occasional summers, following heavy rainfall with extensive flooding. These conditions encourage explosive increases in numbers of water birds, which are the principal vertebrate reservoirs of the virus, and its mosquito vectors, notably *Culex annulirostris.*

St. Louis Encephalitis

St. Louis encephalitis, a member of the mosquito-borne encephalitis complex, is the most potentially explosive mosquito-borne viral disease in the United States—it has a history of sporadic large epidemics involving hundreds to thousands of human cases. The disease in humans may present as aseptic meningitis or encephalitis or even as a benign febrile illness. The overall case-fatality rate is about 8%, but may reach 20% in the elderly. The natural cycle of the virus in western regions of the United States involves *Culex tarsalis* and nesting and juvenile passerine birds; in epidemics the virus is amplified by infection of domestic birds. In eastern and southern regions of the United States, *Culex pipiens* and *Culex quinquefasciatus,* respectively are the most important vectors, although other mosquitoes may become involved as well (Figure 39.3). The virus remains endemic in some regions, producing epidemics when temperature, moisture, and breeding conditions favor vector mosquito species. Breeding sites, such as automobile tire dumps and tree holes, influence vector population density but do not seem to be amenable to vector elimination programs.

Wesselsbron Disease

Wesselsbron virus is the cause of an important disease of sheep in many parts of sub-Saharan Africa. The clinical disease and its epidemiology resemble Rift Valley fever. The disease in sheep is marked by fever, depression, hepatitis with jaundice, and subcutaneous edema. Abortions are frequent and mortality is high in pregnant ewes and newborn lambs. Cattle, horses, and swine are in-

Figure 39.3.

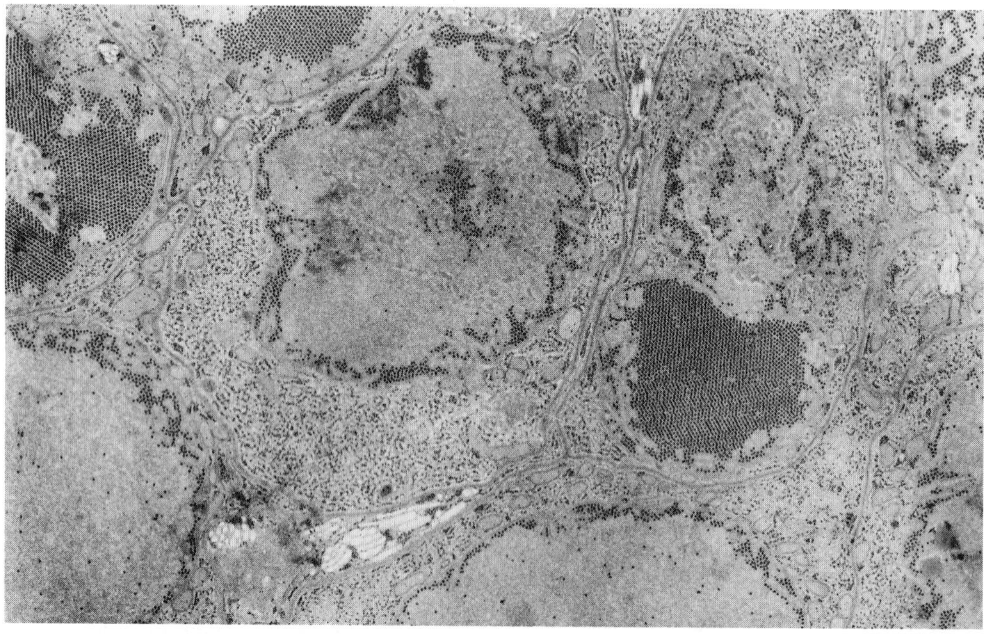

St. Louis encephalitis virus in the salivary gland of a *Culex pipiens* mosquito 26 days postinfection. Massive amounts of virus, some in paracrystalline array, may be seen within the salivary space—transmission to the next vertebrate host occurs when the mosquito injects its saliva (which contains anticoagulants) when taking a blood meal, Magnification: ×21,000.

fected subclinically. The virus is transmitted in summer and autumn by *Aedes* spp. mosquitoes; the disease is a particular problem in low-lying humid areas where mosquito density is greatest. Control involves immunization of lambs with an attenuated virus vaccine that is often combined with Rift Valley fever vaccine. Wesselsbron virus is zoonotic, causing in humans a febrile disease with headache, myalgia, and arthralgia.

Dengue

Dengue has become the most important human arthropod-borne viral disease in the world, with over two billion people at risk and millions of cases annually. The original natural reservoir of the dengue viruses appears to have been African monkeys; reservoirs have also been established in monkeys in southeast Asia. However, the important life cycle of the dengue viruses is mosquito–human–mosquito, involving the urban mosquito *Aedes aegypti. Aedes albopictus* and *A. scutellaris* also serve as efficient vectors. Although dengue has been known for over 200 years, prior to the 1950s outbreaks were rare because of little movement of viremic persons between tropical countries. In recent decades, improvements in transportation and the growth of large cities in the tropics with ubiquitous breeding sites for *A. aegypti* have led to major epidemics involving hundreds of thousands of people. Epidemics have occurred in the Caribbean, South America, Pacific islands, and China as well as in southeast Asia and Africa. Because of the widespread occurrence of *A. aegypti* and the recent extensive spread of *A. albopictus,* dengue is also a threat to southern regions of the United States.

There are four dengue viruses; infection with any one gives lifelong homologous immunity, but there is little cross-protection. The simultaneous circulation of multiple serotypes has led to the appearance of an essentially new disease, dengue hemorrhagic fever. This shock syndrome has become one of the leading causes of hospitalization and death among children in southeast Asia and now is becoming common in the Americas. The prospects for dengue control are poor, although an attenuated virus vaccine containing all four dengue viruses is undergoing clinical trials in southeast Asia, its global use is years away. Mosquito control is the only tool now available, but insecticides sprayed from airplanes or trucks are ineffective because of developing insecticide resistance and because *A. aegypti* lives inside dwellings and is not reached easily by usual environmental spraying methods. Elimination of mosquito breeding sites is theoretically feasible, but increasingly difficult, especially in expanding tropical cities.

West Nile and Kunjin Virus Infections

West Nile virus is maintained in a mosquito–bird–mosquito cycle, involving *Culex* spp. mosquitoes; it also infects ticks. It is endemic in rural Africa, southern Europe, central Asia, India, and the Far East. In humans, the virus causes a dengue-like illness, very rarely encephalitis. The related Kunjin virus is quite common in Australia and occasionally causes encephalitis in humans and, like West Nile virus, can be lethal in horses.

Yellow Fever

Yellow fever has been one of the great plagues throughout history, transported together with its mosquito vector, *Aedes aegypti,* from west Africa to the New World on slave ships. In the 18th and 19th centuries the disease decimated tropical and subtropical cities of South, Central, and North America. Thousands of workers died during the construction of the Panama Canal. In its classical form the human disease begins abruptly, with fever, headache, muscle and back pain, and nausea. The disease is biphasic and, after a short period of remission, there is abdominal pain, jaundice, renal failure, and hemorrhages, most notably the vomiting of blood. Approximately 50% of people who progress to this stage die 7–10 days after onset, with deepening hepatic and renal failure, shock, delirium, and convulsions.

In its jungle habitat, yellow fever virus is maintained in a mosquito–monkey–mosquito cycle. Old World monkeys develop only subclinical infections but New World monkeys often die, reflecting the more recent introduction of the virus to the Americas. Various species of jungle canopy mosquitoes serve as vectors—*Aedes* spp. in Africa and *Haemagogus* spp. in the Americas. These mosquitoes can also transmit the virus to humans; however, it is a mosquito–human–mosquito cycle, involving *A. aegypti* in the Western Hemisphere and *A. africanus* in Africa, that is responsible for urban epidemics. Some 100–300 cases of jungle yellow fever are reported annually in the Western Hemisphere and a few thousand in Africa, but the true incidence is much higher—in Africa, major epidemics occur frequently, involving many thousands of cases with thousands of deaths, but such epidemics oftentimes go unnoticed internationally. In recent years the numbers of *A. aegypti* have increased greatly throughout much of Central and South America and southern regions of the United States, and it is now coming to be appreciated that urban epidemics could recur at any time. Despite this risk, surveillance and diagnostic systems are not well developed—

rapid tests for the detection of antigen and antibody (antigen capture enzyme immunoassay, IgM capture enzyme immunoassay, polymerase chain reaction with assay of amplified products) have been developed but are not available readily in regions at risk. Yellow fever prevention starts with vaccination, using an attenuated virus vaccine, 17D, one of the very best human vaccines ever developed. Prevention also involves *A. aegypti* control—despite proof of the value of this approach gained early in the 20th century in all urban centers of the Western Hemisphere, such programs have proven difficult to sustain in recent years because of cost.

Tick-Borne Encephalitides

Tick-borne encephalitis viruses constitute a complex of 15 related flaviviruses that includes several important zoonotic pathogens, including Russian spring–summer encephalitis virus, central European encephalitis virus, and Omsk hemorrhagic fever virus, all in Eurasia, Kyasanur Forest disease virus in India and recently in the Middle East, and Powassan virus in North America (see Table 39.1). Infected dogs and livestock such as cattle, sheep, and goats are important in the spread of these viruses to humans in Europe and eastern and central Asia; these animals may serve as amplifying hosts for ticks and may also transmit some of the viruses to humans via raw milk (Figure 39.4). The epidemiology of tick-borne flaviviruses is more complex than that of mosquito-borne viruses, as ticks serve as reservoirs of infection as well as acting as vectors. Unlike mosquitoes, ticks live for several years, often longer than the generational time of their reservoir hosts. Ticks are often active from spring through autumn in temperate climates. Ticks develop successively through stages (larva to nymph to

FIGURE 39.4.

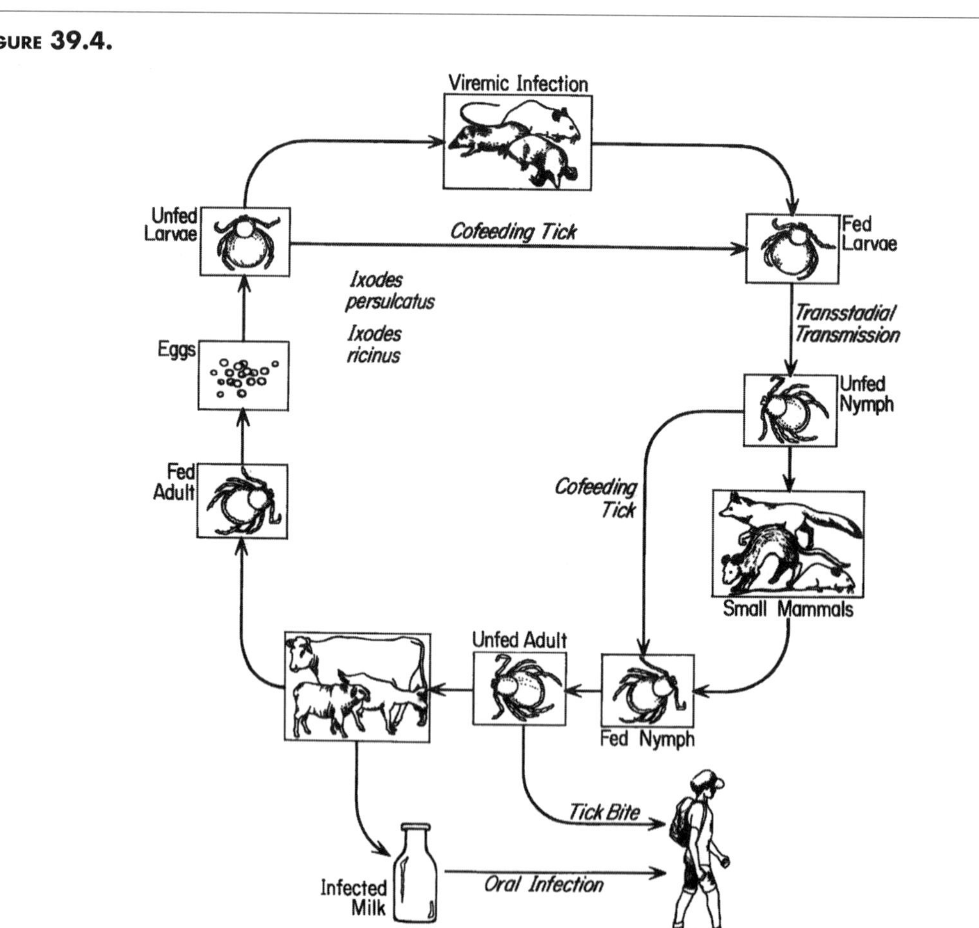

The transmission cycle of viruses of the tick-borne encephalitis complex showing hosts for larval, nymphal, and adult ticks. Virus is passed to succeeding tick stages during molting and is passed transovarially to progeny. Both male and female ticks are involved in transmission. [From T. P. Monath and F. X. Heinz, Flaviviruses. *In* "Fields Virology" (B. N. Fields, D. M. Knipe, P. M. Howley, R. M. Chanock, J. L. Melnick, T. P. Monath, B. Roizman, and S. E. Straus, eds.), 3rd ed., pp. 961–1034. Lippincott-Raven, Philadelphia, PA, 1996.]

adult) and a blood meal is generally required at each stage. Tick-borne flaviviruses are passed from one developmental stage to another (*transstadial transmission*) as well as from one generation of tick to the next (*transovarial transmission*). Some species spend their whole lives on one vertebrate host, whereas others fall off, molt, and then find a different host after each meal. Larvae and nymphs generally feed on birds or small mammals such as rodents, whereas adult ticks prefer larger animals. Inactivated virus vaccines for humans are available for use against tick-borne encephalitis in Europe and eastern Asia, but they are expensive.

Louping Ill

Louping ill is an infectious encephalomyelitis of sheep that occurs in the British Isles and the Iberian peninsula. Louping ill virus is a typical member of the tick-borne virus complex (see earlier discussion). The viral life cycle involves transmission between sheep by the tick *Ixodes ricinus,* with occasional involvement of horses, cattle, deer, and grouse. The disease occurs in spring and summer. Infected sheep develop a prolonged viremia and a biphasic febrile response, the second peak of which coincides with the development of nervous system dysfunction: cerebellar ataxia, tremors, hyperexcitability, and paralysis. The disease gains its name from the peculiar leaping gait of ataxic sheep. Few animals that develop neurologic signs survive, and most of those that do exhibit neurologic deficits as sequelae. Control of the disease involves immunization of lambs, using an inactivated virus vaccine produced in cell culture, dipping of sheep with acaricides, and environmental control of ticks. Louping ill virus is zoonotic, being transmitted to humans by ticks or occupationally by contact with infected sheep and sheep tissues. The human disease is biphasic; the first phase is influenza like and the second phase is a menigoencephalitic syndrome that usually resolves without sequelae in 4 to 10 days.

Diseases Caused by Members of the Genus *Pestivirus*

Bovine Viral Diarrhea

Bovine viral diarrhea and mucosal disease are clinically dissimilar disease syndromes, yet have a common viral etiology. The acute disease is called bovine viral diarrhea; the term mucosal disease is reserved for the chronic disease associated with persistent infection. The virus is an important cause of morbidity, mortality, and economic loss worldwide in dairy and beef cattle.

Clinical Features

The clinical and pathologic manifestations of infection in individual cattle vary with age and pregnancy status. Three situations are considered: postnatal infection in nonpregnant cattle, infection in pregnant cows, and persistent infection in calves and mucosal disease.

Postnatal Infection in Nonpregnant Cattle

Cattle of all ages are susceptible, but infection is most common in animals 8–24 months of age. Although calves may receive antibodies in colostrum, antibody levels decline by 3–8 months of age and animals can then become infected. After an incubation period of 5 to 7 days there is fever and leukopenia, but otherwise the infection is usually trivial. However, some cattle in a susceptible herd may have diarrhea, which may be explosive in character, some may have a nasal and ocular discharge and an erosive stomatitis, and in dairy cows there may be a considerable drop in milk yield. Because of the immunosuppression associated with infection, the disease in calves may be manifested by opportunistic respiratory and intestinal infections.

Infection in Pregnant Cows

Even though infection of susceptible adult cattle is usually of little consequence, transplacental spread of virus to the fetus occurs at a high frequency (Figure 39.5), which may result in any one of several outcomes depending on the age (immunologic maturity) of the fetus and the strain of virus.

Infection very early in pregnancy often results in embryonic death and resorption. Infection at 80–125 days of gestation (before the development of immunologic competence at about 125 days) often results in destructive fetal lesions and retardation in growth, resulting in fetal death or low birth weight ("weak calf syndrome"). Fetal lesions are often manifestations of viral effects on organogenesis and are often most evident as congenital defects in the eye (e.g., retinal dysplasia) and the central nervous system (e.g., cerebellar hypoplasia, cavitation of the cerebrum). Surviving calves that have been infected *in utero* remain infected for life. They never mount an effective immune response to the virus—this is persistent tolerant infection. Such calves, which remain seronegative in all tests, shed large amounts of virus in all body secretions and excretions and are very efficient in transmitting the virus to susceptible cattle in the herd. These animals also have a high probability of developing clinical mucosal disease. Fetuses infected

Figure 39.5.

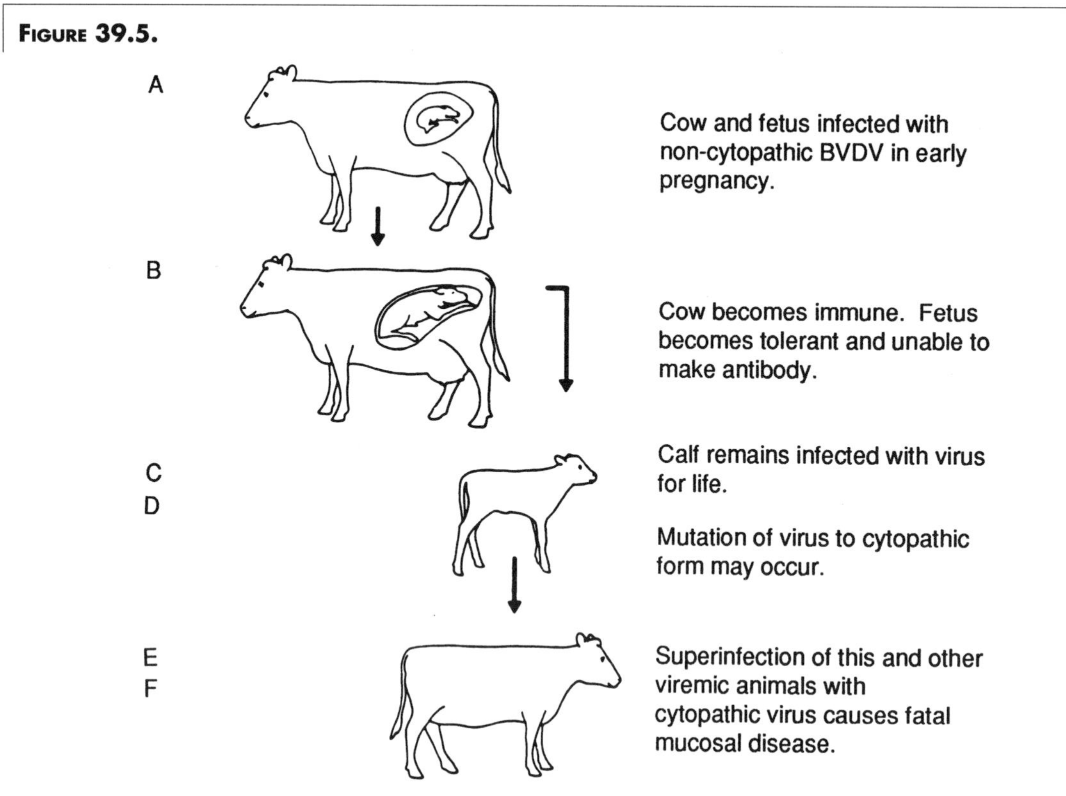

A
Cow and fetus infected with non-cytopathic BVDV in early pregnancy.
B
Cow becomes immune. Fetus becomes tolerant and unable to make antibody.
C
D
Calf remains infected with virus for life.
Mutation of virus to cytopathic form may occur.
E
F
Superinfection of this and other viremic animals with cytopathic virus causes fatal mucosal disease.

The pathogenesis of mucosal disease in cattle. (A) *In utero* infection. (B) Immune tolerance. (C) Persistent viremia. (D) Mutation. (E) Superinfection. (F) Mucosal disease. [Adapted from J. Brownlie, Pathogenesis of mucosal disease and molecular aspects of bovine virus diarrhea virus. *Vet. Microbiol.* **23,** 371–382 (1990).]

after about 125 days of gestation usually survive, whether manifesting pathologic damage or not, and usually develop neutralizing antibody and eliminate the virus.

Persistent Infection in Calves and Mucosal Disease

In susceptible herds in which the virus has been recently introduced, a very high proportion of calves born in the next calving season become persistently infected. Mortality in these calves often reaches 50% in the first year of life due to various manifestations of mucosal disease. Mucosal disease only occurs when two biotypes of bovine viral diarrhea virus are present (see later). The clinical features of mucosal disease mirror bovine viral diarrhea, but with much greater severity. The onset of mucosal disease may be sudden or may extend over several weeks or months with recurrent overt signs. There is fever, anorexia, profuse watery diarrhea, nasal discharge, erosive or ulcerative stomatitis, dehydration and emaciation, and death in a few weeks to a few months.

Pathogenesis, Pathology, and Immunity

In those few cattle that die of acute bovine viral diarrhea virus infection, gross lesions characteristically include erosive or ulcerative lesions extending from the mouth through the esophagus, forestomachs, abomasum, and intestine (Figure 39.6). In the intestine, discoloration of mucosal folds due to hyperemia and hemorrhage may occur, giving a striped appearance to the lumenal surface. Histologic examination confirms the epithelial necrosis seen visibly and also indicates a massive destruction of lymphoid tissue. Necrosis of lymphoid tissues occurs, particularly in the intestine—Peyer's patches become hemorrhagic and necrotic. Destruction of the epithelium of the crypts of Lieberkühn in the small intestine, cecum, and colon is also characteristic of the disease.

Our understanding of the pathogenesis of mucosal disease has been advanced greatly by molecular virology/pathology studies. The usual biotypes of virus isolated when infection occurs for the first time in a herd are noncytopathic. The same biotypes are regularly isolated from persistently infected immunologically tolerant cat-

FIGURE 39.6.

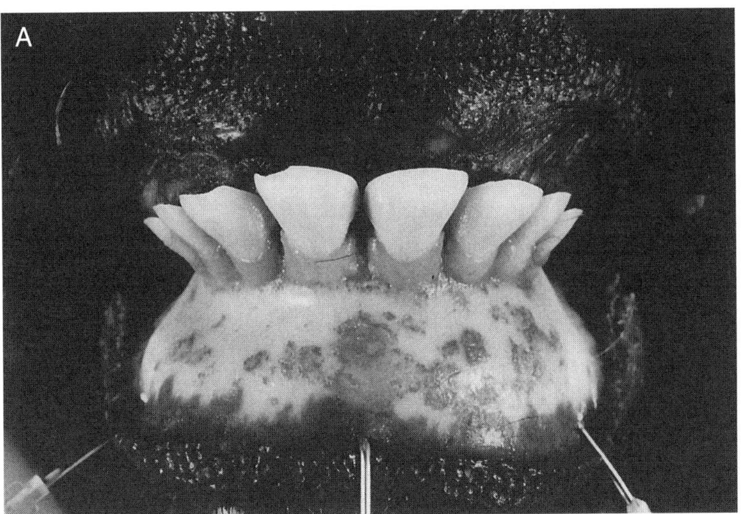

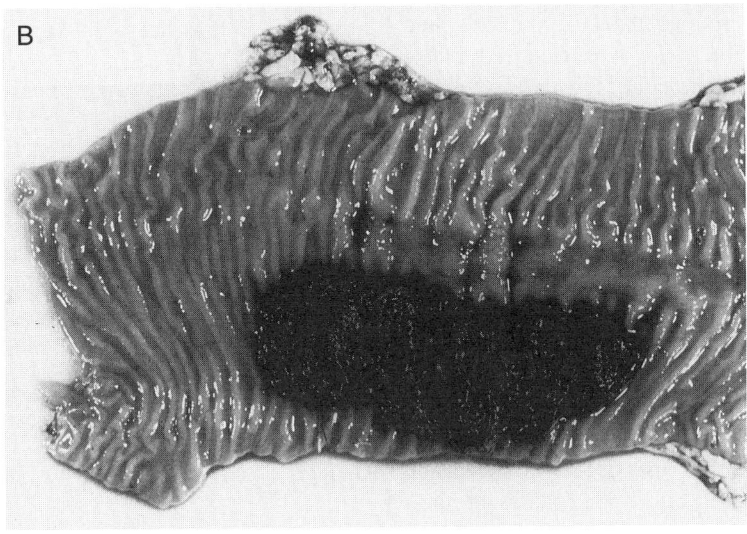

Characteristic lesions in mucosal disease in cattle. (A) Erosive lesions on the dental pad. (B) Large focal necrotic lesion extending through all layers of the duodenum. (Courtesy of V. Moennig and P. Plagemann.)

tle, i.e., cattle that were infected *in utero* before the development of immunologic competence. However, in cattle with mucosal disease, both noncytopathic and cytopathic viral biotypes can be isolated. The very close genetic relationship between the two viral biotypes suggested that cytopathic biotypes might be arising *de novo* by mutation from noncytopathic biotypes. Molecular characterization (genomic sequencing or partial sequencing) of pairs of cytophatic and noncytopathic viral isolates from the same calves revealed this to be the case—remarkably, cytopathic biotypes are generated from noncytopathic biotypes by various mutational events (recombination, insertions of cellular sequences, duplications, deletions, and rearrangements). The mutations all lead to the production of a viral protein that is responsible in a yet unknown way for cytopathology in cell culture and mucosal disease in calves that are already immunologically tolerant to a noncytopathic biotype.

Laboratory Diagnosis

A presumptive diagnosis can be made on the basis of clinical history, examination of herd reproduction records, clinical signs, and gross and microscopic lesions. When present, oral lesions are especially suggestive of this disease. Laboratory diagnosis is based on virus isolation in cell culture, viral antigen detection in tissues, detection of viral RNA in tissues by the reverse transcription–polymerase chain reaction, and serology. Specimens for virus isolation include feces, nasal exudates, blood and tissues collected at necropsy, and aborted fetuses. Immunofluorescence may be used to detect viral antigen in cell cultures and tissues. Paired acute and convalescent sera may be tested by a neutralization test, but interpretation of negative results must be made with an appreciation of the immunologically tolerant state of some cattle.

Epidemiology, Prevention, and Control

Bovine viral diarrhea virus is transmitted easily from animal to animal and from herd to herd by indirect means through feed and fomites contaminated with urine, oral and nasal secretions, feces, or amniotic fluid from infected cattle. The virus is transmitted rather poorly from acutely affected cattle, but very efficiently from persistently infected animals. Because many persistently infected heifers survive to breeding age and give birth to infected, immunologically tolerant calves that are lifelong shedders, viral transmission in a herd may go on for years if husbandry practices remain unchanged. Where infection has been present in a herd for some time and the majority of cattle are immune, the introduction of susceptible animals, typically heifers, results in sporadic losses, again continuing for years in some circumstances. In virus-free herds, the introduction of a persistently infected animal is often followed by dramatic losses. Because the infection also occurs in sheep and goats, as well as swine, deer, bison, and other wild ruminants, these species may also be sources of virus for the initiation of infection in cattle herds.

The economic importance of bovine viral diarrhea is clear, especially in feedlots and in dairy herds, but control is far from satisfactory. The major objective of control measures is to prevent the further occurrence of persistently infected cattle in the herd. This requires the identification and elimination of such animals and the avoidance of further introductions by quarantine—this is expensive, as it requires a serological survey of the herd and attempted virus isolation from seronegative animals. The use of nucleic acid probes and the reverse transcription–polymerase chain reaction may be more sensitive, but is more expensive. An alternative is to allow the introduction of immune adult animals only into the herd.

In most herds, immunization is the only control strategy used (vaccines are administered at 6–10 months of age when colostral immunity has waned). Inactivated virus vaccines produced in cell culture have met with only limited success. Attenuated virus vaccines, also produced in cell culture, are widely used, but there is evidence that vaccination of persistently infected immunologically tolerant animals can result in severe mucosal disease in some cases.

Border Disease

Border disease exists worldwide in sheep. It was first described on farms on the border between England and Wales—hence the name used in Great Britain and North America. Because of its clinical signs, it is known in Australia and New Zealand as "hairy shaker disease." There has been controversy whether the etiologic agent of this disease is a unique pestivirus or really just bovine viral diarrhea virus; it has been shown that among viral isolates from sheep there are two very similar viruses: a bovine viral diarrhea-like virus and true Border disease virus.

Clinical Features

Border disease appears as a congenital disorder of lambs characterized by low birth weight and poor viability, poor conformation, tremors, and an excessively hairy birth coat in normally smooth-coated wool breeds. Kids may also be affected, and a similar condition occasionally occurs in calves.

Pathogenesis, Pathology, and Immunity

In adult sheep the infection is always subclinical, but infection of pregnant ewes results in fetal death or the delivery of dead, deformed, or mummified lambs. Clinical neurologic signs are due to defective myelination of nerve fibers in the central nervous system. In some lambs an immune response to the virus starts *in utero,* while in others there is persistent infection, immunological tolerance, and permanent seronegativity. The latter animals, whether exhibiting clinical signs of infection or not, may become long-term carriers and shed virus continuously in all body secretions and excretions, including semen.

Laboratory Diagnosis

As with bovine viral diarrhea virus infection, a presumptive diagnosis can be made on the basis of clinical history and clinical signs. Laboratory diagnosis is based on virus isolation in cell culture, viral antigen detection in tissues, or serology, the latter done with an appreciation that seronegative animals may be infected and immunologically tolerant.

Epidemiology, Prevention, and Control

In flocks in the first breeding season after the introduction of virus, up to 50% of lambs may be affected; thereafter, the incidence of clinical disease declines while infection becomes endemic, especially when clinically recovered lambs are retained for breeding (in surviving lambs neurologic signs often disappear within 3–4 months of age). Control has been attempted using either inactivated or attenuated virus bovine viral diarrhea virus vaccines, but in most settings no control measures are economically worthwhile.

Hog Cholera

Hog cholera (classical swine fever) is economically the most important contagious disease of swine worldwide. Where the disease is present losses are severe and where immunization or eradication programs are in place there are substantial costs for maintenance of disease control agencies. Hog cholera is diagnosed regularly in Africa, Asia, and South and Central America. The disease has been eliminated from the United States, Canada, Australia, New Zealand, Scandinavian countries, Great Britain, Ireland, and Switzerland, but it still recurs intermittently in many European countries. In the 1990s, there have been repeated large outbreaks in The Netherlands, Belgium, Germany, and Spain—hundreds of thousands of swine have been destroyed either to control transmission or because of quarantines and prohibitions of swine movement and export.

Clinical Features

In its classical form, hog cholera is an acute infection accompanied by high fever, depression, anorexia, and conjunctivitis. These signs appear after an incubation period of 2–4 days and are followed by vomiting, diarrhea and/or constipation, opportunistic bacterial pneumonia, and nervous system dysfunctions such as paresis, paralysis, lethargy, circling, tremors, and occasionally convulsions. Light-skinned swine exhibit a diffuse hyperemia and purpura on the abdomen and ears. There is severe leukopenia, occurring early and reaching levels unmatched in any other disease of swine. In a susceptible herd, clinical signs are usually seen first in a few pigs; then over the course of about 10 days nearly all swine in the herd become sick. Young swine may die peracutely without clinical signs and older pigs may die within a week of onset or later from opportunistic bacterial superinfection. Herd mortality rate may reach 100%.

Less dramatic, subacute and chronic forms of disease have been recognized in which there is a prolonged incubation period, an extended or intermittent course of clinical disease with runting, chronic diarrhea, dermatitis, purpura, secondary bacterial infections, and death occurring weeks or months afterward. These forms of disease have been associated with virus strains of moderate virulence. Swine infected with virus strains of low virulence exhibit few clinical signs or remain healthy. Infection of pregnant sows leads to fetal infection and embryonic death, abortion, fetal mummification, or stillbirth. Newborn piglets may die or survive with tremors, runting, and progressive disease leading to death weeks or months after birth.

Pathogenesis, Pathology, and Immunity

The most common route of viral entry is by ingestion, with the tonsils the site of primary viral replication. Secondary replication occurs in endothelial cells, lymphoid organs, and bone marrow, leading to hemorrhages and profound leukopenia and thrombocytopenia. In peracute cases there may be no gross changes noted at necropsy. In acute cases there are submucosal and subserosal petechial hemorrhages, congestion, and infarction in spleen, liver, bone marrow, and lungs. Infarction of the spleen is considered almost pathognomonic. There is disseminated intravascular coagulation, thrombosis of small vessels, and inflammatory infiltrations into the parenchyma of many organs. Encephalitis with perivascular cuffing is often observed. In subacute or chronic cases there is necrotic ulceration of the mucosa of the large intestine and opportunistic bacterial pneumonia and enteritis. Perhaps the most prominent lesion in swine dying from chronic hog cholera is a general exhaustion of the lymphoid system—complete atrophy of the thymus and germinal centers in the spleen and lymph nodes. Live-born piglets, whether healthy or abnormal, are persistently infected, immunologically tolerant, and lifelong virus shedders. In immunocompetent swine that survive acute infection, immunity develops quickly.

Laboratory Diagnosis

A diagnosis of hog cholera is difficult to make without laboratory confirmation. This is particularly true of the subacute and chronic forms of the disease. In most countries there are regulations in place that require that disease control authorities be notified when the disease is suspected. In such circumstances, tissue specimens (pancreas, lymph nodes, tonsil, spleen, blood) are submitted to an authorized laboratory. Immunofluorescence or immunoperoxidase staining and antigen capture enzyme immunoassay allow rapid detection of viral antigens in tissues. Monoclonal antibodies can be used to distinguish hog cholera virus from other pestiviruses. Virus isolation and neutralizing antibody assays are done in swine cell cultures, but because the virus is not cytopathic, such assays require immunological assays to detect the presence of virus. Serologic methods include neutralization and enzyme immunoassay, with reagents chosen in some cases to differentiate hog cholera virus from bovine viral diarrhea virus. Such differentiation is important in areas where hog cholera eradication programs are in place.

Epidemiology, Prevention, and Control

Hog cholera virus is transmitted by direct contact between swine or indirectly via virus-laden excretions, secretions, and fomites (such as shoes, clothing, and vehicles). Carriage of virus between herds by inapparently infected swine is also important. Garbage and kitchen scrap feeding was at one time an important mode of virus transmission between herds; this was especially important because many swine were slaughtered when they showed the first signs of disease and pork scraps containing high titers of virus were then fed to swine. Garbage-feeding prohibitions and garbage-cooking regulations are now in place in many countries to deal with this risk. Hog cholera virus can also survive in frozen pork and pork products for years; the virus can thus be transported over long distances and can reappear in areas otherwise virus free.

Regional Eradication Programs

For many years, control of hog cholera involved quarantine and immunization. The first immunization schemes employed virulent virus inoculated together with immune serum to prevent clinical disease. Starting in the 1960s attenuated virus vaccines produced in rabbits or cell culture were introduced and were widely used in many countries. Today, in many developed countries this control strategy has given way to a strategy of eradication—by use of "test and slaughter" hog cholera has been eradicated from the United States, Canada, Australia, New Zealand, and several European countries. Eradication programs have been expensive, but very successful. Several factors have contributed to their success:

1. Hog cholera virus infection has been restricted in those countries to domestic swine; the virus has not been transmitted to any important extent by feral swine or wild pig species. Therefore, reintroduction of virus from uncontrollable sources has not been a problem—wild boar in Europe are infected and represent a potential source of reinfection.
2. Effective herd immunity induced by vaccines had reduced the incidence of infection to a level where the amount of slaughtering needed to achieve eradication has been economically feasible.
3. Surveillance of swine populations has been supported by adequate diagnostic techniques and reliable clinical diagnosis.
4. Producers have understood that persistent infections with chronic virus shedding, masked by the presence of vaccine viruses, would always present a risk of reintroductions with consequent great costs; they have therefore supported programs on simple economic grounds.
5. Eradication programs were initiated in many countries in the era when responsibility was assumed by government agencies as a matter of due course—public funding was not a question. Whether such programs could have been started in today's climate of "the user (the producer) pays" is uncertain.

Further Reading

Calisher, C. H. (1994). Medically important arboviruses of the United States and Canada. *Clin. Microbiol. Rev.* 7, 89–116.

Collett, S. (1992). Molecular genetics of pestiviruses. *Comp. Immunol. Microbiol. Infect. Dis.* **15**, 145–154.

Gresíková, M., and Kaluzová, M. (1997). Biology of tick-borne encephalitis viruses. *Acta Virol.* **41**, 115–124.

Karabatsos, N. ed. (1985). "International Catalogue of Arboviruses Including Certain Other Viruses of Vertebrates," 3rd Ed. American Society of Tropical Medicine and Hygiene, San Antonio, Texas (and updates published occasionally in the *American Journal of Tropical Medicine and Hygiene*).

Mackenzie, J. S., and Broom, A. K. (1995). Australian X disease, Murray Valley encephalitis and the French connection. *Vet. Microbiol.* **46**, 79–90.

McMinn, P. C. (1997). The molecular basis of virulence of the encephalitogenic flaviviruses. *J. Gen. Virol.* **78**, 2711–2722.

Monath, T. P., ed. (1988). "The Arboviruses: Epidemiology and Ecology," 5 vol. CRC Press, Boca Raton, FL.

Monath, T. P. (1991). Yellow fever: Victor, Victoria? Conqueror, conquest? Epidemics and research in the last forty years and prospects for the future. *Am. J. Trop. Med. Hyg.* **45**, 1–43.

Monath, T. P., and Heinz, F. X. (1996). Flaviviruses. *In* "Fields Virology" (B. N. Fields, D. M. Knipe, P. M. Howley, R. M. Chanock, J. L. Melnick, T. P. Monath, B. Roizman, and S. E. Straus, eds.), 3rd ed., pp. 961–1034. Lippincott-Raven, Philadelphia, PA.

Rice, C. M. (1996). Flaviviruses: The viruses and their replication. *In* "Fields Virology," (B. N. Fields, D. M. Knipe, P. M. Howley, R. M. Chanock, J. L. Melnick, T. P. Monath, B. Roizman, and S. E. Straus, eds.), 3rd ed., pp. 931–959. Lippincott-Raven, Philadelphia, PA.

Theil, H.-J., Plagemann, P. G. W., and Moennig, V. (1996). Pestiviruses. *In* "Fields Virology," (B. N. Fields, D. M. Knipe, P. M. Howley, R. M. Chanock, J. L. Melnick, T. P. Monath, B. Roizman, and S. E. Straus, eds.), 3rd ed., pp. 1059–1073. Lippincott-Raven, Philadelphia, PA.

CHAPTER 40

Prions: Agents of Transmissible Spongiform Encephalopathies

The term transmissible spongiform encephalopathy is used for several neurodegenerative diseases: scrapie of sheep and goats, bovine spongiform encephalopathy, feline transmissible encephalopathy, transmissible mink encephalopathy, chronic wasting disease of deer and elk and four human diseases, kuru, Creutzfeldt–Jakob disease (including new-variant Creutzfeldt–Jakob disease), Gerstmann–Sträussler–Scheinker syndrome, and fatal familial insomnia. These uniformly fatal diseases are caused by prions, i.e., "infectious proteins" or "rogue proteins." The name prion is an acronym from *pro*teinaceous *i*nfectious particle. In each of these diseases the basic lesion is a spongiform degeneration in the gray matter of the brain and astrogial hypertrophy and proliferation.

The prototype of the prion diseases, scrapie, was first described after the importation of Merino sheep from Spain into England in the 15th century. The name reflects the characteristic scratching behavior of diseased animals. Scrapie is endemic in sheep in all countries except Australia and New Zealand.

In 1963, William Hadlow, a veterinarian working at the Rocky Mountain Laboratory in Montana, United States, proposed that the human disease kuru was similar to scrapie in sheep and that it might be transmissible. Kuru, a fatal neurological disease, occurred only in the Fore tribe in the New Guinea highlands where ritualistic cannibalism was practiced on deceased relatives. Hadlow's idea led to the discovery by Carleton Gajdusek that kuru could be transmitted to chimpanzees, causing a disease indistinguishable from the human counterpart—for this discovery Gajdusek was awarded the Nobel Prize in Medicine. The importance of this discovery became clear when it was shown that more common human diseases, such as Creutzfeldt–Jakob disease, and other animal diseases, such as chronic wasting disease of deer and elk, are also transmissible in the same way.

Bovine spongiform encephalopathy was first detected in 1986 in the United Kingdom. Epidemiological observations suggest that the cattle disease originated in the early 1980s when scrapie prions underwent a "species jump" and became established in cattle; rendered meat-and-bone meal produced from sheep carcasses and offal and fed to cattle is considered the probable source. A less likely alternative is that the cattle disease originated with a spontaneous mutation in a single bovine animal. In any case, as more and more diseased cattle were slaughtered and rendered to produce meat-and-bone meal, a massive multiple point source epidemic followed. Export of meat-and-bone meal from the United Kingdom introduced the disease into Northern Ireland, the Republic of Ireland, Switzerland, France, Germany, The Netherlands, Belgium, and several other European countries, and the same source introduced the disease into zoo animals and cats in the United Kingdom.

In 1996 the British government announced that 10 people had likely become infected with the bovine spongiform encephalopathy prion through exposure to beef: ". . .although there is no direct evidence of a link, on current data and in the absence of any credible alternative, the most likely explanation is that these cases are linked to exposure to bovine spongiform encephalopathy. . . . This is a cause for great concern." By the end of 1998 the number of cases of what is now called new-variant Creutzfeldt–Jakob disease had risen to 34 and epidemiologic, pathologic, and molecular studies had strengthened the causative association between the bovine prion and the human disease. At the heart of this association were research breakthroughs on the nature of prions and the mechanisms of their pathogenicity—in 1997, for his discovery of the bizarre nature of prions and their exceptional pathogenetic pathways, Stanley Prusiner was awarded the Nobel Prize in Medicine.

Properties of Prions

Classification

Prions have not been classified like viruses—there are no families, genera, or species. They first are identified by their host species and disease association (Table 40.1). Then, they are characterized by their molecular and biological properties. Their primary amino acid sequence mainly reflects the host from which they were isolated, but also registers mutations that define inherited variants, e.g., in familial Creutzfeldt–Jakob disease in humans. Full amino acid sequences of virtually all important prion variants have been determined.

Certain biological properties are used to distinguish strains of prions, particularly scrapie strains. Following intracerebral injection of prion-containing material into multiple strains of inbred mice, the following parameters are recorded: (1) incubation period and mortality pattern; (2) distribution and extent of spongiform lesions and prion protein (PrP) plaques in brains (assayed by immunohistochemistry using labeled anti-PrP antibodies); and, in some cases, (3) titer of infectivity in brains. Prion strains "breed true," giving reproducible results in this kind of biological assay system.

For example, prions from cattle, nyala, kudu, and domestic cats behave the same when subjected to this strain characterization protocol, indicating that all have been derived from the same source, namely cattle. Further, mice inoculated in the same way with material from cattle with bovine spongiform encephalopathy and humans with new-variant Creutzfeldt–Jakob disease have behaved the same, yet differently from mice inoculated with material from sporadic cases of Creutzfeldt–Jakob disease or farmers who died of the same disease after working with cattle with bovine spongiform encephalopathy.

Similar results have been recorded by biochemical analysis of prions recovered from various sources: for example, when brain specimens were treated with proteinase K and their protease-resistant residues were subjected to Western blot analysis, four different blot patterns were found. Three patterns represented genetic, sporadic, and iatrogenic Creutzfeldt–Jakob disease in humans; the fourth represented all cases of new-variant Creutzfeldt–Jakob disease, bovine spongiform encephalopathy in cattle, and the similar feline and exotic ungulate diseases.

Prions from animals and humans can also be transmitted to various other animals (hamsters, rats, ferrets, mink, sheep, goats, pigs, cattle, monkeys, and chimpanzees), and again a kind of strain variation is seen. Some donor-recipient pairs lead to short incubation disease, others to longer incubation disease, and yet others no disease even after very long periods of observation or blind passage.

Prion Properties

Prions are normal cellular proteins that have undergone conformational change as a result of posttranslational processing of a normal cellular protein and thereby have become pathogenic. The normal protein, called PrP^C (term for the normal cellular isoform of the prion protein), is composed of about 208 amino acids (M_r 27,000–30,000). It is encoded in the genome of most mammals and is expressed in many tissues, especially in neurons and lymphoreticular cells. The function of PrP^C is unclear; it has been found to bind copper, but knockout mice lacking the gene for the protein appear normal. The amino acid sequence of PrP^C and the abnormal isoform of the protein, called PrP^{SC} (term derived from the scrapie isoform of the prion protein, but in general use for all prion diseases), in a given host are identical. Only the conformation of PrP^{SC} is changed, from a structure made up predominantly of α helices to one made up predominantly of β sheets (Figure 40.1). A monoclonal antibody has been developed that can discriminate between normal and disease-specific forms of PrP. It specifically precipitates bovine, murine, and human PrP^{SC}, but not PrP^C, confirming the presence of an epitope common to prions from different species linked to disease but different from the normal isoform of the protein.

When a given animal prion is passaged in mice or hamsters the amino acid sequence of the recipient PrP^{SC} is that of the PrP^C of the recipient, not the donor. In a particular host, there may be many different mutations in the PrP gene, each resulting in a slightly different PrP^{SC} conformation, each resulting in a different lesion pattern and different incubation and mortality pattern—this is the basis for the different prion strains. For example, prions from new-variant Creutzfeldt–Jakob disease in

TABLE 40.1
Prion Diseases of Animals and Humans

DISEASE	HOST	SOURCE OF INFECTION
Scrapie	Sheep, goats	Not certain, possibly scrapie prion contained in feed, but more likely by direct contact and contamination of pastures by placentas and fetal tissues
Bovine spongiform encephalopathy	Cattle	Bovine spongiform encephalopathy prion contamination of meat-and-bone meal; some vertical transmission from cow to calf
Transmissible mink encephalopathy	Mink	Scrapie prion contamination of sheep carcasses and offal fed to mink
Chronic wasting disease	Mule deer, elk	Unknown in feral animals, possibly scrapie prion contamination of feed or contamination of paddocks in captive animals
Feline spongiform encephalopathy	Cats, felids in zoos	Bovine spongiform encephalopathy prion contamination of meat fed to animals
Exotic ungulate spongiform encephalopathy	Greater kudu, nyala, oryx, and others in zoos	Bovine spongiform encephalopathy prion contamination of meat-and-bone meal
Kuru	Humans	Ritual cannibalism in Fore people
Creutzfeldt–Jakob disease	Humans	Iatrogenic—human prion contamination of dura mater grafts, therapeutic hormones, etc., all derived from cadavers
		Familial—germ line mutation in PrP gene
		Sporadic—unknown cause, perhaps somatic mutation in PrP gene or spontaneous conversion of PrP^{C} into PrP^{SC}
New-variant Creutzfeld–Jakob disease	Humans	Transmission of bovine spongiform encephalopathy prion to humans, unknown route, possibly by eating beef products
Gerstmann–Sträussler–Scheinker syndrome	Humans	Familial—germ line mutation in PrP gene
Fatal familial insomnia	Humans	Familial—germ line mutation in PrP gene

humans have characteristics distinct from those in other types of Creutzfeldt–Jakob disease, but similar to prions isolated from cattle, mice, cats, and macaques infected during the bovine spongiform encephalopathy epidemic in the United Kingdom.

PrP^{SC} protein is very resistant to many environmental insults, chemicals, and physical conditions that would destroy any virus or microorganism (Table 40.2). PrP^{SC} is also resistant to endogenous proteases, which is the key to its accumulation into aggregates, called scrapie-associated fibrils (SAF; term derived from scrapie but in general use for all prion diseases), that form neuronal plaques and cause spongiform damage and neuronal dysfunction.

Other notable characteristics of prions include: (1) they can reach very high titers in the brains of their hosts—laboratory strains passaged in hamsters can reach titers of 10^{11} ID_{50}/g of brain; (2) as measured by ultrafiltration their size seems to be about 30 nm; (2) they are very resistant to UV- and γ-irradiation, having a very small radiation target size (Figure 40.2); (3) they polymerize, forming helically wound filamentous rods 4–6 nm in diameter, called SAF, which are visible by electron microscopy and which make up the plaques seen in neurons (Figure 40.3); and (4) they evoke no inflammatory or immune response in their host.

There are investigators who do not believe that the etiologic role of prions in the spongiform encephalopathies has been proven. They cite alternate, but unproven, hypotheses to explain experimental findings: (1) the virino theory, suggesting that a nucleic acid genome is present that does not code for any protein but regulates the synthesis of a host-coded protein component of the agent, i.e., PrP^{SC}; and (2) the virus theory, suggesting

FIGURE 40.1.

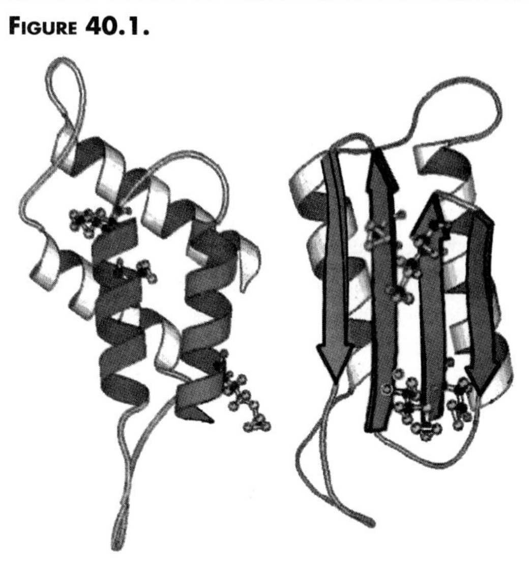

Structure of normal prion protein (PrP^C, the normal isoform of PrP protein) with prominent α helices (left) and PrP^{SC} (the abnormal isoform) with prominent β sheets (right). [From F. Cohen, Structural clues to prion replication. *Science* **273,** 184–189 (1996).]

that because there are viruses that have not yet been visualized or cultivated or had their nucleic acid isolated and characterized it is reasonable that efforts to find a conventional virus may fail despite intensive research efforts.

TABLE 40.2
Effects of Physical and Chemical Treatments on Scrapie Prion Infectivity[a]

TREATMENT	REDUCTION OF INFECTIVITY
1 *M* NaOH	$>10^{6-8}$
Phenol extraction	$>10^6$
0.5% sodium hypochlorite	10^4
Histopathologic processing	$10^{2.6}$
3% formaldehyde	10^2
1% β-propiolactone	10^1
Ether extraction	10^2
Autoclave 132°C for 90 minutes	$>10^{7.4}$
Autoclave 132°C for 60 minutes	$10^{6.5}$
Autoclave 121°C for 90 minutes	$10^{5.6}$
Boiling 100°C for 60 minutes	$10^{3.4}$
Heating 80°C for 60 minutes	10^1

[a]Composite of several studies; therefore no untreated control value given.

Prion Replication

It is the presence of horizontally or perhaps vertically transmitted PrP^{SC} that catalyzes the conversion of normally encoded PrP^C molecules into more PrP^{SC} molecules. While PrP^{SC} acts as the template, the "seed crystal," for the abnormal folding and polymerization of PrP^C—forming a heterodimer with normal cellular PrP^C—there is evidence that another molecule, called protein X, is needed for prion replication when transmission occurs between distant host species. In any case, the process cascades exponentially, with newly formed PrP^{SC} in turn serving as a catalyst for the conversion of more and more PrP^C molecules as they are produced in target cells such as neurons (Figures 40.4A and 40.4B). Eventually, so much PrP^{SC} builds up that it polymerizes, forming fibrillar masses that become visible as plaques and cause neuronal degeneration and neurological dysfunction via mechanisms that are as yet poorly understood. In a like manner, different isoforms of PrP^{SC} "breed true" and are perpetuated even in mixed infections (Figure 40.4C).

Much of our understanding of the prion replicative process has been confirmed by elegant studies using knockout and transgenic mice, i.e., mice lacking the PrP^C gene or mice containing only the PrP^C gene of another species. For example, mice lacking the PrP gene do not get sick when inoculated with the scrapie prion and mice expressing reduced levels of the protein have very long incubation periods. Further, when normal brain explants are grafted into the brains of such knockout mice they develop lesions only in the normal graft tissue. Even more remarkable, transgenic mice, carrying mutated PrP genes mimicking those in human familial spongiform

FIGURE 40.2.

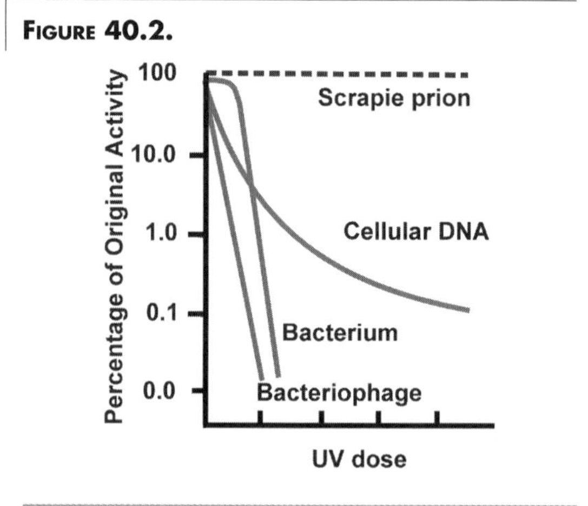

Ultraviolet irradiation decay curves for cellular DNA, a bacterium, a virus (bacteriophage), and the scrapie prion. Data like these provided some of the first insight that the agents of the spongiform encephalopathies are not like microorganisms or viruses.

FIGURE 40.3.

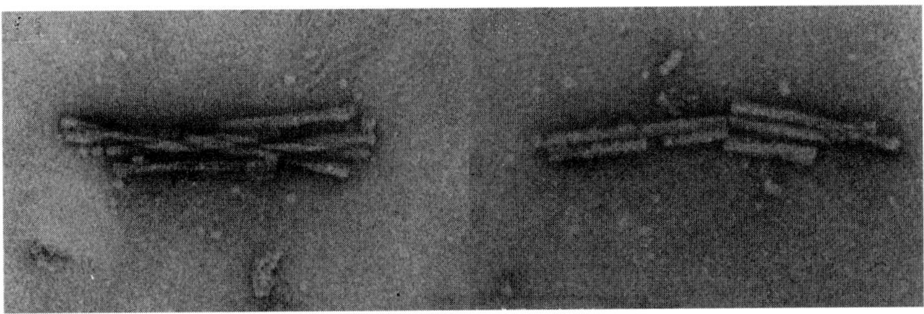

Electron micrographs of extensively purified scrapie-associated fibrils, composed of prion protein, PrP. Negatively stained with uranyl formate. Bar: 100 nm. (Courtesy of S. B. Prusiner.)

encephalopathies, show the neuronal degeneration typical of these diseases even without inoculation of exogenous prions. Finally, transgenic/knockout mice carrying human PrP^C, but not mouse PrP^C, when inoculated with the bovine spongiform encephalopathy prion develop neurologic disease and lesions, starting at about 500 days. This finding has been considered a key element in the association of new-variant Creutzfeldt–Jakob disease with the bovine spongiform encephalopathy prion.

Scrapie

Although recognized as a distinct disease of sheep in many countries for many centuries, scrapie was not understood to be transmissible until an episode in Scotland in 1935. Over 1500 cases of iatrogenic scrapie followed the use of a formalin-inactivated louping ill vaccine prepared from sheep brain. Scrapie is distributed widely in Europe and North America and occurs sporadically in some countries in Africa and Asia. Typically, only a few sheep in a flock are diseased at any given time, but infected flocks suffer losses continuously over many years. In the United Kingdom, some 90 to 95% of cases occur in Suffolk and Hampshire breeds; in the United States, disease occurs almost exclusively in purebred Suffolks. Goats seem to be incidental hosts, with infection following commingling with scrapie-infected sheep or exposure to contaminated pastures.

Clinical Features

The incubation period of scrapie in sheep is 2–5 years and the onset of clinical disease is insidious. Affected sheep become excitable and develop fine tremors of the head and neck, which may be elicited by sudden noise or movement. Shortly thereafter, animals develop intense pruritus, with wool loss and skin rubbed raw. After 1–6 months of progressive deterioration, characterized by emaciation, weakness, weaving gait, staring eyes, ataxia, and hindquarter paralysis, animals invariably die.

Pathogenesis, Pathology, and Immunity

Remarkably, although scrapie spreads within flocks its natural route of infection has not been proven—it is widely considered that sheep acquire the disease by the oral route or from superficial wounds in pastures contaminated by placental tissue or body fluids. Vertical transmission is still disputed—transmission from ewes to lambs may be due to transplacental or postpartum infection. Under experimental conditions, peripheral routes of inoculation (intraperitoneal, subcutaneous, or intravenous) only produce disease after prolonged incubation periods, whereas intracerebral inoculation leads to disease after a much shorter incubation period.

The first appearance of the scrapie prion in experimentally infected lambs occurs in the intestines, tonsils, spleen, and lymph nodes. Sequential infectivity titrations of organs have suggested that following the ingestion of prions, infection is initiated in gut lymphoid tissues and prions produced in these tissues then move to the central nervous system. At death, lesions in the gray matter of the brain include neuronal vacuolation and degeneration and astrocytic hypertrophy and hyperplasia (Figure 40.5). There is no inflammatory reaction or evidence of an immune response.

Laboratory Diagnosis

Diagnosis is based on clinical signs, flock history, and histopathologic examination of the brain of suspect animals. Anti-PrP antibodies are used for immunohistochemical staining of suspect brain specimens and for Western blot assays of solubilized brain extracts and cerebrospinal fluid. The presence of PrP-containing plaques or PrP protein in the cerebrospinal fluid is considered diagnostic. No method is presently available for use on any practicably obtainable antemortem specimen, nor is any method useful in animals before the development of frank clinical signs of disease. However, several promising tests are under study.

Epidemiology, Prevention, and Control

Because the exact mode of transmission of scrapie among sheep in a flock or between flocks is not known, prevention and control strategies remain unproven and, in most places, untried. Most discouraging has been the fact that sheep have developed the disease just by being pastured in fields occupied previously by scrapie-affected sheep. In Iceland, in the most successful eradication program ever attempted, infected flocks have been destroyed and pastures left empty for several years. Scrapie-free sheep have been reintroduced, and in a few instances have developed disease—in these areas the process has been repeated, with an even longer interval before restocking (in some instances land has been turned over to other uses). After years of using this strategy, with fewer and fewer breaks seen, the country is just about to become scrapie free. The question is asked whether this strategy would be feasible in other countries, especially those with large numbers of sheep and a high prevalence of scrapie.

Following its introduction into the United States in 1947 and again in 1952, a scrapie eradication program was established. At first, this involved the identification of affected animals and the destruction of involved flocks as well as other exposed flocks, with owner indemnification from public funds. However, the long incubation period of the disease and the extensive interstate movement of sheep made this program unrealistic. At present, a "certified flock" program is being used: the movement of sheep among certified flocks can be done without risk, while the movement of sheep among other flocks is not constrained. Under the European Union, scrapie has become a notifiable disease, subject to control regulations.

Given the expense and lack of success of these national programs and regulations, programs to exclude scrapie from Australia and New Zealand, with their large sheep populations, based on strict quarantine and control of importations, have been very worthwhile investments.

Bovine Spongiform Encephalopathy

Bovine spongiform encephalopathy was first recognized in the United Kingdom in 1986. By 1989, an alarming increase in the number of cases reported led to a ban on the feeding of meat-and-bone meal derived from ruminant meat or offal; however, the ban was only minimally enforced until some years later. The epidemic, as measured by numbers of cases reported and confirmed, peaked in 1993, at which time more than 300 cases were identified per week. By the end of 1997, more than

FIGURE 40.6.

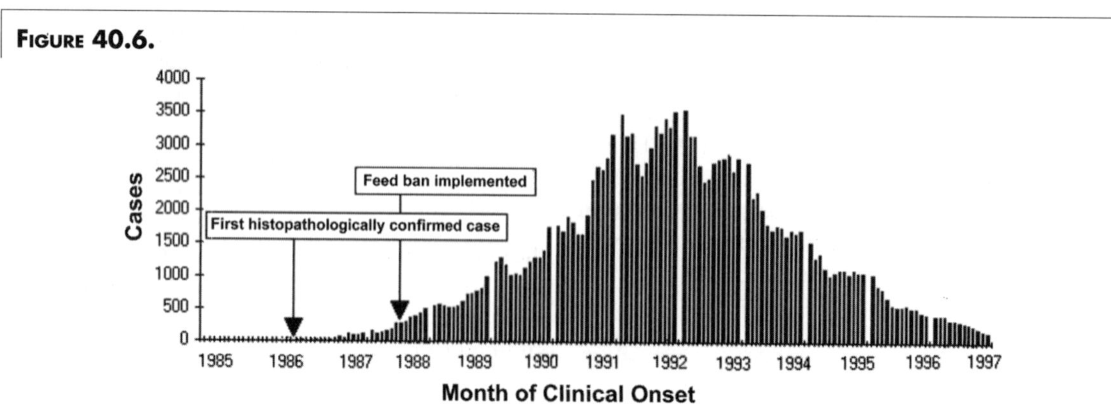

The epidemic curve of bovine spongiform encephalopathy in the United Kingdom. Data are recorded by month of onset of clinical signs; the epidemic curve looks quite different if plotted by quarter or year of onset of clinical signs. (Data from Ministry of Agriculture, Fisheries and Food, United Kingdom.)

FIGURE 40.4.

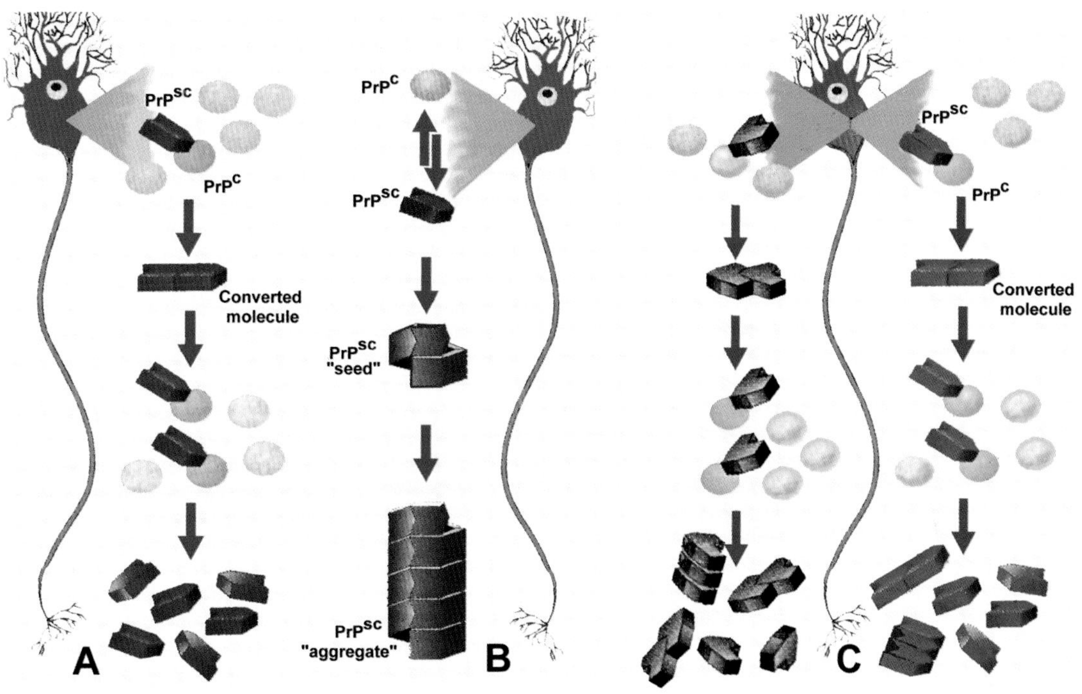

Replication mechanism of prions, as conceived by S. B. Prusiner. (A) The abnormal protein, PrP^{SC}, contacts normal protein, PrP^{C}, and changes its conformation to that of the abnormal form, which eventually leads to neurological disease. (B) A "seed crystal" may be needed to bring about the cascade of transformation of the PrP^{C} protein: the abnormal protein, PrP^{SC}, self-catalyzes rapid aggregation of itself, leading to a buildup of masses of fibrils, which eventually harm neurons. (C) Different prion strains may consist of the same protein misfolded in different ways, i.e., each prion strain, each differently folded version of abnormal protein, PrP^{SC} (left vs right), may transmit its characteristics separately to the normal prion protein, PrP^{C}, by forcing it to fold in its own unique way. [Compiled from four news articles: S. Prusiner, *Science* **273,** 184–189, 274, 2010 (1996); G. C. Telling and S. Prusiner, *Ibid.* **274,** 2079–2082 (1996).]

FIGURE 40.5.

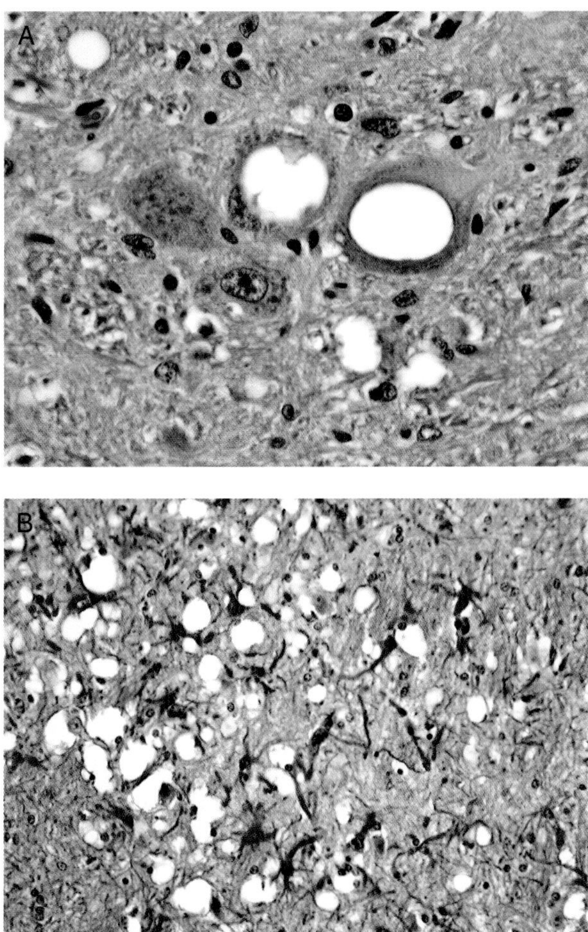

Lesions in the gray matter of the brain of a sheep with scrapie: (A) typical spongiform change in neurons and (B) spongiform change and astrocytic hypertrophy and hyperplasia. (A) Hematoxylin and eosin stain; (B) glial fibrillar acid protein (GFAP) stain. Magnification: ×500. (Courtesy of R. Higgins.)

172,000 cases had been confirmed, involving over 60% of all dairy farms and 14% of beef cow/calf herds (Figure 40.6). Worse still, the number of reported and confirmed cases was dwarfed by the actual number of animals infected and entered into the human food chain because of slaughter before the onset of clinical disease—Roy Anderson and colleagues at Oxford University back-calculated this number to be about 1 million cattle, with a peak in 1988.

Initial studies in the United Kingdom indicated a multiple common source epidemic. It was soon realized that the epidemic was caused by contamination of meat-and-bone meal with a scrapie-like agent. The incidence of the disease has now subsided to a point where its disappearance is predicted to occur by 2005. The economic and social impact of this epidemic has been extraordinary, involving not only the United Kingdom but many European countries. When one realizes that the value of the national cattle herd of the United Kingdom has been estimated to be UK£ 13 billion, the scale of this epidemic becomes all the more clear.

Clinical Features

The onset of disease is insidious, with tremors, hyperaesthesia with kicking during milking, abnormal posture, hindlimb ataxia, progressive apprehensive behavior, aggression and even frenzy, reduced milk yield, and weight loss. The disease is inevitably fatal after a clinical course ranging from 2 to 3 weeks to over a year. Onset is independent of season or stage of lactation. Most cattle affected have been 3–5 years of age; older cattle have been affected and the youngest recorded case was 22 months of age.

Pathogenesis, Pathology, and Immunity

Pathologic changes are seen only in the brain. At death, lesions in the gray matter include neuronal vacuolation, neuronal degeneration and loss, and astrocytic hypertrophy and hyperplasia. There is no inflammatory reaction or evidence of an immune response. Lesions are most prominent in the nuclei of the midbrain, brain stem, and cervical spinal cord with minimal changes in cerebral cortex, cerebellum, hippocampus, and basal nuclei.

Several lines of evidence indicate that there is only a single strain of the bovine spongiform encephalopathy prion; it is unusually species nonspecific, having been shown to cause disease in cats and other ungulates and to be transmitted easily by oral or intracerebral routes to sheep, goats, mink, marmosets, squirrel monkeys, cynomolgus macaques, mice, and hamsters. There is some evidence of vertical transmission in cattle.

Laboratory Diagnosis

Diagnosis is based on clinical signs, herd history, and histopathologic examination of the brain of suspect animals. Standard coronary sections of the most commonly affected areas, i.e., midbrain, brain stem and cervical spinal cord, are examined for routine diagnosis. Anti-PrP antibodies are used for immunohistochemical staining of suspect brain specimens and for Western blot assays of solubilized brain extracts and cerebral spinal fluid. The presence of PrP-containing plaques or PrP protein in the cerebrospinal fluid is considered diagnostic. As in the case of scrapie in sheep, no established method is presently available for use on any practicably obtainable antemortem specimen nor is any method useful in animals before the development of frank clinical signs of disease. However, several methods are in development: for example, an immunoassay for a brain protein (14-3-3, p130-p131) found in the cerebrospinal fluid in human and well as animal spongiform encephalopathies is being advanced for antemortem diagnosis.

Epidemiology, Prevention, and Control

The bovine spongiform encephalopathy epidemic began simultaneously at many geographic locations and was traced solely to contamination of meat-and-bone meal produced from meat and offal from slaughtered and dead sheep. As the epidemic progressed, it was amplified by the feeding of more and more of the same product produced from infected cattle. As noted earlier, several lines of evidence indicate that the source of the bovine prion was the scrapie prion. It is thought that the reason that this species jump occurred at this place and time was that the rendering process was changed in the early 1980s, the use of organic solvents to extract fats being abandoned because of great increases in the cost of petroleum-based solvents. It is thought that the disease was confined mainly to the United Kingdom because of a unique combination of risk factors: (1) a high ratio of sheep to cattle, (2) a relatively high rate of endemic scrapie, and (3) the practice of heavy feeding of meat-and-bone meal of cattle and sheep origin to dairy cattle.

The spread of the disease from the United Kingdom to Northern Ireland, the Republic of Ireland, Switzerland, France, Germany, and other European countries was via exported meat-and-bone meal and breeding cattle. Between 1986 and 1990, more than 57,900 breeding cattle were exported from the United Kingdom to European Union countries, along with thousands of tons of meat-and-bone meal. The spread of the disease to cats (more than 80 cases) and certain exotic zoo animals (greater kudu, eland, nyala, gemsbok, oryx, puma, cheetah, ocelot, rhesus monkey) was via the same means, with protein supplements derived from rendered cattle products being added to animal feed products, including commercial cat food. For example, authorities in Australia, the United States, and other countries initiated surveillance when it was realized that large cats, ungulates, and other zoo animals were being imported from the United Kingdom. Concern followed upon knowledge that meat originating from the death of animals in zoos is fed regularly to other animals. This surveillance did not turn up any evidence of infection in any country.

The control of bovine spongiform encephalopathy in the United Kingdom has rested solely on the exclusion of all meat, offal, and other materials derived from cattle in all cattle feed products. Means to prevent the transfer of the disease into other countries, especially countries of the European Union, have centered on bans against the importation of beef, live bovine animals and embryos, meat-and-bone meal, and other products derived from cattle from the United Kingdom. Beyond this, much of the new international regulation of export/import of beef and other products derived from cattle pertains to concerns over the bovine spongiform encephalopathy prion entering the human food chain.

Biohazard: In 1997, the government of the United Kingdom declared that "the bovine spongiform encephalopathy agent should be considered a human pathogen... those intentionally working with infected material or preparations... should use the same laboratory safety precautions as for Creutzfeldt–Jacob disease."

Transmissible Mink Encephalopathy

This disease was first recognized on mink ranches in Wisconsin in 1947. Carcasses of scrapie-infected sheep were fed to mink, initiating an infection chain that then involved mink-to-mink transmission via fighting and the feeding of mink carcasses back to mink. There seems no doubt that the mink disease was due to the scrapie prion. Clinical signs included hyperirritability, ataxia, compulsive biting, somnolence, coma, and death. Histologic lesions in the brains of affected mink were similar to those in scrapie in sheep. This disease has largely disappeared as mink ranchers have learned not to feed mink any foodstuff derived from sheep or other mink.

Chronic Wasting Disease of Deer and Elk

Chronic wasting disease is a progressive, fatal neurological disease of captive mule deer, mule deer hybrids, black-tailed deer, white-tailed deer, and Rocky Mountain elk. It was first recognized in captive mule deer in 1980 in Colorado; in 1996 a surveillance program in Colorado based on histopathologic examination of hunter-shot animals indicated that 6.5% of deer and 1.5% of the elk were infected. The disease has also been recognized in many other areas of western North America. In recent years the disease has also been found in wild animals that seemingly have lived for many generations far from captive deer and elk facilities. The disease is characterized by abnormal behavior, teeth grinding, polyuria and polydipsia, and marked loss of weight. Death usually occurs within a few months of the appearance of clinical signs. Lesions include widespread spongiform change of the brain, i.e., neuronal vacuolation and astrocytic hypertrophy and hyperplasia. The epidemiology of the disease in deer and elk is unknown; these species are rarely fed meat-and-bone meal supplements but captive animals are often held in facilities previously used for sheep and it is possible that wild animals have occupied land where sheep have grazed in prior years.

Human Prion Diseases

Kuru, Creutzfeldt–Jacob disease, Gerstmann–Sträussler–Scheinker syndrome, and fatal familial insomnia are human prion diseases that are manifested predominantly in middle-aged and older individuals. Usually their onset is indicated by sensory disturbances, confusion, inappropriate behavior, and severe sleeping disorders. Disease progress is marked by myoclonic jerking movements and within 6 months to 1 year progression to frank dementia and ultimately a comatose state and death. There are three major classes of these diseases: sporadic, familial, and iatrogenic:

Creutzfeldt–Jakob disease occurs in all three forms: (1) 85% of cases are sporadic, seemingly with quite long incubation periods, cause unknown; (2) 15% of cases are familial, with very long incubation periods, caused by autosomal dominant mutations in the PrP gene, more than 18 of which have been mapped; and (3) a few hundred cases have been transmitted iatrogenically via contaminated neurosurgical instruments (e.g., implanted stereotactic electroencephalogram electrodes), dura matter and cornea grafts, and hormones, especially growth hormone derived from human cadavers.

New-variant Creutzfeldt–Jakob disease was first described in the United Kingdom in 1996. Ten individuals exhibited features not normally associated with Creutzfeldt–Jakob disease: (1) they were between 19 and 45 years of age when diagnosed (vs average age of 63 years for sporadic cases); (2) the course of their disease was longer than usual (mean 14 months vs 6 months for sporadic cases); (3) their lesions were different than those seen in sporadic cases (prominent florid plaques vs spongiform changes); (4) they initially presented with psychiatric problems (personality changes, depression, fearfulness, paranoia), as well as signs of weakness and dementia as seen in sporadic cases; and (5) late in the course of their disease they exhibited cerebellar syndrome, ataxia, cognitive impairment, and myoclonus as well as dementia and coma as seen terminally in sporadic cases. By the end of 1998, 34 such cases had been recorded.

As described earlier in this chapter, several lines of molecular evidence have linked variant Creutzfeldt–Jakob disease to bovine spongiform encephalopathy and putatively to eating beef or possible other exposure from infected cattle. There are additional epidemiologic and pathogenetic linkages: (1) the variant disease has not been seen in countries other than the United Kingdom (except for one case in France), the same place where the epidemic of bovine spongiform encephalopathy had occurred; (2) the variant disease was first seen about 10 years after the largest number of infected cattle had entered the human food chain; (3) the prion causing bovine spongiform encephalopathy has proven unusually able to infect other species by the oral route; and (4) when transmitted to macaques, the bovine prion has caused the same kind of florid plaques as seen in the variant human disease. Taken together, these observations have been considered to add up to a compelling case for an etiologic relationship between the bovine prion and the variant human disease.

Gerstmann–Sträussler–Scheinker syndrome and fatal familial insomnia are very rare familial diseases caused by autosomal dominant mutations in the PrP gene. In the former there is a single point mutation at codon 102 in the PrP gene that leads to a single amino acid substitution in the normal PrP protein. When this point mutation is introduced into the PrP gene of mice they develop typical spongiform encephalopathy disease and lesions.

Further Reading

Anderson, R. M., Donnelly, C. A., Ferguson, N. M., Woolhouse, M. E. J., Watt, C. J., Udy, H. J., MaWhinney, S., Dunstan, S. P., Southwood, T. R. E., Wilesmith, J. W., Ryan, J. B. M., Hoinville, L. J., Hillerton, J. E., Austin, A. R., and Wells, G. A. H. (1996). Transmission dynamics and epidemiology of BSE in British cattle. *Nature London* **382,** 779–788.

Chesebro, B., and Fields, B. N. (1996). Transmissible spongiform encephalopathies. *In* "Fields Virology" (B. N. Fields, D. M. Knipe, P. M. Howley, R. M. Chanock, J. L. Melnick, T. P. Monath, B. Roizman, and S. E. Straus, eds.), 3rd ed., pp. 2845–2850. Lippincott-Raven, Philadelphia, PA.

Donnelly, C. A., Ghani, A. C., Ferguson, N. M., and Anderson, R. M. (1997). Recent trends in the BSE epidemic. *Nature (London)* **389,** 903.

Hill, A. F., Desbruslais, M., Joiner, S., Sidle, K. C., Gowland, I., Collinge, J., Doey, L. J., and Lantos, P. (1997). The same prion strain causes vCJD and BSE. *Nature (London)* **389,** 448–450.

Ministry of Agriculture, Fisheries and Food of the United Kingdom. BSE Information. Regularly updated. Available at: http://www.maff.gov.uk/animalh/bse/

Nathanson, N., Wilesmith, J., and Griot, C. (1997). Bovine spongiform encephalopathy (BSE): Causes and consequences of a common source epidemic. *Am. J. Epidemiol.* **145,** 959–969.

Prusiner, S. B. (1996). Prions. *In* "Fields Virology" (B. N. Fields, D. M. Knipe, P. M. Howley, R. M. Chanock, J. L. Melnick, T. P. Monath, B. Roizman, and S. E. Straus, eds.), 3rd ed., pp. 2901–22949. Lippincott-Raven, Philadelphia, PA.

Prusiner, S. B. (1997). Prion diseases and the BSE crisis. *Science* **278,** 245–251.

Wells, G. A. H., Hawkins, S. A. C., Green, R. B., Austin, A. R., Dexter, I., Spencer, Y. I., Chaplin, M. J., Stack, M. J., and Dawson, M. (1998). Preliminary observations on the pathogenesis of experimental bovine spongiform encephalopathy (BSE): An update. *Vet. Rec.* **142,** 103–106.

Wilesmith, J. W. (1994). Bovine spongiform encephalopathy: Epidemiological factors associated with the emergence of an important new animal pathogen in Great Britain. *Semin. Virol.* **5,** 179–187.

Will, R. G., Ironside, J. W., Zeidler, M., Cousens, S. N., Estibeiro, K., Alperovitch, A., Poser, S., Pocchiari, M., Hofman, A., and Smith, P. G. (1996). A new variant of Creutzfeldt-Jakob disease in the UK. *Lancet* **347,** 921–925.

CHAPTER 41

Other Viruses: *Hepadnaviridae*, *Deltavirus*

Family *Hepadnaviridae*

Although the prototype virus, hepatitis B virus, is of major importance in human medicine, the viruses of the family *Hepadnaviridae* are of limited importance in veterinary medicine. Viruses closely related to hepatitis B virus have been discovered in Pekin and other ducks, herons, woodchucks (*Marmata monax*), and tree and ground squirrels (*Spermophilus beecheyi*), and there is less well-documented evidence of similar viruses in marsupials, rodents, and cats. There is also a suspicion that there is a similar virus and associated hepatocellular carcinoma of dogs. Given this diversity of member viruses and molecular differences between the viruses, the family has been divided into two genera: *Orthohepadnavirus,* for the mammalian members, and *Avihepadnavirus,* for the avian members.

Although hepadnaviruses are extremely difficult to propagate in cell culture, a great deal is known of their structure and mode of replication, thanks to recombinant DNA technology. Hepadnavirus virions are 42–48 nm in diameter and are composed of a 27- to 30-nm icosahedral nucleocapsid (core) surrounded by an envelope (Figure 41.1). The genome consists of a single molecule of circular (via base pairing of cohesive ends), partially double-stranded, partially single-stranded DNA. The complete strand is negative sense and 3.0–3.3 kb in size; the other strand varies between 1.7 and 2.8 kb, leaving 15–50% of the molecule single stranded. The complete strand contains a nick at a unique site that is different in the orthohepadnaviruses and avihepadnaviruses. The negative-sense genomic strand has a protein molecule covalently attached to its 5′ end; the positive-sense strand has a 5′-19-nucleotide cap.

Hepadnaviruses have a unique and complex mode of replication involving a reverse transcriptase. In the nucleus of hepatocytes the virus genome is converted into a complete circular double-stranded DNA by the DNA polymerase carried in the virion nucleocapsid. The negative-sense strand of this DNA is used as the template for the synthesis of a full-length positive-sense RNA transcript, which is packaged in viral core particles in the cytoplasm of the infected cell. Then, the viral reverse transcriptase transcribes negative-sense DNA from the positive-sense RNA template. As this occurs the positive-sense template is degraded simultaneously. Next, the viral DNA polymerase utilizes the newly formed negative-sense DNA as the template for the synthesis of positive-sense DNA. Newly synthesized double-stranded DNA is packaged into virions before this last step is complete—this is why virion DNA is only partially double stranded. Virion DNA is integrated into the DNA of the host cell, leading to persistent infection and in a yet unknown way to the eventual development of primary hepatocellular carcinoma in humans, ducks, and woodchucks.

Hepadnavirus genomes have three (avian viruses) or four (mammalian viruses) open reading frames. The nucleocapsid is made up of one antigenically distinct protein (expressing HBcAg antigenic specificity); it can be modified, thereby expressing a second antigenic specificity (HBeAg). The envelope is composed of three proteins and some host cell lipid. These constituents also form noninfectious spherical (22 nm in diameter) or

Figure 41.1.

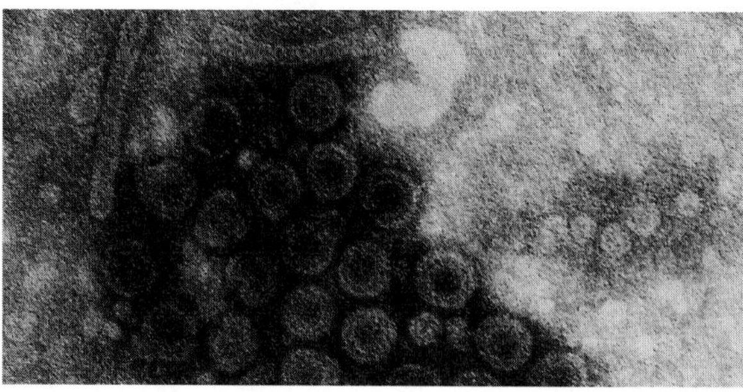

Family *Hepadnaviridae,* genus *Orthohepadnavirus,* hepatitis B virus. Negatively stain electron microscopy. Bar: 100 nm.

filamentous (22 nm in diameter, varying length) particles called hepatitis B surface antigen particles (expressing at least five HBsAg antigenic specificities). Extraordinary numbers of these particles are formed and circulate in the blood of chronically infected humans or woodchucks—up to 10^{13} per milliliter of blood. Each of the antigenic specificities is used in diagnostic tests and in tests to judge the status of human patients in regard to persistent virus carriage, the presage of chronic liver disease and hepatocellular carcinoma. HBsAg, now produced by recombinant DNA technology in yeast or mammalian cells, is the basis for all hepatitis B vaccines.

Hepatitis B virus in humans causes acute hepatitis, chronic hepatitis, liver cirrhosis, and primary hepatocellular carcinoma. Hepatocellular carcinoma is the most common human cancer in the world. Woodchucks infected with the virus specific to this species develop acute hepatitis and, commonly, hepatocellular carcinoma, but not cirrhosis. Pekin ducks infected with the virus specific to this species show few signs of acute hepatitis but do develop hepatocellular carcinoma. Infected ground squirrels rarely develop hepatitis or hepatocellular carcinoma.

Floating Genus *Deltavirus* (Hepatitis D Virus)

Hepatitis D virus, also called hepatitis delta virus, is a satellite virus in that it requires the simultaneous presence of hepatitis B virus for its replication and assembly. This virus is unique among the viruses of vertebrates. On the basis of its unique biological and molecular properties, the virus has been accorded distinct taxonomic status in the floating genus *Deltavirus*. Hepatitis D virions are 36–43 nm in diameter and consist of a shell made of HBsAg surrounding a core containing delta antigen and a circular negative-sense, single-stranded RNA genome, 1.75 kb in size. The genome structure and autocatalytic activities involved in the replication of hepatitis D virus closely resemble those of some viroids and satellite viruses found in plants. In humans infected simultaneously with hepatitis B virus and hepatitis D viruses, disease is more severe with an increased incidence of cirrhosis and increased mortality. The mechanisms involved in this interaction are unknown. Hepatitis delta virus has been transmitted experimentally to woodchucks infected simultaneously with woodchuck hepatitis virus.

Unclassified Arboviruses

Dozens of viruses have been isolated in the course of arbovirus investigations that have been characterized only partially; in most cases they have been passaged in mammalian cell cultures and, in some cases, in experimental animals (mice, hamsters) and in all cases they are available in reference collections. Some molecular data are available as well. However, in general, little is being done to determine whether any of these viruses may be animal pathogens. Such work is only likely to be done in the wake of substantial disease episodes in domestic or important wild animals in settings where public notice is taken and field investigation is feasible and fundable.

Further Reading

Ganem, D. (1996). Hepadnaviridae: The viruses and their replication. *In* "Fields Virology" (B. N. Fields, D. M. Knipe, P. M. Howley, R. M. Chanock, J. L. Melnick, T. P. Monath, B. Roizman, and S. E. Straus, eds.), 3rd ed., pp. 2703–2737. Lippincott-Raven, Philadelphia, PA.

Gerin, J. L., Purcell, R. H., and Rizzetto, M., eds. (1991). "The Hepatitis Delta Virus. Progress in Clinical and Biological Research." Wiley-Liss, New York.

Hollinger, F. B. (1996). Hepatitis B virus. *In* "Fields Virology," (B. N. Fields, D. M. Knipe, P. M. Howley, R. M. Chanock, J. L. Melnick, T. P. Monath, B. Roizman, and S. E. Straus, eds.), 3rd ed., pp. 2738–2808. Lippincott-Raven, Philadelphia, PA.

Taylor, J. M. (1996). Hepatitis delta virus and its replication. *In* "Fields Virology" (B. N. Fields, D. M. Knipe, P. M. Howley, R. M. Chanock, J. L. Melnick, T. P. Monath, B. Roizman, and S. E. Straus, eds.), 3rd ed., pp. 2809–2818. Lippincott-Raven, Philadelphia, PA.

CHAPTER 42

Viral Diseases by Animal Species

In the preceding chapters the contribution of individual viruses to veterinary and zoonotic disease has been examined in the context of the families of viruses. In this final chapter important diseases and syndromes caused by viruses in animal species are listed together with their etiologic associations. The aim is to provide a "bird's eye" view of the commonest viral diseases and syndromes in each animal species. A practicable way of doing this in a concise form is to provide one or two tables for each major domestic animal species and one table each for laboratory animals, fish, and nonhuman primates.

Such a tabulation inevitably involves oversimplification, but page numbers have been provided to direct the reader to appropriate pages for detailed coverage of each of these viral infections. Nevertheless, these tables have attempted to ascribe to each disease a measure of its importance (+ to ++++), as viewed from the perspective of clinical veterinary medicine in countries with modern agricultural practices and veterinary services. When considering diseases that have been eliminated from these countries, we have incorporated into our assessment the relative risk of these exotic diseases should they be introduced/reintroduced. For example, foot-and-mouth disease, which is given a ++++ rating in cattle, is an important disease even in countries in which it does not currently occur because of its potential impact on beef and dairy product exports and the rapidity with which this virus can spread from herd to herd. In contrast, rinderpest, although one of the most important disease of ruminants in countries where it has not been eliminated, is only given a ++ rating because there is little chance of the virus being reintroduced into countries with modern veterinary services and, even if it were to be introduced into these countries, its elimination would present few difficulties.

Had these tables been written from the perspective of the developing countries, then some diseases considered important in areas where intensive husbandry systems predominate would have been rated as inconsequential. For example, infectious bovine rhinotracheitis deserves a high rating in the intensive cattle production environment (dairy or beef), but is not as important in developing countries where herd sizes are small and management systems less intensive.

Some diseases are very difficult to categorize within the context of clinical importance worldwide. The public focus on bovine spongiform encephalopathy and related transmissible encephalopathies of other species is currently intense. The reality is that only in the United Kingdom is bovine spongiform encephalopathy a significant clinical problem. The implications of the epidemic, however, extend far beyond that country because of the worldwide presence of related encephalopathies in other species and the implications of a potential epidemic of new-variant Creutzsfeldt–Jacob disease in humans. The restrictions generated in the international trade of animals and animal products have been enormous, and the ripple effect of the current epidemic in the United Kingdom will almost certainly continue for many years.

There is an arbitrary element in relation to the group of diseases (generalized, respiratory, etc.) to which certain infections are allocated. For example, most generalized skin diseases result from blood-borne infection, but they have been listed as skin diseases. Where viruses cause generalized signs and also signs of particular importance in some system, or in the newborn, they have been entered in both categories. The other headings in the tables have been selected to draw attention to the classification of the causal virus and whether it is persistent, the geographic distribution of the disease, and the availability of vaccines.

TABLE 42.1
Generalized and Respiratory Viral Diseases of Cattle

DISEASE	IMPORTANCE	FAMILY (SUBFAMILY OR GENUS)	VIRUS	NUMBER OF TYPES	GEOGRAPHICAL DISTRIBUTION	VACCINE	PERSISTENCE	PAGES
Generalized diseases (including diseases with central nervous system involvement)								
Bluetongue	++	*Reoviridae* (*Orbivirus*)	Bluetongue viruses	25	Tropics and subtropics, temperate areas of North America	Attenuated but used only in sheep	No, but viremia may last for about 100 days	398
Bovine ephemeral fever	++	*Rhabdoviridae* (*Ephemerovirus*)	Bovine ephemeral fever virus	1	Africa, Asia, and Australia	Inactivated and attenuated	No	441
Bovine leukemia	++	*Retroviridae* (*Deltaretrovirus*)	Bovine leukemia virus	1	Worldwide, Control and eradication programs in some European countries	None	Yes	382
Bovine viral diarrhea	+++	*Flaviviridae* (*Pestivirus*)	Bovine viral diarrhea virus	1	Worldwide	Inactivated and attenuated	Yes	563
Foot-and-mouth disease	++++	*Picornaviridae* (*Aphthovirus*)	Foot-and-mouth disease viruses	7	Eradicated in Europe, North and Central America, Australia, Japan, and most island nations; controlled in several South American countries; common elsewhere	Inactivated	Yes	521
Malignant catarrhal fever (associated with sheep)	+	*Herpesviridae* (*Gammaherpesvirinae*)	Ovine herpesvirus 2	1	Worldwide	None	Yes	322
Malignant catarrhal fever (associated with wildebeest)	+	*Herpesviridae* (*Gammaherpesvirinae*)	Alcelaphine herpesvirus 1	1	Africa and elswhere in association with zoo animals	None	Yes	322
Bovine spongiform encephalopathy	++	BSE prion	BSE prion	NA	Europe, particularly the United Kingdom	None	Yes	576
Rabies	++	*Rhabdoviridae* (*Lyssavirus*)	Rabies virus	Several genotypes	Predominantly in Central and South America in association with vampire bat rabies	Inactivated and attenuated	Yes	432
Rift Valley fever	+++	*Bunyaviridae* (*Phlebovirus*)	Rift Valley fever virus	1	Africa	Attenuated and inactivated	No	473
Rinderpest	++	*Paramyxoviridae* (*Morbillivirus*)	Rinderpest virus	1	Eradicated except for some countries in Africa and parts of Asia	Attenuated	No	421
Respiratory diseases[a]								
Bovine respiratory syncytial disease	+++	*Paramyxoviridae* (*Pneumovirus*)	Bovine respiratory syncytial virus	1	Worldwide	Attenuated	No	426
Infectious bovine rhinotracheitis[b]	+++	*Herpesviridae* (*Alphaherpesvirinae*)	Bovine herpesvirus 1	1	Worldwide	Attenuated	Yes	309
Parainfluenza virus 3 infection	+	*Paramyxoviridae* (*Respirovirus*)	Parainfluenze virus 3	1	Worldwide	Inactivated and attenuated	No	416

[a]Rhinoviruses and adenoviruses have been associated with respiratory disease in cattle, but are of little clinical importance.
[b]Caused by same virus (bovine herpesvirus 1) as infectious pustular vulvovaginitis.

Table 42.2
Viral Diseases of Cattle Affecting Intestinal Tract, Reproductive System, and Skin

Disease	Importance	Family (subfamily or genus)	Virus	Number of types	Geographical distribution	Vaccine	Persistence	Pages
Enteric diseases[a]								
Bovine coronavirus diarrhea	+	*Coronaviridae* (*Coronavirus*)	Bovine coronavirus	1	Worldwide	Inactivated, given to dam	No	501
Bovine rotavirus diarrhea	+++	*Reoviridae* (*Rotavirus*)	Bovine rotaviruses	Several	Worldwide	Attenuated, given to dam	No	402
Bovine viral diarrhea	+++	*Flaviviridae* (*Pestivirus*)	Bovine viral diarrhea virus	2	Worldwide	Inactivated and attenuated	Yes	563
Reproductive and neonatal diseases								
Akabane disease	+	*Bunyaviridae* (*Bunyavirus*)	Akabane virus	1	Africa, Asia, Australia	Inactivated	No	476
Bluetongue	++	*Reoviridae* (*Orbivirus*)	Bluetongue viruses	25	Tropics and subtropics, temperate areas of North America	Attenuated, but used only in sheep	No, but viremia may last for about 100 days	398
Bovine viral diarrhea	+++	*Flaviviridae* (*Pestivirus*)	Bovine viral diarrhea virus	1	Worldwide	Inactivated and attenuated	Yes	563
Infectious pustular vulvovaginitis[b]	+++	*Herpesviridae* (*Alphaherpesvirinae*)	Bovine herpesvirus 1	1	Worldwide	Attenuated	Yes	309
Skin disease (including stomatitis)								
Bovine mammillitis (pseudolumpyskin disease)[c]	+	*Herpesviridae* (*Alphaherpesvirinae*)	Bovine herpesvirus 2	1	Worldwide	None	Yes	311
Bovine papillomatosis	+	*Papovaviridae* (*Papillomavirus*)	Bovine papillomaviruses	6	Worldwide	Inactivated, autogenous	Yes	339
Cowpox	+	*Poxviridae* (*Orthopoxvirus*)	Cowpox virus	1	Europe	None in use	No	282
Lumpyskin disease	+	*Poxviridae* (*Capripoxvirus*)	Lumpyskin disease virus	1	Africa	Attenuated	No	285
Mucosal disease[c]	++	*Flaviviridae* (*Pestivirus*)	Bovine viral diarrhea virus	1	Worldwide	Inactivated and attenuated	Yes	563
Pseudocowpox (milker's nodule)	+	*Poxviridae* (*Parapoxvirus*)	Pseudocowpox virus	1	Worldwide	None	No	292
Vesicular stomatitis	++	*Rhabdoviridae* (*Vesiculovirus*)	Vesicular stomatitis viruses	Several	Americas	Inactivated and attenuated	No	439

[a]Astroviruses, caliciviruses, and toroviruses have been associated with diarrhea in cattle.
[b]Caused by the same virus as infectious bovine rhinotracheitis.
[c]Part of the bovine viral diarrhea/mucosal disease complex.

Table 42.3
Generalized and Respiratory Diseases of Sheep and Goats

Disease	Importance	Family (subfamily or genus)	Virus	Number of types	Geographical distribution	Vaccine	Persistence	Pages
Generalized diseases (including diseases with central nervous system involvement)								
Bluetongue	++	*Reoviridae* (*Orbivirus*)	Bluetongue viruses	25	Tropics and subtropics, temperate areas of North America	Attenuated, but used only in sheep	No, but viremia may last for about 100 days	398
Caprine arthritis-encephalitis	++++	*Retroviridae* (*Lentivirus*)	Caprine arthritis–encephalitis virus	1	Most countries	None	Yes	385
Foot-and-mouth disease	++	*Picornaviridae* (*Aphthovirus*)	Foot-and-mouth disease viruses	7	Eradicated in Europe, North and Central America, Australia, Japan, and most island nations; controlled in several South American countries; common elsewhere	Inactivated	Yes	521
Goatpox	+	*Poxviridae* (*Capripoxvirus*)	Goatpox virus	1	Africa and Asia	Inactivated and attenuated	No	284
Louping ill	+	*Flaviviridae* (*Flavivirus*)	Louping ill virus	1	United Kingdom	Inactivated	No	563
Nairobi sheep disease	+	*Bunyaviridae* (*Nairovirus*)	Nairobi sheep disease	1	Africa	None used	No	477
Peste des petits ruminants	++	*Paramyxoviridae* (*Morbillivirus*)	Peste des petits ruminants virus	1	Africa, Indian subcontinent, and Middle East	Attenuated	No	423
Rift Valley fever	++	*Bunyaviridae* (*Phlebovirus*)	Rift Valley fever virus	1	Africa	Attenuated and inactivated	No	473
Scrapie	++	Scrapie prion	Scrapie prion	NA	Most countries	None	Yes	575
Sheeppox	++	*Poxviridae* (*Capripoxvirus*)	Sheeppox virus	1	Africa and Asia	Inactivated and attenuated	No	284
Respiratory diseases[a]								
Maedi/visna (ovine progressive pneumonia)	++	*Retroviridae* (*Lentivirus*)	Maedi/visna virus	1	Most countries	None	Yes	383
Ovine pulmonary adenomatosis (Jaagsiekte)	++	*Retroviridae* (*Betaretrovirus*)	Ovine pulmonary adenomatosis virus	1	Most countries	None	Yes	378
Parainfluenza virus 3 infection	+	*Paramyoviridae* (*Respirovirus*)	Parainfluenza virus 3	1	Worldwide	Inactivated and attenuated	No	416

[a]Adenoviruses and respiratory syncytial viruses have been associated with respiratory disease in sheep and goats, but are of little clinical importance.

Table 42.4
Viral Diseases of Sheep and Goats Affecting Intestinal Tract, Reproductive System, and Skin

Disease	Importance	Family (subfamily or genus)	Virus	Number of types	Geographical distribution	Vaccine	Persistence	Pages
Enteric diseases[a,b]								
Nairobi sheep disease	+	*Bunyaviridae* (*Nairovirus*)	Nairobi sheep disease	1	Africa	None used	No	477
Peste des petitis ruminants	++	*Paramyxoviridae* (*Morbillivirus*)	Peste des petitis ruminants virus	1	Africa, Indian subcontinent, and Middle East	Attenuated	No	423
Reproductive and neonatal diseases								
Akabane disease	+	*Bunyaviridae* (*Bunyavirus*)	Akabane virus	1	Africa, Asia, and Australia	Inactivated	No	476
Bluetongue	++	*Reoviridae* (*Orbivirus*)	Bluetongue viruses	25	Tropics and subtropics, temperate areas of North America	Attenuated but used only in sheep	No, but viremia may last for about 100 days	398
Border disease	+	*Flaviviridae* (*Pestivirus*)	Border disease virus and bovine viral diarrhea virus	1	Worldwide	None in use	Yes	566
Rift Valley fever	++	*Bunyaviridae* (*Phlebovirus*)	Rift Valley fever virus	1	Africa	Attenuated and inactivated	No	473
Wesselsbron disease	+	*Flaviviridae* (*Flavivirus*)	Wesselsbron virus	1	Africa	Attenuated	No	560
Skin diseases								
Goatpox	+	*Poxviridae* (*Capripoxvirus*)	Goatpox virus	1	Africa and Asia	Inactivated and attenuated	No	284
Orf (contagious pustular dermatitis)	++	*Poxviridae* (*Parapoxvirus*)	Orf virus	1	Worldwide	Wild-type virus, atypical site	No	289
Sheeppox	++	*Poxviridae* (*Capripoxvirus*)	Sheeppox virus	1	Africa and Asia	Inactivated and attenuated	No	284

[a]Rotaviruses, astroviruses, and adenoviruses have been associated with enteric disease in sheep and goats but are of little clinical importance.
[b]Two generalized diseases, which often present as enteric diseases.

Table 42.5
Generalized and Respiratory Viral Diseases of Swine

Disease	Importance	Family (subfamily or genus)	Virus	Number of types	Geographical distribution	Vaccine	Persistence	Pages
Generalized diseases (including diseases with central nervous system involvement)								
African swine fever	++++	*Asfarviridae* (*Asfivirus*)	African swine fever virus	Several genotypes	Sub-Saharan Africa and Sardinia	None	Yes	295
Encephalomyocarditis	+	*Picornaviridae* (*Cardiovirus*)	Encephalomyocarditis virus	1	Worldwide	None	No	531
Foot-and-mouth disease	++	*Picornaviridae* (*Aphthovirus*)	Foot-and-mouth disease viruses	7	Eradicated in Europe, North and Central America, Australia, Japan, and most island nations; controlled in several South American countries; common elsewhere	Inactivated	No	521
Hog cholera	++++	*Flaviviridae* (*Pestivirus*)	Hog cholera virus	1	Eradicated in North and Central America, Australia, and Japan; generally under control in European countries; common elsewhere	Attenuated	Yes	567
Porcine hemagglutinating encephalomyelitis	+	*Coronaviridae* (*Coronavirus*)	Porcine hemagglutinating encephalomyelitis virus	1	Worldwide	None	No	501
Porcine lymphosarcoma	+	*Retroviridae* (*Gammaretrovirus*)	Porcine lymphosarcoma virus	1	Worldwide	None	Yes	381
Porcine polioencephalomyelitis	+	*Picornaviridae* (*Enterovirus*)	Porcine polioencephalomyelitis virus	1	Worldwide	Inactivated, used in eastern Europe	No	529
Porcine reproductive and respiratory syndrome	+++	*Arteriviridae* (*Arterivirus*)	Lelystad virus (porcine reproductive and respiratory syndrome virus)	1	Worldwide except Australia	Attenuated	Yes	513
Postweaning multisystemic wasting syndrome	? Emerging	*Circoviridae* (*Circovirus*)	Porcine circovirus	?	North America and Europe	None	?	361
Pseudorabies	+++	*Herpesviridae* (*Alphaherpesvirinae*)	Suid herpesvirus 1 (pseudorabies virus)	1	Worldwide, except Australia	Inactivated and attenuated	Yes	312
Swine vesicular disease	+	*Picornaviridae* (*Enterovirus*)	Swine vesicular disease virus	1	Sporadic in Asia and Europe	None used	No	528
Vesicular exanthema of swine	NA	*Caliciviridae* (*Vesivirus*)	Vesicular exanthema of swine virus	Many	Eradicated	NA	No	535
Vesicular stomatitis	+	*Rhabdoviridae* (*Vesiculovirus*)	Vesicular stomatitis viruses	Several	Americas	Inactivated	No	439
Respiratory diseases								
Cytomegalic inclusion body disease of swine	+	*Herpesviridae* (*Betaherpesvirinae*)	Swine cytomegalovirus	1	Worldwide	None	Yes	322
Porcine reproductive and respiratory syndrome	+++	*Arterivirus*	Lelystad virus (porcine reproductive and respiratory syndrome virus)	1	Worldwide except Australia	Attenuated	Yes	513
Swine influenza	++	*Orthomyxoviridae* (*Influenzavirus A*)	Swine influenza virus	Several	Worldwide	Inactivated	No	464

Table 42.6
Viral Diseases of Swine Affecting Intestinal Tract, Reproductive System, and Skin

Disease	Importance	Family (Subfamily or Genus)	Virus	Number of Types	Geographical Distribution	Vaccine	Persistence	Pages
Enteric diseases								
Rotavirus gastroenteritis	+++	*Reoviridae* (*Rotavirus*)	Swine rotaviruses	Many	Worldwide	Attenuated, given to dam	No	402
Transmissible gastroenteritis	++	*Coronaviridae* (*Coronavirus*)	Transmissible gastroenteritis virus	1	Worldwide	Attenuated, given to dam	Yes	499
Reproductive and neonatal diseases								
Hog cholera	++++	*Flaviviridae* (*Pestivirus*)	Hog cholera virus	1	Eradicated in North and Central America, Australia, and Japan; generally under control in European countries; common elsewhere	Attenuated	Yes	567
Japanese encephalitis	+	*Flaviviridae* (*Flavivirus*)	Japanese encephalitis virus	1	Asia	Inactivated and attenuated	No	559
Porcine reproductive and respiratory syndrome	+++	*Arterivirus* (*Arterivirus*)	Lelystad virus (porcine reproductive and respiratory syndrome virus)	1	Worldwide except Australia	Attenuated	Yes	513
Pseudorabies	+++	*Herpesviridae* (*Alphaherpesvirinae*)	Suid herpesvirus 1 (pseudorabies virus)	1	Worldwide, except Australia and Japan	Inactivated and attenuated	Yes	312
Swine parvovirus disease	++	*Parvoviridae* (*Parvovirus*)	Swine parvovirus	1	Worldwide	Inactivated	Yes	354
Skin diseases (including stomatitis)								
Swinepox	+	*Poxviridae* (*Suipoxvirus*)	Swinepox virus	1	Worldwide	None used	No	286
Swine vesicular disease	+	*Picornaviridae* (*Enterovirus*)	Swine vesicular disease virus	1	Sporadic in Asia and Europe	None used	No	528
Vesicular exanthema of swine	NA	*Caliciviridae* (*Vesivirus*)	Vesicular exanthema of swine virus	Many	Eradicated	NA	No	535
Vesicular stomatitis	+	*Rhabdoviridae* (*Vesiculovirus*)	Vesicular stomatitis viruses	Several	Americas	Inactivated	No	439

Table 42.7
Generalized and Respiratory Viral Diseases of Horses

Disease	Importance	Family (subfamily or genus)	Virus	Number of types	Geographical distribution	Vaccine	Persistence	Pages
Generalized diseases (including diseases with central nervous system involvement)								
African horse sickness	++	*Reoviridae* (*Orbivirus*)	African horse sickness viruses	9	Africa	Attenuated	No	400
Borna disease	+	*Bornaviridae* (*Bornavirus*)	Borna disease virus	1	Europe	None	Yes	456
Eastern equine encephalitis	++	*Togaviridae* (*Alphavirus*)	Eastern equine encephalitis virus	1	Americas	Inactivated	No	549
Equine arteritis	+	*Arteriviridae* (*Arterivirus*)	Equine arteritis virus	1	Worldwide	Attenuated	Yes	511
Equine encephalosis	+	*Reoviridae* (*Orbivirus*)	Equine encephalosis viruses	Several	South Africa	None	No	402
Equine infectious anemia	+	*Retroviridae* (*Lentivirus*)	Equine infectious anemia virus	1	Worldwide	None	Yes	386
Venezuelan equine encephalitis	++	*Togaviridae* (*Alphavirus*)	Venezuelan equine encephalitis viruses	7	South and Central America	Inactivated and attenuated	No	549
Western equine encephalitis	+	*Togaviridae* (*Alphavirus*)	Western equine encephalitis virus	1	Americas	Inactivated	No	549
Respiratory diseases[a]								
Adenovirus pneumonia	+	*Adenoviridae* (*Mastadenovirus*)	Equine adenoviruses	2	Worldwide	None	Yes	332
Equine influenza	+++	*Orthomyxoviridae* (*Influenzavirus A*)	Equine influenza viruses	2	Worldwide	Inactivated	No	463
Equine rhinopneumonitis	+++	*Herpesviridae* (*Alphaherpesvirinae*)	Equine herpesvirus 4	1	Worldwide	Inactivated and attenuated	Yes	314
Equine abortion	+++	*Herpesviridae* (*Alphaherpesvirinae*)	Equine herpesvirus 1	1	Worldwide	Inactivated and attenuated	Yes	314

[a]Rhinoviruses and equine herpesvirus 2 have been isolated from horses with respiratory disease, but are of uncertain clinical importance.

Table 42.8
Viral Diseases of Horses Affecting Intestinal Tract, Reproductive System, and Skin

Disease	Importance	Family (subfamily or genus)	Virus	Number of types	Geographical distribution	Vaccine	Persistence	Pages
Entric diseases[a]								
Rotavirus gastroenteritis	+++	*Reoviridae* (*Rotavirus*)	Equine rotaviruses	Several	Worldwide	None	No	402
Reproductive and neonatal diseases								
Equine abortion	+++	*Herpesviridae* (*Alphaherpesvirinae*)	Equine herpesvirus 1	1	Worldwide	Inactivated and attenuated	Yes	314
Equine rhinopneumonitis	+	*Herpesviridae* (*Alphaherpesvirinae*)	Equine herpesvirus 4	1	Worldwide	Inactivated and attenuated	Yes	314
Equine arteritis	+	*Arteriviridae* (*Arterivirus*)	Equine arteritis virus	1	Worldwide	Attenuated	Yes	511
Equine coital exanthema	+	*Herpesviridae* (*Alphaherpesvirinae*)	Equine herpesvirus 3	1	Worldwide	None	Yes	315
Skin diseases (including stomatitis)								
Equine papillomatosis	+	*Papovaviridae* (*Papillomavirus*)	Equine papillomaviruses	Several	Worldwide	None	Yes	341
Equine sarcoid	+	*Papovaviridae* (*Papillomavirus*)	Bovine papillomavirus viruses 1 and 2	2	Worldwide	None	Yes	341
Vesicular stomatitis	+	*Rhabdoviridae* (*Vesiculovirus*)	Vesicular stomatitis viruses	Several	Americas	Inactivated	No	439

[a]Toroviruses and coronaviruses have been associated with enteric disease, but are of considered of minor importance.

Table 42.9
Viral Diseases of Dogs

Disease	Importance	Family (subfamily or genus)	Virus	Number of types	Geographical distribution	Vaccine	Persistence	Pages
Generalized diseases (including diseases with central nervous system involvement)								
Canine distemper	+++	*Paramyxoviridae* (*Morbillivirus*)	Canine distemper virus	1	Worldwide	Attenuated	Yes	423
Canine parvovirus disease	++++	*Parvoviridae* (*Parvovirus*)	Canine parvoviruses	2	Worldwide	Attenuated and inactivated	Yes	351
Infectious canine hepatitis	++	*Adenoviridae* (*Mastadenovirus*)	Canine adenovirus 1	1	Worldwide	Attenuated and inactivated	Yes	331
Rabies	+	*Rhabdoviridae* (*Lyssavirus*)	Rabies viruses	Several	Worldwide except some island countries	Inactivated and attenuated	Yes	432
Respiratory disease								
Canine tracheobronchitis	++	*Adenoviridae* (*Mastadenovirus*)	Canine adenovirus 2	1	Worldwide	Attenuated	Yes	331
Parainfluenza virus 2 infection	+	*Paramyxoviridae* (*Rubulavirus*)	Parainfluenza virus 2	1	Worldwide	None	No	418
Enteric diseases								
Canine coronavirus diarrhea	++	*Coronaviridae* (*Coronavirus*)	Canine coronavirus	1	Worldwide	Inactivated	?	503
Canine parvovirus disease	++++	*Parvoviridae* (*Parvovirus*)	Canine parvoviruses	2	Worldwide	Attenuated and inactivated	Yes	351
Reproductive and neonatal diseases								
Hemorrhagic disease of pups	++	*Herpesviridae* (*Alphaherpesvirinae*)	Canine herpesvirus 1	1	Worldwide	None	Yes	315
Skin diseases								
Canine papillomatosis	+	*Papovaviridae* (*Papillomavirus*)	Canine papillomaviruses	Several	Worldwide	None	Yes	341

TABLE 42.10
Viral Diseases of Cats

DISEASE	IMPORTANCE	FAMILY (SUBFAMILY OR GENUS)	VIRUS	NUMBER OF TYPES	GEOGRAPHICAL DISTRIBUTION	VACCINE	PERSISTENCE	PAGES
Generalized diseases (including diseases with central nervous system involvement)								
Feline acquired immunodeficiency syndrome	+++	*Retroviridae* (*Lentivirus*)	Feline immunodeficiency virus	1	Worldwide	None	Yes	387
Feline infectious peritonitis	+++	*Coronaviridae* (*Coronavirus*)	Feline infectious peritonitis virus	1	Worldwide	Attenuated (but of questioned value)	Yes	502
Feline leukemia	++++	*Retroviridae* (*Gammaretrovirus*)	Feline leukemia virus	1	Worldwide	Inactivated subunit	Yes	379
Feline panleukopenia	+++	*Parvoviridae* (*Parvovirus*)	Feline panleukopenia virus	1	Worldwide	Attenuated and inactivated	Yes	348
Rabies	+	*Rhabdoviridae* (*Lyssavirus*)	Rabies viruses	Several	Worldwide except some island countries	Inactivated and attenuated	Yes	432
Respiratory diseases								
Feline calicivirus disease	+++	*Caliciviridae* (*Vesivirus*)	Feline caliciviruses	Several	Worldwide	Attenuated and inactivated	Yes	536
Feline rhinotracheitis	+++	*Herpesviridae* (*Alphaherpesvirinae*)	Feline herpesvirus 1	1	Worldwide	Attenuated and inactivated	Yes	316
Enteric diseases								
Feline panleukopenia	+++	*Parvoviridae* (*Parvovirus*)	Feline panleukopenia virus	1	Worldwide	Attenuated and inactivated	Yes	348
Rotavirus gastroenteritis	+	*Reoviridae* (*Rotavirus*)	Feline rotaviruses	Several	Worldwide	None	No	402
Reproductive and neonatal diseases								
Feline panleukopenia	+++	*Parvoviridae* (*Parvovirus*)	Feline panleukopenia virus	1	Worldwide	Attenuated and inactivated	Yes	348
Skin diseases								
Cowpox virus infection	+	*Poxviridae* (*Orthopoxvirus*)	Cowpox virus	1	Europe	None	No	282

Table 42.11
Viral Diseases of Poultry

Disease	Host species	Importance	Family (subfamily or genus)	Virus	Number of types	Geographical distribution	Vaccine	Persistence	Pages
Generalized diseases (including diseases with central nervous system involvement)									
Adenovirus infection (egg drop syndrome)	Chickens, ducks, and turkeys	+	*Adenoviridae* (*Aviadenovirus*)	Avian adenoviruses 1–12	12	Worldwide	Inactivated	Yes	333
Avian encephalomyelitis	Chickens, ducks, and turkeys	+	*Picornaviridae* (*Enterovirus*)	Avian encephalomyelitis	1	Worldwide	Attenuated	No	530
Avian influenza	Chickens and turkeys	++	*Orthonyxoviridae* (*Influenzavirus A*)	Avian influenza viruses	Many	Worldwide[a]	Inactivated	No	466
Avian leukosis	Chickens	++	*Retroviridae* (*Alpharetrovirus*)	Avian leukosis virus	1	Worldwide	Inactivated and attenuated	Yes	375
Eastern equine encephalitis	Pheasants	+	*Togaviridae* (*Alphavirus*)	Eastern equine encephalitis virus	1	Americas	Inactivated	No	549
Infectious bursal disease	Chickens	++	*Birnaviridae* (*Birnavirus*)	Infectious bursal disease virus	1	Worldwide	Inactivated	No	406
Marek's disease	Chickens	+++	*Herpesviridae* (*Alphaherpesvirinae*)	Gallid herpesvirus 2 (Marek's disease virus)	2	Worldwide	Attenuated	Yes	318
Newcastle disease	Chickens pigeons, and other avian species	++++	*Paramyxoviridae* (*Rubulavirus*)	Newcastle disease virus	1	Worldwide[a]	Attenuated and inactivated	No	419
Respiratory diseases									
Avian infectious bronchitis	Chickens	+++	*Coronaviridae* (*Coronavirus*)	Avian infectious bronchitis virus	Several	Worldwide	Attenuated	Yes	505
Avian reovirus disease	Chickens and other avian species	+	*Reoviridae* (*Orthoreovirus*)	Avian reoviruses	11	Worldwide	None	?	396
Infectious laryngotracheitis	Chickens	+++	*Herpesviridae* (*Alphaherpesvirinae*)	Gallid herpesvirus 1 (infectious laryngotracheitis virus)	1	Worldwide	Attenuated	Yes	317
Enteric disease									
Duck hepatitis	Ducks and turkeys	+	*Picornaviridae* (*Enterovirus*)	Duck hepatitis viruses 1 and 3	2	Worldwide	Attenuated	?	530
Duck plague	Ducks	+	*Herpesviridae* (*Alphaherpesvirinae*)	Anatid herpesvirus 1 (duck plague herpesvirus)	1	Worldwide	None	Yes	321
Skin diseases									
Avian pox	All species	++	*Poxviridae* (*Avipoxvirus*)	Fowlpox and other poxviruses	Several	Worldwide	Attenuated	No	288

[a]Fowl plague (avian influenza) and velogenic Newcastle disease are regarded as exotic viruses in most developed countries.

TABLE 42.12
Viral Diseases of Fish

DISEASE	HOST SPECIES	IMPORTANCE	FAMILY	VIRUS	NUMBER OF TYPES	GEOGRAPHICAL DISTRIBUTION	VACCINE	PAGES
Channel catfish herpesvirus disease	Catfish	+++	*Herpesviridae*	Ictalurid herpesvirus 1	1	North and Central America	No	324
Eel rhabdovirus disease	Eels, trout	+	*Rhabdoviridae*	Eel rhabdovirus	1	America, Japan, and Europe	No	444
Hirame disease	Japanese flounder	+	*Rhabdoviridae*	Hirame disease rhabdovirus	1	Japan	?	444
Infectious hematopoietic necrosis	Salmonids	+++	*Rhabdoviridae*	Infectious hematopoietic necrosis virus	1	North America, Japan, China, France and Italy	Yes	444
Infectious pancreatic necrosis	Salmonids	+++	*Birnaviridae*	Infectious pancreatic necrosis virus	1	Worldwide	Yes	409
Lymphocystis	Many species	++	*Iridoviridae*	Lymphocystis virus	1	Worldwide	No	298
Perch rhabdovirus disease	Perch	+	*Rhabdoviridae*	Perch rhabdovirus	1	Europe	No	444
Pike fry rhabdovirus disease	Northern pike, cyprimids	+	*Rhabdoviridae*	Pike fry rhabdovirus	1	Europe and Russia	No	444
Rio Grande cichlid rhabdovirus disease	Rio Grande cichlid	+	*Rhabdoviridae*	Rio Grande cichlid rhabdovirus	1	United States	No	444
Salmon herpesvirus disease	Salmonids	+	*Herpesviridae*	Salmonid herpesviruses 1–2	2	North America	No	324
Snakehead rhabdovirus disease	Snakehead	+	*Rhabdoviridae*	Snakehead rhabdovirus	1	Southeast Asia	No	444
Spring viremia of carp	Cyprimids	++	*Rhabdoviridae*	Spring viremia of carp virus	1	Europe	No	444
Viral hemorrhagic septicemia	Salmonids	+++	*Rhabdoviridae*	Viral hemorrhagic septicemia virus	1	Europe and west coast of United States	Yes	442

Table 42.13
Viral Diseases of Laboratory Rodents and Lagomorphs

Disease	Host species	Importance	Family (subfamily or genus)	Virus	Number of types	Persistence	Pages
Generalized and respiratory diseases							
Cowpox	Rat	++	*Poxviridae* (*Orthopoxvirus*)	Cowpox virus	1	No	282
Encephalomyocarditis	Mouse and rat	+	*Picornaviridae* (*Cardiovirus*)	Encephalomyocarditis virus	1	No	531
Hantavirus infection	Rat	++	*Bunyaviridae* (*Hantavirus*)	Seoul virus	1	Yes	478
Lactate dehydrogenase-elevating virus infection[a]	Mouse	+	*Arteriviridae* (*Arterivirus*)	Lactic dehydrogenase-elevating virus	1	Yes	514
Lymphocytic choriomeningitis	Mouse	++	*Arenaviridae* (*Arenavirus*)	Lymphocytic choriomeningitis virus	1	Yes	488
Minute virus of mice infection	Mouse	++	*Parvoviridae* (*Parvovirus*)	Minute virus of mice	1	Yes	355
Mouse hepatitis	Mouse	++++	*Coronaviridae* (*Coronavirus*)	Mouse hepatitis viruses	Several	Yes	504
Mousepox (ectromelia)	Mouse	++++	*Poxviridae* (*Orthopoxvirus*)	Ectromelia virus	1	No	283
Murine polyomavirus infection	Mouse	+	*Papovaviridae* (*Polyomavirus*)	Murine polyomavirus	1	Yes	342
Myxomatosis	Rabbit	+++	*Poxviridae* (*Leporivirus*)	Myxoma virus	1	No	286
Pneumonia virus of mice infection	Mouse	++	*Paramyxoviridae* (*Pneumovirus*)	Pneumonia virus of mice	1	Yes	427
Rabbit hemorrhagic disease	Rabbit	++++	*Caliciviridae* (*Lagovirus*)	Rabbit hemorrhagic disease virus	1	No	538
Rabbitpox	Rabbit	++	*Poxviridae* (*Orthopoxvirus*)	Rabbitpox virus	1	No	282
Rat coronavirus infection	Rat	++	*Coronaviridae* (*Coronavirus*)	Rat coronavirus	?	Yes	505
Sendai virus infection	Mouse and other species	++++	*Paramyxoviridae* (*Respirovirus*)	Parainfluenza virus 1	1	No	418
Sialyldacryo-adenitis	Rat	+++	*Coronaviridae* (*Coronavirus*)	Sialyldacryoade-nitis virus	1	Yes	505
Enteric diseases							
Mouse hepatitis	Mouse	++++	*Coronaviridae* (*Coronavirus*)	Mouse hepatitis viruses	Several	Yes	504
Reovirus 3 infection	Mouse and other species	++	*Reoviridae* (*Orthoreovirus*)	Reovirus 3	1	Yes	396
Rotavirus infection (epizootic diarrhea of infant mice)	Mouse	++++	*Reoviridae* (*Rotavirus*)	Rotaviruses	Several	No	402

[a]Usually subclinical; potential contaminants of material collected from rodents and used for experimental studies.

Table 42.14
Viral Diseases of Nonhuman Primates

Disease	Host species	Importance	Family (subfamily or genus)	Virus	Number of types	Persistence	Pages
Adenovirus disease	All species	+	*Adenoviridae* (*Mastadenovirus*)	Adenoviruses	Many	Yes	328
Ateline herpesvirus infection	Spider monkey	?	*Herpesviridae*	Ateline herpesvirus 2	1	Yes	321
B virus infection	*Macaca* spp.	+++	*Herpesviridae* (*Alphaherpesvirinae*, *Varicellovirus*)	B virus (Cercopithecine herpesvirus 1)	1	Yes	316
Baboon herpesvirus infection	Baboon	?	*Herpesviridae* (*Gammaherpesvirinae*)	Cercopithecine herpesvirus 12	1	Yes	321
Chimpanzee herpesvirus infection	Chimpanzee	?	*Herpesviridae* (*Gammaherpesvirinae*)	Pongine herpesvirus 1	1	Yes	321
Cytomegalic inclusion body disease	All species	++	*Herpesviridae* (*Betaherpesvirinae*)	Cytomegaloviruses	Species specific	Yes	322
Monkeypox	All species	+++	*Poxviridae* (*Orthopoxvirus*)	Monkeypox virus	1	No	284
Simian varicella	Old World monkeys	++	*Herpesviridae* (*Alphaherpesvirinae*, *Varicellovirus*)	Cercopithecine herpesviruses 6, 7, and 9	3 (very closely related)	Yes	317
Many other herpesvirus diseases of captive nonhuman primates	All species	++	*Herpesviridae*	Many species-specific herpesviruses	Many	Yes	321

Further Reading

Bhatt, P. N., Jacoby, R. O., Morse, H. C., and New, A. E. (1986). "Viral and Rickettsial Infections of Laboratory Rodents." Academic Press, Orlando, FL.

Blood, D. C., and Radostits, O. M. (1994). "Veterinary Medicine: A Textbook of the Diseases of Cattle, Sheep, Pigs, Goats and Horses," 8th ed. Saunders, Philadelphia, PA.

Blowey, R. W., and Weaver, A. D. (1991). "A Colour Atlas of Diseases and Disorders of Cattle." Wolfe, London.

Calnek, B. N., Barnes, H. J., Beard, C. N., McDougald, L. R., and Saif, Y. M., eds. (1997). "Diseases of Poultry," 10th ed. Iowa State University Press, Ames.

Castro, A. E., and Heuschle, W. P., eds. (1992). "Veterinary Diagnostic Virology—A Practitioner's Guide." Mosby, New York.

Coetzer, J. A. W., Thompson, G. R., and Tustin, R. C., eds. (1994). "Infectious Diseases of Livestock with Special Reference to Southern Africa," 2 Vol. Oxford University Press, Cape Town.

Darai, G., ed. (1987). "Virus Diseases in Laboratory and Captive Animals." Kluwer, Boston, MA.

Ettinger, S. J., and Feldman, E. C. (1995). "Textbook of Veterinary Internal Medicine," 4th ed., 2 vols. Saunders, Philadelphia, PA.

Fowler, M. E., ed. (1986). "Zoo and Wild Animal Medicine," 2nd Ed. Saunders, Philadelphia, PA.

Fraser, C. M. (1998). "The Merck Veterinary Manual: A Handbook of Diagnosis, Therapy, and Disease Prevention and Control for the Veterinarian," 8th ed. Merck, Rahway, NJ.

Gaskell, R. M., and Bennett, M. (1996). "Feline and Canine Infectious Diseases." Blackwell, London.

Gorman, N., ed. (1998). "Canine Medicine and Therapeutics," 4th ed. Blackwell, London.

Greene, C. E., ed. (1998). "Infectious Diseases of the Dog and Cat," 2nd ed. Saunders, Philadelphia, PA.

Horzinek, M. C., ed. (1987–1996). "Virus Infections of Vertebrates," Book Series, Vols. 1–6. Elsevier, Amsterdam.

Howard, J. L., ed. (1992). "Current Veterinary Therapy 3, Food Animal Practice." Saunders, Philadelphia, PA.

Hugh-Jones, M. E., Hubbert, W. T., and Hagstad, H. V. (1995). "Zoonoses: Recognition, Control, and Prevention." Iowa State University Press, Ames.

Johnson-Delaney, C., ed. (1997). "Exotic Companion Medicine Handbook for Veterinarians." Wingers Publishing, Lake Worth, FL.

Leman, A. D., Straw, B. E., Mengeling, W. L., D'Allaire, S., and Taylor, D. J., eds. (1992). "Diseases of Swine." Iowa State University Press, Ames.

Martin, W. B., and Aitkin, I. D., eds. (1991). "Diseases of Sheep," 2nd Ed. Blackwell, London.

National Research Council, National Academy of Sciences of the United States of America. (1991). "Infectious Diseases of Mice and Rats." National Academy Press, Washington, DC.

Pedersen, N. C. (1988). "Feline Infectious Diseases." American Veterinary Publications, Goleta, CA.

Randall, C. J. (1991). "A Colour Atlas of Diseases and Disorders of the Domestic Fowl and Turkey," 2nd ed. Wolfe, London.

Ritchie, B. W. (1995). "Avian Viruses: Function and Control" (Book and CD-ROM). Wingers Publishing, Lake Worth, FL.

Ritchie, B. W., Harrison, G. J., and Harrison, L. R., eds. (1994). "Avian Medicine: Principles and Application" (Book and CD-ROM). Wingers Publishing, Lake Worth, FL.

Smith, W. J., Taylor, D. J., and Penny, R. H. C. (1990). "A Colour Atlas of Diseases and Disorders of the Pig." Wolfe, London.

Timoney, J. F., Gillespie, J. H., Scott, F. N., and Barlough, J. E. (1988). "Hagan and Bruner's Infectious Diseases of Domestic Animals," 8th Ed. Cornell University Press, Ithaca. NY.

Wolf, K. (1988). "Fish Viruses and Fish Viral Diseases." Comstock Publishing Associates (Cornell University Press), Ithaca., NY.

Glossary

abortive infection Viral infection in which some viral genes are expressed but no infectious virus is produced
acetylethyleneimine (or ethyleneimine) One of a group of related alkylating agents used in the preparation of inactivated vaccines
acquired immunity *See* immunity
acquired immunodeficiency syndrome (AIDS) Disease caused by human immunodeficiency viruses 1 or 2 (HIV1 or 2) and resulting in a wide range of adverse immunological and clinical conditions
activator A DNA-binding protein that binds upstream of a gene and activates its transcription
active immunization Specific acquired immunity resulting from immunization with a vaccine (as contrasted with passive immunization resulting from the transfer of antibodies)
Acyclovir A potent and specific antiviral agent against herpesviruses; its inhibitory action results from its selective phosphorylation by the virus-induced thymidine kinase and subsequent inhibition of the virus-encoded DNA polymerase
adjuvant Substance administered with antigen that enhances the immune response nonspecifically
adoptive transfer The transfer of cells, commonly lymphocytes, from an immunized donor to a nonimmune recipient
adsorption *See* attachment
affinity Thermodynamic measure of the strength of binding of an individual Fab fragment of an antibody molecule to an antigenic determinant
affinity maturation Increase in affinity of antibodies associated with mutation/selection of the hypervariable regions of immunoglobulin genes
agammaglobulinemia Complete absence of immunoglobulins (antibodies) in the blood
agarose One of the polysaccharide constituents of agar that is widely used as a support medium for electrophoresis
airborne transmission Method of spread of infection by droplet nuclei or dust
allele One of two or more alternative forms of a gene at the same site or locus in each of a pair of chromosomes that determine alternative characters in inheritance
alternate complement pathway Pathway of complement activation initiated via C3, without previous activation of C1, C4, and C2, as in the classical pathway; does not require antibody
ambisense (applied to single-stranded RNA viral genomes) Part of the nucleotide sequence is of positive sense, part is of negative sense
amino acid Basic building block of proteins that contains amino and carboxyl groups plus a variable side chain that determines the properties of the individual amino acid; 20 amino acids occur commonly in nature
amino acid sequence Linear order of the amino acids in a peptide or protein
amino group (-NH_2) A chemical group, characteristically basic because it tends to bind a proton to form -NH_3^+; the aminoterminus of a polypeptide is the end with a free α-amino group
amphotropic virus Pertaining to a retrovirus that will replicate in the cells of one or more species in addition to those of the original host
anamnestic (secondary) response Rapid rise in antibody and/or cell-mediated immunity following second or subsequent exposure to antigen
anchorage independence Ability of a cell transformed by an oncogenic virus to grow in suspension in liquid or semisolid agar medium
Ångstrom 0.1 nm (10^{-10}m)
antibody (immunoglobulin) A protein produced by B lymphocytes (plasma cells) following exposure to an antigen. Antibody binds specifically to the antigen (or hapten) that elicited its synthesis
antibody–complement-mediated cytotoxicity Cell lysis mediated by antibody and complement, usually via the alternate complement activation pathway
antibody-dependent cell-mediated cytotoxicity (ADCC) Lysis of target cells that express viral antigen on their surface, to which specific antibody binds. Immunologically nonspecific killer cells bind via Fc receptors to the antibody and mediate lysis
anticodon Group of three bases in a tRNA molecule that recognizes (via base pairing) a codon in an mRNA
antigen Substance, usually foreign, that induces an immune response when introduced into an animal. An antigen binds specifically to the antibody so produced
antigenic determinant (epitope) Region of an antigen that binds antibody or is recognized by the T cell receptor in association with MHC proteins
antigenic drift (genetic drift) Point mutation(s) in a gene(s) specifying the surface protein(s) of a virus, resulting in enough antigenic change to allow immune escape
antigenic shift (genetic shift) Genetic reassortment or recombination between viruses resulting in major antigenic change and the emergence of a new variant
antigen-presenting cells Dendritic cells, Langerhans' cells, macrophages, or B lymphocytes that process and present antigenic peptides in association with MHC proteins

Many of the terms have a wide usage in biology; here they are described in terms of virology. For more detailed definitions, see B. W. J. Mahy, "A Dictionary of Virology," Academic Press, San Diego, 1997; D. C. Blood and V. P. Studdert, "Saunders Comprehensive Veterinary Dictionary," 2nd ed. W.B. Saunders, Philadelphia PA, 1999. R. C. King, and W. D. Stansfield, "A Dictionary of Genetics," 5th Ed., Oxford University Press, Oxford, 1996; W. J. Herbert, P. C. Wilkinson, and D. I. Stott, eds., "Dictionary of Immunology," 4th Ed., Academic Press, New York, 1995; J. Swinton, ed., "A Dictionary of Epidemiology," http://epidem13.plantsci.cam.ac.uk/~js/glossary/gloss98.htm

antisense gene A gene in which the orientation of the coding sequence with respect to the promoter has been reversed; RNAs transcribed from such a gene can hybridize with mRNAs transcribed from the normal gene, thereby inhibiting its ultimate translation into protein
antiseptic Chemical antibacterial or antiviral substance for use on skin or mucous membranes
antiserum Serum from an animal exposed to an antigen and containing specific antibodies
apoptosis (programmed cell death) A process that regulates the life span of a cell that involves an endonuclease-directed degradation of chromosomal DNA that leads to death of cells; may occur as a result of virus infection
arbovirus (*ar*thropod-*bo*rne virus) A virus that replicates in an arthropod and is transmitted by bite to a vertebrate host in which it also replicates
assembly units (and subassemblies) Assemblages of structural proteins, forming the most complex units used to assemble viral capsids
attachment (adsorption) Specific adsorption of virus to its receptor on the plasma membrane of the host cell
attenuated Reduced in virulence
autoimmunity Production of an immune response against an organism's own tissues; may involve both humoral and cell-mediated responses
autologous Related to self; belonging to the same organism
autoradiography A technique for the detection of radioactivity in cytological and biochemical preparations, such as gels or membranes, by exposure to photographic film
avidity Measure of the firmness of the binding of antigen to antibody; influenced by affinity and valence
avirulent Lacking in virulence
axenic (Greek, *xenos,* stranger) Totally free of infection with viruses or microorganisms
AZT (azidothymidine) A thymidine analog that blocks DNA replication and is used in the treatment of HIV infection
bacteriophage (or phage) A virus that replicates in a bacterium
base pair A pair of nucleotides held together by hydrogen bonding; double-stranded DNA contains G–C and A–T base pairs and double-stranded RNA contains G–C and A–U base pairs; highly structured, single-stranded RNAs such as tRNA may also contain a variety of additional "non-Watson–Crick" base pairings
benign tumor A circumscribed neoplasm produced by excessive proliferation of cells, but without a tendency for invasiveness or metastasis
bicistronic mRNA A messenger RNA containing two ribosome-binding sites
bioassay Determination of the amount of a virus or a viral product by measuring a biological activity such as infectivity or immunogenicity
biolistics Use of DNA-coated pellets, fired at high speed, usually with an air gun ("Gene Gun") to place DNA into animal cells, as with DNA vaccines
biological control Use of parasites, predators, or pathogens, including viruses, to control pests
biological transmission Transmission of a virus by an arthropod after it has replicated in the tissues of the arthropod
biotechnology Application for industrial purposes of scientific of biological principles, including the use of recombinant DNA technology and genetic engineering to manufacture a wide variety of biologically useful substances such as vaccines, hormones, and cytokines
B lymphocyte (B cell) Lymphocyte derived from the bursa of Fabricius in birds or its equivalent (bone marrow) in mammals. B lymphocytes differentiate into antibody-producing plasma cells
booster Second or subsequent dose of vaccine given to enhance the immune response
budding Process of maturation and release of enveloped virus particles from infected cells in which the viral nucleocapsid associates with an area of the plasma membrane modified by the insertion of viral glycoprotein peplomers and sometimes other viral proteins from which the mature enveloped virus particle is eventually released from the cell
buoyant density Density at which a virus or other macromolecule neither sinks nor floats when suspended in a density gradient (e.g., CsCl or sucrose)
bursa of Fabricius Lymphoid organ in the cloaca of birds that controls the ontogeny of B lymphocytes
burst size Yield of infectious virus particles obtained during the infection of a single host cell
C particle A budding form of retroviruses containing a central core and lipoprotein envelope covered with knob-like peplomers; associated with leukemias and lymphomas and named for the "C shape" of virions in thin section electron microscopy
cachectin Tumor necrosis factor
cancer Vernacular term covering all types of malignant tumors that, if untreated, cause the death of the host
cap (5′-cap) A molecule of 7-methylguanosine present on the 5′ terminus of the genome of some positive-sense, single-stranded RNA viruses or added to the 5′ terminus of RNA transcripts as part of their processing into mRNAs
capsid Icosahedrally symmetrical shell-like structure composed of aggregated protein subunits that surrounds the viral nucleic acid
capsomer Morphological unit from which the virus capsid is built and often consisting of groups of identical protein molecules
carboxyl group COOH A chemical group that is characteristically acidic as a result of the tendency of its proton to dissociate; the carboxy terminus of a polypeptide is the end that carries a free α-carboxyl group (C terminus)
carcinogen Agent (usually chemical) causing cancer
carcinoma Malignant tumor of epithelial cell origin
carrier An individual animal that is infected persistently with a virus but may have no clinical signs of disease; virus may be shed continuously, intermittently, or not at all
case-control study An epidemiological study in which the risk factors of animals with a disease are compared with those without the disease
catalyst Substance that can increase the rate of a chemical reaction without being consumed (e.g., enzymes are biological catalysts)
CD4 A protein complex first identified on human T helper lymphocytes using monoclonal antibodies and subsequently found on other cells; the primary cellular receptor of HIV virus on human lymphocytes; the protein is used as a marker to identify T helper and certain other cells
cell culture *In vitro* growth of cells in suspension or as a monolayer on a solid surface such as the inside surface of a plastic culture flask
cell cycle Cyclical sequence of events in cell division that includes G1, a "resting" phase (G is for gap); S, during which the chromosomes are duplicated (S is for DNA synthesis); G2; and M (which is for mitosis); highly differentiated nondividing cells are said to be in G0

cell fusion Formation of a hybrid cell containing nuclei and cytoplasm from different cells; induced by inactivated paramyxoviruses, viral fusion proteins, or chemicals such as polyethylene glycol

cell-free extract Extract containing subcellular organelles and soluble molecules that is made by cell lysis and removal of large particulate components by centrifugation

cell-mediated immunity Immunity affected predominantly by T lymphocytes (and accessory cells, notably macrophages) rather than by antibody

chemoprophylaxis Drug treatment designed to prevent future occurrences of disease

chemotherapy Drug treatment of a diseased animal

chromosome Self-replicating genetic structure of cells containing the cellular DNA that bears the linear array of genes in its nucleotide sequence. Eukaryotic genomes consist of a number of chromosomes whose DNA is associated with different kinds of proteins. In prokaryotes, chromosomal DNA is circular and the entire genome is carried on one chromosome

chronic infection Infection characterized by continued presence of virus, with or without continuing signs of disease

***cis* and *trans*-acting genetic and molecular actions** In genetics, *cis* refers to linked markers and *trans* to separated markers. In molecular biology, the terms distinguish intermolecular (*trans*) from intramolecular (*cis*) actions. A *trans*-acting controlling effect of a regulatory gene refers to an action on a structural gene at some distance from it (in eukaryotic cells this may be on the same chromosome or on a different chromosome); a *cis*-acting controlling effect of a regulatory gene refers to an action on a structural gene that is adjacent to it

cisternae Membrane-bound channels of vesicles present in normal cells or that proliferate in the cytoplasm of some virus-infected cells

***cis–trans* test** A genetic complementation test used to establish whether two mutations are in the same gene; this test was first used in the genetic mapping of bacteriophage T4 and requires that the wild-type allele be dominant

cistron Basic unit of genetic function, usually a gene or protein-coding sequence

classical complement pathway Series of sequential enzyme–substrate interactions activated by antibody–antigen complexes and involving all complement components

clathrin-coated pits Depressions in plasma membrane coated with clathrin, a fibrous protein, that contain the receptors for viruses undergoing receptor-mediated endocytosis

clone A population of cells or viral particles derived from a single precursor cell or virion and thus having essentially the same genetic constitution

cloning (molecular) Term denoting the isolation and propagation of foreign genes in prokaryotic or eukaryotic cells by recombinant DNA technology

cloning vector Plasmid or viral DNA into which foreign DNA may be inserted to be propagated using recombinant DNA techniques

coat protein External structural protein(s) of a virus

cocarcinogen Two or more agents that may not be carcinogenic separately, but that together induce cancer

coding redundancy Coding of the same amino acid following substitution of one of the four nucleotides for another as the third nucleotide of the triplet (codon)

coding sequence That portion of a nucleic acid that directly specifies the amino acid sequence of a protein product; noncoding sequences may contain various regulatory sequences

codon Triplet of nucleotides that codes for a single amino acid or a translation stop

cohort A subsection of an animal population with a common feature, such as age

cohort study Attempt to identify the cause of a disease by comparing exposed and nonexposed (control) populations in a prospective epidemiological study

cold-adapted mutant Virus that replicates best at lower than body temperature

complement system Series of serum proteins, the first of which binds to any antibody–antigen complex triggering a cascade reaction; cleavage components of the complement proteins either as part of an antibody complex or as soluble components exert a variety of effects, including lysis of microorganisms and infected cells, phagocytosis, chemotaxis, and inflammation

complementary base sequences Polynucleotide sequences that are able to form perfect hydrogen-bonded duplexes, every G base paired with a C and every A base paired with a T or U

complementary determining regions *See* hypervariable regions

complementary DNA (cDNA) A single-stranded DNA molecule that is complementary to the base sequence of the single-stranded template from which it was transcribed; often applied to DNA transcribed from RNA using reverse transcriptase

complementation Occurs in cells that are doubly infected in which one of the viruses provides a gene product that the other requires but cannot make

concatemer Long molecules containing a number of identical monomers linked in a head-to-tail fashion such as DNA or RNA molecules formed as intermediates in the replication of some viruses

conditional lethal mutant Virus that will not replicate under conditions in which the wild-type virus replicates, but will replicate under permissive conditions, such as a different temperature or in another cell line

conformation Overall shape of macromolecules resulting from multiple weak interactions among charged side chains and fewer strong interactions, such as S–S bonds

conformational epitope Epitope composed of nonadjacent amino acids in the same or different polypeptide chains that are brought into proximity in the native protein by folding

congenital infection Infection occurring at or before birth

consensus sequence Archetypal amino acid sequence with which all variants are compared

conserved sequence A nucleotide sequence in a DNA or RNA genome (or an amino acid sequence in a protein) that has remained essentially unchanged throughout evolution

contact inhibition Phenomenon in which cells stop dividing when their cell membranes make contact

core Innermost structure(s) of a virus, the part remaining on removal of the envelope and outer capsid shells

covalent bonds Strong bonds formed by the sharing of electron pairs between atoms; also termed primary bonds

crepuscular Pertaining to animals that become active at twilight and/or at sunrise, such as certain bats, other mammals such as deer, insects, and birds. Contrasts with animals that are nocturnal and diurnal.

critical population size Minimum size of population needed to ensure the endemic status of an infection

cross-protection Protection against virus infection resulting from previous inoculation of the host with a closely related virus

crystallography Science dealing with the study of crystals; such study is the basis for our understanding of the nature of viral proteins and more complex substructures

C terminus End of the peptide with a free α-carboxyl group (traditionally written as the right end)
cup probang Cup on end of flexible rod used for obtaining samples of pharyngeal or esophageal mucus or cells from large animals
cycloheximide Antibiotic isolated from *Streptomyces griseus* that reversibly inhibits eukaryotic (but not prokaryotic) protein biosynthesis
cytocidal (noncytocidal) infection Virus infection resulting in (or not producing) destruction of the infected cell
cytokine Polypeptide that participates in cellular signaling after secretion into the extracellular space and binding to receptors on the same, nearby, or distant target cells (e.g., interferon γ, interleukin 2)
cytolytic Causing cell lysis
cytopathic effect Morphologic changes in cells resulting from viral infection
cytopathogenic Refers to a virus that causes a cytopathic effect
cytoplasm That part of the cell within the cell membrane but outside the nucleus and other organelles
cytoskeleton Intracellular scaffolding and transport system consisting largely of two proteins, tubulin and actin
cytosol Substance of the cytoplasm
cytotoxic Having a deleterious effect on cells
cytotoxic T cell (CTL; Tc) Subset of T lymphocytes capable of antigen-specific lysis of virus-infected cells that express a viral peptide(s) on their surface in association with MHC class I protein
dalton Unit of mass equal to that of a single hydrogen atom. *See* molecular mass
defective interfering virus (or particle) Virus particle with an incomplete genome that may interfere with the replication of infectious virus
defective virus A virus that cannot replicate because it is defective in some way, usually lacking some essential gene; some defective viruses can replicate in mixed infections with a helper virus
delayed hypersentivity T lymphocyte-mediated, antibody-independent, antigen-specific inflammatory reaction; particularly involves Th1 lymphocytes and activated macrophages
deletion mutation Loss of a portion of the viral genetic material ranging in size from a single nucleotide to entire genes
demyelination Destruction of the myelin sheath formed by Schwann cells surrounding peripheral nerve axons or the myelin sheath formed by oligodendrocytes surrounding neuronal processes in the brain
denaturation Loss of the native conformation of a macromolecule due to the breakage of weak bonds (H bonds, etc.); usually results from heat treatment or exposure to extreme pH or certain chemicals
dendritic cell Cell in the skin, lymphoid organs, reticuloendothelial tissues, and other sites that functions in the processing of antigen
density gradient ultracentrifugation Method for separating macromolecules or organelles based on differences in their density through use of a density gradient (usually CsCl or sucrose)
deoxyribonucleoside A purine or pyrimidine base attached by an N–C bond to 2-deoxyribose, a five-carbon sugar
deoxyribonucleotide A deoxyribonucleoside carrying a phosphate group at the 3′ or 5′ position on the ribose sugar
dimer Structure resulting from covalent bonding or aggregation of two subunits; if subunits are identical, a homodimer is formed, if different, a heterodimer is formed
diploid genome Genome that contains two copies of each gene
disinfectant Antibacterial and/or antiviral chemical substance for use on inanimate surfaces
DNA (deoxyribonucleic acid) Polymer of two long chains of deoxyribonucleotides twisted into a double helix and joined by hydrogen bonds between the complementary bases adenine and thymine or cytosine and guanine; carries the genetic information in all cells and some viruses; capable of self-replication and directing the synthesis of RNA
DNA polymerase I *Escherichia coli* enzyme able to catalyze the formation of 3′→5′ phosphodiester bonds in DNA; also possesses 3′→5′ proofreading activity and 3′→5′ double-strand exonuclease activity; it repairs and finishes the replication of DNA
DNA polymerase III *Escherichia coli* enzyme that catalyzes the formation of 3′→5′ phosphodiester bonds at a very rapid rate; also possesses 3′→5′ exonuclease activity for proofreading; its chief role is in DNA replication
DNA-dependent RNA polymerase Enzyme that transcribes RNA from a DNA template; in eukaryotic cells, DNA-dependent RNA polymerase I directs the synthesis of ribosomal RNAs, mRNAs, and tRNAs
DNA–RNA hybrid Double helix containing one strand of DNA hydrogen bonded to one strand of RNA
double-stranded Nucleic acid that occurs as a two-stranded helix
early viral genes Genes that are transcribed before viral nucleic acid replication occurs
eclipse period Interval between viral penetration and appearance of the first progeny virions
ecology Field of science dealing with the mutual relations between organisms, including viruses, and their environment
ecotropic viruses Retroviruses that replicate only in cells from the host species from which they were isolated originally
efficacy An index of the effectiveness of a vaccine or drug (e.g., the percentage of animals that are protected by the vaccine)
electron microscope Instrument that uses a beam of electrons focused by electromagnets to obtain magnified images of specimens; the shorter wavelength of electrons permits greater magnification than is possible with an optical (light) microscope; resolution below 1 nm is attainable
electrophoresis A method of separating large molecules (such as DNA fragments or proteins) from a mixture of similar molecules. An electric current is passed through a medium containing the mixture, and each kind of molecule travels through the medium at a different rate, depending on its electrical charge and size. Separation is based on these differences. Agarose and acrylamide gels are the media commonly used for electrophoresis of proteins and nucleic acids
electroporation Treatment of cells with a high voltage electric current that produces transient pores through which DNA is introduced into the cell
elimination Total control of an infectious disease, usually on a regional scale. Contrast with eradication, which is usually used to denote elimination on a national or global scale
endemic (disease) (1) A term to describe a level of infection in a defined population that does not exhibit wide fluctuations in incidence over time and/or (2) a term to indicate an infection persisting in a population over a long time without reintroduction from outside
endocytosis Uptake by a cell of virus or other material from the environment by invagination of the plasma membrane; it includes both phagocytosis and pinocytosis. Commonly, the full term "receptor-mediated endocytosis" is used when referring to the entry of viruses into cells
endogenous pathway (of viral antigen processing) Production of antigenic peptides by the degradation of endogenously synthesized viral polypeptides and their association with MHC class I proteins and presentation on the cell surface

endogenous virus Virus whose genome is integrated into the germ cell DNA and is thus able to spread by vertical transmission (e.g., certain retroviruses)
endonuclease Enzyme that cleaves DNA or RNA at internal sites in the nucleotide sequence
endoplasmic reticulum Cytoplasmic membrane system of cells involved in the synthesis and intracellular distribution of proteins
endosome Intracellular vesicle formed from the cell membrane that is involved in intracellular transport
enhancer Sequences in genomic DNA that increase the rate of transcription
envelope Lipoprotein outer covering of some viruses, derived from cellular membrane, but containing virus-specific proteins, usually glycoprotein peplomers (some viral envelopes also contain a virus-coded matrix protein)
enzootic Same as endemic, but referring to nonhuman host populations; not used in this book
enzyme A protein (or occasionally an RNA molecule) that acts as a catalyst, speeding the rate at which a biochemical reaction proceeds but not altering the direction or nature of the reaction
enzyme immunoassay (EIA) or enzyme-linked immunosorbent assay (ELISA) Widely used sensitive immunoassay that uses an enzyme linked to an antibody or antigen as a marker for the detection of a specific antigen or antibody. In the most common methods a reagent antigen (or antibody) is immobilized on a solid matrix (often a microtiter well) and the test specimen containing antibody (or antigen) is added. Binding of the antibody (or antigen) to the matrix is recognized by the addition of a detector (e.g., an antibody specific for the suspect antibody or an antibody specific for the suspect antigen)—the detector is conjugated to an enzyme that produces a colored product when its substrate is added. This colored product indicates a positive reaction
eosinophilic Staining readily with eosin, producing a pink color
epidemic Major increase in disease incidence affecting either a large number of animals or spreading over a large area
epidemiology Study of the role of various factors that determine the incidence and distribution of infectious diseases over time and place
episome Autonomous extra-chromosomal genetic element (which may later become integrated into chromosomal DNA or may remain separate). *See* plasmid
epithelial tissue Cells making up the exterior and interior surfaces of tissues and organs
epitope *See* antigenic determinant
epizootic Same as epidemic, but referring to nonhuman host populations; not used in this book
eradication Elimination of an infectious disease, usually on a national or global scale
etiology Cause(s) of disease
eukaryote Organisms that have (1) a genome divided among multiple chromosomes contained within a nuclear envelope, (2) a cytoplasm containing membrane-bound organelles and 80 S ribosomes, and (3) a biochemistry differentiating them from prokaryote cells (i.e., bacteria and blue-green algae)
evolution Gradual change of organisms and viruses over time due to the selection of favorable genetic mutations
excision Release of an integrated provirus; reversal of integration (also called induction or activation); also removal of mismatched or damaged nucleotides from DNA molecules
exocytosis Discharge from a cell of particles that are too large to diffuse through the plasma membrane; the opposite of endocytosis
exogenous pathway (of viral antigen processing) Production of antigenic peptides by degradation of antigens that are phagocytosed by antigen-presenting cells and their association with MHC class I proteins and presentation on the cell surface
exogenous retroviruses Horizontally transmitted retroviruses
exon A sequence of nucleotides, contiguous or not, in DNA that encodes a protein(s). In eukaryotic cells, the DNA sequences encoding primary RNA transcripts are usually not contiguous; instead, coding sequences must be spliced together (i.e., introns must be excised) to form functional mRNA
exotic virus Virus not normally occurring in a particular country. Often used in veterinary medicine in the context of "foreign animal diseases"
explant Tissue taken from the body and grown in an artificial medium without dissociation of individual cells
expression vector *See* cloning vector
extrinsic Of external origin
extrinsic incubation period Interval between the feeding by an arthropod on a viremic host and the development of infectious virus in the arthropod so that it may then transmit virus to another host
Fab ("fragment antigen-binding") That portion of an immunoglobulin molecule produced by papain digestion that comprises the variable domains of the light and heavy chains (containing the antigen-binding site), as well as the constant domain of the light chain and part of the constant domain of the heavy chain
Fc ("fragment crystallizable") That portion of an immunoglobulin molecule produced by papain digestion that comprises the major part of the constant domains of the heavy chains; this fragment does not bind to antigen but is responsible for effector functions
Fc receptor Receptor present on various leukocytes that binds immunoglobulin via its Fc segment
filamentous Having a long thread-like structure; used to describe some viruses such as filoviruses
flow cytometry Technique used to identify and separate different types of cells, based on detecting (and in some cases separating) cells with bound fluorescent labels using a laser light beam (and a high throughput droplet collector)
fluorescent antibody (immunofluorescence) Antibody conjugated to a fluorescent dye and used in combination with a fluorescence microscope to detect the presence of viral antigens in cells
focus Cluster of morphologically transformed or damaged cells in a monolayer culture, initiated by a single virus particle. Foci may be quantitated (e.g., focus-forming units)
fomite Inanimate object that may be contaminated with virus and become the vehicle for transmission
frameshift mutation Mutation caused by the insertion or deletion of one or more nucleotide or slippage of a polymerase during transcription, the effect of which is to change the reading frame starting at the affected codon
framework region Four relatively conserved regions located on either side of the hypervariable regions in the variable domains of immunoglobulins and T cell receptors
freeze fracture Technique for the preparation of specimens for electron microscopy in which rapidly frozen samples are broken and the exposed surfaces are etched to reveal structural details
fusion Process by which some enveloped viruses become incorporated into the cell membrane and thus enter the cell. Also the mechanism by which such viruses bring about the fusion of adjacent cell membranes to form multinucleated cells or syncytia
β-galactosidase Enzyme catalyzing the hydrolysis of lactose into glucose plus galactose; its absence is a key element in the pathophysiology of viral diarrhea

gamma globulin Fraction of serum proteins that contains antibodies

gel filtration Type of column chromatography that separates molecules on the basis of size

genetic code Sequence of nucleotides, coded in triplets (codons) along the mRNA, that determines the sequence of amino acids in protein synthesis. The DNA sequence of a gene can be used to predict the mRNA sequence, and the genetic code can, in turn, be used to predict the amino acid sequence

genetic drift (antigenic drift) Point mutation(s) in gene(s) specifying the surface protein(s) of a virus, resulting in enough antigenic change to allow immune escape

genetic map Graphic representation of the linear arrangement of genes within a genome or chromosome; in virology usually determined by nucleotide sequencing, but other methods are used when longer sequences are involved, as in eukaryotic chromosomes

genetic shift (antigenic shift) Genetic reassortment or recombination between viruses resulting in major antigenic change and the emergence of a new variant

genome Complete set of genes of a virus or organism

genomic library A collection of clones made from a set of randomly generated overlapping DNA fragments representing the entire genome of a virus or organism

genotype Genetic constitution of a virus or organism, as distinguished from its physical appearance or phenotype

germ-line transmission Transmission of a virus by egg or sperm

glycolipids Lipids that are linked covalently to polysaccharides

glycoprotein Polypeptide to which at least one carbohydrate residue is attached covalently

gnotobiotic An animal whose infection status is known. Often used in the context of "germ-free" or "specific pathogen-free" animals

Golgi complex (or Golgi apparatus) Subcellular organelle consisting of flattened, parallel membranes derived from the endoplasmic reticulum and playing a role in intracellular transport

group-specific antigen Antigen specific to (shared by) a group of viruses

Guarnieri bodies Inclusion bodies in vaccinia virus-infected cells

hairpin Double-helical regions resulting from the base pairing of contiguous, largely complementary stretches of nucleotides on DNA or RNA strands

haploid genome Genome that contains one copy of each gene—all viruses except retroviruses have haploid genomes

HeLa cells An established line of human cervical carcinoma cells often used in research and diagnostics—susceptible to infection by many viruses

helical symmetry Configuration of a viral nucleocapsid in which the nucleic acid and protein structural units are arranged as a helix

helicase An enzyme involved in DNA replication, responsible for unwinding the double helix

helix Spiral structure with a repeating pattern; it is the natural conformation of many regular biological polymers (e.g., polypeptides, DNA, RNA, and the nucleocapsids of some viruses)

helper T cells (Th cells) T lymphocytes, which when stimulated by antigen presented in association with MHC class II molecules, are able to enhance the function of themselves, other lymphocytes, and other cells, notably macrophages; there are two classes of such cells, Th1 and Th2, distinguished by their cytokine profiles

helper virus A virus which, in a mixed infection with a defective virus, provides some factor(s) that enables the defective virus to replicate

hemadsorption Adsorption of erythrocytes to the surface of virus-infected cells (mediated by bound viral proteins or virions)

hemagglutination Agglutination of red blood cells (mediated by bound viral proteins or virions)

hemagglutinin One of the viral glycoprotein peplomers of orthomyxoviruses and most paramyxoviruses

herd immunity Immune status of a population that affects viral transmission rates. Often used in describing the elimination of a virus from a population when there are too few susceptible hosts remaining to sustain a transmission chain

heteroduplex Double-stranded nucleic acid in which the two strands are not completely complementary

heterologous Derived from a species with a different genetic constitution

hexon (hexamer) In an icosahedral capsid, those capsomers having six neighboring capsomers

histones Proteins rich in basic amino acids (e.g., lysine and arginine) found in the nucleus of eukaryotic cells in association with DNA

holoenzyme Active (complete) form of an enzyme

homology Degree of relatedness between two nucleic acid or amino acid sequences

horizontal transmission Transfer of infectious virus from one animal to another by any means other than vertical transmission

host range Range of species of animals (or cells derived therefrom) susceptible to a particular virus

hot spots Sites in a genome at which mutations occur and are selected for with exceptionally high frequency

humoral immunity Immunity mediated by antibodies

hybrid cell Cell created by the fusion of two unrelated cells through the action of certain viruses or other substances

hybridization Formation of stable duplexes between complementary RNA or DNA sequences by means of Watson–Crick base pairing; in classical genetics and breeding, the formation of a novel diploid organism by normal sexual processes or cell fusion

hybridoma Antibody-secreting cell line formed by the fusion of a non-antibody-producing myeloma tumor cell with a particular clone of antigen-primed B lymphocytes

hydrophilic Chemical groups with ability to form hydrogen bonds, thus having an affinity for water and similar solvents (e.g., $-OH$, $=O$, $-NH$)

hydrophobic Chemical groups unable to form hydrogen bonds, thus lacking affinity for water (e.g., benzene and other aromatic rings, aliphatic hydrocarbons)

hyperimmunization Repeated immunization against a particular virus or antigen

hypervariable regions (complementary determining regions) One of three regions within the variable domain of each immunoglobulin heavy and light chain and the variable regions of the α and β chains of the T cell receptor, i.e., subject to most variation and contributes most to antigen specific binding

iatrogenic Pertaining to a disease caused directly by professional veterinary or medical intervention

icosahedron Configuration of a virion in which capsomers are assembled into a symmetrical polyhedron having 20 equilateral triangular faces and 12 vertices

idiotype An epitope (immunogenic site) on the variable regions of an antibody molecule—antibodies may be raised against such sites that can bind specifically to the particular antibody molecule (anti-idiotypic antibody)

immune complexes Antibody–antigen complexes

immune response (Ir) genes Genes influencing the immune response to a given antigen; they map within the major histocompatibility complex (MHC) genetic locus

immune surveillance Monitoring function of the immune system whereby it recognizes and reacts against aberrant cells arising within the body
immunity (1) A state in which a host is not susceptible to infection or disease or (2) the mechanism(s) by which this is achieved. Immunity is achieved by one of three means: natural or innate (genetically inherited) immunity, passively acquired immunity (via transfer of antibody, usually from dam to offspring), and actively acquired immunity (through vaccination)
immunofluorescence A method of determining the location of antigen (or antibody) in a tissue section or smear using a specific antibody (or antigen) conjugated to a fluorochrome
immunogen An antigen that stimulates a protective immune response
immunogenicity Capacity of a vaccine to stimulate an immune response, as measured by the proportion of individual animals in a population that produce specific antibody or T cells
immunoglobulin Set of proteins produced by B lymphocytes (plasma cells) during the immune response; in many species, nine classes of immunoglobulins are distinguished on the basis of differences in their heavy chains: IgG1, 2, 3, 4, IgA1, 2, IgM, IgD, and IgE
immunologic memory Capacity of an animal that has been exposed to a particular antigen to respond more rapidly and effectively on reexposure to that antigen
immunologic tolerance Specific unresponsiveness to a particular antigen
immunology Study of the immune system and immunity
immunopathology Damage to the host caused by its own immune response
immunosuppression A reduction in the normal level of responsiveness of the immune system caused by infection (e.g., lentivirus infections), drugs, irradiation, pregnancy, malnutrition, etc. Immunosuppressed animals are also referred to as immunocompromised
inapparent infection Subclinical infection
incidence rate (or attack rate) A measure of the occurrence of infection or disease in a population over time; it refers to the proportion of a population contracting a particular disease during a specified period
inclusion bodies Microscopically distinct sites of virus synthesis ("viral factories") or accumulation of virions or viral products in virus-infected cells
incubation period Interval between the time of infection and the onset of clinical signs
induction Initiation of virus production in a lysogenic or latently infected cell
infection Invasion and replication of a virus within a host where it may cause disease
infection cycle Time between infection of a cell and the shedding of virions
infectious dose 50 (ID_{50}) Dose of virus required to infect 50% of inoculated hosts or cells
infectious period Time period during which infected animals are able to transmit a virus to a susceptible host or vector; the infectious period may not necessarily be associated with clinical signs
initiation (start) codon Trinucleotide in a mRNA at which ribosomes begin the process of translation, thereby establishing the reading frame; usually AUG (which encodes methionine), but may be GUG (valine) in prokaryote cells
initiation factors Specific proteins required for ribosome binding and the initiation of mRNA translation
insertion sequences Short (300–1000 nucleotides) DNA sequences able to integrate themselves at new positions within the genome without any sequence similarity to the target locus; related to transposons
***in situ* hybridization** Use of a DNA or RNA probe to detect the presence of the complementary DNA sequence in a preparation of cloned virus or other specimen of interest
integrase An enzyme involved in the integration of some viruses, such as bacteriophage lambda (λ), retroviruses, and some transposons into host cell chromosomal DNA
integration Insertion of a smaller DNA into a larger DNA; integration of a viral DNA into the host genome usually requires a virus-encoded enzyme, integrase
intercalation Insertion of planar molecules (e.g., ethidium bromide) between adjacent base pairs in DNA or RNA
interference Prevention of the replication of one virus by another virus or by products (e.g., interferons) produced by cells as a result of viral infection
interferons Family of cellular proteins (cytokines) produced and secreted in response to foreign nucleic acid (especially viral RNA or DNA) that protect other cells against viral infection; a particular class of cytokines
intergrins A group of heterodimeric cell adhesion molecules present on the surface of endothelial cells; some serve as receptors for viruses
interleukins *("acting between leukocytes")* Soluble substances (cytokines) produced by leukocytes that stimulate the growth or activities of other leukocytes
intron (intervening sequence) Sequence of DNA that has no coding function and is excised in processing of an RNA transcript to produce mRNA
in vitro Literally, "in glass"; a biologic or biochemical process occurring outside a living organism. For example, a virological experiment done in cell culture rather than in living animal hosts
in vivo Literally, "in life"; a biologic or biochemical process occurring within a living organism. For example, a virological experiment done in an experimental animal model.
isoelectric point pH value of a solution in which a macromolecule has no net surface charge and fails to move in an electric field
isolate Sample of a virus (or other infectious gent) from a single defined source
isometric Of equal dimensions
isometric virions Virions that are symmetrical in three dimensions; some isometric virions may appear spherical but their capsids have icosahedral symmetry
kappa chain One of the two light chains (the other is lambda) of immunoglobulin molecules
killer (K) cell Non B, non T, lymphocyte-like cell (also called null cell); lacking B and T cell surface markers, but having Fc receptors; responsible for antibody-dependent cellular cytotoxicity
kinase Any enzyme catalyzing a phosphorylation reaction
Kleinschmidt technique Method in which nucleic acid molecules are spread on an air–water interface in a monolayer; after heavy metal shadowing, the molecules are visualized by electron microscopy
Koch's postulates Classic set of criteria to assess the role of a given virus or microorganism as the etiologic agent of a particular disease. The original postulates are often difficult to prove in viral infections, so additional criteria have been established by Evans (see Chapter 2).
lambda chain One of the two light chains (the other is kappa) of immunoglobulin molecules

Langerhans' cell Dendritic cell in the skin that functions in the processing of antigen. *See* dendritic cell
late viral genes Genes transcribed after viral nucleic acid replication
latent infection Persistent infection in which little or no infectious virus is detectable, despite the continued presence of the viral genome
leader sequence Nontranslated region of mRNA extending from its 5′ end to the start codon; contains regulatory signals
leader sequence peptide Sequence of 15–20 amino acids at the N terminus of eukaryotic proteins that determines its ultimate destination
lectins Plant glycoproteins that bind specifically to sugar residues in cell membrane glycoproteins and thereby act as mitogens
lethal dose 50 (LD_{50}) Dose of virus required to kill 50% of inoculated animals or cells
leukemia Neoplastic proliferation of leukocytes manifest by an increased number of leukocytes in the blood
leukosis Neoplasia in which there is an abnormal increase in the number of leukocytes
ligand (1) Receptor-binding molecule on the surface of a virion or (2) nonviral molecules involved in receptor–ligand interactions
ligase An enzyme that repairs single-strand nicks in duplex DNA and covalently joins DNA fragments with complementary, overlapping (called also cohesive or sticky) ends or, less efficiently, with blunt ends
ligation Process of joining the 5′ and 3′ termini of linear nucleic acid molecule via a phosphodiester bond
lipid bilayer Model for the structure of cell membranes and viral envelopes based on the hydrophobic interactions between phospholipids; the polar head groups face the inner and outer surface of the membrane, whereas the hydrophobic tails are contained within the body of the membrane
lipids Hydrophobic bioorganic molecules; includes steroids, fats, fatty acids, phospholipids, and water-insoluble vitamins
lipopolysaccharides Molecules rich in lipids and sugars
liposome Artificially constructed lipid vesicle into which viral proteins or other substances may be incorporated
long terminal repeats (LTRs) Sequences at the termini of the genome and proviral DNA of retroviruses, containing promoters and enhancers necessary for efficient viral replication
lymphocytes White blood cells involved in the immune response; B lymphocytes (which mature to become plasma cells) produce antibodies and T lymphocytes are responsible for cell-mediated immunity
lymphokine Soluble mediator produced by lymphocytes that influences the function of other cells; a subclass of cytokines
lymphoma Solid tumor of lymphoid tissue
lyophilization A stable preparation of a biological substance produced by rapid freezing and dehydration of the frozen product under high vacuum, also called freeze-drying
lysis Rupture of a cell caused by the destruction of the cell membrane
lysogenic virus Virus (generally a bacteriophage) that can become stably established within its host: either by integration into the host cell genome or by plasmid formation
lysosome Cytoplasmic organelle containing hydrolytic enzymes that play an important role in the degradation of material ingested by phagocytosis or endocytosis
lytic infection *See* cytocidal infection
macromolecule Molecule with molecular weight ranging from a few thousand to hundreds of millions of daltons
macrophage White blood cell that phagocytoses and destroys foreign particles or debris and processes and presents antigenic peptides on its surface in association with MHC class II protein
major histocompatability complex (MHC) Chromosomal region containing the genes for histocompatibility antigens and some other genes involved in the immune response
malignant tumor Invasive tumor resulting from uncontrolled proliferation of abnormal (transformed) cells
Marek's disease A lymphoproliferative disease of birds caused by an avian alphaherpesvirus
marker rescue Phenomenon in which cells that are infected/transfected mixedly with active virus and inactivated virus or viral DNA yield progeny that contain some gene(s) from the inactivated virus or viral DNA
maternal immunity Transfer of maternal antibody to the fetus, the embryonating egg, or the newborn
mathematical model (epidemiological) A means to convey quantitative information about a host–virus interaction, such as an epidemic or an emerging disease episode, by the construction of a set of predictive mathematical algorithms. Models may provide (1) an indication of the dynamics of the interaction between the virus and the host, (2) an indication of the mode and rate of transmission of the virus between individual animals, and (3) an indication of the host population at risk (numbers of animals, population density, age distribution, etc.) and the possible future spread of infection and disease
matrix protein Protein lining the inner surface of the envelope of many enveloped viruses
maturation phase Period toward the end of the viral replication cycle during which progeny virions are being assembled
mechanical transmission Transmission of a virus by an arthropod, without replication of the virus in the vector—likened to a "flying needle"
melting temperature (TM) Temperature at which a double-stranded DNA or RNA molecule denatures into separate single strands or the temperature at which the secondary structure of a single-stranded nucleic acid is lost; influenced by the G + C content of the nucleic acid and the salt concentration of the solution
memory cells Expanded clones T and B lymphocytes that persist after primary and subsequent immunization
messenger RNA (mRNA) A single-stranded, positive-sense molecule of RNA produced by transcription from the viral or host genome, which, after processing, is translated on ribosomes to make protein; the genome of certain RNA viruses can act directly as mRNA
metastasis Spread of cells from a primary malignant tumor to other parts of the body, usually via the bloodstream or lymphatic system
MHC restriction Recognition of foreign antigen by T lymphocytes occurs only when that antigen is presented on a cell surface as a peptide in association with an MHC protein
microsomes Fraction of a cell homogenate obtained by ultracentrifugation that contains ribosomes and small vesicles derived from the rough endoplasmic reticulum
mitogen A substance that induces cell proliferation
mitomycin C Antibiotic that selectively inhibits DNA replication by cross-linking the strands
mitosis That part of the cell cycle (M phase) of eukaryotic somatic cells that ends with cell division
molecular cloning *See* cloning
molecular mass (M_r) Molecular mass (relative) is a dimensionless number representing the ratio of the mass of an entity to one-twelfth the mass of an atom of ^{12}C. When indicating the mass of viruses or other biologically complex entities containing different kinds of molecules, the molecular mass, not molecular weight, should be used. When indicating the mass of proteins, carbohydrates, or other large molecules the term M_r is also preferred, but molecular weight (MW) may be used. It is acceptable to use the mass

unit, the dalton, with the term molecular mass, but not with the term molecular weight or relative molecular mass (M_r). For example, "the M_r of poliovirus protein VP1 is 33,521"

molecular mimicry Similar nucleotide or amino acid sequences found in disparate organisms, such as in a virus and its host

molecular weight Number representing the sum of the atomic weights of the constituent atoms in a molecule (see molecular mass)

monocistronic mRNA A mRNA encoding a single polypeptide

monoclonal antibody Highly specific antibodies produced by specifically selected cell clones (hybridoma cells) obtained by fusing antibody-producing B lymphocytes with myleoma cells. *See* hybridoma

monolayer cells Animal cells grown in culture while attached to a solid surface, in contrast to cells grown in suspension culture

monomer Basic subunit from which, by repetition of a single type of reaction, polymers are made, e.g., amino acids (monomers) are linked to yield polypeptides or proteins (polymers)

morbidity rate Percentage of animals in a population that develop clinical disease attributable to a particular virus over a defined period of time

mortality rate Percentage of animals in a population that die from a particular disease over a defined period of time. The case-fatality rate represents the percentage of animals with a particular disease that die from the disease

M_r See molecular mass

multicistronic mRNA mRNA carrying the information for the synthesis of two or more proteins

multiplex polymerase chain reaction A modification of the polymerase chain reaction in which the detection of more than one nucleic acid sequence in a mixture is accomplished in a single run by the addition of more than one set of oligonucleotide primer pairs

multiplicity of infection (MOI) Number of infectious units of virus inoculated per cell

mutagens Physical or chemical agents (e.g., radiation, heat, and alkylating or deaminating agents) that raise the frequency of genetic mutation above the spontaneous rate

mutation Heritable change in the nucleotide sequence of the genome of an organism or virus

myeloma B lymphocyte tumor

N terminus End of the polypeptide chain that carries a free α-amino group (by convention the left end)

natural killer (NK) cell Non B, non T, lymphocyte-like cell (null cell); lacking B and T cell surface markers and lacking antigen-specific receptors. It serves one particularly important function: it lyses cells in which MHC expression is down-regulated (as occurs in many viral infections); this is important in the early removal of virus-infected cells and probably in the elimination of many potentially neoplastic cells

negative stain (negative contrast) electron microscopy Method used in electron microscopy; employs an electron-opaque material such as potassium phosphotungstate to "stain" the background around particles of interest. Used to visualize virions and viral subunits in exquisite detail

negative sense Nucleotide sequence that is complementary to that of mRNA, which by convention represents the positive sense

neoplasm Cellular proliferation leading to malignant tumors

nested set transcription A hallmark of the replication strategy of coronaviruses, toroviruses, and arteriviruses, in which a nested set of subgenomic mRNAs are generated having an identical 5′ leader sequence and a common 3′ terminus, but because of discontinuous transcription, each mRNA has a unique coding sequence and is transcribed into a unique viral protein

nested-set polymerase chain reaction A variation of the usual polymerase chain reaction method in which the primers used in the first round of amplification are replaced with different primers for the second and subsequent rounds of amplification; this increases the specificity of the reaction

neuraminic acid Nine-carbon sugar derivative that is part of the cellular receptor recognized by the orthomyxovirus hemagglutinin

neutralization Inactivation of a virus by the binding of antibodies to sites required for adsorption and entry into the host cell

nonionic detergent Detergent with no net charge (e.g., Triton X-100 and Nonidet P-40)

nonpermissive cells Cells that do not allow a complete virus replication cycle

nonsense mutation Mutation that produces one of the three stop codons, resulting in premature termination of the growing polypeptide chain

nonstructural protein Virus-coded protein found in infected cells but not part of the structure of the virion. Some so-called "nonstructural" proteins, such as polymerases, may be incorporated in the virion.

Northern blot (laboratory jargon derived by analogy with Southern blot) A method in which RNA fragments of interest are transferred from a polyacrylamide gel to a membrane by blotting; the membrane is then probed with labeled complementary DNA to determine the nature of the RNA fragments

nosocomial Pertaining to hospital-acquired (or veterinary clinic-acquired) infection

notifiable disease Diseases whose occurrence is required by law to be made known to a government authority

nucleases Enzymes that cleave the phosphodiester bonds of nucleic acid chains

nucleocapsid Viral nucleic acid surrounded by its protein coat

nucleoprotein Virion protein that is tightly associated with the viral nucleic acid; in the case of helically symmetrical RNA viruses, the nucleoprotein coats the RNA forming the nucleocapsid

nucleosomes Basic structural subunit of chromatin, consisting of approximately 200 base pairs of DNA and a histone protein octamer

nucleotide A subunit of DNA or RNA consisting of a nitrogenous base (adenine, guanine, thymine, or cytosine in DNA; adenine, guanine, uracil, or cytosine in RNA), a phosphate molecule, and a sugar molecule (deoxyribose in DNA and ribose in RNA). Thousands of nucleotides are linked to form a DNA or RNA molecule

nude mouse Strain of hairless mouse that is congenitally without a thymus gland

Okazaki fragments Short (1000–2000 nucleotide) DNA fragments made in the course of discontinuous DNA replication and later joined together to form an intact strand

oligonucleotide A polymer made up of a few nucleotides

oligopeptide Short chain of amino acids

oligosaccharides Short sugar polymers that, in viruses, are usually attached to asparagine residues in proteins and contain mannose, glucosamine, fucose, sialic acid, etc.

oncogene Cellular (c-*onc*) or virus (v-*onc*) gene whose products are able to transform eukaryotic cells so that they begin to grow like tumor cells

oncogenesis (carcinogenesis, tumorigenesis) Multistep process leading to the development of a tumor

oncogenic Giving rise to tumors or causing tumor formation; said especially of tumor-inducing viruses

open reading frame (ORF) Nucleic acid sequence between start and stop codons that encodes a protein or a polyprotein

operator Site on DNA that interacts with a specific repressor protein, thereby controlling the functioning of an adjacent operon
operon Group of adjacent genes under the joint control of an operator and a repressor; unit of bacterial gene expression and regulation
organelle Particulate subcellular structures in eukaryotic cells such as the nucleus, mitochondria, Golgi apparatus, and ribosomes
orphan virus Usually enteroviruses or reoviruses that have no known disease attributed to them
palindrome DNA sequence that is the same when one strand is read left to right and the other is read right to left, i.e., a sequence consisting of adjacent inverted repeats
pancreatic ribonuclease A Endonuclease that cleaves RNA only at the 3′ site of pyrimidine nucleotides
pandemic Worldwide epidemic
papilloma A small neoplasm on the skin caused by a papilloma virus; also called a wart
passage Serial transfer and recovery of a virus in cell cultures or animals; often done to adapt a new isolate to grow faster and to higher titer in the laboratory
passive immunization (passive protection) Transfer of antibodies to a nonimmune animal, either by maternal transfer (via the placenta or in colostrum and milk) or by administration of plasma or serum
pathogen Any disease-causing virus or microorganism
pathogenicity An expression of the absolute harm done to a host by a virus. Contrasted with the term virulence, which is used to express the relative level of harm done to a host
penetration Entry of a virus particle into a host cell
penton (pentamer) Twelve structural units located at the vertices of icosahedral virions; each has five neighbors
peplomer (spike) Oligomer of viral glycoproteins forming the projections that typically extend from a viral envelope; usually contains the ligand that is responsible for viral attachment to the host cell
peptide Two or more amino acids joined by a peptide bond
peptidoglycan Glycopeptide constituent of the bacterial cell wall
perforin A protein in cytotoxic T lymphocytes that creates transmembrane pores that act as ion channels in the target cell; related structurally and chemically to C9 protein of complement, which performs a similar function
perivascular cuffing Infiltration of lymphocytes around blood vessels; most notable in the brain but can occur in any organ, classic evidence of an inflammatory response to certain viral infections
permissive temperature (or permissive cell) Temperature or cell type that permits the replication of a conditional lethal viral mutant
persistent infection In animals and cells, infection that persists for a prolonged period (months, years) after the primary infection
phage display A method for defining antibody-binding epitopes on a protein by cloning fragments of the gene encoding the protein into a bacteriophage coat protein gene, which then expresses the epitope as a component of the bacteriophage capsid
phagocytosis Engulfment of particles by cells, particularly by macrophages and polymorphonuclear cells
phenotype Biologic properties of an organism or virus resulting from expression of its genotype but modified by environmental factors
phenotypic mixing A phenomenon in which viruses exchange their outside envelopes or coats, thus the genome of one virus may be encapsidated in the external membrane or coat of the other
phosphodiester bond Linkage of phosphoric acid with the 3′-hydroxyl group of one ribosome or deoxyribose molecule and the 5′-hydroxyl group of the next ribose or deoxyribose molecule in a polynucleotide
phosphokinase *See* kinase
phospholipids Lipids that contain charged phosphate groups, thus showing both hydrophobic and hydrophilic properties; they are a primary component of cell membranes
phosphoproteins Proteins containing phosphate groups, most commonly attached to serine, threonine, or tyrosine residues
phosphorylation Process of esterifying a molecule with phosphoric acid; generally catalyzed by a kinase using ATP
pinocytosis Uptake of water, solutes, or particles by internalization of fluid-filled vacuoles; also called viropexis
plaque assay Assay based on the number of plaques produced when a viral suspension is inoculated on a cell monolayer
plaque Localized region of cell lysis resulting from cell-to-cell spread of virus replicating in a cell monolayer, usually under agar
plasma cell Antibody-secreting cell; the end stage of differentiation of a B lymphocyte
plasma membrane Membrane that makes up the cell surface and encloses the cytoplasm; it is semipermeable and composed largely of phospholipids and proteins
plasmid Autonomously replicating, extrachromosomal circular DNA molecule, nonessential for cell survival under nonselective conditions. Some plasmids are capable of integrating into the host genome. Bacteria may contain 1 to more than 100 copies of particular plasmids. A number of artificially constructed plasmids are used as cloning vectors
plating efficiency Proportion of a population of virions that successfully infects a particular cell culture, usually detected by plaque assay
point mutation Alteration (deletion, substitution, etc.) in a single nucleotide in a genome
polarity (1) Of single-stranded DNA or RNA, expressed as either positive sense (i.e., the same sense as messenger RNA) or negative sense (i.e., the complementary sense) or (2) of cells, referring to differences between apical and basolateral surfaces of epithelial cells
poly(A) tail (polyadenylated RNA) Sequence of 50–300 adenylate residues present in the genome of some single-stranded RNA viruses or added enzymatically to the 3′ terminus of RNA transcripts in the process of formation of mRNA
poly(A), poly(U), poly(G) Polyribonucleotides containing a single type of base; the 3′ ends of most eukaryotic mRNAs contain up to 300 adenosine nucleotides that are added enzymatically after transcription
polyacrylamide gel electrophoresis (PAGE) Electrophoresis in a hydrophilic polyacrylamide matrix; separation usually depends on the molecular size of molecules; used commonly to estimate the relative molecular sizes of proteins and nucleic acids; denaturation of proteins with sodium dodecyl sulfate (SDS-PAGE) provides a uniform charge to all molecules and favors separations based on size alone
polycistronic Representing several genes
polyclonal antibody Preparation containing antibodies against more than one epitope on an antigen; antibodies obtained from whole animals are always polyclonal
polyhedrin Matrix protein comprising the major component of occlusion bodies produced by nuclear polyhedrosis virus and cytoplasmic polyhedrosis virus
polyhedrosis Disease caused by invertebrate (e.g., insect) viruses that lead to tissue breakdown and accumulation of virions embedded in polyhedral crystals in the cytoplasm or nucleus
polykaryocyte Cell with multiple nuclei (synonyms: syncytium or syncytial cell, multinucleate giant cell)
polymer Regular covalently bonded chain of monomeric subunits

polymerase (DNA polymerase, RNA polymerase) An enzyme that catalyzes the synthesis of nucleic acids from preexisting nucleic acid templates, assembling RNA from ribonucleotides or DNA from deoxyribonucleotides

polymerase chain reaction (PCR) A method for amplifying a DNA nucleotide sequence using a heat-stable polymerase and two oligonucleotide primers, one complementary to the positive DNA strand at one end of the sequence to be amplified and the other complementary to the negative DNA strand at the other end. The DNA of interest (template) and primers are subjected to repeated cycles of heating to separate (melt) double-stranded DNA and cooling in the presence of nucleotides and DNA polymerase such that the template sequence is copied over and over. There are many variations in use, some of which are used to detect the existence of viral genome sequences in diagnostic specimens

polynucleotide Linear nucleic acid polymer in which the 3′ position of the sugar of a nucleotide is linked through a phosphate group to the 5′ position on the sugar of the adjacent molecule

polynucleotide phosphorylase Enzyme catalyzing the polymerization of ribonucleoside diphosphates to yield free phosphate and polynucleotides (e.g., RNA)

polypeptide Polymer of amino acids linked together by peptide bonds

polyploid More than one copy of the genome present; a characteristic of some neoplastic cells

polyprotein Large primary translation product from which individual mature functional proteins are subsequently formed by posttranslational or cotranslational proteolytic cleavage

polysaccharide Carbohydrate (sugar) polymer; in viruses often mannose, galactose, fucose, sialic acid, and glucosamine

polysome (or polyribosome) Complex that contains a mRNA molecule and attached ribosomes actively engaged in polypeptide synthesis; the number of attached ribosomes depends on the size of the mRNA

prevalence Ratio, at a particular point in time, of the number of cases currently present in the population divided by the number of animals in the population; it is a snapshot of the occurrence of infection or disease at a given time

primary cell culture Culture of cells directly obtained from a multicellular organism without passage

primary immune response Immune response following the first contact of an animal with an antigen

primary structure Nucleotide sequence of an RNA or DNA molecule or the amino acid sequence of a polypeptide

primer Structure that serves as a growing point for polymerization, e.g., a small oligonucleotide with a free 3′-hydroxyl group necessary for the initiation of DNA (and occasionally RNA) synthesis

prion Infectious agents composed of abnormally folded protein, with no nucleic acid. Prions are the cause of the spongiform encephalopathies (e.g., bovine spongiform encephalopathy, scrapie); the word is derived from "proteinaceous infectious particle"

probe Single-stranded DNA or RNA molecules of specific base sequence, labeled either radioactively or immunologically, that are used to detect the complementary base sequence by hybridization

processing (1) Of RNA transcripts: series of posttranscriptional alterations to primary RNA transcripts, which lead to the formation of mRNA. (2) Of proteins: changes subsequent to translation of polypeptide, such as cleavage, glycosylation, or phosphorylation. (3) Of antigens: cleavage of polypeptides within cells to form peptides that are presented on the surface of cells in association with MHC molecules

prodrug Chemotherapeutic agent that depends on a viral enzyme to convert it to its active form

productive (or nonproductive) infection Infection of a permissive (or nonpermissive) cell by a virus resulting in the production (or failure of production) of infectious progeny virions

prokaryote Unicellular organism, such as bacteria or blue-green algae, that lacks a nuclear membrane and membrane-bound organelles

promoter Region of nucleic acid molecule to which RNA polymerase binds in order to initiate transcription

prospective study Attempt to identify the cause of a disease by observing populations that are exposed to the infection over a period of time

protein subunits The most elemental units of folded polypeptide chains specified by the viral genome that begin to form the major structural units of the viral capsid

proteosome A large multifunctional protease complex responsible for intracellular proteolysis, i.e., the sequential degradation of proteins

protomer Single polypeptide chains (either identical or nonidentical) of a multimeric protein

protooncogene A gene in a normal eukaryotic cell that is believed to have given rise to an oncogene in a transforming virus

provirus Viral genome integrated covalently into a host cell chromosome and thus transmissible from a cell to its daughter cells

pseudoreplica technique Method used in negative stain electron microscopy where virions or viral substructures are captured in a very thin plastic film

pseudotype Virus particle containing the genome of one virus and the capsid or envelope of another. *See* phenotypic mixing

pulse-chase experiment Experimental technique in which a radioactively labeled compound is added to living cells or a cell extract (pulse) and then, a short time later, an excess of unlabeled compound is added to dilute out the labeled compound and samples are then collected at various times after the pulse to follow the course of the label as the compound is metabolized (chased)

purine A nitrogen-containing, single-ring, basic compound that occurs in nucleic acids. Purines in DNA and RNA are adenine and guanine

puromycin An antibiotic that mimics a charged tRNA and inhibits protein synthesis

pyknosis Shrinkage and condensation of the nucleus of a cell

pyrimidine A nitrogen-containing, double-ring, basic compound that occurs in nucleic acids. Pyrimidines in DNA are cytosine and thymine; in RNA, cytosine and uracil

quantitative polymerase chain reaction (quantitative PCR) A means for quantifying the amount of a template DNA present in a sample; usually achieved by the addition of a known amount of target sequence that is amplified by the same primer set but can be differentiated, usually by size, at the end of the reaction

quarantine A period (originally 40 days) of detention for animals, plants, or people coming from a place where a disease is known to exist

quasi-species A cluster (or cloud or swarm) of variant viruses that arise from mutations over time within a viral isolate, even a cloned isolate. Seen particularly with RNA viruses because of the inherently high mutation rate caused by copy errors during replication by RNA-dependent RNA polymerase and the absence of proofreading in RNA replication

radioimmunoassay Very sensitive assay for viral antigen or antibody that utilizes radioactive labeling of either the antigen or the antibody

reactivation Activation of a virus (e.g., herpesvirus) from a latent stage

reading frame A nucleotide sequence that starts with an initiation (start) codon, partitions the subsequent nucleotides into amino acid-encoding triplets, and ends with a termination (stop) codon
readthrough Translation of mRNA through a stop codon
reannealing Reassociation of single-stranded nucleic acids after denaturation to restore the H-bonded, double-stranded structure
reassortment Genetic recombination between viruses with segmented genomes, whereby some progeny of a doubly infected cell acquire genome segments from each parental virus
receptor Structure on surface of cell that is recognized by a specific extracellular molecule or structure (ligand) or virus that binds to it
receptor-mediated endocytosis Uptake of virions (or other entities) following attachment to a specific receptor on the plasma membrane and subsequent endocytosis through clathrin-coated pits
recombinant DNA molecule A combination of DNA molecules of different origin that are joined using recombinant DNA technologies
recombinant DNA technology The many procedures used to join together DNA segments to produce genes of interest and the procedures to introduce such recombinant DNA molecules into expression systems (such as bacterial culture systems, cell culture systems, or transgenic animal systems) for the large-scale production of proteins (or DNA) of interest
recombination (intramolecular) Exchange of nucleic acid sequences between molecules derived from different parents, giving rise to progeny with a different genotype
repeat (reiterated) sequence Nucleotide sequence present in more than one copy (usually many copies)
replicase Enzyme involved in the replication of the viral genomic nucleic acids, e.g., RNA-dependent RNA replicase (or polymerase)
replication Duplication of the genomic DNA or RNA of a virus
replication fork Y-shaped region of a DNA genome that is the growing point during DNA replication
replicative form (RF) Structure of a nucleic acid at the time of its replication; the term used most frequently to refer to double-helical intermediates in the replication of single-stranded DNA and RNA viruses
replicative intermediate (RI) Intermediate in the replication of viral nucleic acid, consisting of one complete (template) strand on which one or several nascent strands of opposite sense are being replicated simultaneously by a polymerase molecule at each growing point
repressor Regulatory protein that binds to operator sites on a DNA, thereby preventing the transcription of adjacent sequences into RNA
reproductive ratio (R_o) Average number of secondary cases of infection to which one primary case gives rise throughout its infectious period in a defined population consisting solely of susceptible animals
reservoir host Animal species constituting the source of virus in nature
restriction endonuclease Enzyme that recognizes short specific palindromic sequences in double-stranded DNA and cleaves the duplex (usually at the recognition site, but sometimes elsewhere); components of the bacterial restriction–modification systems that protect the bacterial cell against invasion by foreign nucleic acids
restriction fragment length polymorphism (RFLP) Method for assessing viral variants as determined by differences in DNA fragment sizes cut by specific restriction enzymes. Different RFLP profiles are caused by mutation at restriction enzyme cutting sites. In animal genetics, polymorphic sequences that result in RFLPs are used as markers to build physical maps and genetic linkage maps, including maps pertaining to variation in susceptibility/resistance to viral diseases
reticulocyte Immature red blood cell (or erythrocyte) that is able to synthesize hemoglobin; cell-free rabbit reticulocyte extracts are often used to study protein synthesis *in vitro*
retrospective study Attempt to identify the cause of a disease by comparing the presence or absence of suspected etiologic factors in animals with a certain disease to their occurrence in animals without that disease
reverse genetics Genetic studies that proceed from the recognition of a gene to the function of its product
ribonuclease Enzyme that hydrolyzes (cleaves) the phosphodiester bonds of RNA
ribonucleotide Compound consisting of a purine or pyrimidine base bound to ribose, which in turn is esterified with phosphoric acid
ribosomes Small (~20 nm in diameter) subcellular ribonucleoprotein particles that are made up of two subparticles and are responsible for the translation of mRNAs into proteins
ribozymes RNA molecules having the ability to catalyze a variety of intra- and/or intermolecular reactions
rifampicin Synthetic antibiotic that binds to certain prokaryotic RNA polymerases, thereby inhibiting RNA synthesis
RNA (ribonucleic acid) A polymer of ribonucleotides, found in all living cells and many viruses, consisting of a long, usually single-stranded chain of alternating phosphate and ribose units with the bases adenine, guanine, cytosine, and uracil bonded to the ribose
rolling circle replication Mechanism for nucleic acid replication in which the template is a circular molecule (either DNA or RNA); the newly synthesized strand may either be released as a single copy or, more commonly, continue on to form a concatamer of progeny molecules before cleavage to unit length molecules for packaging into viral capsids
S phase Stage of cell cycle when DNA synthesis occurs
S1 mapping A method for mapping precursor or mature mRNA to particular DNA sequences using the enzyme S1 nuclease
sarcoma Malignant tumor of cells of mesenchymal origin
secondary cells Cells arising from proliferation of cultured primary cells; unless they become transformed, such cells are able to divide only a finite number of times
secondary immune response *See* anamnestic response
secondary structure Features of a macromolecular structure that are maintained by hydrogen bonds and other weak interactions: for proteins, secondary structural features include α helixes and β-pleated sheets; for nucleic acids, the G–C and A–T(U) base-pairing interactions
secular trend (distribution) Trend (occurrence) of a disease over time (usually years)
sedimentation coefficient Rate at which a macromolecule sediments under a defined gravitational force; influenced by both the molecular weight and the shape of a macromolecule; the basic unit is the Svedberg (S)
semiconservative replication DNA replication mechanism in which both strands of a double-stranded DNA are used as templates and the two resulting progeny duplexes each contain one parental and one newly synthesized strand
sense Polarity of a nucleic acid; positive sense is that found in messenger RNA, negative sense is that which is complementary to that in messenger RNA
sensitivity (of a test) Ability of a test to give positive results on animals known to have the infection—in contrast to false positives
sentinel study Investigation of the circulation of arboviruses by testing for specific antibodies in exposed "sentinel" animals
sequencing Determination of the order of nucleotides (base sequences) in a DNA or RNA molecule or the order of amino acids in a protein

seroprevalence rate Proportion of animals in a population that are seropositive

serotype A set of viruses or microorganisms that can be distinguished from all others on the basis of antigenic properties

shadow casting Technique used to prepare virus specimens for electron microscopy; shadows outlining the virions are created by the accumulation of heavy metal atoms (e.g., platinum) deposited in a vacuum

sigla (acronym) Name formed from a few letters, often initial letters of descriptive words (e.g., ***Reo****viridae* = *r*espiratory, *e*nteric, *o*rphan viruses)

signal sequence N-terminal sequence of 16–30 amino acids of a protein that initiates transport across membranes; subsequently cleaved off

signal transduction A cascade of biochemical events triggered at the cell surface by the binding of a ligand to a cell surface receptor that is transmitted to the nucleus and results in altered patterns of gene expression

silent gene (message) Gene that is not expressed because a potential ribosome-binding site is blocked/unavailable

single stranded Nucleic acid that occurs as a single-stranded helix

site-directed mutagenesis Introduction of a particular point mutation or deletion at a predetermined position

slow infection Infection with a prolonged preclinical phase (incubation period) that is followed by a slowly progressive disease

sodium dodecyl sulfate (SDS) A strong anionic detergent, often used to disrupt enveloped viruses and to denature proteins

somatic mutation (1) A change in the DNA sequence that occurs in somatic cells, i.e., not gametes. (2) The mechanism underlying the generation of diversity of antigen recognition by immunoglobulins and T cell receptor molecules. (3) The fundamental cause of cancer in which the mutation occurs spontaneously or is induced by a carcinogen such as sunlight, chemicals, or viruses

Southern blot Transfer of electrophoretically separated DNA fragments from an agarose gel to a nylon membrane by blotting so that fragments can be detected and analyzed by hybridization with radioactively labeled complementary nucleic acid probes; named after its inventor, Edward Southern

species jumping Referring to a virus that derives from an ancient reservoir life cycle in one host, but has subsequently established a new life cycle in another and no longer uses the first host as its reservoir

specificity (of a test) Ability of a test to give negative results on animals known not to have the infection; in contrast to false negatives

splicing Process of excision of introns and splicing of exons from RNA transcripts to form mRNA

spongiform encephalopathy (or transmissible spongiform encephalopathy, TSE) Term describing the disease and degenerative changes that occur in the brains of animals (or humans) infected with prions: e.g., scrapie, bovine spongiform encephalopathy, chronic wasting disease of deer and elk, and so on

start (initiation) codon Group of three adjacent ribonucleotides (AUG) in a mRNA where translation is initiated; preceded by base sequences that have a high affinity for ribosomes

steady-state infection Persistent infection in which all cells are infected and produce noncytocidal virus

stop (termination) codon Ribonucleotide triplet (UGA, UAG, UAA) in an mRNA signaling the termination of translation of a polypeptide chain

structural proteins Virus-coded proteins that are an essential part of the structure of a virion

structural units Assemblages of protein subunits, usually forming structures of intermediate complexity, which are then assembled into viral capsids

subclinical infection An infection in which clinical signs are inapparent; diagnosis involves laboratory methods

subgenomic RNA Less than genome length RNA found in infected cells that may serve as mRNA and is occasionally encapsidated

sucrose density gradient centrifugation Technique in which particles having different sedimentation coefficients are separated by sedimentation through a continuous or discontinuous gradient of sucrose solution

supercoiling Coiling of a covalently closed circular, double-stranded DNA molecule such that it crosses over its own axis; the structure results from the action of DNA gyrase and other proteins

superinfection Attempt to infect a host with a second virus; may result in interference, synergism, recombination, or phenotypic mixing

suppressor mutation Compensating mutation, generally in another gene, that restores wild-type phenotype without affecting the mutant gene

suppressor-sensitive mutation Point mutation creating a termination codon that tends to be misread by a suppressor tRNA

surveillance Organized collection, collation, and analysis of data on disease incidence or prevalence

susceptibility Measure of sensitivity of a host cell or organism to infection

symptom A condition reported by an individual when suffering from a disease; because animals cannot express objectively how they feel, this term is not used in veterinary medicine. Instead, the term clinical sign is used

syncytium A multinucleate cellular mass produced by the fusing of cells

synergism A situation in which the clinical signs caused by coinfection with two viruses are more severe than the sum of those caused by the individual viruses

systemic infection Infection resulting from the spread of virus from the site of infection to most or all parts of the body

T cell receptor Antigen (peptide)-specific heterodimer, either α/β or γ/δ receptor molecule on the surface of T cell that recognizes the antigenic peptide in association with MHC protein

T cell Thymus-derived lymphocytes responsible for cell-mediated immunity and for immune regulation

***Taq* polymerase** A polymerase such as that obtained from the bacterium *Thermus aquaticus*; used commonly in the polymerase chain reaction and DNA sequencing reactions

TATA box Consensus sequence TATAAAA that starts about 30 bases upstream from the cap site that directs RNA polymerase II to begin synthesis at the cap site

temperature-sensitive mutation Mutation resulting in a gene product that is nonfunctional at a certain nonpermissive temperature but functional at a permissive temperature

template Nucleic acid molecule from which a complementary nucleic acid molecule is synthesized

terminal redundancy Presence of identical sequences at both ends of a DNA or RNA molecule, such as a viral genome

termination (stop) codon Ribonucleotide triplet (UGA, UAG, UAA) in a mRNA signaling the termination of translation of a polypeptide chain

tissue culture infectious dose 50 ($TCID_{50}$) Median tissue culture infectious dose; that amount of a pathogenic agent that will produce pathological change in 50% of inoculated animals or cell cultures

topoisomerase Enzyme that can change the linking number (i.e., the degree of supercoiling) of a DNA molecule

***trans* and *cis*-acting genetic and molecular actions** *See cis-* and *trans*-acting genetic and molecular actions

transcapsidation *See* phenotypic mixing

transcriptase RNA polymerase responsible for transcription

transcription Synthesis of a complementary RNA strand from a DNA or RNA template; the first step in gene expression
transcription unit Region of a genome extending from the transcription initiation site to transcription termination site including all introns and exons; may include more than one gene
transduction Transfer by a virus of cellular genes from one organism or cell to another
transfection Introduction of foreign DNA or RNA into a cell
transfer RNA (tRNA) Small (~ 75 nucleotide) RNAs responsible for decoding the genetic information in mRNA; each species of tRNA is able to combine covalently with a specific amino acid and to hydrogen bond with at least one mRNA nucleotide triplet
transformation (1) Transfer of genetic information into a cell via free DNA. (2) Infectious process in which a virus does not kill the host cell, but induces genetic changes in it that lead to changes in growth characteristics and sometimes to tumor formation
transgenesis Transfer of genes from one individual into the genome of another, which may then transmit them to successive generations
transgenic Product of transgenesis
transitional mutation Mutation in which one pyrimidine (purine) is substituted for the other (in contrast to transversion)
translation Process whereby the genetic information present in a mRNA molecule directs the synthesis of proteins from amino acids
translocation Movement of maternal immunoglobulins across the wall of the intestinal tract of newborn animals
translocation cutoff Time at which translocation of maternal immunoglobulins across the wall of the intestinal tract of the newborn animal ceases
transmission Process by which a pathogen is shed from one host and infects the next
transovarial transmission Transmission of virus from one generation to the next through the egg
transposition Movement of genes from one chromosome site to another or to an extrachromosomal genetic element (episome, plasmid), usually mediated by another genetic element such as a transposon
transposon A DNA molecule that is able to insert itself into unrelated DNA sequences within the cell; the ends of transposons usually contain inverted repeat sequences
transstadial transmission Transmission of virus from one developmental stage of an arthropod to the next stage
transversional mutation Mutation in which a purine is replaced by a pyrimidine or vice versa
trypsin Proteolytic enzyme that is secreted by the pancreas and cleaves only on the carboxyl side of the basic amino acids, arginine and lysine; its nonenzymatic precursor is trypsinogen
tubulin Important protein component of the cytoskeleton, aggregating in the form of microtubules that are essential in many cellular functions (e.g., mitosis)
tumor (T) antigens Virus-specific proteins found in transformed cells; some are required to maintain transformation
tumor-associated transplantation antigen Antigens found on the surface of tumor cells that are undetectable on normal cells of adult individuals and that act as transplantation antigens
tumor necrosis factors (tumor necrosis factors α and β, TNF α and β) Two related cytokines produced by macrophages (TNF α) and some T lymphocytes (TNF β); they are cytotoxic for tumor cells but not for normal cells and play a role in inflammatory responses
tumor promoter Substance or agent that helps the progression of a transformed cell
tumor virus Virus that induces the formation of a tumor; also called oncogenic virus
ultracentrifuge High-speed centrifuge that can attain speeds in excess of 70,000 rpm and centrifugal fields up to 500,000 times gravity and thus is capable of rapidly sedimenting viruses and macromolecules
ultraviolet (UV) light Electromagnetic radiation with wavelengths of 40–400 nm; damages nucleic acids, thus causing mutations and chromosome breaks; also used in chemical analyses and in fluorescence microscopy
vaccination Administration of a vaccine; immunization
vacuole Intracytoplasmic liquid-containing vesicle
vector (1) Intermediate host (e.g., arthropod) that transmits the causative agent of disease from infected to noninfected hosts. (2) Plasmid or viral DNA employed in recombinant DNA technology to clone a foreign gene in prokaryotic or eukaryotic cells. (3) Virus used to incorporate a gene for a protective antigen from another virus to study of its function or use as a vaccine (e.g., vaccinia-vectored rabies vaccine)
vertical transmission Transmission of virus from parent to progeny through the genome, sperm, or ovum or extracellularly (e.g., through colostrum or across the placenta)
vesicle Intracellular compartment enclosed by membranes derived from the endoplasmic reticulum
viral core Innermost structure of complex virions containing the viral nucleic acid and associated proteins
viremia Presence of virus in the bloodstream, either free (plasma viremia) or in infected leukocytes (cell-associated viremia)
virgin-soil epidemic Epidemic occurring in a totally nonimmune (naive) population
virion Complete virus particle
viroid The smallest known nucleic acid-containing infectious agent, consisting of a small circular RNA molecule only 300–400 nucleotides in size. Viroids replicate entirely by means of host cell machinery. Viroids cause a number of important diseases of plants but they have not been identified in animals
virokine Cytokine coded for by a viral gene
viroplasm (virus factory) Intracellular focus of active virus synthesis and/or maturation
virulence An expression of the relative level of harm done to a host by a virus as opposed to the term pathogenicity, which is used to express an absolute level of harm done to a host (e.g., "virus A is more virulent than virus B")
virulent virus A virus causing particularly severe disease
viruria Presence of virus in the urine
virus factory (viroplasm) Intracellular focus of active virus synthesis and/or maturation
VPg Small virus-encoded protein attached through a phosphodiester linkage to the 5′ terminus of a viral genome; abbreviation for *v*irion *p*rotein *g*enome-linked; found on the genome of picornaviruses
Western blot (laboratory jargon derived by analogy with Southern blot) Method for detecting and identifying individual proteins in a mixture of proteins following electrophoretic separation. Proteins are transferred from a gel to a substrate (usually a nitrocellulose sheet) which is then flooded with radiolabeled- or enzyme-conjugated antibody to the protein(s) of interest. This is a valuable method for assessing the presence of individual proteins of viruses
wild type The putative original strain of virus circulating in nature, the parent type from which mutants arise
xenotransplantation Transplantation of organs or tissues from one species to another, e.g., the transplantation of the liver of a pig into a human
xenotropic viruses Retroviruses that replicate only in cells from animals other than the species from which they were derived
zoonosis Disease transmitted naturally to humans from an ongoing reservoir life cycle in animals or arthropods, without the permanent establishment of a new life cycle in humans

INDEX